S A U N D E R S

PHARMACEUTICAL
WORD
BOOK

2009

ELLEN DRAKE, CMT, FAAMT
RANDY DRAKE, MS

S A U N D E R S

PHARMACEUTICAL WORD BOOK

2009

SAUNDERS

ELSEVIER

SAUNDERS
ELSEVIER

11830 Westline Industrial Drive
St. Louis, Missouri 63146

SAUNDERS PHARMACEUTICAL WORD BOOK 2009 ISBN: 978-1-4160-3768-2

Previous editions copyrighted 2008, 2007, 2006, 2005, 2004, 2003, 2002, 2001, 2000, 1999, 1998, 1997, 1996, 1995, 1994, 1992

ISSN: 1072-7779
ISBN: 978-1-4160-3768-2

Working together to grow
libraries in developing countries

www.elsevier.com | www.bookaid.org | www.sabre.org

ELSEVIER   BOOK AID International   Sabre Foundation

Printed in the United States of America

Last digit is the print number: 9   8   7   6   5   4   3   2   1

Contents

Preface

This is a professional medical reference. It was written *by* medical professionals *for* medical professionals. It has been published by the world's largest publisher of professional medical references. You can rely on the information in this book.

This edition is being published simultaneously in print and on CD-ROM. The electronic edition has a new interface and, in response to users' comments, has added features and is easier to use than last year's edition. It contains our complete drug database, including all 27,376 entries in this print edition, plus more than 10,000 entries that do not appear in the book.

The electronic edition will be updated each month via free Web downloads. The updates for the 2009 edition will be available through December 2009 and will contain all the latest new drugs, new doseforms, new strengths, and new indications. The downloads will be incorporated into the database on *your* computer, so every search you perform will include all the latest information. We've provided multiple ways to access the information via searches and hotlinks:

- Browse the entire database, beginning at any point.
- Search for drug names (includes wildcard searching).
- Search for drug names phonetically (a "sound-alike" search).
- Search by indications, using a wildcard search or a comprehensive indications list.
- Optionally limit searches to only Rx drugs, only OTC drugs, or only generic drugs.
- Include or exclude medicinal herbs and natural remedies in your searches.
- Find brand names that contain a certain generic drug.
- Find other brands that contain the same generics as the brand displayed.
- Find devices, such as *in vitro* testing kits, by name or by indication.
- Find unique doseforms, delivery forms, and packaging names.
- Find chemotherapy protocols by name or by drugs contained in the protocol.
- Find chemotherapy drugs by the types of cancer treated.
- Find hazardous materials (HazMat) by name or by hazard category.
- Find other HazMats in the same category as the HazMat displayed.
- Find HazMats used specifically for bioterrorism, chemical weapons, and WMDs.
- Find the "street slang" for illicit drugs, and cross-reference it to the actual drug name.
- Find old brand names for current products.
- Find brands that were discontinued or withdrawn from the market many years ago.
- Find drugs that have been given "orphan" status by the FDA.
- Find drugs that are experimental, investigational, and/or pending FDA approval.
- See when an entry was added to our database and when it was last updated.

To order the *Saunders Pharmaceutical Word Book 2009* on CD-ROM, please contact Elsevier customer service toll-free at 800-545-2522, or visit them online at www.elsevierhealth.com and search with keyword **Drake**.

For bulk CD sales, contact Beverly Folgliani at Elsevier Health Sciences Division, Special Markets, 11830 Westline Industrial Drive, St. Louis MO 63146-3313. Phone: 800-325-4177 ext 4545. Fax: 314-453-4318. E-mail: b.fogliani@elsevier.com

For site licensing, contact Bryan Mee at Elsevier Health Sciences Division, Licensing/Business Development, 1600 John F. Kennedy Blvd., Suite 1800, Philadelphia PA 19103-2899. Phone: 215-239-3276. Fax: 215-239-3286. E-mail: H.Licensing@elsevier.com

The *Saunders Pharmaceutical Word Book* series has been compiled primarily with the medical transcriptionist in mind, although it will certainly appeal to coders, quality assurance personnel, nurses, ward clerks, students of all allied health professions—anyone who has a need for a quick, easy-to-use drug reference that gives more information than just the spelling. Even physicians may find it useful to get quick information on medications their patients may be using for conditions outside their specialty. The "Notes on Using the Text" will show you the format of generic and brand name entries, explain the variety of information this book contains, and give tips on how to find that information.

We think you will find this edition more complete and more valuable than ever; however, no book is ever perfect. Although we have tried to be as accurate and comprehensive as possible, we certainly welcome your comments regarding additions, inconsistencies, or inaccuracies. Please send them to us via e-mail at the address below, or via regular mail to Elsevier Saunders, 11830 Westline Industrial Drive, St. Louis, MO 63146-3313. We welcome your suggestions.

Authors' e-mail address:
    authors@spwb.com
Authors' web site:
    spwb.com

ELLEN DRAKE, CMT, FAAMT
RANDY DRAKE, MS
Atlanta, Georgia

Notes on Using the Text

The purpose of the *Saunders Pharmaceutical Word Book* is to provide the medical transcriptionist (as well as medical record administrators and technicians, coders, nurses, ward clerks, court reporters, legal secretaries, medical assistants, allied health students, physicians, and even pharmacists) a quick, easy-to-use reference that gives not only the correct spellings and capitalizations of drugs, but the designated uses of those drugs, the cross-referencing of brand names to generics, and the usual methods of administration (e.g., capsule, IV, cream). The indication of the preferred nonproprietary (generic) names and the agencies adopting these names (e.g., USAN, USP) should be particularly useful to those writing for publication. The reader will also find various trademarked or proprietary names (e.g., Spansule, Dosepak) that are not drugs but are closely associated with the packaging or administration of drugs.

There are four different ways to refer to drugs. One of these ways is not the name of the drug itself but the class to which it belongs—aminoglycosides, for example. Inexperienced transcriptionists sometimes confuse these classes with the names of drugs. We have included over 350 drug classes in the main list, with a brief description of the therapeutic use and/or method of action common to drugs in the class. Beyond a class description, each drug has three names. The first is the *chemical name*, which describes its chemical composition and how the molecules are arranged. It is often long and complex, sometimes containing numbers, Greek letters, italicized letters, and hyphens between elements. This name is rarely used in dictation except in research hospitals and sometimes in the laboratory section when the blood or urine is examined for traces of the drug. The second name for a drug is the *nonproprietary* or *generic name*. This is a name chosen by the discovering manufacturer or agency and submitted to a nomenclature committee (the United States Adopted Names Council, for example). The name is simpler than the chemical name but often reflects the chemical entity. It is arrived at by using guidelines provided by the nomenclature committee—beta-blockers must end in "olol," for example—and must be unique. There is increasing emphasis on the adoption of the same nonproprietary name by various nomenclature committees worldwide (see the list on page xi). The third name for a drug is the *trade* or *brand name*. There may be several trade names for the same generic drug, each marketed by a different company. These are the ones that are highly advertised and sometimes have unusual capitalization.

We have included many foreign names of drugs for our Canadian friends, and also because we have so many visitors to the United States from other countries (and they get sick, too). The international and British spellings of generic drugs are cross-referenced to the American spellings, and vice versa. Occasionally there will be three different spellings—one American, one international, and another British—which are all cross-referenced to each other. Other special features that may be useful, especially for students, are the commonly used prescribing abbreviations and the sound-alike lists that are found in the appendices. The Therapeutic Drug Levels and Most Prescribed Drugs appendices will be useful as well.

This information was compiled using a variety of sources including direct communication with over 500 drug companies. The orphan entries are taken directly from the latest list issued by the FDA. When sources differed, we ranked our sources as to reliability and went with what we thought was the most reliable source. We recognize that there may be several published ways in which to type a single drug, but we have chosen to use only one of those ways. In the instance of internal capitalization (e.g., pHisoHex), it should be recognized that in most instances it is acceptable to type such words with initial capitalization only (Phisohex).

How the Book Is Arranged

While other pharmaceutical references have separate listings for brand names and generics, or put entries into separate sections by body system or therapeutic use, we have chosen to list all entries in one comprehensive alphabetical listing. Therefore, it is not necessary to know if the term sought is a brand name, a generic, a drug class, a chemotherapy protocol, approved or investigational, or slang; what it's used for; or which body system it affects. If it's given to a patient, it's in "the list." In addition to strict pharmaceuticals, we have included other "consumable" products, such as *in vitro* testing kits, radiographic contrast and other imaging agents, wound dressings, etc.

All entries are in alphabetical order by word. Initial numbers, chemical prefixes (*N-*, *p-*, L-, D-, etc.), and punctuation (prime, hyphens, etc.) are ignored. For example, L-dopa would be alphabetized under "dopa," but levodopa under "levo."

We have indicated brand names with initial capital letters unless an unusual combination of capitals and lowercase has been designated by the manufacturer (e.g., pHisoHex, ALternaGEL). Generic names are rendered in lowercase. Where the same name can be either generic or brand, both have been included.

The general format of a *generic* entry is:

entry council(s) *designated use* [other references] dosages 👂 sound-alike(s)

| #1 | #2 | #3 | #4 | #5 | #6 |

1. The name of the drug (in bold).
2. The various agencies that have approved the name, shown in small caps, which may be any or all of the following:

USAN	United States Adopted Name Council
USP	United States Pharmacopeial Convention
NF	National Formulary
FDA	U.S. Food and Drug Administration
INN	International Nonproprietary Name (a project of the World Health Organization)
BAN	British Approved Name
JAN	Japanese Accepted Name

3. The indications, sometimes referred to as the drug's "designated use," "approved use," or "therapeutic action." This is provided only for official FDA-approved names or other names for the same substance (e.g., the British name of an official U.S. generic). This entry is always in italics.
4. The entry in brackets is one of four cross-references:

see:	refers the reader to the "official" name(s).
now:	for an older generic name no longer used, refers reader to the current official name(s).
also:	a substance that has two or more different names, each officially recognized by one of the above groups, will cross-reference the other name(s).
q.v.	Latin for *quod vide*; which see. Used exclusively for abbreviations, it invites the reader to turn to the reference in parentheses.

   If there is more than one cross reference, alternate names will follow the order of the above agency list; i.e., U.S. names, then international names, then British and Japanese names. The first cross-reference will always be to the approved U.S. name, unless the entry itself is the U.S. name.
5. Dosage information, including the delivery form(s), is given for medications that may be dispensed generically. No dosage information appears for drugs dispensed only under the brand name. Some drugs may be available in more than one strength, indicated by a comma in the dosage field:

   erythromycin stearate USP, BAN *macrolide antibiotic* 250, 500 mg oral

   A semicolon in the dosage field separates different delivery forms, such as:

   nitroglycerin USP *coronary vasodilator; antianginal; antihypertensive* [also: glyceryl trinitrate] 0.3, 0.4, 0.6 mg sublingual; 2.5, 6.5, 9 mg oral; 5 mg/mL injection; 0.1, 0.2, 0.4, 0.6 mg/hr. transdermal; 2% topical

   (Note that some delivery forms come in multiple strengths.)
6. Sound-alike drugs follow the "ear" icon. Listen again to make sure you've found the drug actually being dictated.

The general format for a *brand name* entry is:

Entry Ⓒᴬᴺ form(s) ℞/OTC *designated use* [generics] dosages ② sound-alike(s)
| #1 | #2 | #3 | #4 | #5 | #6 | #7 | #8 |

1. The drug name (in bold), which almost always starts with a capital letter.
2. If a brand is not marketed in the U.S., an icon designates the country where it is available. Canadian brands are designated by Ⓒᴬᴺ, European brands by Ⓔᵁᴿ.
3. The form of administration; e.g., tablets, capsules, syrup. (Sometimes these words are slurred by the dictator, causing confusion regarding the name.)
4. The ℞ or OTC status. A few drugs may be either ℞ or OTC depending on strength or various state laws.
5. The designated use in italics as for generics. These are more complete or less complete as supplied by the individual drug companies.
6. The brackets that follow contain the generic names of the active ingredients to which the reader may refer for further information.
7. Dosage information follows the generics. For multi-ingredient drugs, a bullet separates the dosages of each ingredient, listed in the same order as the generics. For example,

   > **Darvon Compound 65** Pulvules (capsules) ℞ *narcotic analgesic; antipyretic* [propoxyphene HCl; aspirin; caffeine] 65•389•32.4 mg

   shows a three-ingredient product containing 65 mg propoxyphene HCl, 389 mg aspirin, and 32.4 mg caffeine.

   Some drugs may have more than one strength, indicated by a comma in the dosage field:

   > **Norpace** capsules ℞ *antiarrhythmic* [disopyramide phosphate] 100, 150 mg

   A semicolon in the dosage field separates either different products listed together, such as:

   > **Pred Mild; Pred Forte** eye drop suspension ℞ *corticosteroidal anti-inflammatory* [prednisolone acetate] 0.12%; 1%

   or different delivery forms:

   > **Phenergan** tablets, suppositories, injection ℞ *antihistamine; sedative; antiemetic; motion sickness relief* [promethazine HCl] 12.5, 25, 50 mg; 12.5, 25 mg; 25, 50 mg/mL

   (Note that all three delivery forms of Phenergan come in multiple strengths.)

   Liquid delivery forms show the strength per usual dose where appropriate. Thus injectables and drops are usually shown per milliliter (mL), with oral liquids and syrups shown per 5 mL or 15 mL.

   The ≟ symbol indicates that dosage information has not been supplied by the manufacturer for one or more ingredients.

   The ± symbol is used when a value *cannot* be given because the generic entry refers to multiple ingredients.
8. Sound-alike drugs follow the "ear" icon.

Experimental, Investigational, and Orphan Drugs

Before a drug can be advertised or sold in the United States, it must first be approved for marketing by the U.S. Food and Drug Administration. With a few exceptions, FDA approval is contingent solely upon the manufacturer demonstrating that the proposed drug is both safe and effective.

To provide such proof, the manufacturer undertakes a series of tests. Preclinical (before human) research is done through computer simulation, then *in vitro* (L. "in glass," meaning laboratory) tests, then in animals. In most cases neither the public nor the general medical community hears about "experimental drugs" in this stage of testing. Neither are they listed in this reference.

If safety and efficacy are successfully demonstrated during the preclinical stage, an Investigational New Drug (IND) application is filed with the FDA. There are three phases of clinical trials, designated Phase I, Phase II, and Phase III. After each phase, the FDA will review the findings and approve or deny further testing.

An orphan drug is a drug or biological product for the diagnosis, treatment, or prevention of a rare disease or condition. A rare disease is one that affects fewer than 200,000 persons or for which there is no reasonable expectation that the cost of development will be recovered through U.S. sales of the product. Federal subsidies are provided to the manufacturer for the development of orphan drugs.

A Brief Note on the Transcription of Drugs

Many references are available describing several acceptable ways to transcribe drug information when dictated. We offer the following only as brief guidelines.

The generally accepted style today for the transcription of medical reports for hospital and doctors' office charts (see the American Medical Association *Manual of Style*[1] for publications) is to capitalize the initial letter of brand name drugs and lowercase generic name drugs. The institution may also designate that brand name drugs with unusual capitalization may be typed with initial capital letter only, or typed using the manufacturer's scheme.

The Institute for Safe Medication Practices (ISMP) has issued a list of *Error-Prone Abbreviations, Symbols, and Dose Designations* that should be avoided in prescribing instructions. The Joint Commission for Accreditation of Health Organizations (JCAHO) has mandated a graduated implementation of the ISMP list and has placed certain ISMP abbreviations in a "Do Not Use" list, directing healthcare organizations to add at least three more abbreviations to the JCAHO list. This mandate essentially means that each institution may have its own "Do Not Use" list that differs from other institutions. For that reason, it may be simpler for medical transcriptionists and MTSOs to simply adopt the entire ISMP list as a "Do Not Use" list, assuming, of course, that doing so is acceptable to the originator or client.

Because many of the abbreviations on the ISMP "error-prone" list are Latin or pseudo-Latin abbreviations, many MTs have chosen to translate all Latin abbreviations into English, although this practice is by no means universal. In fact, in its discussion of drug-related terminology, *The Book of Style for Medical Transcription*[2] provides a list of Latin abbreviations for which it says "do not translate." If Latin dosing and dosage abbreviations are used, they should be transcribed in lowercase with periods.

Commas are omitted between the drug name, the dosage, and the instructions for purposes of simplification. Items in a series may be separated by either commas (if no internal commas are used) or semicolons. A simple series might be typed:

Procardia, nitroglycerin sublingual, and Tolinase

or

Procardia 10 mg 3 times a day, nitroglycerin 0.4 mg p.r.n., and Tolinase 250 mg twice a day.

or

Procardia 10 mg t.i.d., nitroglycerin 0.4 mg p.r.n., and Tolinase 250 mg b.i.d.

A more complex or lengthy list of medications, or a list with internal commas, may require the use of semicolons to separate the items in a series. The use of numerals, even for numbers less than ten, is recommended to make dosing information stand out. When two numbers are adjacent to each other, write out one number and use a numeral for the other (e.g., Tylenol No. 3 one q. 4–6 h. p.r.n.). Occasionally, physicians may dictate the number of pills or capsules to be dispensed. When they do, the number should be set off by commas as it is for oxycodone with APAP in this example:

Vigamox 0.5% 1 drop OS; EconoPred 1% 1 drop OS (shake well); atropine 1% 1 drop OS 3 days only (each 5 minutes apart, given at 9 a.m., 1 p.m., 5 p.m., and 9 p.m.); and oxycodone with APAP 5/325, #5, no refills, 1 tablet every 4-6 hours p.r.n. ["#5, no refills" could also be placed in parentheses]

The typing of chemicals with superscripts or subscripts, italics, small capitals, and Greek letters often presents a problem to the transcriptionist. In general, Greek letters are written out (alpha-, beta-, gamma-, etc.). Italics and small capitals are written as standard letters followed by a hyphen (dl-alpha-tocopherol, L-dopa).

When typing nonproprietary (generic) isotope names, element symbols should be included with the name. It may appear to be redundant, but it is the correct form. Therefore, we would type sodium pertechnetate Tc 99m, iodohippurate sodium I 131, or sodium iodide I 125. Occasionally the physician may simply dictate isotopes such as Tc 99m, iodine 131 or I 131, or sodium iodide I 125, and unless he is indicating a trademarked name, it should be typed with a space, no hyphen, and no superscript. This reference indicates proper capitalization, spacing, and hyphenation of isotope entries.

Other combinations of letters and numbers are usually written without spaces or hyphens (OKT1, OKT3, T101, SC1), but this is a complex subject and is dealt with extensively in the AMA Manual of Style.

---

[1] AMA Manual of Style: A Guide for Authors and Editors, 10th ed. New York: Oxford Press; 2007.

[2] The Book of Style for Medical Transcription, 3rd ed. Modesto, California: Association for Healthcare Documentation Integrity (formerly AAMT); 2008.

A (vitamin A) [q.v.]

A and D ointment OTC *moisturizer; emollient* [fish liver oil (vitamins A and D); cholecalciferol; lanolin]

A and D Medicated ointment OTC *diaper rash treatment* [zinc oxide; vitamins A and D]

A + D (ara-C, daunorubicin) *chemotherapy protocol*

A1cNOW fingerstick test kit for home use ℞ *in vitro diagnostic aid for glycosylated hemoglobin levels* ⑤ A.C.N.; Yocon

A-200 shampoo concentrate OTC *pediculicide for lice* [pyrethrins; piperonyl butoxide] 0.33%•4%

AA (ara-C, Adriamycin) *chemotherapy protocol*

AA (arachadonic acid) [q.v.]

AAD (adaptive aerosol delivery) system [see: I-neb AAD; Prodose AAD]

a-(3-aminophthalimido) glutaramide *investigational (orphan) agent for lupus nephritis*

AaT (alpha₁-antitrypsin) [q.v.]

abacavir succinate USAN *antiviral nucleoside reverse transcriptase inhibitor for HIV infection*

abacavir sulfate USAN *antiviral nucleoside reverse transcriptase inhibitor (NRTI) for HIV infection*

abacavir sulfate & lamivudine & zidovudine *nucleoside reverse transcriptase inhibitor (NRTI) combination for HIV and AIDS* 300•150•300 mg oral

abafilcon A USAN *hydrophilic contact lens material*

abamectin USAN, INN *antiparasitic*

abanoquil INN, BAN

abaperidone INN

abarelix USAN *GnRH antagonist to suppress LH and FSH, leading to the cessation of testosterone production (medical castration, androgen ablation); treatment for prostate cancer*

Abarelix-Depot-M (name changed to **Plenaxis** upon marketing release in 2004)

abatacept *selective T-cell co-stimulation modulator for rheumatoid arthritis (RA) and juvenile idiopathic arthritis*

abavca & perthon *investigational (Phase I/II) plant derivative combination for HIV and AIDS*

Abbokinase powder for IV or intra-coronary artery infusion ℞ *thrombolytic enzymes for pulmonary embolism or coronary artery thrombosis* [urokinase] 250 000 IU/vial

Abbo-Pac (trademarked packaging form) *unit dose package*

Abbott TestPack Plus hCG-Urine Plus test kit for professional use ℞ *in vitro diagnostic aid; urine pregnancy test* [monoclonal antibody-based enzyme immunoassay]

ABC (Adriamycin, BCNU, cyclophosphamide) *chemotherapy protocol*

ABC to Z tablets OTC *vitamin/mineral/iron supplement* [multiple vitamins & minerals; ferrous fumarate; folic acid; biotin] ≜•18 mg•0.4 mg•30 mcg

abciximab USAN, INN *monoclonal antibody to glycoprotein (GP) IIb/IIIa receptors; antithrombotic/antiplatelet agent for PTCA and acute arterial occlusive disorders*

ABCM (Adriamycin, bleomycin, cyclophosphamide, mitomycin) *chemotherapy protocol*

ABD (Adriamycin, bleomycin, DTIC) *chemotherapy protocol*

ABDIC (Adriamycin, bleomycin, DIC, [CCNU, prednisone]) *chemotherapy protocol*

ABDV (Adriamycin, bleomycin, DTIC, vinblastine) *chemotherapy protocol*

ABE (antitoxin botulism equine) [see: botulism equine antitoxin, trivalent]

abecarnil INN *anxiolytic*

Abelcet suspension for IV infusion ℞ *systemic polyene antifungal for aspergillosis and other resistant fungal infections (orphan)* [amphotericin B lipid complex (ABLC)] 100 mg/20 mL

Abelmoschus moschatus medicinal herb [see: ambrette]

abetimus INN

abetimus sodium USAN *investigational (NDA filed, orphan) oligonucleotide immunosuppressant for systemic lupus erythematosus–associated nephritis*

Abilify tablets, oral solution, IM injection ℞ *novel (atypical) quinolinone antipsychotic for schizophrenia and manic episodes of a bipolar disorder; adjunctive treatment for major depression* [aripiprazole] 2, 5, 10, 15, 20, 30 mg; 1 mg/mL; 7.5 mg/mL

Abilify Discmelt (orally disintegrating tablets) ℞ *novel (atypical) quinolinone antipsychotic for schizophrenia and manic episodes of a bipolar disorder; adjunctive treatment for major depression* [aripiprazole] 10, 15 mg

ABIP (amphotericin B inhalation powder) [q.v.]

ABLC (amphotericin B lipid complex) [q.v.]

ablukast USAN, INN *antiasthmatic; leukotriene antagonist*

ablukast sodium USAN *antiasthmatic; leukotriene antagonist*

abortifacients *a class of agents that stimulate uterine contractions sufficient to produce uterine evacuation*

ABP (Adriamycin, bleomycin, prednisone) *chemotherapy protocol*

ABPP (aminobromophenylpyrimidinone) [see: bropirimine]

Abraxane suspension of albumin-bound microspheres for IV infusion ℞ *antineoplastic for metastatic breast cancer* [paclitaxel; human albumin] 100•900 mg/dose

Abreva cream OTC *antiviral for cold sores and fever blisters* [docosanol] 10%

abrineurin USAN *treatment for amyotrophic lateral sclerosis (ALS)*

Abrus precatorius medicinal herb [see: precatory bean]

absinthe; absinthites; absinthium *medicinal herb* [see: wormwood]

absorbable cellulose cotton [see: cellulose, oxidized]

absorbable collagen sponge [see: collagen sponge, absorbable]

absorbable dusting powder [see: dusting powder, absorbable]

absorbable gelatin film [see: gelatin film, absorbable]

absorbable gelatin powder [see: gelatin powder, absorbable]

absorbable gelatin sponge [see: gelatin sponge, absorbable]

absorbable surgical suture [see: suture, absorbable surgical]

Absorbase OTC *ointment base* [water-in-oil emulsion of cholesterolized petrolatum and purified water]

absorbent gauze [see: gauze, absorbent]

Absorbine Antifungal Foot aerosol powder (discontinued 2007) OTC *antifungal* [miconazole nitrate; alcohol 10%] 2%

Absorbine Arthritis Strength Liquid with Capsaicin topical liquid OTC *mild anesthetic; antipruritic; counterirritant; analgesic* [menthol; capsaicin] 4%•0.025%

Absorbine Athlete's Foot cream OTC *antifungal* [tolnaftate] 1%

Absorbine Footcare spray liquid OTC *antifungal* [tolnaftate] 1%

Absorbine Jr. liniment OTC *mild anesthetic; antipruritic; counterirritant* [menthol] 1.27%, 4%

Absorbine Jr. Extra Strength topical liquid OTC *mild anesthetic; antipruritic; counterirritant* [menthol] 4%

Abthrax *investigational (orphan) treatment for anthrax exposure* [PA MAb]

abunidazole INN

ABV (actimomycin D, bleomycin, vincristine) *chemotherapy protocol*

ABV (Adriamycin, bleomycin, vinblastine) *chemotherapy protocol for Kaposi sarcoma*

ABV (Adriamycin, bleomycin, vincristine) *chemotherapy protocol for Kaposi sarcoma*

ABVD (Adriamycin, bleomycin, vinblastine, dacarbazine) *chemotherapy protocol for Hodgkin lymphoma*

ABVD/MOPP (alternating cycles of ABVD and MOPP) *chemotherapy protocol*

AC (Adriamycin, carmustine) *chemotherapy protocol*

AC (Adriamycin, CCNU) *chemotherapy protocol*

AC (Adriamycin, cisplatin) *chemotherapy protocol for bone sarcoma*

AC; A-C (Adriamycin, cyclophosphamide) *chemotherapy protocol for breast cancer and pediatric neuroblastoma*

AC/paclitaxel, sequential (Adriamycin, cyclophosphamide; paclitaxel) *chemotherapy protocol for breast cancer*

ACA125 *investigational (orphan) agent for epithelial ovarian cancer*

acacia NF, JAN *suspending agent; emollient; demulcent*

acacia (Acacia senegal; A. verek) gum *medicinal herb for colds, cough, periodontal disease, and wound healing*

acadesine USAN, INN, BAN *platelet aggregation inhibitor*

acamprosate INN

acamprosate calcium GABA/*taurine analogue for the treatment of alcoholism*

acamylophenine [see: camylofin]

Acanthopanax senticosus medicinal herb [see: eleuthero]

Acapodene *investigational (Phase III) antiestrogen antineoplastic for adjunctive treatment of advanced prostate cancer* [toremifene citrate]

acaprazine INN

acarbose USAN, INN, BAN *antidiabetic agent for type 2 diabetes; alpha-glucosidase inhibitor that delays the digestion of dietary carbohydrates* 25, 50, 100 mg oral

ACaT (acylCoA transferase) inhibitors *a class of antihyperlipidemics that lower serum cholesterol levels* ② ACT

Accolate film-coated tablets ℞ *leukotriene receptor antagonist (LTRA) for prevention and chronic treatment of asthma* [zafirlukast] 10, 20 mg ② Equilet

Accretropin injection ℞ *growth hormone for children and adults with congenital or endogenous growth hormone deficiency (GHD), short bowel syndrome, or AIDS-wasting syndrome; for children with Turner syndrome, Prader-Willi syndrome, or renal-induced growth failure* [somatropin] 5 mg/mL

Accu-Chek Advantage reagent strips for home use OTC *in vitro diagnostic aid for blood glucose*

AccuHist oral drops OTC *decongestant; antihistamine; for children 6–36 months* [pseudoephedrine HCl; chlorpheniramine maleate] 9•0.8 mg/mL

AccuHist DM Pediatric oral drops ℞ *antitussive; antihistamine; decongestant; for children 1–24 months* [dextromethorphan hydrobromide; brompheniramine maleate; pseudoephedrine HCl] 4•1•15 mg/mL

AccuHist DM Pediatric syrup (discontinued 2007) OTC *decongestant; antihistamine; antitussive; expectorant; for children 2–11 years* [dextromethorphan hydrobromide; pseudoephedrine HCl; brompheniramine maleate; guaifenesin] 5•30•2•50 mg/5 mL

AccuHist LA sustained-release caplets (discontinued 2006) ℞ *decongestant; antihistamine; anticholinergic to dry mucosal secretions* [phenylephrine HCl; chlorpheniramine maleate; hyoscyamine sulfate; atropine sulfate; scopolamine hydrobromide] 20•8•0.19•0.04•0.01 mg

AccuHist PDX oral drops ℞ *antitussive; antihistamine; decongestant; for children 6–36 months* [dextromethorphan hydrobromide; chlorpheniramine maleate; pseudoephedrine HCl] 3•0.8•9 mg/mL

AccuHist PDX syrup ℞ *antitussive; antihistamine; decongestant; expectorant* [dextromethorphan hydrobromide; brompheniramine maleate; phenylephrine HCl; guaifenesin] 5•2•5•50 mg/5 mL

AccuNeb solution for inhalation ℞ *sympathomimetic bronchodilator for children 2–12 years* [albuterol sulfate] 0.021%, 0.042% (0.63, 1.25 mg/3 mL)

Accu-Pak (trademarked packaging form) *unit dose blister pack*

Accupep HPF powder OTC *enteral nutritional therapy for GI impairment*

Accupril film-coated tablets ℞ *antihypertensive; angiotensin-converting enzyme (ACE) inhibitor; adjunctive treatment for congestive heart failure* [quinapril HCl] 5, 10, 20, 40 mg

Accurbron syrup (discontinued 2008) ℞ *antiasthmatic; bronchodilator* [theophylline; alcohol 7.5%] 150 mg/15 mL

Accuretic film-coated tablets ℞ *antihypertensive; angiotensin-converting enzyme (ACE) inhibitor; diuretic* [quinapril HCl; hydrochlorothiazide] 10•12.5, 20•12.5, 20•25 mg

Accutane capsules ℞ *keratolytic for severe recalcitrant cystic acne; investigational (Phase III) for neuroblastoma* [isotretinoin] 10, 20, 40 mg

Accuzyme ointment, spray ℞ *proteolytic enzyme for debridement of necrotic tissue; vulnerary* [papain; urea] 830 000 IU/g•10%

Accuzyme SE spray ℞ *proteolytic enzyme for debridement of necrotic tissue; vulnerary* [papain; urea] 830 000 IU/g•10%

ACD solution (acid citrate dextrose; anticoagulant citrate dextrose) [see: anticoagulant citrate dextrose solution]

ACD whole blood [see: blood, whole]

ACe (Adriamycin, cyclophosphamide) *chemotherapy protocol for breast cancer*

ACE (Adriamycin, cyclophosphamide, etoposide) *chemotherapy protocol for small cell lung cancer (SCLC)* [also: CAE]

ACE inhibitors (angiotensin-converting enzyme inhibitors) [q.v.]

acebrochol INN

aceburic acid INN

acebutolol USAN, INN, BAN *antihypertensive; antianginal; antiarrhythmic; antiadrenergic (β-receptor)* [also: acebutolol HCl]

acebutolol HCl JAN *antihypertensive; antianginal; antiarrhythmic for premature ventricular contractions (PVCs); antiadrenergic (β-blocker)* [also: acebutolol] 200, 400 mg oral

acecainide INN *antiarrhythmic* [also: acecainide HCl]

acecainide HCl USAN *investigational (orphan) antiarrhythmic* [also: acecainide]

acecarbromal INN *CNS depressant; sedative; hypnotic*

aceclidine USAN, INN *cholinergic*

aceclofenac INN, BAN

acedapsone USAN, INN, BAN *antimalarial; antibacterial; leprostatic*

acediasulfone sodium INN

acedoben INN

acefluranol INN, BAN

acefurtiamine INN

acefylline clofibrol INN

acefylline piperazine INN [also: acepifylline]

aceglaton JAN [also: aceglatone]

aceglatone INN [also: aceglaton]

aceglutamide INN *antiulcerative* [also: aceglutamide aluminum]

aceglutamide aluminum USAN, JAN *antiulcerative* [also: aceglutamide]

ACEIs (angiotensin-converting enzyme inhibitors) [q.v.]

acellular pertussis vaccine [see: diphtheria & tetanus toxoids & acellular pertussis (DTaP) vaccine, adsorbed]

acemannan USAN, INN *hydrogel wound dressing*

acemetacin INN, BAN, JAN

acemethadone [see: methadyl acetate]

aceneuramic acid INN

acenocoumarin [see: acenocoumarol]

acenocoumarol NF, INN [also: nicoumalone]

Aceon tablets ℞ *angiotensin-converting enzyme (ACE) inhibitor for hypertension and stable coronary artery disease (CAD)* [perindopril erbumine] 2, 4, 8 mg ② Aczone; Ocean

aceperone INN ② aspirin; azaperone; Easprin; esuprone

Acephen suppositories OTC *analgesic; antipyretic* [acetaminophen] 120, 325, 650 mg ② Asaphen; Ucephan

acephenazine dimaleate [see: acetophenazine maleate]

acepifylline BAN [also: acefylline piperazine]

acepromazine INN, BAN *veterinary sedative* [also: acepromazine maleate]

acepromazine maleate USAN *veterinary sedative* [also: acepromazine]

aceprometazine INN

acequinoline INN

acerola (*Malpighia glabra; M. punicifolia*) fruit *natural dietary source of vitamin C* ② azarole

acesulfame INN, BAN

Aceta tablets, elixir (discontinued 2008) OTC *analgesic; antipyretic* [acetaminophen] 325, 500 mg; 120 mg/5 mL ② ICE-T

Aceta with Codeine tablets ℞ *narcotic analgesic; antitussive; antipyretic* [codeine phosphate; acetaminophen] 30•300 mg

Acetadote IV injection ℞ *antidote to severe acetaminophen overdose (orphan)* [acetylcysteine] 20% in 30 mL single-dose vials

Aceta-Gesic tablets (discontinued 2007) OTC *analgesic; antipyretic; antihistamine; sleep aid* [acetaminophen; phenyltoloxamine citrate] 325•30 mg

p-**acetamidobenzoic acid** [see: acedoben]

6-acetamidohexanoic acid [see: acexamic acid]

4-acetamidophenyl acetate [see: diacetamate]

acetaminocaproic acid [see: acexamic acid]

acetaminophen USP *analgesic; antipyretic* [also: paracetamol] 80, 325, 500 mg oral; 160, 166.6 mg/5 mL oral; 120, 325, 650 mg rectal

acetaminophen & caffeine & butalbital *analgesic; barbiturate sedative* 325•40•50, 500•40•50 mg oral

acetaminophen & caffeine & butalbital & codeine phosphate *analgesic; barbiturate sedative; narcotic antitussive* 325•40•50•30 mg oral

acetaminophen & caffeine & dihydrocodeine bitartrate *analgesic; narcotic antitussive* 712.8•60•32 mg

acetaminophen & codeine *narcotic analgesic; narcotic antitussive* 300•15, 300•30, 300•60 mg oral; 30•12 mg/5 mL oral

acetaminophen & hydrocodone bitartrate *analgesic; narcotic antitussive* 325•5, 325•10, 500•2.5, 500•10, 650•7.5, 650•10, 750•7.5, 750•10 mg oral; 325•10, 500•7.5 mg/15 mL oral

acetaminophen & isometheptene mucate & dichloralphenazone *cerebral vasoconstrictor and analgesic for vascular and tension headaches; "possibly effective" for migraine headaches* 325•65•100 mg oral

acetaminophen & oxycodone HCl *narcotic analgesic* 325•7.5, 325•10, 500•7.5, 650•10 mg oral

acetaminophen & pentazocine HCl *narcotic analgesic* 650•25 mg oral

acetaminophen & propoxyphene napsylate *narcotic analgesic* 500•100, 650•100 mg oral

acetaminophenol [see: acetaminophen]

acetaminosalol INN

acetanilid (or acetanilide) NF

acetannin [see: acetyltannic acid]

acetarsol INN, BAN [also: acetarsone]

acetarsone NF [also: acetarsol]

acetarsone salt of arecoline [see: drocarbil]

Acetasol ear drops ℞ *antibacterial; antifungal; antiseptic* [acetic acid; benzethonium chloride] 2%•0.02%

Acetasol HC ear drops ℞ *corticosteroidal anti-inflammatory; antibacterial; antifungal; acidifying agent* [hydrocortisone; acetic acid; benzethonium chloride] 1%•2%•0.02%

acetazolamide USP, INN, BAN, JAN *carbonic anhydrase inhibitor; diuretic for edema and glaucoma; anticonvulsant for centrencephalic epilepsies; treatment for acute mountain sickness* 125, 250 mg oral; 500 mg injection

acetazolamide sodium USP, JAN *carbonic anhydrase inhibitor; diuretic; anticonvulsant; antiglaucoma; treatment for acute mountain sickness*

acetcarbromal [see: acecarbromal]

acet-dia-mer-sulfonamide (sulfacetamide, sulfadiazine & sulfamerazine) [q.v.]

acetergamine INN

Acetest reagent tablets for professional use ℞ *in vitro diagnostic aid for acetone (ketones) in the urine or blood*

acetiamine INN

acetic acid NF, JAN *acidifying agent* 0.25%

acetic acid, aluminum salt [see: aluminum acetate]

acetic acid, calcium salt [see: calcium acetate]

acetic acid, diluted NF *bladder irrigant*

acetic acid, ethyl ester [see: ethyl acetate]

acetic acid, glacial USP, INN *acidifying agent*

acetic acid, potassium salt [see: potassium acetate]

acetic acid, sodium salt trihydrate [see: sodium acetate]

acetic acid, zinc salt dihydrate [see: zinc acetate]

Acetic Acid 2% and Aluminum Acetate Otic ear drops ℞ *antibacterial; antifungal; antiseptic; astringent* [acetic acid; aluminum acetate] 2%• ②

acetic acid & hydrocortisone *acidifying agent; corticosteroid; anti-inflammatory* 2%•1% otic solution

acetic acid 5-nitrofurfurylidenehydrazide [see: nihydrazone]

Acetic Acid Otic ear drops ℞ *antibacterial; antifungal; antiseptic* [acetic acid; benzethonium chloride] 2%•0.02%

aceticyl [see: aspirin]

acetilum acidulatum [see: aspirin]

acetiromate INN

acetohexamide USAN, USP, INN, BAN, JAN *sulfonylurea antidiabetic that stimulates insulin secretion in the pancreas*

acetohydroxamic acid (AHA) USAN, USP, INN *urease enzyme inhibitor for chronic urea-splitting urinary infections*

acetol [see: aspirin]

acetomenaphthone BAN

acetomeroctol

acetone NF *solvent; antiseptic* ② Istin

acetophen [see: aspirin]

acetophenazine INN *antipsychotic* [also: acetophenazine maleate]

acetophenazine maleate USAN, USP *antipsychotic* [also: acetophenazine]

p-acetophenetidide (*withdrawn from market*) [see: phenacetin]

acetophenetidin (*withdrawn from market*) [now: phenacetin]

acetorphan *investigational enkephalinase inhibitor for acute diarrhea, opioid withdrawal, and gastroesophageal reflux disease (GERD)*

acetorphine INN, BAN *enkephalinase inhibitor for acute diarrhea; investigational for opioid withdrawal and GERD*

acetosal [see: aspirin]

acetosalic acid [see: aspirin]

acetosalin [see: aspirin]

acetosulfone sodium USAN *antibacterial; leprostatic* [also: sulfadiasulfone sodium]

acetoxyphenylmercury [see: phenylmercuric acetate]

acetoxythymoxamine [see: moxisylyte]

acetphenarsine [see: acetarsone]

acetphenetidin *(withdrawn from market)* [now: phenacetin]

acetphenolisatin [see: oxyphenisatin acetate]

acetrizoate sodium USP [also: sodium acetrizoate]

acetrizoic acid USP

acetryptine INN

acetsalicylamide [see: salacetamide]

acet-theocin sodium [see: theophylline sodium acetate]

aceturate USAN, INN *combining name for radicals or groups*

acetyl adalin [see: acetylcarbromal]

N-acetyl cysteine (NAC) *natural source of cysteine; promotes an increase in the endogenous antioxidant glutathione*

acetyl sulfisoxazole [see: sulfisoxazole acetyl]

***l*-acetyl-α-methadol (LAAM)** [see: levomethadyl acetate]

***p*-acetylaminobenzaldehyde thiosemicarbazone** [see: thioacetazone; thiacetazone]

acetylaminobenzene [see: acetanilid]

N-acetyl-*p*-aminophenol (APAP; NAPA) [see: acetaminophen]

acetylaniline [see: acetanilid]

acetylated polyvinyl alcohol *viscosity-increasing agent*

acetyl-bromo-diethylacetylcarbamide [see: acecarbromal]

acetylcarbromal [see: acecarbromal]

acetylcholine chloride USP, INN, BAN, JAN *cardiac depressant; cholinergic; miotic; peripheral vasodilator*

acetylcholinesterase (AChE) inhibitors *a class of drugs that alter acetylcholine neurotransmitters, used as a cognition adjuvant in Alzheimer dementia* [also called: cholinesterase inhibitors]

N-acetylcysteinate lysine *investigational (orphan) for cystic fibrosis*

acetylcysteine (N-acetylcysteine) USAN, USP, INN, BAN *mucolytic inhaler; antidote to severe acetaminophen overdose (orphan); investigational (orphan) for acute liver failure* [also: N-acetyl-L-cysteine; NAC] 10%, 20% oral

acetylcysteine sodium *mucolytic inhaler* 10%, 20% inhalation

N-acetyl-D-glucosamine *natural remedy for osteoarthritis*

acetyldigitoxin (α-acetyldigitoxin) NF, INN

acetyldihydrocodeinone [see: thebacon]

N-acetyl-DL-leucine [see: acetylleucine]

acetylin [see: aspirin]

acetylkitasamycin JAN *antibacterial* [also: kitasamycin; kitasamycin tartrate]

acetyl-L-carnitine (ALC; ALCAR) *natural protector of neurologic and cardiac function; biologically active amino acid that transports fatty acids into the cellular mitochondria for increased energy output; acetylated form of L-carnitine*

N-acetyl-L-cysteine JAN *mucolytic inhaler* [also: acetylcysteine]

N-acetyl-L-cysteine salicylate [see: salnacedin]

acetylleucine (N-acetyl-DL-leucine) INN

acetylmethadol INN *narcotic analgesic* [also: methadyl acetate]

acetyloleandomycin [see: troleandomycin]

2-acetyloxybenzoic acid [see: aspirin]

acetylpheneturide JAN [also: pheneturide]

acetylphenylisatin [see: oxyphenisatin acetate]

N-acetyl-procainamide (NAPA) [see: acecainide HCl]

acetylpropylorvinol [see: acetorphine]

acetylresorcinol [see: resorcinol monoacetate]

acetylsal [see: aspirin]

N-acetylsalicylamide [see: salacetamide]

acetylsalicylate aluminum [see: aspirin aluminum]

acetylsalicylic acid (ASA) [now: aspirin]

acetylsalicylic acid, phenacetin & caffeine [see: APC]

acetylspiramycin JAN *macrolide antibiotic* [also: spiramycin]

acetylsulfamethoxazole JAN *broad-spectrum sulfonamide bacteriostatic* [also: sulfamethoxazole; sulphamethoxazole; sulfamethoxazole sodium]

acetyltannic acid USP

acetyltannin [see: acetyltannic acid]

acevaltrate INN

acexamic acid INN

ACFUCY (actinomycin D, fluoro-uracil, cyclophosphamide) *chemotherapy protocol*

AChE (acetylcholinesterase) inhibitors [q.v.]

Achillea millefolium medicinal herb [see: yarrow]

aciclovir INN, JAN *antiviral* [also: acyclovir]

acid acriflavine [see: acriflavine HCl]

acid alpha-glucosidase, human [see: alglucosidase alfa]

acid citrate dextrose (ACD) [see: anticoagulant citrate dextrose solution]

acid histamine phosphate [see: histamine phosphate]

Acid Jelly OTC *antibacterial; acidity modifier; moisturizer/lubricant* [acetic acid; oxyquinoline sulfate; ricinoleic acid; glycerin] 0.921%•0.025%• 0.7%•5%

Acid Mantle cream base (name changed to **A-Mantle** in 2007)

Acid Reducer 200 film-coated tablets OTC *histamine H_2 antagonist for episodic heartburn and acid indigestion* [cimetidine] 200 mg

acid sphingomyelinase *investigational (orphan) agent for Niemann-Pick disease type B*

acid trypaflavine [see: acriflavine HCl]

acidogen [see: glutamic acid HCl]

acidol HCl [see: betaine HCl]

Acidophilus capsules, wafers OTC *natural intestinal bacteria; probiotic; dietary supplement; fever blister treatment* [*Lactobacillus acidophilus*] >100 million CFU; 20 million CFU

acidophilus (*Lactobacillus acidophilus*) *natural bacteria for replenish-ment of normal flora in the gastrointestinal tract and vagina; not generally regarded as safe and effective as an antidiarrheal*

Acidophilus with Bifidus wafers OTC *natural intestinal bacteria; probiotic; dietary supplement* [*Lactobacillus acidophilus; L. bifidus*] >100 billion CFU•25 mg

acidulated phosphate fluoride (sodium fluoride & hydrofluoric acid) *dental caries prophylactic*

acidum acetylsalicylicum [see: aspirin]

Acid-X tablets OTC *analgesic; antipyretic; antacid* [acetaminophen; calcium carbonate] 500•250 mg

acifran USAN, INN *antihyperlipoproteinemic* ② Isovorin

aciglumin [see: glutamic acid HCl]

Aci-jel vaginal jelly (discontinued 2005) OTC *antiseptic; acidity modifier; moisturizer/lubricant* [acetic acid; oxyquinoline sulfate; ricinoleic acid; glycerin] 0.921%•0.025%•0.7%•5%

acinitrazole BAN *veterinary antibacterial* [also: nithiamide; aminitrozole]

Aciphex enteric-coated delayed-release tablets ℞ *proton pump inhibitor for duodenal ulcers, erosive or ulcerative gastroesophageal reflux disease (GERD), H. pylori infection, and other gastroesophageal disorders* [rabeprazole sodium] 20 mg

acipimox INN, BAN

acistrate INN *combining name for radicals or groups*

acitemate INN

acitretin USAN, INN, BAN *second generation retinoid; retinoic acid analogue; systemic antipsoriatic*

acivicin USAN, INN *antineoplastic*

ackee (*Blighia sapida*) *fruit medicinal herb for colds, fever, edema, and epilepsy; not generally regarded as safe and effective as seeds and unripened fruit are highly toxic*

aclacinomycin A [now: aclarubicin]

aclantate INN

Aclaro emulsion (discontinued 2007)
R̥ *hyperpigmentation bleaching agent*
[hydroquinone] 4% ☒ Acular

aclarubicin USAN, INN, BAN *antibiotic
antineoplastic* [also: aclarubicin HCl]

aclarubicin HCl JAN *antibiotic antineoplastic* [also: aclarubicin]

Aclasta ⓒ ⓔ (Canadian and European
name for U.S. product **Reclast**)

aclatonium napadisilate INN, BAN, JAN

Aclovate ointment, cream R̥ *corticosteroidal anti-inflammatory* [alclomet-
asone dipropionate] 0.05%

**ACM (Adriamycin, cyclophospha-
mide, methotrexate)** *chemotherapy
protocol*

A.C.N. tablets OTC *vitamin supplement*
[vitamins A, B₃, and C] 25 000 IU•
25 mg•250 mg ☒ A1cNOW; Yocon

Acne Clear gel OTC *keratolytic for acne*
[benzoyl peroxide] 10%

Acne Lotion 10 OTC *antiseptic and keratolytic for acne* [colloidal sulfur] 10%

Acno lotion OTC *antiseptic and keratolytic for acne* [sulfur] 3% ☒ Yocon;
A1cNOW

Acno Cleanser topical liquid OTC
cleanser for acne [isopropyl alcohol]
60%

Acnomel; Adult Acnomel cream
OTC *antiseptic, antifungal, and keratolytic for acne* [sulfur; resorcinol; alco-
hol] 8%•2%•11%

Acnotex lotion OTC *antiseptic, antifungal, and keratolytic for acne* [sulfur;
resorcinol; isopropyl alcohol] 8%•
2%•20%

**ACNU (1-(4-amino-2-methyl-5-pyri-
midnyl)-methyl-3-(2-chloroethyl)-
3-nitrosourea)** [see: nimustin]

acodazole INN *antineoplastic* [also: acodazole HCl]

acodazole HCl USAN *antineoplastic*
[also: acodazole]

Acomplia ⓔ (available in 7 European
countries) *investigational (NDA filed)
selective cannabinoid CB₁ blocker for
smoking cessation, weight loss, increasing HDL, increasing insulin sensitivity,*
*and decreasing C-reactive protein
(CRP) levels* [rimonabant] 20 mg

aconiazide INN *investigational (orphan)
agent for tuberculosis*

aconite (Aconitum napellus) plant
and root *medicinal herb for fever,
hypertension, and neuralgia; not generally regarded as safe and effective as it
is highly toxic*

aconitine USP ☒ Akineton

**ACOP (Adriamycin, cyclophos-
phamide, Oncovin, prednisone)**
chemotherapy protocol

**ACOPP; A-COPP (Adriamycin,
cyclophosphamide, Oncovin,
procarbazine, prednisone)** *chemotherapy protocol*

acortan [see: corticotropin]

Acorus calamus medicinal herb [see:
calamus]

acoxatrine INN

**9-acridinamine monohydrochlo-
ride** [see: aminacrine HCl]

acridinyl anisidide [see: amsacrine]

**acridinylamine methanesulfon ani-
sidide (AMSA)** [see: amsacrine]

acridorex INN

acrids *a class of agents that have a pun-
gent taste or cause heat and irritation
when applied to the skin*

acriflavine NF

acriflavine HCl NF [also: acriflavinium chloride]

acriflavinium chloride INN [also:
acriflavine HCl]

acrihellin INN

acrinol JAN [also: ethacridine lactate;
ethacridine]

acrisorcin USAN, USP, INN *antifungal*

acrivastine USAN, INN, BAN *antihistamine*

acrocinonide INN

acronine USAN, INN *antineoplastic*

acrosoxacin BAN *antibacterial* [also:
rosoxacin]

AcryDerm Strands wound dressing
*high-exudate absorbent dressing for
cavitated wounds*

ACT oral rinse OTC *dental caries preventative* [sodium fluoride; alcohol 7%] 0.05%

ACT (actinomycin) [see: cactinomycin; dactinomycin]

ACT (activated cellular therapy) [q.v.]

Actaea alba; A. pachypoda; A. rubra medicinal herb [see: white cohosh]

Actaea racemosa medicinal herb [see: black cohosh]

actagardin INN

actaplanin USAN, INN, BAN *veterinary growth stimulant*

actarit INN

Actemra investigational (NDA filed) interleukin-6 blocker for moderate to severe rheumatoid arthritis [tocilizumab]

ACTH (adrenocorticotropic hormone) [see: corticotropin]

Acthar Gel [see: H.P. Acthar Gel]

ActHIB powder for injection ℞ *vaccine for H. influenzae type b (HIB) infections in children 2–18 months and invasive diseases caused by HIB infections in children 15–18 months* [Haemophilus b conjugate vaccine; tetanus toxoid] 10•24 mcg/0.5 mL ⊠ AK-Tob

ActHIB/Tripedia IM injection ℞ *vaccine for children younger than 5 months* [Hemophilus b conjugate vaccine; diphtheria & tetanus toxoids & acellular pertussis (DTaP) vaccine] 10 mcg•6.7 LfU•5 LfU•46.8 mcg per 0.5 mL

Acthrel IV infusion ℞ *diagnostic aid for adrenocorticotropic hormone (ACTH)-dependent Cushing syndrome (orphan)* [corticorelin ovine triflutate] 100 mcg ⊠ AK-Trol

ActiBath effervescent tablets OTC *moisturizer; emollient* [colloidal oatmeal] 20%

Acticin cream ℞ *pediculicide for lice; scabicide* [permethrin] 5%

Acticort 100 lotion ℞ *corticosteroidal anti-inflammatory* [hydrocortisone] 1%

Actidose with Sorbitol oral suspension OTC *adsorbent antidote for poisoning; reduces intestinal transit time* [activated charcoal; sorbitol] 25•⅔ g/120 mL; 50•⅔ g/240 mL

Actidose-Aqua oral suspension OTC *adsorbent antidote for poisoning* [activated charcoal] 25 g/120 mL, 50 g/240 mL

Actifed Cold & Allergy tablets OTC *decongestant; antihistamine* [phenylephrine HCl; chlorpheniramine maleate] 10•4 mg

Actifed Cold & Sinus caplets (discontinued 2007) OTC *decongestant; antihistamine; analgesic; antipyretic* [pseudoephedrine HCl; chlorpheniramine maleate; acetaminophen] 30•2•500 mg

Actigall capsules ℞ *naturally occurring bile acid for primary biliary cirrhosis (orphan); gallstone preventative and dissolving agent* [ursodiol] 300 mg

Actimid *investigational (orphan) agent for lupus nephritis and multiple myeloma* [a-(3-aminophthalimido) glutaramide]

Actimmune subcu injection ℞ *immunoregulator for chronic granulomatous disease (orphan) and severe malignant osteopetrosis (orphan); investigational (orphan) for renal cell carcinoma and pulmonary fibrosis* [interferon gamma-1b] 100 mcg (2 million IU) per 0.5 mL

actinium *element (Ac)*

actinomycin C BAN *antibiotic antineoplastic* [also: cactinomycin]

actinomycin D JAN *antibiotic antineoplastic* [also: dactinomycin]

actinoquinol INN *ultraviolet screen* [also: actinoquinol sodium]

actinoquinol sodium USAN *ultraviolet screen* [also: actinoquinol]

actinospectocin [see: spectinomycin]

Actiq "lollipops" ℞ *oral transmucosal narcotic analgesic for breakthrough pain in cancer patients* [fentanyl citrate] 200, 400, 600, 800, 1200, 1600 mcg

Actisite periodontal fiber (discontinued 2004) ℞ *oral antibiotic for periodontitis* [tetracycline] 12.7 mg/23 cm

actisomide USAN, INN *antiarrhythmic*
  ⑨ octazamide

Activase powder for IV infusion ℞ *tissue plasminogen activator (tPA) for acute myocardial infarction, acute ischemic stroke, or pulmonary embolism; investigational (orphan) for intraventricular hemorrhage with intracerebral hemorrhage* [alteplase] 50, 100 mg/vial (29, 58 million IU/vial)

Activase Cathflo [see: Cathflo Activase]

activated attapulgite [see: attapulgite, activated]

activated carbon

activated cellular therapy (ACT) *investigational (Phase II) agent for AIDS*

activated charcoal [see: charcoal, activated]

activated 7-dehydrocholesterol [see: cholecalciferol]

activated ergosterol [see: ergocalciferol]

activated prothrombin complex BAN

Activella film-coated tablets (in packs of 28) ℞ *a mixture of natural and synthetic hormones; hormone replacement therapy for postmenopausal symptoms* [estradiol; norethindrone acetate] 1•0.5, 0.5•0.1 mg

actodigin USAN, INN *cardiotonic*

Actonel film-coated tablets ℞ *bisphosphonate bone resorption inhibitor for Paget disease and corticosteroid-induced or age-related osteoporosis in men and women* [risedronate sodium] 5, 30, 35, 75, 150 mg

Actonel with Calcium monthly dosepak (28 film-coated tablets) ℞ *bisphosphonate bone resorption inhibitor for postmenopausal osteoporosis in women; calcium supplement* [risedronate sodium; calcium (as carbonate)] 35•0 mg × 4 tablets; 0•500 mg × 24 tablets

Actonel with Calcium weekly dosepak (7 film-coated tablets) (discontinued 2007) ℞ *bisphosphonate bone resorption inhibitor for postmenopausal osteoporosis in women; calcium supple-ment* [risedronate sodium; calcium (as carbonate)] 35•0 mg × 1 tablet; 0•500 mg × 6 tablets

ACTOplus met film-coated tablets ℞ *combination antidiabetic agent for type 2 diabetes that decreases hepatic glucose production and increases cellular response to insulin without increasing insulin secretion* [pioglitazone HCl; metformin HCl] 15•500, 15•850 mg

ACTOplus met XR *investigational (NDA filed) extended-release combination antidiabetic agent for type 2 diabetes* [pioglitazone HCl; metformin HCl]

Actos tablets ℞ *antidiabetic for type 2 diabetes that increases cellular response to insulin without increasing insulin secretion* [pioglitazone HCl] 15, 30, 45 mg

Act-O-Vial (trademarked packaging form) *vial system*

ACU-dyne ointment, perineal wash concentrate, prep solution, skin cleanser, prep swabs, swabsticks OTC *broad-spectrum antimicrobial* [povidone-iodine]

ACU-dyne Douche vaginal concentrate OTC *antiseptic/germicidal cleanser and deodorizer* [povidone-iodine]

Acular; Acular LS; Acular PF eye drops ℞ *nonsteroidal anti-inflammatory drug (NSAID) for allergic conjunctivitis, cataract extraction, and corneal refractive surgery* [ketorolac tromethamine] 0.5%; 0.4%; 0.5% ⑨ Aclaro

Acurox *investigational (Phase III) analgesic for moderate-to-severe pain with a low risk of dependency*

AcuTect ℞ *radiopharmaceutical diagnostic aid for acute venous thrombosis* [technetium Tc 99m apcitide]

acycloguanosine [see: acyclovir]

acyclovir USAN, USP, BAN *oral antiviral for herpes simplex virus type 2 (HSV-2, genital herpes), herpes zoster (shingles), and adult-onset varicella (chickenpox); prophylaxis of viral infections in immunocompromised patients* [also: aciclovir] 200, 400, 800 mg oral; 200/5 mL oral

acyclovir redox [see: redox-acyclovir]

acyclovir sodium USAN *parenteral antiviral for herpes simplex virus types 1 and 2 (HSV-1 and HSV-2), herpes simplex encephalitis, and neonatal HSV infections; prophylaxis of viral infections in immunocompromised patients* 50 mg/mL injection

acylCoA transferase (ACaT) inhibitors *a class of antihyperlipidemics that lower serum cholesterol levels*

acylpyrin [see: aspirin]

Aczone gel ℞ *antibacterial for acne vulgaris* [dapsone] 5% ☒ Aceon; Ocean

AD (Adriamycin, dacarbazine) *chemotherapy protocol for soft tissue sarcoma*

ad5CMV-p53 [see: adenoviral p53 gene]

ADA (adenosine deaminase) [see: pegademase bovine; pegademase]

Adacel IM injection ℞ *active immunizing agent for diphtheria, tetanus, and pertussis; Tdap (tetanus predominant) booster vaccine used in adults and children* ≥ 11 *years* [diphtheria toxoid; tetanus toxoid; detoxified pertussis toxins] 2 LfU•5 LfU•2.5 mcg per 0.5 mL dose

adafenoxate INN

Adagen IM injection ℞ *adenosine deaminase (ADA) enzyme replacement for severe combined immunodeficiency disease (orphan)* [pegademase bovine] 250 U/mL

Adalat capsules (discontinued 2008) ℞ *calcium channel blocker for angina* [nifedipine] 10, 20 mg

Adalat CC film-coated sustained-release tablets ℞ *calcium channel blocker for hypertension; also used for anal fissures* [nifedipine] 30, 60, 90 mg

adalimumab INN *recombinant human immunoglobulin G1 (rhIgG1); tumor necrosis factor-α (TNF-α) blocker; DMARD for moderate to severe rheumatoid arthritis (RA), psoriatic arthritis, and ankylosing spondylitis; immunostimulant for Crohn disease*

adamantanamine [see: amantadine]

adamantanamine HCl [see: amantadine HCl]

adamexine INN

adapalene USAN, INN, BAN *synthetic retinoid analogue for topical treatment of acne*

Adapettes solution OTC *rewetting solution for hard contact lenses*

Adapettes Especially for Sensitive Eyes solution OTC *rewetting solution for soft contact lenses*

adaprolol maleate USAN *ophthalmic antihypertensive (β-blocker)*

adaptive aerosol delivery (AAD) system [see: I-neb AAD; Prodose AAD]

adatanserin INN *anxiolytic; antidepressant* [also: adatanserin HCl]

adatanserin HCl USAN *anxiolytic; antidepressant* [also: adatanserin]

AdatoSil 5000 intraocular injection ℞ *retinal tamponade for retinal detachment* [polydimethylsiloxane] 10, 15 mL

Adavite tablets OTC *vitamin supplement* [multiple vitamins; folic acid; biotin] ±•400•35 mcg ☒ Advate

Adavite-M tablets OTC *vitamin/mineral/iron supplement* [multiple vitamins & minerals; iron; folic acid; biotin] ±•27 mg•0.4 mg•30 mcg

ADBC (Adriamycin, DTIC, bleomycin, CCNU) *chemotherapy protocol*

ADC with Fluoride pediatric oral drops ℞ *vitamin supplement; dental caries preventative* [vitamins A, C, and D; fluoride] 1500 IU•35 mg•400 IU•0.5 mg per mL

Adderall tablets ℞ *CNS stimulant for attention-deficit/hyperactivity disorder (ADHD), narcolepsy, and obesity* [amphetamine aspartate; amphetamine sulfate; dextroamphetamine sulfate; dextroamphetamine saccharate] 5, 7.5, 10, 12.5, 15, 20, 30 mg total amphetamines (25% of each)

Adderall XR capsules containing extended-release spheres ℞ *CNS stimulant for attention-deficit/hyperactivity disorder (ADHD); once-daily doseform* [amphetamine aspartate; amphetamine sulfate; dextroamphetamine sulfate; dextroamphetamine saccharate] 5, 10, 15, 20, 25, 30 mg total amphetamines (25% of each)

adder's mouth *medicinal herb* [see: chickweed]

adder's tongue (*Erythronium americanum*) bulb and leaves *medicinal herb used as an emetic, antiscrofulous agent, and emollient*

ADD-Vantage (trademarked delivery device) *intravenous drug admixture device* ⑨ Advantage 24

ADE (ara-C, daunorubicin, etoposide) *chemotherapy protocol*

Adeflor M pediatric tablets (discontinued 2004) ℞ *vitamin supplement; dental caries preventative* [multiple vitamins; fluoride; calcium; iron] ± • 1•250•30 mg

adefovir dipivoxil USAN *nucleotide analogue reverse transcriptase inhibitor for chronic hepatitis B virus (HBV) infection*

ADEKs chewable tablets OTC *vitamin/mineral supplement* [multiple vitamins & minerals; folic acid; biotin] ± • 200•50 mcg ⑨ Adoxa; Edex; Iodex

ADEKs pediatric oral drops OTC *vitamin/mineral supplement* [multiple vitamins & minerals; biotin] ± •15 mcg ⑨ Adoxa; Edex; Iodex

adelmidrol INN

ademetionine INN

adenazole [see: tocladesine]

adenine USP, JAN *amino acid*

adenine arabinoside (ara-A) [see: vidarabine]

adeno-associated viral vector containing the gene for human coagulation Factor IX *investigational (orphan) agent for moderate to severe hemophilia*

adeno-associated viral-based vector cystic fibrosis gene therapy *investigational (orphan) for cystic fibrosis*

adeno-associated virus alpha₁-antitrypsin vector, recombinant (rAAV-AaT) *investigational (orphan) for alpha₁-antitrypsin deficiency*

Adenocard IV injection ℞ *antiarrhythmic* [adenosine] 3 mg/mL

Adenoscan IV infusion ℞ *cardiac diagnostic aid; cardiac stressor; adjunct to thallium 201 myocardial perfusion scintigraphy* [adenosine] 3 mg/mL

adenosine USAN, BAN *antiarrhythmic for paroxysmal supraventricular tachycardia; also used as a diagnostic aid for coronary artery disease; investigational (orphan) for brain tumors* 3 mg/mL injection

adenosine deaminase (ADA) [see: pegademase bovine; pegademase]

adenosine monophosphate (AMP) [see: adenosine phosphate]

adenosine phosphate USAN, INN, BAN *nutrient; treatment for varicose veins and herpes infections*

adenosine triphosphate (aTP) disodium JAN

S-adenosyl-L-methionine (SAMe) *natural amino acid derivative used to treat depression and protect the liver from toxic overload; regenerates liver function and restores hepatic glutathione levels when taken with B vitamins; investigational (orphan) for AIDS-related myelopathy*

adenoviral p53 gene *investigational (Phase III) gene therapy for head and neck cancer* [also: p53 adenoviral gene]

adenovirus-based vector Factor VIII complementary DNA to somatic cells *investigational (orphan) agent for hemophilia A*

adenovirus-mediated herpes simplex virus-thymidine kinase gene *investigational (orphan) agent for malignant glioma*

5'-adenylic acid [see: adenosine phosphate]

adepsine oil [see: mineral oil]

adhesive bandage [see: bandage, adhesive]

adhesive tape [see: tape, adhesive]

adibendan INN

A-DIC (Adriamycin, dacarbazine) *chemotherapy protocol*

adicillin INN, BAN

adimolol INN

adinazolam USAN, INN, BAN *antidepressant; sedative*

adinazolam mesylate USAN *antidepressant*

Adipex-P capsules, tablets ℞ *anorexiant; CNS stimulant* [phentermine HCl] 37.5 mg

adiphenine INN *smooth muscle relaxant* [also: adiphenine HCl]

adiphenine HCl USAN *smooth muscle relaxant* [also: adiphenine]

adipiodone INN, JAN *parenteral radiopaque contrast medium* [also: iodipamide]

adipiodone meglumine JAN *parenteral radiopaque contrast medium (49.42% iodine)* [also: iodipamide meglumine]

aditeren INN

aditoprim INN

Adlea topical liquid *investigational highly purified natural product used during surgery to block pain receptors* [capsaicin]

adnephrine [see: epinephrine]

ADOAP (Adriamycin, Oncovin, ara-C, prednisone) *chemotherapy protocol* ⧈ EDAP; UDIP

Adolph's Salt Substitute OTC *salt substitute* [potassium chloride] 64 mEq K/5 g; 35 mEq K/5 g

ADOP (Adriamycin, Oncovin, prednisone) *chemotherapy protocol* ⧈ EDAP; UDIP

adosopine INN

Adoxa film-coated tablets ℞ *tetracycline antibiotic* [doxycycline monohydrate] 50, 75, 100, 150 mg ⧈ ADEKs; Edex; Iodex

adozelesin USAN, INN *antineoplastic*

Adprin-B coated tablets (discontinued 2007) OTC *analgesic; antipyretic; antiinflammatory; antirheumatic* [aspirin (buffered with calcium carbonate, magnesium oxide, and magnesium carbonate)] 325, 500 mg

ADR (Adriamycin) [see: Adriamycin; doxorubicin HCl]

adrafinil INN

adrenal [see: epinephrine]

adrenal cortical steroids *a class of steroid hormones that stimulate the adrenal cortex*

Adrenalin Chloride nasal spray (discontinued 2006) ℞ *nasal decongestant* [epinephrine HCl] 0.1%

Adrenalin Chloride nose drops ℞ *nasal decongestant; vasopressor for shock* [epinephrine HCl] 0.1% (1 mg/mL or 1:1000)

Adrenalin Chloride solution for inhalation ℞ *sympathomimetic bronchodilator; vasopressor for shock* [epinephrine HCl] 1:100, 1:1000 (10, 1 mg/mL)

Adrenalin Chloride subcu, IV, IM or intracardiac injection ℞ *sympathomimetic bronchodilator for bronchial asthma, bronchospasm, and COPD; vasopressor for shock* [epinephrine HCl] 1:1000 (1 mg/mL)

adrenaline BAN *vasoconstrictor; sympathomimetic bronchodilator; topical antiglaucoma agent; vasopressor for shock* [also: epinephrine]

adrenaline bitartrate [see: epinephrine bitartrate]

adrenaline HCl [see: epinephrine HCl]

adrenalone USAN, INN *ophthalmic adrenergic*

adrenamine [see: epinephrine]

adrenergic agonists *a class of bronchodilators that relax the bronchial muscles, reducing bronchospasm; a class of cardiac agents that increase myocardial contractility, causing a vasopressor effect to counteract shock (inadequate tissue perfusion)* [also called: sympathomimetics]

adrenine [see: epinephrine]

adrenochromazone [see: carbazochrome salicylate]

adrenochrome [see: carbazochrome salicylate]

adrenochrome guanylhydrazone mesilate JAN

adrenochrome monoaminoguanidine sodium methylsulfonate [see: adrenochrome guanylhydrazone mesilate]

adrenochrome monosemicarba-zone sodium salicylate [see: carbazochrome salicylate]

adrenocorticotrophin [see: corticotropin]

adrenocorticotropic hormone (ACTH) [see: corticotropin]

adrenone [see: adrenalone]

Adria + BCNU (Adriamycin, BCNU) *chemotherapy protocol*

Adria-L-PAM (Adriamycin, L-phenylalanine mustard) *chemotherapy protocol*

Adriamycin PFS (preservative-free solution) IV injection ℞ *anthracycline antibiotic antineoplastic* [doxorubicin HCl] 2 mg/mL

Adriamycin RDF (rapid dissolution formula) powder for IV injection ℞ *anthracycline antibiotic antineoplastic* [doxorubicin HCl] 10, 20, 50, 150 mg/vial

Adria-Oncoline Chemo-Pin (trademarked delivery form)

adrogolide INN

adrogolide HCl USAN *dopamine D_1 receptor agonist for Parkinson disease*

Adrucil IV injection ℞ *antimetabolite antineoplastic for colorectal (orphan), esophageal (orphan), breast, stomach, and pancreatic cancers; investigational (orphan) for glioblastoma multiforme; also used for several other cancers* [fluorouracil] 50 mg/mL

ADS (azodisal sodium) [now: olsalazine sodium]

adsorbed diphtheria toxoid [see: diphtheria toxoid, adsorbed]

Adsorbocarpine eye drops ℞ *antiglaucoma agent; direct-acting miotic* [pilocarpine HCl] 1%, 2%, 4%

Adsorbonac eye drops OTC *corneal edema-reducing agent* [sodium chloride (hypertonic saline solution)] 2%, 5%

ADT (trademarked dosage form) *alternate-day therapy*

Adult Acnomel [see: Acnomel]

Advagraf ⓔ extended-release form of **Prograf** (approved in Europe) *investigational (NDA filed) once-daily*

immunosuppressant for liver, kidney, and heart transplants [tacrolimus]

Advair Diskus 100/50; Advair Diskus 250/50; Advair Diskus 500/50 powder for inhalation ℞ *corticosteroidal anti-inflammatory and bronchodilator combination for chronic asthma and chronic obstructive pulmonary disease (COPD) with chronic bronchitis* [fluticasone propionate; salmeterol xinafoate] 100•50 mcg; 250•50 mcg; 500•50 mcg

Advair HFA 45/21; Advair HFA 115/21; Advair HFA 230/21 inhalation aerosol in a metered-dose inhaler ℞ *corticosteroidal anti-inflammatory and bronchodilator combination for chronic asthma and chronic obstructive pulmonary disease (COPD) with chronic bronchitis* [fluticasone propionate; salmeterol xinafoate] 45•21 mcg; 115•21 mcg; 230•21 mcg

Advance test stick for home use OTC *in vitro diagnostic aid; urine pregnancy test*

Advanced Care Cholesterol Test kit for home use OTC *in vitro diagnostic aid for cholesterol in the blood*

Advanced Eye Relief eye drops OTC *moisturizer/lubricant* [propylene glycol] 0.95%

"Advanced Formula" products [see under product name]

Advanced-RF Natal Care tablets ℞ *vitamin/mineral/calcium/iron supplement; stool softener* [multiple vitamins & minerals; calcium; iron; folic acid; docusate sodium] ≛•200•90•1•50 mcg

Advantage 24 vaginal gel OTC *spermicidal contraceptive (for use with a diaphragm)* [nonoxynol 9] 3.5% ②

ADD-Vantage

Advantage Invisible Acne Patch topical liquid OTC *keratolytic* [salicylic acid] 2%

Advate powder for IV injection ℞ *systemic hemostatic; antihemophilic for the prevention and control of bleeding in classical hemophilia (hemophilia A) and von Willebrand disease (orphan)* [antihemophilic factor VIII, recombinant] 250, 500, 1000, 1500, 2000, 3000 U/vial ⧉ Adavite

Advera oral liquid OTC *enteral nutritional therapy for HIV and AIDS patients* [lactose-free formula] 240 mL

Advexin *investigational (Phase III) gene therapy for head and neck cancer* [p53 adenoviral gene]

Advia Centaur HBc IgM test kit for professional use ℞ *in vitro diagnostic aid to detect IgM antibodies to hepatitis B core (HBc) antigen*

Advicor caplets ℞ *combination treatment for hypercholesterolemia and mixed dyslipidemia: HMG-CoA reductase inhibitor to lower LDL and total cholesterol plus niacin to raise HDL and lower triglycerides* [lovastatin; extended-release niacin] 20•500, 20•1000, 40•1000 mg

Advil tablets, Liqui-Gels (liquid-filled gelcaps) OTC *analgesic; antiarthritic; antipyretic; nonsteroidal anti-inflammatory drug (NSAID) for mild to moderate pain, migraine headaches, and primary dysmenorrhea* [ibuprofen] 200 mg

Advil, Children's chewable tablets, oral suspension OTC *analgesic; antipyretic; nonsteroidal anti-inflammatory drug (NSAID) for minor aches and pains* [ibuprofen] 50 mg; 100 mg/5 mL

Advil, Junior Strength chewable tablets OTC *analgesic; antipyretic; nonsteroidal anti-inflammatory drug (NSAID) for minor aches and pains* [ibuprofen] 100 mg

Advil Allergy Sinus caplets OTC *decongestant; antihistamine; analgesic; antipyretic* [pseudoephedrine HCl; chlorpheniramine maleate; ibuprofen] 30•2•200 mg

Advil Cold, Children's oral suspension (discontinued 2007) OTC *decongestant; analgesic; antipyretic* [pseudoephedrine HCl; ibuprofen] 15•100 mg/5 mL

Advil Cold & Sinus Liqui-gels (liquid-filled gelcaps), caplets OTC *decongestant; analgesic; antipyretic* [pseudoephedrine HCl; ibuprofen] 30•200 mg

Advil Flu & Body Ache caplets (discontinued 2007) OTC *decongestant; analgesic; antipyretic* [pseudoephedrine HCl; ibuprofen] 30•200 mg

Advil Migraine liquid-filled capsules OTC *analgesic; antipyretic; nonsteroidal anti-inflammatory drug (NSAID) for mild to moderate pain of migraine headaches* [ibuprofen] 200 mg

Advil Pediatric Drops oral suspension OTC *analgesic; antipyretic; nonsteroidal anti-inflammatory drug (NSAID) for minor aches and pains* [ibuprofen] 100 mg/2.5 mL

Advil PM caplets OTC *analgesic; antipyretic; antihistaminic sleep aid* [ibuprofen; diphenhydramine citrate] 200•38 mg

AE-941 *investigational (Phase III) shark cartilage–based angiogenesis inhibitor for osteoarthritis, rheumatoid arthritis, and various cancers; investigational (orphan) for renal cell carcinoma*

AEDs (anti-epileptic drugs) [see: anticonvulsants]

A-E-R pads OTC *emollient; astringent* [hamamelis water (witch hazel)] 50%

Aeroaid spray OTC *antiseptic; antibacterial; antifungal* [thimerosal; alcohol 72%] 1:1000 ⧉ Aredia; Award; Euro-D

AeroBid; AeroBid-M oral inhalation aerosol ℞ *corticosteroidal anti-inflammatory for chronic asthma* [flunisolide] 250 mcg/dose ⧉ EryPed

AeroCaine aerosol solution (discontinued 2007) OTC *anesthetic; antiseptic* [benzocaine; benzethonium chloride] 13.6%•0.5% ⧉ argon; Ircon

AeroChamber (trademarked delivery device) *aerosol holding chamber*

Aerodine aerosol (discontinued 2004) OTC *broad-spectrum antimicrobial* [povidone-iodine] ⧉ Arduan

Aerofreeze topical spray OTC *refrigerant anesthetic* [trichloromonofluoromethane; dichlorodifluoromethane]

Aerohist extended-release tablets ℞ *antihistamine; anticholinergic to dry mucosal secretions* [chlorpheniramine maleate; methscopolamine nitrate] 8•2.5 mg

AeroHist Plus extended-release caplets ℞ *decongestant; antihistamine; anticholinergic to dry mucosal secretions* [phenylephrine HCl; chlorpheniramine maleate; methscopolamine nitrate] 20•8•2.5 mg

AeroKid syrup ℞ *decongestant; antihistamine; anticholinergic to dry mucosal secretions* [phenylephrine HCl; chlorpheniramine maleate; methscopolamine nitrate] 10•4•1.25 mg/5 mL

Aerolate Sr.; Aerolate Jr.; Aerolate III timed-action capsules ℞ *antiasthmatic; bronchodilator* [theophylline] 260 mg; 130 mg; 65 mg

Aerolizer (trademarked delivery device) *oral inhaler for encapsulated dry powder*

Aeropin *investigational (orphan) for cystic fibrosis* [heparin, 2-0-desulfated]

Aeroseb-Dex aerosol spray ℞ *corticosteroidal anti-inflammatory* [dexamethasone] 0.01%

aerosol OT [see: docusate sodium]

aerosolized pooled immune globulin [see: globulin, aerosolized pooled immune]

AeroSpan oral inhalation aerosol ℞ *corticosteroidal anti-inflammatory for chronic asthma* [flunisolide hemihydrate] 80 mcg/dose ⊡ erizepine

AeroTherm aerosol solution (discontinued 2004) OTC *anesthetic; antiseptic* [benzocaine; benzethonium chloride] 13.6%•0.5%

Aerotrol (trademarked delivery form) *inhalation aerosol* ⊡ Urotrol

AeroTuss 12 oral suspension ℞ *antitussive* [dextromethorphan tannate] 30 mg/5 mL ⊡ Artiss; Ertaczo

AeroZoin topical spray OTC *skin protectant; antiseptic* [benzoin; isopropyl alcohol 44.8%] 30% ⊡ Orasone; Ureacin-10

AERx *investigational (Phase III) insulin inhalation system for diabetes management*

Aesculus hippocastanum; A. californica; A. glabra *medicinal herb* [see: horse chestnut]

Aethusa cynapium *medicinal herb* [see: dog poison]

aethylis chloridum [see: ethyl chloride]

afalanine INN

Afeditab CR extended-release tablets ℞ *calcium channel blocker for hypertension; also used for anal fissures* [nifedipine] 30, 60 mg

Affinitac *investigational (Phase III) antisense agent for lung cancer*

Afinitor (available in Europe as **Certican**) *investigational (NDA filed) once-daily oral antineoplastic for kidney and neuroendocrine cancer* [everolimus]

afloqualone INN, JAN

Afluria suspension for IM injection in multidose vials ℞ *vaccine for influenza virus types A and B for patients ≥ 18 years* [influenza split-virus vaccine (with thiomersal preservative)] 0.5 mL/dose (mercury 24.5 mcg/dose)

Afluria suspension for IM injection in prefilled syringes ℞ *vaccine for influenza virus types A and B for patients ≥ 18 years* [influenza split-virus vaccine (preservative free)] 0.5 mL/dose

AFM (Adriamycin, fluorouracil, methotrexate [with leucovorin rescue]) *chemotherapy protocol*

afovirsen INN *antisense antiviral*

afovirsen sodium USAN *antisense antiviral*

AFP (alpha fetoprotein) [q.v.]

AFP-Scan *investigational (orphan) for diagnostic aid for AFP-producing tumors, hepatoblastoma, and hepatocellular carcinoma* [monoclonal antibodies to human alpha-fetoprotein (AFP), murine, radiolabeled with technetium Tc 99m]

Afresa *investigational (Phase III) orally inhaled insulin for diabetes* [insulin]

African ginger *medicinal herb* [see: ginger]

African pepper; African red pepper *medicinal herb* [see: cayenne]

Afrin 12-Hour Original nasal spray, pump spray OTC *nasal decongestant* [oxymetazoline HCl] 0.05%

Afrin Children's Pump Mist nasal spray OTC *nasal decongestant* [phenylephrine HCl] 0.25%

Afrin Moisturizing Saline Mist solution OTC *nasal moisturizer* [sodium chloride (saline solution)] 0.64%

Afrin No-Drip 12-Hour; Afrin No-Drip 12-Hour Extra Moisturizing; Afrin No-Drip 12-Hour Severe Congestion with Menthol nasal spray OTC *nasal decongestant* [oxymetazoline HCl] 0.05%

Afrin Severe Congestion with Menthol nasal spray OTC *nasal decongestant* [oxymetazoline HCl] 0.05%

Afrin Sinus nasal spray OTC *nasal decongestant* [oxymetazoline HCl] 0.05%

Afrin Sinus with Vapornase; Afrin No-Drip Sinus with Vapornase nasal spray OTC *nasal decongestant* [oxymetazoline HCl] 0.05%

Aftate for Athlete's Foot spray powder, spray liquid OTC *antifungal* [tolnaftate] 1%

Aftate for Jock Itch spray powder OTC *antifungal* [tolnaftate] 1%

afurolol INN

A/G Pro tablets OTC *dietary supplement* [protein hydrolysate; multiple vitamins & minerals; multiple amino acids] 542•≛ mg ☑ AKPro

agalsidase alfa USAN *investigational (NDA filed, orphan) enzyme replacement therapy for Fabry disease*

agalsidase beta *enzyme replacement therapy for Fabry disease (orphan)*

agalsidase beta & ceramide trihexosidase (CTH) *investigational (orphan) enzyme replacement therapy for Fabry disease*

aganodine INN

agar NF, JAN *suspending agent* ☑ Icar

agar-agar [see: agar]

Agathosma betulina medicinal herb [see: buchu]

agave (*Agave americana*) plant *medicinal herb used as an antiseptic, diuretic, and laxative and for jaundice and liver disease, pulmonary tuberculosis, and syphilis; also used to combat putrefactive bacteria in the stomach and intestines*

age cross-link breakers *a class of investigational antiaging compounds that break age-mediated bonds between proteins*

Agenerase capsules, oral solution (discontinued 2008) ℞ *protease inhibitor antiviral for HIV infection* [amprenavir; vitamin E] 50 mg•36 IU; 15 mg•46 IU per mL

Aggrastat IV infusion ℞ *platelet aggregation inhibitor for acute coronary syndrome, unstable angina, myocardial infarction, and cardiac surgery* [tirofiban HCl] 50, 250 mcg/mL

aggregated albumin [see: albumin, aggregated]

aggregated radio-iodinated I 131 serum albumin [see: albumin, aggregated iodinated I 131 serum]

Aggrenox dual-release capsules ℞ *platelet aggregation inhibitor to reduce the risk of stroke* [dipyridamole (extended release); aspirin (immediate release)] 200•25 mg

Agilect (name changed to **Azilect** upon marketing release in 2006)

aglepristone INN

agofollin [see: estradiol]

agomelatine *agonist to melatonin* MT_1 *and* MT_2 *receptors and antagonist to serotonin* 5-HT_{2c} *receptors; investigational (Phase III) oral treatment for major depressive disorder (MDD)*

Agoral oral liquid OTC *stimulant laxative* [sennosides] 25 mg/15 mL ☑ Aquoral

agrimony (*Agrimonia eupatoria*) plant *medicinal herb for diarrhea, gastroenteritis, jaundice, kidney stones, liver disorders, mucous membrane inflammation with discharge; also used topically as an astringent and antiseptic*

agrimony, hemp *medicinal herb* [see: hemp agrimony]

Agropyron repens medicinal herb [see: couch grass]

Agrylin capsules ℞ *thrombolytic and antiplatelet agent for essential thrombocytopenia (orphan); investigational (orphan) for thrombocytosis and polycythemia vera* [anagrelide HCl] 0.5, 1 mg

ague tree *medicinal herb* [see: sassafras]

agurin [see: theobromine sodium acetate]

AHA (acetohydroxamic acid) [q.v.]

AHA (alpha hydroxy acids) [see: glycolic acid]

AH-chew Ultra Tannate oral suspension ℞ *decongestant; antihistamine; anticholinergic to dry mucosal secretions* [phenylephrine tannate; chlorpheniramine tannate; methscopolamine nitrate] 10•2•1.5 mg/5 mL

AH-chew D chewable tablets ℞ *nasal decongestant* [phenylephrine HCl] 10 mg

AH-chew D oral suspension ℞ *nasal decongestant* [phenylephrine tannate] 10 mg/5 mL

AH-chew Ultra chewable tablets ℞ *decongestant; antihistamine; anticholinergic to dry mucosal secretions* [phenylephrine HCl; chlorpheniramine maleate; methscopolamine nitrate] 10•2•1.25 mg

AHF (antihemophilic factor) [q.v.]

AHG (antihemophilic globulin) [see: antihemophilic factor]

A-Hydrocort IV or IM injection ℞ *corticosteroid; anti-inflammatory* [hydrocortisone sodium succinate] 100, 250, 500, 1000 mg/vial

AIDS vaccine (several different compounds are included in this general category; e.g., gp120, rgp160, rgp160 MN, rp24) *investigational (Phase I–III) antiviral for HIV and AIDS treatment and prophylaxis* [also: gp120; rgp160; rp24]

AIDSVax *investigational (Phase III) bivalent HIV vaccine* [gp120 antigens]

AIIRAs (angiotensin II receptor antagonists) [q.v.]

air, compressed [see: air, medical]

air, medical USP *medicinal gas*

Airet solution for inhalation ℞ *sympathomimetic bronchodilator* [albuterol sulfate] 0.083%

AI-RSA *investigational (orphan) agent for autoimmune uveitis*

ajmaline JAN

Akarpine eye drops ℞ *antiglaucoma agent; direct-acting miotic* [pilocarpine HCl] 1%, 2%, 4%

AKBeta eye drops ℞ *antiglaucoma agent (β-blocker)* [levobunolol HCl] 0.25%, 0.5%

AK-Chlor eye drops, ophthalmic ointment (discontinued 2005) ℞ *antibiotic* [chloramphenicol] 5 mg/mL; 10 mg/g ⊠ OcuClear

AK-Cide eye drop suspension, ophthalmic ointment (discontinued 2004) ℞ *corticosteroidal anti-inflammatory; antibiotic* [prednisolone acetate; sulfacetamide sodium] 0.5%•10% ⊠ Axid

AK-Con eye drops ℞ *decongestant; vasoconstrictor* [naphazoline HCl] 0.1%

AK-Dex eye drops (discontinued 2004) ℞ *corticosteroidal anti-inflammatory* [dexamethasone sodium phosphate] 0.1%

AK-Dilate eye drops ℞ *decongestant; vasoconstrictor; mydriatic* [phenylephrine HCl] 2.5%, 10%

AK-Fluor antecubital venous injection ℞ *ophthalmic diagnostic agent* [fluorescein] 10%, 25%

Akineton IV or IM injection ℞ *anticholinergic; antiparkinsonian* [biperiden lactate] 5 mg/mL ⊠ aconitine

Akineton tablets ℞ *anticholinergic; antiparkinsonian* [biperiden HCl] 2 mg ⊠ aconitine

aklomide USAN, INN, BAN *coccidiostat for poultry* ⊠ iogulamide

AK-NaCl eye drops, ophthalmic ointment OTC *corneal edema-reducing agent* [sodium chloride (hypertonic saline solution)] 5%

Akne-Mycin ointment ℞ *antibiotic for acne* [erythromycin] 2%

AK-Pentolate eye drops ℞ *mydriatic; cycloplegic* [cyclopentolate HCl] 1%

AK-Poly-Bac ophthalmic ointment ℞ *antibiotic* [polymyxin B sulfate; bacitracin zinc] 10 000●500 U/g

AK-Pred eye drops (discontinued 2006) ℞ *corticosteroidal anti-inflammatory* [prednisolone sodium phosphate] 0.125%, 1%

AKPro eye drops ℞ *antiglaucoma agent* [dipivefrin HCl] 0.1% ▣ A/G Pro

AK-Rinse ophthalmic solution OTC *extraocular irrigating solution* [sterile isotonic solution]

AK-Spore eye drops ℞ *antibiotic* [polymyxin B sulfate; neomycin sulfate; gramicidin] 10 000 U●1.75 mg●0.025 mg per mL ▣ Exubera

AK-Spore ophthalmic ointment ℞ *antibiotic* [polymyxin B sulfate; neomycin sulfate; bacitracin zinc] 10 000 U●5 mg●400 U per g ▣ Exubera

AK-Spore H.C. ear drop solution, ear drop suspension (discontinued 2004) ℞ *corticosteroidal anti-inflammatory; antibiotic* [hydrocortisone; neomycin sulfate; polymyxin B sulfate] 1%●5 mg●10 000 U per mL

AK-Spore H.C. ophthalmic ointment ℞ *corticosteroidal anti-inflammatory; antibiotic* [hydrocortisone; neomycin sulfate; bacitracin zinc; polymyxin B sulfate] 1%●0.35%●400 U/g●10 000 U/g

AK-Sulf eye drops, ophthalmic ointment ℞ *antibiotic* [sulfacetamide sodium] 10% ▣ Ocusulf-10

AK-Tob eye drops ℞ *aminoglycoside antibiotic* [tobramycin] 0.3%

AK-Tracin ophthalmic ointment ℞ *bactericidal antibiotic* [bacitracin] 500 U/g ▣ Ocutricin

AK-Trol eye drop suspension (discontinued 2004) ℞ *corticosteroidal anti-inflammatory; antibiotic* [dexamethasone; neomycin sulfate; polymyxin B sulfate] 0.1%●0.35%●10 000 U/mL

AK-Trol ophthalmic ointment ℞ *corticosteroidal anti-inflammatory; antibiotic* [dexamethasone; neomycin sulfate; polymyxin B sulfate] 0.1%●0.35%●10 000 U/g

Akwa Tears eye drops OTC *moisturizer/lubricant* [polyvinyl alcohol] 1.4%

Akwa Tears ophthalmic ointment OTC *moisturizer/lubricant* [white petrolatum; mineral oil]

ALA (alpha lipoic acid) *natural antioxidant* [q.v.]

ALA; 5-ALA HCl [see: aminolevulinic acid HCl]

alacepril INN, JAN

Alacol syrup, oral drops ℞ *decongestant; antihistamine; drops for children 2–5 years* [phenylephrine HCl; brompheniramine maleate] 5●2 mg/5 mL; 1●0.4 mg/mL

Alacol DM syrup, oral drops ℞ *antitussive; antihistamine; decongestant* [dextromethorphan hydrobromide; brompheniramine maleate; phenylephrine HCl] 10●2●5 mg/5 mL; 5●1●2.5 mg/2.5 mL

Ala-Cort cream, lotion ℞ *corticosteroidal anti-inflammatory* [hydrocortisone] 1%

Alacramyn *investigational (orphan) antitoxin for scorpion stings* [centruroides immune Fab 2]

alafosfalin INN, BAN

Alamag oral suspension OTC *antacid* [aluminum hydroxide; magnesium hydroxide] 225●200 mg/5 mL

Alamag Plus oral suspension OTC *antacid; antiflatulent* [aluminum hydroxide; magnesium hydroxide; simethicone] 225●200●25 mg/5 mL

Alamast eye drops ℞ *mast cell stabilizer for allergic conjunctivitis* [pemirolast potassium] 0.1%

alamecin USAN *antibacterial*

alanine (L-alanine) USAN, USP, INN *nonessential amino acid; symbols: Ala, A*

alanine nitrogen mustard [see: melphalan]

alanosine INN

alaproclate USAN, INN *antidepressant*

Ala-Quin cream ℞ *corticosteroidal anti-inflammatory; antifungal; antibacterial* [hydrocortisone; clioquinol] 0.5%• 3% ⊠ Alcaine; Elocon; elucaine

Ala-Scalp lotion ℞ *corticosteroidal anti-inflammatory* [hydrocortisone] 2%

AlaSTaT lab test for professional use ℞ *test for allergic reaction to latex* ⊠ Elestat

Alasulf vaginal cream ℞ *broad-spectrum antibiotic; antiseptic; moisturizer/lubricant* [sulfanilamide; aminacrine HCl; allantoin] 15%•0.2%•2% ⊠ alusulf

alatrofloxacin mesylate USAN *broad-spectrum fluoroquinolone antibiotic*

Alavert orally disintegrating tablets OTC *nonsedating antihistamine for allergic rhinitis; also used for chronic idiopathic urticaria* [loratadine] 10 mg

Alavert Children's syrup OTC *nonsedating antihistamine for allergic rhinitis* [loratadine] 5 mg/5 mL

Alavert D-12 Hour, Allergy & Sinus extended-release tablets OTC *nonsedating antihistamine; decongestant* [loratadine; pseudoephedrine HCl] 5•120 mg

Alaway eye drops OTC *antihistamine and mast cell stabilizer for allergic conjunctivitis* [ketotifen] 0.025%

alazanine triclofenate INN

Albalon eye drops ℞ *decongestant; vasoconstrictor; moisturizer/lubricant* [naphazoline HCl; polyvinyl alcohol] 0.1%•1.4%

Albamycin capsules (discontinued 2004) ℞ *bacteriostatic antibiotic* [novobiocin sodium] 250 mg

Albatussin oral liquid OTC *antitussive; decongestant; antihistamine; sleep aid* [dextromethorphan hydrobromide; phenylephrine HCl; pyrilamine maleate] 15•5•12.5 mg/5 mL

Albatussin SR extended-release capsules (discontinued 2007) ℞ *antitussive; antihistamine; sleep aid; decongestant; expectorant* [dextromethorphan hydrobromide; pyrilamine maleate; phenylephrine HCl; potassium guaiacolsulfonate] 40•25•20•600 mg

Albay subcu or IM injection ℞ *venom sensitivity testing (subcu); venom desensitization therapy (IM)* [extracts of honeybee, yellow jacket, yellow hornet, white-faced hornet, mixed vespid, and wasp venom] ⊠ Eye-Lube-A

albendazole USAN, INN, BAN *anthelmintic for neurocysticercosis (tapeworm) and cestode-induced hydatid cyst disease (orphan)*

albendazole oxide INN, BAN

Albenza Tiltab (film-coated tablets) ℞ *anthelmintic for neurocysticercosis (tapeworm) and cestode-induced hydatid cyst disease (orphan)* [albendazole]

Alberta Lens ℞ *contact lens* [sulfocon B]

Albright solution (sodium citrate and citric acid) *urine alkalizer; compounding agent*

albucid [see: sulfacetamide]

albumin, aggregated USAN *lung imaging aid (with technetium Tc 99m)*

albumin, aggregated iodinated I 131 serum USAN, USP *radioactive agent*

albumin, chromated Cr 51 serum USAN *radioactive agent*

albumin, human USP *blood volume expander for shock, burns, and hypoproteinemia* 5%, 25% injection

albumin, iodinated (^{125}I) human serum INN *radioactive agent; blood volume test* [also: albumin, iodinated I 125 serum]

albumin, iodinated (^{131}I) human serum INN, JAN *radioactive agent; intrathecal imaging agent; blood volume test* [also: albumin, iodinated I 131 serum]

albumin, iodinated I 125 USP *radioactive agent; blood volume test*

albumin, iodinated I 125 serum USAN, USP *radioactive agent; blood volume test* [also: iodinated (^{125}I) human serum albumin]

22   albumin, iodinated I 131

albumin, iodinated I 131 USP *radioac-*
tive agent; intrathecal imaging agent;
blood volume test

albumin, iodinated I 131 serum
USAN, USP *radioactive agent; intrathe-*
cal imaging agent; blood volume test
[also: iodinated (^{131}I) human serum
albumin]

albumin, normal human serum
[now: albumin, human]

Albuminar-5; Albuminar-25 IV
infusion ℞ *blood volume expander for*
shock, burns, and hypoproteinemia
[human albumin] 5%; 25%

Albunex injection ℞ *ultrasound heart*
imaging agent [human albumin, soni-
cated] 5%

Albustix reagent strips for professional
use ℞ *in vitro diagnostic aid for albu-*
min (protein) in the urine

Albutein 5%; Albutein 25% IV
infusion ℞ *blood volume expander for*
shock, burns, and hypoproteinemia
[human albumin] 5%; 25%

albuterol USAN, USP *sympathomimetic*
bronchodilator; investigational (orphan)
to prevent paralysis caused by spinal
cord injury [also: salbutamol] 90 mcg
inhalation

Albuterol HFA inhalation aerosol
with a CFC-free propellant (discontinued 2007) ℞ *sympathomimetic*
bronchodilator [albuterol] 90 mcg/dose

albuterol sulfate USAN, USP *sympatho-*
mimetic bronchodilator [also: salbutamol sulfate] 2, 4, 8 mg oral; 2 mg/5
mL oral; 0.021%, 0.042%, 0.083%,
0.5% (0.625, 1.25, 2.5, 15 mg/3 mL)
inhalation solution

albuterol sulfate & ipratropium
bromide *bronchodilator combination*
for bronchospasm, emphysema, and
chronic obstructive pulmonary disease
(COPD) 0.083%•0.017% (3•0.5
mg/dose) inhaler

albutoin USAN, INN *anticonvulsant*

ALC (acetyl-ʟ-carnitine) [q.v.]

Alcaine Drop-Tainers (eye drops) ℞
topical anesthetic [proparacaine HCl]
0.5% ⊉ Ala-Quin; Elocon; elucaine

alcanna *medicinal herb* [see: henna
(Alkanna)]

ALCAR (acetyl-ʟ-carnitine) [q.v.]

Alcare foam OTC *antiseptic* [ethyl alco-
hol] 62% ⊉ Allegra

Alchemilla xanthochlora; A. vulgaris
medicinal herb [see: lady's mantle]

alclofenac USAN, INN, BAN, JAN *anti-*
inflammatory

alclometasone INN, BAN *topical corti-*
costeroidal anti-inflammatory [also:
alclometasone dipropionate]

alclometasone dipropionate USAN,
USP, JAN *topical corticosteroidal anti-*
inflammatory [also: alclometasone]
0.05% topical

alcloxa USAN, INN *astringent; kerato-*
lytic [also: aluminum chlorohydroxy
allantoinate]

Alco-Gel OTC *antiseptic for instant sani-*
tation of hands [ethyl alcohol] 60%

alcohol USP *topical anti-infective/anti-*
septic; astringent; solvent; a widely
abused "legal street drug" used to pro-
duce euphoria [also: ethanol]

alcohol, dehydrated USP *antidote*
[also: ethanol, dehydrated]

alcohol, diluted NF *solvent*

alcohol, rubbing USP, INN *rubefacient*

5% Alcohol and 5% Dextrose in
Water; 10% Alcohol and 5% Dex-
trose in Water IV infusion ℞ *for*
caloric replacement and rehydration
[dextrose; alcohol] 5%•5%; 10%•5%

Alcon Saline Especially for Sensi-
tive Eyes solution OTC *rinsing/storage*
solution for soft contact lenses [sodium
chloride (preserved saline solution)]

Alcortin gel ℞ *corticosteroidal anti-*
inflammatory; antimicrobial [hydro-
cortisone; iodoquinol] 2%•1%

alcuronium chloride USAN, INN,
BAN, JAN *skeletal muscle relaxant*

Aldactazide tablets ℞ *antihypertensive;*
diuretic [spironolactone; hydrochlo-
rothiazide] 25•25, 50•50 mg

Aldactone tablets ℞ *antihypertensive;*
potassium-sparing diuretic [spironolac-
tone] 25, 50, 100 mg

Aldara cream ℞ *immunomodulator for external genital and perianal warts (condylomata acuminata), actinic keratoses, and superficial basal cell carcinoma (sBCC)* [imiquimod] 5% in 250 mg single-use packets

alder, spotted *medicinal herb* [see: witch hazel]

alder, striped *medicinal herb* [see: winterberry; witch hazel]

alder buckthorn; European black alder *medicinal herb* [see: buckthorn]

alderlin [see: pronethalol]

aldesleukin USAN, INN, BAN *immunostimulant; biological response modifier; antineoplastic for metastatic melanoma and renal cell carcinoma (orphan); investigational (Phase III, orphan) for immunodeficiency diseases and acute myelogenous leukemia (AML); investigational (Phase II) for non-Hodgkin lymphoma*

aldesulfone sodium INN *antibacterial; leprostatic* [also: sulfoxone sodium]

Aldex AN chewable tablets ℞ *antihistamine; sleep aid* [doxylamine succinate] 5 mg

Aldex DM Tannate oral suspension ℞ *antitussive; antihistamine; sleep aid; decongestant* [dextromethorphan hydrobromide; pyrilamine maleate; phenylephrine HCl] 15•16•5 mg/5 mL

aldioxa USAN, INN, JAN *astringent; keratolytic*

Aldoclor-150; Aldoclor-250 film-coated tablets (discontinued 2007) ℞ *antihypertensive* [chlorothiazide; methyldopa] 150•250 mg; 250•250 mg

aldocorten [see: aldosterone]

Aldomet; Aldomet Ester HCl IV injection ℞ *antihypertensive* [methyldopate HCl] 50 mg/mL

Aldoril 15; Aldoril 25; Aldoril D30; Aldoril D50 film-coated tablets (discontinued 2007) ℞ *antihypertensive; diuretic* [hydrochlorothiazide; methyldopa] 15•250 mg; 25•250 mg; 30•500 mg; 50•500 mg

aldosterone INN, BAN

Aldurazyme powder for IV infusion ℞ *enzyme replacement therapy for mucopolysaccharidosis I (MPS I) (orphan)* [laronidase] 2.9 mg/vial

Alec *investigational (orphan) agent to prevent or treat neonatal respiratory distress syndrome* [colfosceril palmitate; phosphatidylglycerol]

alefacept USAN *immunosuppressant; recombinant human LFA-3/IgG1 (leukocyte function–associated antigen, type 3/immunoglobulin G1) fusion protein for chronic plaque psoriasis*

alemcinal USAN, INN *motilin agonist to stimulate gastrointestinal peristaltic action*

alemtuzumab *humanized monoclonal antibody (huMAb); immunosuppressant for B-cell chronic lymphocytic leukemia (orphan); also used for rheumatoid arthritis and multiple sclerosis*

Alenaze-D; Alenaze-D NR oral liquid ℞ *decongestant; antihistamine* [phenylephrine HCl; brompheniramine maleate] 7.5•2 mg/5 mL; 7.5•4 mg/5 mL

alendronate sodium USAN *bisphosphonate bone resorption inhibitor for Paget disease and corticosteroid-induced or age-related osteoporosis in men and women; investigational (orphan) for bone manifestations of Gaucher disease and pediatric osteogenesis imperfecta* 5, 10, 35, 40, 70, 75 mg oral

alendronic acid INN, BAN

Alenic Alka chewable tablets (discontinued 2007) OTC *antacid* [aluminum hydroxide; magnesium trisilicate] 80•20 mg

Alenic Alka oral liquid OTC *antacid* [aluminum hydroxide; magnesium carbonate] 31.7•137.3 mg/5 mL

Alenic Alka, Extra Strength chewable tablets (discontinued 2007) OTC *antacid* [aluminum hydroxide; magnesium carbonate] 160•105 mg

alentemol INN *antipsychotic; dopamine agonist* [also: alentemol hydrobromide]

alentemol hydrobromide USAN *antipsychotic; dopamine agonist* [also: alentemol]

alepride INN

Alesse tablets (in packs of 28) ℞ *monophasic oral contraceptive* [levonorgestrel; ethinyl estradiol] 0.1 mg• 20 mcg × 21 days; counters × 7 days

alestramustine INN

aletamine HCl USAN *antidepressant* [also: alfetamine]

Aletris farinosa medicinal herb [see: star grass]

Aleurites moluccana; A. cordata medicinal herb [see: tung seed]

Aleve tablets, capsules, gelcaps OTC *analgesic; nonsteroidal anti-inflammatory drug (NSAID) for osteoarthritis, rheumatoid arthritis, juvenile arthritis, ankylosing spondylitis, primary dysmenorrhea, bursitis/tendinitis, and other mild to moderate pain* [naproxen sodium] 220 mg (200 mg base) ⑨ Aluvia; ELF; olive

Aleve Cold & Sinus; Aleve Sinus & Headache extended-release caplets OTC *decongestant; analgesic; antipyretic* [pseudoephedrine HCl; naproxen sodium] 120•220 mg

alexidine USAN, INN *antibacterial* ⑨ aloxidone

alexitol sodium INN, BAN

alexomycin USAN *veterinary growth promoter for poultry and swine*

alfacalcidol (1α-hydroxycholecalciferol; 1α-hydroxyvitamin D₃) INN, BAN, JAN *vitamin D precursor (converted to calcifediol in the body); calcium regulator for treatment of hypocalcemia and osteodystrophy from chronic renal dialysis*

alfadex INN

alfadolone INN [also: alphadolone]

alfalfa (Medicago sativa) leaves and flowers *medicinal herb for anemia, appetite stimulation, arthritis, atherosclerosis, blood cleansing, diabetes, hemorrhages, kidney cleansing, lowering cholesterol levels, nausea, pituitary disorders, and peptic ulcers*

alfaprostol USAN, INN, BAN *veterinary prostaglandin*

alfaxalone INN, JAN [also: alphaxalone]

Alfenta IV or IM injection ℞ *narcotic analgesic; primary anesthetic for surgery* [alfentanil HCl] 500 mcg/mL ⑨ Alphanate

alfentanil INN, BAN *narcotic analgesic* [also: alfentanil HCl]

alfentanil HCl USAN *narcotic analgesic; primary anesthetic for surgery* [also: alfentanil] 500 mcg/mL injection

Alferon N intralesional injection ℞ *immunomodulator and antiviral for condylomata acuminata; investigational (Phase III) cytokine for HIV, AIDS, and ARC* [interferon alfa-n3] 5 million IU/mL

alfetamine INN *antidepressant* [also: aletamine HCl]

alfetamine HCl [see: aletamine HCl]

alfimeprase *investigational (Phase III) fibrinolytic for dissolving clots that cause acute peripheral arterial occlusion*

alfuzosin INN, BAN *alpha₁-adrenergic blocker for hypertension and benign prostatic hyperplasia (BPH)* [also: alfuzosin HCl]

alfuzosin HCl USAN *alpha₁-adrenergic blocker for hypertension and benign prostatic hyperplasia (BPH)* [also: alfuzosin]

algeldrate USAN, INN *antacid*

algestone INN *anti-inflammatory* [also: algestone acetonide]

algestone acetonide USAN, BAN *anti-inflammatory* [also: algestone]

algestone acetophenide USAN *progestin*

algin [see: sodium alginate]

alginic acid NF, BAN *tablet binder and emulsifying agent*

alginic acid, sodium salt [see: sodium alginate]

alglucerase USAN, INN, BAN *glucocerebrosidase enzyme replacement for Gaucher disease type I (orphan); investigational (orphan) for types II and III*

alglucosidase alfa *exogenous source of the acid alpha-glucosidase enzyme; enzyme replacement therapy for patients* with Pompe disease (glycogenosis type 2; glycogen storage disease type II; GSDII) (orphan)

alglucosidase alfa, highly phosphorylated *exogenous source of the acid alpha-glucosidase enzyme; investigational (orphan) enzyme replacement therapy for patients with Pompe disease (glycogenosis type 2; glycogen storage disease type II; GSDII)*

alibendol INN

alicaforsen sodium USAN, INN *antiinflammatory; antisense inhibitor of intercellular adhesion molecule 1 (ICAM-1); investigational (Phase III) injection for Crohn disease; investigational (Phase II) suppository for ulcerative colitis; investigational (Phase II) topical treatment of psoriasis*

aliconazole INN

alidine dihydrochloride [see: anileridine]

alidine phosphate [see: anileridine]

alifedrine INN

aliflurane USAN, INN *inhalation anesthetic*

Align capsules OTC *natural probiotic supplement* [Bifidobacterium infantis] 4 mg (10⁹ live cultures) ☒ Ala-Quin; Alcaine; aloin; Elocon; elucaine

alimadol INN

alimemazine INN *phenothiazine antihistamine; antipruritic* [also: trimeprazine tartrate; trimeprazine; alimemazine tartrate]

alimemazine tartrate JAN *phenothiazine antihistamine; antipruritic* [also: trimeprazine tartrate; alimemazine; trimeprazine]

Alimentum ready-to-use oral liquid OTC *hypoallergenic infant food* [casein protein formula]

Alimentum Advance ready-to-use oral liquid OTC *hypoallergenic infant food with omega-3 and omega-6 fatty acids* [casein protein formula; iron; docosahexaenoic acid (DHA); arachidonic acid (AA)]

Alimta powder for IV infusion ℞ *folic acid antagonist; antineoplastic for malig-*

nant pleural mesothelioma (orphan) and non–small cell lung cancer (NSCLC) [pemetrexed disodium] 100, 500 mg/dose ☒ Elimite

Alinia tablets, powder for oral suspension ℞ *antiprotozoal for pediatric diarrhea due to* Cryptosporidium parvum *and* Giardia lamblia *infections (orphan)* [nitazoxanide] 500 mg; 100 mg/5 mL ☒ aloin

alinidine INN, BAN

alipamide USAN, INN, BAN *diuretic; antihypertensive*

alisactide [see: alsactide]

aliskiren hemifumarate *oral direct renin inhibitor for hypertension*

alisobumal [see: butalbital]

Alista cream *investigational (Phase III) treatment for female sexual arousal disorder* [alprostadil]

alitame USAN *sweetener*

alitretinoin USAN, INN *second generation retinoid; topical treatment of cutaneous lesions of AIDS-related Kaposi sarcoma (orphan); investigational (Phase III, orphan) oral treatment for acute promyelocytic leukemia (APL); investigational (orphan) to prevent retinal detachment*

alizapride INN

Alka-Mints chewable tablets OTC *antacid* [calcium carbonate] 850 mg

Alkanna tinctoria *medicinal herb* [see: henna]

Alka-Seltzer; Alka-Seltzer Lemon Lime effervescent tablets OTC *antacid; analgesic; antipyretic* [sodium bicarbonate; citric acid; aspirin; phenylalanine] 1700•1000•325•9 mg

Alka-Seltzer, Extra Strength effervescent tablets OTC *antacid; analgesic; antipyretic* [sodium bicarbonate; citric acid; aspirin] 1985•1000•500 mg

Alka-Seltzer, Original effervescent tablets OTC *antacid; analgesic; antipyretic* [sodium bicarbonate; citric acid; aspirin] 1916•1000•325 mg

Alka-Seltzer Gold effervescent tablets OTC *antacid* [sodium bicarbonate;

potassium bicarbonate; citric acid]
1050•344•1000 mg

Alka-Seltzer Heartburn Relief effervescent tablets OTC *antacid* [sodium bicarbonate; citric acid; phenylalanine] 1940•1000•5.6 mg

Alka-Seltzer Plus Cold & Cough Liqui-Gels (liquid-filled gelcaps), effervescent tablets, oral liquid OTC *antitussive; antihistamine; decongestant; analgesic; antipyretic* [dextromethorphan hydrobromide; chlorpheniramine maleate; phenylephrine HCl; acetaminophen] 10•2•30•325 mg; 10•2•5•250 mg; 10•2•5•325 mg/10 mL

Alka-Seltzer Plus Cold & Flu; Alka-Seltzer Plus Flu Medicine Liqui-Gels (liquid-filled gelcaps) (discontinued 2007) OTC *antitussive; decongestant; analgesic; antipyretic* [dextromethorphan hydrobromide; pseudoephedrine HCl; acetaminophen] 10•30•325 mg

Alka-Seltzer Plus Cold Medicine Liqui-Gels (liquid-filled gelcaps) OTC *decongestant; antihistamine; analgesic; antipyretic* [pseudoephedrine HCl; chlorpheniramine maleate; acetaminophen] 30•2•325 mg

Alka-Seltzer Plus Cold Medicine; Alka-Seltzer Plus Regular Seltzer Multi-Symptom Cold Relief effervescent tablets OTC *decongestant; antihistamine; analgesic; antipyretic* [phenylephrine HCl; chlorpheniramine maleate; acetaminophen] 5•2•250 mg

Alka-Seltzer Plus Cold & Sinus effervescent tablets (name changed to **Alka-Seltzer Plus Sinus** in 2008)

Alka-Seltzer Plus Cold & Sinus Liqui-Gels (liquid-filled gelcaps) (discontinued 2007) OTC *decongestant; analgesic; antipyretic* [pseudoephedrine HCl; acetaminophen] 30•325 mg

Alka-Seltzer Plus Day & Night Cold effervescent tablets OTC *antitussive; decongestant; analgesic; antipyretic; antihistamine/sleep aid added* PM [dextromethorphan hydrobromide; phenylephrine HCl; acetaminophen; doxylamine succinate (PM)] 10•5•250 mg AM; 10•5•250•6.25 mg PM

Alka-Seltzer Plus Day & Night Cold Liqui-Gels (liquid-filled gelcaps) OTC *antitussive; analgesic; antipyretic; decongestant added* AM; *antihistamine/sleep aid added* PM [dextromethorphan hydrobromide; acetaminophen; phenylephrine HCl (AM); doxylamine succinate (PM)] 10•325•5 mg AM; 15•325•6.25 mg PM

Alka-Seltzer Plus Day Non-Drowsy Cold oral liquid OTC *antitussive; decongestant; analgesic; antipyretic* [dextromethorphan hydrobromide; phenylephrine HCl; acetaminophen] 10•5•325 mg/10 mL

Alka-Seltzer Plus Flu effervescent tablets OTC *antitussive; antihistamine; analgesic; antipyretic* [dextromethorphan hydrobromide; chlorpheniramine maleate; aspirin] 15•2•500 mg

Alka-Seltzer Plus Night Cold Liqui-Gels (liquid-filled gelcaps) OTC *antitussive; antihistamine; sleep aid; analgesic; antipyretic* [dextromethorphan hydrobromide; doxylamine succinate; acetaminophen] 15•6.25•325 mg

Alka-Seltzer Plus Night Cold oral liquid OTC *antitussive; decongestant; antihistamine; sleep aid; analgesic; antipyretic* [dextromethorphan hydrobromide; phenylephrine HCl; doxylamine succinate; acetaminophen] 10•5•6.25•325 mg/10 mL

Alka-Seltzer Plus Night-Time Cold effervescent tablets OTC *antitussive; decongestant; antihistamine; sleep aid; analgesic; antipyretic* [dextromethorphan hydrobromide; phenylephrine HCl; doxylamine succinate; acetaminophen] 10•5•6.25•250 mg

Alka-Seltzer Plus Nose & Throat effervescent tablets (discontinued 2007) OTC *antitussive; decongestant; antihistamine; analgesic; antipyretic* [dextromethorphan hydrobromide;

phenylephrine HCl; chlorpheniramine maleate; acetaminophen] 10•
5•2•250 mg

Alka-Seltzer Plus Sinus effervescent
tablets OTC *decongestant; analgesic;
antipyretic* [phenylephrine HCl; aspi-
rin] 5•250 mg

Alka-Seltzer PM effervescent tablets
OTC *antihistaminic sleep aid; analgesic;
antipyretic* [diphenhydramine citrate;
aspirin] 38•325 mg

Alka-Seltzer Wake-Up Call effervescent tablets OTC *analgesic; antipyretic; anti-inflammatory* [aspirin; caf-
feine] 500•65 mg

Alka-Seltzer with Aspirin effervescent tablets OTC *antacid; analgesic;
antipyretic* [sodium bicarbonate; citric
acid; aspirin] 1700•1200•325, 1900•
1000•325, 1900•1000•500 mg

**alkavervir (Veratrum viride alka-
loids)**

Alkavite extended-release tablets OTC
*vitamin/mineral supplement for alcohol-
related deficiencies* [multiple vitamins
& minerals; calcium carbonate; iron
sulfate; folic acid; biotin] ≛•68.5•
60•1•0.03 mg

Alkeran film-coated tablets, powder
for IV infusion ℞ *nitrogen mustard-
type alkylating antineoplastic for multiple myeloma (orphan) and ovarian
cancer; investigational (orphan) for
metastatic melanoma; also used for
breast and testicular cancers and bone
marrow transplantation* [melphalan] 2
mg; 50 mg

Alkets chewable tablets (discontinued
2005) OTC *antacid* [calcium carbon-
ate] 500, 750 mg

alkyl aryl sulfonate *surfactant/wetting
agent*

alkylade *investigational (Phase III)
AGT inhibitor for brain cancer*

alkylamines *a class of antihistamines*

**alkylbenzyldimethylammonium
chloride** [see: benzalkonium chloride]

**alkyldimethylbenzylammonium
chloride** [see: benzalkonium chloride]

alkylpolyaminoethylglycine JAN

alkylpolyaminoethylglycine HCl JAN

All Clear eye drops OTC *decongestant;
vasoconstrictor; moisturizer/lubricant*
[naphazoline HCl; polyethylene
300] 0.012%•0.2%

All Clear AR eye drops OTC *decongestant; vasoconstrictor; moisturizer/lubri-
cant* [naphazoline HCl; hydroxypropyl methylcellulose] 0.012%•0.5%

Allanderm-T ointment OTC *proteolytic
enzyme for debridement of necrotic tissue; vulnerary* [trypsin; Peruvian bal-
sam] 90 U•87 mg

AllanEnzyme ointment ℞ *proteolytic
enzyme for debridement of necrotic tissue; vulnerary* [papain; urea] 830 000
U/g•10% (note: one of two products
with the same name)

AllanEnzyme ointment ℞ *proteolytic
enzyme for debridement of necrotic tissue; vulnerary; wound deodorant*
[papain; urea; chlorophyllin copper
complex] 521 700 U/g•10%•0.5%
(note: one of two products with the
same name)

AllanEnzyme spray ℞ *proteolytic
enzyme for debridement of necrotic tissue; vulnerary* [papain; urea] 830 000
IU/g•10%

AllanfillEnzyme spray ℞ *proteolytic
enzyme for debridement of necrotic tissue; vulnerary; wound deodorant*
[papain; urea; chlorophyllin copper
complex] ≥ 521 700 U/g•10%•0.5%

AllanHist PDX oral drops ℞ *antitussive; antihistamine; decongestant; for
children 1–24 months* [dextromethor-
phan hydrobromide; brompheniramine maleate; pseudoephedrine
HCl] 3•1•12.5 mg/mL

allantoin USAN, BAN *topical vulnerary;
moisturizer; investigational (orphan) for
skin blistering and erosions associated
with inherited epidermolysis bullosa*

AllanVan-DM B.I.D. oral suspension
℞ *antitussive; antihistamine; sleep aid;
decongestant* [dextromethorphan tannate; pyrilamine tannate; phenylephrine tannate] 25•30•12.5 mg/5 mL

AllanVan-S B.I.D. oral suspension ℞ *decongestant; antihistamine; sleep aid* [phenylephrine tannate; pyrilamine tannate] 12.5•30 mg/5 mL

Allbee C-800 film-coated tablets OTC *vitamin supplement* [multiple B vitamins; vitamins C and E] ≜•800•45 mg

Allbee C-800 plus Iron film-coated tablets OTC *vitamin/iron supplement* [ferrous fumarate; multiple B vitamins; vitamins C and E; folic acid] 27 mg•≜•800 mg•45 IU•0.4 mg

Allbee with C caplets OTC *vitamin supplement* [multiple B vitamins; vitamin C] ≜•300 mg

Allbee-T tablets OTC *vitamin supplement* [multiple B vitamins; vitamin C] ≜•500 mg

Allegra capsules (discontinued 2007) ℞ *nonsedating antihistamine for allergic rhinitis and chronic idiopathic urticaria* [fexofenadine HCl] 60 mg 🔁 agar; Alcare; Icar

Allegra film-coated tablets, oral suspension ℞ *nonsedating antihistamine for allergic rhinitis and chronic idiopathic urticaria* [fexofenadine HCl] 30, 60, 180 mg; 30 mg/5 mL 🔁 agar; Alcare; Icar

Allegra ODT (orally disintegrating tablets) ℞ *nonsedating antihistamine for allergic rhinitis* [fexofenadine HCl] 30 mg 🔁 Eligard

Allegra-D 12-Hour; Allegra-D 24-Hour dual-release film-coated tablets ℞ *nonsedating antihistamine; decongestant* [fexofenadine HCl (immediate release); pseudoephedrine HCl (extended release)] 60•120 mg; 180•240 mg

allegron [see: nortriptyline]

Allent sustained-release capsules ℞ *decongestant; antihistamine* [pseudoephedrine HCl; brompheniramine maleate] 120•12 mg

AllePak Dose Pack tablets ℞ *anticholinergic to dry mucosal secretions; decongestant added* AM; *antihistamine added* PM [methscopolamine nitrate; pseudoephedrine HCl (AM); chlorpheniramine maleate (PM)] 2.5•120 mg AM; 2.5•8 mg PM

Aller-Chlor tablets, syrup OTC *antihistamine* [chlorpheniramine maleate] 4 mg; 2 mg/5 mL

Allercreme Skin lotion (discontinued 2004) OTC *moisturizer; emollient*

Allercreme Ultra Emollient cream (discontinued 2004) OTC *moisturizer; emollient*

Allerest eye drops (discontinued 2006) OTC *decongestant; vasoconstrictor* [naphazoline HCl] 0.012%

Allerest tablets OTC *decongestant; antihistamine* [pseudoephedrine HCl; chlorpheniramine maleate] 30•2 mg

Allerest Allergy & Sinus Relief tablets (discontinued 2007) OTC *decongestant; analgesic; antipyretic* [pseudoephedrine HCl; acetaminophen] 30•325 mg

Allerest PE tablets OTC *decongestant; antihistamine* [phenylephrine HCl; chlorpheniramine maleate] 10•4 mg

Allerfrim film-coated tablets, syrup OTC *decongestant; antihistamine* [pseudoephedrine HCl; triprolidine HCl] 60•2.5 mg; 60•2.5 mg/10 mL

Allergan Enzymatic tablets OTC *enzymatic cleaner for soft contact lenses* [papain]

Allergan Hydrocare [see: Hydrocare]

Allergen Ear Drops ℞ *anesthetic; analgesic* [benzocaine; antipyrine] 1.4%•5.4%

allergenic extracts *a class of agents derived from various biological sources containing antigens that possess immunologic activity*

allergenic extracts (aqueous, glycerinated, or alum-precipitated) *over 900 allergens available for diagnosis of and desensitization to specific allergies*

Allergy tablets OTC *antihistamine* [chlorpheniramine maleate] 4 mg

Allergy DN tablets ℞ *anticholinergic to dry mucosal secretions; decongestant added* AM; *antihistamine added* PM [methscopolamine nitrate; pseudoephedrine HCl (AM); chlorpheniramine maleate (PM)] 2.5•120 mg AM; 2.5•8 mg PM

Allergy Drops eye drops (discontinued 2006) OTC *decongestant; vasoconstrictor* [naphazoline HCl] 0.012%; 0.03%

Allergy Relief tablets OTC *antihistamine* [chlorpheniramine maleate] 4 mg

AllerMax caplets, oral liquid OTC *antihistamine; sleep aid* [diphenhydramine HCl] 50 mg; 12.5 mg/5 mL

Allermist (name changed to **Veramyst** upon marketing release in 2007)

AllerTan oral suspension ℞ *decongestant; antihistamine; sleep aid* [phenylephrine tannate; chlorpheniramine tannate; pyrilamine tannate] 15•8•12.5 mg/5 mL

AlleRx oral suspension (discontinued 2007) ℞ *decongestant; antihistamine* [phenylephrine tannate; chlorpheniramine tannate] 22.5•9 mg/15 mL ② Alrex

AlleRx Dose Pack controlled-release tablets ℞ *anticholinergic to dry mucosal secretions; decongestant added AM; antihistamine added PM* [methscopolamine nitrate; pseudoephedrine HCl (AM); chlorpheniramine maleate (PM)] 2.5•120 mg AM; 2.5•8 mg PM

AlleRx-D controlled-release caplets (discontinued 2007) ℞ *decongestant; anticholinergic to dry mucosal secretions* [pseudoephedrine HCl; methscopolamine nitrate] 120•2.5 mg

alletorphine BAN, INN

Allfen sustained-release tablets (discontinued 2004) ℞ *expectorant* [guaifenesin] 1000 mg ② Alophen

Allfen C extended-release caplets (discontinued 2007) ℞ *antitussive; expectorant* [carbetapentane citrate; guaifenesin] 5•1000 mg

Allfen DM sustained-release tablets ℞ *antitussive; expectorant* [dextromethorphan hydrobromide; guaifenesin] 58•1000 mg

Allfen Jr. tablets ℞ *expectorant* [guaifenesin] 400 mg

all-heal *medicinal herb* [see: mistletoe; valerian]

Alli capsules OTC *lipase inhibitor for weight loss in overweight adults ≥ 18 years* [orlistat] 60 mg

Allium cepa *medicinal herb* [see: onion]

Allium porrum *medicinal herb* [see: leek]

Allium sativum *medicinal herb* [see: garlic]

All-Nite oral liquid (discontinued 2007) OTC *antitussive; antihistamine; sleep aid; decongestant; analgesic; antipyretic* [dextromethorphan hydrobromide; doxylamine succinate; acetaminophen; alcohol 10%] 30•12.6•1000 mg/30 mL

All-Nite Children's Cold/Cough Relief oral liquid (discontinued 2007) OTC *antitussive; antihistamine; decongestant; for children 6–11 years* [dextromethorphan hydrobromide; chlorpheniramine maleate; pseudoephedrine HCl] 15•2•30 mg/15 mL

allobarbital USAN, INN *hypnotic*

allobarbitone [see: allobarbital]

alloclamide INN

allocupreide sodium INN

AlloMap lab test for professional use ℞ *blood test for heart transplant rejection markers*

allomethadione INN [also: aloxidone]

allopurinol USAN, USP, INN, BAN, JAN *xanthine oxidase inhibitor for gout and hyperuricemia; antineoplastic adjunct for reducing uric acid levels following chemotherapy for leukemia, lymphoma, and solid-tumor malignancies (orphan)* 100, 300 mg oral

allopurinol riboside *investigational (orphan) agent for Chagas disease and for cutaneous and visceral leishmaniasis*

allopurinol sodium *antineoplastic adjunct for reducing uric acid levels following chemotherapy for leukemia, lymphoma, and solid tumor malignancies (orphan); investigational (orphan) for ex vivo preservation of organs for transplant* 500 mg injection

Allovectin-7 *investigational (Phase II/III, orphan) for invasive and meta-*

static melanoma [HLA-B7/beta2M DNA lipid complex]

Allpyral subcu or IM injection ℞ *allergenic sensitivity testing (subcu); allergenic desensitization therapy (IM)* [allergenic extracts, alum-precipitated]

allspice (*Eugenia pimenta; Pimenta dioica; P. officinalis*) unripe fruit and leaves *medicinal herb for diarrhea and gas; also used as a purgative and tonic*

all-*trans*-retinoic acid [see: tretinoin]

allyl isothiocyanate USAN, USP

allylamines *a class of antifungals*

allylbarbituric acid [now: butalbital]

allylestrenol INN, JAN [also: allyloestrenol]

allyl-isobutylbarbituric acid [see: butalbital]

allylisopropylmalonylurea [see: aprobarbital]

4-allyl-2-methoxyphenol [see: eugenol]

N-allylnoretorphine [see: alletorphine]

N-allylnoroxymorphone HCl [see: naloxone HCl]

allyloestrenol BAN [also: allylestrenol]

allylprodine INN, BAN

5-allyl-5-*sec*-butylbarbituric acid [see: talbutal]

allylthiourea INN

allypropymal [see: aprobarbital]

Almacone chewable tablets, oral liquid OTC *antacid; antiflatulent* [aluminum hydroxide; magnesium hydroxide; simethicone] 200•200•20 mg; 200•200•20 mg/5 mL

Almacone II oral liquid OTC *antacid; antiflatulent* [aluminum hydroxide; magnesium hydroxide; simethicone] 400•400•40 mg/5 mL

almadrate sulfate USAN, INN *antacid*

almagate USAN, INN *antacid*

almagodrate INN

almasilate INN, BAN

Almebex Plus B$_{12}$ oral liquid OTC *vitamin supplement* [multiple B vitamins]

almecillin INN

almestrone INN

alminoprofen INN, JAN

almitrine INN, BAN *respiratory stimulant* [also: almitrine mesylate]

almitrine mesylate USAN *respiratory stimulant* [also: almitrine]

almokalant INN *antiarrhythmic*

almond (*Prunus amygdalus*) kernels *medicinal herb used as a demulcent, emollient, and pectoral*

almond oil NF *emollient and perfume; oleaginous vehicle*

Almora tablets OTC *magnesium supplement* [magnesium gluconate dihydride] 500 mg (27 mg Mg)

almotriptan USAN, INN *vascular serotonin 5-HT$_{1B/1D/1F}$ receptor agonist for the acute treatment of migraine*

almotriptan malate USAN *vascular serotonin 5-HT$_{1B/1D/1F}$ receptor agonist for the acute treatment of migraine*

almoxatone INN

alnespirone INN

alniditan dihydrochloride USAN *serotonin 5-HT$_{1D}$ agonist for migraine*

Alnus glutinosa *medicinal herb* [see: black alder]

Alocril eye drops ℞ *mast cell stabilizer for allergic conjunctivitis* [nedocromil sodium] 2%

Alodox Convenience Kit tablets ℞ *tetracycline antibiotic* [doxycycline (as hyclate)] 20 mg

aloe USP

aloe (*Aloe vera* and more than 500 other species) leaves and juice *medicinal herb for burns, hemorrhoids, insect bites, and scalds; also used as a deodorant and to aid digestion and limit scarring; not generally regarded as safe and effective as a cathartic*

Aloe Grande lotion OTC *moisturizer; emollient; skin protectant* [vitamins A and E; aloe] 3333.3•50• $\underline{?}$ U/g

Aloe Vesta lotion OTC *emollient/protectant* [dimethicone; aloe vera gel] 3%• $\underline{?}$

Aloe Vesta spray OTC *emollient/protectant* [petrolatum; mineral oil; aloe extract] 36%• $\underline{?}$ • $\underline{?}$

Aloe Vesta Perineal solution OTC
emollient/protectant [propylene glycol;
aloe vera gel]

alofilcon A USAN *hydrophilic contact
lens material*

alogliptin *investigational (NDA filed)
dipeptidyl peptidase-4 (DPP-4) inhibitor oral antidiabetic that enhances the
function of the body's incretin system to
increase insulin production in the pancreas and reduce glucose production in
the liver*

aloin BAN ▢ Align

**ALOMAD (Adriamycin, Leukeran,
Oncovin, methotrexate, actinomycin D, dacarbazine)** *chemotherapy protocol*

Alomide Drop-Tainers (eye drops) ℞
*antiallergic for vernal keratoconjunc-
tivitis (orphan)* [lodoxamide trometh-
amine] 0.1%

alonacic INN

alonimid USAN, INN *sedative; hypnotic*

Alophen enteric-coated tablets OTC
stimulant laxative [bisacodyl] 5 mg ▢
Allfen

Aloprim powder for IV infusion ℞
*antineoplastic adjunct for reducing uric
acid levels following chemotherapy for
leukemia, lymphoma, and solid-tumor
malignancies (orphan); investigational
(orphan) for ex vivo preservation of
organs for transplant* [allopurinol
sodium] 500 mg

Alor 5/500 tablets ℞ *narcotic analgesic; antipyretic* [hydrocodone bitartrate; aspirin] 5•500 mg

Alora transdermal patch ℞ *estrogen
replacement therapy for the treatment
of postmenopausal symptoms and prevention of postmenopausal osteoporosis*
[estradiol] 25, 50, 75, 100 mcg/day

aloracetam INN

alosetron INN, BAN *antiemetic; serotonin 5-HT₃ receptor antagonist for
diarrhea-predominant irritable bowel
syndrome (IBS) in women* [also: alosetron HCl] ▢ Elestrin

alosetron HCl USAN *antiemetic; serotonin 5-HT₃ receptor antagonist for diarrhea-predominant irritable bowel syndrome (IBS) in women* (base=89%)
[also: alosetron]

alovudine USAN, INN *antiviral*

Aloxi IV injection, capsules ℞ *antiemetic to prevent chemotherapy-
induced and postoperative nausea and
vomiting* [palonosetron HCl] 0.05
mg/mL; 0.5 mg ▢ I-L-X; Olux

aloxidone BAN [also: allomethadione]
▢ alexidine

aloxiprin INN, BAN

aloxistatin INN

Aloysiatriphylla **spp.** *medicinal herb*
[see: lemon verbena]

alozafone INN

alpertine USAN, INN *antipsychotic*

alpha amylase (α-amylase) USAN
anti-inflammatory

**alpha fetoprotein, recombinant
human (rhAFP)** *investigational
(orphan) for myasthenia gravis*

alpha hydroxy acids (AHA) [see:
glycolic acid]

alpha interferon-2A [see: interferon
alfa-2A]

alpha interferon-2B [see: interferon
alfa-2B]

alpha interferon-N1 [see: interferon
alfa-N1]

alpha interferon-N3 [see: interferon
alfa-N3]

Alpha Keri Moisturizing Soap bar
(discontinued 2004) OTC *therapeutic
skin cleanser*

Alpha Keri Shower & Bath OTC
bath emollient

Alpha Keri Spray (discontinued
2004) OTC *bath emollient*

Alpha Keri Therapeutic Bath Oil
(name changed to **Alpha Keri
Shower & Bath** in 2008)

alpha lipoic acid (ALA) *natural antioxidant that is both fat- and water-soluble and readily crosses cell membranes;
used in the treatment of AIDS, diabetes, liver ailments, oxidative stress
injuries, and various cancers*

d-alpha tocopherol *fat-soluble vitamin; antioxidant; platelet aggregation inhibitor; topical emollient* (relative potency: 100%) [see also: vitamin E]

dl-alpha tocopherol *fat-soluble vitamin; antioxidant; platelet aggregation inhibitor; topical emollient* (relative potency: 74%) [see also: vitamin E]

d-alpha tocopheryl acetate *fat-soluble vitamin; antioxidant; platelet aggregation inhibitor; topical emollient* (relative potency: 91%) [see also: vitamin E]

dl-alpha tocopheryl acetate *fat-soluble vitamin; antioxidant; platelet aggregation inhibitor; topical emollient* (relative potency: 67%) [see also: vitamin E]

d-alpha tocopheryl acid succinate *fat-soluble vitamin; antioxidant; platelet aggregation inhibitor; topical emollient* (relative potency: 81%) [see also: vitamin E]

dl-alpha tocopheryl acid succinate *fat-soluble vitamin; antioxidant; platelet aggregation inhibitor; topical emollient* (relative potency: 60%) [see also: vitamin E]

alpha$_1$ PI (alpha$_1$-proteinase inhibitor) [q.v.]

alpha$_1$-acid glycoprotein *investigational (orphan) antidote to tricyclic antidepressant and cocaine overdose*

alpha$_1$-adrenergic blockers *a class of agents that block the alpha$_1$ adrenergic receptors, used for the treatment of hypertension and benign prostatic hyperplasia (BPH) also called: antiadrenergics*

alpha$_1$-antitrypsin, recombinant (rAaT) *investigational (orphan) for alpha$_1$-antitrypsin deficiency in the ZZ phenotype population, cystic fibrosis, and to delay the progression of emphysema and chronic obstructive pulmonary disease*

alpha$_1$-antitrypsin, transgenic human *investigational (Phase II, orphan) for emphysema secondary to alpha$_1$-antitrypsin deficiency*

alpha$_1$-proteinase inhibitor (alpha$_1$ PI) *enzyme replacement therapy for hereditary alpha$_1$ PI deficiency, which leads to progressive panacinar emphysema (orphan)*

alpha-2,6-sialyltransferase adenoviral gene therapy

alphacemethadone [see: alphacetylmethadol]

alphacetylmethadol BAN, INN

alpha-chymotrypsin [see: chymotrypsin]

alpha-cypermethrin BAN

α-D-galactopyranose [see: galactose]

alpha-D-galactosidase *digestive enzyme*

alphadolone BAN [also: alfadolone]

alpha-estradiol [see: estradiol]

alpha-estradiol benzoate [see: estradiol benzoate]

alpha-ethyltryptamine (alpha-EtT) *a hallucinogenic street drug chemically related to MDMA* [see also: MDMA; alpha-methyltryptamine]

alphafilcon A USAN *hydrophilic contact lens material*

alpha-galactosidase A [see: agalsidase alfa; agalsidase beta]

Alphagan *eye drops (discontinued 2004)* ℞ *selective α_2 agonist for open-angle glaucoma and ocular hypertension; investigational (orphan) for anterior ischemic optic neuropathy* [brimonidine tartrate] 0.2%

Alphagan P *eye drops* ℞ *selective α_2 agonist for open-angle glaucoma and ocular hypertension; investigational (orphan) for anterior ischemic optic neuropathy* [brimonidine tartrate] 0.1%, 0.15%

alpha-glucosidase, human acid [see: alglucosidase alfa]

alpha-glucosidase inhibitors *a class of antidiabetic agents for type 2 diabetes that delay the digestion of dietary carbohydrates*

alpha-hypophamine [see: oxytocin]

alpha-L-iduronidase [now: laronidase]

alpha-melanocyte stimulating hormone investigational (orphan) agent for the prevention and treatment of acute renal failure due to ischemia

alphameprodine INN, BAN

alphamethadol INN, BAN

alpha-methyldopa [now: methyldopa]

alpha-methyltryptamine (alpha-MeT) a hallucinogenic street drug chemically related to MDMA [see also: MDMA; alpha-ethyltryptamine]

Alphanate powder for IV injection ℞ systemic hemostatic; antihemophilic for the prevention and control of bleeding in classical hemophilia (hemophilia A) and von Willebrand disease (orphan) [antihemophilic factor concentrate, human] (actual number of AHF units is indicated on the vial) ☑ Alfenta

AlphaNine SD powder for IV injection ℞ systemic hemostatic; antihemophilic for factor IX deficiency (hemophilia B; Christmas disease) (orphan) [factor IX, solvent/detergent treated] (actual number of units is indicated on the vial)

alpha-phenoxyethyl penicillin, potassium [see: phenethicillin potassium]

alphaprodine INN, BAN [also: alphaprodine HCl]

alphaprodine HCl USP [also: alphaprodine]

17 alpha-progesterone (17P) naturally occurring progesterone; investigational (NDA filed) hormonal intervention to prevent preterm births

alphasone acetophenide [now: algestone acetonide]

Alphatrex cream (discontinued 2004) ℞ corticosteroidal anti-inflammatory [betamethasone dipropionate] 0.05%

alphaxalone BAN [also: alfaxalone]

alpidem USAN, INN, BAN anxiolytic

Alpinia officinarum; A. galanga medicinal herb [see: galangal]

Alpinia oxyphylla; A. fructus medicinal herb [see: bitter cardamom]

Alpinia speciosa medicinal herb for edema, fungal infections, hypertension, and thrombosis

alpiropride INN

alprafenone INN

alprazolam USAN, USP, INN, BAN, JAN benzodiazepine anxiolytic; sedative; treatment for panic disorders and agoraphobia 0.25, 0.5, 1, 2, 3 mg oral

Alprazolam Intensol oral drops ℞ benzodiazepine anxiolytic; sedative [alprazolam] 1 mg/mL

alprenolol INN, BAN antiadrenergic (β-receptor) [also: alprenolol HCl]

alprenolol HCl USAN, JAN antiadrenergic (β-receptor) [also: alprenolol]

alprenoxime HCl USAN antiglaucoma agent

alprostadil USAN, USP, INN, BAN, JAN vasodilator for erectile dysfunction; platelet aggregation inhibitor; investigational (orphan) for peripheral arterial occlusive disease; investigational (Phase III) topical treatment for female sexual arousal disorder

alprostadil alfadex BAN

alprostadil lipid emulsion vasodilator; platelet aggregation inhibitor; investigational (orphan) for acute respiratory distress syndrome (ARDS) and ischemic ulcerations due to peripheral arterial disease

alrestatin INN aldose reductase enzyme inhibitor [also: alrestatin sodium]

alrestatin sodium USAN aldose reductase enzyme inhibitor [also: alrestatin]

Alrex eye drop suspension ℞ corticosteroidal anti-inflammatory [loteprednol etabonate] 0.2% ☑ AlleRx

alsactide INN

alseroxylon JAN antihypertensive; rauwolfia derivative

Altabax ointment ℞ pleuromutilin antibiotic for impetigo caused by Staphylococcus aureus and Streptococcus pyogenes infections [retapamulin] 1%

Altacaine eye drops ℞ topical anesthetic [tetracaine HCl] 0.5%

Altace tablets, capsules ℞ antihypertensive; angiotensin-converting enzyme

(ACE) inhibitor; treatment for myocardial infarction (MI), congestive heart
failure (CHF), and stroke [ramipril]
1.25, 2.5, 5, 10 mg ⊡ Yelets

Altafrin eye drops OTC decongestant
[phenylephrine HCl] 0.12%] (note:
the ℞ product has the same name,
but a different strength)

Altafrin eye drops ℞ decongestant;
vasoconstrictor; mydriatic [phenyleph-
rine HCl] 2.5%, 10% (note: the OTC
product has the same name, but a
different strength)

altanserin INN serotonin antagonist
[also: altanserin tartrate]

altanserin tartrate USAN serotonin
antagonist [also: altanserin]

altapizone INN

Altarussin syrup OTC expectorant [guai-
fenesin] 100 mg/5 mL

Altarussin-PE oral liquid OTC decongestant; expectorant [pseudoephedrine
HCl; guaifenesin] 60•200 mg/10 mL

Altaryl Children's Allergy oral liquid
OTC antihistamine; sleep aid [diphen-
hydramine HCl] 12.5 mg/5 mL

Altastaph investigational (orphan) prophylaxis against S. aureus infections in
low birthweight neonates [Staphylococ-
cus aureus immune globulin, human]

Altazine eye drops OTC decongestant;
vasoconstrictor [tetrahydrozoline HCl]
0.05% ⊡ Ilotycin

Altazine Irritation Relief eye drops
OTC decongestant; astringent [tetrahy-
drozoline HCl; zinc sulfate] 0.05%•
0.25%

Altazine Moisture Relief eye drops
OTC decongestant; vasoconstrictor;
moisturizer/lubricant [tetrahydrozoline
HCl; polyethylene glycol 400; povi-
done] 0.05%•1%•1%

alteconazole INN

alteplase USAN, INN, BAN, JAN tissue
plasminogen activator (tPA) for acute
myocardial infarction, acute ischemic
stroke, or pulmonary embolism; investigational (orphan) for intraventricular
hemorrhage with intracerebral hemorrhage

alteratives a class of agents that produce
gradual beneficial changes in the body,
usually by improving nutrition, without
having any marked specific effect

ALternaGEL oral liquid OTC antacid
[aluminum hydroxide gel] 600 mg/
5 mL

Althaea officinalis medicinal herb [see:
marsh mallow]

althiazide USAN antihypertensive [also:
altizide]

Altinac cream (discontinued 2004) ℞
keratolytic for acne [tretinoin]
0.025%, 0.05%, 0.1% ⊡ eltenac

altinicline INN

altinicline maleate USAN nicotinic
acetylcholine receptor agonist

altizide INN antihypertensive [also: alth-
iazide]

Altocor (name changed to **Altoprev**
in 2004)

Altoprev extended-release tablets ℞
HMG-CoA reductase inhibitor for
hyperlipidemia, mixed dyslipidemia,
atherosclerosis, and the prevention and
treatment of coronary heart disease
(CHD) [lovastatin] 10, 20, 40, 60 mg

altoqualine INN

Altracin investigational (orphan) antibiotic for pseudomembranous enterocolitis [bacitracin]

altrenogest USAN, INN, BAN veterinary
progestin

altretamine USAN, INN, BAN antineoplastic for advanced ovarian adenocarcinoma (orphan)

altumomab USAN, INN monoclonal
antibody to carcinoembryonic antigen
(CEA)

altumomab pentetate USAN monoclonal antibody to carcinoembryonic antigen (CEA) [also: indium In 111 altumomab pentetate]

Alu-Cap capsules (discontinued 2006)
OTC antacid [aluminum hydroxide
gel] 400 mg

Aludrox oral suspension OTC antacid;
antiflatulent [aluminum hydroxide;
magnesium hydroxide; simethicone]
307•103• ⊡ mg/5 mL

alukalin [see: kaolin]

alum, ammonium USP *topical astringent*

alum, potassium USP *topical astringent*
[also: aluminum potassium sulfate]

alum root (Geranium maculatum)
*medicinal herb used as an astringent,
hemostatic, and antiseptic*

alumina & magnesia USP *antacid*

**aluminopara-aminosalicylate cal-
cium (alumino p-aminosalicylate
calcium)** JAN

**aluminosilicic acid, magnesium salt
hydrate** [see: silodrate]

aluminum *element (Al)*

aluminum, micronized *astringent*

aluminum acetate USP *topical astringent; Burow solution*

aluminum aminoacetate [see: dihydroxyaluminum aminoacetate]

**aluminum ammonium sulfate
dodecahydrate** [see: alum, ammo-
nium]

aluminum bismuth oxide [see: bismuth aluminate]

aluminum carbonate, basic USAN,
USP *antacid*

aluminum chlorhydroxide [now:
aluminum chlorohydrate]

**aluminum chlorhydroxide alcohol
soluble complex** [now: aluminum
chlorohydrex]

aluminum chloride USP *topical astringent for hyperhidrosis* 20% topical

aluminum chloride, basic [see: aluminum sesquichlorohydrate]

aluminum chloride hexahydrate
[see: aluminum chloride]

**aluminum chloride hydroxide
hydrate** [see: aluminum chlorohy-
drate]

aluminum chlorohydrate USAN *anhidrotic*

aluminum chlorohydrex USAN *topical astringent*

**aluminum chlorohydrol propylene
glycol complex** [now: aluminum
chlorohydrex]

**aluminum chlorohydroxy allanto-
inate** JAN *astringent; keratolytic* [also:
alcloxa]

aluminum clofibrate INN, BAN, JAN

aluminum dihydroxyaminoacetate
[see: dihydroxyaluminum aminoace-
tate]

aluminum flufenamate JAN

aluminum glycinate, basic [see:
dihydroxyaluminum aminoacetate]

aluminum hydroxide gel USP *antacid*
320, 450, 600 mg/5 mL oral

aluminum hydroxide gel, dried USP,
JAN *antacid*

aluminum hydroxide glycine [see:
dihydroxyaluminum aminoacetate]

aluminum hydroxide hydrate [see:
algeldrate]

aluminum hydroxychloride [now:
aluminum chlorohydrate]

**aluminum magnesium carbonate
hydroxide dihydrate** [see: almagate]

**aluminum magnesium hydroxide
carbonate hydrate** [see: hydrotal-
cite]

**aluminum magnesium hydroxide
oxide sulfate** [see: almadrate sulfate]

**aluminum magnesium hydroxide
oxide sulfate hydrate** [see: almadrate sulfate]

**aluminum magnesium hydroxide
sulfate** [see: magaldrate]

**aluminum magnesium hydroxide
sulfate hydrate** [see: magaldrate]

aluminum monostearate NF, JAN

aluminum oxide

Aluminum Paste ointment OTC
occlusive skin protectant [metallic alu-
minum] 10%

aluminum phosphate gel USP *antacid
(disapproved for use as an antacid in
1989)*

aluminum potassium sulfate JAN *topical astringent* [also: alum, potassium]

**aluminum potassium sulfate dodeca-
hydrate** [see: alum, potassium]

aluminum sesquichlorohydrate
USAN *anhidrotic*

aluminum silicate, natural JAN

aluminum silicate, synthetic JAN

**aluminum sodium carbonate
hydroxide** [see: dihydroxyaluminum sodium carbonate]

aluminum subacetate USP *topical astringent*

aluminum sulfate USP *anhidrotic*

aluminum sulfate hydrate [see: aluminum sulfate]

aluminum zirconium glycine tetrachloro hydrate complex [see: aluminum zirconium tetrachlorohydrex gly]

aluminum zirconium glycine trichloro hydrate complex [see: aluminum zirconium trichlorohydrex gly]

aluminum zirconium octachlorohydrate USP *anhidrotic*

aluminum zirconium octachlorohydrex gly USP *anhidrotic*

aluminum zirconium pentachlorohydrate USP *anhidrotic*

aluminum zirconium pentachlorohydrex gly USP *anhidrotic*

aluminum zirconium tetrachlorohydrate USP *anhidrotic*

aluminum zirconium tetrachlorohydrex gly USAN, USP *anhidrotic*

aluminum zirconium trichlorohydrate USP *anhidrotic*

aluminum zirconium trichlorohydrex gly USAN, USP *anhidrotic*

Alupent inhalation aerosol powder, solution for inhalation ℞ *sympathomimetic bronchodilator* [metaproterenol sulfate] 0.65 mg/dose; 0.4%, 0.6%, 5%

Alurate elixir (discontinued 2004) ℞ *sedative; hypnotic* [aprobarbital] 40 mg/5 mL ② yellow root

Alustra cream ℞ *hyperpigmentation bleaching agent* [hydroquinone; tretinoin (in a base containing glycolic acid and vitamins C and E)] 4%• 0.1%

alusulf INN ② Alasulf

Alu-Tab film-coated tablets (discontinued 2008) OTC *antacid* [aluminum hydroxide gel] 500 mg

Aluvia (foreign name for U.S. product **Kaletra**) ② Aleve; ELF; olive

ALVAC-120TMG *investigational (Phase II) vaccine for HIV* [also: VCP 205]

alvameline INN

alverine INN, BAN *anticholinergic* [also: alverine citrate]

alverine citrate USAN, NF *anticholinergic* [also: alverine]

Alvesco inhalation aerosol ℞ *once-daily corticosteroidal anti-inflammatory for persistent asthma* [ciclesonide] 80, 160 mcg/activation

alvimopan *peripherally acting opioid receptor antagonist for postoperative ileus (POI); restores normal bowel function after surgery*

alvircept sudotox USAN, INN *antiviral*

Alwextin *investigational (orphan) vulnerary for skin blistering and erosions associated with inherited epidermolysis bullosa* [allantoin]

Alzhemed *investigational (Phase III) amyloid-beta antagonist to reduce plaque formation in Alzheimer disease* [tramiprosate]

amabevan [see: carbarsone]

amacetam HCl [now: pramiracetam HCl]

amacetam sulfate [now: pramiracetam sulfate]

amadinone INN *progestin* [also: amadinone acetate]

amadinone acetate USAN *progestin* [also: amadinone]

amafolone INN, BAN

amalgucin ② imiloxan

Amanita muscaria **mushrooms** *a species that produces muscarine and ibotenic acid, a psychotropic substance ingested as a street drug*

amanozine INN ② Aminess N

amantadine INN, BAN *antiviral for influenza A virus; dopaminergic antiparkinson agent* [also: amantadine HCl]

amantadine HCl USAN, USP, JAN *antiviral for influenza A infections; dopaminergic antiparkinson agent* [also: amantadine] 100 mg oral; 50 mg/5 mL oral

amantanium bromide INN

A-Mantle OTC *cream base*

amantocillin INN

amara; amargo *medicinal herb* [see: quassia]

amaranth (*Amnaranthus* spp.) leaves and flowers *medicinal herb for diarrhea, dysentery, excessive menstruation, and nosebleeds*

amaranth (FD&C Red No. 2) USP

amargo; amara *medicinal herb* [see: quassia]

amarsan [see: acetarsone]

Amaryl tablets ℞ *once-daily sulfonylurea antidiabetic that stimulates insulin secretion in the pancreas* [glimepiride] 1, 2, 4 mg

ambamustine INN

ambasilide INN *antiarrhythmic*

ambazone INN, BAN 🔊 amipizone; ampyzine

ambenonium chloride USP, INN, BAN, JAN *anticholinesterase muscle stimulant*

ambenoxan INN, BAN

amber; amber touch-and-heal *medicinal herb* [see: St. John wort]

Ambi 10 bar OTC *therapeutic skin cleanser* 🔊 AMPA

Ambi 60/580 caplets ℞ *decongestant; expectorant* [pseudoephedrine HCl; guaifenesin] 60•580 mg 🔊 AMPA

Ambi 60/580/30 extended-release caplets ℞ *decongestant; expectorant; antitussive* [pseudoephedrine HCl; guaifenesin; dextromethorphan hydrobromide] 60•580•30 mg 🔊 AMPA

Ambi 80/700/40; Ambi 80/780/40 extended-release caplets (discontinued 2007) ℞ *decongestant; expectorant; antitussive* [pseudoephedrine HCl; guaifenesin; dextromethorphan hydrobromide] 80•700•40 mg; 80•780•40 mg 🔊 AMPA

Ambi 600; Ambi 800; Ambi 1000; Ambi 1200 sustained-release caplets (discontinued 2004) ℞ *expectorant* [guaifenesin] 600 mg; 800 mg; 1000 mg; 1200 mg 🔊 AMPA

Ambi 1000/5 caplets ℞ *expectorant; antitussive* [guaifenesin; carbetapentane citrate] 1000•5 mg 🔊 AMPA

Ambi 1000/55 extended-release tablets ℞ *expectorant; antitussive* [guaifenesin; dextromethorphan hydrobromide] 1000•55 mg 🔊 AMPA

ambicromil INN, BAN *prophylactic antiallergic* [also: probicromil calcium]

ambicromil calcium [see: probicromil calcium]

Ambien film-coated tablets ℞ *imidazopyridine sedative and hypnotic for the short-term treatment of insomnia* [zolpidem tartrate] 5, 10 mg

Ambien CR controlled-release bilayered tablets ℞ *imidazopyridine sedative and hypnotic for the short-term treatment of insomnia* [zolpidem tartrate] 6.25, 12.5 mg

Ambifed-G DM extended-release caplets ℞ *antitussive; decongestant; expectorant* [dextromethorphan hydrobromide; pseudoephedrine HCl; guaifenesin] 30•60•1000 mg

AmBisome powder for IV infusion ℞ *systemic polyene antifungal for cryptococcal meningitis, visceral leishmaniasis, and histoplasmosis (orphan)* [amphotericin B lipid complex (ABLC)] 50 mg/vial

ambomycin USAN, INN *antineoplastic*

ambrette (*Abelmoschus moschatus*) seeds and oil *medicinal herb for gastric cancer, gonorrhea, hysteria, and respiratory disorders; also used as a fragrance in cosmetics and a flavoring in alcoholic beverages, bitters, and coffees; not generally regarded as safe and effective for medicinal uses*

ambrisentan *endothelin receptor antagonist (ERA) vasodilator for pulmonary arterial hypertension (PAH)*

ambroxol INN [also: ambroxol HCl]

ambroxol HCl JAN [also: ambroxol]

ambruticin USAN, INN *antifungal*

ambucaine INN

ambucetamide INN, BAN

ambuphylline USAN *diuretic; smooth muscle relaxant* [also: bufylline]

ambuside USAN, INN, BAN *diuretic*

ambuterol [see: mabuterol]

ambutonium bromide BAN

ambutoxate [see: ambucaine]

amcinafal USAN, INN *anti-inflammatory*

amcinafide USAN, INN *anti-inflammatory*

amcinonide USAN, USP, INN, BAN, JAN *topical corticosteroidal anti-inflammatory* 0.1% topical

Amcort IM injection (discontinued 2006) ℞ *corticosteroid; anti-inflammatory* [triamcinolone diacetate] 40 mg/mL ⊘ Emo-Cort

amdinocillin USAN, USP *aminopenicillin antibiotic* [also: mecillinam]

amdinocillin pivoxil USAN *antibacterial* [also: pivmecillinam; pivmecillinam HCl]

amdoxovir USAN *investigational (Phase II) nucleoside analog antiviral for HIV-1 and hepatitis B infections*

Amdry-D extended-release caplets ℞ *decongestant; anticholinergic to dry mucosal secretions* [pseudoephedrine HCl; methscopolamine nitrate] 120•2.5 mg

ameban [see: carbarsone]

amebarsone [see: carbarsone]

amebicides *a class of drugs that kill amoebae*

amebucort INN

amechol [see: methacholine chloride]

amedalin INN *antidepressant* [also: amedalin HCl] ⊘ imidoline; omidoline

amedalin HCl USAN *antidepressant* [also: amedalin]

amediplase INN

ameltolide USAN, INN, BAN *anticonvulsant*

Amen tablets (discontinued 2004) ℞ *synthetic progestin for secondary amenorrhea, abnormal uterine bleeding, and endometrial hyperplasia* [medroxyprogesterone acetate] 10 mg

amenozine [see: amanozine]

Amerge film-coated tablets ℞ (available OTC in Europe as **Triptan**) *vascular serotonin 5-HT$_{1D}$ receptor agonist for the acute treatment of migraine* [naratriptan HCl] 1, 2.5 mg

Americaine ointment, anorectal ointment, aerosol spray (discontinued 2007) OTC *anesthetic* [benzocaine] 20%

Americaine Anesthetic Lubricant gel (discontinued 2007) ℞ *anesthetic lubricant for upper GI procedures* [benzocaine] 20%

Americaine First Aid ointment OTC *anesthetic* [benzocaine] 20%

Americaine Otic ear drops (discontinued 2004) ℞ *anesthetic* [benzocaine] 20%

American angelica *medicinal herb* [see: angelica]

American aspen *medicinal herb* [see: poplar]

American centaury (Sabatia angularis) *plant medicinal herb used as a bitter tonic, emmenagogue, febrifuge, and vermifuge*

American elder *medicinal herb* [see: elderberry]

American elm *medicinal herb* [see: slippery elm]

American foxglove *medicinal herb* [see: feverweed]

American ginseng (Panax quinquefolia) *medicinal herb* [see: ginseng]

American hellebore (Veratrum viride) [see: hellebore]

American ivy (Parthenocissus quinquefolia) *bark and twigs medicinal herb used as an alterative, astringent, and expectorant*

American nightshade *medicinal herb* [see: pokeweed]

American pepper; American red pepper *medicinal herb* [see: cayenne]

American saffron *medicinal herb* [see: safflower]

American valerian *medicinal herb* [see: lady's slipper]

American vegetable tallow tree; American vegetable wax *medicinal herb* [see: bayberry]

American woodbine *medicinal herb* [see: American ivy]

Americet tablets ℞ *barbiturate sedative; analgesic; antipyretic* [butalbital; aspirin; caffeine] 50•325•40 mg

americium *element (Am)*

Amerifed oral liquid (discontinued 2007) OTC *decongestant; antihistamine* [pseudoephedrine HCl; chlorpheniramine maleate] 80•4 mg/5 mL

Amerigel lotion, ointment OTC *emollient; diaper rash treatment*

Amerituss AD oral liquid (discontinued 2007) ℞ *antitussive; antihistamine; decongestant* [dextromethorphan hydrobromide; chlorpheniramine maleate; phenylephrine HCl] 30•6•20 mg/10 mL

amesergide USAN, INN *serotonin antagonist; antidepressant*

ametantrone INN *antineoplastic* [also: ametantrone acetate]

ametantrone acetate USAN *antineoplastic* [also: ametantrone]

ametazole BAN [also: betazole HCl; betazole]

A-Methapred powder for injection ℞ *corticosteroid; anti-inflammatory; immunosuppressant* [methylprednisolone sodium succinate] 40, 125 mg/vial

amethocaine BAN *topical anesthetic* [also: tetracaine]

amethocaine HCl BAN *local anesthetic* [also: tetracaine HCl]

amethopterin [now: methotrexate]

Amevive powder for IM injection ℞ *immunosuppressant for chronic plaque psoriasis* [alefacept] 15 mg/dose

Amevive powder for IV injection (discontinued 2006) ℞ *immunosuppressant for chronic plaque psoriasis* [alefacept] 7.5 mg/dose

amezepine INN ⦰ amicibone

amezinium metilsulfate INN, JAN

amfebutamone INN *aminoketone antidepressant; non-nicotine aid to smoking cessation* [also: bupropion HCl; bupropion]

amfebutamone HCl [see: bupropion HCl]

amfecloral INN, BAN *anorectic* [also: amphecloral]

amfenac INN, BAN *anti-inflammatory* [also: amfenac sodium]

amfenac sodium USAN, JAN *anti-inflammatory* [also: amfenac]

amfepentorex INN

amfepramone INN *anorexiant* [also: diethylpropion HCl; diethylpropion]

amfepramone HCl *anorexiant* [see: diethylpropion HCl]

amfetamine INN *CNS stimulant* [also: amphetamine sulfate; amphetamine]

amfetaminil INN

amfilcon A USAN *hydrophilic contact lens material*

amflutizole USAN, INN *gout suppressant*

amfodyne [see: imidecyl iodine]

amfomycin INN *antibacterial* [also: amphomycin]

amfonelic acid USAN, INN, BAN *CNS stimulant*

AMG 706 *investigational (Phase II) multikinase inhibitor (MKI) for advanced gastrointestinal stromal tumors (GISTs)*

amibiarson [see: carbarsone]

Amicar tablets, syrup, IV infusion ℞ *systemic hemostatic to control excessive bleeding* [aminocaproic acid] 500, 1000 mg; 250 mg/mL; 250 mg/mL ⦰ Omacor

amicarbalide INN, BAN

amicibone INN ⦰ amezepine

amicloral USAN *veterinary food additive*

amicycline USAN, INN *antibacterial*

amidantel INN, BAN

amidapsone USAN, INN *antiviral for poultry*

Amidate IV injection ℞ *rapid-acting nonbarbiturate general anesthetic* [etomidate] 2 mg/mL

amidefrine mesilate INN *adrenergic* [also: amidephrine mesylate; amidephrine]

amidephrine BAN *adrenergic* [also: amidephrine mesylate; amidefrine mesilate]

amidephrine mesylate USAN *adrenergic* [also: amidefrine mesilate; amidephrine]

amidofebrin [see: aminopyrine]

amidol [see: dimepheptanol]

amidone HCl [see: methadone HCl]

amidopyrazoline [see: aminopyrine]

amidopyrine [now: aminopyrine]

amidotrizoate sodium [see: diatrizoate sodium]

amidotrizoic acid JAN *radiopaque con-trast medium* [also: diatrizoic acid]

amiflamine INN

amifloverine INN

amifloxacin USAN, INN, BAN *broad-spectrum fluoroquinolone antibiotic*

amifloxacin mesylate USAN *broad-spectrum fluoroquinolone antibiotic*

amifostine USAN, INN, BAN *chemopro-tective agent for cisplatin and paclitaxel chemotherapy (orphan); treatment for moderate to severe xerostomia following postoperative radiation therapy (orphan); investigational (orphan) for cyclophos-phamide-induced granulocytopenia* 500 mg injection

Amigesic film-coated tablets, film-coated caplets, capsules ℞ *analgesic; antipyretic; anti-inflammatory; anti-rheumatic* [salsalate] 500 mg; 750 mg; 500 mg

amiglumide INN

amikacin USP, INN, BAN *aminoglycoside antibiotic; investigational (Phase II) liposomal formulation for complicated urinary tract infections and AIDS-related Mycobacterial infection*

amikacin sulfate USAN, USP, JAN *ami-noglycoside antibiotic* 50, 250 mg/mL injection

amikhelline INN ⊡ Amoclan

Amikin IV or IM injection, pediatric injection ℞ *aminoglycoside antibiotic* [amikacin sulfate] 250 mg/mL; 50 mg/mL

amilomer INN

amiloride INN, BAN *antihypertensive; potassium-sparing diuretic* [also: amil-oride HCl]

amiloride HCl USAN, USP *antihyper-tensive; potassium-sparing diuretic; investigational (orphan) inhalant for cystic fibrosis* [also: amiloride]

amiloxate USAN *ultraviolet B sunscreen*

aminacrine BAN *topical antiseptic* [also: aminacrine HCl; aminoacridine]

aminacrine HCl USAN *vaginal antisep-tic* [also: aminoacridine; aminacrine]

aminarsone [see: carbarsone]

amindocate INN

amine resin [see: polyamine-methyl-ene resin]

amineptine INN

Aminess 5.2% IV infusion ℞ *nutri-tional therapy for renal failure* [multi-ple essential amino acids]

Aminess N film-coated tablets ℞ *nutritional therapy for dialysis patients* [multiple essential amino acids] ⊡ amanozine

aminicotin [see: niacinamide]

aminitrozole INN *veterinary antibacte-rial* [also: nithiamide; acinitrazole]

2-amino-2-deoxyglucose [see: gluco-samine]

aminoacetic acid JAN *nonessential amino acid; urologic irrigant; symbols: Gly, G* [also: glycine]

aminoacridine INN *topical antiseptic* [also: aminacrine HCl; aminacrine]

aminoacridine HCl [see: aminacrine HCl]

9-aminoacridine monohydrochlo-ride [see: aminacrine HCl]

ρ-aminobenzenearsonic acid [see: arsanilic acid]

ρ-aminobenzenesulfonamide [see: sulfanilamide]

ρ-aminobenzene-sulfonylacetylim-ide [see: sulfacetamide]

aminobenzoate potassium USP *water-soluble vitamin; analgesic; "possibly effective" for scleroderma and other skin diseases and Peyronie disease* 500 mg oral

aminobenzoate sodium USP *analgesic*

ρ-aminobenzoic acid [see: aminoben-zoic acid]

aminobenzoic acid (4-aminobenzoic acid) USP *water-soluble vitamin; ultra-violet screen; "possibly effective" for scleroderma and other skin diseases and Peyronie disease*

aminobenzylpenicillin [see: ampi-cillin]

γ-amino-β-hydroxybutyric acid JAN

aminobromophenylpyrimidinone (ABPP) [see: bropirimine]

γ-aminobutyric acid (GABA) JAN *inhibitory neurotransmitter*

aminocaproic acid USAN, USP, INN, BAN *systemic hemostatic; investigational (orphan) topical treatment for traumatic hyphema of the eye* [also: ε-aminocaproic acid] 250 mg oral; 250 mg/mL oral; 250 mg/mL injection

ε-aminocaproic acid JAN *systemic hemostatic* [also: aminocaproic acid]

aminocardol [see: aminophylline]

Amino-Cerv vaginal cream ℞ *emollient; antifungal; anti-inflammatory* [urea; sodium propionate; methionine; cystine; inositol] 8.34%•0.5%•0.83%•0.35%•0.83%

aminodeoxykanamycin [see: bekanamycin]

2-aminoethanethiol [see: cysteamine]

2-aminoethanethiol HCl [see: cysteamine HCl]

2-aminoethanol [see: monoethanolamine]

aminoethyl nitrate (2-aminoethyl nitrate) INN

amino-ethyl-propanol [see: ambuphylline]

aminoethylsulfonic acid JAN [also: taurine]

Aminofen; Amnofen Max tablets OTC *analgesic; antipyretic* [acetaminophen] 325 mg; 500 mg

aminoform [see: methenamine]

2-aminoglutaramic acid [see: glutamine]

aminoglutethimide USP, INN, BAN *adrenal steroid inhibitor; antisteroidal antineoplastic*

aminoglycosides *a class of bactericidal antibiotics effective against gram-negative organisms* [also called: "mycins"]

aminoguanidine monohydrochloride [see: pimagedine HCl]

6-aminohexanoic acid [see: aminocaproic acid]

aminohippurate sodium USP *diagnostic aid for renal function* [also: p-aminohippurate sodium] 20% injection

p-aminohippurate sodium JAN *renal function test* [also: aminohippurate sodium]

aminohippuric acid (p-aminohippuric acid) USP

aminohydroxypropylidene diphosphonate (APD) [see: pamidronate disodium]

aminoisobutanol [see: ambuphylline]

3-(4'-aminoisoindoline-1'-one)-1-piperidine-2,6-dione *investigational (orphan) for multiple myeloma*

aminoisometradine [see: methionine]

aminoketones *a class of oral antidepressants*

5-aminolevulinic acid HCl (5-ALA HCl) USAN *photosensitizer for photodynamic therapy of precancerous actinic keratoses of the face and scalp (for use with the BLU-U Blue Light Photodynamic Therapy Illuminator)*

aminometradine INN, BAN

Amino-Min-D capsules OTC *dietary supplement* [calcium carbonate; multiple minerals; vitamin D] 250 mg•±•100 IU

aminonat [see: protein hydrolysate]

Amino-Opti-C sustained-release tablets OTC *vitamin C supplement with multiple bioflavonoids* [vitamin C; lemon bioflavonoids; rose hips; rutin; hesperidin] 1000•250•±•±•± mg

aminopenicillins *a subclass of penicillins (q.v.)*

aminopentamide sulfate [see: dimevamide]

aminophenazone INN [also: aminopyrine]

aminophenazone cyclamate INN

p-aminophenylarsonic acid [see: arsanilic acid]

aminophylline USP, INN, BAN, JAN *smooth muscle relaxant; bronchodilator* (theophylline=79%) 100, 200 mg oral; 25 mg/mL injection

aminopromazine INN [also: proquamezine]

aminopterin sodium INN, BAN *antifolate antineoplastic*

4-aminopyridine [see: fampridine]

aminopyrine NF, JAN [also: aminophenazone]

aminoquin naphthoate [see: pamaquine naphthoate]

aminoquinol INN

aminoquinoline [see: aminoquinol]

4-aminoquinoline [see: chloroquine phosphate]

8-aminoquinoline [see: primaquine phosphate]

aminoquinuride INN

aminorex USAN, INN, BAN *anorectic*

aminosalicylate calcium USP [also: calcium para-aminosalicylate]

aminosalicylate potassium USP

aminosalicylate sodium (p-aminosalicylate sodium) USP *bacteriostatic; tuberculosis retreatment agent; investigational (orphan) for Crohn disease*

aminosalicylic acid (4-aminosalicylic acid; p-aminosalicylic acid) USP *antibacterial; tuberculostatic (orphan); investigational (orphan) for ulcerative colitis*

5-aminosalicylic acid (5-ASA) [see: mesalamine]

aminosalyle sodium [see: aminosalicylate sodium]

aminosidine *investigational (orphan) agent for tuberculosis,* Mycobacterium avium *complex (MAC), and visceral leishmaniasis*

aminosidine sulfate [see: paromomycin sulfate]

21-aminosteroids *a class of potent antioxidants that can protect against oxygen radical–mediated lipid peroxidation and progressive neuronal degeneration following brain or spinal trauma, subarachnoid hemorrhage, or stroke* [also called: lazaroids]

aminosuccinic acid [see: aspartic acid]

Aminosyn 3.5% (5%, 7%, 8.5%, 10%); Aminosyn (pH6) 10%; Aminosyn II 3.5% (5%, 7%, 8.5%, 10%, 15%); Aminosyn-PF 7% (10%) IV infusion ℞ *total parenteral nutrition (except 3.5%); peripheral parenteral nutrition (all)* [multiple essential and nonessential amino acids] ② amanozine

Aminosyn 3.5% M; Aminosyn II 3.5% M IV infusion ℞ *peripheral parenteral nutrition* [multiple essential and nonessential amino acids; electrolytes]

Aminosyn 7% (8.5%) with Electrolytes; Aminosyn II 7% (8.5%, 10%) with Electrolytes IV infusion ℞ *total parenteral nutrition; peripheral parenteral nutrition* [multiple essential and nonessential amino acids; electrolytes] ② amanozine

Aminosyn II 3.5% in 5% (25%) Dextrose; Aminosyn II 4.25% in 10% (20%, 25%) Dextrose; Aminosyn II 5% in 25% Dextrose IV infusion ℞ *total parenteral nutrition (except 3.5% in 5%); peripheral parenteral nutrition (not 20% and 25%)* [multiple essential and nonessential amino acids; dextrose]

Aminosyn II 3.5% M in 5% Dextrose; Aminosyn II 4.25% M in 10% Dextrose IV infusion ℞ *total parenteral nutrition (4.25% in 10% only); peripheral parenteral nutrition (both)* [multiple essential and nonessential amino acids; electrolytes; dextrose]

Aminosyn-HBC 7% IV infusion ℞ *nutritional therapy for high metabolic stress* [multiple branched-chain essential and nonessential amino acids; electrolytes]

Aminosyn-RF 5.2% IV infusion ℞ *nutritional therapy for renal failure* [multiple essential amino acids]

aminothiazole INN

aminotrate phosphate [see: trolnitrate phosphate]

aminoxaphen [see: aminorex]

Aminoxin enteric-coated tablets OTC *vitamin B_6 supplement* [pyridoxal-5'-phosphate] 20 mg

aminoxytriphene INN

aminoxytropine tropate HCl [see: atropine oxide HCl]

Amio-Aqueous *investigational (orphan) antiarrhythmic for incessant ventricular tachycardia* [amiodarone]

amiodarone USAN, INN, BAN *antiar-rhythmic for acute ventricular tachycardia and fibrillation (orphan)*

amiodarone HCl *ventricular antiar-rhythmic for acute ventricular tachycardia and fibrillation (orphan)* 200, 400 mg oral; 50 mg/mL injection

amiperone INN ② Empirin

amiphenazole INN, BAN

amipizone INN ② ambazone; ampyzine

amipramidine [see: amiloride HCl]

amiprilose INN *synthetic monosaccharide anti-inflammatory* [also: amiprilose HCl]

amiprilose HCl USAN *investigational (NDA filed) synthetic monosaccharide anti-inflammatory for rheumatoid arthritis* [also: amiprilose]

amiquinsin INN *antihypertensive* [also: amiquinsin HCl]

amiquinsin HCl USAN *antihypertensive* [also: amiquinsin]

amisometradine NF, INN, BAN

amisulpride INN

amiterol INN ② Emetrol

amithiozone [see: thioacetazone; thiacetazone]

amitivir USAN, INN *influenza vaccine* ② emitefur

Amitiza softgels ℞ *selective chloride channel activator to increase fluid secretion in the small intestine for the treatment of chronic idiopathic constipation in adults and irritable bowel syndrome with constipation (IBS-C) in women* [lubiprostone] 8, 24 mcg

Amitone chewable tablets (discontinued 2005) OTC *antacid* [calcium carbonate] 350 mg ② emetine; iometin

amitraz USAN, INN, BAN *scabicide*

amitriptyline (AMT) INN, BAN *tricyclic antidepressant* [also: amitriptyline HCl]

amitriptyline HCl USP, JAN *tricyclic antidepressant* [also: amitriptyline] 10, 25, 50, 75, 100, 150 mg oral

amitriptylinoxide INN

amixetrine INN ② amogastrin

AmLactin cream, lotion OTC *moisturizer; emollient* [ammonium lactate] 12%

AmLactin AP cream OTC *local anesthetic; moisturizer; emollient* [pramoxine HCl; lactic acid] 1%•12%

AmLactin XL lotion OTC *moisturizer; emollient* [ammonium lactate; potassium lactate; sodium lactate]

amlexanox USAN, INN, JAN *anti-inflammatory for aphthous ulcers; topical histamine and leukotriene inhibitor*

amlintide USAN *antidiabetic for type 1 diabetes* [see also: pramlintide acetate]

amlodipine INN, BAN *antianginal; antihypertensive; calcium channel blocker* [also: amlodipine besylate]

amlodipine besylate USAN *antianginal; antihypertensive; calcium channel blocker* [also: amlodipine] 2.5, 5, 10 mg oral

amlodipine besylate & benazepril HCl *antihypertensive; angiotensin-converting enzyme (ACE) inhibitor; calcium channel blocker* 2.5•10, 5•10, 5•20, 10•20 mg

amlodipine maleate USAN *antianginal; antihypertensive*

ammi (Ammi majus; A. visnaga) dried ripe fruits *medicinal herb for angina, bronchial asthma, diabetes, diuresis, kidney and bladder stones, psoriasis, respiratory diseases, and vitiligo*

ammoidin [see: methoxsalen]

[¹³N] ammonia [see: ammonia N 13]

ammonia [see: ammonia spirit, aromatic]

ammonia N 13 USAN, USP *radioactive diagnostic aid for cardiac and liver imaging* 30–300 mCi/8 mL injection

ammonia solution, strong NF *solvent; source of ammonia* [also: ammonia water]

ammonia spirit, aromatic USP *respiratory stimulant*

ammonia water JAN *solvent; source of ammonia* [also: ammonia solution, strong]

ammoniated mercury [see: mercury, ammoniated]

ammonio methacrylate copolymer NF *coating agent*

ammonium alum [see: alum, ammonium]

ammonium benzoate USP

ammonium carbonate NF *source of ammonia*

ammonium chloride USP, JAN *urinary acidifier; diuretic; expectorant* 486, 500 mg oral; 5 mEq/mL (26.75%) injection

ammonium 2-hydroxypropanoate [see: ammonium lactate]

ammonium ichthosulfonate [see: ichthammol]

ammonium lactate (lactic acid neutralized with ammonium hydroxide) USAN *antipruritic; emollient for xerosis* 12% topical

ammonium mandelate USP

ammonium molybdate USP *dietary molybdenum supplement* 25 mcg/mL injection

ammonium molybdate tetrahydrate [see: ammonium molybdate]

ammonium phosphate NF *pharmaceutic aid*

ammonium salicylate NF

ammonium tetrathiomolybdate *investigational (orphan) for Wilson disease*

ammonium valerate NF

Ammonul IV infusion ℞ *adjunctive therapy (rescue agent) to prevent and treat hyperammonemia due to urea cycle enzymopathy (orphan)* [sodium benzoate; sodium phenylacetate] 101•100 mg/mL

ammophyllin [see: aminophylline]

Amnaranthus spp. *medicinal herb* [see: amaranth]

Amnesteem capsules ℞ *keratolytic for severe recalcitrant cystic acne* [isotretinoin] 10, 20, 40 mg

AMO Endosol; AMO Endosol Extra ophthalmic solution ℞ *intraocular irrigating solution* [sodium chloride (balanced saline solution)]

AMO Vitrax intraocular injection ℞ *viscoelastic agent for ophthalmic surgery* [hyaluronate sodium] 30 mg/mL

amobarbital USP, INN, JAN *sedative; hypnotic; anticonvulsant; also abused as a street drug* [also: amylobarbitone]

amobarbital sodium USP, JAN *hypnotic; sedative; anticonvulsant; also abused as a street drug*

amocaine chloride [see: amolanone HCl]

amocarzine INN

Amoclan powder for oral suspension ℞ *aminopenicillin antibiotic plus synergist* [amoxicillin; clavulanate potassium] 200•28.5, 400•57 mg/5 mL ⊠ amikhelline

amodiaquine USP, INN, BAN *antiprotozoal*

amodiaquine HCl USP *antimalarial*

amogastrin INN, JAN ⊠ amixetrine

amolanone INN

amolanone HCl [see: amolanone]

amonafide INN *antineoplastic*

amoproxan INN

amopyroquine INN

amorolfine USAN, INN, BAN *antimycotic*

Amorphophallus konjac *medicinal herb* [see: glucomannan]

Amosan powder OTC *oral antibacterial* [sodium peroxyborate monohydrate] ⊠ E-Mycin

amoscanate INN

amosulalol INN [also: amosulalol HCl]

amosulalol HCl JAN [also: amosulalol]

amotriphene [see: aminoxytriphene]

amoxapine USAN, USP, INN, BAN, JAN *tricyclic antidepressant* 25, 50, 100, 150 mg oral

amoxecaine INN

Amoxicilin Pulsys oral *investigational (NDA filed) once-daily aminopenicillin antibiotic for tonsillitis and pharyngitis due to streptococcal infections* [amoxicillin]

amoxicillin USAN, USP, JAN *aminopenicillin antibiotic* [also: amoxicilline; amoxycillin] 125, 200, 250, 400, 500, 875 mg oral; 125, 200, 250, 400 mg/5 mL oral

amoxicillin & clavulanate potassium *aminopenicillin antibiotic plus synergist* 200•28.5, 250•125, 400•57, 500•125, 875•125 mg oral; 200•28.5, 400•57, 600•42.9 mg/5 mL oral

amoxicillin sodium USAN *aminopenicillin antibiotic*

amoxicillin trihydrate [see: amoxicillin]

amoxicilline INN *aminopenicillin antibiotic* [also: amoxicillin; amoxycillin]

Amoxil chewable tablets (discontinued 2008) ℞ *aminopenicillin antibiotic* [amoxicillin] 200, 400 mg

Amoxil film-coated caplets, capsules, powder for oral suspension, pediatric oral drops ℞ *aminopenicillin antibiotic* [amoxicillin] 875 mg; 500 mg; 125, 200 mg/5 mL; 50 mg/mL

amoxycillin BAN *aminopenicillin antibiotic* [also: amoxicillin; amoxicilline]

amoxydramine camsilate INN [also: amoxydramine camsylate]

amoxydramine camsylate [also: amoxydramine camsilate]

AMP; A₅MP (adenosine monophosphate) [see: adenosine phosphate]

AMPA (α-amino-3-hydroxy-5-methyl-4-isoxazolepropionic acid) ⊉ Ambi 10

ampakines *a class of drugs that modulate neurotransmitters by affecting the AMPA-glutamate receptors (AMPA-GluR) in the brain, enhancing cognition and memory; investigational treatment for Alzheimer and other dementias*

amperozide INN, BAN *antipsychotic*

Amphadase solution for injection ℞ *adjuvant to increase the absorption and dispersion of injected drugs, hypodermoclysis, and subcutaneous urography; investigational (NDA filed) agent to clear vitreous hemorrhage; also used for diabetic retinopathy* [hyaluronidase (bovine)] 150 U/mL

amphecloral USAN *anorectic* [also: amfecloral]

amphenidone INN

amphetamine BAN *CNS stimulant; widely abused as a street drug, which causes strong psychic dependence* [also: amphetamine sulfate; amfetamine]

d-amphetamine [see: dextroamphetamine]

(+)-amphetamine [see: dextroamphetamine]

l-amphetamine [see: levamphetamine]

(−)-amphetamine [see: levamphetamine]

amphetamine aspartate *CNS stimulant*

amphetamine complex (resin complex of amphetamine & dextroamphetamine) [q.v.]

amphetamine phosphate, dextro [see: dextroamphetamine phosphate]

Amphetamine Salt Combo tablets ℞ *CNS stimulant mixture for attention-deficit/hyperactivity disorder (ADHD)* [amphetamine aspartate; amphetamine sulfate; dextroamphetamine sulfate; dextroamphetamine saccharate] 5, 10, 20, 30 mg total amphetamines (25% of each)

amphetamine succinate, levo [see: levamphetamine succinate]

amphetamine sulfate USP *CNS stimulant; widely abused as a street drug, which causes strong psychic dependence* [also: amfetamine; amphetamine]

amphetamine sulfate, dextro [see: dextroamphetamine sulfate]

amphetamines *a class of CNS stimulants that includes amphetamine, dextroamphetamine, levamphetamine, methamphetamine, and their salts*

amphetamines, mixed (equal parts amphetamine aspartate, amphetamine sulfate, dextroamphetamine sulfate, and dextroamphetamine saccharate) *CNS stimulant for attention-deficit/hyperactivity disorder (ADHD), narcolepsy, and obesity; also abused as a street drug, which causes strong psychic dependence* [5, 10, 20, 30 mg oral]

Amphocin powder for IV infusion ℞ *systemic polyene antifungal* [amphotericin B deoxycholate] 50 mg/vial

amphocortrin [see: amphomycin]

Amphojel oral suspension (discontinued 2004) OTC *antacid* [aluminum hydroxide gel] 320 mg/5 mL

Amphojel tablets OTC *antacid* [aluminum hydroxide gel] 300, 600 mg

amphomycin USAN, BAN *antibacterial* [also: amfomycin]

amphotalide INN

Amphotec powder for IV infusion ℞ *systemic polyene antifungal for invasive aspergillosis* [amphotericin B cholesteryl sulfate] 50, 100 mg/vial

amphotericin B USP, INN, BAN, JAN *polyene antifungal*

amphotericin B cholesteryl *systemic polyene antifungal for invasive aspergillosis*

amphotericin B deoxycholate *systemic polyene antifungal* 50 mg injection

amphotericin B inhalation powder (ABIP) *investigational (Phase I, orphan) polyene antifungal for the prevention of pulmonary aspergillosis and other fungal infections in immunocompromised patients*

amphotericin B lipid complex (ABLC) *systemic polyene antifungal for meningitis, leishmaniasis, histoplasmosis, and other invasive infections (orphan)*

ampicillin USAN, USP, INN, BAN, JAN *aminopenicillin antibiotic* 250, 500 mg oral

ampicillin sodium USAN, USP, JAN *aminopenicillin antibiotic* 250, 500 mg, 1, 2 g injection

ampicillin sodium & sulbactam sodium *aminopenicillin antibiotic plus synergist* 1•0.5, 2•1, 10•5 g injection

ampiroxicam INN, BAN

Amplicor Chlamydia test kit for professional use ℞ *in vitro diagnostic aid for* Chlamydia trachomatis [DNA amplification test]

Amplicor HIV-1 Monitor test kit for professional use ℞ *in vitro diagnostic aid for HIV-1 in blood* [polymerase chain reaction (PCR) test]

Amplicor MTB test kit for professional use ℞ *in vitro diagnostic aid for* Mycobacterium *tuberculosis* [polymerase chain reaction (PCR) test]

Ampligen *investigational (Phase III, orphan) RNA synthesis inhibitor and immunomodulator for AIDS, renal cell carcinoma, metastatic melanoma, and chronic fatigue syndrome* [poly I: poly C12U]

amprenavir USAN, INN *protease inhibitor antiviral for HIV infection*

amprocidum [see: amprolium]

amprolium USP, INN, BAN *coccidiostat for poultry*

amprotropine phosphate

ampyrimine INN ② embramine; imipramine

ampyzine INN *CNS stimulant* [also: ampyzine sulfate] ② ambazone; amipizone

ampyzine sulfate USAN *CNS stimulant* [also: ampyzine]

amquinate USAN, INN *antimalarial*

amrinone INN, BAN *cardiotonic* [also: inamrinone]

amrinone lactate [now: inamrinone lactate]

Amrix extended-release capsules ℞ *once-daily skeletal muscle relaxant* [cyclobenzaprine HCl] 15, 30 mg

amrubicin INN

AMSA; *m*-AMSA (acridinylamine methanesulfon anisidide) [see: amsacrine]

amsacrine USAN, INN, BAN *investigational (NDA filed, orphan) antineoplastic for acute adult leukemias (AML, APL, and ALL) and lymphomas*

Amsidyl *investigational (NDA filed, orphan) antineoplastic for acute adult leukemias (AML, APL, and ALL) and lymphomas* [amsacrine]

amsonate INN, BAN *combining name for radicals or groups*

AMT (amitriptyline HCl) [q.v.]

amtolmetin guacil INN

Amvaz tablets (discontinued 2007) ℞ *antianginal; antihypertensive; calcium* *channel blocker* [amlodipine] 2.5, 5, 10 mg

Amvisc; Amvisc Plus intraocular injection ℞ *viscoelastic agent for ophthalmic surgery* [hyaluronate sodium] 12 mg/mL; 16 mg/mL

amyl alcohol, tertiary [see: amylene hydrate]

amyl nitrite USP, JAN *coronary vasodilator; antianginal; also abused as a euphoric street drug and sexual stimulant* 0.3 mL inhalant

amylase *digestive enzyme (digests carbohydrates)* [100 IU/mg in pancrelipase; 25 IU/mg in pancreatin]

amylase [see: alpha amylase]

amylene hydrate NF *solvent*

amylin *a naturally occurring neuroendocrine hormone synthesized in the pancreas in the postprandial period* [see: amlintide; pramlintide acetate]

amylmetacresol INN, BAN

amylobarbitone BAN *sedative; hypnotic; anticonvulsant* [also: amobarbital]

amylocaine BAN

amylopectin sulfate, sodium salt [see: sodium amylosulfate]

amylosulfate sodium [see: sodium amylosulfate]

Amytal Sodium powder for injection ℞ *sedative; hypnotic; anxiolytic; anticonvulsant; also abused as a street drug* [amobarbital sodium]

anabolic steroids *a class of hormones derived from or closely related to testosterone that increase anabolic (tissue-building) and decrease catabolic (tissue-depleting) processes*

anacetrapib *investigational (Phase III) antihyperlipidemic; cholesterol ester transfer protein (CETP) inhibitor that raises HDL cholesterol*

Anacin caplets, tablets OTC *analgesic; antipyretic; anti-inflammatory* [aspirin; caffeine] 400•32 mg; 400•32, 500•32 mg ☒ Enzone; inosine; Unasyn

Anacin Advanced Headache tablets OTC *analgesic; antipyretic; anti-inflammatory* [acetaminophen; aspirin; caffeine] 250•250•65 mg

Anacin Aspirin Free tablets, caplets, gelcaps (discontinued 2008) OTC *analgesic; antipyretic* [acetaminophen] 500 mg

Anacin P.M., Aspirin Free film-coated caplets OTC *antihistaminic sleep aid; analgesic; antipyretic* [diphenhydramine HCl; acetaminophen] 25•500 mg

Anadrol-50 tablets ℞ *anabolic steroid for anemia; also abused as a street drug* [oxymetholone] 50 mg ☒ Inderal

anafebrina [see: aminopyrine]

Anafranil capsules ℞ *tricyclic antidepressant for obsessive-compulsive disorders* [clomipramine HCl] 25, 50, 75 mg

anagestone INN *progestin* [also: anagestone acetate]

anagestone acetate USAN *progestin* [also: anagestone]

anagrelide INN *antithrombotic/antiplatelet agent* [also: anagrelide HCl]

anagrelide HCl USAN *antithrombotic/antiplatelet agent for essential thrombocythemia (orphan); investigational (orphan) for thrombocytosis and polycythemia vera* [also: anagrelide] 0.5, 1 mg oral

anakinra USAN, INN *interleukin-1 receptor antagonist (IL-1ra); nonsteroidal anti-inflammatory drug (NSAID) for rheumatoid arthritis; investigational (orphan) for juvenile rheumatoid arthritis and graft-versus-host disease*

analeptics *a class of central nervous system stimulants used to maintain or improve alertness*

Analgesia Creme OTC *analgesic* [trolamine salicylate] 10%

Analgesic Balm OTC *analgesic; mild anesthetic; antipruritic; counterirritant* [methyl salicylate; menthol]

Analgesic Balm-GRX OTC *analgesic; mild anesthetic; antipruritic; counterirritant* [methyl salicylate; menthol] 14%•6%

analgesics *a class of drugs that relieve pain or reduce sensitivity to pain without causing loss of consciousness*

analgesine [see: antipyrine]

Analpram-HC anorectal cream, lotion ℞ *corticosteroidal anti-inflammatory; local anesthetic* [hydrocortisone acetate; pramoxine] 1%•1%, 2.5%•1%; 2.5%•1%

AnaMantle HC; AnaMantle HC 2.5% cream ℞ *corticosteroidal anti-inflammatory; anesthetic* [hydrocortisone acetate; lidocaine] 0.5%•3%; 2.5%•3%

Anamirta cocculus; A. paniculata medicinal herb [see: levant berry]

ananain *investigational (orphan) proteolytic enzymes for debridement of severe burns*

Ananas comosus medicinal herb [see: pineapple]

Anaphalis margaritacea; Gnaphalium polycephalum; G. uliginosum medicinal herb [see: everlasting]

anaphrodisiacs *a class of agents that reduce sexual desire or potency*

Anaplex-DM Cough syrup ℞ *antitussive; antihistamine; decongestant* [dextromethorphan hydrobromide; brompheniramine maleate; pseudoephedrine HCl] 30•4•60 mg/5 mL

Anaplex DMX oral suspension ℞ *antitussive; antihistamine; decongestant* [dextromethorphan tannate; brompheniramine tannate; pseudoephedrine tannate] 60•8•90 mg/5 mL

Anaplex HD oral liquid ℞ *narcotic antitussive; antihistamine; decongestant* [hydrocodone bitartrate; brompheniramine maleate; pseudoephedrine HCl] 1.7•2•30 mg/5 mL

Anaprox; Anaprox DS film-coated tablets ℞ *analgesic; nonsteroidal anti-inflammatory drug (NSAID) for osteoarthritis, rheumatoid arthritis, juvenile arthritis, ankylosing spondylitis, primary dysmenorrhea, bursitis/tendinitis, and other mild to moderate pain* [naproxen sodium] 275 mg (250 mg base); 550 mg (500 mg base)

anarel [see: guanadrel sulfate]

anaritide INN, BAN *antihypertensive; diuretic* [also: anaritide acetate]

anaritide acetate USAN *antihypertensive; diuretic; investigational (orphan) for acute renal failure and renal transplants*

Anaspaz tablets ℞ *GI/GU antispasmodic; antiparkinsonian; anticholinergic "drying agent" for allergic rhinitis and hyperhidrosis* [hyoscyamine sulfate] 0.125 mg

anastrozole USAN, INN, BAN *aromatase inhibitor; estrogen antagonist; antineoplastic for advanced breast cancer; also used as an adjunct to testosterone replacement therapy for postandropausal symptoms*

Anatrast oral/rectal paste ℞ *radiopaque contrast medium for esophageal imaging (oral) or defecography (rectal)* [barium sulfate] 100% ⊡ IntraSite

Anatrofin brand name for stenbolone acetate, an anabolic steroid abused as a street drug ⊡ Entrophen

anatumomab mafenatox INN

Anavar brand name for oxandrolone, an anabolic steroid abused as a street drug

anaxirone INN

anayodin [see: chiniofon]

anazocine INN

anazolene sodium USAN, INN *blood volume and cardiac output test* [also: sodium anoxynaphthonate]

Anbesol topical liquid, oral gel OTC *mucous membrane anesthetic; antipruritic; counterirritant; antiseptic* [benzocaine; phenol; alcohol 70%] 6.3%• 0.5%

Anbesol, Baby oral gel OTC *mucous membrane anesthetic* [benzocaine] 7.5%

Anbesol, Maximum Strength topical liquid, oral gel OTC *mucous membrane anesthetic* [benzocaine; alcohol 50%] 20%

Anbesol Cold Sore Therapy oral ointment OTC *mucous membrane anesthetic; vulnerary; antipruritic/counterirritant; emollient* [benzocaine; allantoin; camphor; petrolatum] 20%•1%•3%•65%

ancarolol INN

Ancef powder or frozen premix for IV or IM injection (discontinued 2007)

Rx *first-generation cephalosporin antibiotic* [cefazolin sodium] 0.5, 1, 5, 10 g

ancestim USAN, INN *recombinant-methionyl human stem cell factor (r-metHuSCF); hematopoietic growth factor; investigational (NDA filed, orphan) myelosuppressive and myeloablative therapy for non-Hodgkin lymphoma, breast and ovarian cancer, and multiple myeloma*

Ancet topical liquid OTC *soap-free therapeutic skin cleanser*

anchusa *medicinal herb* [see: henna (Alkanna)]

ancitabine INN [also: ancitabine HCl] ☑ enocitabine

ancitabine HCl JAN [also: ancitabine]

Ancobon capsules Rx *systemic antifungal* [flucytosine] 250, 500 mg

ancrod USAN, INN, BAN *anticoagulant enzyme derived from the venom of the Malayan pit viper; investigational (orphan) for cardiopulmonary bypass in heparin-intolerant patients*

Andehist DM NR oral drops (discontinued 2007) Rx *antitussive; antihistamine; decongestant; for children 1–24 months* [dextromethorphan hydrobromide; carbinoxamine maleate; pseudoephedrine HCl] 4•1•15 mg/mL

Andehist DM NR syrup Rx *antitussive; antihistamine; decongestant* [dextromethorphan hydrobromide; brompheniramine maleate; pseudoephedrine HCl] 15•4•45 mg/5 mL

Andehist NR oral drops (discontinued 2007) Rx *decongestant; antihistamine* [pseudoephedrine HCl; carbinoxamine maleate] 15•1 mg/mL

Andehist NR syrup Rx *decongestant; antihistamine* [pseudoephedrine HCl; brompheniramine maleate] 45•4 mg/5 mL

andolast INN

andrachne (Andrachne aspera; A. cordifolia; A. phyllanthoides) *root medicinal herb for eye inflammation; not generally regarded as safe and effective*

Androcur *investigational (orphan) anti-androgen for severe hirsutism* [cyproterone acetate]

Androderm transdermal patch (for nonscrotal area) Rx *androgen for hypogonadism or testosterone deficiency in men; hormone replacement therapy (HRT) for postandropausal symptoms; investigational (Phase III) for AIDS-wasting syndrome* [testosterone] 2.5, 5 mg/day (12.2, 24.3 mg total)

AndroGel single-use packets, metered-dose pump Rx *androgen for hypogonadism or testosterone deficiency in men; hormone replacement therapy (HRT) for postandropausal symptoms; investigational (Phase II, orphan) for AIDS-wasting syndrome* [testosterone; alcohol 67%] 1% (25, 50 mg/pkt.; 12.5 mg/pump)

Androgel-DHT *investigational (Phase III) transdermal testosterone replacement therapy for postandropausal symptoms; investigational (Phase II, orphan) for AIDS-wasting syndrome* [dihydrotestosterone]

androgens *a class of sex hormones responsible for the development of the male sex organs and secondary sex characteristics*

Androgyn [see: depAndrogyn]

Android capsules (discontinued 2007) Rx *androgen for hypogonadism or testosterone deficiency in men, delayed puberty in boys, and metastatic breast cancer in women; hormone replacement therapy for postandropausal symptoms; also abused as a street drug* [methyltestosterone] 10 mg ☑ Inderide 40/25

Andropogon citratus *medicinal herb* [see: lemongrass]

androstanazole [now: stanozolol]

androstane [see: androstanolone; stanolone]

androstanolone INN *anabolic steroid; investigational (orphan) for AIDS-wasting syndrome* [also: stanolone]

androtest P [see: testosterone propionate]

Androvite tablets OTC *vitamin/mineral/
iron supplement* [multiple vitamins &
minerals; iron; folic acid; biotin] ± •
3•0.06• ± mg

Androxy tablets ℞ *oral androgen for
hypogonadism or testosterone deficiency
in men, delayed puberty in boys, and
metastatic breast cancer in women;
hormone replacement therapy (HRT)
for postandropausal symptoms* [fluoxy-
mesterone] 10 mg ⑨ Ondrox

anecortave INN *angiostatic steroid for
neovascularization of the eye to preserve vision in patients with wet age-
related macular degeneration* [also:
anecortave acetate]

anecortave acetate USAN *investigational (NDA filed) angiostatic steroid
for neovascularization of the eye to preserve vision in patients with wet age-
related macular degeneration* [also:
anecortave]

Anectine IV or IM injection, Flo-Pack
(powder for injection) ℞ *muscle relaxant; anesthesia adjunct* [succinylcholine
chloride] 20 mg/mL; 500, 1000 mg

Anemagen gelcaps (discontinued
2004) ℞ *hematinic; vitamin/iron supplement* [multiple vitamins; ferrous
fumarate] ± •200 mg

Anemagen OB gelcaps ℞ *vitamin/cal-
cium/iron supplement* [multiple vitamins; calcium; ferrous fumarate;
folic acid] ± •200•27•1 mg

Anemone patens medicinal herb [see:
pasque flower]

anertan [see: testosterone propionate]

Anestacon oral jelly ℞ *mucous membrane anesthetic* [lidocaine HCl] 2%

Anestafoam topical foam OTC *anesthetic* [lidocaine HCl] 4%

anesthesin [see: benzocaine]

anesthetics *a class of agents that abolish
the sensation of pain*

anesthrone [see: benzocaine]

anethaine [see: tetracaine HCl]

anethole NF *flavoring agent* ⑨ Intal

anetholtrithion JAN

Anethum foeniculum medicinal herb
[see: fennel]

Anethum graveolens medicinal herb
[see: dill]

aneurine HCl [see: thiamine HCl]

**Anexsia; Anexsia 5/500; Anexsia
7.5/650; Anexsia 10/660** tablets ℞
narcotic analgesic; antipyretic [hydro-
codone bitartrate; acetaminophen]
5•325, 7.5•325 mg; 5•500 mg; 7.5•
650 mg; 10•660 mg

Anextuss extended-release tablets ℞
antitussive; decongestant; expectorant
[dextromethorphan hydrobromide;
phenylephrine HCl; guaifenesin]
60•40•600 mg

angelica (*Angelica atropurpurea*)
root *medicinal herb for appetite stimulation, bronchial disorders, colds, colic,
cough, exhaustion, gas, heartburn, and
rheumatism; also used as a tonic* ⑨
one.click

Angelica levisticum medicinal herb [see:
lovage]

*Angelica polymorpha; A. sinensis; A.
dahurica* medicinal herb [see: dong
quai]

Angeliq film-coated tablets (in packs
of 28) ℞ *monophasic oral contraceptive* [drospirenone; estradiol] 0.5•1
mg ⑨ one.click

Angiomax powder for IV injection ℞
*anticoagulant thrombin inhibitor for
percutaneous coronary intervention
(PCI), percutaneous transluminal coronary angioplasty (PTCA), or heparin-
induced thrombocytopenia (HIT); used
with aspirin therapy* [bivalirudin] 250
mg/vial

angiotensin 1-7 *investigational (orphan)
agent for myelodysplastic syndrome and
neutropenia due to bone marrow transplantation*

angiotensin II INN

**angiotensin II receptor antagonists
(AIIRAs)** *a class of antihypertensives
that reduce the vasoconstricting effects
of angiotensin II by blocking the angiotensin II receptor sites in the vascular
smooth muscles* [compare to: angiotensin-converting enzyme inhibitors;
renin inhibitors]

angiotensin amide USAN, NF, BAN *vasoconstrictor* [also: angiotensin-amide]

angiotensinamide INN *vasoconstrictor* [also: angiotensin amide]

angiotensin-converting enzyme inhibitors (ACEIs) *a class of antihypertensives that reduce the vasoconstricting effects of angiotensin II by blocking the enzyme (kininase II) that converts angiotensin I to angiotensin II* [compare to: angiotensin II receptor antagonists; renin inhibitors]

anhidrotics *a class of agents that reduce or suppress perspiration* [also called: anidrotics; antihydrotics]

anhydrohydroxyprogesterone [now: ethisterone]

anhydrous lanolin [see: lanolin, anhydrous]

anidoxime USAN, INN, BAN *analgesic*

anidrotics *a class of agents that reduce or suppress perspiration* [also called: anhidrotics; antihydrotics]

anidulafungin USAN, INN *echinocandin antifungal for candidemia of the internal organs, esophageal candidiasis, and other serious fungal infections*

anilamate INN

anileridine USP, INN, BAN *narcotic analgesic*

anileridine HCl USP *narcotic analgesic*

anilopam INN *analgesic* [also: anilopam HCl]

anilopam HCl USAN *analgesic* [also: anilopam]

Animal Shapes chewable tablets OTC *vitamin supplement* [multiple vitamins; folic acid] ±•0.3 mg

Animal Shapes + Iron chewable tablets OTC *vitamin/iron supplement* [multiple vitamins; iron; folic acid] ±•15•0.3 mg

Animi-3 capsules OTC *dietary supplement* [omega-3 fatty acids (source of DHA and EPA); vitamins B₆ and B₁₂; folic acid] 500 (350+35)•12.5•0.5•1 mg

anion exchange resin [see: polyamine-methylene resin]

anipamil INN

aniracetam USAN, INN *mental performance enhancer*

anirolac USAN, INN *anti-inflammatory; analgesic*

anisacril INN

anisatil USAN *combining name for radicals or groups* ⊕ inositol

anise (Pimpinella anisum) *oil and seeds medicinal herb for colic, convulsions, cough, gas, intestinal cleansing, iron-deficiency anemia, mucous discharge, promoting expectoration, and psoriasis; also used as an antibacterial, antimicrobial, and antiseptic* ⊕ Uni-Ace

anise oil NF ⊕ Anusol; Enisyl; Enseal; Unisol

anise root; sweet anise *medicinal herb* [see: sweet cicely]

anisindione NF, INN, BAN *indanedione-derivative anticoagulant*

anisopirol INN

anisopyradamine [see: pyrilamine maleate]

anisotropine methylbromide USAN, JAN *anticholinergic; peptic ulcer adjunct* [also: octatropine methylbromide] 50 mg oral

anisoylated plasminogen streptokinase activator complex (APSAC) [see: anistreplase]

anisperimus INN

anistreplase USAN, INN, BAN *fibrinolytic; thrombolytic enzyme for acute myocardial infarction*

Anisum officinarum; A. vulgare *medicinal herb* [see: anise]

anitrazafen USAN, INN *topical anti-inflammatory*

anodynes *a class of agents that lessen or relieve pain*

anodynine [see: antipyrine]

anodynon [see: ethyl chloride]

anorectics *a class of central nervous system stimulants that suppress the appetite* [also called: anorexiants; anorexigenics]

anorexiants *a class of central nervous system stimulants that suppress the* *appetite* [also called: anorectics; anorexigenics]

anorexigenics *a class of central nervous system stimulants that suppress the appetite* [also called: anorexiants; anorectics]

anovlar [see: norethindrone & ethinyl estradiol]

anoxomer USAN *antioxidant; food additive*

anoxynaphthonate sodium [see: anazolene sodium]

anpirtoline INN

Ansaid film-coated tablets ℞ *analgesic; nonsteroidal anti-inflammatory drug (NSAID) for osteoarthritis and rheumatoid arthritis* [flurbiprofen] 50, 100 mg

ansamycin [see: rifabutin]

ansoxetine INN

Answer One-Step; Answer Plus; Answer Quick & Simple test kit for home use OTC *in vitro diagnostic aid; urine pregnancy test*

Answer Ovulation test kit for home use OTC *in vitro diagnostic aid to predict ovulation time*

Antabuse tablets ℞ *deterrent to alcohol consumption* [disulfiram] 250, 500 mg

Antacid chewable tablets OTC *antacid* [calcium carbonate] 500, 750 mg

Antacid oral suspension OTC *antacid* [aluminum hydroxide; magnesium hydroxide] 225•200 mg/5 mL

antacids *a class of drugs that neutralize gastric acid*

antafenite INN

Antagon subcu injection (discontinued 2004) ℞ *gonadotropin-releasing hormone (GnRH) antagonist for infertility* [ganirelix acetate] 250 mcg/0.5 mL

Antara capsules ℞ *antihyperlipidemic for primary hypercholesterolemia, hypertriglyceridemia, and mixed dyslipidemia; also used for hyperuricemia* [fenofibrate] 43, 130 mg

antastan [see: antazoline HCl]

antazoline INN, BAN [also: antazoline HCl]

antazoline HCl USP [also: antazoline]

antazoline phosphate USP *antihistamine*

antazoline phosphate & naphazoline HCl *topical ocular antihistamine and decongestant* 0.5%•0.05%

antazonite INN

Antegren (name changed to **Tysabri** upon marketing release in 2004)

antelmycin INN *anthelmintic* [also: anthelmycin]

anterior pituitary

anthelmintics *a class of drugs effective against parasitic infections* [also called: vermicides; vermifuges]

anthelmycin USAN *anthelmintic* [also: antelmycin]

Anthemis nobilis medicinal herb [see: chamomile]

anthiolimine INN

Anthoxanthum odoratum medicinal herb [see: sweet vernal grass]

anthracyclines *a class of antibiotic antineoplastics*

Anthra-Derm ointment (discontinued 2006) ℞ *antipsoriatic* [anthralin] 0.1%, 0.25%, 0.5%, 1%

anthralin USP *topical antipsoriatic* [also: dithranol] 1% topical

anthramycin USAN *antineoplastic* [also: antramycin]

anthraquinone of cascara [see: cascara sagrada]

anthrax test [see: Rapid Anthrax Test]

anthrax vaccine, adsorbed (AVA) *active bacterin derived from an attenuated strain of* Bacillus anthracis

Anthriscus cerefolium medicinal herb [see: chervil]

anti-A blood grouping serum USP *in vitro blood testing*

antiadrenergics *a class of agents that block the alpha$_1$ adrenergic receptors in the sympathetic nervous system, used for the treatment of hypertension and benign prostatic hyperplasia (BPH)* [also called: sympatholytics; alpha$_1$-adrenergic blockers]

antiandrogens *a class of hormonal antineoplastics*

antiangiogenic agents extracted from marine cartilage [see: AE-941; Neovastat]

antib [see: thioacetazone; thiacetazone]

anti-B blood grouping serum USP *in vitro blood testing*

antibason [see: methylthiouracil]

AntibiŌtic ear drop suspension (discontinued 2006) ℞ *corticosteroidal anti-inflammatory; antibiotic* [hydrocortisone; neomycin sulfate; polymyxin B sulfate] 1%•5 mg•10 000 U per mL

AntibiŌtic ear drops ℞ *corticosteroidal anti-inflammatory; antibiotic* [hydrocortisone; neomycin sulfate; polymyxin B sulfate] 1%•5 mg•10 000 U per mL

Antibiotic Ear Solution ℞ *corticosteroidal anti-inflammatory; antibiotic* [hydrocortisone; neomycin sulfate; polymyxin B sulfate] 1%•5 mg•10 000 U per mL

Antibiotic Ear Suspension ℞ *corticosteroidal anti-inflammatory; antibiotic* [hydrocortisone; neomycin sulfate; polymyxin B sulfate] 1%•5 mg•10 000 U per mL

antibiotics *a class of agents that destroy or arrest the growth of micro-organisms*

antibromics *a class of agents that mask undesirable or offensive odors* [also called: deodorants]

anti-C blood grouping serum [see: blood grouping serum, anti-C]

anti-c blood grouping serum [see: blood grouping serum, anti-c]

anticholinergics *a class of agents that block parasympathetic nerve impulses, producing antiemetic, antinausea, and antispasmodic effects; also used to dry mucosal secretions*

anticoagulant citrate dextrose (ACD) solution USP *anticoagulant for storage of whole blood and during cardiac surgery*

anticoagulant citrate phosphate dextrose adenine solution USP *anticoagulant for storage of whole blood*

anticoagulant citrate phosphate dextrose solution USP *anticoagulant for storage of whole blood*

anticoagulant heparin solution USP *anticoagulant for storage of whole blood*

anticoagulant sodium citrate solution USP *anticoagulant for plasma and for blood for fractionation*

anticoagulants *a class of therapeutic agents that inhibit or inactivate blood clotting factors*

anticonvulsants *a class of drugs that prevent seizures by suppressing abnormal neuronal discharges in the central nervous system* [also called: anti-epileptic drugs (AEDs)]

Anticort *investigational (Phase II) for HIV infection* [procaine HCl]

anti-D antibodies [see: Rh$_O$(D) immune globulin]

antidopaminergics *a class of anti-emetic drugs*

antidotes *a class of drugs that counteract the effects of toxic doses of other drugs or toxic substances*

anti-E blood grouping serum [see: blood grouping serum, anti-E]

anti-e blood grouping serum [see: blood grouping serum, anti-e]

antiemetics *a class of agents that prevent or alleviate nausea and vomiting* [also called: antinauseants]

antienite INN

antiepilepsirine [now: ilepcimide]

anti-epileptic drugs (AEDs) *a class of drugs that prevent seizures by suppressing abnormal neuronal discharges in the central nervous system* [also called: anticonvulsants]

antiestrogen [see: tamoxifen citrate]

antiestrogens *a class of hormonal antineoplastics*

antifebriles *a class of agents that relieve or reduce fever* [also called: antipyretics; antithermics; febricides; febrifuges]

antifebrin [see: acetanilide]

antifolic acid [see: methotrexate]

antiformin, dental JAN [also: sodium hypochlorite, diluted]

antigen-presenting cells pulsed with tumor immunoglobulin idiotype *investigational (orphan) agent for multiple myeloma*

anti–growth and differentiation factor 8 antibody, recombinant human (anti-GDF8) *investigational (orphan) for Duchenne and Becker muscular dystrophies*

antihemophilic factor (AHF; FVIII) USP *systemic hemostatic; antihemophilic for the prevention and control of bleeding in classical hemophilia (hemophilia A) and von Willebrand disease (orphan)*

Antihemophilic Factor (Porcine) Hyate:C powder for IV injection ℞ *antihemophilic to correct coagulation deficiency* [antihemophilic factor VIII:C] 400–700 porcine units/vial

antihemophilic factor, human [now: antihemophilic factor]

antihemophilic factor, recombinant (rFVIII) *antihemophilic for treatment of hemophilia A and presurgical prophylaxis for hemophiliacs (orphan)*

antihemophilic factor A [see: antihemophilic factor]

antihemophilic factor B [see: factor IX complex]

antihemophilic globulin (AHG) [see: antihemophilic factor]

antihemophilic human plasma [now: plasma, antihemophilic human]

antihemophilic plasma, human [now: plasma, antihemophilic human]

antiheparin [see: protamine sulfate]

antihistamines *a class of drugs that counteract the effect of histamine*

antihydrotics *a class of agents that reduce or suppress perspiration* [also called: anhidrotics; anidrotics]

antihyperlipidemic agents *a class of drugs that lower serum lipid levels* [also called: antilipemics]

anti-inhibitor coagulant complex *antihemophilic*

anti-interferon-gamma Fab from goats *investigational (orphan) immunologic for corneal allograft rejection*

Anti-Itch cream OTC *poison ivy treatment* [diphenhydramine HCl; zinc acetate] 2%•0.1%

Anti-Itch gel OTC *poison ivy treatment* [camphor; alcohol 37%] 0.45%

antilipemics *a class of drugs that lower serum lipid levels* [also called: antihyperlipidemics]

Antilirium IV or IM injection ℞ *cholinergic to reverse anticholinergic overdose; investigational (orphan) for Friedreich and other inherited ataxias* [physostigmine salicylate] 1 mg/mL

antilithics *a class of agents that prevent the formation of stone or calculus* [see also: litholytics]

antilymphocyte immunoglobulin BAN

antimelanoma antibody XMMME-001-DTPA 111 indium *investigational (orphan) imaging aid for systemic and nodal melanoma metastasis*

antimelanoma antibody XMMME-001-RTA *investigational (orphan) agent for stage III melanoma*

Antiminth oral suspension (discontinued 2004) OTC *anthelmintic for ascariasis (roundworm) and enterobiasis (pinworm)* [pyrantel pamoate] 50 mg/mL

antimony *element (Sb)*

antimony potassium tartrate USP *antischistosomal*

antimony sodium tartrate USP, JAN *antischistosomal*

antimony sodium thioglycollate USP

antimony sulfide [see: antimony trisulfide colloid]

antimony trisulfide colloid USAN *pharmaceutic aid*

antimonyl potassium tartrate [see: antimony potassium tartrate]

antimuscarinics *a class of anticholinergic agents*

antinauseants *a class of agents that prevent or alleviate nausea and vomiting* [also called: antiemetics]

antineoplastics *a class of chemotherapeutic agents capable of selective action on neoplastic (abnormally proliferating) tissues*

antineoplastons *a class of naturally occurring peptides that suppress cancer oncogenes and stimulate the body's cancer suppressor genes*

Antiox capsules OTC *vitamin supplement* [vitamins C and E; beta carotene] 120 mg•100 IU•25 mg 🄐 Entex

anti-pellagra vitamin [see: niacin]

antiperiodics *a class of agents that prevent periodic or intermittent recurrence of symptoms, as in malaria*

anti-pernicious anemia principle [see: cyanocobalamin]

antiphlogistics *a class of agents that reduce inflammation and fever*

antipsychotics *a class of psychotropic agents that are used to treat schizophrenia and other psychiatric illnesses; further classified as conventional (typical) antipsychotics and novel (atypical) antipsychotics* [q.v.]

antipyretics *a class of agents that relieve or reduce fever* [also called: antifebriles; antithermics; febricides; febrifuges]

antipyrine USP, JAN *analgesic; investigational (orphan) diagnostic agent to determine hepatic drug metabolizing activity* [also: phenazone]

Antipyrine and Benzocaine Otic ear drops R *anesthetic; analgesic* [benzocaine; antipyrine] 1.4%•5.4%

N-antipyrinylnicotinamide [see: nifenazone]

antirabies serum (ARS) USP *passive immunizing agent*

anti-Rh antibodies [see: Rh$_O$(D) immune globulin]

anti-Rh typing serums [now: blood grouping serums]

antiscorbutic vitamin [see: ascorbic acid]

antiscorbutics *a class of agents that are sources of vitamin C and are effective in the prevention or relief of scurvy*

antiscrofulous herbs *a class of agents that counteract scrofuloderma (tuberculous cervical lymphadenitis)*

antisense 20-mer phosphorothiolate oligonucleotide *investigational (orphan) agent for renal cell carcinoma*

antisense C-myb oligodeoxynucleotide *investigational (orphan) for chronic myelogenous leukemia*

antisense drugs *a class of antiviral drugs that interfere with the replication of viral protein*

Antiseptic Wound & Skin Cleanser topical liquid OTC *antiseptic wound and skin cleanser* [benzethonium chloride] 0.1%

antiseptics *a class of agents that inhibit the growth and development of microorganisms, usually on a body surface, without necessarily killing them* [see also: disinfectants; germicides]

Antispas IM injection (discontinued 2008) R *gastrointestinal anticholinergic/antispasmodic for irritable bowel syndrome (IBS)* [dicyclomine HCl] 10 mg/mL

Antispasmodic elixir R *GI/GU anticholinergic/antispasmodic; sedative* [atropine sulfate; scopolamine hydrobromide; hyoscyamine sulfate; phenobarbital] 0.0194•0.0065•0.1037•16.2 mg/5 mL

antispasmodics *a class of agents that relieve spasms or cramps, usually of gastrointestinal tract or blood vessels*

antisterility vitamin [see: vitamin E]

anti-T lymphocyte immunotoxin XMMLY-H65-RTA [now: zolimomab aritox]

anti-tac, humanized; SMART anti-tac [now: daclizumab]

anti-tap-72 immunotoxin *investigational (orphan) for metastatic colorectal adenocarcinoma*

antithermics *a class of agents that relieve or reduce fever* [also called: antifebriles; antipyretics; febricides; febrifuges]

antithrombin III (aT-III) INN, BAN *agent for thrombosis and pulmonary emboli of congenital aT-III deficiency (orphan); investigational (Phase III, orphan) for heparin deficiency in patients undergoing surgical or obstetrical procedures and for aT-III-dependent heparin resistance*

antithrombin III, human [see: antithrombin III]

antithrombin III, recombinant human (rhaTIII) [see: antithrombin III]

antithrombin III concentrate [see: antithrombin III]

antithymocyte globulin (aTG) *treatment for aplastic anemia; passive immunizing agent to prevent allograft rejection of renal transplants (orphan); investigational (orphan) for other solid organ and bone marrow transplants; investigational (orphan) for myelodysplastic syndrome (MDS)* [also: lymphocyte immune globulin (LIG)]

antithymocyte serum [see: antithymocyte globulin]

antitoxin botulism equine (ABE) [see: botulism equine antitoxin, trivalent]

antitoxins *a class of drugs used for passive immunization that consist of antibodies which combine with toxins to neutralize them*

anti–transforming growth factor B1,2,3 *investigational (orphan) for idiopathic pulmonary fibrosis* [compare: monoclonal antibody to transforming growth factor beta 1]

α_1-antitrypsin [see: alpha$_1$-antitrypsin]

antituberculous agents *a class of antibiotics, divided into primary and retreatment agents*

Anti-Tuss syrup (discontinued 2004) OTC *expectorant* [guaifenesin; alcohol 3.5%] 100 mg/5 mL

Antitussive Hydrocodone Bitartrate and Homatropine Methylbromide tablets ℞ *narcotic antitussive; anticholinergic* [hydrocodone bitartrate; homatropine methylbromide] 5•1.5 mg

antitussives *a class of drugs that prevent or relieve cough*

antivenin (Crotalidae) polyvalent (equine) USP *passive immunizing agent for pit viper (rattlesnake, copperhead, and cottonmouth moccasin) bites*

antivenin (Crotalidae) polyvalent immune Fab (equine) *investigational (orphan) treatment for pit viper (rattlesnake, copperhead, and cottonmouth moccasin) bites*

antivenin (Crotalidae) polyvalent immune Fab (ovine) *treatment for pit viper (rattlesnake, copperhead, and cottonmouth moccasin) bites (orphan)*

antivenin (Crotalidae) purified (avian) *investigational (orphan) treatment for pit viper (rattlesnake, copperhead, and cottonmouth moccasin) bites*

antivenin (Latrodectus mactans) (equine) USP *passive immunizing agent for black widow spider bites* $\geq$ 6000 U/vial

antivenin (Micrurus fulvius) USP *passive immunizing agent for coral snake bites*

antivenins *a class of drugs used for passive immunization against or treatment for venomous bites and stings*

Antivert; Antivert/25; Antivert/50 tablets ℞ *anticholinergic; antihistamine; antivertigo agent; motion sickness preventative* [meclizine HCl] 12.5 mg; 25 mg; 50 mg

Antivipmyn *investigational (orphan) treatment for pit viper (rattlesnake, copperhead, and cottonmouth moccasin) bites* [antivenin (Crotalidae) polyvalent immune Fab (equine)]

antivirals *a class of drugs effective against viral infections*

antixerophthalmic vitamin [see: vitamin A]

Antizol injection ℞ *alcohol dehydrogenase inhibitor for methanol or ethylene glycol poisoning (orphan)* [fomepizole] 1 g/mL

antler (deer and elk) *natural remedy for aging, energy, hormone balancing, impotence, infertility, and longevity*

antrafenine INN

antramycin INN *antineoplastic* [also: anthramycin]

Antril *investigational (orphan) nonsteroidal anti-inflammatory drug (NSAID) for juvenile rheumatoid arthritis and graft vs. host disease* [anakinra]

Antrizine tablets ℞ *anticholinergic; antihistamine; antivertigo agent;*

motion sickness preventative [mecli-zine HCl] 12.5 mg

Antrocol elixir ℞ gastrointestinal anti-cholinergic/antispasmodic; sedative [atropine sulfate; phenobarbital] 0.195•16 mg/5 mL

Antrypol (available only from the Centers for Disease Control and Prevention) ℞ antiparasitic for African trypanosomiasis and onchocerciasis [suramin sodium]

antrypol [see: suramin sodium]

Anturane tablets, capsules ℞ urico-suric for gout [sulfinpyrazone] 100 mg; 200 mg ⊡ Intron A

Anucort HC rectal suppositories ℞ corticosteroidal anti-inflammatory [hydrocortisone acetate] 25 mg

Anu-Med rectal suppositories OTC temporary relief of hemorrhoidal symp-toms [phenylephrine HCl] 0.25%

Anumed HC rectal suppositories ℞ corticosteroidal anti-inflammatory [hydrocortisone acetate] 10 mg

Anusol anorectal ointment (name changed to **Tucks** in 2006) ⊡ anise oil; Enisyl; Enseal; Unisol

Anusol rectal suppositories (name changed to **Tucks** in 2005) ⊡ anise oil; Enisyl; Enseal; Unisol

Anusol-HC anorectal cream ℞ corti-costeroidal anti-inflammatory [hydro-cortisone] 2.5%

Anusol-HC rectal suppositories ℞ cor-ticosteroidal anti-inflammatory [hydro-cortisone acetate] 25 mg

Anusol-HC 1 ointment (name changed to **Tucks** in 2005)

Anzemet film-coated tablets, IV injection ℞ antiemetic to prevent nau-sea and vomiting following chemother-apy or surgery; also used to prevent radiation-induced nausea and vomiting [dolasetron mesylate] 50, 100 mg; 20 mg/mL

AOPA (ara-C, Oncovin, predni-sone, asparaginase) chemotherapy protocol

AOPE (Adriamycin, Oncovin, prednisone, etoposide) chemother-apy protocol

Aosept + Aodisc solution + tablet OTC two-step chemical disinfecting sys-tem for soft contact lenses [hydrogen peroxide–based] ⊡ Azopt

AP (Adriamycin, Platinol) chemo-therapy protocol for ovarian and endo-metrial cancer

AP-1903 investigational (orphan) agent for graft-versus-host disease

Apacet chewable tablets, drops (discon-tinued 2008) OTC analgesic; antipyretic [acetaminophen] 80 mg; 100 mg/mL

apafant USAN, INN platelet activating factor antagonist for allergies, asthma, and acute pancreatitis

apalcillin sodium USAN, INN antibac-terial

APAP film-coated tablets OTC analge-sic; antipyretic [acetaminophen] 325, 500 mg ⊡ ABP

APAP (N-acetyl-p-aminophenol) [see: acetaminophen]

Apap 500 oral liquid OTC analgesic; antipyretic [acetaminophen] 500 mg/ 5 mL ⊡ ABP

APAP Plus tablets OTC analgesic; anti-pyretic [acetaminophen; caffeine] 500•65 mg

Apatate chewable tablets, oral liquid (discontinued 2004) OTC vitamin supplement [vitamins B_1, B_6, and B_{12}] 15•0.5•0.025 mg; 15•0.5•0.025 mg/5 mL

Apatate with Fluoride pediatric oral liquid ℞ vitamin supplement; dental caries preventative [vitamins B_1, B_6, and B_{12}; fluoride] 15•0.5•0.025•0.5 mg/5 mL

apaxifylline USAN, INN selective adeno-sine A_1 antagonist for cognitive deficits

apazone USAN anti-inflammatory [also: azapropazone]

APC (AMSA, prednisone, chlor-ambucil) chemotherapy protocol

APC (aspirin, phenacetin & caf-feine) [q.v.]

apcitide [see: technetium Tc 99m apc-
itide]

**APD (aminohydroxypropylidene
diphosphonate)** [see: pamidronate
disodium]

**APE (Adriamycin, Platinol, etopo-
side)** *chemotherapy protocol*

**APE (aminophylline, phenobarbi-
tal, ephedrine)**

APE (ara-C, Platinol, etoposide)
chemotherapy protocol

Apep *investigational (orphan) antineoplastic for non-Hodgkin lymphoma*
[mitoguazone]

aperients *a class of agents that have a
mild purgative or laxative effect* [see
also: aperitives]

aperitives *a class of agents that stimulate
the appetite or have a mild purgative or
laxative effect* [see also: aperients]

Apetil *oral liquid* OTC *vitamin/mineral
supplement* [multiple B vitamins;
multiple minerals] ⊘ Epitol

ApexiCon *ointment* ℞ *corticosteroidal
anti-inflammatory* [diflorasone diace-
tate] 0.05%

ApexiCon E *cream* ℞ *corticosteroidal
anti-inflammatory; emollient* [diflora-
sone diacetate] 0.05%

aphrodisiacs *a class of agents that arouse
or increase sexual desire or potency*

Aphrodyne *tablets* ℞ *alpha$_2$-adrenergic
blocker for impotence and orthostatic
hypotension; sympatholytic; mydriatic;
may have aphrodisiac activity; no FDA-
sanctioned indications* [yohimbine
HCl] 5.4 mg ⊘ avridine

Aphthaid *investigational (orphan) for
severe aphthous stomatitis in terminally
immunocompromised patients* [lactic
acid]

Aphthasol *oral paste* ℞ *anti-inflammatory for aphthous ulcers; topical histamine and leukotriene inhibitor* [amlex-
anox] 5% ⊘ efetozole

apicillin [see: ampicillin]

apicycline INN

Apidra *subcu or IV injection in vials
and OptiClik cartridges* ℞ *rapid-
onset, short-acting insulin analogue for*

diabetes [insulin glulisine, human
(rDNA)] 100 IU/mL; 300 U/3 mL

apiquel fumarate [see: aminorex]

Apium graveolens medicinal herb [see:
celery]

apixaban *factor Xa coagulation inhibitor; investigational (Phase III) antithrombotic for deep vein thrombosis
(DVT), venous thromboembolism
(VTE), and stroke prevention*

A.P.L. *powder for IM injection* (discontinued 2004) ℞ *hormone for prepubertal cryptorchidism or hypogonadism; ovulation stimulant* [chorionic
gonadotropin] 500, 1000, 2000 U/mL
⊘ apple; E-Pilo-1; IPOL; OPAL

APL 400-020 V-Beta DNA vaccine
*investigational (orphan) agent for cuta-
neous T-cell lymphoma*

Aplenzin *extended-release tablets* ℞
*aminoketone antidepressant for major
depression* [bupropion hydrobromide]
174, 348, 522 mg

Aplidin *investigational (orphan) antineoplastic for multiple myeloma* [plitidep-
sin]

Apligraf ℞ *living skin construct for diabetic foot ulcers and pressure sores*
[graftskin]

Aplisol *intradermal injection tuberculosis skin test* [tuberculin purified protein derivative (PPD)] 5 U/0.1 mL

aplonidine HCl [see: apraclonidine
HCl]

**APO (Adriamycin, prednisone,
Oncovin)** *chemotherapy protocol*

*Apocynum androsaemifolium medicinal
herb* [see: dogbane]

apodol [see: anileridine HCl]

Apokinon ® (French name for U.S.
product **Apokyn**)

Apokyn *subcu injection* ℞ *dopamine
agonist for hypomobility episodes of
late-stage Parkinson disease (orphan)*
[apomorphine HCl] 10 mg/mL ⊘
Opcon-A

Apomate *investigational (orphan) radiodiagnostic aid to assess the rejection status of heart and lung transplants* [tech-
netium Tc 99m rh-Annexin V]

apomorphine BAN *dopamine D$_1$ agonist for Parkinson disease* [also: apomorphine HCl]

apomorphine HCl USP *dopamine D$_1$ agonist for hypomobility episodes of late-stage Parkinson disease (orphan)* [also: apomorphine]

apovincamine INN

appetizers *a class of agents that stimulate the appetite* [see also: aperitives]

APPG (aqueous penicillin G procaine) [see: penicillin G procaine]

apple (Pyrus malus) *fruit medicinal herb for constipation and diarrhea, dysentery, fever, heart ailments, scurvy, and warts* 🔁 A.P.L.; E-Pilo-1; IPOL; OPAL

apple, ground *medicinal herb* [see: chamomile]

apple, hog; Indian apple; May apple *medicinal herb* [see: mandrake]

Appli-Kit (trademarked device) *ointment and adhesive dosage covers*

Appli-Ruler (trademarked device) OTC *dose-determining pads*

Appli-Tape (trademarked device) OTC *dosage covers*

Apra *investigational (Phase II, orphan) antineoplastic for soft tissue sarcomas and malignant mesothelioma* [CT-2584 mesylate (code name—generic name not yet assigned)]

Apra, Children's *oral liquid* OTC *analgesic; antipyretic* [acetaminophen] 160 mg/5 mL

apraclonidine INN, BAN *topical adrenergic for glaucoma* [also: apraclonidine HCl]

apraclonidine HCl USAN *topical adrenergic for glaucoma* [also: apraclonidine]

apramycin USAN, INN, BAN *antibacterial*

Apreia *investigational (Phase III) treatment for postmenopausal osteoporosis and vasomotor symptoms* [bazedoxifene; conjugated estrogens]

aprepitant USAN *neurokinin NK$_1$ receptor antagonist; antiemetic for chemotherapy-induced and postoperative nausea and vomiting*

Apresazide 25/25; Apresazide 50/50; Apresazide 100/50 capsules (dis-

continued 2007) ℞ *antihypertensive; vasodilator; diuretic* [hydralazine HCl; hydrochlorothiazide] 25•25 mg; 50•50 mg; 100•50 mg

Apresoline tablets ℞ *antihypertensive; vasodilator* [hydralazine HCl] 10, 25, 50, 100 mg

Apri tablets (in packs of 28) ℞ *monophasic oral contraceptive* [desogestrel; ethinyl estradiol] 0.15 mg•30 mcg × 21 days; counters × 7 days

apricot (Prunus armeniaca) *fruit, seeds, and kernel oil medicinal herb for asthma, constipation, cough, eye inflammation, hemorrhage, infertility, spasm, and vaginal infections; not generally regarded as safe and effective as apricot kernel ingestion causes cyanide poisoning*

apricot kernel water JAN

aprikalim INN *antianginal*

aprindine USAN, INN, BAN *antiarrhythmic*

aprindine HCl USAN, JAN *antiarrhythmic*

aprobarbital NF, INN *sedative*

Aprodine tablets, syrup OTC *decongestant; antihistamine* [pseudoephedrine HCl; triprolidine HCl] 60•2.5 mg; 60•2.5 mg/10 mL

aprofene INN

aprosulate sodium INN

aprotinin USAN, INN, BAN, JAN *systemic hemostatic for coronary artery bypass graft (CABG) surgery (orphan); protease inhibitor*

A.P.S. (aspirin, phenacetin & salicylamide) [q.v.]

APSAC (anisoylated plasminogen streptokinase activator complex) [see: anistreplase]

aptazapine INN *antidepressant* [also: aptazapine maleate]

aptazapine maleate USAN *antidepressant* [also: aptazapine]

aptiganel HCl USAN *NMDA ion channel blocker for stroke and traumatic brain injury*

Aptivus softgels, oral solution ℞ *antiviral; HIV protease inhibitor; must be used* *with* **Norvir** (ritonavir) [tipranavir disodium] 250 mg; 100 mg/mL

aptocaine INN, BAN

Aptosyn *investigational (NDA filed, orphan) apoptosis modulator for adenomatous polyposis coli (APC); investigational (Phase III) for lung cancer* [exisulind]

apyron [see: magnesium salicylate]

Aqua Glycolic Face; Aqua Glycolic Hand & Body lotion OTC *moisturizer; emollient; exfoliant* [glycolic acid; hyaluronic acid]

AquaBalm cream OTC *moisturizer; emollient*

Aqua-Ban enteric-coated tablets OTC *diuretic* [ammonium chloride; caffeine] 325•100 mg

Aqua-Ban, Maximum Strength tablets OTC *diuretic* [pamabrom] 50 mg

Aqua-Ban Plus enteric-coated tablets OTC *diuretic; iron supplement* [ammonium chloride; caffeine; ferrous sulfate] 650•200•6 mg

Aquabase OTC *ointment base* ☒ Equipoise; ICaps

Aquacare cream, lotion OTC *moisturizer; emollient; keratolytic* [urea] 10%

Aquachloral Supprettes (suppositories) ℞ *nonbarbiturate sedative and hypnotic* [chloral hydrate] 324, 648 mg

aquaday [see: menadione]

Aqua-E oral liquid OTC *vitamin supplement* [vitamin E] 32 mg (30 mg tocopherols; 2 mg tocotrienols)

aquakay [see: menadione]

AquaMEPHYTON IM or subcu injection (discontinued 2007) ℞ *coagulant to correct anticoagulant-induced prothrombin deficiency; vitamin K supplement* [phytonadione] 2, 10 mg/mL

Aquanil lotion OTC *moisturizer; emollient* ☒ Equanil

Aquanil Cleanser lotion OTC *soap-free therapeutic skin cleanser*

Aquaphilic OTC *ointment base*

Aquaphilic with Carbamide OTC *ointment base* [urea] 10%, 20%

Aquaphor OTC *ointment base*

Aquaphyllin syrup (discontinued 2004) ℞ *antiasthmatic; bronchodilator* [theophylline] 80 mg/15 mL

AquaSite eye drops (discontinued 2004) OTC *moisturizer/lubricant* [polyethylene glycol 400] 0.2% ☒ wax, white

Aquasol A IM injection ℞ *vitamin deficiency therapy* [vitamin A] 50 000 IU/mL ☒ wax, yellow

Aquasol E oral drops OTC *vitamin supplement* [vitamin E (as *dl*-alpha tocopherol acetate)] 15 IU/0.3 mL ☒ wax, yellow

Aquatab C extended-release tablets (discontinued 2007) ℞ *antitussive; decongestant; expectorant* [dextromethorphan hydrobromide; pseudoephedrine HCl; guaifenesin] 60•60•1200 mg

Aquatab D extended-release tablets (discontinued 2007) ℞ *decongestant; expectorant* [pseudoephedrine HCl; guaifenesin] 75•1200 mg

Aquatab D Dose Pack sustained-release tablets (discontinued 2007) ℞ *decongestant; expectorant* [pseudoephedrine HCl; guaifenesin] 60•600 mg

Aquatab DM tablets, syrup (discontinued 2007) ℞ *antitussive; expectorant* [dextromethorphan hydrobromide; guaifenesin] 60•1200 mg; 10•200 mg/5 mL

Aquatensen tablets (discontinued 2008) ℞ *antihypertensive; diuretic* [methyclothiazide] 5 mg

Aquavan injection *investigational anesthetic* [fospropofol disodium]

Aquavit-E oral drops OTC *vitamin supplement* [vitamin E (as *dl*-alpha tocopheryl acetate)] 15 IU/0.3 mL ☒ Ocuvite

aqueous penicillin G procaine (APPG) [see: penicillin G procaine]

Aquilegia vulgaris medicinal herb [see: columbine]

aquinone [see: menadione]

Aquoral throat spray ℞ *saliva substitute* [lipid-based formula] ☒ Agoral

ara-A (adenine arabinoside) [see: vidarabine]

ara-AC (azacytosine arabinoside) [see: fazarabine]

arabinofuranosylcytosine [see: cytarabine]

9-β-D-arabinofuranosylguanine (ara-G) *antineoplastic*

arabinogalactans *a class of dietary fiber used as an immune booster; stimulates macrophages, increases levels of natural killer (NK) cells, interferon-gamma (IFN-γ), tumor necrosis factor-alpha (TNF-α), and interleukin-1 beta (IL-1 β)* [see also: larch]

arabinoluranosylcytosine HCl [see: cytarabine HCl]

arabinosyl cytosine [see: cytarabine]

ara-C (cytosine arabinoside) [see: cytarabine]

ara-C + 6-TG (ara-C, thioguanine) *chemotherapy protocol*

ara-C + ADR (ara-C, Adriamycin) *chemotherapy protocol*

ara-C + DNR + PRED + MP (ara-C, daunorubicin, prednisolone, mercaptopurine) *chemotherapy protocol*

ARAC-DNR (ara-C, daunorubicin) *chemotherapy protocol for acute myelocytic leukemia (AML)*

arachadonic acid (AA) *natural omega-6 fatty acid*

arachis oil [see: peanut oil]

ara-C-HU (ara-C, hydroxyurea) *chemotherapy protocol* ☒ ERYC

Aracmyn *investigational (orphan) treatment for black widow spider bites [Latrodectus immune F(ab)2]*

ara-cytidine [see: cytarabine]

ara-G (9-β-D-arabinofuranosylguanine) *antineoplastic* ☒ ERYC

Aralast *powder for IV infusion ℞ enzyme replacement therapy for hereditary alpha₁-proteinase inhibitor deficiency, which leads to progressive panacinar emphysema* [alpha₁-proteinase inhibitor] ≥ 16 mg/mL (400, 800 mg/vial)

Aralen HCl *IM injection ℞ antimalarial; amebicide* [chloroquine HCl] 50 mg/mL

Aralen Phosphate *film-coated tablets ℞ antimalarial; amebicide* [chloroquine phosphate] 500 mg

Aralia racemosa *medicinal herb* [see: spikenard]

Aralia spp. *medicinal herb* [see: ginseng]

Aramine *IV, subcu or IM injection ℞ vasopressor for acute hypotensive shock, anaphylaxis, or traumatic shock* [metaraminol bitartrate] 10 mg/mL (1%) ☒ Orimune

Aranelle *tablets (in packs of 28) ℞ triphasic oral contraceptive* [norethindrone; ethinyl estradiol]
Phase 1 (7 days): 0.5 mg•35 mcg;
Phase 2 (9 days): 1 mg•35 mcg;
Phase 3 (5 days): 0.5 mg•35 mcg

Aranesp *IV or subcu injection, prefilled syringes ℞ erythropoiesis-stimulating agent (ESA); recombinant human erythropoietin for anemia associated with chronic renal failure or chemotherapy for nonmyeloid malignancies* [darbepoetin alfa] 25, 40, 60, 100, 200, 300, 500 mcg/mL; 25, 40, 60, 100, 150, 200, 300, 500 mcg/dose

Aranesp SureClick *prefilled self-injector ℞ hematopoietic; recombinant erythropoietin analogue for anemia associated with chronic renal failure* [darbepoetin alfa]

aranidipine INN

aranotin USAN, INN *antiviral*

araprofen INN

Arava *film-coated tablets ℞ anti-inflammatory for rheumatoid arthritis (RA)* [leflunomide] 10, 20, 100 mg

ARBs (angiotensin II receptor blockers) [see: angiotensin II receptor antagonists]

arbaprostil USAN, INN *gastric antisecretory*

arbekacin INN

arberry *medicinal herb* [see: uva ursi]

arbutamine INN, BAN *cardiac stressor for diagnosis of coronary artery disease* [also: arbutamine HCl]

arbutamine HCl USAN *cardiac stressor for diagnosis of coronary artery disease* [also: arbutamine]

Arbutus uva ursi medicinal herb [see: uva ursi]

Arcalyst subcu injection ℞ *immunosuppressant for cryopyrin-associated periodic syndrome (CAPS), familial cold autoinflammatory syndrome (FCAS), and Muckle-Wells syndrome (MWS); investigational (Phase II) for chronic gout* [rilonacept] 220 mg/dose

archangel medicinal herb [see: angelica]

arcitumomab USAN *investigational (orphan) imaging agent for detection of recurrent or metastatic thyroid cancers; investigational (Phase III) for lung cancer*

arclofenin USAN, INN *hepatic function test*

Arcobee with C caplets OTC *vitamin supplement* [multiple B vitamins; vitamin C] ± • 300 mg

Arcoxia tablets *investigational (NDA filed) COX-2 inhibitor for osteoarthritis, rheumatoid arthritis, musculoskeletal pain, and gout* [etoricoxib] 60, 90, 10 mg

Arctium lappa; A. majus; A. minus medicinal herb [see: burdock]

Arctostaphylos uva ursi medicinal herb [see: uva ursi]

ardacin INN

ardeparin sodium USAN, INN *a low molecular weight heparin–type anticoagulant and antithrombotic for the prevention of deep vein thrombosis (DVT) following knee replacement surgery*

Arduan powder for IV injection (discontinued 2004) ℞ *nondepolarizing neuromuscular blocking agent; muscle relaxant; adjunct to general anesthesia* [pipecuronium bromide] 10 mg/vial ⑨ Aerodine

arecoline acetarsone salt [see: drocarbil]

arecoline hydrobromide NF

Aredia powder for IV infusion ℞ *bisphosphonate bone resorption inhibitor for Paget disease, hypercalcemia of malig-*

nancy (HCM), and bone metastases of breast cancer and multiple myeloma; also used for postmenopausal osteoporosis* [pamidronate disodium] 30, 90 mg/vial ⑨ Aeroaid; Award; Euro-D

Arestin sustained-release microspheres for subgingival injection ℞ *tetracycline antibiotic for periodontitis* [minocycline HCl] 1 mg

arfalasin INN

arfendazam INN

arformoterol tartrate *long-acting beta$_2$ agonist; sympathomimetic bronchodilator for chronic obstructive pulmonary disease (COPD), bronchitis, and emphysema* (base=68%)

argatroban USAN, INN, JAN *anticoagulant for heparin-induced thrombocytopenia (HIT) and thrombosis syndrome (HITTS); prevention of HIT or HITTS in percutaneous coronary intervention (PCI)* 250 mg/vial injection

Argesic cream (discontinued 2004) OTC *analgesic; counterirritant* [methyl salicylate; trolamine] ⑨ Urogesic

Argesic-SA tablets ℞ *analgesic; anti-inflammatory* [salsalate] 500 mg

argimesna INN

Arginaid Extra oral liquid OTC *enteral nutritional treatment for wound healing* [whey protein–based]

L-argininamide [see: iseganan HCl]

arginine (L-arginine) USP, INN *nonessential amino acid; ammonia detoxicant; diagnostic aid for pituitary function; symbols: Arg, R*

arginine butanoate [see: arginine butyrate]

arginine butyrate (L-arginine butyrate) USAN *investigational (orphan) for beta-hemoglobinopathies, beta-thalassemia, and sickle cell disease*

arginine deiminase, pegylated *investigational (orphan) treatment for hepatocellular carcinoma and invasive malignant melanoma*

arginine glutamate (L-arginine L-glutamate) USAN, BAN, JAN *ammonia detoxicant*

arginine HCl USAN, USP, JAN *ammonia detoxicant; pituitary (growth hormone) function diagnostic aid*

L-arginine monohydrochloride [see: arginine HCl]

8-L-arginine vasopressin [see: vasopressin]

8-arginineoxytocin [see: argiprestocin]

8-L-argininevasopressin tannate [see: argipressin tannate]

argipressin INN, BAN *antidiuretic* [also: argipressin tannate]

argipressin tannate USAN *antidiuretic* [also: argipressin]

argiprestocin INN

argon *element (Ar)* ⊠ AeroCaine; Ircon

argyn [see: silver protein, mild]

Aricept tablets, oral drops ℞ *reversible acetylcholinesterase (AChE) inhibitor; cognition adjuvant for Alzheimer dementia; also used for vascular dementia, post-stroke aphasia, and memory improvement in multiple sclerosis patients* [donepezil HCl] 5, 10 mg; 1 mg/mL ⊠ Orasept

Aricept ODT (orally disintegrating tablets) ℞ *reversible acetylcholinesterase (AChE) inhibitor; cognition adjuvant for Alzheimer dementia; also used for vascular dementia, post-stroke aphasia, and memory improvement in multiple sclerosis patients* [donepezil HCl] 5, 10 mg

Aridex Pediatric oral drops (discontinued 2007) ℞ *antitussive; antihistamine; decongestant* [carbetapentane citrate; carbinoxamine maleate; phenylephrine HCl] 4•1•2 mg/mL

Aridex-D pediatric oral drops (discontinued 2007) ℞ *decongestant; antihistamine* [phenylephrine HCl; carbinoxamine maleate] 2•1 mg/mL

arildone USAN, INN *antiviral*

Arimidex film-coated tablets ℞ *aromatase inhibitor; estrogen antagonist; antineoplastic for advanced breast cancer; also used as an adjunct to testosterone replacement therapy for postandropausal symptoms* [anastrozole] 1 mg

arimoclomol *investigational (orphan) for amyotrophic lateral sclerosis (ALS)*

aripiprazole USAN *novel (atypical) quinolinone antipsychotic for schizophrenia and manic episodes of a bipolar disorder; adjunctive treatment for major depression; dopamine D_2 and serotonin $5\text{-}HT_1$ and $5\text{-}HT_2$ agonist*

Aristocort ointment, cream ℞ *corticosteroidal anti-inflammatory* [triamcinolone acetonide] 0.1%, 0.5%; 0.025%, 0.1%, 0.5%

Aristocort tablets (discontinued 2008) ℞ *corticosteroid; anti-inflammatory* [triamcinolone] 1, 2, 4, 8 mg

Aristocort A ointment, cream ℞ *corticosteroidal anti-inflammatory* [triamcinolone acetonide in a water-washable base] 0.1%; 0.025%, 0.1%, 0.5%

Aristocort Forte IM injection (discontinued 2004) ℞ *corticosteroid; anti-inflammatory* [triamcinolone diacetate] 40 mg/mL

Aristocort Intralesional injection (discontinued 2006) ℞ *corticosteroid; anti-inflammatory* [triamcinolone diacetate] 25 mg/mL

Aristolochia clematitis *medicinal herb* [see: birthwort]

Aristospan Intra-articular injection ℞ *corticosteroidal anti-inflammatory* [triamcinolone hexacetonide] 20 mg/mL

Aristospan Intralesional injection ℞ *corticosteroidal anti-inflammatory* [triamcinolone hexacetonide] 5 mg/mL

Arixtra subcu injection in prefilled syringes ℞ *selective factor Xa inhibitor; antithrombotic for prevention of deep vein thrombosis (DVT) and acute pulmonary embolism (PE) following abdominal or orthopedic surgery; investigational (NDA filed) for acute coronary syndrome (ACS)* [fondaparinux sodium] 2.5 mg/0.5 mL, 5 mg/0.4 mL, 7.5 mg/0.6 mL, 10 mg/0.8 mL

Arm-A-Med (trademarked packaging form) *single-dose plastic vial*

Arm-A-Vial (trademarked packaging form) *single-dose plastic vial*

armodafinil *analeptic for excessive daytime sleepiness due to narcolepsy (orphan), obstructive sleep apnea, or shift work sleep disorder (SWSD); isomer of modafinil*

Armoracia rusticana; A. lapathiofolia *medicinal herb* [see: horseradish]

Armour Thyroid tablets ℞ *natural thyroid replacement for hypothyroidism or thyroid cancer* [thyroid, desiccated (porcine)] 15, 30, 60, 90, 120, 180, 240, 300 mg

arnica (*Arnica montana; A. cordifolia; A. fulgens*) *flowers medicinal herb used as a topical counterirritant and vulnerary for acne, bruises, rashes, and other dermal lesions; not generally regarded as safe and effective taken internally as it is highly toxic*

arnolol INN

arofylline USAN *phosphodiesterase IV inhibitor for asthma*

Aromasin tablets ℞ *aromatase inhibitor; antihormonal antineoplastic for advanced breast cancer in postmenopausal women (orphan)* [exemestane] 25 mg

aromatase inhibitors *a class of antihormonal antineoplastics which block the conversion of androgens to estrogens, effectively depriving hormone-dependent tumors of estrogen in postmenopausal women*

aromatic ammonia spirit [see: ammonia spirit, aromatic]

aromatic cascara fluidextract [see: cascara fluidextract, aromatic]

aromatic cascara sagrada [see: cascara fluidextract, aromatic]

aromatic elixir NF *flavored and sweetened vehicle*

aromatics *a class of agents that have an agreeable odor and stimulating qualities; also, substances with a specific molecular structure in organic chemistry*

aronixil INN

arotinolol INN [also: arotinolol HCl]

arotinolol HCl JAN [also: arotinolol]

arprinocid USAN, INN, BAN *coccidiostat*

arpromidine INN

Arranon IV infusion ℞ *antineoplastic for T-cell acute lymphoblastic leukemia (T-ALL; orphan) and T-cell lymphoblastic lymphoma (T-LBL; orphan)* [nelarabine] 5 mg/mL (250 mg/vial)

arrow wood; Indian arrow wood; Indian arrow *medicinal herb* [see: wahoo]

ARS (antirabies serum) [q.v.]

arsambide [see: carbarsone]

arsanilic acid INN, BAN *investigational (Phase I/II, orphan) immunomodulator for AIDS*

arseclor [see: dichlorophenarsine HCl]

arsenic *element (As)* 🔢 Orazinc

arsenic acid, sodium salt [see: sodium arsenate]

arsenic trioxide (AsO$_3$) JAN *antineoplastic for acute promyelocytic leukemia (orphan); investigational (orphan) for other leukemias, multiple myeloma, myelodysplastic syndromes, liver cancer, and malignant glioma*

arsenobenzene [see: arsphenamine]

arsenobenzol [see: arsphenamine]

arsenphenolamine [see: arsphenamine]

Arsobal (available only from the Centers for Disease Control) ℞ *investigational anti-infective for trypanosomiasis* [melarsoprol]

arsphenamine USP

arsthinenol [also: arsthinol]

arsthinol INN [also: arsthinenol]

arteflene USAN, INN *antimalarial*

artegraft USAN *arterial prosthetic aid*

artemether INN

Artemisia absinthium *medicinal herb* [see: wormwood]

Artemisia dracunculus *medicinal herb* [see: tarragon]

Artemisia vulgaris *medicinal herb* [see: mugwort]

artemisinin INN *natural herbal drug for malaria*

artemotil INN

artenimol INN

arterenol [see: norepinephrine bitartrate]

artesunate INN *antimalarial; investigational (NDA filed, orphan) rectal sup-*

positories for emergency treatment of malaria

Artha-G tablets OTC *analgesic; anti-inflammatory* [salsalate] 750 mg ⊡ Oretic; Wartec

ArthriCare, Double Ice gel OTC *mild anesthetic; antipruritic; counterirritant* [menthol; camphor] 4%•3.1%

ArthriCare, Odor Free rub OTC *mild anesthetic; antipruritic; counterirritant; analgesic* [menthol; methyl nicotinate; capsaicin] 1.25%•0.25%•0.025%

ArthriCare Triple Medicated gel OTC *mild anesthetic; antipruritic; counterirritant* [methyl salicylate; menthol; methyl nicotinate] 30%• 1.5%•0.7%

"Arthritis Formula"; "Arthritis Strength" products [see under product name]

Arthritis Hot Creme OTC *analgesic; mild anesthetic; antipruritic; counterirritant* [methyl salicylate; menthol] 15%•10%

Arthritis Pain Formula caplets OTC *analgesic; antipyretic; anti-inflammatory; antirheumatic* [aspirin (buffered with magnesium hydroxide and aluminum hydroxide)] 500 mg

Arthropan IM injection (discontinued 2007) ℞ *analgesic; antipyretic; anti-inflammatory; antirheumatic* [choline salicylate] 870 mg/5 mL

Arthrotec film-coated tablets ℞ *analgesic; nonsteroidal anti-inflammatory drug (NSAID) for osteoarthritis, rheumatoid arthritis, and ankylosing spondylitis with a coating to protect gastric mucosa* [diclofenac sodium (enteric-coated core); misoprostol (coating)] 50•0.2, 75•0.2 mg

articaine INN *amide local anesthetic for dentistry* [also: carticaine]

articaine HCl USAN *amide local anesthetic for dentistry* [also: articaine; carticaine]

artichoke *(Cynara scolymus)* flower heads *medicinal herb for albuminuria, bile stimulation, diabetes, diuresis, dys-*

pepsia, jaundice, liver diseases, and postoperative anemia

Articoat bandages OTC *antimicrobial dressings*

Articulose L.A. IM injection ℞ *corticosteroid; anti-inflammatory* [triamcinolone diacetate] 40 mg/mL

Artificial Tears eye drops OTC *moisturizer/lubricant*

Artificial Tears ophthalmic ointment OTC *ocular moisturizer/lubricant* [white petrolatum; mineral oil; lanolin]

Artificial Tears Plus eye drops OTC *moisturizer/lubricant* [polyvinyl alcohol] 1.4%

artilide INN *antiarrhythmic* [also: artilide fumarate]

artilide fumarate USAN *antiarrhythmic* [also: artilide]

Artiss topical liquid, powder for topical liquid ℞ *kit to adhere autologous skin grafts to wounds from burns; the sealant and thrombin are mixed just before applying to the graft, and it "sets" in about 60 seconds* [fibrin sealant, human; thrombin, human] 96–125 mg/mL; 2.5–6.5 IU/mL ⊡ AeroTuss 12; Ertaczo

Arxxant *investigational (Phase III) protein kinase C beta (PKC-β) inhibitor for diabetic retinopathy* [ruboxistaurin]

Arzol Silver Nitrate applicators ℞ *antiseptic* [silver nitrate; potassium nitrate] 75%•25%

arzoxifene INN *selective estrogen receptor modulator (SERM) for breast cancer, uterine fibroids, endometriosis, and dysfunctional uterine bleeding* [also: arzoxifene HCl]

arzoxifene HCl USAN *selective estrogen receptor modulator (SERM) for breast cancer, uterine fibroids, endometriosis, and dysfunctional uterine bleeding* [also: arzoxifene]

AS-013 [see: prostaglandin E_1 enol ester]

^{74}As [see: sodium arsenate As 74]

5-ASA (5-aminosalicylic acid) [see: mesalamine]

ASA (acetylsalicylic acid) [see: aspirin]

Asacol delayed-release tablets ℞ *anti-inflammatory for active ulcerative colitis, proctosigmoiditis, and proctitis* [mesalamine (5-aminosalicylic acid)] 400 mg ⊠ Isocal; Os-Cal 500

asafetida; asafoetida *(Ferula assafoetida; F. foetida; F. rubricaulis)* gum resin from dried roots and rhizomes *medicinal herb for abdominal tumors, amenorrhea, asthma, colic, convulsions, corns and calluses, edema; also used as an expectorant; not generally regarded as safe and effective in children as it may induce methemoglobinemia*

asafoetida *medicinal herb* [see: asafetida]

Asarum canadense medicinal herb [see: wild ginger]

ASC Lotionized topical liquid OTC *medicated cleanser for acne* [triclosan] 0.3%

Asclepias geminata medicinal herb [see: gymnema]

Asclepias syriaca medicinal herb [see: milkweed]

Asclepias tuberosa medicinal herb [see: pleurisy root]

Ascocaps capsules OTC *vitamin C supplement* [ascorbic acid] 500 mg

Ascocid granules for oral solution OTC *vitamin supplement* [vitamin C (as calcium ascorbate)] 4 g/tsp.

Ascomp with Codeine capsules ℞ *barbiturate sedative; narcotic analgesic; antipyretic* [butalbital; codeine phosphate; aspirin; caffeine] 50•30•325•40 mg

Ascor L 500 injection ℞ *vitamin C supplement* [ascorbic acid] 500 mg/mL ⊠ ozagrel

ascorbic acid (L-ascorbic acid; vitamin C) USP, INN, BAN, JAN *water-soluble vitamin; antiscorbutic; urinary acidifier; topical sunscreen* 250, 500, 1000, 1500 mg oral; 240 mg/tsp. oral; 500 mg/5 mL oral; 500 mg/mL injection

L-ascorbic acid, monosodium salt [see: sodium ascorbate]

L-ascorbic acid 6-palmitate [see: ascorbyl palmitate]

ascorbyl gamolenate INN, BAN

ascorbyl palmitate NF *antioxidant*

Ascriptin caplets OTC *analgesic; antipyretic; anti-inflammatory; antirheumatic* [aspirin (buffered with magnesium hydroxide, aluminum hydroxide, and calcium carbonate)] 500 mg

Ascriptin; Ascriptin A/D coated caplets OTC *analgesic; antipyretic; anti-inflammatory; antirheumatic* [aspirin (buffered with magnesium hydroxide, aluminum hydroxide, and calcium carbonate)] 500 mg; 325 mg

asenapine *investigational (NDA filed) novel (atypical) serotonin 5-HT$_{2A}$ and dopamine D$_2$ receptor antagonist antipsychotic for schizophrenia and manic episodes of a bipolar disorder*

Asendin tablets (discontinued 2006) ℞ *tricyclic antidepressant* [amoxapine] 25, 50, 100, 150 mg

aseptichrome [see: merbromin]

ash, bitter *medicinal herb* [see: quassia; wahoo]

ash, mountain; American mountain ash; European mountain ash *medicinal herb* [see: mountain ash]

ash, poison *medicinal herb* [see: fringe tree]

ASHAP; A-SHAP (Adriamycin, Solu-Medrol, high-dose ara-C, Platinol) *chemotherapy protocol* ⊠ ESHAP

Asimina triloba medicinal herb [see: pawpaw]

Asmalix elixir (discontinued 2008) ℞ *antiasthmatic; bronchodilator* [theophylline] 80 mg/15 mL

Asmanex Twisthaler (powder for oral inhalation) ℞ *corticosteroidal anti-inflammatory for chronic asthma; not indicated for acute attacks* [mometasone furoate] 200 mcg/adult dose, 100 mcg/pediatric dose

AsO$_3$ (arsenic trioxide) [q.v.]

asobamast INN, BAN

asocainol INN

Aspalathus linearis; A. contaminata; Borbonia pinifolia medicinal herb [see: red bush tea]

asparaginase (L-asparaginase) USAN, JAN antineoplastic adjunct for acute lymphocytic leukemia [also: colaspase]

asparagine (L-asparagine) nonessential amino acid; symbols: Asn, N ⑨
esproquine

L-asparagine amidohydrolase [see: asparaginase]

asparagus (*Asparagus officinalis*) roots, seeds medicinal herb for acne, constipation, contraception, edema, neuritis, parasites, rheumatism, stimulating hair growth, and toothache

aspartame USAN, NF, INN, BAN sweetener

L-aspartate potassium JAN

aspartic acid (L-aspartic acid) USAN, INN nonessential amino acid; symbols: Asp, D

L-aspartic acid insulin [see: insulin aspart]

aspartocin USAN, INN antibacterial

A-Spas S/L sublingual tablets (discontinued 2006) ℞ GI/GU antispasmodic; anticholinergic [hyoscyamine sulfate] 0.125 mg ⑨ isobuzole

aspen, European medicinal herb [see: black poplar]

aspen poplar; American aspen; quaking aspen medicinal herb [see: poplar]

Aspercreme; Aspercreme with Aloe cream OTC analgesic [trolamine salicylate] 10%

Aspercreme Rub lotion OTC analgesic [trolamine salicylate] 10%

Aspergillus oryase **proteinase** [see: asperkinase]

Aspergum chewing gum tablets OTC analgesic; antipyretic; anti-inflammatory; antirheumatic [aspirin] 227.5 mg

asperkinase

asperlin USAN antibacterial; antineoplastic

Asperula odorata medicinal herb [see: sweet woodruff]

aspidium (*Dryopteris filix-mas*) plant medicinal herb for bloody nose, menor-rhagia, worm infections including tapeworm and ringworm, and wound healing; not generally regarded as safe and effective for internal use as it is highly toxic

aspidosperma USP

aspirin USP, BAN, JAN analgesic; antipyretic; anti-inflammatory; antirheumatic 325, 500, 650, 975 mg oral; 120, 200, 300, 600 mg suppositories ⑨ aceperone; azaperone; Easprin; esuprone

aspirin, buffered USP analgesic; antipyretic; anti-inflammatory; antirheumatic 325, 500 mg oral

aspirin aluminum NF, JAN

aspirin & butalbital & caffeine analgesic; barbiturate sedative 325•50•40 mg oral

aspirin & codeine phosphate antipyretic; analgesic; narcotic antitussive 15•325 mg oral

aspirin & codeine phosphate & carisoprodol narcotic analgesic; skeletal muscle relaxant 325•16•200 mg oral

aspirin DL-lysine JAN investigational (orphan) for pain and fever due to sickle cell disease

Aspirin Free Excedrin caplets, geltabs OTC analgesic; antipyretic [acetaminophen; caffeine] 500•65 mg

Aspirin with Codeine No. 3 and No. 4 tablets ℞ narcotic antitussive; analgesic; antipyretic [codeine phosphate; aspirin] 30•325 mg; 60•325 mg

ASPIRINcheck urine test kit for professional use ℞ in vitro diagnostic aid for antiplatelet metabolites of aspirin

Aspirin-Free Pain Relief tablets, caplets (discontinued 2008) OTC analgesic; antipyretic [acetaminophen] 325, 500 mg; 500 mg

Aspirol (trademarked delivery form) crushable ampule for inhalation ⑨ Isuprel

aspogen [see: dihydroxyaluminum aminoacetate]

aspoxicillin INN, JAN

Asprimox Extra Protection for Arthritis Pain tablets, caplets OTC analgesic; antipyretic; anti-inflammatory; antirheumatic [aspirin (buffered with aluminum hydroxide, magnesium hydroxide, and calcium carbonate)] 325 mg

aspro [see: aspirin]

astatine *element (At)*

Astelin Ready-Spray nasal spray in a metered-dose pump ℞ *peripherally selective phthalazinone antihistamine and mast cell stabilizer for allergic and vasomotor rhinitis* [azelastine HCl] 137 mcg/spray

astemizole USAN, INN, BAN *antiallergic; second-generation piperidine antihistamine*

astifilcon A USAN *hydrophilic contact lens material*

astragalus (Astragalus membranaceus) root *medicinal herb for cancer, chronic fatigue, and Epstein-Barr syndrome; also used to strengthen the immune system, especially after chemotherapy and HIV treatments*

Astramorph PF (preservative free) IV, IM, or subcu injection ℞ *narcotic analgesic* [morphine sulfate] 0.5, 1 mg/mL

astringents *a class of agents that contract tissue, reducing secretions or discharges* [see also: hemostatics; styptics]

Astroglide vaginal gel OTC *moisturizer/lubricant* [glycerin; propylene glycol] ⊡ Oystercal-D 250

astromicin INN *antibacterial* [also: astromicin sulfate]

astromicin sulfate USAN, JAN *antibacterial* [also: astromicin]

aT-1001 *investigational (orphan) treatment for Fabry disease*

aT-III (antithrombin III) [q.v.]

Atacand tablets ℞ *antihypertensive; angiotensin II receptor antagonist; treatment for heart failure* [candesartan cilexetil] 4, 8, 16, 32 mg

Atacand HCT 16-12.5; Atacand HCT 32-12.5 tablets ℞ *antihypertensive; angiotensin II receptor antagonist; diuretic* [candesartan cilexetil; hydrochlorothiazide] 16•12.5; 32•12.5 mg

atamestane INN *investigational (Phase III) aromatase inhibitor for breast cancer*

ataprost INN

ataquimast INN

Atarax tablets, syrup (discontinued 2004) ℞ *anxiolytic; minor tranquilizer* [hydroxyzine HCl] 10, 25, 50, 100 mg; 10 mg/5 mL

Atarax 100 tablets (discontinued 2004) ℞ *anxiolytic; minor tranquilizer; antihistamine for allergic pruritus* [hydroxyzine HCl] 100 mg

atarvet [see: acepromazine]

atazanavir sulfate *antiviral; azapeptide protease inhibitor for HIV-1 infection*

atenolol USAN, INN, BAN, JAN *antihypertensive; antiadrenergic (β-receptor)* 25, 50, 100 mg oral

atenolol & chlorthalidone *antihypertensive; antiadrenergic (β-receptor); diuretic* 50•25, 100•25 mg oral

atevirdine INN *antiviral* [also: atevirdine mesylate] ⊡ etofuradine

atevirdine mesylate USAN *non-nucleoside reverse transcriptase inhibitor (NNRTI) antiviral* [also: atevirdine]

aTG (antithymocyte globulin) [q.v.]

Atgam IV infusion ℞ *treatment for aplastic anemia; immunizing agent to prevent allograft rejection of renal transplants* [antithymocyte globulin, equine] 50 mg/mL

athyromazole [see: carbimazole]

atipamezole USAN, INN, BAN α_2-receptor antagonist

atiprimod dihydrochloride USAN *immunomodulator; anti-inflammatory; antiarthritic*

atiprimod dimaleate USAN *immunomodulator; anti-inflammatory; antiarthritic*

atiprosin INN *antihypertensive* [also: atiprosin maleate]

atiprosin maleate USAN *antihypertensive* [also: atiprosin]

Ativan IV or IM injection ℞ *benzodiazepine anxiolytic; preanesthetic sedative; anticonvulsant* [lorazepam] 2, 4 mg/mL

atizoram USAN, INN

atlafilcon A USAN *hydrophilic contact lens material*

aTnativ *investigational (orphan) agent for congenital aT-III deficiency in patients undergoing surgical or obstetrical procedures* [antithrombin III]

atolide USAN, INN *anticonvulsant*

Atolone tablets (discontinued 2008) ℞ *corticosteroid; anti-inflammatory* [triamcinolone] 4 mg

atomoxetine HCl *selective norepinephrine reuptake inhibitor; non-stimulant treatment for attention-deficit/hyperactivity disorder (ADHD); investigational (orphan) for Tourette syndrome*

atorolimumab INN

atorvastatin calcium USAN *HMG-CoA reductase inhibitor for hypercholesterolemia, dysbetalipoproteinemia, hypertriglyceridemia, mixed dyslipidemia, and the prevention of cardiovascular disease and stroke in high-risk patients*

atosiban USAN, INN *oxytocin antagonist* ⊡ etazepine

atovaquone USAN, INN, BAN *antimalarial; antiprotozoal for AIDS-related Pneumocystis pneumonia (orphan); investigational (orphan) for AIDS-related Toxoplasma gondii encephalitis*

aTP (adenosine triphosphate) [see: adenosine triphosphate disodium]

aTPase (adenosine triphosphatase) inhibitors *a class of gastric antisecretory agents that inhibit the aTPase "proton pump" within the gastric parietal cell* [also called: proton pump inhibitors; substituted benzimidazoles] ⊡ WOWtabs

atracurium besilate INN *skeletal muscle relaxant; nondepolarizing neuromuscular blocker; adjunct to anesthesia* [also: atracurium besylate]

atracurium besylate USAN, BAN *skeletal muscle relaxant; nondepolarizing neuromuscular blocker; adjunct to anesthesia* [also: atracurium besilate] 10 mg/mL injection

Atralin gel ℞ *keratolytic for acne* [tretinoin] 0.05% ⊡ iotrolan

atrasentan HCl USAN *investigational (NDA filed) endothelin-A (EtA; ETA; ET_A) receptor antagonist to retard the progression of metastatic prostate cancer by reducing its proliferative effects in bone and prostate tissue*

atreleuton USAN *5-lipoxygenase inhibitor for asthma*

Atretol tablets (discontinued 2004) ℞ *anticonvulsant; analgesic for trigeminal neuralgia; antipsychotic* [carbamazepine] 200 mg

Atridox controlled-release gel for subgingival injection ℞ *antibiotic for periodontal disease* [doxycycline hyclate] 10%

Atrigel (trademarked dosage form) *sustained-release gel*

Atrigel Depot (trademarked dosage form) *sustained-release subcu injection*

atrimustine INN

atrinositol INN

Atripla film-coated caplets ℞ *antiviral non-nucleoside reverse transcriptase inhibitor (NNRTI) and nucleoside reverse transcriptase inhibitor (NRTI) combination therapy for HIV infection in adults* [efavirenz; emtricitabine; tenofovir disoproxil fumarate] 600•200•300 mg

atromepine INN

Atropa belladonna *medicinal herb* [see: belladonna]

AtroPen auto-injector (automatic IM injection device) ℞ *antidote for organophosphorous or carbamate insecticides* [atropine sulfate] 0.5, 1, 2 mg/0.7 mL dose

atropine USP, BAN *anticholinergic*

Atropine Care eye drops (discontinued 2004) ℞ *mydriatic; cycloplegic* [atropine sulfate] 1%

atropine methonitrate INN, BAN *anticholinergic* [also: methylatropine nitrate]

atropine methylnitrate [see: methylatropine nitrate]

atropine oxide INN *anticholinergic* [also: atropine oxide HCl]

atropine oxide HCl USAN *anticholinergic* [also: atropine oxide]

atropine propionate [see: prampine]

atropine sulfate USP, JAN *GI/GU antispasmodic; antiparkinsonian; bronchodilator; cycloplegic; mydriatic; antidote to insecticide poisoning* [also: atropine sulphate] 0.4, 0.6 mg oral; 1%, 2% eye drops; 0.05, 0.1, 0.3, 0.4, 0.5, 0.8, 1 mg/mL injection

atropine sulphate BAN *GI/GU antispasmodic; antiparkinsonian; bronchodilator; cycloplegic; mydriatic* [also: atropine sulfate]

Atropine-1 eye drops ℞ *mydriatic; cycloplegic* [atropine sulfate] 1%

Atrosept sugar-coated tablets ℞ *urinary antibiotic; analgesic; antispasmodic; acidifier* [methenamine; phenyl salicylate; atropine sulfate; methylene blue; hyoscyamine sulfate; benzoic acid] 40.8•18.1•0.03•5.4•0.03•4.5 mg

Atrovent nasal spray, inhalation aerosol ℞ *anticholinergic bronchodilator for bronchospasm, emphysema, and chronic obstructive pulmonary disease (COPD); antisecretory for rhinorrhea* [ipratropium bromide] 0.03%, 0.06% (21, 42 mcg/dose); 18 mcg/dose

Atrovent solution for inhalation (discontinued 2005) ℞ *anticholinergic bronchodilator for bronchospasm, emphysema, and chronic obstructive pulmonary disease (COPD)* [ipratropium bromide] 0.02%

Atrovent HFA inhalation aerosol with a CFC-free propellant ℞ *anticholinergic bronchodilator for bronchospasm, emphysema, and chronic obstructive pulmonary disease (COPD)* [ipratropium bromide] 17 mcg/dose

A/T/S topical solution, gel ℞ *antibiotic for acne* [erythromycin; alcohol 66%–92%] 2% ☒ oats

Attain oral liquid OTC *enteral nutritional therapy* [lactose-free formula] ☒ 8 in 1

attapulgite, activated USP *suspending agent; GI adsorbent*

Attenuvax powder for subcu injection ℞ *measles vaccine* [measles virus vaccine, live attenuated] 0.5 mL

Atuss DM syrup (discontinued 2005) ℞ *antitussive; antihistamine; decongestant* [dextromethorphan hydrobromide; chlorpheniramine maleate; phenylephrine HCl] 15•2•10 mg/5 mL

Atuss DS Tannate oral suspension ℞ *antitussive; antihistamine; decongestant* [dextromethorphan tannate; chlorpheniramine tannate; pseudoephedrine tannate] 60•8•60 mg/5 mL

Atuss EX syrup (discontinued 2004) ℞ *narcotic antitussive; expectorant* [hydrocodone bitartrate; potassium guaiacolsulfonate] 5•240 mg/10 mL

Atuss G syrup (discontinued 2007) ℞ *narcotic antitussive; decongestant; expectorant* [hydrocodone bitartrate; phenylephrine HCl; guaifenesin] 4•20•200 mg/10 mL

Atuss HC; Atuss MS oral liquid (discontinued 2007) ℞ *narcotic antitussive; antihistamine; decongestant* [hydrocodone bitartrate; chlorpheniramine maleate; phenylephrine HCl] 5•4•20 mg/10 mL; 10•4•20 mg/10 mL

Atuss HD dual-release capsules ℞ *narcotic antitussive; antihistamine; decongestant* [hydrocodone bitartrate (immediate release); chlorpheniramine maleate (extended release); pseudoephedrine HCl (extended release)] 5•2•30 mg

Atuss HD oral liquid (discontinued 2005) ℞ *narcotic antitussive; antihistamine; decongestant* [hydrocodone bitartrate; chlorpheniramine maleate; phenylephrine HCl] 2.5•4•10 mg/5 mL

Atuss HS oral suspension ℞ *narcotic antitussive; antihistamine; decongestant* [hydrocodone tannate; chlorpheniramine tannate; pseudoephedrine tannate] 10•8•60 mg/5 mL

Atuss HX dual-release capsules ℞ *narcotic antitussive; expectorant* [hydrocodone bitartrate (extended release); guaifenesin (immediate release)] 5• 100 mg

Atuss-12 DM extended-release oral suspension (discontinued 2007) ℞ *antitussive; antihistamine; decongestant* [dextromethorphan polistirex; chlorpheniramine polistirex; pseudoephedrine polistirex] 30•6•30 mg/5 mL

Atuss-12 DX extended-release oral suspension (discontinued 2007) ℞ *antitussive; expectorant* [dextromethorphan hydrobromide; guaifenesin] 30•200 mg/5 mL

"atypical" antipsychotics [see: novel antipsychotics]

198Au [see: gold Au 198]

augmented betamethasone dipropionate *topical corticosteroid*

Augmentin film-coated tablets, chewable tablets, powder for oral suspension ℞ *aminopenicillin antibiotic plus synergist* [amoxicillin; clavulanate potassium] 250•125, 500•125, 875•125 mg; 250•62.5, 400•57 mg; 125•31.25, 250•62.5, 400•57 mg/5 mL

Augmentin ES-600 powder for oral suspension ℞ *aminopenicillin antibiotic plus synergist* [amoxicillin; clavulanate potassium] 600•42.9 mg/5 mL

Augmentin XR extended-release film-coated tablets ℞ *aminopenicillin antibiotic plus synergist* [amoxicillin; clavulanic acid] 1000•62.5 mg

augmerosen *investigational (NDA filed, orphan) antineoplastic for malignant melanoma; investigational (Phase III, orphan) for multiple myeloma and chronic lymphocytic leukemia (CLL)*

Auralgan ear drops ℞ *anesthetic; analgesic* [benzocaine; antipyrine; acetic acid; polycosanol] 1.4%•5.4%•0.01%•0.01%

auranofin USAN, INN, BAN, JAN *antirheumatic (29% gold)*

aureoquin [now: quinetolate]

Auriculin *investigational (orphan) for acute renal failure and renal transplants* [anaritide acetate]

Auro Ear Drops OTC *cerumenolytic to emulsify and disperse ear wax* [carbamide peroxide] 6.5% ⃝ E-R-O Ear Drops

Auro-Dri ear drops OTC *antiseptic; astringent* [boric acid] 2.75% ⃝ Ear-Dry

Auroguard Otic ear drops ℞ *anesthetic; analgesic* [benzocaine; antipyrine] 1.4%•5.4%

Aurolate IM injection ℞ *antirheumatic* [gold sodium thiomalate] 50 mg/mL ⃝ Oralet

aurolin [see: gold sodium thiosulfate]

auropin [see: gold sodium thiosulfate]

aurosan [see: gold sodium thiosulfate]

aurothioglucose USP *antirheumatic (50% gold)* 50 mg/mL injection

aurothioglycanide INN

aurothiomalate disodium [see: gold sodium thiomalate]

aurothiomalate sodium [see: gold sodium thiomalate]

Auroto Otic ear drops (discontinued 2004) ℞ *anesthetic; analgesic* [antipyrine; benzocaine] 1.4%•5.4%

Australian tea tree *medicinal herb* [see: tea tree oil]

Autohaler (delivery device) *breath-activated metered-dose inhaler*

auto-injector (delivery device) *automatic IM injection device*

autologous cell (AC) vaccine *investigational (Phase III, orphan) therapeutic vaccine for adjuvant treatment of ovarian cancer*

autolymphocyte therapy (ALT) *investigational (orphan) for metastatic renal cell carcinoma*

Autoplex T IV injection or drip (discontinued 2006) ℞ *antihemophilic to correct factor VIII deficiency and coagulation deficiency* [anti-inhibitor coagulant complex, heat treated] (each bottle is labeled with dosage)

autoprothrombin I [see: factor VII]

autoprothrombin II [see: factor IX]

autumn crocus (Colchicum autumnale; C. speciosum; C. vernum) plant and corm *medicinal herb for* edema, gonorrhea, gout, prostate enlargement, and rheumatism; not generally regarded as safe and effective as it is highly toxic because of its colchicine content

AV (Adriamycin, vincristine) chemotherapy protocol

AVA (anthrax vaccine, adsorbed) [q.v.]

Avage cream ℞ retinoid pro-drug; adjuvant treatment for facial wrinkles, hyper- and hypopigmentation, and benign lentigines [tazarotene] 0.1%

Avail tablets OTC vitamin/mineral/iron supplement [multiple vitamins & minerals; iron; folic acid] ± • 18 • 0.4 mg

Avalide tablets ℞ combination angiotensin II receptor antagonist and diuretic for hypertension [irbesartan; hydrochlorothiazide] 150 • 12.5, 300 • 12.5, 300 • 25 mg

Avamys ⓔ (European name for U.S. product **Veramyst**)

Avandamet film-coated tablets ℞ antidiabetic combination for type 2 diabetes that decreases hepatic glucose production and increases cellular response to insulin without increasing insulin secretion [rosiglitazone maleate; metformin HCl] 2 • 500, 2 • 1000, 4 • 500, 4 • 1000 mg

Avandaryl tablets ℞ antidiabetic combination for type 2 diabetes that increases cellular response to insulin and stimulates insulin secretion in the pancreas [rosiglitazone maleate; glimepiride] 4 • 1, 4 • 2, 4 • 4, 8 • 2, 8 • 4 mg

Avandia film-coated tablets ℞ antidiabetic for type 2 diabetes that increases cellular response to insulin without increasing insulin secretion [rosiglitazone maleate] 2, 4, 8 mg

Avapro tablets ℞ angiotensin II receptor antagonist for hypertension; treatment to delay the progression of diabetic nephropathy [irbesartan] 75, 150, 300 mg

Avar cleanser, gel ℞ antibiotic and keratolytic for acne [sulfacetamide sodium; sulfur] 10% • 5%

Avar Green gel (tinted for "color correction") (discontinued 2008) ℞ antibiotic and keratolytic for acne [sulfacetamide sodium; sulfur] 10% • 5%

Avar-e Emollient; Avar-e Green cream (Green is tinted for "color correction") ℞ antibiotic and keratolytic for acne [sulfacetamide sodium; sulfur; glycerin] 10% • 5% • ²

avasimibe USAN, INN acylCoA transferase (ACaT) inhibitor for hyperlipidemia and atherosclerosis

Avastin IV infusion ℞ antineoplastic; angiogenesis inhibitor for metastatic colorectal cancer, HER2-negative breast cancer, and non–small cell lung cancer (NSCLC); investigational (Phase III) for cervical, renal, prostate, and pancreatic cancers [bevacizumab] 25 mg/mL

Aveeno lotion OTC moisturizer; emollient [colloidal oatmeal] 1% ☒ Aviane; Iophen

Aveeno Anti-Itch cream OTC poison ivy treatment [calamine; pramoxine HCl] 3% • 1%

Aveeno Cleansing bar OTC soap-free therapeutic skin cleanser [colloidal oatmeal] 51%

Aveeno Cleansing for Acne-Prone Skin bar OTC medicated cleanser for acne [salicylic acid; colloidal oatmeal]

Aveeno Moisturizing cream OTC moisturizer; emollient [colloidal oatmeal] 1%

Aveeno Oilated Bath packets OTC bath emollient [colloidal oatmeal; mineral oil] 43% • ²

Aveeno Regular Bath packets OTC bath emollient [colloidal oatmeal] 100%

Aveeno Shave gel OTC moisturizer; emollient [oatmeal flour]

Aveeno Shower & Bath oil OTC bath emollient [colloidal oatmeal] 5%

Avelox film-coated tablets, IV infusion ℞ broad-spectrum fluoroquinolone antibiotic [moxifloxacin HCl] 400 mg; 400 mg/bag ☒ Euflex; I-Valex-1

Avena sativa medicinal herb [see: oats]

Aventyl HCl oral solution (discontinued 2005) ℞ *tricyclic antidepressant* [nortriptyline HCl] 10 mg/5 mL

Aventyl HCl Pulvules (capsules) ℞ *tricyclic antidepressant* [nortriptyline HCl] 25 mg

avertin [see: tribromoethanol]

avian flu vaccine [see: influenza virus vaccine, H5N1]

Aviane tablets (in packs of 28) ℞ *monophasic oral contraceptive* [levonorgestrel; ethinyl estradiol] 0.1 mg• 20 mcg × 21 days; counters × 7 days ② Aveeno; Iophen

avicatonin INN

Avicine *investigational (Phase III) theraccine for cervical and pancreatic cancer* [CTP-37 (code name—generic name not yet assigned)]

avilamycin USAN, INN, BAN *antibacterial*

avinar [see: uredepa]

Avinza dual-release (immediate- plus extended-release) capsules ℞ *once-daily narcotic analgesic for treatment of chronic pain* [morphine sulfate] 30, 60, 90, 120 mg

Avita cream, gel ℞ *keratolytic for acne* [tretinoin] 0.025%

Avitene Hemostat nonwoven web ℞ *topical hemostat for surgery* [microfibrillar collagen hemostat]

avitriptan fumarate USAN *serotonin 5-HT₁ agonist for migraine*

avizafone INN, BAN

avobenzone USAN, INN *sunscreen*

avocado *(Persea americana; P. gratissima)* fruit and seed *medicinal herb for diarrhea, dysentery, inducing menstruation, lowering total cholesterol and improving overall lipid profile, promoting hair growth, and stimulating wound healing; also used as an aphrodisiac*

avocado sugar extract *natural weight-loss agent used to diminish carbohydrate cravings* [see also: D-mannoheptulose]

Avodart capsules ℞ *5α-reductase blocker for benign prostatic hyperplasia (BPH); investigational (Phase III) for prostate cancer* [dutasteride] 0.5 mg

Avolean capsules OTC *natural weight-loss agent used to diminish carbohydrate cravings* [avocado sugar extract] 50 mg ② Iophylline

Avonex single-dose vials and prefilled syringes for IM injection ℞ *immunomodulator for relapsing remitting multiple sclerosis (orphan); investigational (orphan) for non-A, non-B hepatitis, juvenile rheumatoid arthritis, Kaposi sarcoma, brain tumors, and various other cancers* [interferon beta-1a] 30 mcg (6.6 MIU)

avoparcin USAN, INN, BAN *glycopeptide antibiotic*

AVP (actinomycin D, vincristine, Platinol) *chemotherapy protocol*

avridine USAN, INN *antiviral* ② Aphrodyne

Award *hydrophilic contact lens material* [hilafilcon A] ② Aeroaid; Aredia; Euro-D

axamozide INN

axerophthol [see: vitamin A]

Axert tablets ℞ *vascular serotonin HT₁B/1D/1F receptor agonist for the acute treatment of migraine* [almotriptan malate] 6.25, 12.5 mg

axetil USAN, INN *combining name for radicals or groups*

Axid Pulvules (capsules); oral liquid ℞ *histamine H₂ antagonist for gastric and duodenal ulcers and gastroesophageal reflux disease (GERD); also used to prevent NSAID-induced gastric ulcers* [nizatidine] 150, 300 mg; 15 mg/mL ② AK-Cide

Axid AR ("acid reducer") tablets OTC *histamine H₂ antagonist for acid indigestion and heartburn* [nizatidine] 75 mg

axitinib *investigational (Phase III) vascular endothelial growth factor (VEGF) receptor inhibitor for thyroid and pancreatic cancer*

axitirome USAN, INN *antihyperlipidemic*

Axocet caplets (discontinued 2004) ℞ *barbiturate sedative; analgesic; antipyretic* [butalbital; acetaminophen] 50•650 mg

Axsain cream OTC *analgesic; counterirritant* [capsaicin] 0.25%

Aygestin tablets ℞ *synthetic progestin for amenorrhea, abnormal uterine bleeding, and endometriosis* [norethindrone acetate] 5 mg ⊇ Extina

Ayr Mentholated Vapor Inhaler OTC *antiseptic; mild anesthetic; antipruritic; counterirritant; emollient* [eucalyptus oil; menthol; lavender oil]

Ayr Saline nasal mist, nose drops, nasal gel OTC *nasal moisturizer* [sodium chloride (saline solution)] 0.65%

5-AZA (5-azacitidine) [see: azacitidine]

5-aza-2′-deoxycytidine *investigational (orphan) for acute leukemia*

azabon USAN, INN *CNS stimulant* ⊇ Isopan

azabuperone INN

azacitidine (5-AZA; 5-AZC) USAN, INN *demethylating antineoplastic for myelodysplastic syndrome (orphan); also used for acute lymphocytic leukemia and acute myelogenous leukemia*

azaclorzine INN *coronary vasodilator* [also: azaclorzine HCl]

azaclorzine HCl USAN *coronary vasodilator* [also: azaclorzine]

azaconazole USAN, INN *antifungal* ⊇ isoconazole

azacosterol INN *avian chemosterilant* [also: azacosterol HCl]

azacosterol HCl USAN *avian chemosterilant* [also: azacosterol]

AZA-CR [see: azacitidine]

Azactam powder for IV or IM injection ℞ *monobactam bactericidal antibiotic* [aztreonam] 0.5, 1, 2 g

azacyclonol INN, BAN [also: azacyclonol HCl]

azacyclonol HCl NF [also: azacyclonol]

5-azacytosine arabinoside (ara-AC) [see: fazarabine]

5-aza-2′-deoxycytidine *investigational (orphan) for acute leukemia*

Azadirachta indica medicinal herb [see: neem tree]

azaftozine INN

azalanstat dihydrochloride USAN *hypolipidemic*

azaline B [now: prazarelix acetate]

azalomycin INN, BAN

azaloxan INN *antidepressant* [also: azaloxan fumarate]

azaloxan fumarate USAN *antidepressant* [also: azaloxan]

azamethiphos BAN

azamethonium bromide INN, BAN

azamulin INN ⊇ azumolene

azanator INN *bronchodilator* [also: azanator maleate]

azanator maleate USAN *bronchodilator* [also: azanator]

azanidazole USAN, INN, BAN *antiprotozoal*

azaperone USAN, INN, BAN *antipsychotic* ⊇ aceperone; aspirin; Easprin; esuprone

azapetine BAN ⊇ Aseptone 1; isobutane

azapetine phosphate [see: azapetine]

azaprocin INN ⊇ isoprazone

azapropazone INN, BAN *anti-inflammatory* [also: apazone]

azaquinzole INN ⊇ isoconazole

azaribine USAN, INN, BAN *antipsoriatic*

azarole USAN *immunoregulator* ⊇ acerola

Azasan tablets ℞ *immunosuppressant for organ transplantation (orphan) and rheumatoid arthritis* [azathioprine] 25, 50, 75, 100 mg

azaserine USAN, INN *antifungal*

azasetron INN

AzaSite eye drops ℞ *macrolide antibiotic for bacterial conjunctivitis* [azithromycin] 1%

azaspirium chloride INN

azaspirones *a class of anxiolytics*

azastene

azatadine INN, BAN *piperidine antihistamine for allergic rhinitis and chronic urticaria* [also: azatadine maleate]

azatadine maleate USAN, USP *piperidine antihistamine for allergic rhinitis and chronic urticaria* [also: azatadine]

azatepa INN *antineoplastic* [also: azetepa]

azathioprine USAN, USP, INN, BAN, JAN *immunosuppressant for organ transplantation (orphan) and rheumatoid arthritis; investigational (orphan)* *graft-versus-host (GVH) disease of the oral mucosa* 50 mg oral

azathioprine sodium USP *immunosuppressant for organ transplantation (orphan) and rheumatoid arthritis* 100 mg injection

5-AZC (5-azacitidine) [see: azacitidine]

Azdone tablets ℞ *narcotic analgesic; antipyretic* [hydrocodone bitartrate; aspirin] 5•500 mg

azdU (3'-azido-2',3'-dideoxyuridine) [see: azidouridine]

azelaic acid USAN, INN *topical antimicrobial and keratolytic for acne and rosacea*

azelastine INN, BAN *peripherally selective phthalazinone antihistamine for allergic and vasomotor rhinitis; mast cell stabilizer; antiasthmatic* [also: azelastine HCl]

azelastine HCl USAN, JAN *peripherally selective phthalazinone antihistamine for allergic and vasomotor rhinitis; mast cell stabilizer; antiasthmatic* [also: azelastine]

Azelex cream ℞ *antimicrobial and keratolytic for inflammatory acne vulgaris* [azelaic acid] 20%

azelnidipine INN

azepexole INN, BAN

azephine [see: azapetine phosphate]

azepinamide [see: glypinamide]

azepindole USAN, INN *antidepressant*

azetepa USAN, BAN *antineoplastic* [also: azatepa]

azetirelin INN

azidamfenicol INN, BAN

3'-azido-2',3'-dideoxyuridine (azdU) [see: azidouridine]

azidoamphenicol [see: azidamfenicol]

azidocillin INN, BAN

azidothymidine (AZT) [now: zidovudine]

azidouridine (azdU) *investigational (orphan) antiviral for HIV and AIDS*

Azilect tablets ℞ *once-daily monoamine oxidase B (MAO-B) inhibitor for Parkinson disease* [rasagiline] 0.5, 1 mg

azimexon INN

azimilide dihydrochloride USAN *investigational (NDA filed) antiarrhythmic and antifibrillatory*

azintamide INN

azinthiamide [see: azintamide]

azipramine INN *antidepressant* [also: azipramine HCl]

azipramine HCl USAN *antidepressant* [also: azipramine]

aziridinyl benzoquinone [see: diaziquone]

azithromycin USAN, USP, INN, BAN *macrolide antibiotic* 250, 500, 600 mg oral; 100, 200 mg/5 mL oral; 500 mg injection ⊠ astromicin

azlocillin USAN, INN, BAN *penicillin antibiotic*

azlocillin sodium USP *penicillin antibiotic*

Azmacort oral inhalation aerosol ℞ *corticosteroidal anti-inflammatory for chronic asthma; not indicated for chronic attacks* [triamcinolone acetonide] 75 mcg/dose

Azo Standard tablets ℞ *urinary tract analgesic for relief of pain, burning, urgency, and frequency due to mucosal irritation from surgery, catheterization, endoscopic procedures, or trauma; adjunct to antibacterial agents for urinary tract infection (UTI)* [phenazopyridine HCl] 97.5 mg

Azo Test Strips reagent strips for home use OTC *in vitro diagnostic aid for urinary tract infections*

azoconazole [now: azaconazole]

azodisal sodium (ADS) [now: olsalazine sodium]

"azoles" *a class of fungicides that include all with generic names ending in "azole," such clotrimazole, fluconazole, etc.*

azolimine USAN, INN *diuretic*

Azopt eye drop suspension ℞ *carbonic anhydrase inhibitor for glaucoma* [brinzolamide] 1% ⊠ Aosept + Aodisc

Azor tablets ℞ *combination calcium channel blocker and angiotensin II receptor antagonist for hypertension* [amlodipine (as besylate); olmesartan medoxomil] 5•20, 5•40, 10•20, 10•40 mg

azosemide USAN, INN, JAN *diuretic*

Azo-Standard tablets OTC *urinary tract analgesic for relief of pain, burning,* urgency, and frequency due to mucosal irritation from surgery, catheterization, endoscopic procedures, or trauma; adjunct to antibacterial agents for urinary tract infection (UTI) [phenazopyridine HCl] 95 mg

Azostix reagent strips for professional use ℞ *in vitro diagnostic aid to estimate the amount of BUN in whole blood*

Azo-Sulfisoxazole tablets (discontinued 2008) ℞ *urinary anti-infective; urinary analgesic* [sulfisoxazole; phenazopyridine HCl] 500•50 mg

azotomycin USAN, INN *antibiotic antineoplastic*

azovan blue BAN *blood volume test* [also: Evans blue]

azovan sodium [see: Evans blue]

AZT (azidothymidine) [now: zidovudine]

Aztec controlled release *investigational (Phase III) antiviral for early HIV and AIDS* [zidovudine]

aztreonam USAN, USP, INN, BAN, JAN *monobactam bactericidal antibiotic; investigational (orphan) inhalation therapy for cystic fibrosis*

azulene sulfonate sodium JAN [also: sodium gualenate]

Azulfidine tablets ℞ *anti-inflammatory for ulcerative colitis; also used for ankylosing spondylitis, Crohn disease, and regional enteritis* [sulfasalazine] 500 mg

Azulfidine EN-tabs enteric-coated delayed-release tablets ℞ *anti-inflammatory for ulcerative colitis, rheumatoid arthritis (RA), and juvenile rheumatoid arthritis (JRA); also used for ankylosing spondylitis, Crohn disease, and regional enteritis* [sulfasalazine] 500 mg

azumolene INN *skeletal muscle relaxant* [also: azumolene sodium] 🔃 azamulin

azumolene sodium USAN *skeletal muscle relaxant* [also: azumolene]

azure A carbacrylic resin [see: azuresin]

azuresin NF, BAN

1,4-B (1,4-butanediol) *a precursor to gamma hydroxybutyrate (GHB); a formerly legal alternative to GHB, now also illegal (Schedule I)* [see: gamma hydroxybutyrate (GHB)]

B Complex + C timed-release tablets OTC *vitamin supplement* [multiple B vitamins; vitamin C] ≜•500 mg 🔃 B-Complex

B Complex with C and B-12 injection ℞ *parenteral vitamin supplement* [multiple vitamins] 🔃 B-Complex with B-12

B Complex-50 sustained-release tablets OTC *vitamin supplement* [multiple B vitamins; folic acid; biotin] ≜• 400•50 mcg 🔃 B-Complex

B Complex-150 sustained-release tablets OTC *vitamin supplement* [multiple B vitamins; folic acid; biotin] ≜• 400•150 mcg 🔃 B-Complex

B & O Supprettes No. 15A; B & O Supprettes No. 16A suppositories ℞ *narcotic analgesic* [belladonna extract; opium] 16.2•30 mg; 16.2• 60 mg

B vitamins [see: vitamin B]

B_1 (vitamin B_1) [see: thiamine HCl]

B_2 (vitamin B_2) [see: riboflavin]

B_3 (vitamin B_3) [see: niacin; niacinamide]

B_5 (vitamin B_5) [see: calcium pantothenate]

B_6 (vitamin B_6) [see: pyridoxine HCl]

B_8 (vitamin B_8) [see: adenosine phosphate]

B_{12} (vitamin B_{12}) [see: cyanocobalamin]

B₁₂ₐ (vitamin B₁₂ₐ) [see: hydroxoco-
balamin]

B₁₂ᵦ (vitamin B₁₂ᵦ) [see: hydroxoco-
balamin]

B-50 tablets OTC *vitamin supplement*
[multiple B vitamins; folic acid; bio-
tin] ±•100•50 mcg

B-100 tablets, timed-release tablets
OTC *vitamin supplement* [multiple B
vitamins; folic acid; biotin] ±•100•
100 mcg; ±•400•50 mcg

Bᶜ (vitamin Bᶜ) [see: folic acid]

Bₜ (vitamin Bₜ) [see: carnitine]

Babee Teething oral lotion OTC
*mucous membrane anesthetic; antisep-
tic* [benzocaine; cetalkonium chlo-
ride] 2.5%•0.02%

baby brain I *chemotherapy protocol for
pediatric brain tumors* [see: COPE]

Baby Vitamin drops OTC *vitamin supplement* [multiple vitamins]

Baby Vitamin with Iron drops OTC
vitamin/iron supplement [multiple
vitamins; iron] ±•10 mg/mL

BabyBIG powder for IV infusion ℞
*treatment for infant botulism type A or
B (orphan)* [botulism immune globulin (BIG)] 100 mg/vial

Babylax [see: Fleet Babylax]

Baby's Bliss Gripe Water oral drops
OTC *natural product to relieve colic,
stomach cramps, hiccups, and gas in
infants* [ginger; fennel; sodium bicarbonate; fructose]

**BAC (BCNU, ara-C, cyclophos-
phamide)** *chemotherapy protocol*

BAC (benzalkonium chloride) [q.v.]

bacampicillin INN, BAN *aminopenicillin
antibiotic* [also: bacampicillin HCl]

bacampicillin HCl USAN, USP, JAN
aminopenicillin antibiotic [also: bacam-
picillin]

bachelor's buttons *medicinal herb* [see:
cornflower; feverfew; tansy; buttercup]

Bacid capsules OTC *probiotic; dietary
supplement; fever blister treatment; not
generally regarded as safe and effective
as an antidiarrheal* [Lactobacillus acido-
philus] 500 million CFU

Baci-IM powder for IM injection ℞
bactericidal antibiotic [bacitracin]
50 000 U

**bacillus Calmette-Guérin (BCG)
vaccine** [see: BCG vaccine]

bacitracin USP, INN, BAN, JAN *bactericidal antibiotic; investigational (orphan)
for pseudomembranous enterocolitis*
500 U/g topical; 500 U/g ophthalmic; 50 000 U/vial injection

bacitracin zinc USP, BAN *bactericidal
antibiotic*

**bacitracin zinc & neomycin sulfate
& polymyxin B sulfate** *topical
antibiotic* 400 U•5 mg•10 000 U per
g ophthalmic

**bacitracin zinc & polymyxin B sul-
fate** *topical antibiotic* 500•10 000
U/g ophthalmic

bacitracins zinc complex [see: bacitracin zinc]

**Backache Maximum Strength
Relief** film-coated caplets OTC *analgesic; antirheumatic* [magnesium sali-
cylate] 467 mg

Back-Pack (trademarked packaging
form) *unit-of-use package*

baclofen (L-baclofen) USAN, USP,
INN, BAN, JAN *skeletal muscle relaxant
for intractable spasticity due to multiple
sclerosis or spinal cord injury (orphan);
investigational (orphan) for trigeminal
neuralgia, cerebral palsy, spinal cord
disease, and dystonia* 10, 20 mg oral

bacmecillinam INN

Bacmin tablets ℞ *vitamin/mineral/iron
supplement* [multiple vitamins &
minerals; iron; folic acid; biotin] ±•
27•0.8•0.15 mg

**BACOD (bleomycin, Adriamycin,
CCNU, Oncovin, dexametha-
sone)** *chemotherapy protocol* ⊡
BCAD 2; BCD; pokeweed

**BACON (bleomycin, Adriamycin,
CCNU, Oncovin, nitrogen mus-
tard)** *chemotherapy protocol* ⊡ BiCNU

**BACOP (bleomycin, Adriamycin,
cyclophosphamide, Oncovin,
prednisone)** *chemotherapy protocol*

⑫ BCAP; BCOP; BCP; BEACOPP; PCP

BACT (BCNU, ara-C, cyclophosphamide, thioguanine) *chemotherapy protocol*

bactericidal and permeability-increasing (BPI) protein, recombinant *investigational (Phase III, orphan) treatment for gram-negative sepsis, hemorrhagic shock, and meningococcemia*

bacteriostatic sodium chloride [see: sodium chloride]

Bacteriostatic Sodium Chloride Injection ℞ *IV diluent* [sodium chloride (normal saline solution)] 0.9% (normal)

Bacti-Cleanse topical liquid OTC *soap-free therapeutic skin cleanser* [benzalkonium chloride]

Bactigen B Streptococcus-CS slide test for professional use ℞ *in vitro diagnostic aid for Group B streptococcal antigens in vaginal and cervical swabs*

Bactigen Meningitis Panel slide test for professional use ℞ *in vitro diagnostic aid for H. influenzae, N. meningitidis, and S. pneumoniae in various fluids* [latex agglutination test]

Bactigen N. meningitidis slide test for professional use (discontinued 2004) ℞ *in vitro diagnostic aid for Neisseria meningitidis* [latex agglutination test]

Bactigen Salmonella-Shigella slide test for professional use ℞ *in vitro diagnostic aid for salmonella and shigella* [latex agglutination test]

Bactine Antiseptic Anesthetic topical liquid, topical spray OTC *anesthetic; antiseptic* [lidocaine HCl; benzalkonium chloride] 2.5%•0.13%

Bactine Hydrocortisone; Maximum Strength Bactine cream OTC *corticosteroidal anti-inflammatory* [hydrocortisone] 0.5%; 1%

Bactine Pain Relieving Cleansing Spray OTC *anesthetic; antiseptic* [lidocaine HCl; benzalkonium chloride] 2.5%•0.13%

Bactine Pain Relieving Cleansing Wipes OTC *anesthetic; antiseptic* [pramoxine HCl; benzalkonium chloride] 1%•0.13%

BactoShield aerosol foam, solution OTC *broad-spectrum antimicrobial; germicidal* [chlorhexidine gluconate; alcohol 4%] 4%

BactoShield 2 solution OTC *broad-spectrum antimicrobial; germicidal* [chlorhexidine gluconate; alcohol 4%] 2%

Bactrim; Bactrim DS tablets ℞ *anti-infective; antibacterial* [trimethoprim; sulfamethoxazole] 80•400 mg; 160•800 mg

Bactrim IV infusion ℞ *anti-infective; antibacterial* [trimethoprim; sulfamethoxazole] 80•400 mg/5 mL

Bactrim Pediatric oral suspension ℞ *anti-infective; antibacterial* [trimethoprim; sulfamethoxazole] 40•200 mg/5 mL

Bactroban cream ℞ (available OTC in Canada) *antibiotic* [mupirocin calcium] 2.15% (2% base)

Bactroban ointment ℞ *antibiotic for impetigo* [mupirocin] 2%

Bactroban Nasal ointment in single-use tubes ℞ *antibiotic for iatrogenic methicillin-resistant* Staphylococcus aureus *(MRSA) infections* [mupirocin calcium] 2.15% (2% base)

Bagshawe protocol, modified *chemotherapy protocol* [see: CHAMOCA]

bakeprofen INN

baker's yeast *natural source of protein and B-complex vitamins*

BAL (British antilewisite) [now: dimercaprol]

BAL in Oil deep IM injection ℞ *chelating agent for arsenic, gold, and mercury poisoning; adjunct to lead poisoning* [dimercaprol in peanut oil] 10% ⑫ bolenol

Balacet 325 film-coated caplets ℞ *narcotic analgesic; antipyretic* [propoxyphene napsylate; acetaminophen] 100•325 mg

balafilcon A USAN *hydrophilic contact lens material*

balaglitazone *investigational (Phase III) peroxisome proliferator–activated receptor (PPAR) agonist for type 2 diabetes*

Balamine DM syrup, oral drops (discontinued 2007) ℞ *antitussive; antihistamine; decongestant; drops for children 1–18 months* [dextromethorphan hydrobromide; carbinoxamine maleate; pseudoephedrine HCl] 12.5•4• 60 mg/5 mL; 3.5•2•25 mg/mL

balipramine BAN [also: depramine]

balm *medicinal herb* [see: lemon balm]

balm, eye; eye root *medicinal herb* [see: goldenseal]

balm, mountain *medicinal herb* [see: yerba santa]

balm, squaw; squaw mint *medicinal herb* [see: pennyroyal]

balm of Gilead *(Populus balsamifera; P. candicans)* buds *medicinal herb used as an antiscorbutic, balsamic, diuretic, stimulant, and vulnerary*

Balmex ointment, cream OTC *astringent; moisturizer; emollient* [zinc oxide] 11.3%

Balmex Baby powder OTC *diaper rash treatment* [zinc oxide; Peruvian balsam; cornstarch]

Balmex Emollient lotion OTC *moisturizer; emollient*

balmony *medicinal herb* [see: turtlebloom]

Balneol Hygienic Cleansing lotion OTC *emollient/protectant* [mineral oil; lanolin]

Balneol Perianal Cleansing lotion (name changed to **Balneol Hygienic Cleansing** in 2008)

Balnetar bath oil OTC *antipsoriatic; antipruritic; emollient* [coal tar] 2.5%

balsalazide INN, BAN *gastrointestinal anti-inflammatory for ulcerative colitis* [also: balsalazide disodium]

balsalazide disodium USAN *gastrointestinal anti-inflammatory for ulcerative colitis* [also: balsalazide] 750 mg oral

balsalazide sodium [see: balsalazide disodium]

balsalazine [see: balsalazide disodium; balsalazide]

balsam apple; balsam pear *medicinal herb* [see: bitter melon]

balsam Peru [see: peruvian balsam; balsam tree]

balsam poplar *medicinal herb* [see: balm of Gilead]

balsam tree *medicinal herb* [see: Peruvian balsam]

balsamics; balsams *a class of agents that soothe or heal; balms; also, certain resinous substances of vegetable origin*

Balsamodendron myrrha medicinal herb [see: myrrh]

balsan [see: peruvian balsam]

Baltussin syrup (discontinued 2005) ℞ *narcotic antitussive; antihistamine; decongestant* [dihydrocodeine bitartrate; chlorpheniramine maleate; phenylephrine HCl] 3•2•20 mg/5 mL

Baltussin HC oral liquid (discontinued 2007) ℞ *narcotic antitussive; antihistamine; decongestant* [hydrocodone bitartrate; chlorpheniramine maleate; phenylephrine HCl] 5•4• 10 mg/10 mL

Balziva tablets (in packs of 28) ℞ *monophasic oral contraceptive* [norethindrone; ethinyl estradiol] 0.4 mg• 35 mcg × 21 days; counters × 7 days

bamaluzole INN

bambermycin INN, BAN *antibacterial antibiotic* [also: bambermycins]

bambermycins USAN *antibacterial antibiotic* [also: bambermycin]

bambuterol INN, BAN

bamethan INN, BAN *vasodilator* [also: bamethan sulfate] ⊞ pimetine

bamethan sulfate USAN, JAN *vasodilator* [also: bamethan]

bamifylline INN, BAN *bronchodilator* [also: bamifylline HCl] ⊞ pimefylline

bamifylline HCl USAN *bronchodilator* [also: bamifylline]

bamipine INN, BAN

bamnidazole USAN, INN *antiprotozoal (Trichomonas)* ⊞ pimonidazole

BAMON (bleomycin, Adriamycin, methotrexate, Oncovin, nitrogen

mustard) *chemotherapy protocol* ⑨
Pamine

Banadyne-3 topical solution OTC *mucous membrane anesthetic; antipruritic; counterirritant; antiseptic* [lidocaine; menthol; alcohol 45%] 4%•1%

Banalg lotion OTC *analgesic; mild anesthetic; antipruritic; counterirritant* [methyl salicylate; camphor; menthol] 4.9%•2%•1%

Banalg Hospital Strength lotion OTC *analgesic; mild anesthetic; antipruritic; counterirritant* [methyl salicylate; menthol] 14%•3%

Bancap HC capsules ℞ *narcotic analgesic; antipyretic* [hydrocodone bitartrate; acetaminophen] 5•500 mg ⑨ Pancof-HC

bandage, adhesive USP *surgical aid*

bandage, gauze USP *surgical aid*

Banflex IV or IM injection ℞ *skeletal muscle relaxant; analgesic; anticholinergic* [orphenadrine citrate] 30 mg/mL

banocide [see: diethylcarbamazine citrate]

Banophen caplets, capsules OTC *antihistamine; sleep aid* [diphenhydramine HCl] 25 mg

Banophen Allergy elixir OTC *antihistamine; sleep aid* [diphenhydramine HCl] 12.5 mg/5 mL

bapineuzumab *investigational (Phase III) monoclonal antibody against amyloid plaque in the brain, used to treat mild-to-moderate Alzheimer disease*

Baptisia tinctoria medicinal herb [see: wild indigo]

baquiloprim INN, BAN

Baraclude film-coated tablets, oral solution ℞ *nucleoside reverse transcriptase inhibitor (NRTI); antiviral for chronic hepatitis B virus (HBV) infection* [entecavir] 0.5, 1 mg; 0.05 mg/mL ⑨ pergolide

Barbados aloe *medicinal herb* [see: aloe]

barbenyl [see: phenobarbital]

barberry (Berberis vulgaris) bark *medicinal herb for bacteria-associated diarrhea, blood cleansing, cough, fever,* indigestion, jaundice, liver disorders, sciatica, and sore throat

barberry, California *medicinal herb* [see: Oregon grape]

barbexaclone INN

Barbidonna; Barbidonna No. 2 tablets (discontinued 2008) ℞ *GI/GU anticholinergic/antispasmodic; sedative* [atropine sulfate; scopolamine hydrobromide; hyoscyamine hydrobromide; phenobarbital] 0.025•0.0074•0.1286•16 mg; 0.025•0.0074•0.1286•32 mg

barbiphenyl [see: phenobarbital]

barbital NF, INN, JAN [also: barbitone]

barbital, soluble [now: barbital sodium]

barbital sodium NF, INN [also: barbitone sodium]

barbitone BAN [also: barbital]

barbitone sodium BAN [also: barbital sodium]

barbiturates *a class of sedative/hypnotics that produce a wide range of mood alteration; also widely abused as addictive street drugs*

bardana *medicinal herb* [see: burdock]

Baricon powder for oral suspension ℞ *radiopaque contrast medium for gastrointestinal imaging* [barium sulfate] 98% ⑨ Paracaine; procaine; Puregon; pyrrocaine

Baridium tablets ℞ *urinary tract analgesic for the relief of pain, burning, urgency, and frequency due to mucosal irritation from surgery, catheterization, endoscopic procedures, or trauma; adjunct to antibacterial agents for urinary tract infection (UTI)* [phenazopyridine HCl] 100 mg ⑨ Perdiem; Prodium; Pyridium

barium *element (Ba)* ⑨ broom

barium hydroxide lime USP *carbon dioxide absorbent*

barium sulfate USP, JAN *oral/rectal radiopaque contrast medium for gastrointestinal imaging*

barley (Hordeum vulgare) juice powder *medicinal herb for anemia, arthritis, blood cleansing, boils, bronchitis, cancer, metal poisoning, poor circula-*

tion, and reducing total and LDL cholesterol and increasing HDL cholesterol ☒ Paral; perilla; Prelu-2

barley malt soup extract *bulk laxative*

barmastine USAN, INN *antihistamine*

BarnesHind Saline for Sensitive Eyes solution OTC *rinsing/storage solution for soft contact lenses* [sodium chloride (preserved saline solution)]

barnidipine INN ☒ pranidipine

Barobag powder for oral/rectal suspension ℞ *radiopaque contrast medium for gastrointestinal imaging* [barium sulfate] 95% ☒ Boropak; Propac

Baro-cat oral suspension ℞ *radiopaque contrast medium for gastrointestinal imaging* [barium sulfate] 1.5% ☒ Pro-Cute

Baros effervescent granules ℞ *adjunct to gastrointestinal imaging* [sodium bicarbonate; tartaric acid] 460•420 mg/g

Barosma betulina; B. cenulata; B. serratifolia medicinal herb [see: buchu]

barosmin [see: diosmin]

Barosperse powder for oral/rectal suspension ℞ *radiopaque contrast medium for gastrointestinal imaging* [barium sulfate] 95%

Barosperse, Liquid oral suspension ℞ *radiopaque contrast medium for gastrointestinal imaging* [barium sulfate] 60%

Bar-test tablets ℞ *radiopaque contrast medium for gastrointestinal imaging* [barium sulfate] 650 mg

barucainide INN

BAS (benzyl analogue of serotonin) [see: benanserin HCl]

base [def.] *The active part of a compound. In naproxen sodium, for example, the base is naproxen.* [compare to: salt]

basic aluminum acetate [see: aluminum subacetate]

basic aluminum aminoacetate [see: dihydroxyaluminum aminoacetate]

basic aluminum carbonate [see: aluminum carbonate, basic]

basic aluminum chloride [see: aluminum sesquichlorohydrate]

basic aluminum glycinate [see: dihydroxyaluminum aminoacetate]

basic bismuth carbonate [see: bismuth subcarbonate]

basic bismuth gallate [see: bismuth subgallate]

basic bismuth nitrate [see: bismuth subnitrate]

basic bismuth potassium bismuthotartrate [see: bismuth potassium tartrate]

basic bismuth salicylate [see: bismuth subsalicylate]

basic fibroblast growth factor (bFGF) [see: ersofermin]

basic fuchsin [see: fuchsin, basic]

basic zinc acetate [see: zinc acetate, basic]

basifungin USAN, INN *antifungal*

basil (Ocimum basilicum) leaves *medicinal herb for colds, headache, indigestion, insect and snake bites, and whooping cough*

basiliximab USAN *immunosuppressant; IL-2 receptor antagonist for the prevention of acute rejection of renal transplants (orphan)*

basswood; bast tree *medicinal herb* [see: linden tree]

bastard hemp *medicinal herb* [see: hemp nettle]

bastard saffron *medicinal herb* [see: safflower]

batanopride INN *antiemetic* [also: batanopride HCl]

batanopride HCl USAN *antiemetic* [also: batanopride]

batebulast INN

batelapine INN *antipsychotic* [also: batelapine HCl]

batelapine maleate USAN *antipsychotic* [also: batelapine]

batilol INN

batimastat USAN, INN *antineoplastic; matrix metalloproteinase (MMP) inhibitor*

batoprazine INN ☒ butaperazine

batroxobin INN, JAN

batyl alcohol [see: batilol]

batylol [see: batilol]

BAVIP (bleomycin, Adriamycin, vinblastine, imidazole carboxa-

mide, prednisone) *chemotherapy protocol* 🔲 BVAP; BVPP; PVB; PVP

baxitozine INN

bay; bay laurel; bay tree; Indian bay; sweet bay *medicinal herb* [see: laurel]

bay, holly; red bay; white bay *medicinal herb* [see: magnolia]

bayberry (Myrica cerifera) bark, berries, root bark *medicinal herb for cholera, diarrhea, dysentery, glands, goiter, indigestion, jaundice, excessive menstruation, scrofuloderma, and uterine hemorrhage; not generally regarded as safe and effective because of its high tannin content* 🔲 Pap-Urea

Bayer Arthritis Regimen delayed-release enteric-coated tablets OTC *analgesic; antipyretic; anti-inflammatory; antirheumatic* [aspirin] 500 mg

Bayer Aspirin, Genuine; Maximum Bayer Aspirin film-coated tablets, film-coated caplets OTC *analgesic; antipyretic; anti-inflammatory; antirheumatic* [aspirin] 325 mg; 500 mg

Bayer Aspirin Regimen delayed-release enteric-coated tablets and caplets OTC *analgesic; antipyretic; anti-inflammatory; antirheumatic* [aspirin] 81, 325 mg

Bayer Back & Body Pain caplets OTC *analgesic; antipyretic; anti-inflammatory; antirheumatic* [aspirin; caffeine] 500•32.5 mg

Bayer Children's Aspirin chewable tablets OTC *analgesic; antipyretic; anti-inflammatory* [aspirin] 81 mg

Bayer Muscle & Joint Cream OTC *analgesic; mild anesthetic; antipruritic; counterirritant* [methyl salicylate; menthol; camphor] 30%•10%•4%

Bayer Plus caplets OTC *analgesic; antipyretic; anti-inflammatory; antirheumatic* [aspirin (buffered with calcium carbonate, magnesium carbonate, and magnesium oxide)] 500 mg 🔲 propolis

Bayer PM Aspirin Plus Sleep Aid caplet OTC *analgesic; antipyretic; anti-inflammatory; antirheumatic; antihista-*

minic sleep aid [aspirin; diphenhydramine HCl] 500•25 mg

Bayer Select Backache caplets OTC *analgesic; antipyretic; anti-inflammatory; antirheumatic* [magnesium salicylate] 580 mg

Bayer Timed Release, 8-Hour caplets OTC *analgesic; antipyretic; anti-inflammatory; antirheumatic* [aspirin] 650 mg

Bayer Women's Aspirin Plus Calcium caplets OTC *analgesic; antipyretic; anti-inflammatory; antirheumatic; calcium supplement* [aspirin; calcium] 81•300 mg

BayGam IM injection (name changed to **GamaSTAN S/D** in 2007) 🔲 PCM

BayHep B IM injection (name changed to **HyperHEP B S/D** in 2007)

BayRab IM injection (name changed to **HyperRab S/D** in 2007)

BayRho-D Full Dose IM injection in prefilled syringes ℞ *immunizing agent for antenatal or postpartum prophylaxis of Rh hemolytic disease of the newborn* [Rh$_O$(D) immune globulin, solvent/detergent treated] 300 mcg

BayRho-D Mini Dose IM injection (name changed to **HyperRHO S/D Mini-Dose** in 2006)

BayTet IM injection ℞ *passive immunizing agent for post-exposure tetanus prophylaxis in patients with incomplete or uncertain pre-exposure immunization with tetanus toxoids* [tetanus immune globulin, solvent/detergent treated] 250 U

bazedoxifene *second-generation selective estrogen receptor modulator (SERM); investigational (NDA filed) for the prevention and treatment of postmenopausal osteoporosis*

bazinaprine INN

BBVP-M (BCNU, bleomycin, VePesid, prednisone, methotrexate) *chemotherapy protocol*

B$_c$ (vitamin B$_c$) [see: folic acid]

BC Allergy, Sinus, Headache oral powder OTC *decongestant; antihista-*

mine; *analgesic; antipyretic* [pseudo-ephedrine HCl; chlorpheniramine maleate; acetaminophen] 60•4•650 mg/pkt.

BC Arthritis Strength oral powder OTC *analgesic; antipyretic; anti-inflammatory* [aspirin; salicylamide; caffeine] 742•222•38 mg

BC Fast Pain Relief oral powder OTC *analgesic; antipyretic; anti-inflammatory* [aspirin; salicylamide; caffeine] 650•195•33.3 mg/pkt.

B-C with Folic Acid tablets ℞ *vitamin supplement* [multiple B vitamins; vitamin C; folic acid] ≛•500•0.5 mg

B-C with Folic Acid Plus tablets ℞ *vitamin/mineral/iron supplement* [multiple vitamins & minerals; ferrous fumarate; folic acid; biotin] ≛•27•0.8•0.15 mg

BCAA (branched-chain amino acids) [see: isoleucine; leucine; valine]

BCAD 2 powder OTC *enteral nutritional therapy for maple syrup urine disease (MSUD)* ▣ BACOD; BCD; pokeweed

BCAP (BCNU, cyclophosphamide, Adriamycin, prednisone) *chemotherapy protocol* ▣ BACOP; BCOP; BCP; BEACOPP; PCP

BCAVe; B-CAVe (bleomycin, CCNU, Adriamycin, Velban) *chemotherapy protocol for Hodgkin lymphoma* ▣ PCV

B-C-Bid caplets (discontinued 2005) OTC *vitamin supplement* [multiple B vitamins; vitamin C] ≛•300 mg

BCD (bleomycin, cyclophosphamide, dactinomycin) *chemotherapy protocol*

BCG Vaccine powder for multiple dermal puncture device ℞ *active bacterin for tuberculosis prevention* [BCG vaccine, Tice strain] 50 mg (1–8 × 10^8 CFU)

BCG vaccine (bacillus Calmette-Guérin) USP *active bacterin for tuberculosis prevention; antineoplastic for urinary bladder cancer*

B-CHOP (bleomycin, Cytoxin, hydroxydaunomycin, Oncovin, prednisone) *chemotherapy protocol* ▣ BACOP; BCAP; BCOP; BCP; BEACOPP; PCP

BCMF (bleomycin, cyclophosphamide, methotrexate, fluorouracil) *chemotherapy protocol*

BCNU (bis-chloroethyl-nitrosourea) [see: carmustine]

B-Complex elixir OTC *vitamin supplement* [multiple B vitamins] ▣ B Complex + C

B-Complex and B-12 tablets OTC *vitamin supplement* [multiple B vitamins; protease] ≛•10 mg

B-Complex with B-12 tablets OTC *vitamin supplement* [multiple B vitamins] ▣ B Complex with C and B-12

B-Complex/Vitamin C caplets OTC *vitamin supplement* [multiple B vitamins; vitamin C] ≛•300 mg

BCOP (BCNU, cyclophosphamide, Oncovin, prednisone) *chemotherapy protocol* ▣ BACOP; BCAP; BCP; BEACOPP; PCP

BCP (BCNU, cyclophosphamide, prednisone) *chemotherapy protocol*

BCVP (BCNU, cyclophosphamide, vincristine, prednisone) *chemotherapy protocol*

BCVPP (BCNU, cyclophosphamide, vinblastine, procarbazine, prednisone) *chemotherapy protocol for Hodgkin lymphoma*

B-D glucose chewable tablets OTC *blood glucose elevating agent for hypoglycemia* [glucose] 5 g

BDNF (brain-derived neurotrophic factor) [see: methionyl neurotropic factor, brain-derived]

BDO (1,4-butanediol) *a precursor to gamma hydroxybutyrate (GHB); a formerly legal alternative to GHB, now also illegal (Schedule I)* [see: gamma hydroxybutyrate (GHB)]

B-DOPA (bleomycin, DTIC, Oncovin, prednisone, Adriamycin) *chemotherapy protocol*

BDP (beclomethasone dipropionate) [q.v.]

BEAC (BCNU, etoposide, ara-C, cyclophosphamide) *chemotherapy protocol*

BEACOPP (bleomycin, etoposide, Adriamycin, cyclophosphamide, Oncovin, procarbazine, prednisone, [filgrastim]) *chemotherapy protocol for Hodgkin lymphoma* ② BACOP; BCAP; BCOP; BCP; PCP

BEAM (BCNU, etoposide, ara-C, melphalan) *chemotherapy protocol*

bean herb *medicinal herb* [see: summer savory]

bean trefoil *medicinal herb* [see: buckbean]

Beano oral liquid, tablets OTC *digestive aid* [alpha-D-galactosidase enzyme]

bearberry *medicinal herb* [see: uva ursi]

beard, old man's *medicinal herb* [see: fringe tree; woodbine]

Bear-E-Bag Pediatric rectal suspension (discontinued 2004) ℞ *radiopaque contrast medium for gastrointestinal imaging* [barium sulfate] 95%

Bear-E-Yum CT oral suspension ℞ *radiopaque contrast medium for gastrointestinal imaging* [barium sulfate] 1.5%

Bear-E-Yum GI oral suspension ℞ *radiopaque contrast medium for gastrointestinal imaging* [barium sulfate] 60% ② Promega

bear's grape *medicinal herb* [see: uva ursi]

bear's weed *medicinal herb* [see: yerba santa]

bearsfoot *medicinal herb* [see: hellebore]

Beaumont root *medicinal herb* [see: Culver root]

beaver tree *medicinal herb* [see: magnolia]

Bebulin VH powder for IV injection ℞ *systemic hemostatic; antihemophilic for factor IX deficiency (hemophilia B; Christmas disease) (orphan)* [coagulation factors II, IX, and X, heat treated] (actual number of units is indicated on the vial)

becanthone HCl USAN *antischistosomal* [also: becantone]

becantone INN *antischistosomal* [also: becanthone HCl]

becantone HCl [see: becanthone HCl]

becaplermin USAN *recombinant platelet-derived growth factor B for chronic diabetic foot ulcers*

beciparcil INN

beclamide INN, BAN

becliconazole INN

beclobrate INN, BAN

beclometasone INN *corticosteroidal inhalant for asthma; intranasal steroid* [also: beclomethasone dipropionate; beclomethasone; beclometasone dipropionate]

beclometasone dipropionate JAN *corticosteroidal inhalant for asthma; intranasal steroid* [also: beclomethasone dipropionate; beclomethasone; beclometasone]

beclomethasone BAN *corticosteroidal anti-inflammatory for chronic asthma* [also: beclomethasone dipropionate; beclometasone; beclometasone dipropionate]

beclomethasone dipropionate (BDP) USAN, USP *corticosteroidal anti-inflammatory for chronic asthma and rhinitis; investigational (Phase III, orphan) oral treatment for intestinal graft vs. host disease* [also: beclometasone; beclomethasone; beclometasone dipropionate]

beclotiamine INN

Beconase nasal inhalation aerosol (discontinued 2004) ℞ *corticosteroidal anti-inflammatory for seasonal or perennial rhinitis* [beclomethasone dipropionate] 42 mcg/dose

Beconase AQ nasal spray ℞ *corticosteroidal anti-inflammatory for seasonal or perennial rhinitis* [beclomethasone dipropionate] 0.042% (42 mcg/dose)

bectumomab USAN *monoclonal antibody IgG$_{2a}$ to B cell, murine* [also: technetium Tc 99m bectumomab]

bedstraw (Galium aparine; G. verum) plant *medicinal herb used as an anti-*

spasmodic, aperient, diaphoretic, diuretic, and vulnerary

bee balm *medicinal herb* [see: lemon balm]

bee pollen *natural remedy for anemia, bodily weakness, cerebral hemorrhage, colitis, constipation, enteritis, and weight loss; also used as an anti-aging agent and prenatal nutritional supplement; not generally regarded as safe and effective because of widespread allergic reactions*

bee venom (derived from Apis mellifera) *natural remedy for arthritis and multiple sclerosis, and for hyposensitization of persons highly sensitive to bee stings*

beechwood creosote [see: creosote carbonate]

beef tallow JAN

Beelith tablets OTC *dietary supplement* [vitamin B_6; magnesium oxide] 20•362 mg

bee's nest plant *medicinal herb* [see: carrot]

beeswax, white JAN [also: wax, white]

beeswax, yellow JAN [also: wax, yellow]

Bee-Zee tablets OTC *vitamin/zinc supplement* [multiple vitamins; zinc] ±•22.5 mg

befiperide INN

Be-Flex Plus capsules R *antihistamine; sleep aid; analgesic; antipyretic* [phenyltoloxamine citrate; acetaminophen; salicylamide] 20•300•200 mg

befloxatone INN

befunolol INN [also: befunolol HCl] ⊡ pafenolol

befunolol HCl JAN [also: befunolol]

befuraline INN ⊡ bufrolin

behenyl alcohol [see: docosanol]

behepan [see: cyanocobalamin]

bekanamycin INN *antibiotic* [also: bekanamycin sulfate]

bekanamycin sulfate JAN *antibiotic* [also: bekanamycin]

belarizine INN ⊡ plauracin

belfosdil USAN, INN *antihypertensive; calcium channel blocker*

Belganyl (available only from the Centers for Disease Control) R *antiparasitic for African trypanosomiasis and onchocerciasis* [suramin sodium] ⊡ Plaquenil

belimumab *investigational (Phase III) human monoclonal antibody to B-lymphocyte for active systemic lupus erythematosus (SLE)*

Bellacane elixir (discontinued 2008) R *GI/GU anticholinergic/antispasmodic; sedative* [atropine sulfate; scopolamine hydrobromide; hyoscyamine sulfate; phenobarbital] 0.0194•0.0065•0.1037•16.2 mg/5 mL ⊡ bulaquine; Pilagan; Polocaine

Bellacane tablets (discontinued 2008) R *GI/GU anticholinergic/antispasmodic; sedative* [hyoscyamine sulfate; phenobarbital] 0.125•15 mg ⊡ bulaquine; Pilagan; Polocaine

Bellacane SR sustained-release tablets (discontinued 2008) R *GI/GU anticholinergic/antispasmodic; sedative; analgesic* [belladonna alkaloids; phenobarbital; ergotamine tartrate] 0.2•40•0.6 mg

belladonna (Atropa belladonna) leaves, tops, and berries *medicinal herb used as an antispasmodic, calmative, diaphoretic, diuretic, and narcotic* ⊡ Paladin; Polydine

belladonna alkaloids *a class of GI/GU anticholinergic/antispasmodics that includes atropine sulfate, scopolamine hydrobromide, hyoscyamine hydrobromide, and hyoscyamine sulfate*

belladonna alkaloids & phenobarbital *GI/GU anticholinergic/antispasmodic; sedative* 0.13•16.2 mg oral

belladonna extract USP *GI/GU anticholinergic/antispasmodic; antiparkinsonian; respiratory antisecretory* 27–33 mg/100 mL oral

Bellahist-D LA sustained-release caplets R *decongestant; antihistamine; anticholinergic to dry mucosal secretions* [phenylephrine HCl; chlorpheniramine maleate; hyoscyamine sulfate;

atropine sulfate; scopolamine hydrobromide] 20•8•0.19•0.04•0.01 mg

Bellamine tablets ℞ *GI/GU anticholinergic/antispasmodic; sedative; analgesic* [belladonna alkaloids; phenobarbital; ergotamine tartrate] 0.2•40•0.6 mg

Bell/ans tablets OTC *antacid* [sodium bicarbonate] 520 mg ◙ polyenes

Bellatal tablets ℞ *long-acting barbiturate sedative, hypnotic, and anticonvulsant* [phenobarbital] 16.2 mg ◙ Pletal

Bellergal·S tablets (discontinued 2008) ℞ *GI/GU anticholinergic/antispasmodic; sedative; analgesic* [belladonna extract; phenobarbital; ergotamine tartrate] 0.2•40•0.6 mg

Bellis perennis medicinal herb [see: wild daisy]

bells, May medicinal herb [see: lily of the valley]

beloxamide USAN, INN *antihyperlipoproteinemic*

beloxepin USAN *norepinephrine uptake inhibitor for depression*

Bel-Phen-Ergot SR sustained-release tablets ℞ *GI/GU anticholinergic/antispasmodic; sedative; analgesic* [belladonna alkaloids; phenobarbital; ergotamine tartrate] 0.2•40•0.6 mg

bemarinone INN *cardiotonic; positive inotropic; vasodilator* [also: bemarinone HCl]

bemarinone HCl USAN *cardiotonic; positive inotropic; vasodilator* [also: bemarinone]

bemegride USP, INN, BAN, JAN

bemesetron USAN, INN *antiemetic*

bemetizide INN, BAN

Beminal 500 tablets OTC *vitamin supplement* [multiple B vitamins; vitamin C] ±•500 mg

bemitradine USAN, INN *antihypertensive; diuretic*

bemoradan USAN, INN *cardiotonic*

BEMP (bleomycin, Eldisine, mitomycin, Platinol) *chemotherapy protocol* ◙ B-MOPP; BMP; BOMP; POMP

benactyzine INN, BAN

benactyzine HCl *mild antidepressant; anticholinergic*

Benadryl IV or IM injection ℞ *antihistamine; motion sickness preventative; sleep aid* [diphenhydramine HCl] 50 mg/mL

Benadryl; Benadryl 2% cream, spray OTC *antihistamine* [diphenhydramine HCl] 1%; 2%

Benadryl Allergy Liqui-Gels (liquid-filled gelcaps), Kapseals (sealed capsules), Ultratabs (tablets), chewable tablets OTC *antihistamine; sleep aid* [diphenhydramine HCl] 25 mg; 25 mg; 25 mg; 12.5 mg

Benadryl Allergy & Cold caplets OTC *decongestant; antihistamine; sleep aid; analgesic* [phenylephrine HCl; diphenhydramine HCl; acetaminophen] 5•12.5•325 mg

Benadryl Allergy Quick Dissolve Strips OTC *antihistamine; sleep aid* [diphenhydramine HCl] 25 mg

Benadryl Allergy & Sinus tablets, oral liquid (discontinued 2007) OTC *decongestant; antihistamine; sleep aid* [pseudoephedrine HCl; diphenhydramine HCl] 60•25 mg; 60•25 mg/10 mL

Benadryl Allergy & Sinus Fastmelt (orally dissolving tablets) (discontinued 2007) OTC *decongestant; antihistamine; sleep aid* [pseudoephedrine HCl; diphenhydramine citrate] 30•19 mg

Benadryl Allergy & Sinus Headache caplets OTC *decongestant; antihistamine; sleep aid; analgesic; antipyretic* [phenylephrine HCl; diphenhydramine HCl; acetaminophen] 5•12.5•325 mg

Benadryl Allergy & Sinus Headache gelcaps (discontinued 2007) OTC *decongestant; antihistamine; sleep aid; analgesic; antipyretic* [phenylephrine HCl; diphenhydramine HCl; acetaminophen] 5•12.5•500 mg

Benadryl Children's Allergy oral liquid OTC *antihistamine; sleep aid* [diphenhydramine HCl] 12.5 mg/5 mL

Benadryl Children's Allergy & Cold Fastmelt (orally dissolving tablets) (discontinued 2007) OTC *decongestant; antihistamine; sleep aid* [pseudoephedrine HCl; diphenhydramine citrate] 30•19 mg

Benadryl Children's Allergy Fastmelt (orally disintegrating tablets) OTC *antihistamine; sleep aid* [diphenhydramine citrate] 19 mg

Benadryl Children's Allergy & Sinus oral liquid OTC *decongestant; antihistamine; sleep aid* [pseudoephedrine HCl; diphenhydramine citrate] 30•19 mg/5 mL

Benadryl Decongestant Allergy film-coated tablets OTC *decongestant; antihistamine; sleep aid* [pseudoephedrine HCl; diphenhydramine HCl] 60•25 mg

Benadryl Itch Relief spray, cream, stick OTC *antihistamine; astringent* [diphenhydramine HCl; zinc acetate] 2%•0.1%

Benadryl Itch Relief, Children's spray, cream OTC *antihistamine; astringent* [diphenhydramine HCl; zinc acetate] 1%•0.1%

Benadryl Itch Stopping Gel; Benadryl Itch Stopping Gel Children's Formula OTC *antihistamine; astringent* [diphenhydramine HCl; zinc acetate] 2%•1%; 1%•1%

Benadryl Itch Stopping Spray OTC *antihistamine; astringent* [diphenhydramine HCl; zinc acetate; alcohol] 1%•0.1%•73.6%, 2%•0.1%•73.5%

Benadryl Severe Allergy & Sinus Headache caplets OTC *decongestant; antihistamine; sleep aid; analgesic; antipyretic* [phenylephrine HCl; diphenhydramine HCl; acetaminophen] 5•25•325 mg

Benadryl-D Allergy & Sinus tablets OTC *decongestant; antihistamine; sleep aid* [phenylephrine HCl; diphenhydramine HCl] 10•25 mg

Benadryl-D Children's Allergy & Sinus oral liquid OTC *decongestant; antihistamine; sleep aid* [pseudoephedrine HCl; diphenhydramine HCl] 30•12.5 mg

benafentrine INN

benanserin HCl

benapen [see: benethamine penicillin]

benaprizine INN *anticholinergic* [also: benapryzine HCl; benapryzine]

benapryzine BAN *anticholinergic* [also: benapryzine HCl; benaprizine]

benapryzine HCl USAN *anticholinergic* [also: benaprizine; benapryzine]

benaxibine INN 🔲 pinoxepin

benazepril INN, BAN *antihypertensive; angiotensin-converting enzyme (ACE) inhibitor* [also: benazepril HCl]

benazepril HCl USAN *antihypertensive; angiotensin-converting enzyme (ACE) inhibitor; also used for nondiabetic neuropathy* [also: benazepril] 5, 10, 20, 40 mg oral

benazepril HCl & amlodipine besylate *antihypertensive; calcium channel blocker; angiotensin-converting enzyme (ACE) inhibitor* 10•2.5, 10•5, 20•5, 20•10 mg

benazepril HCl & hydrochlorothiazide *antihypertensive; angiotensin-converting enzyme (ACE) inhibitor; diuretic* 5•6.25, 10•12.5, 20•12.5, 20•25 mg oral

benazeprilat USAN, INN *antihypertensive; angiotensin-converting enzyme (ACE) inhibitor*

bencianol INN

bencisteine INN

benclonidine INN

bencyclane INN [also: bencyclane fumarate]

bencyclane fumarate JAN [also: bencyclane]

bendacalol mesylate USAN *antihypertensive*

bendamustine HCl INN *purine analogue; alkylating antineoplastic for chronic lymphocytic leukemia (orphan); derivative of mechlorethamine HCl; investigational (NDA filed, orphan) for non-Hodgkin lymphoma*

bendazac USAN, INN, BAN, JAN *antiinflammatory*

bendazol INN ② panidazole

benderizine INN

bendrofluazide BAN *diuretic; antihypertensive* [also: bendroflumethiazide]

bendroflumethiazide USP, INN *diuretic; antihypertensive* [also: bendrofluazide]

bendroflumethiazide & nadolol *antihypertensive; diuretic; β-blocker* 5•40, 5•80 mg oral

bendroflumethiazide & rauwolfia serpentina *antihypertensive; diuretic; peripheral antiadrenergic* 4•50 mg oral

Benefiber powder for oral solution OTC *dietary fiber supplement* [guar gum] 3 g fiber per pkt. or tbsp.

BeneFin *investigational (Phase III, orphan) angiogenesis inhibitor for the treatment of solid tumors* [squalamine (shark cartilage powder)]

BeneFIX ("Factor IX") powder for IV injection Ɍ *systemic hemostatic; antihemophilic for factor IX deficiency (hemophilia B; Christmas disease) (orphan)* [nonacog alfa (synthetic coagulation factor IX)] 250, 500, 1000, 2000 U

benethamine penicillin INN, BAN

benexate INN

benexate HCl JAN

benfluorex INN

benfosformin INN

benfotiamine INN, JAN *lipophilic form of vitamin B_1 (thiamine)* [compare: thiamine; thiamine HCl]

benfurodil hemisuccinate INN

bengal gelatin [see: agar]

Ben-Gay, Arthritis Formula cream OTC *analgesic; mild anesthetic; antipruritic; counterirritant* [methyl salicylate; menthol] 30%•8%

Ben-Gay Original ointment OTC *analgesic; mild anesthetic; antipruritic; counterirritant* [methyl salicylate; menthol] 18.3%•16%

Ben-Gay Patch OTC *mild anesthetic; antipruritic; counterirritant* [menthol] 1.4%

Ben-Gay Regular Strength cream OTC *analgesic; mild anesthetic; antipru-*

ritic; counterirritant [methyl salicylate; menthol] 15%•10%

Ben-Gay SPA cream (discontinued 2004) OTC *mild anesthetic; antipruritic; counterirritant* [menthol] 10%

Ben-Gay Ultra Strength cream OTC *analgesic; mild anesthetic; antipruritic; counterirritant* [methyl salicylate; menthol; camphor] 30%•10%•4%

Ben-Gay Vanishing Scent gel OTC *mild anesthetic; antipruritic; counterirritant* [menthol; camphor] 3%• ②

benhepazone INN

Benicar film-coated tablets Ɍ *antihypertensive; angiotensin II receptor antagonist* [olmesartan medoxomil] 5, 20, 40 mg ② Penecare

Benicar HCT film-coated tablets Ɍ *antihypertensive; angiotensin II receptor antagonist; diuretic* [olmesartan medoxomil; hydrochlorothiazide] 20•12.5, 40•12.5, 40•25 mg

benidipine INN

benmoxin INN

benolizime INN

Benoquin cream Ɍ *depigmenting agent for vitiligo* [monobenzone] 20%

benorilate INN [also: benorylate]

benorterone USAN, INN *antiandrogen*

benorylate BAN [also: benorilate]

benoxafos INN

benoxaprofen USAN, INN, BAN *antiinflammatory; analgesic*

benoxinate HCl USP *topical ophthalmic anesthetic* [also: oxybuprocaine; oxybuprocaine HCl]

benpenolisin INN

benperidol USAN, INN, BAN *antipsychotic*

benproperine INN [also: benproperine phosphate]

benproperine phosphate JAN [also: benproperine]

benrixate INN

Bensal HP ointment Ɍ *antifungal; keratolytic* [benzoic acid; salicylic acid] 6%•3%

bensalan USAN, INN *disinfectant*

benserazide USAN, INN, BAN *decarboxylase inhibitor; antiparkinsonian adjunct* [also: benserazide HCl]

benserazide HCl JAN *decarboxylase inhibitor; antiparkinsonian adjunct* [also: benserazide]

bensuldazic acid INN, BAN

Bensulfoid cream OTC *antiseptic, antifungal, and keratolytic for acne* [colloidal sulfur; resorcinol; alcohol] 8%•2%•12%

bensylyte HCl [see: phenoxybenzamine HCl]

Ben-Tann oral suspension R *antihistamine; sleep aid* [diphenhydramine tannate] 25 mg/5 mL ⓈPanitone-500

bentazepam USAN, INN *sedative*

bentemazole INN

bentiamine INN

bentipimine INN

bentiromide USAN, INN, BAN, JAN *diagnostic aid for pancreas function*

bentonite NF, JAN *suspending agent*

bentoquatam USAN *topical skin protectant for allergic contact dermatitis and poison ivy exposure*

Bentyl capsules, tablets, syrup, IM injection R *gastrointestinal anticholinergic/antispasmodic for irritable bowel syndrome (IBS)* [dicyclomine HCl] 10 mg; 20 mg; 10 mg/5 mL; 10 mg/mL Ⓢ peanut oil

benurestat USAN, INN *urease enzyme inhibitor*

Benylin Adult oral liquid (discontinued 2006) OTC *antitussive* [dextromethorphan hydrobromide] 15 mg/5 mL

Benylin Expectorant oral liquid (discontinued 2007) OTC *antitussive; expectorant* [dextromethorphan hydrobromide; guaifenesin] 20•400 mg/20 mL

Benylin Pediatric oral liquid (discontinued 2006) OTC *antitussive* [dextromethorphan hydrobromide] 7.5 mg/5 mL

Benz 42 *hydrophilic contact lens material* [hefilcon A] Ⓢ Pannaz

Benza topical solution OTC *antiseptic* [benzalkonium chloride] 1:750 Ⓢ Pannaz

Benzac 5; Benzac 10 gel R *keratolytic and antiseptic for acne* [benzoyl peroxide; alcohol] 5%•12%; 10%•12%

Benzac AC 2½; Benzac W 2½; Benzac AC 5; Benzac W 5; Benzac AC 10; Benzac W 10 gel R *keratolytic for acne* [benzoyl peroxide] 2.5%; 2.5%; 5%; 5%; 10%; 10%

Benzac AC Wash 2½; Benzac AC Wash 5; Benzac W Wash 5; Benzac AC Wash 10; Benzac W Wash 10 topical liquid R *keratolytic for acne* [benzoyl peroxide] 2.5%; 5%; 5%; 10%; 10%

BenzaClin gel R *antibiotic and keratolytic for acne* [clindamycin phosphate; benzoyl peroxide] 1%•5%

Benzagel Wash gel R *keratolytic and antiseptic for acne* [benzoyl peroxide; alcohol] 10%•14%

benzaldehyde NF *flavoring agent*

benzalkonium chloride (BAC) NF, INN, BAN, JAN *preservative; bacteriostatic antiseptic; surfactant/wetting agent* 17% topical

Benzamine (trademarked ingredient) *antioxidant; a proprietary blend of the nutritional supplements aminobenzoic acid, vitamin E, and alpha lipoic acid (ALA); also known as* **Primorine**

Benzamycin gel R *antibiotic and keratolytic for acne* [erythromycin; benzoyl peroxide; alcohol 20%] 3%•5%

benzaprinoxide INN

benzarone INN

benzathine benzylpenicillin INN *natural penicillin antibiotic* [also: penicillin G benzathine; benzathine penicillin; benzylpenicillin benzathine]

benzathine penicillin BAN *natural penicillin antibiotic* [also: penicillin G benzathine; benzathine benzylpenicillin; benzylpenicillin benzathine]

benzathine penicillin G [see: penicillin G benzathine]

benzatropine INN *antiparkinsonian; anticholinergic* [also: benztropine mesylate; benztropine]

benzazoline HCl [see: tolazoline HCl]

benzbromaron JAN *uricosuric* [also: benzbromarone]

benzbromarone USAN, INN, BAN *uricosuric* [also: benzbromaron]

benzchinamide [see: benzquinamide]

benzchlorpropamide [see: beclamide]

Benzedrex inhaler ℞ *nasal decongestant* [propylhexedrine] 250 mg

benzene ethanol [see: phenylethyl alcohol]

benzene hexachloride, gamma [now: lindane]

benzeneacetic acid, sodium salt [see: sodium phenylacetate]

benzenebutanoic acid, sodium salt [see: sodium phenylbutyrate]

1,3-benzenediol [see: resorcinol]

benzenemethanol [see: benzyl alcohol]

benzestrofol [see: estradiol benzoate]

benzestrol USP, INN, BAN

benzethacil [see: penicillin G benzathine]

benzethidine INN, BAN

benzethonium chloride USP, INN, BAN, JAN *topical anti-infective; preservative*

benzetimide INN *anticholinergic* [also: benzetimide HCl]

benzetimide HCl USAN *anticholinergic* [also: benzetimide]

benzfetamine INN *anorexiant; CNS stimulant* [also: benzphetamine HCl; benzphetamine]

benzhexol BAN *anticholinergic; antiparkinsonian* [also: trihexyphenidyl HCl; trihexyphenidyl]

N-benzhydryl-N-methylpiperazine [see: cyclizine HCl]

benzilone bromide [see: benzilonium bromide]

benzilonium bromide USAN, INN, BAN *anticholinergic*

benzimidavir *investigational (Phase II) DNA inhibitor for AIDS-related cytomegalovirus infection*

2-benzimidazolepropionic acid [see: procodazole]

benzimidazoles, substituted *a class of gastric antisecretory agents that inhibit the aTPase "proton pump" within the* cell [also called: proton pump inhibitors; aTPase inhibitors]

benzin, petroleum JAN

benzindamine HCl [see: benzydamine HCl]

benzindopyrine INN *antipsychotic* [also: benzindopyrine HCl]

benzindopyrine HCl USAN *antipsychotic* [also: benzindopyrine]

benzinoform [see: carbon tetrachloride]

benziodarone INN, BAN

Benziq; Benziq LS gel ℞ *keratolytic for acne* [benzoyl peroxide] 5.25%; 2.75%

Benziq Wash ℞ *keratolytic for acne* [benzoyl peroxide] 5.25%

benzisoxazoles *a class of novel (atypical) antipsychotic agents*

benzmalecene INN

benzmethoxazone [see: chlorthenoxazine]

benznidazole INN

benzoaric acid [see: ellagic acid]

benzoate & phenylacetate [see: sodium benzoate & sodium phenylacetate]

benzobarbital INN

benzocaine USP, INN, BAN *topical anesthetic; mucous membrane anesthetic; nonprescription diet aid* [also: ethyl aminobenzoate] 5% topical

benzoclidine INN

benzoctamine INN, BAN *sedative; muscle relaxant* [also: benzoctamine HCl]

benzoctamine HCl USAN, INN *sedative; muscle relaxant* [also: benzoctamine]

Benzodent oral ointment OTC *mucous membrane anesthetic* [benzocaine] 20%

benzodepa USAN, INN *antineoplastic*

benzodiazepine HCl [see: medazepam HCl]

benzodiazepines *a class of nonbarbiturate sedative/hypnotics and anticonvulsants*

benzododecinium chloride INN

benzogynestryl [see: estradiol benzoate]

benzoic acid USP, JAN *antifungal; urinary acidifier*

benzoic acid, phenylmethyl ester [see: benzyl benzoate]

benzoic acid, potassium salt [see: potassium benzoate]

benzoic acid, sodium salt [see: sodium benzoate]

benzoin USP, JAN *topical protectant*

Benzoin Compound tincture OTC *skin protectant; antiseptic* [benzoin; aloe; alcohol 74–80%]

benzol [see: benzene ...]

benzonatate USP, INN, BAN *antitussive* 100, 200 mg oral

benzophenone

benzopyrrolate [see: benzopyrronium]

benzopyrronium bromide INN

benzoquinamide HCl *post-anesthesia antiemetic*

benzoquinone amidoinohydrazone thiosemicarbazone hydrate [see: ambazone]

benzoquinonium chloride

benzorphanol [see: levophenacylmorphan]

Benz-O-Sthetic aerosol spray, gel OTC *anesthetic* [benzocaine] 20%

benzosulfinide [see: saccharin]

benzosulphinide sodium [see: saccharin sodium]

benzothiazepines *a class of calcium channel blockers*

benzothiozon [see: thioacetazone; thiacetazone]

benzotript INN

benzoxiquine USAN, INN *antiseptic/disinfectant*

benzoxonium chloride INN

benzoyl *p*-aminosalicylate (B-PAS) [see: benzoylpas calcium]

benzoyl peroxide USAN, USP *keratolytic* 2.5%, 5%, 10% topical

benzoyl peroxide & erythromycin *keratolytic and antibiotic for acne* 5%• 3% topical

***m*-benzoylhydratropic acid** [see: ketoprofen]

benzoylmethylecgonine [see: cocaine]

benzoylpas calcium USAN, USP *antibacterial; tuberculostatic* [also: calcium benzamidosalicylate]

benzoylsulfanilamide [see: sulfabenzamide]

benzoylthiamindisulfide [see: bisbentiamine]

benzoylthiaminmonophosphate [see: benfotiamine]

benzphetamine BAN *anorexiant; CNS stimulant* [also: benzphetamine HCl; benzfetamine]

benzphetamine chloride [see: benzphetamine HCl]

benzphetamine HCl NF *anorexiant; CNS stimulant* [also: benzfetamine; benzphetamine] 50 mg oral

benzpiperylon [see: benzpiperylone]

benzpiperylone INN

benzpyrinium bromide NF, INN

benzquercin INN

benzquinamide USAN, INN, BAN *post-anesthesia antinauseant and antiemetic*

benzthiazide USP, INN, BAN *diuretic; antihypertensive*

benztropine BAN *anticholinergic; antiparkinsonian* [also: benztropine mesylate; benzatropine]

benztropine mesylate USP *anticholinergic; antiparkinsonian* [also: benzatropine; benztropine] 0.5, 1, 2 mg oral

benztropine methanesulfonate [see: benztropine mesylate]

benzydamine INN, BAN *analgesic; antipyretic; anti-inflammatory* [also: benzydamine HCl]

benzydamine HCl USAN, JAN *analgesic; antipyretic; anti-inflammatory; investigational (orphan) radioprotectant for oral mucosa following radiation therapy for head and neck cancer* [also: benzydamine]

benzydroflumethiazide [see: bendroflumethiazide]

benzyl alcohol NF, INN, JAN *antimicrobial agent; antiseptic; local anesthetic*

benzyl analogue of serotonin (BAS) [see: benanserin HCl]

benzyl antiserotonin [see: benanserin HCl]

benzyl benzoate USP, JAN

benzyl carbinol [see: phenylethyl alcohol]

***S*-benzyl thiobenzoate** [see: tibenzate]

benzylamide [see: beclamide]

benzylamines *a class of antifungals structurally related to the allylamines*

N-benzylanilinoacetamidoxime [see: cetoxime]

2-benzylbenzimidazole [see: bendazol]

benzyldimethyltetradecylammonium chloride [see: miristalkonium chloride]

benzyldodecyldimethylammonium chloride [see: benzododecinium chloride]

0-6-benzylguanine [see: alkylade]

benzylhexadecyldimethylammonium [see: cetalkonium]

benzylhexadecyldimethylammonium chloride [see: cetalkonium chloride]

benzylhydrochlorothiazide JAN

p-benzyloxyphenol [see: monobenzone]

benzylpenicillin INN, BAN *natural penicillin antibiotic; investigational (orphan) for penicillin hypersensitivity assessment*

benzylpenicillin benzathine JAN *natural penicillin antibiotic* [also: penicillin G benzathine; benzathine benzylpenicillin; benzathine penicillin]

benzylpenicillin potassium BAN, JAN *natural penicillin antibiotic* [also: penicillin G potassium]

benzylpenicillin procaine *natural penicillin antibiotic* [see: penicillin G procaine]

benzylpenicillin sodium BAN *natural penicillin antibiotic* [also: penicillin G sodium]

benzylpenicilloic acid [see: benzylpenicillin]

benzylpenicilloyl polylysine USP *diagnostic aid for penicillin sensitivity*

benzylpenilloic acid [see: benzylpenicillin]

benzylsulfamide INN

benzylsulfanilamide [see: benzylsulfamide]

BEP (bleomycin, etoposide, Platinol) *chemotherapy protocol for testicular cancer and germ cell tumors*

bepafant INN

bepanthen [see: panthenol]

beperidium iodide INN

bephene oxinaphthoate [see: bephenium hydroxynaphthoate]

bephenium embonate [see: bephenium hydroxynaphthoate]

bephenium hydroxynaphthoate USP, INN, BAN

bepiastine INN

bepridil INN, BAN *vasodilator; antianginal; calcium channel blocker* [also: bepridil HCl]

bepridil HCl USAN *vasodilator; antianginal; calcium channel blocker* [also: bepridil]

beractant USAN *pulmonary surfactant for neonatal respiratory distress syndrome or respiratory failure (orphan)*

beraprost USAN, INN *platelet aggregation inhibitor; peripheral vasodilator; prostacyclin analogue; investigational (orphan) for pulmonary arterial hypertension (PAH)*

beraprost sodium USAN *platelet aggregation inhibitor*

berberine chloride JAN

berberine sulfate JAN

berberine tannate JAN

Berberis vulgaris *medicinal herb* [see: barberry]

berculon A [see: thioacetazone; thiacetazone]

berefrine USAN, INN *mydriatic*

bergamot, scarlet *medicinal herb* [see: Oswego tea]

bergamot, wild *medicinal herb* [see: wild bergamot]

bergamot oil (Citrus aurantium; C. bergamia) *fruit peel medicinal herb used in conjunction with long-wave UV light therapy for psoriasis and vitiligo; not generally regarded as safe and effective because of its photosensitizing properties*

bergenin JAN

Berinert-P *investigational (orphan) agent to prevent or treat acute attacks of angioedema* [C1-esterase-inhibitor, human]

berkelium *element (Bk)* ⊗ brooklime

berlafenone INN

bermastine [see: barmastine]

bermoprofen INN

Berocca tablets ℞ *vitamin supplement* [multiple B vitamins; vitamin C; folic acid] ± • 500•0.5 mg ⓡ Pro-Q

Berocca Plus tablets ℞ *vitamin/mineral/iron supplement* [multiple vitamins & minerals; ferrous fumarate; folic acid; biotin] ± •27•0.8•0.15 mg

bertosamil INN

beryllium *element (Be)*

berythromycin USAN, INN *antiamebic; antibacterial*

besigomsin INN

besilate INN *combining name for radicals or groups* [also: besylate]

besipirdine INN *cognition enhancer for Alzheimer disease* [also: besipiridine HCl]

besipirdine HCl USAN *cognition enhancer for Alzheimer disease* [also: besipiridine]

besulpamide INN

besunide INN

besylate USAN *combining name for radicals or groups* [also: besilate]

beta alethine *investigational (orphan) antineoplastic and immunostimulant multiple myeloma and metastatic melanoma*

beta blockers (β-blockers) *a class of cardiac agents characterized by their antihypertensive, antiarrhythmic, and antianginal actions; a class of topical antiglaucoma agents* [also called: beta-adrenergic antagonists]

beta carotene USAN, USP *vitamin A precursor* [also: betacarotene] 15 mg (25 000 IU) oral

beta cyclodextrin (β-cyclodextrin) [now: betadex]

betacarotene INN *vitamin A precursor* [also: beta carotene]

betacetylmethadol INN, BAN

betadex USAN, INN *sequestering agent*

beta-D-galactosidase *digestive enzyme* [see: tilactase]

Betadine aerosol, gauze pads, lubricating gel, cream, ointment, skin cleanser, foam, solution, swab, swabsticks OTC *broad-spectrum antimicrobial* [povidone-iodine] 5%; 10%; 5%; 5%; 10%; 7.5%; 7.5%; 10%; 10%; 10%

Betadine shampoo OTC *broad-spectrum antimicrobial for dandruff* [povidone-iodine] 7.5%

Betadine 5% Sterile Ophthalmic Prep solution ℞ *broad-spectrum antimicrobial for eye surgery* [povidone-iodine] 5%

Betadine First Aid Antibiotics Plus Moisturizer ointment OTC *antibiotic* [polymyxin B sulfate; bacitracin zinc] 10 000•500 IU/g

Betadine Medicated vaginal suppositories, vaginal gel OTC *antiseptic/germicidal cleanser and deodorant* [povidone-iodine] 10%

Betadine Medicated Douche; Betadine Medicated Disposable Douche; Betadine Premixed Medicated Disposable Douche vaginal solution OTC *antiseptic/germicidal cleanser and deodorant* [povidone-iodine] 10%

Betadine Plus First Aid Antibiotics and Pain Reliever ointment OTC *antibiotic; anesthetic* [polymyxin B sulfate; bacitracin zinc; pramoxine HCl] 10 000 IU•500 IU•10 mg per g

Betadine PrepStick swab OTC *broad-spectrum antimicrobial* [povidone-iodine] 10%

Betadine PrepStick Plus swab OTC *broad-spectrum antimicrobial* [povidone-iodine; alcohol] 10%• ±

beta-estradiol [see: estradiol]

beta-estradiol benzoate [see: estradiol benzoate]

betaeucaine HCl [now: eucaine HCl]

Betagan Liquifilm eye drops ℞ *antiglaucoma agent* (β-blocker) [levobunolol HCl] 0.25%, 0.5%

Betagen ointment, solution, surgical scrub OTC *broad-spectrum antimicrobial* [povidone-iodine] 1%; 10%; 7.5% ⓡ butacaine

beta-glucocerebrosidase [see: alglucerase]

betahistine INN, BAN *vasodilator* [also: betahistine HCl; betahistine mesilate]

betahistine HCl USAN *vasodilator; treatment for vertigo due to Meniere syndrome* [also: betahistine; betahistine mesilate]

betahistine mesilate JAN *vasodilator* [also: betahistine HCl; betahistine]

beta-hypophamine [see: vasopressin]

betaine HCl USP *electrolyte replenisher for homocystinuria* (orphan)

Betaject 3 (trademarked delivery device) *automatic subcutaneous self-injector for* **Betaseron**

beta-lactams *a class of antibiotics*

beta-lactone [see: propiolactone]

betameprodine INN, BAN

betamethadol INN, BAN

betamethasone USAN, USP, INN, BAN, JAN *corticosteroidal anti-inflammatory*

betamethasone acetate USP, JAN *corticosteroidal anti-inflammatory*

betamethasone acibutate INN, BAN *corticosteroidal anti-inflammatory*

betamethasone benzoate USAN, USP, BAN *topical corticosteroidal anti-inflammatory*

betamethasone dipropionate USAN, USP, BAN, JAN *topical corticosteroidal anti-inflammatory* 0.05% topical

betamethasone dipropionate, augmented *topical corticosteroidal anti-inflammatory* 0.05% topical

betamethasone dipropionate & clotrimazole *corticosteroidal anti-inflammatory; broad-spectrum antifungal* 0.05%•1% topical

betamethasone sodium phosphate USP, BAN, JAN *corticosteroidal anti-inflammatory*

betamethasone valerate USAN, USP, BAN, JAN *topical corticosteroidal anti-inflammatory; mousse for scalp psoriasis* 0.1% topical

betamicin INN *antibacterial* [also: betamicin sulfate]

betamicin sulfate USAN *antibacterial* [also: betamicin]

betamipron INN

betanaphthol NF

betanidine INN *antihypertensive* [also: bethanidine sulfate; bethanidine; betanidine sulfate]

betanidine sulfate JAN *antihypertensive* [also: bethanidine sulfate; betanidine; bethanidine]

Betapace tablets ℞ *antiarrhythmic (β-blocker) for life-threatening ventricular arrhythmias* (orphan) [sotalol HCl] 80, 120, 160, 240 mg

Betapace AF tablets ℞ *antiarrhythmic (β-blocker) for atrial fibrillation or atrial flutter* [sotalol HCl] 80, 120, 160 mg

betaprodine INN, BAN

beta-propiolactone [see: propiolactone]

beta-pyridylcarbinol [see: nicotinyl alcohol]

BetaRx *investigational* (orphan) *antidiabetic for type 1 patients on immunosuppression* [porcine islet preparation, encapsulated]

Betasept *topical liquid* OTC *broad-spectrum antimicrobial; germicidal* [chlorhexidine gluconate; alcohol 4%] 4%

Betaseron *powder for subcu injection* ℞ *immunomodulator for relapsing-remitting multiple sclerosis* (orphan); *investigational* (orphan) *for AIDS* [interferon beta-1b] 0.25 mg (8 MIU)/dose

BetaTan *oral suspension* ℞ *antitussive; antihistamine; decongestant* [carbetapentane tannate; brompheniramine tannate; phenylephrine tannate] 30•4•7.5 mg/5 mL

Betathine *investigational* (orphan) *antineoplastic and immunostimulant for multiple myeloma and metastatic melanoma* [beta alethine]

Beta-Val *cream, lotion* ℞ *corticosteroidal anti-inflammatory* [betamethasone valerate] 0.1%

BetaVent *syrup* ℞ *antitussive; expectorant* [carbetapentane citrate; guaifenesin] 20•100 mg/5 mL

betaxolol INN, BAN *topical antiglaucoma agent; β-blocker for hypertension; antianginal* [also: betaxolol HCl]

betaxolol HCl USAN, USP *topical antiglaucoma agent; β-blocker for hyper-*

tension; *antianginal* [also: betaxolol]
10, 20 mg oral; 0.5% eye drops

Betaxon eye drops ℞ *antiglaucoma
agent (β-blocker)* [levobetaxolol HCl]
0.5% ② butikacin

betazole INN [also: betazole HCl;
ametazole]

betazole HCl USP [also: betazole;
ametazole]

betazolium chloride [see: betazole
HCl]

betel nut (*Areca catechu*) leaves and
quids (a mixture of tobacco, powdered or sliced areca nut, and slaked
lime wrapped in a *Piper betel* leaf)
*medicinal herb used as a digestive aid
and mild stimulant; not generally
regarded as safe and effective as it
causes leukoplakia and oral cancer*

beth root *medicinal herb* [see: birthroot]

bethanidine sulfate *investigational
(orphan) prevention and treatment of
primary ventricular fibrillation*

bethanechol chloride USP, BAN, JAN
*cholinergic urinary stimulant for post-
surgical and postpartum urinary retention* 5, 10, 25, 50 mg oral

bethanidine BAN *antihypertensive* [also:
bethanidine sulfate; betanidine;
betanidine sulfate]

bethanidine sulfate USAN *antihypertensive; investigational (orphan) agent
for the prevention and treatment of primary ventricular fibrillation* [also:
betanidine; bethanidine; betanidine
sulfate]

betiatide USAN, INN, BAN *pharmaceutic
aid*

Betimol eye drops ℞ *antiglaucoma
agent (β-blocker)* [timolol hemihy-
drate] 0.25%, 0.5%

Betonica officinalis *medicinal herb*
[now: *Stachys officinalis*] [see: betony]

betony (*Stachys officinalis*) plant
*medicinal herb for anxiety, delirium,
diarrhea, fever, jaundice, liver and
spleen sclerosis, migraine headache,
mouth or throat irritation, nervousness,
palpitations, and toothache; also used*

as a purgative and emetic agent ② biotin; Bitin; butane; P-Tanna 12

Betoptic; Betoptic S Drop-Tainers
(eye drops) ℞ *antiglaucoma agent (β-
blocker)* [betaxolol HCl] 0.5%; 0.25%

betoxycaine INN

betoxycaine HCl [see: betoxycaine]

betula oil [see: methyl salicylate]

Betula spp. *medicinal herb* [see: birch]

Betuline lotion OTC *analgesic; mild
anesthetic; antipruritic; counterirritant*
[methyl salicylate; camphor; menthol]

bevacizumab *recombinant humanized
monoclonal antibody to vascular endothelial growth factor (VEGF); angiogenesis inhibitor for colorectal, breast, and
non–small cell lung cancers (NSCLC);
investigational (Phase III) for cervical,
renal, and pancreatic cancers*

bevantolol INN, BAN *antianginal; antihypertensive; antiarrhythmic* [also:
bevantolol HCl]

bevantolol HCl USAN *antianginal;
antihypertensive; antiarrhythmic* [also:
bevantolol]

bevirimat *Syzygium claviflorum derivative; investigational cellular replication
inhibitor for HIV*

bevonium methylsulphate BAN
[also: bevonium metilsulfate]

bevonium metilsulfate INN [also:
bevonium methylsulphate]

bexarotene USAN, INN *synthetic retinoid analogue antineoplastic for cutaneous T-cell lymphoma (orphan); investigational (Phase III) for lung cancer*

bexlosteride USAN, INN *antineoplastic
5α-reductase inhibitor for prostate cancer*

Bextra film-coated caplets (withdrawn
from the market in 2005 due to
safety concerns) ℞ *COX-2 inhibitor;
nonsteroidal anti-inflammatory drug
(NSAID) for osteoarthritis (OA),
rheumatoid arthritis (RA), and primary
dysmenorrhea* [valdecoxib] 10, 20 mg

Bexxar Dosimetric Package IV infusion ℞ *first of two steps in the radiotherapeutic treatment of non-Hodgkin
lymphoma (NHL)* [tositumomab;

iodine I 131 tositumomab] 450•35 mg (5 mCi of radiation)

Bexxar Therapeutic Package IV infusion ℞ *second of two steps in the radiotherapeutic treatment of non-Hodgkin lymphoma (orphan)* [tositumomab; iodine I 131 tositumomab] 450•35 mg (delivers 65–75 cGy of radiation)

bezafibrate USAN, INN, BAN, JAN *antihyperlipidemic*

bezitramide INN, BAN

bezomil INN *combining name for radicals or groups*

bFGF (basic fibroblast growth factor) [see: ersofermin]

B.F.I. Antiseptic powder OTC *antiseptic* [bismuth-formic-iodide] 16%

BHA (butylated hydroxyanisole) [q.v.]

BHAPs (bisheteroarylpiperazines) *a class of antiviral drugs*

BHD (BCNU, hydroxyurea, dacarbazine) *chemotherapy protocol*

BHDV; BHD-V (BCNU, hydroxyurea, dacarbazine, vincristine) *chemotherapy protocol*

BHT (butylated hydroxytoluene) [q.v.]

bialamicol INN, BAN *antiamebic* [also: bialamicol HCl]

bialamicol HCl USAN *antiamebic* [also: bialamicol]

biallylamicol [see: bialamicol]

biantrazole [now: losoxantrone HCl]

biapenem USAN, INN *antibacterial*

Biavax II powder for subcu injection ℞ *rubella and mumps vaccine* [rubella & mumps virus vaccine, live; neomycin] 1000 U•20 000 U•25 mcg/ 0.5 mL dose

Biaxin Filmtabs (film-coated tablets), granules for oral suspension ℞ *macrolide antibiotic* [clarithromycin] 250, 500 mg; 125, 250 mg/5 mL ⊡ Bicozene; pecazine

Biaxin XL film-coated extended-release tablets ℞ *once-daily macrolide antibiotic* [clarithromycin] 500 mg

bibapcitide USAN *glycoprotein (GP) IIb/IIIa receptor antagonist; investigational (Phase III) diagnostic imaging aid for deep vein thrombosis*

bibenzonium bromide INN, BAN

bibrocathin [see: bibrocathol]

bibrocathol INN

bicalutamide USAN, INN, BAN *antiandrogen antineoplastic for prostatic cancer*

bicalutamide + LHRH-A (bicalutamide, goserelin acetate [Zoladex subcu implant]) *chemotherapy protocol for prostate cancer*

bicalutamide + LHRH-A (bicalutamide, leuprolide acetate [Lupron Depot injection]) *chemotherapy protocol for prostate cancer*

Bichloracetic Acid topical liquid ℞ *cauterant; keratolytic* [dichloroacetic acid] 10 mL

bicifadine INN *analgesic* [also: bicifadine HCl]

bicifadine HCl USAN *analgesic* [also: bicifadine]

Bicillin C-R; Bicillin C-R 900/300 Tubex (cartridge-needle unit) for deep IM injection ℞ *natural penicillin antibiotic* [penicillin G benzathine; penicillin G procaine] 300 000•300 000, 600 000•600 000, 1 200 000• 1 200 000 U; 900 000•300 000 U

Bicillin L-A Tubex (cartridge-needle unit) for deep IM injection ℞ *natural penicillin antibiotic* [penicillin G benzathine] 600 000, 1 200 000, 2 400 000 U

biciromab USAN, INN, BAN *monoclonal antibody to fibrin*

Bicitra oral solution ℞ *urinary alkalinizing agent* [sodium citrate; citric acid] 500•334 mg/5 mL ⊡ Posture

biclodil INN *antihypertensive; vasodilator* [also: biclodil HCl]

biclodil HCl USAN *antihypertensive; vasodilator* [also: biclodil]

biclofibrate INN

biclotymol INN

BiCNU powder for IV injection ℞ *nitrosourea-type alkylating antineoplastic for brain tumors, multiple myeloma,*

Hodgkin disease and non-Hodgkin lymphomas [carmustine] 100 mg/dose ⍰ BACON

bicozamycin INN

Bicozene cream OTC *anesthetic; antifungal* [benzocaine; resorcinol] 6%•1.67% ⍰ Biaxin; pecazine

bicyclomycin [see: bicozamycin]

bidCAP (trademarked dosage form) *twice-daily capsule*

Bidex-A extended-release tablets ℞ *antitussive; expectorant* [dextromethorphan hydrobromide; guaifenesin] 25•600 mg ⍰ Pediox

Bidex-DMI tablets OTC *antitussive; expectorant* [dextromethorphan hydrobromide; guaifenesin] 20•400 mg/10 mL

Bidhist extended-release tablets ℞ *antihistamine* [brompheniramine maleate] 6 mg ⍰ PD-Hist D

Bidhist-D extended-release tablets ℞ *decongestant; antihistamine* [pseudoephedrine HCl; brompheniramine maleate] 45•6 mg ⍰ PD-Hist D

BiDil film-coated tablets (discontinued 2007) ℞ *vasodilator combination for heart failure in black patients* [hydralazine HCl; isosorbide dinitrate] 37.5•20 mg

bidimazium iodide INN, BAN

bidisomide USAN, INN *antiarrhythmic*

Biebrich scarlet red [see: scarlet red]

Biebrich scarlet-picroaniline blue

bietamiverine INN

bietamiverine HCl [see: bietamiverine]

bietaserpine INN

bifemelane INN [also: bifemelane HCl]

bifemelane HCl JAN [also: bifemelane]

bifepramide INN

bifeprofen INN

bifeprunox *dopamine agonist; investigational (NDA filed) novel (atypical) antipsychotic for schizophrenia; investigational (Phase III) for bipolar disorder*

Bifidobacterium longum infantis 35624 *investigational (orphan) agent for pediatric Crohn disease*

Bifidobacterium sp. [see also: lactic acid bacteria]

bifluranol INN, BAN

bifonazole USAN, INN, BAN, JAN *antifungal*

Big Shot B-12 tablets OTC *vitamin B_{12} supplement* [cyanocobalamin] 5 mg

Bignonia sempervirens medicinal herb [see: gelsemium]

biguanides *a class of antidiabetic agents that decrease hepatic glucose production and increase cellular response to insulin*

bilastine INN

bilberry (Myrtilli fructus; Vaccinium myrtillus) *fruit medicinal herb for cold hands and feet, diarrhea, edema, increasing microvascular blood flow, gastroenteritis, mucous membrane inflammation, night blindness, and varicose veins* ⍰ Bluboro

bile acid sequestrants *a class of antihyperlipidemic agents*

bile acids, conjugated *investigational (orphan) for steatorrhea in short bowel syndrome*

bile acids, oxidized [see: dehydrocholic acid]

bile salts BAN *digestive enzymes; laxative*

BiliCheck (breath analyzer device) *in vitro diagnostic aid for infant jaundice*

Bili-Labstix reagent strips *in vitro diagnostic aid for multiple urine products*

Biltricide film-coated tablets ℞ *anthelmintic for schistosomiasis (flukes)* [praziquantel] 600 mg

bimakalim INN

bimatoprost *topical prostamide analogue for glaucoma and ocular hypertension*

bimazol [see: carbimazole]

bimethadol [see: dimepheptanol]

bimethoxycaine lactate

bimosiamose disodium USAN *antiinflammatory for asthma, psoriasis, and reperfusion injury following transplants or coronary revascularization*

bindarit USAN, INN *antirheumatic; investigational (orphan) for lupus nephritis*

bindazac [see: bendazac]

binedaline INN ⍰ pinadoline

binetrakin USAN, INN *immunomodulator for gastrointestinal carcinoma and rheumatoid arthritis*

binfloxacin USAN, INN *veterinary anti-bacterial*

binifibrate INN ⍰ ponfibrate

biniramycin USAN, INN *antibacterial antibiotic*

binizolast INN

binodaline [see: binedaline]

binospirone INN *anxiolytic* [also: binospirone mesylate]

binospirone mesylate USAN *anxiolytic* [also: binospirone]

bioallethrin BAN *pediculicide*

Biobrane wound dressing *nylon fabric matrix bound to a silicon film* ⍰ piperine

Biobrane-L light adherence wound dressing *nylon fabric matrix bound to a silicon film*

Biocef capsules, powder for oral suspension (discontinued 2007) ℞ *first-generation cephalosporin antibiotic* [cephalexin] 500 mg; 250 mg/5 mL

Bioclate powder for IV injection (discontinued 2008) ℞ *systemic hemostatic; antihemophilic for the prevention and control of bleeding in classical hemophilia (hemophilia A) and von Willebrand disease (orphan)* [antihemophilic factor concentrate, recombinant] 250, 500, 1000 IU

Biocult-GC culture paddles for professional use ℞ *in vitro diagnostic aid for Neisseria gonorrhoeae*

Biodine Topical solution OTC *broad-spectrum antimicrobial* [povidone-iodine] 1%

Bio-E-Gel *investigational (NDA filed) bioidentical human estrogen transdermal gel for postmenopausal symptoms* [estradiol]

bioflavonoids (vitamin P) *a class of more than 4000 natural substances with widespread biological activity, including anthelmintic, antimicrobial, antimalarial, antineoplastic, antioxidant, anti-inflammatory, and antiviral activity; historically named "vitamin P"*

biogastrone [see: carbenoxolone]

Biohist-LA sustained-release tablets (discontinued 2007) ℞ *decongestant;*

antihistamine [pseudoephedrine HCl; chlorpheniramine maleate] 120•12 mg

biological indicator for dry-heat sterilization USP *sterilization indicator*

biological indicator for ethylene oxide sterilization USP *sterilization indicator*

biological indicator for steam sterilization USP *sterilization indicator*

Bion Tears eye drops OTC *moisturizer/lubricant* [hydroxypropyl methylcellulose] 0.3%

Bionect cream, gel, topical spray ℞ *wound healing agent for skin irritations, dermal ulcers, wounds, and burns* [hyaluronate sodium] 0.2%

bioral [see: carbenoxolone]

Bio-Rescue *investigational (orphan) chelating agent for acute iron poisoning* [dextran; deferoxamine]

bioresmethrin INN

bios I [see: inositol]

bios II [see: biotin]

Biosafe HbA1c (hemoglobin A1c) test kit for home use OTC *in vitro diagnostic aid for glycemic control*

Biosafe PSA (prostate-specific antigen) test kit for home use OTC *in vitro diagnostic aid for prostate function*

Biosafe Total Cholesterol (only) test kit for home use OTC *in vitro diagnostic aid for hypercholesterolemia*

Biosafe Total Cholesterol Panel (includes HDL, LDL, and triglycerides) test kit for home use OTC *in vitro diagnostic aid for hypercholesterolemia and hypertriglyceridemia*

Biosafe TSH (thyroid-stimulating hormone) test kit for home use OTC *in vitro diagnostic aid for thyroid function*

biosimilar [def.] *a generic version of a biological medicine, such as a monoclonal antibody; for example,* **Reditux** *contains biosimilar* **rituximab** *and sells for half the price of the original drug,* **Rituxan**

Biosynject *investigational (orphan) for newborn hemolytic disease and ABO blood incompatibility of organ or bone* *marrow transplants* [trisaccharides A and B]

biosynthetic human parathyroid hormone (1-34) [see: teriparatide]

BioTears gelcaps OTC *nutritional support to increase tear production for symptomatic relief of chronic dry eyes* [vitamins A, B₆, C, D₃, and E; magnesium (from sulfate); omega-3 and -6 EFAs; mucopolysaccharides; turmeric; lactoferrin] 500 IU•4 mg•50 mg•25 IU•16 IU•10 mg•401 mg•125 mg•50 mg•5 mg ☒ bitters

Biotel kidney reagent strips *in vitro diagnostic aid for urine hemoglobin, RBCs, and albumin (predictor of kidney diseases)*

Bioténe with Calcium mouthwash OTC

biotexin [see: novobiocin]

Bio-Throid capsules ℞ *natural thyroid replacement for hypothyroidism or thyroid cancer* [thyroid, desiccated (porcine)] 7.5, 15, 30, 60, 90, 120, 150, 180, 240 mg

biotin USP, INN, JAN *B complex vitamin; vitamin H* ☒ betony; Bitin; butane; P-Tanna 12

Biotin Forte tablets OTC *vitamin supplement* [multiple B vitamins; vitamin C; folic acid; biotin] ≜•200•0.8•3 mg, ≜•100•0.8•5 mg

BioTropin *investigational (orphan) for cachexia due to AIDS* [somatropin]

Biotuss oral liquid ℞ *antitussive; decongestant; expectorant* [dextromethorphan hydrobromide; phenylephrine HCl; guaifenesin] 15•10•300 mg/5 mL

BIP (bleomycin, ifosfamide [with mesna rescue], Platinol) *chemotherapy protocol for cervical cancer*

bipenamol INN *antidepressant* [also: bipenamol HCl]

bipenamol HCl USAN *antidepressant* [also: bipenamol]

biperiden USP, INN, BAN, JAN *anticholinergic; antiparkinsonian*

biperiden HCl USP, BAN, JAN *anticholinergic; antiparkinsonian*

biperiden lactate USP, BAN, JAN *anticholinergic; antiparkinsonian*

biphasic insulin [see: insulin, biphasic]

biphenamine HCl USAN *topical anesthetic; antibacterial; antifungal* [also: xenysalate]

biprofenide [see: bifepramide]

birch (*Betula* spp.) bark and leaves *medicinal herb for bladder problems, blood cleansing, and eczema* ☒ Berocca; Portia; Pro-Q

birch oil, sweet [see: methyl salicylate]

bird flu vaccine [see: influenza virus vaccine, H5N1]

bird lime *medicinal herb* [see: mistletoe]

bird pepper *medicinal herb* [see: cayenne]

bird's nest root *medicinal herb* [see: carrot]

biricodar dicitrate USAN *multi-drug–resistance inhibitor*

biriperone INN

birthroot (*Trillium erectum; T. grandiflorum; T. pendulum*) plant *medicinal herb for insect and snake bites, stimulating menses and diaphoresis, and stopping bleeding after childbirth; also used as an antiseptic and astringent*

birthwort (*Aristolochia clematitis*) root and flowering plant *medicinal herb used as a diaphoretic, emmenagogue, febrifuge, oxytocic, and stimulant*

Bisac-Evac enteric-coated tablets, suppositories OTC *stimulant laxative* [bisacodyl] 5 mg; 10 mg

bisacodyl USP, INN, BAN, JAN *stimulant laxative* 5 mg oral; 10 mg suppositories

bisacodyl tannex USAN *stimulant laxative*

Bisa-Lax enteric-coated tablets, suppositories OTC *stimulant laxative* [bisacodyl] 5 mg; 10 mg

bisantrene INN *antineoplastic* [also: bisantrene HCl]

bisantrene HCl USAN *antineoplastic* [also: bisantrene]

bisaramil INN

bisatin [see: oxyphenisatin acetate]

bisbendazole INN

bisbentiamine INN, JAN

bisbutiamine [see: bisbutitiamine]

bisbutitiamine JAN

bis-chloroethyl-nitrosourea (BCNU) [see: carmustine]

bisdequalinium diacetate JAN

bisfenazone INN

bisfentidine INN

*bis***(4-fluorophenyl)phenylacetamide** *investigational (orphan) for sickle cell disease*

bisheteroarylpiperazines (BHAPs) *a class of antiviral drugs*

bishop's wort *medicinal herb* [see: nutmeg; betony]

bishydroxycoumarin [now: dicumarol]

bisibutiamine JAN [also: sulbutiamine]

Bismatrol chewable tablets, oral liquid OTC *antidiarrheal; antinauseant* [bismuth subsalicylate] 262 mg; 524 mg/5 mL

bismucatebrol [see: bibrocathol]

bismuth *element (Bi)*

bismuth, milk of USP *antacid; astringent*

bismuth aluminate USAN

bismuth betanaphthol USP

bismuth carbonate USAN

bismuth carbonate, basic [see: bismuth subcarbonate]

bismuth citrate USP

bismuth cream [see: bismuth, milk of]

bismuth gallate, basic [see: bismuth subgallate]

bismuth glycollylarsanilate BAN [also: glycobiarsol]

bismuth hydroxide [see: bismuth, milk of]

bismuth hydroxide nitrate oxide [see: bismuth subnitrate]

bismuth magma [now: bismuth, milk of]

bismuth magnesium aluminosilicate JAN

bismuth oxycarbonate [see: bismuth subcarbonate]

bismuth potassium tartrate NF

bismuth sodium triglycollamate USP

bismuth subcarbonate USAN, JAN *antacid; GI adsorbent*

bismuth subcitrate potassium *antacid; GI adsorbent*

bismuth subgallate USAN, USP *antacid; GI adsorbent; systemic deodorizer for ostomy and incontinence odors*

bismuth subnitrate USP, JAN *skin protectant*

bismuth subsalicylate (BSS) USAN, JAN *antiperistaltic; antacid; GI adsorbent*

bisnafide dimesylate USAN *antineoplastic; DNA and RNA synthesis inhibitor*

bisobrin INN *fibrinolytic* [also: bisobrin lactate] ☒ buspirone

bisobrin lactate USAN *fibrinolytic* [also: bisobrin]

Bisolvon *investigational (orphan) agent for keratoconjunctivitis sicca of Sjögren syndrome* [bromhexine HCl]

bisoprolol USAN, INN, BAN *β-blocker for hypertension*

bisoprolol fumarate USAN, JAN *β-blocker for hypertension* 5, 10 mg oral

bisoprolol fumarate & hydrochlorothiazide *antihypertensive; β-blocker; diuretic* 2.5•6.5, 5•6.5, 10•6.5 mg oral

bisorcic INN

bisoxatin INN, BAN *laxative* [also: bisoxatin acetate]

bisoxatin acetate USAN *laxative* [also: bisoxatin]

bisphosphonates *a class of calcium-regulating agents that inhibit normal and abnormal bone resorption*

bispyrithione magsulfex USAN *antibacterial; antidandruff; antifungal*

bistort (Polygonum bistorta) *root medicinal herb for bleeding, cholera, cuts, diarrhea, dysentery, gum disease (mouthwash), and hemorrhoids*

bis-tropamide [now: tropicamide]

Bi-Tann DP oral suspension ℞ *decongestant; antihistamine* [pseudoephedrine tannate; dexchlorpheniramine tannate] 75•5 mg/2.5 mL

Bite Rx solution OTC *astringent wet dressing (Burow solution) for insect bites* [aluminum acetate] 0.5% ☒ Pitrex

bithionol NF, INN, BAN, JAN *anti-infec-*
tive for paragonimiasis and fascioliasis
(available only from the Centers for
Disease Control and Prevention) ⑨
Botanol; Patanol

bithionolate sodium USAN *topical anti-*
infective [also: sodium bitionolate]

bithionoloxide INN

Bitin (available only from the Centers
for Disease Control) ℞ *anti-infective*
for paragonimiasis and fascioliasis
[bithionol] ⑨ betony; biotin; butane;
P-Tanna 12

bitipazone INN

bitolterol INN, BAN *sympathomimetic*
bronchodilator [also: bitolterol mesylate; bitolterol mesilate]

bitolterol mesilate JAN *sympathomi-*
metic bronchodilator [also: bitolterol
mesylate; bitolterol]

bitolterol mesylate USAN *sympathomi-*
metic bronchodilator [also: bitolterol;
bitolterol mesilate]

bitoscanate INN

bitter ash *medicinal herb* [see: quassia;
wahoo]

bitter ash; bitter quassia; bitter
wood *medicinal herb* [see: quassia]

bitter buttons *medicinal herb* [see: tansy]

bitter cardamom (Alpinia fructus;
A. oxyphylla) *medicinal herb for*
dementia, excessive water loss, and
gastric lesions

bitter cucumber *medicinal herb* [see:
bitter melon]

bitter dogbane *medicinal herb* [see:
dogbane]

bitter grass *medicinal herb* [see: star
grass]

bitter herb *medicinal herb* [see: centaury]

bitter melon (Momordica charantia)
fruit, leaves, seeds, oil *medicinal herb*
used as an antimicrobial and hypoglyce-
mic; also used to reduce fertility in both
males and females, and can act as an
abortifacient

bitter quassia; bitter ash; bitter wood
medicinal herb [see: quassia tree]

bitter tonics; bitters *a class of agents*
that have a bitter taste, used as tonics,
alteratives, or appetizers

bitter wintergreen *medicinal herb* [see:
pipsissewa]

bitter wood; bitter ash; bitter quas-
sia *medicinal herb* [see: quassia tree]

bitterroot; bitterwort *medicinal herb*
[see: dogbane; gentian]

bitters; bitter tonics *a class of agents*
that have a bitter taste, used as tonics,
alteratives, or appetizers ⑨ BioTears

bittersweet herb; bittersweet twigs
medicinal herb [see: bittersweet night-
shade]

bittersweet nightshade (Solanum
dulcamara) *medicinal herb for topical*
application on abrasions and felons; not
generally regarded as safe and effective
for internal use as it is highly toxic

bitterweed *medicinal herb* [see: fleabane; horseweed]

bitterwort; bitterroot *medicinal herb*
[see: gentian]

bivalirudin USAN *anticoagulant throm-*
bin inhibitor for percutaneous coronary
intervention (PCI), percutaneous trans-
luminal coronary angioplasty (PTCA),
or heparin-induced thrombocytopenia
(HIT); used with aspirin therapy

bizelesin USAN, INN *antineoplastic* ⑨
pecilocin

B-Ject-100 injection (discontinued
2006) ℞ *parenteral vitamin therapy*
[multiple B vitamins]

black alder (Alnus glutinosa) bark
and leaves *medicinal herb used as an*
astringent, demulcent, emetic, hemo-
static, and tonic

black alder dogwood *medicinal herb*
[see: buckthorn; cascara sagrada]

black birch *medicinal herb* [see: birch]

black cherry; poison black cherry
medicinal herb [see: belladonna]

black choke *medicinal herb* [see: wild
black cherry]

black cohosh (Cimicifuga racemosa)
root and rhizome *medicinal herb for*
asthma, bronchitis, dysmenorrhea, dys-
pepsia, epilepsy, hypertension, hormone

imbalance, lung disorders, menopause, rheumatism, snake bite, sore throat, St. Vitus dance, and tuberculosis

black currant (Ribes nigrum) *medicinal herb* [see: currant]

black dogwood *medicinal herb* [see: buckthorn; cascara sagrada]

black elder *medicinal herb* [see: elderberry]

black false hellebore (Veratrum niger) [see: hellebore]

black ginger *medicinal herb* [see: ginger]

black hellebore (Helleborus niger) [see: hellebore]

black mulberry (Morus nigra) *medicinal herb* [see: mulberry]

black oak (Quercus tinctoria) *medicinal herb* [see: white oak]

black poplar (Populus nigra; P. tremula) *buds medicinal herb used as a diaphoretic, diuretic, expectorant, and vulnerary*

black root *medicinal herb* [see: Culver root]

black sanicle *medicinal herb* [see: sanicle]

black snakeroot *medicinal herb* [see: black cohosh; sanicle]

black walnut (Juglans nigra) *hulls and leaves medicinal herb for parasites, ringworm, skin rashes, and stopping lactation; also used as an external antiseptic*

black widow spider antivenin [see: antivenin (Latrodectus mactans)]

black willow (Salix nigra) *medicinal herb* [see: willow]

blackberry (Rubus fructicosus; R. villosus) *berries, leaves, and root bark medicinal herb for bleeding, cholera, diarrhea in children, dysentery, sinus drainage, and vomiting*

Black-Draught *tablets, chewable tablets, granules OTC stimulant laxative* [sennosides] 6 mg; 10 mg; 20 mg/5 mL

blackwort *medicinal herb* [see: comfrey]

bladder fucus; bladderwrack *medicinal herb* [see: kelp (Fucus)]

bladderpod *medicinal herb* [see: lobelia]

Blairex Lens Lubricant *solution OTC rewetting solution for soft contact lenses*

Blairex Sterile Saline *aerosol solution OTC rinsing/storage solution for soft contact lenses* [sodium chloride (saline solution)]

blastomycin NF

blazing star *medicinal herb* [see: star grass]

blazing star (Liatris scariosa; L. spicata; L. squarrosa) *root medicinal herb used as a diuretic*

Blenoxane *powder for IM, IV, subcu, or intrapleural injection* ℞ *glycopeptide antibiotic antineoplastic for Hodgkin and non-Hodgkin lymphomas, testicular and squamous cell carcinomas, and malignant pleural effusion (orphan); investigational (orphan) for pancreatic cancer* [bleomycin sulfate] 15, 30 U

BLEO-COMF (bleomycin, cyclophosphamide, Oncovin, methotrexate, fluorouracil) *chemotherapy protocol*

bleomycin (BLM) INN, BAN *glycopeptide antibiotic antineoplastic* [also: bleomycin sulfate; bleomycin HCl] ⚇ **paulomycin; peliomycin**

bleomycin HCl JAN *glycopeptide antibiotic antineoplastic* [also: bleomycin sulfate; bleomycin]

bleomycin sulfate USAN, USP, JAN *glycopeptide antibiotic antineoplastic for Hodgkin and non-Hodgkin lymphomas, testicular and squamous cell carcinomas, and malignant pleural effusion (orphan); investigational (orphan) for pancreatic cancer* [also: bleomycin; bleomycin HCl] 15, 30 U injection

Bleph-10 *eye drops, ophthalmic ointment* ℞ *antibiotic* [sulfacetamide sodium] 10%

Blephamide *eye drop suspension, ophthalmic ointment* ℞ *corticosteroidal anti-inflammatory; antibiotic* [prednisolone acetate; sulfacetamide sodium] 0.2%•10%

blessed cardus; holy thistle *medicinal herb* [see: blessed thistle]

blessed thistle (*Cnicus benedictus*) plant *medicinal herb for blood cleansing, digestive disorders, headache, hormonal imbalance, lactation disorders, liver and gallbladder ailments, menstrual disorders, poor circulation, and strengthening heart and lungs*

Blighia sapida *medicinal herb* [see: ackee]

blind nettle (*Lamium album*) plant and flowers *medicinal herb used as an antispasmodic, astringent, expectorant, and styptic*

Blinx ophthalmic solution OTC *extraocular irrigating solution* [sterile isotonic solution]

BlisterGard topical liquid OTC *skin protectant*

Blistex ointment OTC *antipruritic/counterirritant; mild local anesthetic; vulnerary* [camphor; phenol; allantoin] 0.5%•0.5%•1%

Blistik lip balm OTC *antipruritic/counterirritant; mild local anesthetic; skin protectant; sunscreen (SPF 10)* [camphor; phenol; allantoin; dimethicone; padimate O; oxybenzone] 0.5%•0.5%•1%•2%•6.6%•2.5%

Blis-To-Sol topical liquid OTC *antifungal; keratolytic* [tolnaftate] 1%

Blis-To-Sol topical powder OTC *antifungal* [zinc undecylenate] 12%

BLM (bleomycin) [q.v.]

Blocadren tablets ℞ *antihypertensive; antianginal; migraine preventative; β-blocker* [timolol maleate] 5, 10, 20 mg

blood, whole USP *blood replenisher*

blood, whole human [now: blood, whole]

blood cells, human red [now: blood cells, red]

blood cells, red USP *blood replenisher*

blood group specific substances A, B & AB USP *blood neutralizer*

blood grouping serum, anti-A [see: anti-A blood grouping serum]

blood grouping serum, anti-B [see: anti-B blood grouping serum]

blood grouping serum, anti-C USP *for in vitro blood testing*

blood grouping serum, anti-c USP *for in vitro blood testing*

blood grouping serum, anti-D USP *for in vitro blood testing*

blood grouping serum, anti-E USP *for in vitro blood testing*

blood grouping serum, anti-e USP *for in vitro blood testing*

blood mononuclear cells, allogenic peripheral *investigational (orphan) agent for pancreatic cancer*

blood staunch *medicinal herb* [see: fleabane; horseweed]

blood volume expanders *a class of therapeutic blood modifiers used to increase the volume of circulating blood* [also called: plasma expanders]

bloodroot (*Sanguinaria canadensis*) root and rhizome *medicinal herb for diuresis, fever, inducing emesis, nasal polyps, rheumatism, sedation, skin cancer, stimulating menstrual flow, and warts; also used in toothpaste and mouthwash; not generally regarded as safe and effective for internal use*

BLP-25 liposome vaccine *investigational (Phase III) antineoplastic vaccine against MUC-1 for the treatment of non–small cell lung cancer*

Bluboro powder packets (discontinued 2008) OTC *astringent wet dressing (modified Burow solution)* [aluminum sulfate; calcium acetate] ⊡ bilberry

blue cohosh (*Caulophyllum thalictroides*) root *medicinal herb for cramps, epilepsy, induction of labor, menstrual flow stimulant, nerves, and chronic uterine problems*

blue curls *medicinal herb* [see: woundwort]

blue flag (*Iris versicolor*) root *medicinal herb used as a cathartic, diuretic, laxative, sialagogue, and vermifuge*

Blue Gel Muscular Pain Reliever gel OTC *mild anesthetic; antipruritic; counterirritant* [menthol]

blue ginseng *medicinal herb* [see: blue cohosh]

blue gum tree *medicinal herb* [see: eucalyptus]

Blue Ice gel OTC *mild anesthetic; antipruritic; counterirritant* [menthol] 2% ⊠ Boil-Ease; PALS

blue mountain tea *medicinal herb* [see: goldenrod]

blue pimpernel; blue skullcap *medicinal herb* [see: skullcap]

blue vervain *(Verbena hastata)* plant *medicinal herb for asthma, bladder and bowel disorders, bronchitis, colds, convulsions, cough, fever, insomnia, pulmonary tuberculosis, stomach upset, and worms*

blueberry *medicinal herb* [see: bilberry; blue cohosh]

bluebonnet; bluebottle *medicinal herb* [see: cornflower]

blue-green algae (Chloroplast membrane sulfolipids) *nutritional supplement for boosting the immune system*

bluensomycin INN *antibiotic*

BLU-U Blue Light PhotoDynamic Illuminator (device) *used with Levulan* (5-aminolevulinic acid HCl) *for photodynamic therapy of precancerous actinic keratoses of the face and scalp*

BLyS (B lymphocyte stimulating) protein *investigational (orphan) natural immunostimulant for common variable immunodeficiency (CVI, CVID), autoimmune diseases, and B-cell tumors*

B-MOPP (bleomycin, nitrogen mustard, Oncovin, procarbazine, prednisone) *chemotherapy protocol* ⊠ BEMP; BMP; BOMP; POMP

BMP (BCNU, methotrexate, procarbazine) *chemotherapy protocol*

BMS 234475 *investigational (Phase II) second-generation protease inhibitor for HIV infection*

BMY-45622 *investigational (orphan) antineoplastic for ovarian cancer*

BOAP (bleomycin, Oncovin, Adriamycin, prednisone) *chemotherapy protocol*

Bo-Cal tablets OTC *dietary supplement* [calcium; vitamin D; magnesium] 250 mg•100 IU•125 mg

boceprevir *investigational (Phase III) oral hepatitis C protease inhibitor for chronic hepatitis C infections*

Body Fortress Natural Amino tablets OTC *protein supplement* [protein; lactalbumin hydrolysate] 1.67•1.5 g

boforsin [see: colforsin]

bofumustine INN

bogbean; bog myrtle *medicinal herb* [see: buckbean]

Boil-Ease ointment OTC *anesthetic* [benzocaine] 20% ⊠ Blue Ice; PALS

bolandiol INN *anabolic* [also: bolandiol dipropionate] ⊠ Plendil

bolandiol dipropionate USAN, JAN *anabolic* [also: bolandiol]

bolasterone USAN, INN *anabolic steroid; also abused as a street drug*

bolazine INN

BOLD (bleomycin, Oncovin, lomustine, dacarbazine) *chemotherapy protocol*

Boldea fragrans *medicinal herb* [see: boldo]

boldenone INN, BAN *veterinary anabolic steroid; also abused as a street drug* [also: boldenone undecylenate]

boldenone undecylenate USAN *veterinary anabolic steroid; also abused as a street drug* [also: boldenone]

boldo *(Peumus boldus)* plant and leaves *medicinal herb for bile stimulation, colds, constipation, digestive disorders, earache, edema, gallstones, gonorrhea, gout, liver disease, rheumatism, syphilis, and worms*

Boldu boldus *medicinal herb* [see: boldo]

bolenol USAN, INN *anabolic* ⊠ BAL in Oil

bolmantalate USAN, INN, BAN *anabolic*

bolus alba [see: kaolin]

Bombay aloe *medicinal herb* [see: aloe]

bometolol INN ⊠ pamatolol

BOMP (bleomycin, Oncovin, Matulane, prednisone) *chemotherapy protocol* ⊠ BEMP; B-MOPP; BMP; POMP

BOMP; CLD-BOMP (bleomycin, Oncovin, mitomycin, Platinol)

chemotherapy protocol for cervical cancer ⊠ BEMP; B-MOPP; BMP; POMP

Bonamil Infant Formula with Iron powder, oral liquid OTC *total or supplementary infant feeding* 453 g; 384, 946 mL

bone ash [see: calcium phosphate, tribasic]

Bone Assure capsules OTC *vitamin/mineral/calcium supplement to maintain bone mineral density* [calcium (from bis-glycinate); magnesium (from oxide); zinc (from citrate); manganese (from citrate); trimethylglycine; multiple vitamins and minerals] 1000•320•12•3•100• ± per 6 capsules

Bone Meal tablets OTC *dietary supplement* [calcium; phosphorus] 236•118 mg

bone powder, purified [see: calcium phosphate, tribasic]

Bonefos ⓒⒶⓃ capsules, IV infusion (available in Canada) *investigational (orphan) bisphosphonate bone resorption inhibitor for hypercalcemia and osteolysis of malignancy* [clodronate disodium tetrahydrate] 400 mg; 60 mg/mL

boneset (Eupatorium perfoliatum) plant *medicinal herb for chills, colds, constipation, dengue fever, edema, fever, flu, pneumonia, and rheumatism* ⊠ Panacet 5/500; poinsettia

Bone-Up capsules OTC *vitamin/mineral/calcium supplement to maintain bone mineral density* [calcium (hydroxyapatite); protein; magnesium (oxide); zinc (monomethionine); manganese; glucosamine HCl; multiple vitamins and minerals] 1000•1000•600•10•5•300• ± per 6 capsules

Bonine chewable tablets OTC *antiemetic; motion sickness preventative* [meclizine HCl] 25 mg

Bonine for Kids chewable tablets OTC *antiemetic; motion sickness preventative* [cyclizine HCl] 25 mg

Bonisara tablets ℞ *nutritional supplement for osteoporosis* [strontium gluconate; Ranamine (q.v.)] 680•30 mg

Boniva once-daily film-coated tablets, once-monthly tablets, once-quarterly IV injection ℞ *bisphosphonate bone resorption inhibitor for the prevention and treatment of postmenopausal osteoporosis in women; also used for metastatic bone disease in breast cancer* [ibandronate (as sodium)] 2.5 mg; 150 mg; 3 mg/3 mL dose

Boniva extended-release (3 month) tablets *investigational (NDA filed) doseform for postmenopausal osteoporosis* [ibandronate sodium]

Bontril slow-release capsules ℞ *anorexiant; CNS stimulant* [phendimetrazine tartrate] 105 mg

Bontril PDM tablets ℞ *anorexiant; CNS stimulant* [phendimetrazine tartrate] 35 mg

Bonviva ⓔⓤⓡ (European name for U.S. product **Boniva**)

bookoo *medicinal herb* [see: buchu]

Boost oral liquid, pudding OTC *enteral nutritional therapy* [milk-based formula] 237 mL ⊠ Bucet

Boost Glucose Control oral liquid OTC *enteral nutritional therapy formulated for low blood glucose response* [milk-based formula] 8 oz.

Boostrix IM injection ℞ *active immunizing agent for tetanus, diphtheria, and pertussis; Tdap (tetanus predominant) booster vaccine used in adolescents 10–18 years old* [diphtheria toxoid; tetanus toxoid; inactivated pertussis toxins] 2.5 LfU•5 LfU•8 mcg per 0.5 mL dose

BOP (BCNU, Oncovin, prednisone) *chemotherapy protocol*

BOPAM (bleomycin, Oncovin, prednisone, Adriamycin, mechlorethamine, methotrexate) *chemotherapy protocol*

bopindolol INN

BOPP (BCNU, Oncovin, procarbazine, prednisone) *chemotherapy protocol*

boracic acid [see: boric acid]

borage (Borago officinalis) leaves *medicinal herb for bronchitis, colds, eye* inflammation, hay fever, strengthening of heart, lactation stimulation, rashes, rheumatism, ringworm; not generally regarded as safe and effective ⍰ Berocca; Pro-Q; Purge

borax [see: sodium borate]

Borbonia pinifolia medicinal herb [see: red bush tea]

boric acid NF, JAN *acidifying agent; ophthalmic emollient; antiseptic; astringent* 10% topical ⍰ BrachySeed I-125

2-bornanone [see: camphor]

bornaprine INN, BAN ⍰ pirenperone

bornaprolol INN

bornelone USAN, INN *ultraviolet screen* ⍰ pyrinoline

bornyl acetate USAN

borocaptate sodium B 10 USAN *antineoplastic; radioactive agent* [also: sodium borocaptate (^{10}B)]

Borocell *investigational (orphan) for boron neutron capture therapy (BNCT) for glioblastoma multiforme* [sodium monomercaptoundecahydro-closo-dodecaborate]

Borofair Otic ear drops ℞ *antibacterial; antifungal; antiseptic; astringent* [acetic acid; aluminum acetate] 2%•⍰

Borofax Skin Protectant ointment OTC *astringent* [zinc oxide] 15%

boroglycerin NF

boron *element (B); trace mineral for enhancing mental acuity and improving alertness; not generally regarded as safe and effective as it is highly toxic if taken internally or absorbed through broken skin* ⍰ bryony

Boropak powder packets (discontinued 2006) OTC *astringent wet dressing (modified Burow solution)* [aluminum sulfate; calcium acetate] ⍰ Barobag; Propac

bortezomib *proteasome inhibitor; antineoplastic for multiple myeloma (orphan) and mantle cell (non-Hodgkin) lymphoma; also used for myelomatous pleural effusion*

bosentan USAN, INN *endothelin receptor antagonist (ERA) for pulmonary arte-rial hypertension (orphan); also used to prevent digital ulcers in systemic sclerosis*

Boston Advance Cleaner; Boston Cleaner solution OTC *cleaning solution for rigid gas permeable contact lenses*

Boston Advance Comfort Formula solution OTC *disinfecting/wetting/soaking solution for rigid gas permeable contact lenses*

Boston Conditioning Solution OTC *disinfecting/wetting/soaking solution for rigid gas permeable contact lenses*

Boston Rewetting Drops OTC *rewetting solution for rigid gas permeable contact lenses*

Boston Simplicity Multi-Action solution OTC *disinfecting/wetting/soaking solution for rigid gas permeable contact lenses*

Boswellia serrata medicinal herb [see: frankincense]

botiacrine INN

Botox; Botox Cosmetic powder for injection ℞ *neurotoxin complex for blepharospasm and strabismus of dystonia (orphan), cervical dystonia (orphan), axillary hyperhidrosis, and cosmetic wrinkle treatments; investigational (orphan) for pediatric cerebral palsy* [botulinum toxin, type A] 100 U/vial

BottomBetter ointment OTC *diaper rash treatment*

botulinum toxin, type A *neurotoxin complex derived from Clostridium botulinum; treatment for blepharospasm and strabismus of dystonia (orphan), cervical dystonia (orphan), and cosmetic wrinkle treatments; investigational (orphan) for pediatric cerebral palsy*

botulinum toxin, type B *neurotoxin complex derived from Clostridium botulinum, type B; symptomatic treatment of cervical dystonia (orphan)*

botulinum toxin, type F *investigational (orphan) neurotoxin for cervical dystonia and essential blepharospasm*

botulism antitoxin USP *passive immunizing agent*

botulism equine antitoxin, trivalent *passive immunizing agent*

botulism immune globulin intravenous (BIG-IV) *treatment for infant botulism type A or B (orphan)*

Bounty Bears chewable tablets OTC *vitamin supplement* [multiple vitamins; folic acid] ±•0.3 mg

Bounty Bears Plus Iron chewable tablets OTC *vitamin/iron supplement* [multiple vitamins; iron; folic acid] ±•15•0.3 mg

bourbonal [see: ethyl vanillin]

bovactant BAN

bovine colostrum [see: *Cryptosporidium parvum* bovine colostrum IgG concentrate]

bovine fibrin BAN

bovine immunoglobulin concentrate [see: *Cryptosporidium parvum* bovine colostrum IgG concentrate]

bovine superoxide dismutase (bSOD) [see: orgotein]

bovine whey protein concentrate [see: *Cryptosporidium parvum* bovine colostrum IgG concentrate]

bower, virgin's *medicinal herb* [see: woodbine]

Bowman's root *medicinal herb* [see: Culver root]

box, mountain *medicinal herb* [see: uva ursi]

boxberry *medicinal herb* [see: wintergreen]

boxidine USAN, INN *antihyperlipoproteinemic*

Boyol salve OTC *anti-infective; anesthetic* [ichthammol; benzocaine] 10%• ?

BP Poly-650 tablets ℞ *analgesic; antipyretic; antihistamine; sleep aid* [acetaminophen; phenyltoloxamine citrate] 650•60 mg

B-PAS (benzoyl para-aminosalicylate) [see: benzoylpas calcium]

BPD-MA (benzoporphyrin derivative) [see: verteporfin]

BPI (bactericidal and permeability-increasing) protein [q.v.]

B-Plex tablets ℞ *vitamin supplement* [multiple B vitamins; vitamin C; folic acid] ±•500•0.5 mg

BPM Pseudo 6/45 extended-release tablets ℞ *antihistamine; decongestant* [brompheniramine maleate; pseudoephedrine HCl] 6•45 mg

BrachySeed I-125 implants ℞ *radioactive brachytherapy* [iodine I 125 ceramic beads] 0.19–0.65 mCi (7–24.1 MBq) ? boric acid

BrachySeed Pd-103 ceramic bead implants ℞ *radioactive "seeds" for ultrasound-guided brachytherapy for adenocarcinoma of the prostate* [palladium Pd 103] 1.0–1.8 mCi (37–66.6 MBq)

brain-derived neurotrophic factor (BDNF) [see: methionyl neurotropic factor, brain-derived]

brallobarbital INN

bramble *medicinal herb* [see: blackberry]

BranchAmin 4% IV infusion ℞ *nutritional therapy for high metabolic stress* [multiple branched-chain essential amino acids]

branched-chain amino acids (BCAA) *investigational (orphan) for amyotrophic lateral sclerosis* [see: isoleucine; leucine; valine]

brandy mint *medicinal herb* [see: peppermint]

Brasivol cream OTC *abrasive cleanser for acne* [aluminum oxide]

brasofensine maleate USAN *dopamine reuptake inhibitor*

Brassica alba *medicinal herb* [see: mustard]

Bravavir *investigational (NDA filed) antiviral for herpes zoster (orphan) and varicella zoster infections in immunocompromised patients* [sorivudine]

Bravelle powder for subcu or IM injection ℞ *follicle-stimulating hormone (FSH); ovulation stimulant for polycystic ovary disease and assisted reproductive technologies (ART)* [urofollitropin] 75 IU ? Prefill

brazergoline INN

Breathe Free nasal spray OTC *nasal moisturizer* [sodium chloride (saline solution)] 0.65%

Breezee Mist Aerosol powder OTC *antifungal; mild anesthetic; antipruri-*

tic; anhidrotic [undecylenic acid; menthol; aluminum chlorohydrate]

Breezee Mist Antifungal powder OTC *antifungal* [tolnaftate] 1% (note: one of two different products with the same name)

Breezee Mist Antifungal powder (discontinued 2007) OTC *antifungal for tinea pedis, tinea cruris, and tinea corporis* [miconazole nitrate] 2% (note: one of two different products with the same name)

Breezee Mist Foot Powder OTC *anhidrotic* [talc; aluminum chlorohydrate]

brefonalol INN

bremazocine INN

bremelanotide *investigational (Phase II) for erectile dysfunction*

brequinar INN *antineoplastic* [also: brequinar sodium]

brequinar sodium USAN *antineoplastic* [also: brequinar]

bretazenil USAN, INN *anxiolytic*

Brethine tablets, IV or subcu injection ℞ *sympathomimetic bronchodilator for asthma and bronchospasm; also used as a tocolytic to stop preterm labor* [terbutaline sulfate] 2.5, 5 mg; 1 mg/mL ⊡ Pre-Attain; protein A

bretylium tosilate INN *antiadrenergic; antiarrhythmic* [also: bretylium tosylate]

bretylium tosylate USAN, BAN *antiadrenergic; antiarrhythmic* [also: bretylium tosilate] 500, 1000 mg/vial injection

Brevibloc; Brevibloc Double Strength IV infusion ℞ *antiarrhythmic; β-blocker for supraventricular tachycardia* [esmolol HCl] 10, 250 mg/mL; 20 mg/mL

Brevicon tablets (in Wallettes of 28) ℞ *monophasic oral contraceptive* [norethindrone; ethinyl estradiol] 0.5 mg•35 mcg × 21 days; counters × 7 days ⊡ parvaquone; porofocon A

Brevital Sodium powder for IV injection ℞ *barbiturate general anesthetic* [methohexital sodium] 2.5 g

Brevoxyl Cleansing Lotion ℞ *keratolytic for acne* [benzoyl peroxide] 4%, 8%

Brevoxyl-4; Brevoxyl-8 gel ℞ *keratolytic for acne* [benzoyl peroxide] 4%; 8%

Brevoxyl-4 Creamy Wash; Brevoxyl-8 Creamy Wash topical liquid ℞ *keratolytic for acne* [benzoyl peroxide] 4%; 8%

brewer's yeast *natural source of protein and B-complex vitamins*

Bridion ⊞ (approved in Europe) *investigational (NDA filed) selective relaxation binding agent (SRBA) to reverse the effects of strong muscle relaxants, used for postanesthesia "stir-up"* [sugammadex]

brifentanil INN *narcotic analgesic* [also: brifentanil HCl]

brifentanil HCl USAN *narcotic analgesic* [also: brifentanil]

Brigham tea; Brigham Young weed *medicinal herb* [see: ephedra]

Brik-Paks (trademarked delivery form) *ready-to-use liquid containers*

brimonidine INN *ophthalmic α_2-adrenergic agonist for open-angle glaucoma and ocular hypertension* [also: brimonidine tartrate] ⊡ bromindione

brimonidine tartrate USAN *selective α_2 agonist for open-angle glaucoma and ocular hypertension; investigational (orphan) for anterior ischemic optic neuropathy* [also: brimonidine] 0.2% eye drops

brinaldix [see: clopamide]

brinase INN [also: brinolase]

brinazarone INN

brindoxime INN

brineurin [now: abrineurin]

brinolase USAN *fibrinolytic enzyme* [also: brinase]

brinzolamide USAN, INN *topical carbonic anhydrase inhibitor for glaucoma*

Bristoject (trademarked delivery form) *prefilled disposable syringe*

Brite Eyes II eye drops OTC *antioxidant and anti-glycation agent to prevent free radical damage in the lens;*

moisturizer/lubricant [N-acetyl-L-carnitine; glycerin; carboxymethylcellulose sodium] 1%•1%•0.3% ☒ Pretz; protease

British antilewisite (BAL) [now: dimercaprol]

British tobacco *medicinal herb* [see: coltsfoot]

brivudine INN

brobactam INN

brobenzoxaldine [see: broxaldine]

broclepride INN

brocresine USAN, INN, BAN *histidine decarboxylase inhibitor*

brocrinat USAN, INN *diuretic*

brodimoprim INN

brofaromine INN *reversible/selective MAO inhibitor*

Brofed oral liquid (discontinued 2007) Ŗ *decongestant; antihistamine* [pseudoephedrine HCl; brompheniramine maleate] 60•8 mg/10 mL

brofezil INN, BAN

brofoxine USAN, INN *antipsychotic*

brolaconazole INN

brolamfetamine INN

bromacrylide INN

bromadel [see: carbromal]

Bromadine-DX syrup (discontinued 2005) Ŗ *antitussive; decongestant; antihistamine* [dextromethorphan hydrobromide; pseudoephedrine HCl; brompheniramine maleate] 10•30•2 mg/5 mL

bromadoline INN *analgesic* [also: bromadoline maleate]

bromadoline maleate USAN *analgesic* [also: bromadoline]

bromamid INN

Bromanate pediatric elixir (discontinued 2007) OTC *decongestant; antihistamine* [pseudoephedrine HCl; brompheniramine maleate] 30•2 mg/10 mL

Bromanate DM Cold & Cough elixir (discontinued 2007) OTC *antitussive; antihistamine; decongestant* [dextromethorphan hydrobromide; brompheniramine maleate; pseudoephedrine HCl] 5•1•15 mg/5 mL

bromanylpromide [see: bromamid]

Bromatan Plus oral suspension Ŗ *antitussive; antihistamine; decongestant* [dextromethorphan tannate; dexchlorpheniramine tannate; pseudoephedrine tannate] 30•3.5•45 mg/5 mL

Bromatan-DM oral suspension Ŗ *antitussive; antihistamine; decongestant* [dextromethorphan tannate; brompheniramine tannate; phenylephrine tannate] 20•8•20 mg/5 mL

Bromatane DX syrup (discontinued 2007) Ŗ *antitussive; antihistamine; decongestant* [dextromethorphan hydrobromide; brompheniramine maleate; pseudoephedrine HCl; alcohol 1%] 20•4•60 mg/10 mL

bromauric acid NF

bromazepam USAN, INN, BAN, JAN *benzodiazepine anxiolytic; minor tranquilizer* ☒ premazepam

bromazine INN *antihistamine* [also: bromodiphenhydramine HCl; bromodiphenhydramine] ☒ Pramosone; primycin; promazine; puromycin

bromazine HCl [see: bromodiphenhydramine HCl]

brombenzonium [see: bromhexine HCl]

bromchlorenone USAN, INN *topical anti-infective*

bromebric acid INN, BAN

bromelain JAN *anti-inflammatory; proteolytic enzymes* [also: bromelains]

bromelains USAN, INN, BAN *anti-inflammatory; proteolytic enzymes* [also: bromelain]

bromelin [see: bromelains]

bromerguride INN

Brometane-DX Cough syrup Ŗ *antitussive; antihistamine; decongestant* [dextromethorphan hydrobromide; brompheniramine maleate; pseudoephedrine HCl] 10•2•30 mg/5 mL

brometenamine INN

bromethol [see: tribromoethanol]

Bromfed extended-release capsules (discontinued 2007) Ŗ *decongestant;*

antihistamine [phenylephrine HCl; brompheniramine maleate] 15•12 mg

Bromfed syrup (discontinued 2007) OTC *decongestant; antihistamine* [pseudoephedrine HCl; brompheniramine maleate] 60•4 mg/10 mL

Bromfed tablets (discontinued 2007) ℞ *decongestant; antihistamine* [pseudoephedrine HCl; brompheniramine maleate] 60•4 mg

Bromfed DM Cough syrup (discontinued 2007) ℞ *antitussive; antihistamine; decongestant* [dextromethorphan hydrobromide; brompheniramine maleate; pseudoephedrine HCl] 20•4•60 mg/10 mL

Bromfed-PD extended-release pediatric capsules (discontinued 2007) ℞ *decongestant; antihistamine* [phenylephrine HCl; brompheniramine maleate] 7.5•6 mg

bromfenac INN *long-acting nonsteroidal anti-inflammatory drug (NSAID); analgesic; antipyretic* [also: bromfenac sodium]

bromfenac sodium USAN *long-acting nonsteroidal anti-inflammatory drug (NSAID); analgesic; antipyretic; ocular treatment following cataract extraction surgery* [also: bromfenac]

Bromfenex extended-release capsules ℞ *decongestant; antihistamine* [pseudoephedrine HCl; brompheniramine maleate] 120•12 mg

Bromfenex PD extended-release capsules ℞ *decongestant; antihistamine* [pseudoephedrine HCl; brompheniramine maleate] 60•6 mg

bromhexine INN, BAN *expectorant; mucolytic* [also: bromhexine HCl] ⊘ pramoxine

bromhexine HCl USAN, JAN *expectorant; mucolytic; investigational (orphan) for keratoconjunctivitis sicca of Sjögren syndrome* [also: bromhexine]

Bromhist-DM oral drops ℞ *antitussive; antihistamine; decongestant; for children 1–24 months* [dextromethorphan hydrobromide; bromphenir-

amine maleate; pseudoephedrine HCl] 4•3•30 mg/mL

Bromhist-DM Pediatric syrup ℞ *antitussive; decongestant; antihistamine; expectorant* [dextromethorphan hydrobromide; pseudoephedrine HCl; brompheniramine maleate; guaifenesin] 5•30•2•50 mg/5 mL

Bromhist-NR; Bromhist Pediatric oral drops ℞ *decongestant; antihistamine; for children 1–24 months* [pseudoephedrine HCl; brompheniramine maleate] 12.5•1 mg/mL; 15•1 mg/mL

Bromhist-PDX oral drops ℞ *antitussive; antihistamine; decongestant; for children 1–24 months* [dextromethorphan hydrobromide; brompheniramine maleate; pseudoephedrine HCl] 3•1•12.5 mg/mL

Bromhist-PDX syrup ℞ *antitussive; decongestant; antihistamine; expectorant* [dextromethorphan hydrobromide; phenylephrine HCl; brompheniramine maleate; guaifenesin] 5•5•2•50 mg/5 mL

bromindione USAN, INN, BAN *anticoagulant* ⊘ brimonidine

bromine *element (Br)*

bromisoval INN [also: bromisovalum; bromvalerylurea; bromovaluree]

bromisovalum NF [also: bromisoval; bromvalerylurea; bromovaluree]

2-bromo-α-ergocryptine [see: bromocriptine]

bromocamphor [see: camphor, monobromated]

bromociclen INN [also: bromocyclen]

bromocriptine USAN, INN, BAN *dopamine agonist for Parkinson disease; lactation inhibitor; treatment for acromegaly, infertility, and hypogonadism*

bromocriptine mesilate JAN *dopamine agonist for Parkinson disease; lactation inhibitor; treatment for acromegaly, infertility, and hypogonadism* [also: bromocriptine mesylate]

bromocriptine mesylate USAN, USP *dopamine agonist for Parkinson disease; lactation inhibitor; treatment for acromegaly, infertility, and hypogonad-*

ism [also: bromocriptine mesilate] 2.5, 5 mg oral

bromocyclen BAN [also: bromociclen]

bromodeoxyuridine [now: broxuridine]

bromodiethylacetylurea [see: carbromal]

bromodiphenhydramine BAN *antihistamine; sleep aid* [also: bromodiphenhydramine HCl; bromazine]

bromodiphenhydramine HCl USP *antihistamine; sleep aid* [also: bromazine; bromodiphenhydramine]

bromofenofos INN

bromoform USP

bromofos INN ☑ Premphase

1-bromoheptadecafluorooctane [see: perflubron]

bromoisovaleryl urea (BVU) [see: bromisovalum]

bromophenol blue

bromophin [see: apomorphine HCl]

bromophos [see: bromofos]

bromopride INN

Bromo-Seltzer effervescent granules OTC *antacid; analgesic; antipyretic* [sodium bicarbonate; citric acid; acetaminophen] 2781•2224•325 mg/dose

bromotheophyllinate aminoisobutanol [see: pamabrom]

bromotheophyllinate pyranisamine [see: pyrabrom]

bromotheophyllinate pyrilamine [see: pyrabrom]

8-bromotheophylline [see: pamabrom]

bromovaluree [also: bromisovalum; bromisoval; bromvalerylurea]

11-bromovincamine [see: brovincamine]

bromovinyl arabinosyluracil (BV-araU) [see: sorivudine]

bromoxanide USAN, INN *anthelmintic*

bromperidol USAN, INN, BAN, JAN *antipsychotic*

bromperidol decanoate USAN, BAN *antipsychotic*

Bromphenex DM oral liquid ℞ *antitussive; antihistamine; decongestant* [dextromethorphan hydrobromide;

brompheniramine maleate; pseudoephedrine HCl] 30•4•60 mg/5 mL

Bromphenex HD oral liquid ℞ *narcotic antitussive; antihistamine; decongestant* [hydrocodone bitartrate; brompheniramine maleate; pseudoephedrine HCl] 1.7•2•30 mg/5 mL

brompheniramine INN, BAN *alkylamine antihistamine* [also: brompheniramine maleate]

brompheniramine maleate USP *alkylamine antihistamine* [also: brompheniramine] 10 mg/mL injection

brompheniramine maleate & pseudoephedrine HCl *antihistamine; decongestant* 4•60 mg/5 mL oral

brompheniramine maleate & pseudoephedrine HCl & hydrocodone bitartrate *antihistamine; decongestant; narcotic antitussive* 3•30•2.5 mg/5 mL oral

brompheniramine tannate *alkylamine antihistamine* 12 mg oral; 12 mg/5 mL oral

Bromplex HD oral liquid ℞ *narcotic antitussive; antihistamine; decongestant* [hydrocodone bitartrate; brompheniramine maleate; pseudoephedrine HCl] 1.7•2•30 mg/5 mL

Brompton's Cocktail; Brompton's Mixture (refers to any oral narcotic/alcoholic solution containing morphine and either cocaine or a phenothiazine derivative) *prophylaxis for chronic, severe pain*

bromvalerylurea JAN [also: bromisovalum; bromisoval; bromovaluree]

Bronchial capsules (discontinued 2007) ℞ *antiasthmatic; bronchodilator; expectorant* [theophylline; guaifenesin] 150•90 mg ☑ periwinkle

Bronchitol *investigational (orphan) mucolytic for bronchiectasis and cystic fibrosis* [mannitol]

Broncholate syrup ℞ *bronchodilator; decongestant; expectorant* [ephedrine HCl; guaifenesin] 12.5•200 mg/10 mL

Broncotron-D oral suspension ℞ *antitussive; decongestant; expectorant*

[dextromethorphan hydrobromide; phenylephrine HCl; guaifenesin] 20•5•200 mg/5 mL

Brondelate elixir (discontinued 2007) R̶ *antiasthmatic; bronchodilator; expectorant* [theophylline; guaifenesin] 192•150 mg/15 mL

Bronkaid Dual Action caplets OTC *bronchodilator; decongestant; expectorant* [ephedrine sulfate; guaifenesin] 25•400 mg

Bronkids oral drops R̶ *antitussive; antihistamine; decongestant; for children 6–24 months* [dextromethorphan hydrobromide; chlorpheniramine maleate; phenylephrine HCl] 2.75•0.6•1.5 mg/mL

Bronkodyl capsules (discontinued 2008) R̶ *antiasthmatic; bronchodilator* [theophylline] 100, 200 mg

bronopol INN, BAN, JAN

brook bean *medicinal herb* [see: buckbean]

brooklime *(Veronica beccabunga)* plant *medicinal herb used as a diuretic, emmenagogue, and febrifuge* ⸮ berkelium

broom *(Cytisus scoparius)* plant and bloom *medicinal herb for inducing bowel evacuation, diuresis, and emesis; also used as a homeopathic remedy for arrhythmias, diphtheria, and head and throat congestion* ⸮ barium

broom, butcher's *medicinal herb* [see: butcher's broom]

broom, dyer's; green broom *medicinal herb* [see: dyer's broom]

broparestrol INN

broperamole USAN, INN *anti-inflammatory*

bropirimine USAN, INN *antineoplastic; antiviral*

broquinaldol INN

brosotamide INN

brosuximide INN

brotianide INN, BAN

brotizolam USAN, INN, BAN, JAN *hypnotic*

Brovana inhalation solution for nebulization R̶ *twice-daily bronchodilator*

for chronic obstructive pulmonary disease (COPD), bronchitis, and emphysema [arformoterol tartrate] 15 (22) mcg per 2 mL dose ⸮ paraffin; Preven; Privine; Profen II

brovanexine INN

brovavir [see: sorivudine]

BröveX oral suspension R̶ *antihistamine* [brompheniramine tannate] 12 mg/5 mL

BröveX CT chewable tablets R̶ *antihistamine* [brompheniramine tannate] 12 mg

BröveX D oral suspension (discontinued 2007) R̶ *decongestant; antihistamine* [phenylephrine tannate; brompheniramine tannate] 20•12 mg/5 mL

BröveX PD oral suspension R̶ *decongestant; antihistamine* [pseudoephedrine HCl; brompheniramine maleate] 30•6 mg/5 mL

BröveX SR extended-release capsules R̶ *decongestant; antihistamine* [pseudoephedrine HCl; brompheniramine maleate] 90•9 mg

brovincamine INN [also: brovincamine fumarate]

brovincamine fumarate JAN [also: brovincamine]

brown algae *medicinal herb* [see: kelp *(Laminaria)*]

brownwort *medicinal herb* [see: woundwort]

broxaldine INN

broxaterol INN

Broxine *investigational (NDA filed, orphan) radiosensitizer for primary brain tumors* [broxuridine]

broxitalamic acid INN

broxuridine INN *investigational (NDA filed, orphan) radiosensitizer for primary brain tumors*

broxyquinoline INN

brucine sulfate NF

bruisewort *medicinal herb* [see: comfrey; soapwort]

bryony *(Bryonia alba; B. dioica)* root *medicinal herb used as a pectoral and purgative; not generally regarded as* *safe and effective as root is poisonous in high doses (ingestion of as few as 40 berries can be fatal in adults, 15 in children)* ⌕ boron

bryostatin-1 *investigational (orphan) agent for esophageal cancer; investigational (Phase I) for AIDS-related lymphomas*

B-Salt Forte ophthalmic solution (discontinued 2004) ℞ *intraocular irrigating solution* [sodium chloride (balanced saline solution)]

bSOD (bovine superoxide dismutase) [see: orgotein]

BSS (bismuth subsalicylate) [q.v.]

BSS; BSS Plus ophthalmic solution ℞ *intraocular irrigating solution* [sodium chloride (balanced saline solution)]

BTA Rapid Urine Test test kit for professional use ℞ *in vitro diagnostic aid for bladder tumor analytes in the urine*

BTA Stat Test test kit for home use OTC *in vitro diagnostic aid for bladder tumor analytes in the urine* [rapid immunoassay (RIA)]

bucainide INN *antiarrhythmic* [also: bucainide maleate]

bucainide maleate USAN *antiarrhythmic* [also: bucainide]

bucco *medicinal herb* [see: buchu]

Bucet capsules ℞ *barbiturate sedative; analgesic; antipyretic* [butalbital; acetaminophen] 50•650 mg ⌕ Boost

bucetin INN, BAN, JAN

buchu *(Agathosma betulina; Barosma betulina; B. cenulata; B. serratifolia)* leaves *medicinal herb for edema, gas, gout, inflammation, kidney and urinary tract infections, and prostatitis; also used as a douche for leukorrhea and vaginal yeast infections*

buciclovir INN

bucillamine INN, JAN

bucindolol INN, BAN *antihypertensive* [also: bucindolol HCl]

bucindolol HCl USAN *antihypertensive* [also: bucindolol]

buckbean *(Menyanthes trifoliata)* leaves *medicinal herb used as a tonic,*

cathartic, diuretic, anthelmintic, and emetic

buckeye; California buckeye; Ohio buckeye *medicinal herb* [see: horse chestnut]

buckhorn brake *(Osmunda cinnamomea; O. regalis)* root *medicinal herb used as a demulcent and tonic*

Buckley's Chest Congestion oral liquid OTC *expectorant* [guaifenesin] 100 mg/5 mL

Buckley's Cough Mixture oral liquid OTC *antitussive* [dextromethorphan hydrobromide] 12.5 mg/5 mL

buckthorn *(Rhamnus cathartica; R. frangula)* bark and berries *medicinal herb for bleeding, bowel disorders, chronic constipation, fever, gallstones, lead poisoning, and liver disorders* [see also: cascara sagrada] ⌕ buquiterine; picotrin

bucku *medicinal herb* [see: buchu]

bucladesine INN [also: bucladesine sodium]

bucladesine sodium JAN [also: bucladesine]

buclizine INN, BAN *antinauseant; antiemetic; anticholinergic; motion sickness relief* [also: buclizine HCl]

buclizine HCl USAN *antinauseant; antiemetic; anticholinergic; motion sickness relief* [also: buclizine]

buclosamide INN, BAN

bucloxic acid INN

bucolome INN, JAN

bucricaine INN

bucrilate INN *tissue adhesive* [also: bucrylate]

bucromarone USAN, INN *antiarrhythmic*

bucrylate USAN *tissue adhesive* [also: bucrilate]

bucumolol INN [also: bucumolol HCl]

bucumolol HCl JAN [also: bucumolol]

Budeprion SR sustained-release (12-hour) film-coated tablets ℞ *aminoketone antidepressant; also used for attention deficit/hyperactivity disorder (ADHD), neuropathic pain, and weight loss* [bupropion HCl] 100, 150 mg

Budeprion XL sustained-release (24-hour) film-coated tablets ℞ *aminoketone antidepressant; also used for attention deficit/hyperactivity disorder (ADHD), neuropathic pain, and weight loss* [bupropion HCl] 300 mg

budesonide USAN, INN, BAN, JAN *topical corticosteroidal anti-inflammatory; oral inhalation aerosol for chronic asthma; nasal aerosol for allergic rhinitis; rectal treatment for inflammatory bowel disease*

budipine INN

budotitane INN

budralazine INN, JAN

bufenadine [see: bufenadrine]

bufenadrine INN

bufeniode INN

bufetolol INN [also: bufetolol HCl]

bufetolol HCl JAN [also: bufetolol]

bufexamac INN, BAN, JAN

bufezolac INN

buffered aspirin [see: aspirin, buffered]

Bufferin coated tablets, coated caplets OTC *analgesic; antipyretic; anti-inflammatory; antirheumatic* [aspirin (buffered with calcium carbonate, magnesium oxide, and magnesium carbonate)] 325, 500 mg

Bufferin AF Nite Time tablets OTC *antihistaminic sleep aid; analgesic; antipyretic* [diphenhydramine HCl; acetaminophen] 30•500 mg

bufilcon A USAN *hydrophilic contact lens material*

buflomedil INN, BAN

bufogenin INN

buformin USAN, INN *antidiabetic*

bufrolin INN, BAN ☑ befuraline

bufuralol INN, BAN

bufylline BAN *diuretic; smooth muscle relaxant* [also: ambuphylline] ☑ Pavulon

bugbane *medicinal herb* [see: hellebore; black cohosh]

bugleweed (Lycopus virginicus) plant *medicinal herb for cough, excessive menses, nervous indigestion, and other nervous disorders*

bugloss *medicinal herb* [see: borage]

Bugs Bunny Complete chewable tablets OTC *vitamin/mineral/calcium/iron supplement* [multiple vitamins & minerals; calcium; iron; folic acid; biotin] ≛•100•18•0.4•0.04 mg

Bugs Bunny Plus Iron chewable tablets OTC *vitamin/iron supplement* [multiple vitamins; iron; folic acid] ≛•15•0.3 mg

Bugs Bunny with Extra C Children's chewable tablets OTC *vitamin supplement* [multiple vitamins; folic acid] ≛•0.3 mg

bugwort *medicinal herb* [see: black cohosh]

buku *medicinal herb* [see: buchu]

bulaquine INN ☑ Bellacane; Pilagan; Polocaine

Bulk Forming Fiber Laxative film-coated tablets OTC *bulk laxative; antidiarrheal* [calcium polycarbophil] 625 mg

bulk-producing laxatives *a subclass of laxatives that work by increasing the hydration and volume of stool to stimulate peristalsis; also form an emollient gel to ease the movement of stool through the intestines* [see also: laxatives]

bull's foot *medicinal herb* [see: coltsfoot]

bumadizone INN

bumecaine INN

bumepidil INN

bumetanide USAN, USP, INN, BAN, JAN *loop diuretic* 0.5, 1, 2 mg oral; 0.25 mg/mL injection

bumetrizole USAN, INN *ultraviolet screen*

Bumex IV or IM injection (discontinued 2004) ℞ *loop diuretic* [bumetanide] 0.25 mg/mL

Bumex tablets ℞ *loop diuretic* [bumetanide] 0.5, 1, 2 mg

Buminate 5%; Buminate 25% IV infusion ℞ *blood volume expander for shock, burns, and hypoproteinemia* [human albumin] 5%; 25%

bunaftine INN

bunamidine INN, BAN *anthelmintic* [also: bunamidine HCl]

bunamidine HCl USAN *anthelmintic* [also: bunamidine]

bunamiodyl INN [also: buniodyl]

bunamiodyl sodium [see: bunamiodyl; buniodyl]

bunaprolast USAN, INN *antiasthmatic; 5-lipoxygenase inhibitor*

bunapsilate INN *combining name for radicals or groups*

bunazosin INN [also: bunazosin HCl]

bunazosin HCl JAN [also: bunazosin]

bundlin [now: sedecamycin]

buniodyl BAN [also: bunamiodyl] ⑳ Panadol

bunitrolol INN [also: bunitrolol HCl]

bunitrolol HCl JAN [also: bunitrolol]

bunolol INN *antiadrenergic (β-receptor)* [also: bunolol HCl]

bunolol HCl USAN *antiadrenergic (β-receptor)* [also: bunolol]

Bupap caplets ℞ *barbiturate sedative; analgesic; antipyretic* [butalbital; acetaminophen] 50•650 mg

buparvaquone INN, BAN

buphenine INN, BAN *peripheral vasodilator* [also: nylidrin HCl]

Buphenyl tablets, powder for oral solution ℞ *antihyperammonemic for urea cycle disorders (orphan); investigational (orphan) for various sickling disorders* [sodium phenylbutyrate] 500 mg; 3 g/tsp., 8.6 g/tbsp.

bupicomide USAN, INN *antihypertensive*

bupivacaine INN, BAN *injectable local anesthetic* [also: bupivacaine HCl]

bupivacaine HCl USAN, USP, JAN *injectable local anesthetic* [also: bupivacaine] 0.25%, 0.5%, 0.75%

bupivacaine HCl & epinephrine *injectable local anesthetic; vasoconstrictor* 0.25%•1:200 000, 0.5%•1:200 000, 0.75%•1:200 000

Bupivicaine Spinal injection ℞ *local anesthetic for obstetric use* [bupivacaine HCl; dextrose] 0.75%•8.25%

bupranol [see: bupranolol]

bupranolol INN [also: bupranolol HCl]

bupranolol HCl JAN [also: bupranolol]

Buprenex IV or IM injection ℞ *narcotic agonist-antagonist analgesic* [buprenorphine HCl] 0.3 mg/mL

buprenorphine INN, BAN *narcotic agonist-antagonist analgesic* [also: buprenorphine HCl]

buprenorphine HCl USAN, JAN *narcotic agonist-antagonist analgesic for inpatient treatment of opiate dependence (orphan)* [also: buprenorphine] 0.3 mg/mL injection

bupropion BAN *aminoketone antidepressant; non-nicotine aid to smoking cessation* [also: bupropion HCl; amfebutamone]

bupropion HCl USAN *aminoketone antidepressant; non-nicotine aid to smoking cessation; also used for attention-deficit/hyperactivity disorder (ADHD), neuropathic pain, and weight loss* [also: amfebutamone; bupropion] 75, 100, 150, 200, 300 mg oral

bupropion hydrobromide *aminoketone antidepressant*

buquineran INN, BAN

buquinolate USAN, INN *coccidiostat for poultry*

buquiterine INN ⑳ picotrin

buramate USAN, INN *anticonvulsant; antipsychotic* ⑳ PowerMate

burdock (Arctium lappa; A. majus; A. minus) root *medicinal herb for arthritis, blood cleansing, dandruff, eczema, edema, fever, gout, kidney and lung disorders, rheumatism, skin diseases, and tumors; also used as an antimicrobial and diaphoretic* ⑳ Pred-G

burefrine [now: berefrine]

burnet (Pimpinella magna; P. saxifrage) root *medicinal herb used as an antispasmodic, astringent, carminative, diaphoretic, diuretic, stimulant, and stomachic* ⑳ Parnate; Pronto

burning bush *medicinal herb* [see: fraxinella; wahoo]

Burn-O-Jel gel OTC *anesthetic* [lidocaine] 0.5%

burodiline INN ⑳ Predalone 50

Buro-Sol solution (discontinued 2004) OTC *astringent wet dressing (Burow solution)* [aluminum sulfate] 0.23% ⑳ parsley; ProSol 20%

Burow solution [see: aluminum acetate]

Burow's Otic ear drops ℞ *antibacterial; antifungal; antiseptic; astringent* [acetic acid; aluminum acetate] 2%• <u>2</u>

burr seed; turkey burr seed; clotbur; hareburr; hurr-burr; thorny burr *medicinal herb* [see: burdock]

burrage *medicinal herb* [see: borage]

buserelin INN, BAN *hormonal antineoplastic; gonad-stimulating principle; luteinizing hormone-releasing hormone analogue* [also: buserelin acetate]

buserelin acetate USAN, JAN *hormonal antineoplastic; gonad-stimulating principle; luteinizing hormone-releasing hormone analogue* [also: buserelin]

BuSpar tablets ℞ *nonsedating azaspirone anxiolytic* [buspirone HCl] 5, 10, 15, 30 mg

buspirone INN, BAN *nonsedating azaspirone anxiolytic* [also: buspirone HCl] ② bisobrin

buspirone HCl USAN *nonsedating azaspirone anxiolytic* [also: buspirone] 5, 7.5, 10, 15, 30 mg oral

busulfan USP, INN, JAN *alkylating antineoplastic for chronic myelogenous leukemia (CML); pretreatment for bone marrow or stem cell transplants (orphan); investigational (orphan) for neoplastic meningitis and primary brain malignancies* [also: busulphan]

Busulfex IV infusion ℞ *alkylating antineoplastic for chronic myelogenous leukemia (CML); pretreatment for bone marrow or stem cell transplants (orphan)* [busulfan] 6 mg/mL

busulphan BAN *alkylating antineoplastic* [also: busulfan]

butabarbital USP *sedative; hypnotic* [also: secbutobarbitone]

butabarbital sodium USP *sedative; hypnotic* [also: secbutabarbital sodium] 15, 30 mg oral

butacaine INN, BAN [also: butacaine sulfate]

butacaine sulfate USP [also: butacaine]

butacetin USAN *analgesic; antidepressant*

butacetoluide [see: butanilicaine]

butaclamol INN *antipsychotic* [also: butaclamol HCl]

butaclamol HCl USAN *antipsychotic* [also: butaclamol]

butadiazamide INN

butafosfan INN, BAN

butalamine INN, BAN

butalbital USAN, USP, INN *barbiturate sedative*

butalbital & acetaminophen & caffeine *barbiturate sedative; analgesic; antipyretic* 50•325•40, 50•500•40 mg oral

butalbital & acetaminophen & caffeine & codeine phosphate *barbiturate sedative; analgesic; narcotic antitussive* 50•325•40•30 mg oral

butalbital & aspirin & caffeine *analgesic; barbiturate sedative* 50•325•40 mg oral

Butalbital Compound tablets, capsules ℞ *barbiturate sedative; analgesic; antipyretic* [butalbital; aspirin; caffeine] 50•325•40 mg

butalgin [see: methadone HCl]

butallylonal NF

butamben USAN, USP *topical anesthetic*

butamben picrate USAN *topical anesthetic* 1% topical

butamirate INN *antitussive* [also: butamirate citrate; butamyrate]

butamirate citrate USAN *antitussive* [also: butamirate; butamyrate]

butamisole INN *veterinary anthelmintic* [also: butamisole HCl]

butamisole HCl USAN *veterinary anthelmintic* [also: butamisole]

butamiverine [see: butaverine]

butamoxane INN

butamyrate BAN *antitussive* [also: butamirate citrate; butamirate]

butane (n-butane) NF *aerosol propellant* ② betony; biotin; Bitin; P-Tanna 12

1,4-butanediol (1,4-B; BDO); butane-1,4-diol *precursor to gamma hydroxybutyrate (GHB); a formerly legal alternative to GHB, now also illegal (Schedule I)* [see: gamma hydroxybutyrate (GHB)]

butanilicaine INN, BAN

butanixin INN
butanserin INN
butantrone INN
butaperazine USAN, INN *antipsychotic*
  ⑨ batoprazine
butaperazine maleate USAN *antipsychotic*
butaprost USAN, INN, BAN *bronchodilator*
butaverine INN
butaxamine INN *antidiabetic; antihyperlipoproteinemic* [also: butoxamine HCl; butoxamine]
butcher's broom (*Ruscus aculeatus*) rhizomes *medicinal herb for atherosclerosis, circulatory disorders, hemorrhoids, thrombosis, varicose veins, and venous insufficiency; not generally regarded as safe and effective*
butedronate tetrasodium USAN *bone imaging aid*
butedronic acid INN
butelline [see: butacaine sulfate]
butenafine *benzylamine antifungal*
butenafine HCl USAN *topical benzylamine antifungal*
butenemal [see: vinbarbital]
buteprate INN *former combining name for radicals or groups (name rescinded by the USAN)* [now: probutate]
buterizine USAN, INN *peripheral vasodilator* ⑨ Pitressin
Butesin Picrate ointment (discontinued 2004) OTC *anesthetic* [butamben picrate] 1%
butetamate INN [also: butethamate]
butethal NF [also: butobarbitone]
butethamate BAN [also: butetamate]
butethamine HCl NF
butethanol [see: tetracaine]
Butex Forte capsules ℞ *barbiturate sedative; analgesic; antipyretic* [butalbital; acetaminophen] 50•650 mg
buthalital sodium INN [also: buthalitone sodium]
buthalitone sodium BAN [also: buthalital sodium]
buthiazide USAN *diuretic; antihypertensive* [also: butizide]
Butibel tablets, elixir ℞ *GI/GU anticholinergic/antispasmodic; sedative* [belladonna extract; butabarbital sodium] 15•15 mg; 15•15 mg/5 mL
butibufen INN
butidrine INN
butikacin USAN, INN, BAN *antibacterial* ⑨ Betaxon
butilfenin USAN, INN *hepatic function test*
butinazocine INN
butinoline INN
butirosin INN *antibacterial antibiotic* [also: butirosin sulfate; butirosin sulphate] ⑨ Pitressin
butirosin sulfate USAN *antibacterial antibiotic* [also: butirosin; butirosin sulphate]
butirosin sulphate BAN *antibacterial antibiotic* [also: butirosin sulfate; butirosin]
Butisol Sodium tablets, elixir ℞ *sedative; hypnotic* [butabarbital sodium] 30, 50 mg; 30 mg/5 mL
butixirate USAN, INN *analgesic; antirheumatic*
butixocort INN
butizide INN *diuretic; antihypertensive* [also: buthiazide]
butobarbitone BAN [also: butethal]
butobendine INN
butoconazole INN, BAN *topical antifungal* [also: butoconazole nitrate]
butoconazole nitrate USAN, USP *topical antifungal* [also: butoconazole]
butocrolol INN
butoctamide INN [also: butoctamide semisuccinate]
butoctamide semisuccinate JAN [also: butoctamide]
butofilolol INN
butonate USAN, INN *anthelmintic*
butopamine USAN, INN *cardiotonic*
butopiprine INN
butoprozine INN *antiarrhythmic; antianginal* [also: butoprozine HCl] ⑨ batoprazine
butoprozine HCl USAN *antiarrhythmic; antianginal* [also: butoprozine]
butopyrammonium iodide INN
butopyronoxyl USP

butorphanol USAN, INN, BAN *analgesic; antitussive*

butorphanol tartrate USAN, USP, BAN, JAN *narcotic agonist-antagonist analgesic; antitussive* 10 mg nasal spray; 1, 2 mg/mL injection

butoxamine BAN *antidiabetic; antihyperlipoproteinemic* [also: butoxamine HCl; butaxamine]

butoxamine HCl USAN *antidiabetic; antihyperlipoproteinemic* [also: butaxamine; butoxamine]

2-butoxyethyl nicotinate [see: nicoboxil]

butoxylate INN

butoxyphenylacethydroxamic acid [see: bufexamac]

butriptyline INN, BAN *antidepressant* [also: butriptyline HCl]

butriptyline HCl USAN *antidepressant* [also: butriptyline]

butropium bromide INN, JAN

butterbur *(Petasites hybridus)* leaves and root *medicinal herb used as an analgesic for migraines and as an antispasmodic for asthma, cough, and gastrointestinal and urinary tract disorders; not generally regarded as safe and effective due to organ damage and carcinogenic properties*

buttercup *(Ranunculus acris; R. bulbosus; R. sceleratus)* plant *medicinal herb used as an acrid, anodyne, antispasmodic, diaphoretic, and rubefacient*

butterfly weed *medicinal herb* [see: pleurisy root]

butternut *(Juglans cinerea)* bark, leaves, flowers *medicinal herb used as an anthelmintic, antiseptic, cathartic, cholagogue, and nervine*

butterweed *medicinal herb* [see: fleabane; horseweed]

butydrine [see: butidrine]

butyl alcohol NF *solvent*

butyl aminobenzoate (butyl p-aminobenzoate) [now: butamben]

butyl p-aminobenzoate picrate [see: butamben picrate]

butyl chloride NF

butyl 2-cyanoacrylate [see: enbucrilate]

butyl DNJ (deoxynojirimycin) [see: deoxynojirimycin]

butyl p-hydroxybenzoate [see: butylparaben]

butyl methoxydibenzoylmethane [see: avobenzone]

butyl nitrite; isobutyl nitrite *amyl nitrite substitutes, sold as euphoric street drugs, which produce a quick but short-lived "rush"* [see also: amyl nitrite; volatile nitrites]

butyl parahydroxybenzoate JAN *antifungal agent* [also: butylparaben]

p-butylaminobenzoyldiethylaminoethyl HCl JAN

butylated hydroxyanisole (BHA) NF, BAN *antioxidant*

butylated hydroxytoluene (BHT) NF, BAN *antioxidant*

α-butylbenzyl alcohol [see: fenipentol]

1-butylbiguanide [see: buformin]

N-butyl-deoxynojirimycin [see: deoxynojirimycin]

1,4-butylene glycol (1,4-BG) *precursor to gamma hydroxybutyrate (GHB); a formerly legal alternative to GHB, now also illegal (Schedule I)* [see: gamma hydroxybutyrate (GHB)]

1,5-(butylimino)-1,5-dideoxy-D-glucitol *investigational (orphan) for Fabry disease and Gaucher disease*

butylmesityl oxide [see: butopyronoxyl]

butylparaben NF *antifungal agent* [also: butyl parahydroxybenzoate]

butylphenamide

butylphenylsalicylamide [see: butylphenamide]

butylscopolamine bromide JAN

butynamine INN

butyrate propionate [see: probutate; buteprate]

butyrophenones *a class of dopamine receptor antagonists with conventional (typical) antipsychotic activity* [also called: phenylbutylpiperadines]

butyrylcholesterinase *investigational (orphan) agent for reduction and clear-*

ance of serum cocaine levels and post-surgical apnea

butyrylperazine [see: butaperazine]

O-butyrylthiamine disulfide [see: bisbutitiamine]

butyvinyl [see: vinylbital]

buzepide metiodide INN

BVAP (BCNU, vincristine, Adriamycin, prednisone) *chemotherapy protocol* ⊇ BAVIP; BVPP; PVB; PVP

BV-araU (bromovinyl arabinosyluracil) [see: sorivudine]

BVCPP (BCNU, vinblastine, cyclophosphamide, procarbazine, prednisone) *chemotherapy protocol*

BVDS (bleomycin, Velban, doxorubicin, streptozocin) *chemotherapy protocol*

B-Vex D oral suspension ℞ *decongestant; antihistamine* [phenylephrine tannate; brompheniramine tannate] 20•12 mg/5 mL

BVPP (BCNU, vincristine, procarbazine, prednisone) *chemotherapy protocol* ⊇ BAVIP; BVAP; PVB; PVP

BVU (bromoisovaleryl urea) [see: bromisovalum]

BW 12C *investigational (orphan) agent for sickle cell disease*

Byclomine capsules, tablets ℞ *gastrointestinal anticholinergic/antispasmodic for irritable bowel syndrome (IBS)* [dicyclomine HCl] 10 mg; 20 mg ⊇ picolamine

Byetta subcu injection in prefilled pen injector ℞ *incretin mimetic antidiabetic for type 2 diabetes that improves the body's normal glucose-sensing mechanisms and slows gastric emptying; investigational for once-weekly dosing* [exenatide] 5, 10 mcg/dose

Bystolic tablets ℞ *cardioselective β-blocker for hypertension* [nebivolol HCl] 2.5, 5, 10 mg

C (vitamin C) [see: ascorbic acid]

C & E softgels OTC *vitamin supplement* [vitamins C and E] 500•400 mg

C Factors "1000" Plus tablets OTC *vitamin C supplement with multiple bioflavonoids* [vitamin C; rose hips; citrus bioflavonoids; rutin; hesperidin] 1000•25•250•50•25 mg

C vitamin [see: ascorbic acid]

^{14}C urea *diagnostic aid for H. pylori in the stomach* [also: carbon C 14 urea]

C1-esterase-inhibitor, recombinant human *investigational (Phase III, orphan) agent to prevent or treat acute attacks of angioedema*

CA (cyclophosphamide, Adriamycin) *chemotherapy protocol*

CA (cytarabine, asparaginase) *chemotherapy protocol for acute myelocytic leukemia (AML)*

^{45}Ca [see: calcium chloride Ca 45]

^{47}Ca [see: calcium chloride Ca 47]

cabastine INN

cabbage, cow *medicinal herb* [see: masterwort; white pond lily]

cabbage, meadow; swamp cabbage *medicinal herb* [see: skunk cabbage]

cabbage, water *medicinal herb* [see: white pond lily]

cabergoline USAN, INN *dopamine agonist for hyperprolactinemia* 0.5 mg oral

cabis bromatum [see: bibrocathol]

CABO (cisplatin, Abitrexate, bleomycin, Oncovin) *chemotherapy protocol for head and neck cancer*

CABOP; CA-BOP (Cytoxin, Adriamycin, bleomycin, Oncovin, prednisone) *chemotherapy protocol* ⊇ CAP-BOP; CPOB; cubeb; Q-Pap

CABS (CCNU, Adriamycin bleomycin, streptozocin) *chemotherapy protocol*

cabufocon A USAN *hydrophobic contact lens material*

cabufocon B USAN *hydrophobic contact lens material*

CAC (cisplatin, ara-C, caffeine) *chemotherapy protocol*

cacao butter JAN ⑨ cocoa butter

Cachexon *investigational (orphan) for AIDS-related cachexia* [L-glutathione, reduced]

cactinomycin USAN, INN *antibiotic antineoplastic* [also: actinomycin C]

CAD (cyclophosphamide, Adriamycin, dacarbazine) *chemotherapy protocol*

CAD (cytarabine [and] daunorubicin) *chemotherapy protocol*

cade oil [see: juniper tar]

cadexomer INN

cadexomer iodine USAN, INN, BAN *antiseptic; antiulcerative wound dressing*

cadmium *element (Cd)*

cadralazine INN, BAN, JAN

Ca-DTPA (calcium pentetate) [see: pentetate calcium trisodium]

Caduet *film-coated tablets* ℞ *combination calcium channel blocker and HMG-CoA reductase inhibitor for coronary artery disease (CAD), hypertension, chronic unstable angina, and hyperlipidemia* [amlodipine besylate; atorvastatin (as calcium)] 2.5•10, 2.5•20, 2.5•40, 5•10, 5•20, 5•40, 5•80, 10•10, 10•20, 10•40, 10•80 mg

CAE (cyclophosphamide, Adriamycin, etoposide) *chemotherapy protocol for small cell lung cancer (SCLC)* [also: ACE]

CAF (cyclophosphamide, Adriamycin, fluorouracil) *chemotherapy protocol for breast cancer*

cafaminol INN

Cafatine *suppositories (discontinued 2008)* ℞ *migraine-specific vasoconstrictor* [ergotamine tartrate; caffeine] 2•200 mg

Cafatine-PB *tablets* ℞ *migraine treatment; vasoconstrictor; anticholinergic; sedative* [ergotamine tartrate; caffeine; pentobarbital sodium; belladonna extract] 1•100•30•0.125 mg

Cafcit *oral solution, injectable* ℞ *analeptic; CNS stimulant for apnea of prematurity (orphan)* [caffeine citrate] 20 mg/mL

cafedrine INN, BAN

Cafergot *suppositories (discontinued 2008)* ℞ *migraine treatment; vasoconstrictor* [ergotamine tartrate; caffeine] 2•100 mg

Cafergot *tablets* ℞ *migraine treatment; vasoconstrictor* [ergotamine tartrate; caffeine] 1•100 mg

Caffedrine *tablets* OTC *CNS stimulant; analeptic* [caffeine] 200 mg

caffeic acid phenethyl ester (CAPE) *antimicrobial substance found in bee propolis*

caffeine USP, BAN, JAN *methylxanthine analeptic; CNS stimulant; diuretic; treatment for apnea of prematurity (orphan); potentiator of various NSAIDs* ⑨ C-Phen; Kuvan

caffeine citrate *methylxanthine analeptic; CNS stimulant for apnea of prematurity (orphan)* 10, 20 mg/mL oral; 10, 20 mg/mL injection

caffeine monohydrate [see: caffeine, citrated]

caffeine nut *medicinal herb* [see: kola nut]

caffeine & sodium benzoate *analeptic for respiratory depression due to an overdose of CNS depressants* 250 mg/mL injection

CAFP (cyclophosphamide, Adriamycin, fluorouracil, prednisone) *chemotherapy protocol* ⑨ CAV/EP; CCVPP; CFP; CH1VPP; CHVP; CVB; CVEB; CVP

CAFTH (cyclophosphamide, Adriamycin, fluorouracil, tamoxifen, Halotestin) *chemotherapy protocol*

CAFVP (cyclophosphamide, Adriamycin, fluorouracil, vincristine, prednisone) *chemotherapy protocol*

Cal Carb-HD *powder for oral solution* OTC *calcium supplement* [calcium carbonate] 2.5 g Ca/pkt.

Caladryl *cream (discontinued 2007)* OTC *antihistamine; astringent; antipru-*

ritic; emollient [diphenhydramine HCl; calamine] 1%•8%

Caladryl lotion OTC *poison ivy treatment* [calamine; pramoxine HCl; alcohol 2.2%] 8%•1%

Caladryl Clear lotion OTC *poison ivy treatment* [pramoxine HCl; zinc acetate; alcohol 2%] 1%•0.1%

Calafol tablets R̶ *vitamin/calcium supplement* [vitamins B_6 and B_{12}; folic acid; vitamin D_3; calcium] 25 mg• 425 mcg•1.6 mg•400 IU•400 mg ⧆ clove oil

Cala-gen lotion (discontinued 2004) OTC *antipruritic; anesthetic; antihistamine* [diphenhydramine HCl; alcohol 2%] 1% ⧆ collagen; Glaucon; Glyquin; Qualaquin

calamine USP, JAN *topical protectant; antipruritic; astringent; poison ivy treatment* ⧆ Chlo-Amine; gallamine

Calamine, Phenolated lotion OTC *poison ivy treatment* [calamine; zinc oxide; phenol] 8%•8%•1%

Calamine Lotion OTC *poison ivy treatment* [calamine; zinc oxide] 6.97%• 6.97%

calamint (Calamintha officinalis) *medicinal herb* [see: summer savory]

Calamintha hortensis medicinal herb [see: summer savory]

Calamintha montana medicinal herb [see: winter savory]

calamus (Acorus calamus) rhizome *medicinal herb for anxiety, bad breath from smoking, colic, digestive disorders, fever, gas, irritated throat, and promoting wound healing; not generally regarded as safe and effective and is prohibited in the U.S. as a food additive or supplement*

Calamycin lotion OTC *antihistamine; astringent; anesthetic; antiseptic* [pyrilamine maleate; zinc oxide; calamine; benzocaine; chloroxylenol; alcohol 2%]

Calan film-coated tablets R̶ *antianginal; antiarrhythmic; antihypertensive; calcium channel blocker* [verapamil HCl] 40, 80, 120 mg ⧆ Clenia; kaolin; khellin

Calan SR film-coated sustained-release tablets R̶ *antihypertensive; antianginal; antiarrhythmic; calcium channel blocker* [verapamil HCl] 120, 180, 240 mg

calanolide A *investigational (Phase I/II) non-nucleoside reverse transcriptase inhibitor (NNRTI) for HIV infection*

Calcarb 600 with Vitamin D tablets OTC *calcium supplement* [calcium carbonate; vitamin D] 1.5 g (600 mg Ca)•125 IU

Cal-Carb Forte chewable tablets, caplets OTC *antacid; calcium supplement* [calcium carbonate] 1250 mg (500 mg Ca)

Cal-C-Caps capsules OTC *calcium supplement* [calcium citrate] 825 mg (180 mg Ca) ⧆ gelcaps

Cal-Cee tablets OTC *calcium supplement* [calcium citrate] 1150 mg (250 mg Ca) ⧆ Colace; K-Lease

Calcet tablets OTC *dietary supplement* [calcium; vitamin D] 150 mg•100 IU ⧆ Gelhist; Glyset

Calcet Plus tablets OTC *vitamin/calcium/iron supplement* [multiple vitamins; calcium; iron; folic acid] ≛• 152.8•18•0.8 mg

Calcibind powder for oral solution R̶ *antiurolithic to prevent stone formation in absorptive calciuria type I* [cellulose sodium phosphate] 300 g bulk pack

CalciCaps tablets OTC *dietary supplement* [dibasic calcium phosphate; calcium gluconate; calcium carbonate; vitamin D] 125 mg (Ca)•60 mg (P) •67 IU

CalciCaps with Iron tablets OTC *dietary supplement* [dibasic calcium phosphate; calcium gluconate; calcium carbonate; vitamin D; ferrous gluconate] 125 mg (Ca)•60 mg (P)• 67 IU•7 mg

Calci-Chew chewable tablets OTC *calcium supplement* [calcium carbonate] 1250 mg (500 mg Ca)

calcidiol [see: calcifediol]

calcifediol (25-hydroxycholecalcif-erol; 25-hydroxyvitamin D₃) USAN, USP, INN *vitamin D precursor (converted to calcitriol in the body); calcium regulator for treatment of metastatic bone disease or hypocalcemia associated with chronic renal dialysis*

Calciferol IM injection (discontinued 2005) ℞ *vitamin deficiency therapy for refractory rickets, familial hypophosphatemia, and hypoparathyroidism* [ergocalciferol (vitamin D₂)] 500 000 IU/mL

calciferol [now: ergocalciferol]

Calciferol Drops for oral or IM administration OTC *vitamin supplement; vitamin deficiency therapy for refractory rickets, familial hypophosphatemia, and hypoparathyroidism* [ergocalciferol (vitamin D₂)] 8000 IU/mL

Calcijex injection ℞ *vitamin D therapy for hypoparathyroidism and hypocalcemia of chronic renal dialysis* [calcitriol] 1 mcg/mL

Calcimar subcu or IM injection (discontinued 2006) ℞ *calcium regulator for Paget disease (orphan), hypercalcemia, and postmenopausal osteoporosis* [calcitonin (salmon)] 200 IU/mL

Calci-Mix capsules OTC *calcium supplement* [calcium carbonate] 1250 mg (500 mg Ca)

Calcionate syrup OTC *calcium supplement* [calcium glubionate] 1.8 g/5 mL ② Cleocin T

calcipotriene USAN *topical antipsoriatic* [also: calcipotriol] 0.005% topical

calcipotriol INN, BAN *topical antipsoriatic* [also: calcipotriene]

Calciquid syrup OTC *calcium supplement* [calcium glubionate] 1.8 g/5 mL

calcitonin (human) USAN, INN, BAN, JAN *calcium regulator for symptomatic Paget disease (osteitis deformans) (orphan)*

calcitonin (salmon) USAN, INN, BAN *calcium regulator for Paget disease (orphan), hypercalcemia, and postmenopausal osteoporosis*

calcitonin salmon (synthesis) JAN *synthetic analogue of calcitonin (salmon); calcium regulator* [also: salcatonin]

Cal-Citrate tablets, capsules OTC *calcium supplement* [calcium citrate] 250 mg Ca; 225 mg Ca

calcitriol (1α,25-dihydroxycholecalciferol; 1,25-hydroxyvitamin D₃; 1,25 [OH]₂D₃) USAN, INN, BAN, JAN *physiologically active form of vitamin D; calcium regulator for hypoparathyroidism and hypocalcemia due to chronic renal dialysis; also used to decrease the severity of psoriatic lesions* 0.25, 0.5 mcg oral; 1 mcg/mL oral; 1, 2 mcg injection

calcium *element (Ca)*

calcium, oyster shell [see: calcium carbonate]

Calcium 600 tablets OTC *calcium supplement* [calcium carbonate] 1500 mg (600 mg Ca)

Calcium 600 + D tablets OTC *dietary supplement* [calcium; vitamin D] 600 mg•125 IU ② galosemide

Calcium 600 with Vitamin D tablets OTC *dietary supplement* [calcium; vitamin D] 600 mg•100 IU

calcium acetate USP, JAN *dietary calcium supplement (25% elemental calcium); buffering agent for hyperphosphatemia of end-stage renal disease (orphan)* 667 mg (169 mg Ca) oral

calcium alginate fiber *topical hemostatic*

calcium aminacyl B-PAS (benzoyl para-aminosalicylate) [see: benzoylpas calcium]

calcium 4-aminosalicylate trihydrate [see: aminosalicylate calcium]

calcium amphomycin [see: amphomycin]

calcium antagonists *a class of coronary vasodilators that inhibit cardiac muscle contraction and slow cardiac electrical conduction velocity* [also called: calcium channel blockers; slow channel blockers]

calcium ascorbate (vitamin C) USP *water-soluble vitamin; antiscorbutic* 500 mg oral; 3256 mg/tsp. oral

calcium benzamidosalicylate INN, BAN *antibacterial; tuberculostatic* [also: benzoylpas calcium]

calcium benzoyl *p*-aminosalicylate (B-PAS) [see: benzoylpas calcium]

calcium benzoylpas [see: benzoylpas calcium]

calcium bis-dioctyl sulfosuccinate [see: docusate calcium]

calcium bis-glycinate *dietary calcium supplement*

calcium bromide JAN

calcium carbimide INN [also: cyanamide]

calcium carbonate USP *antacid; dietary calcium supplement (40% elemental calcium); investigational (orphan) for hyperphosphatemia of end-stage renal disease* [also: precipitated calcium carbonate] 500, 600, 650, 1250 mg oral; 1250 mg/5 mL oral

calcium carbonate, precipitated [now: calcium carbonate]

calcium carbophil *bulk laxative*

calcium caseinate *dietary calcium supplement; infant formula modifier*

calcium channel blockers *a class of coronary vasodilators that inhibit cardiac muscle contraction and slow cardiac electrical conduction velocity* [also called: calcium antagonists; slow channel blockers]

calcium chloride USP, JAN *calcium replenisher*

calcium chloride Ca 45 USAN *radioactive agent*

calcium chloride Ca 47 USAN *radioactive agent*

calcium chloride dihydrate [see: calcium chloride]

calcium citrate USP *dietary calcium supplement (22% elemental calcium)* 1.2, 4.5 g oral; 3.6 g/5 mL oral

calcium citrate tetrahydrate [see: calcium citrate]

calcium clofibrate INN

calcium cyanamide [see: calcium carbimide]

calcium D-glucarate tetrahydrate [see: calcium saccharate]

calcium D-gluconate lactobionate monohydrate [see: calcium glubionate]

calcium dioctyl sulfosuccinate [see: docusate calcium]

calcium disodium edathamil [see: edetate calcium disodium]

calcium disodium edetate JAN *heavy metal chelating agent* [also: edetate calcium disodium; sodium calcium edetate; sodium calciumedetate]

Calcium Disodium Versenate IM, IV, or subcu injection ℞ *chelating agent for acute or chronic lead poisoning and lead encephalopathy* [edetate calcium disodium] 200 mg/mL

calcium dobesilate INN

calcium doxybensylate [see: calcium dobesilate]

calcium DTPA [see: pentetate calcium trisodium]

calcium edetate sodium [see: edetate calcium disodium]

calcium EDTA (ethylene diamine tetraacetic acid) [see: edetate calcium disodium]

calcium folinate INN, BAN, JAN *antianemic; folate replenisher; antidote to folic acid antagonist* [also: leucovorin calcium]

calcium glubionate USAN, INN *dietary calcium supplement*

calcium gluceptate USP *parenteral calcium replenisher* [also: calcium glucoheptonate] 1100 mg/5 mL injection

calcium glucoheptonate INN *parenteral calcium replenisher* [also: calcium gluceptate]

calcium gluconate (calcium D-gluconate) USP *dietary calcium supplement (8% elemental calcium); investigational (orphan) wash for hydrofluoric acid burns* 500, 650, 975, 1000 mg oral; 3.85 g/15 mL oral; 10% injection

calcium glycerinophosphate [see: calcium glycerophosphate]

calcium glycerophosphate NF, JAN

calcium hopantenate JAN

calcium hydroxide USP *astringent*

calcium hydroxide phosphate [see: calcium phosphate, tribasic]

calcium hydroxylapatite *subcu collagen production stimulant for HIV-related facial lipoatrophy and moderate to severe facial wrinkles and folds*

calcium hypophosphite NF

calcium iodide *expectorant*

calcium iododocosanoate [see: iodobehenate calcium]

calcium lactate USP, JAN *dietary calcium supplement (13% elemental calcium)* 325, 650, 770 mg oral

calcium lactate hydrate [see: calcium lactate]

calcium lactate pentahydrate [see: calcium lactate]

calcium lactobionate USP *dietary calcium supplement*

calcium lactobionate dihydrate [see: calcium lactobionate]

calcium lactophosphate NF

calcium L-aspartate JAN

calcium levofolinate [see: levoleucovorin calcium]

calcium levulate [see: calcium levulinate]

calcium levulinate USP *dietary calcium supplement*

calcium levulinate dihydrate [see: calcium levulinate]

calcium mandelate USP

calcium oxide [see: lime]

calcium pangamate [now: dimethylglycine HCl]

calcium pantothenate (calcium D-pantothenate; vitamin B₅) USP, INN, JAN *water-soluble vitamin; coenzyme A precursor* [also: pantothenic acid] 100, 218, 545 mg oral

calcium pantothenate, racemic (calcium DL-pantothenate) USP *water-soluble vitamin; enzyme cofactor*

calcium para-aminosalicylate JAN [also: aminosalicylate calcium]

calcium phosphate, dibasic USP, JAN *dietary calcium supplement; tablet base*

calcium phosphate, monocalcium [see: calcium phosphate, dibasic]

calcium phosphate, tribasic NF *dietary calcium supplement (39% elemental calcium)* [also: durapatite; hydroxyapatite]

calcium polycarbophil USAN, USP *bulk laxative; antidiarrheal*

calcium polystyrene sulfonate JAN *ion exchange resin for hyperkalemia*

calcium polysulfide & calcium thiosulfate [see: lime, sulfurated]

calcium saccharate USP, INN *stabilizer*

calcium silicate NF *tablet excipient*

calcium sodium ferriclate INN *hematinic* [also: ferriclate calcium sodium]

calcium stearate NF, JAN *tablet and capsule lubricant*

calcium sulfate NF *tablet and capsule diluent*

calcium tetracemine disodium [see: edetate calcium disodium]

calcium trisodium pentetate INN, BAN *plutonium chelating agent* [also: pentetate calcium trisodium]

calcium 10-undecenoate [see: calcium undecylenate]

calcium undecylenate USAN *antifungal*

calciumedetate sodium [see: edetate calcium disodium]

Calderol capsules (discontinued 2005) ℞ *vitamin D therapy for metastatic bone disease or hypocalcemia associated with chronic renal dialysis* [calcifediol] 20, 50 mcg

Caldesene ointment OTC *moisturizer; emollient; astringent* [cod liver oil (vitamins A and D); zinc oxide; lanolin] ⊡ clodazon

Caldesene topical powder OTC *antifungal* [calcium undecylenate] 10% ⊡ clodazon

caldiamide INN *pharmaceutic aid* [also: caldiamide sodium]

caldiamide sodium USAN, BAN *pharmaceutic aid* [also: caldiamide]

Calel D tablets OTC *dietary supplement* [calcium carbonate; cholecalciferol] 500 mg•200 IU

Calendula officinalis *medicinal herb* [see: marigold]

CALF (cyclophosphamide, Adriamycin, leucovorin [rescue], fluorouracil) *chemotherapy protocol*

calfactant USAN *surface-active extract of saline lavage of calf lungs, used for prevention of respiratory distress syndrome (RDS) in premature infants (orphan)*

CALF-E (cyclophosphamide, Adriamycin, leucovorin [rescue], fluorouracil, ethinyl estradiol) *chemotherapy protocol*

Cal-G capsules OTC *calcium supplement* [calcium gluconate] 700 mg (50 mg Ca)

CAL-G (cyclophosphamide, asparaginase, leurocristine, daunorubicin, prednisone) *chemotherapy protocol for acute lymphocytic leukemia*

Cal-Gest chewable tablets OTC *calcium supplement* [calcium carbonate] 500 mg (200 mg Ca)

Calgonate wash *investigational (orphan) emergency treatment for hydrofluoric acid burns* [calcium gluconate]

California barberry *medicinal herb* [see: Oregon grape]

California buckthorn *medicinal herb* [see: buckthorn; cascara sagrada]

California false hellebore (*Veratrum californicum*) [see: hellebore]

californium *element* (Cf)

calioben [see: calcium iodobehenate]

Cal-Lac capsules OTC *calcium supplement* [calcium lactate] 500 mg

Calluna vulgaris *medicinal herb* [see: heather]

calmatives *a class of soothing agents that reduce excitement, nervousness, distress, or irritation* [also called: sedatives]

Calmol 4 rectal suppositories OTC *emollient; astringent* [cocoa butter; zinc oxide] 80%•10%

Calmoseptine ointment OTC *astringent; mild anesthetic; antipruritic; counterirritant* [zinc oxide; menthol] 20.6%•0.44%

Calm-X tablets OTC *anticholinergic; antiemetic; antivertigo agent; motion sickness preventative* [dimenhydrinate] 50 mg

Cal-Nate tablets ℞ *vitamin/mineral/calcium/iron supplement; stool softener* [multiple vitamins & minerals; calcium; iron; folic acid; docusate sodium] ±•125•27•1•50 mg 🔁 kola nut

calomel NF

CaloMist nasal spray ℞ *once-daily maintenance administration following intramuscular vitamin B$_{12}$ therapy* [cyanocobalamin] 25 mcg/0.1 mL dose

Calphosan IV injection ℞ *calcium replacement* [calcium glycerophosphate; calcium lactate] 50•50 mg/10 mL (0.08 mEq Ca/mL) 🔁 clofezone

Calphron tablets ℞ *calcium supplement; buffering agent for hyperphosphatemia in end-stage renal failure (orphan)* [calcium acetate] 667 mg (169 mg Ca) 🔁 Claforan; Kolephrin

calteridol INN *pharmaceutic aid* [also: calteridol calcium]

calteridol calcium USAN, BAN *pharmaceutic aid* [also: calteridol]

Caltha palustris *medicinal herb* [see: cowslip]

Caltrate 600 film-coated tablets OTC *calcium supplement* [calcium carbonate] 1500 mg (600 mg Ca)

Caltrate 600 + D tablets OTC *dietary supplement* [calcium carbonate; vitamin D] 600 mg•200 IU

Caltrate 600 + Iron/Vitamin D film-coated tablets OTC *dietary supplement* [calcium carbonate; ferrous fumarate; vitamin D] 600 mg•18 mg•125 IU

Caltrate Plus tablets OTC *dietary supplement* [calcium carbonate; vitamin D; multiple minerals] 600 mg•200 IU•±

Caltro tablets OTC *dietary supplement* [calcium; vitamin D] 250 mg•125 IU 🔁 coal tar; Kaletra

calumba; calumba root; calumbo *medicinal herb* [see: colombo]

calusterone USAN, INN *antineoplastic*

Calypte test kit for professional use ℞ *urine test for HIV-1 antibodies*

CAM (cyclophosphamide, Adriamycin, methotrexate) *chemotherapy protocol*

Cama Arthritis Pain Reliever tablets (discontinued 2007) OTC *analgesic; antipyretic; anti-inflammatory; antirheumatic* [aspirin (buffered with magnesium oxide and aluminum hydroxide)] 500 mg

camazepam INN

CAMB (Cytoxin, Adriamycin, methotrexate, bleomycin) *chemotherapy protocol* ⊡ C-MOPP; COMB

cambendazole USAN, INN, BAN *anthelmintic*

CAMELEON (cytosine arabinoside, methotrexate, Leukovorin, Oncovin) *chemotherapy protocol*

camellia oil JAN

Camellia sinensis medicinal herb [see: green tea]

CAMEO (cyclophosphamide, Adriamycin, methotrexate, etoposide, Oncovin) *chemotherapy protocol*

Cameo Oil OTC *bath emollient* ⊡ COMLA

CAMF (cyclophosphamide, Adriamycin, methotrexate, folinic acid) *chemotherapy protocol* ⊡ CMF; CMV; COMF

camiglibose USAN, INN *antidiabetic*

Camila tablets (in packs of 28) ℞ *oral contraceptive (progestin only)* [norethindrone] 0.35 mg ⊡ COMLA

camiverine INN

camomile *medicinal herb* [see: chamomile]

camonagrel INN

camostat INN [also: camostat mesilate]

camostat mesilate JAN [also: camostat]

cAMP (cyclic adenosine monophosphate) [see: adenosine phosphate]

CAMP (cyclophosphamide, Adriamycin, methotrexate, procarbazine HCl) *chemotherapy protocol for non–small cell lung cancer (NSCLC)* ⊡ C-MOPP; COMB

Campath IV infusion ℞ *immunosuppressant for B-cell chronic lymphocytic leukemia (orphan); also used for rheumatoid arthritis and multiple sclerosis* [alemtuzumab] 30 mg/mL ⊡ Compete

camphetamide [see: camphotamide]

Campho-Phenique topical liquid, gel OTC *mild anesthetic; anti-infective; counterirritant* [camphor; phenol; eucalyptus oil] 10.8%•4.7%• ⅔

Campho-Phenique Cold Sore Treatment and Scab Relief cream OTC *anesthetic for cold sores and fever blisters* [pramoxine HCl; petrolatum] 1%•30%

camphor (d-camphor; dl-camphor) USP, JAN *topical antipruritic; mild local anesthetic; counterirritant* [also: trans-π-oxocamphor] ⊡ comfrey

camphor, monobromated USP

camphorated opium tincture [now: paregoric]

camphorated parachlorophenol [see: parachlorophenol, camphorated]

camphoric acid USP

camphotamide INN

Campral enteric-coated delayed-release tablets ℞ *GABA/taurine analogue for the treatment of alcoholism* [acamprosate calcium] 333 mg

Camptosar IV infusion ℞ *topoisomerase I inhibitor; antineoplastic for metastatic colorectal cancer* [irinotecan HCl] 20 mg/mL

camptothecin-11 (CPT-11) [see: irinotecan]

camsilate INN *combining name for radicals or groups* [also: camsylate]

camsylate USAN, BAN *combining name for radicals or groups* [also: camsilate]

Camvirex *investigational (orphan) for pancreatic cancer and pediatric HIV/AIDS infections* [rubitecan]

camylofin INN

Canada fleabane *medicinal herb* [see: fleabane; horseweed]

Canada pitch tree *medicinal herb* [see: hemlock]

Canada root *medicinal herb* [see: pleurisy root]

Canada tea *medicinal herb* [see: winter-green]

canaigre (Rumex hymenosepalus) *medicinal herb for a variety of disease states and used as a purported substitute for ginseng; not generally regarded as safe and effective because of high tannin content and possible mutagenic effect when used internally* ☑ ginger

Canasa suppositories ℞ *anti-inflammatory for active ulcerative colitis, proctosigmoiditis, and proctitis* [mesalamine (5-aminosalicylic acid)] 1000 mg

canbisol INN

Cancidas powder for IV infusion ℞ *antifungal for candidiasis, candidemia, invasive aspergillosis and other resistant fungal infections* [caspofungin acetate] 50, 70 mg/vial

candesartan USAN, INN *antihypertensive; angiotensin II receptor antagonist*

candesartan cilexetil USAN *antihypertensive; angiotensin II receptor antagonist; treatment for heart failure*

candicidin USAN, USP, INN, BAN *polyene antifungal*

Candida albicans skin test antigen *diagnostic aid for diminished cellular immunity; test for HIV patients to assess TB antigen response*

CandidaSure reagent slides for professional use ℞ *in vitro diagnostic aid for Candida albicans in the vagina*

Candin intradermal injection ℞ *diagnostic aid for diminished cellular immunity; test for HIV patients to assess TB antigen response* [Candida albicans skin test antigen] 0.1 mL ☑ quinidine

candleberry; candleberry myrtle *medicinal herb* [see: bayberry; tung seed]

candocuronium iodide INN

candoxatril USAN, INN, BAN *antihypertensive*

candoxatrilat USAN, INN, BAN *antihypertensive*

Cankaid oral solution OTC *anti-inflammatory; antiseptic* [carbamide peroxide] 10%

cankerroot *medicinal herb* [see: gold thread]

canna; channa *medicinal herb* [see: kanna]

cannabidinol (CBD) INN, BAN *a nonpsychoactive derivative of the Cannabis sativa (marijuana) plant; approved in Canada as an analgesic for pain associated with cancer and multiple sclerosis*

Cannabis sativa (marijuana; marihuana; hashish) *euphoric/hallucinogenic street drug made from the resin or dried leaves and flowering tops of the cannabis plant; medicinal herb for asthma, analgesia, leprosy, and loss of appetite*

canrenoate potassium USAN *aldosterone antagonist* [also: canrenoic acid; potassium canrenoate]

canrenoic acid INN, BAN *aldosterone antagonist* [also: canrenoate potassium; potassium canrenoate]

canrenone USAN, INN *aldosterone antagonist*

cantharides JAN

cantharidin *topical keratolytic*

Cantil tablets ℞ GI *antispasmodic; anticholinergic; peptic ulcer adjunct* [mepenzolate bromide] 25 mg

Canvaxin *investigational (Phase III) theraccine for malignant melanoma*

CAO (cyclophosphamide, Adriamycin, Oncovin) *chemotherapy protocol*

CAP (cellulose acetate phthalate) [q.v.]

CAP (cyclophosphamide, Adriamycin, Platinol) *chemotherapy protocol for non–small cell lung cancer (NSCLC)*

CAP (cyclophosphamide, Adriamycin, prednisone) *chemotherapy protocol*

CAP; CAP-I (cyclophosphamide, Adriamycin, Platinol) *chemotherapy protocol*

CAP-II (cyclophosphamide, Adriamycin, high-dose Platinol) *chemotherapy protocol*

Capastat Sulfate powder for IM injection ℞ *tuberculostatic* [capreomycin sulfate] 1 g/vial

CAP-BOP (cyclophosphamide, Adriamycin, procarbazine, bleomycin, Oncovin, prednisone) *chemotherapy protocol* ☒ CABOP; CPOB; cubeb; Q-Pap

CAPE (caffeic acid phenethyl ester) *antimicrobial substance found in bee propolis*

Cape aloe *medicinal herb* [see: aloe]

cape gum *medicinal herb* [see: acacia]

capecitabine USAN, INN *oral fluoropyrimidine (a 5-FU prodrug) antineoplastic for metastatic breast and colorectal cancer; investigational (Phase III) for pancreatic cancer*

capers (*Capparis spinosa*) flower buds and leaves *medicinal herb for skin disorders and for reducing the effects of enlarged capillaries*

Capex shampoo ℞ *corticosteroidal antiinflammatory; antiseborrheic* [fluocinolone acetonide] 0.01% ☒ Copegus

capimorelin tartrate [see: capromorelin tartrate]

Capital with Codeine oral suspension ℞ *narcotic antitussive; analgesic; antipyretic* [codeine phosphate; acetaminophen] 12•120 mg/5 mL

Capitrol shampoo ℞ *antibacterial and antifungal for seborrheic dermatitis* [chloroxine] 2% ☒ Gabitril

caplet (dosage form) *capsule-shaped tablet* ☒ cobalt

capmul 8210 [see: monoctanoin]

capobenate sodium USAN *antiarrhythmic*

capobenic acid USAN, INN *antiarrhythmic*

Capoten tablets ℞ *antihypertensive; angiotensin-converting enzyme (ACE) inhibitor; treatment for congestive heart failure (CHF) and diabetic nephropathy* [captopril] 12.5, 25, 50, 100 mg

Capozide 25/15; Capozide 25/25; Capozide 50/15; Capozide 50/25 tablets ℞ *antihypertensive; angiotensin-converting enzyme (ACE) inhibi-*tor; *diuretic* [captopril; hydrochlorothiazide] 25•15 mg; 25•25 mg; 50•15 mg; 50•25 mg

Capparis spinosa *medicinal herb* [see: capers]

CAPPr (cyclophosphamide, Adriamycin, Platinol, prednisone) *chemotherapy protocol* ☒ copper; Keppra

capreomycin INN, BAN *bactericidal antibiotic; tuberculostatic* [also: capreomycin sulfate]

capreomycin sulfate USAN, USP, JAN *bactericidal antibiotic; tuberculostatic* [also: capreomycin]

Caprogel *investigational (orphan) topical treatment for traumatic hyphema of the eye* [aminocaproic acid]

capromab INN *monoclonal antibody; imaging adjunct for prostate cancer and its metastases* [also: capromab pendetide]

capromab pendetide USAN *monoclonal antibody; after on-site radiolabeling with indium In 111, it becomes **indium In 111 capromab**, a radiodiagnostic imaging agent for new or recurrent prostate cancer and its metastases* [also: capromab]

capromorelin tartrate USAN *growth hormone secretagogue for anti-aging, congestive heart failure, and catabolic illness*

caproxamine INN, BAN

capsaicin *topical analgesic; counterirritant; investigational (orphan) for erythromelalgia and painful HIV-related neuropathy* 0.025%, 0.075% topical

Capsella bursa-pastoris *medicinal herb* [see: shepherd's purse]

Capsicum frutescens; C. annuum *medicinal herb* [see: cayenne]

capsicum oleoresin *topical analgesic; counterirritant*

Capsin lotion OTC *analgesic; counterirritant* [capsaicin] 0.025%, 0.075% ☒ Cubicin; kebuzone; quipazine

Capsulets (trademarked dosage form) *sustained-release caplet*

captab (dosage form) *capsule-shaped tablet*

captamine INN *depigmentor* [also: capt-amine HCl]

captamine HCl USAN *depigmentor* [also: captamine]

captodiame INN, BAN

captodiame HCl [see: captodiame]

captodiamine HCl [see: captodiame]

captopril USAN, USP, INN, BAN, JAN *antihypertensive; angiotensin-convert-ing enzyme (ACE) inhibitor; treatment for congestive heart failure (CHF) and diabetic nephropathy* 12.5, 25, 50, 100 mg oral

captopril & hydrochlorothiazide *antihypertensive; angiotensin-converting enzyme (ACE) inhibitor; diuretic* 25•15, 25•25, 50•15, 50•25 mg oral

capuride USAN, INN *hypnotic* ☒ Key-Pred

Capzasin-HP cream OTC *analgesic; counterirritant* [capsaicin] 0.1%

Capzasin-P cream OTC *analgesic; coun-terirritant* [capsaicin] 0.035%

Carac cream ℞ *antineoplastic for actinic keratoses (AK)* [fluorouracil] 0.5% ☒ Coreg; Kuric

caracemide USAN, INN *antineoplastic*

Carafate tablets, oral suspension ℞ *treatment for duodenal ulcer* [sucral-fate] 1 g; 1 g/10 mL ☒ Geravite

caramel NF *coloring agent* ☒ Gerimal

caramiphen INN, BAN *antitussive*

caramiphen edisylate *antitussive*

caramiphen HCl [see: caramiphen]

caraway (Carum carvi) NF *seeds medicinal herb for acid indigestion, appetite stimulation, colic, gas, gastro-intestinal spasms, and uterine cramps*

caraway oil NF ☒ coral; Kerol

carazolol INN, BAN ☒ Kerasal AL

Carb PSE 12 DM oral suspension ℞ *antitussive; antihistamine; decongestant* [dextromethorphan tannate; carbi-noxamine tannate; pseudoephedrine tannate] 27.5•3.2•45.2 mg/5 mL

Carb Pseudo-Tan oral suspension ℞ *antitussive; decongestant* [carbetapen-tane tannate; pseudoephedrine tan-nate] 25•75 mg/5 mL

carbacephems *a class of bactericidal antibiotics similar to second-generation cephalosporins (q.v.)*

carbachol USP, INN, BAN, JAN *ophthal-mic cholinergic; miotic for surgery; antiglaucoma agent* [also: carbacho-line chloride]

carbacholine chloride *ophthalmic cho-linergic; miotic for surgery; antiglau-coma agent* [also: carbachol]

carbacrylamine resins

carbadipimidine HCl [see: carpipra-mine dihydrochloride]

carbadox USAN, INN, BAN *antibacterial*

carbaldrate INN

carbamate choline chloride [see: carbachol]

carbamazepine USAN, USP, INN, BAN, JAN *iminostilbene anticonvulsant; anal-gesic for trigeminal neuralgia; antipsy-chotic for manic episodes of a bipolar disorder; also used for restless legs syn-drome (RLS), alcohol withdrawal, and postherpetic neuralgia* 100, 200 mg oral; 100 mg/5 mL oral

carbamide [see: urea]

carbamide peroxide USP *topical dental antiseptic; cerumenolytic to emulsify and disperse ear wax*

N-carbamoylarsanilic acid [see: car-barsone]

carbamoylcholine chloride [see: car-bachol]

O-carbamoylsalicylic acid lactam [see: carsalam]

carbamylcholine chloride [see: car-bachol]

carbamylglutamic acid *investigational (orphan) treatment for N-acetylgluta-mate synthetase deficiency*

carbamylmethylcholine chloride [see: bethanechol chloride]

carbantel INN *anthelmintic* [also: car-bantel lauryl sulfate]

carbantel lauryl sulfate USAN *anthel-mintic* [also: carbantel]

carbapenems *a class of broad-spectrum antibiotics that are effective against both gram-positive and gram-negative bacteria* [also called: "penems"]

Carbaphen 12 oral liquid ℞ *antitus-sive; antihistamine; decongestant* [car-betapentane tannate; chlorphenir-amine tannate; phenylephrine tannate] 60•8•20 mg/5 mL

carbaril INN [also: carbaryl]

carbarsone USP, INN

carbaryl BAN [also: carbaril]

carbasalate calcium INN *analgesic* [also: carbaspirin calcium]

carbaspirin calcium USAN *analgesic* [also: carbasalate calcium]

Carbastat solution ℞ *direct-acting miotic for ophthalmic surgery* [carba-chol] 0.01%

Carbatab-12 tablets ℞ *antitussive; decongestant; expectorant* [carbeta-pentane citrate; phenylephrine HCl; guaifenesin] 60•15•600 mg

Carbatrol extended-release capsules ℞ *iminostilbene anticonvulsant; analgesic for trigeminal neuralgia; also used for restless legs syndrome (RLS), alcohol withdrawal, and postherpetic neuralgia* [carbamazepine] 100, 200, 300 mg

Carbatuss CL oral liquid (discontin-ued 2007) ℞ *antitussive; decongestant; expectorant* [carbetapentane citrate; phenylephrine HCl; potassium guai-acolsulfonate] 20•10•100 mg/5 mL

Carbaxefed RF oral drops (discontin-ued 2007) ℞ *decongestant; antihista-mine* [pseudoephedrine HCl; carbi-noxamine maleate] 15•1 mg/mL

carbazeran USAN, INN *cardiotonic*

carbazochrome INN, JAN

carbazochrome salicylate INN

carbazochrome sodium sulfonate INN

carbazocine INN

carbenicillin INN, BAN *extended-spec-trum penicillin antibiotic* [also: carbeni-cillin disodium; carbenicillin sodium]

carbenicillin disodium USAN, USP *extended-spectrum penicillin antibiotic* [also: carbenicillin; carbenicillin sodium]

carbenicillin indanyl sodium USAN, USP *extended-spectrum penicillin antibi-otic* (base=76.4%) [also: carindacillin]

carbenicillin phenyl sodium USAN *antibacterial* [also: carfecillin]

carbenicillin potassium USAN *anti-bacterial*

carbenicillin sodium JAN *antibacterial* [also: carbenicillin disodium; carben-icillin]

carbenoxolone INN, BAN *corticoster-oid; anti-inflammatory* [also: carben-oxolone sodium]

carbenoxolone sodium USAN *cortico-steroid; anti-inflammatory* [also: car-benoxolone]

carbenzide INN

carbesilate INN *combining name for radicals or groups*

carbetapentane citrate NF *antitussive* [also: pentoxyverine]

carbetapentane tannate *antitussive*

Carbetaplex oral liquid (discontinued 2007) ℞ *antitussive; decongestant; expectorant* [carbetapentane citrate; phenylephrine HCl; guaifenesin] 20•15•100 mg/5 mL

carbetimer USAN, INN *antineoplastic*

carbetocin INN, BAN *uterotonic agent to prevent postpartum hemorrhage fol-lowing cesarean section*

Carbex tablets ℞ *monoamine oxidase inhibitor (MAOI); dopaminergic for Parkinson disease* [selegiline HCl] 5 mg

Carbic DS pediatric syrup (discontin-ued 2007) ℞ *decongestant; antihista-mine* [pseudoephedrine HCl; carbi-noxamine maleate] 25•2 mg/5 mL

carbidopa USAN, USP, INN, BAN, JAN *decarboxylase inhibitor; levodopa potentiator for Parkinson disease (no effect when given alone)*

carbidopa & levodopa *dopamine pre-cursor plus potentiator for Parkinson disease (orphan)* 10•100, 25•100, 25•250, 50•200 mg oral

carbifene INN *analgesic* [also: carbi-phene HCl; carbiphene]

carbimazole INN, BAN

carbinoxamine INN, BAN *antihistamine for allergic rhinitis* [also: carbinoxa-mine maleate]

Carbinoxamine syrup, oral drops (discontinued 2007) ℞ *decongestant; antihistamine* [pseudoephedrine HCl; carbinoxamine maleate] 60•4 mg/5 mL; 25•2 mg/mL

Carbinoxamine Compound syrup, pediatric oral drops (discontinued 2004) ℞ *antitussive; antihistamine; decongestant* [dextromethorphan hydrobromide; carbinoxamine maleate; pseudoephedrine HCl] 15•4•60 mg/5 mL; 4•2•25 mg/mL

carbinoxamine maleate USP *antihistamine for allergic rhinitis* [also: carbinoxamine] 4 mg oral; 4 mg/5 mL oral

carbinoxamine maleate & carbinoxamine tannate *antihistamine for allergic rhinitis* 2•6 mg/5 mL oral

carbinoxamine maleate & hydrocodone bitartrate & pseudoephedrine HCl *antihistamine; antitussive; decongestant* 2•5•30 mg/5 mL oral

carbinoxamine maleate & pseudoephedrine HCl *antihistamine; decongestant* 4•60 mg/5 mL oral; 2•25 mg/mL oral

carbinoxamine tannate *antihistamine for allergic rhinitis*

carbinoxamine tannate & carbinoxamine maleate *antihistamine for allergic rhinitis* 6•2 mg/5 mL oral

carbiphene BAN *analgesic* [also: carbiphene HCl; carbifene]

carbiphene HCl USAN *analgesic* [also: carbifene; carbiphene]

Carbocaine injection ℞ *local anesthetic* [mepivacaine HCl] 1%, 1.5%, 2%, 3%

Carbocaine with Neo-Cobefrin injection ℞ *local anesthetic; vasoconstrictor* [mepivacaine HCl; levonordefrin] 2%•1:20 000

carbocisteine INN, BAN *mucolytic* [also: carbocysteine]

carbocloral USAN, INN, BAN *hypnotic*

carbocromen INN *coronary vasodilator* [also: chromonar HCl]

carbocysteine USAN *mucolytic* [also: carbocisteine]

Carbodex DM oral drops (discontinued 2007) ℞ *antitussive; antihistamine; decongestant; for children 1–18 months* [dextromethorphan hydrobromide; carbinoxamine maleate; pseudoephedrine HCl] 4•2•15 mg/mL

Carbodex DM syrup (discontinued 2007) ℞ *antitussive; antihistamine; decongestant* [dextromethorphan hydrobromide; brompheniramine maleate; pseudoephedrine HCl] 15•4•45 mg/5 mL

carbodimid calcium [see: calcium carbimide]

Carbofed DM oral drops (discontinued 2007) ℞ *antitussive; antihistamine; decongestant; for children 1–24 months* [dextromethorphan hydrobromide; carbinoxamine maleate; pseudoephedrine HCl] 4•1•15 mg/mL

Carbofed DM syrup ℞ *antitussive; antihistamine; decongestant* [dextromethorphan hydrobromide; brompheniramine maleate; pseudoephedrine HCl] 15•4•45 mg/5 mL

carbofenotion INN [also: carbophenothion]

carbol-fuchsin solution (or paint) USP *antifungal*

carbolic acid [see: phenol]

carbolin [see: carbachol]

carbolonium bromide BAN [also: hexcarbacholine bromide]

carbomer INN, BAN *emulsifying and suspending agent* [also: carbomer 910]

carbomer 1342 NF *emulsifying and suspending agent*

carbomer 910 USAN, NF *emulsifying and suspending agent* [also: carbomer]

carbomer 934 USAN, NF *emulsifying and suspending agent*

carbomer 934P USAN, NF *emulsifying and suspending agent*

carbomer 940 USAN, NF *emulsifying and suspending agent*

carbomer 941 USAN, NF *emulsifying and suspending agent*

carbomycin INN

carbon *element* (C)

carbon, activated

carbon C 13 urea *diagnostic aid for detection of* H. pylori *in the stomach*

carbon C 14 urea *diagnostic aid for* H. pylori *in the stomach* [also: ^{14}C urea]

carbon dioxide (CO_2) USP *respiratory stimulant*

carbon tetrachloride NF *solvent*

carbonic acid, calcium salt [see: calcium carbonate]

carbonic acid, dilithium salt [see: lithium carbonate]

carbonic acid, dipotassium salt [see: potassium carbonate]

carbonic acid, disodium salt [see: sodium carbonate]

carbonic acid, magnesium salt [see: magnesium carbonate]

carbonic acid, monoammonium salt [see: ammonium carbonate]

carbonic acid, monopotassium salt [see: potassium bicarbonate]

carbonic acid, monosodium salt [see: sodium bicarbonate]

carbonic anhydrase inhibitors *a class of diuretic agents that reduce the rate of aqueous humor formation, resulting in decreased intraocular pressure; available in both systemic (tablets) and topical (eye drops) forms*

carbonis detergens, liquor (LCD) [see: coal tar]

carbonyl iron *hematinic; iron supplement (100% elemental iron as microparticles)*

carbophenothion BAN [also: carbofenotion]

carboplatin USAN, INN, BAN *alkylating antineoplastic for ovarian and other cancers* 10 mg/mL, 50, 150, 450 mg/ dose injection

carboplatin & etoposide & paclitaxel *chemotherapy protocol for primary adenocarcinoma and small cell lung cancer (SCLC)*

carboplatin & gemcitabine *chemotherapy protocol for non–small cell lung cancer (NSCLC)*

carboprost USAN, INN, BAN *oxytocic*

carboprost methyl USAN *oxytocic*

carboprost trometanol BAN *oxytocic; prostaglandin-type abortifacient* [also: carboprost tromethamine]

carboprost tromethamine USAN, USP *oxytocic; prostaglandin-type abortifacient* [also: carboprost trometanol]

Carboptic Drop-Tainers (eye drops) ℞ *antiglaucoma agent; direct-acting miotic* [carbachol] 3%

carboquone INN

carbose D [see: carboxymethylcellulose sodium]

Carbo-Tax (carboplatin, Taxol) *chemotherapy protocol for ovarian cancer* [also: CaT]

carbovir *investigational (orphan) agent for AIDS and symptomatic HIV infections*

carboxyimamidate [see: carbetimer]

carboxymethylcellulose calcium NF *tablet disintegrant*

carboxymethylcellulose sodium USP *bulk laxative; suspending and viscosity-increasing agent; ophthalmic moisturizer; tablet excipient* [also: carmellose; carmellose sodium]

carboxymethylcellulose sodium 12 NF *suspending and viscosity-increasing agent*

carboxypeptidase G2 *investigational (orphan) for methotrexate toxicity*

carbromal NF, INN

carbubarb INN

carbubarbital [see: carbubarb]

carburazepam INN

carbutamide INN, BAN

carbuterol INN, BAN *bronchodilator* [also: carbuterol HCl]

carbuterol HCl USAN *bronchodilator* [also: carbuterol]

carcainium chloride INN

carcinoembryonic antigen (CEA)

cardamom seed NF

cardamom [see: bitter cardamom]

Cardec syrup ℞ *decongestant; antihistamine* [phenylephrine HCl; chlorpheniramine maleate] 12.5•4 mg/5 mL

Cardec DM oral drops ℞ *antitussive; antihistamine; decongestant; for children 6–24 months* [dextromethorphan hydrobromide; chlorpheniramine maleate; phenylephrine HCl] 3•1•3.5 mg/mL

Cardec-DM syrup (discontinued 2004) ℞ *antitussive; antihistamine; decongestant* [dextromethorphan hydrobromide; carbinoxamine maleate; pseudoephedrine HCl] 15•60•4 mg/5 mL

Cardec-S oral liquid (discontinued 2004) ℞ *decongestant; antihistamine* [pseudoephedrine HCl; carbinoxamine maleate] 60•4 mg/5 mL 🄳 Kerodex #51; Kredex

Cardene capsules ℞ *vasodilator for chronic stable angina; calcium channel blocker for hypertension* [nicardipine HCl] 20, 30 mg

Cardene I.V. injection ℞ *calcium channel blocker for the short-term treatment of hypertension* [nicardipine HCl] 2.5 mg/mL

Cardene SR sustained-release capsules ℞ *calcium channel blocker for hypertension* [nicardipine HCl] 30, 45, 60 mg 🄳 Gordon's Urea 40%

cardiac glycosides *a class of cardiovascular drugs that increase the force of cardiac contractions* [also called: digitalis glycosides]

Cardiac T test *in vitro diagnostic aid for troponin T (indicator of cardiac damage) in whole blood*

cardiacs *a class of agents that stimulate or otherwise affect the heart (a term used in folk medicine)* 🄳 Kerodex; Kredex

cardiamid [see: nikethamide]

cardin *medicinal herb* [see: blessed thistle]

Cardio-Green (CG) powder for IV injection (discontinued 2004) ℞ *in vivo diagnostic aid for cardiac output, hepatic function, and ophthalmic angiography* [indocyanine green] 25, 50 mg

Cardiolite injection ℞ *myocardial perfusion agent for cardiac SPECT imaging* [technetium Tc 99m sestamibi] 5 mL

Cardi-Omega 3 capsules OTC *dietary supplement* [omega-3 fatty acids; multiple vitamins & minerals] 1000• ≜ mg

cardioplegic solution (calcium chloride, magnesium chloride, potassium chloride, sodium chloride) [q.v.]

cardioprotective agents *a class of potent intracellular chelating agents which protect the heart from the effects of doxorubicin*

Cardiotek Rx coated tablets ℞ *dietary supplement* [vitamins B_6 and B_{12}; folic acid; L-arginine HCl] 50•0.5• 2• ≜ mg

Cardizem IV injection (discontinued 2008) ℞ *calcium channel blocker for atrial fibrillation or paroxysmal supraventricular tachycardia (PSVT)* [diltiazem HCl] 5 mg/mL

Cardizem Lyo-Ject (prefilled syringe) ℞ *calcium channel blocker for atrial fibrillation or paroxysmal supraventricular tachycardia (PSVT)* [diltiazem HCl] 25 mg

Cardizem tablets ℞ *antianginal; antihypertensive; antiarrhythmic; calcium channel blocker* [diltiazem HCl] 30, 60, 90, 120 mg

Cardizem CD sustained-release capsules ℞ *antihypertensive; antianginal; antiarrhythmic; calcium channel blocker* [diltiazem HCl] 120, 180, 240, 300, 360 mg

Cardizem LA extended-release caplets ℞ *antihypertensive; antianginal; calcium channel blocker* [diltiazem HCl] 120, 180, 240, 300, 360, 420 mg

Cardizem SR sustained-release capsules (discontinued 2004) ℞ *antihypertensive; antianginal; antiarrhythmic; calcium channel blocker* [diltiazem HCl] 60, 90, 120 mg

cardophyllin [see: aminophylline]

Cardura tablets ℞ *α_1-adrenergic blocker for hypertension and benign prostatic hyperplasia (BPH)* [doxazosin mesylate] 1, 2, 4, 8 mg

Cardura XL extended-release tablets ℞ *α_1-adrenergic blocker for benign prostatic hyperplasia (BPH)* [doxazosin mesylate] 4, 8 mg

carebastine INN

carena [see: aminophylline]

carfecillin INN, BAN *antibacterial* [also: carbenicillin phenyl sodium]

carfenazine INN *antipsychotic* [also: carphenazine maleate; carphenazine]

carfentanil INN *narcotic analgesic* [also: carfentanil citrate]

carfentanil citrate USAN *narcotic analgesic* [also: carfentanil]

carfimate INN ⊡ crufomate

cargentos [see: silver protein]

cargutocin INN

cariabamate *investigational (Phase III) anticonvulsant*

Carica papaya *medicinal herb* [see: papaya]

Carimune NF powder for IV infusion ℞ *passive immunizing agent for HIV and idiopathic thrombocytopenic purpura (ITP); investigational (orphan) for Guillain-Barré syndrome* [immune globulin (IVIG)] 1, 3, 6, 12 g/dose

carindacillin INN, BAN *extended-spectrum penicillin antibiotic* [also: carbenicillin indanyl sodium]

carisoprodol USP, INN, BAN *skeletal muscle relaxant* 350 mg oral

carisoprodol & aspirin & codeine phosphate *skeletal muscle relaxant; narcotic analgesic* 200•325•16 mg oral

carline thistle (*Carlina acaulis*) root *medicinal herb used as a carminative, diaphoretic, digestive, diuretic, febrifuge, and, in large doses, an emetic and purgative*

carmantadine USAN, INN *antiparkinsonian*

carmellose INN *suspending agent; tablet excipient* [also: carboxymethylcellulose sodium; carmellose sodium]

carmellose sodium BAN *suspending agent; tablet excipient* [also: carboxymethylcellulose sodium; carmellose]

carmetizide INN

carminatives *a class of agents that relieve flatulence*

carminomycin HCl [now: carubicin HCl]

carmofur INN

Carmol 10 lotion OTC *moisturizer; emollient; keratolytic* [urea] 10% ⊡ Gerimal

Carmol 20 cream OTC *moisturizer; emollient; keratolytic* [urea] 20% ⊡ Gerimal

Carmol 40 cream, gel ℞ *moisturizer; emollient; keratolytic* [urea] 40% ⊡ Gerimal

Carmol HC cream ℞ *corticosteroidal anti-inflammatory; moisturizer; emollient* [hydrocortisone acetate; urea] 1%•10%

Carmol Scalp Treatment lotion ℞ *antibiotic; keratolytic* [sulfacetamide sodium; urea] 10%•10%

carmoxirole INN

carmustine USAN, INN, BAN *nitrosourea-type alkylating antineoplastic for brain tumors, multiple myeloma, Hodgkin disease, and non-Hodgkin lymphomas; polymer implant for recurrent malignant glioma (orphan)*

Carnation Follow-Up oral liquid, powder for oral liquid OTC *total or supplementary infant feeding*

Carnation Good Start [see: Good Start]

carnauba wax [see: wax, carnauba]

carnidazole USAN, INN, BAN *antiprotozoal*

carnitine INN *vitamin B_t*

L-carnitine [see: levocarnitine]

Carnitor tablets, oral solution, IV injection or infusion ℞ *dietary amino acid for primary and secondary genetic carnitine deficiency (orphan) and end-stage renal disease (orphan); investigational (orphan) for pediatric cardiomyopathy* [levocarnitine] 330 mg; 100 mg/mL; 500 mg/2.5 mL, 1 g/5 mL

Carnitor SF sugar-free oral solution ℞ *dietary amino acid for primary and secondary genetic carnitine deficiency (orphan) and end-stage renal disease (orphan); investigational (orphan) for pediatric cardiomyopathy* [levocarnitine] 100 mg/mL

carnosine *natural anti-carbonylation agent that prevents cross-linking of protein and collagen; antioxidant; dipeptide of β-alanine and L-histidine*

carocainide INN
Caroid enteric-coated tablets OTC *stimulant laxative* [bisacodyl] 5 mg
β-carotene [see: beta carotene]
caroverine INN
caroxazone USAN, INN *antidepressant*
carpenter's herb *medicinal herb* [see: woundwort]
carpenter's square *medicinal herb* [see: figwort]
carperidine INN, BAN
carperone INN
carphenazine BAN *antipsychotic* [also: carphenazine maleate; carfenazine]
carphenazine maleate USAN, USP *antipsychotic* [also: carfenazine; carphenazine]
carpindolol INN
carpipramine INN
carpipramine dihydrochloride [see: carpipramine]
carpolene [now: carbomer 934P]
carprazidil INN
carprofen USAN, INN, BAN *nonsteroidal anti-inflammatory drug (NSAID); analgesic; antipyretic; approved for humans, but currently marketed only for veterinary use* 25, 50, 100 mg oral
carpronium chloride INN
Carpuject (trademarked delivery form) *prefilled syringe*
Carpuject Smartpak (trademarked delivery form) *prefilled cartridge-needle unit package*
CarraFoam; CarraWash topical liquid OTC *skin cleanser for incontinence care* [aloe vera; acemannan] ☒ Geravim; Kerafoam
carrageenan NF *suspending and viscosity-increasing agent*
CarraKlenz topical liquid OTC *wound cleanser for intact skin* [aloe vera; acemannan]
CarraSmart gel OTC *hydrogel wound dressing* [acemannan]
Carrasyn; Carrasyn V gel OTC *hydrogel wound dressing* [acemannan] ☒ chrysin; garcinia
carrot (*Daucus carota*) oil from the dried seed and root *medicinal herb for*

edema, gas, and worms; also used as a nutritional and vitamin supplement and stimulant; may possibly protect the heart and liver ☒ Geriot
carsalam INN, BAN
carsatrin INN *cardiotonic* [also: carsatrin succinate]
carsatrin succinate USAN *cardiotonic* [also: carsatrin]
cartazolate USAN, INN *antidepressant*
carteolol INN, BAN *topical antiglaucoma agent; β-blocker for hypertension* [also: carteolol HCl]
carteolol HCl USAN *topical antiglaucoma agent; β-blocker for hypertension* [also: carteolol] 1%
Carthamus tinctorius *medicinal herb* [see: safflower]
Cartia XT extended-release capsules ℞ *antihypertensive; antianginal; antiarrhythmic; calcium channel blocker* [diltiazem HCl] 120, 180, 240, 300 mg
carticaine BAN *amide local anesthetic for dentistry* [also: articaine] ☒ Corticaine
Cartrix (delivery form) *prefilled syringe*
Cartrol Filmtabs (film-coated tablets) OTC *β-blocker for hypertension* [carteolol HCl] 2.5, 5 mg
carubicin INN *antineoplastic* [also: carubicin HCl]
carubicin HCl USAN *antineoplastic* [also: carubicin]
Carum carvi NF *medicinal herb* [see: caraway]
carumonam INN, BAN *antibacterial* [also: carumonam sodium] ☒ germanium
carumonam sodium USAN *antibacterial* [also: carumonam]
carvedilol USAN, INN, BAN, JAN *α- and β-blocker for hypertension, congestive heart failure (CHF), and left ventricular dysfunction (LVD) following myocardial infarction (MI); also used for chronic angina pectoris and idiopathic cardiomyopathy* 3.125, 6.25, 12.5, 25 mg oral
carvedilol phosphate *α- and β-blocker for hypertension, congestive heart failure (CHF), and left ventricular dysfunction (LVD) following myocardial infarction*

(MI); also used for chronic angina pectoris and idiopathic cardiomyopathy

carvotroline HCl USAN *antipsychotic*

Caryophyllus aromaticus medicinal herb [see: cloves]

carzelesin USAN *antineoplastic*

carzenide INN

casanthranol USAN, USP *stimulant laxative*

Cascara Aromatic oral liquid OTC *stimulant laxative* [cascara sagrada; alcohol 18%]

cascara fluidextract, aromatic USP *stimulant laxative; investigational (orphan) to speed the evacuation of an oral drug overdose* 2–6 mL oral

cascara sagrada USP *stimulant laxative* 325 mg oral

cascara sagrada (Frangula purshiana; Rhamnus purshiana) bark *medicinal herb for constipation, cough, and gallbladder, intestinal, and liver disorders; chronic use can cause hypokalemia and melanosis coli* [see also: buckthorn]

cascarin [see: casanthranol]

Casec powder OTC *protein supplement* [calcium caseinate]

Casodex film-coated tablets ℞ *antiandrogen antineoplastic for prostatic cancer* [bicalutamide] 50 mg

casopitant *investigational (NDA filed) NK-1 receptor antagonist for the prevention of chemotherapy-induced nausea and vomiting*

caspofungin acetate USAN *systemic echinocandin antifungal for candidiasis, candidemia, invasive aspergillosis and other resistant fungal infections*

Cassia acutifolia; C. angustifolia; C. senna medicinal herb [see: senna]

cassia oil [see: cinnamon oil]

CAST (Color Allergy Screening Test) reagent sticks *for professional use* ℞ *in vitro diagnostic aid for immunoglobulin E in serum*

Castaderm topical liquid OTC *antifungal; astringent; antiseptic* [resorcinol; boric acid; acetone; basic fuchsin; phenol; alcohol 9%]

Castel Minus; Castel Plus topical liquid OTC *antifungal; antiseptic* [resorcinol; acetone; basic fuchsin; alcohol 11.5%]

Castellani Paint Modified topical solution ℞ *antifungal; antibacterial; keratolytic* [basic fuchsin; phenol; resorcinol]

Castellani's paint [see: carbol-fuchsin solution]

Castile soap

castor oil USP *stimulant laxative*

CaT (carboplatin, Taxol) *chemotherapy protocol for adenocarcinoma, non–small cell lung cancer (NSCLC), and ovarian cancer* [also: Carbo-Tax]

CaT (cytarabine, Adriamycin, thioguanine) *chemotherapy protocol*

Cataflam tablets ℞ *analgesic; nonsteroidal anti-inflammatory drug (NSAID) for osteoarthritis, rheumatoid arthritis, ankylosing spondylitis, and dysmenorrhea* [diclofenac potassium] 50 mg

Catapres tablets ℞ *antihypertensive* [clonidine HCl] 0.1, 0.2, 0.3 mg

Catapres-TTS-1; Catapres-TTS-2; Catapres-TTS-3 7-day transdermal patch ℞ *antihypertensive* [clonidine HCl] 0.1 mg/day (2.5 mg); 0.2 mg/day (5 mg); 0.3 mg/day (7.5 mg)

Catatrol *investigational (orphan) bicyclic antidepressant for cataplexy and narcolepsy* [viloxazine HCl]

catchfly *medicinal herb* [see: dogbane]

catchweed *medicinal herb* [see: bedstraw]

catechins *a class of natural polyphenolic antioxidants found in green tea and grape seed extract, used for their anti-carcinogenic, anti-inflammatory, and antiatherosclerotic properties and to promote thermogenesis* [see also: epicatechins; kunecatechins]

catechol-O-methyltransferase (COMT) [see: COMT inhibitors]

catgut suture [see: absorbable surgical suture]

Catha edulis the plant from which cathinone, a naturally occurring stimulant, is derived [see also: cathinone; methcathinone]

Catharanthus roseus medicinal herb [see: periwinkle]

cathartics a class of agents that cause vigorous evacuation of the bowels by increasing bulk, stimulating peristaltic action, etc. [also called: purgatives]

Cathflo Activase powder for intra-catheter instillation ℞ tissue plasminogen activator (tPA) thrombolytic to keep open (TKO) central venous access devices (CVADs) (not therapeutic) [alteplase] 2.2 mg/vial

cathine INN ᵈ Kao-Tin; K-Tan

cathinone INN an extract of the Catha edulis plant, a naturally occurring stimulant [see also: Catha edulis; methcathinone] ᵈ cotinine

cathomycin sodium [see: novobiocin sodium]

catkins willow medicinal herb [see: willow]

catmint medicinal herb [see: catnip]

catnip (*Nepeta cataria*) plant medicinal herb for colds, colic, convulsions, diarrhea, digestion, fever, flu, gas, hives, nervous conditions, and stimulating delayed menses

Catrix Correction cream OTC moisturizer; emollient

catrup medicinal herb [see: catnip]

cat's claw (*Uncaria guianensis*; *U. tomentosa*) inner bark medicinal herb for cancer, Candida infections, chronic fatigue, contraception, Crohn disease, diverticulitis, hypertension, irritable bowel, lupus, parasites, PMS, ulcers, and viral infections; also used as immune booster ᵈ Guiatuss AC

catswort medicinal herb [see: catnip]

Caucasian walnut medicinal herb [see: English walnut]

Caulophyllum thalictroides medicinal herb [see: blue cohosh]

caustics a class of escharotic or corrosive agents that destroy living tissue [also called: cauterants]

cauterants a class of escharotic or corrosive agents that destroy living tissue [also called: caustics]

CAV (cyclophosphamide, Adriamycin, vinblastine) chemotherapy protocol

CAV (cyclophosphamide, Adriamycin, vincristine) chemotherapy protocol for small cell lung cancer (SCLC) [also: VAC]

CAVe; CA-Ve (CCNU, Adriamycin, vinblastine) chemotherapy protocol

CAVE (cyclophosphamide, Adriamycin, vincristine, etoposide) chemotherapy protocol for small cell lung cancer (SCLC)

CAV/EP (cyclophosphamide, Adriamycin, vincristine, etoposide, Platinol) chemotherapy protocol for small cell lung cancer (SCLC) ᵈ CAFP; CCVPP; CFP; CH1VPP; CHVP; CVB; CVEB; CVP

Caverject intracavernosal injection, Luer-lock single-use autoinjector ℞ vasodilator for erectile dysfunction [alprostadil] 5, 10, 20, 40 mcg/mL

Caverject Impulse powder for intra-cavernosal injection in prefilled syringe ℞ vasodilator for erectile dysfunction [alprostadil] 10, 20 mcg/0.5 mL dose

CA-VP16; CAVP16 (cyclophosphamide, Adriamycin, VP-16) chemotherapy protocol for small cell lung cancer (SCLC) ᵈ CAFP; CCVPP; CFP; CH1VPP; CHVP; CVB; CVEB; CVP

cayenne (*Capsicum annuum*; *C. frutescens*) fruit medicinal herb for arthritis, bleeding, cold feet, diabetes, high blood pressure, kidney disorders, rheumatism, poor circulation, strokes, topical neuritis syndromes, tumors, and ulcers

CBD (cannabidinol) [q.v.]

CBV (cyclophosphamide, BCNU, VePesid) chemotherapy protocol

CBV (cyclophosphamide, BCNU, VP-16-213) chemotherapy protocol

CC (carboplatin, cyclophosphamide) chemotherapy protocol for ovarian cancer

CC-Galactosidase investigational (orphan) enzyme replacement therapy for Fabry disease [agalsidase alfa]

CCM (cyclophosphamide, CCNU, methotrexate) *chemotherapy protocol*

CCNU (chloroethyl-cyclohexyl-nitrosourea) [see: lomustine]

CCV-AV (CCNU, cyclophosphamide, vincristine [alternates with] Adriamycin, vincristine) *chemotherapy protocol*

CCVPP (CCNU, cyclophosphamide, Velban, procarbazine, prednisone) *chemotherapy protocol* ⊠ CAFP; CAV/EP; CFP; CH1VPP; CHVP; CVB; CVEB; CVP

CD (cytarabine, daunorubicin) *chemotherapy protocol*

CD4, recombinant soluble human (rCD4) *investigational (Phase II, orphan) antiviral for AIDS*

CD4 human truncated 369 AA polypeptide *investigational (orphan) treatment for AIDS*

CD4 immunoglobulin G, recombinant human *investigational (orphan) for AIDS*

CD5-T lymphocyte immunotoxin *investigational (orphan) for graft vs. host disease following bone marrow transplants*

CD-33 [see: ricin (blocked) conjugated murine MCA myeloid cells]

CdA (2-chloro-2'-deoxyadenosine) [see: cladribine]

CDB (cisplatin, dacarbazine, BCNU) *chemotherapy protocol for malignant melanoma*

CDC (carboplatin, doxorubicin, cyclophosphamide) *chemotherapy protocol*

CDDP; C-DDP (cis-diamminedichloroplatinum) [see: cisplatin]

CDDP/VP; CDDP/VP-16 (CDDP, VP-16) *chemotherapy protocol for pediatric brain tumors*

CDE (cyclophosphamide, doxorubicin, etoposide [filgrastim]) *chemotherapy protocol for HIV-related non-Hodgkin lymphoma*

CDP-571 *investigational (Phase III, orphan) anti-TNFα (tumor necrosis factor alpha) antibody CB-0010 for steroid-dependent Crohn disease*

CDP-cholin [see: citicoline]

CEA (carcinoembryonic antigen)

CEA-Cide Y-90 *investigational (orphan) antineoplastic for colorectal, pancreatic, ovarian, and small cell lung cancer (SCLC)* [yttrium Y 90 labetuzumab]

Ceanothus americanus *medicinal herb* [see: New Jersey tea]

CEA-Scan *powder for injection investigational (orphan) imaging agent for detection of recurrent or metastatic thyroid cancers; investigational (Phase III) for lung cancer* [arcitumomab] 1.25 mg

CEA-Vac *investigational (Phase III) vaccine for breast cancer*

CEB (carboplatin, etoposide, bleomycin) *chemotherapy protocol*

CECA (cisplatin, etoposide, cyclophosphamide, Adriamycin) *chemotherapy protocol*

Ceclor Pulvules (capsules), powder for oral suspension ℞ *second-generation cephalosporin antibiotic* [cefaclor] 250 mg; 125, 187, 250, 375 mg/5 mL

Ceclor CDpak extended-release tablets (in compliance packs of 14) ℞ *second-generation cephalosporin antibiotic* [cefaclor] 500 mg

Cecon oral drops OTC *vitamin C supplement* [ascorbic acid] 100 mg/mL

Cedax capsules, powder for oral suspension ℞ *third-generation cephalosporin antibiotic* [ceftibuten] 400 mg; 90 mg/5 mL ⊠ ciadox; Cidex; Sudex

cedefingol USAN *antipsoriatic; antineoplastic adjunct*

cedelizumab USAN *monoclonal antibody; prophylaxis of rejection of solid organ allograft; immunomodulator for autoimmune diseases*

CEE (conjugated equine estrogen) [see: estrogens, conjugated]

CeeNu capsules, dose pack ℞ *nitrosourea-type alkylating antineoplastic for brain tumors and Hodgkin disease* [lomustine] 10, 40, 100 mg; 2 × 100 mg + 2 × 40 mg + 2 × 10 mg

CEF (cyclophosphamide, epirubicin, fluorouracil, [co-trimoxazole]) *chemotherapy protocol for breast cancer*

cefacetrile INN *antibacterial* [also: cephacetrile sodium]

cefacetrile sodium [see: cephacetrile sodium]

cefaclor USAN, USP, INN, BAN, JAN *second-generation cephalosporin antibiotic* 250, 375, 500 mg oral; 125, 187, 250, 375 mg/5 mL oral

cefadroxil USAN, USP, INN, BAN *first-generation cephalosporin antibiotic* 500, 1000 mg oral

cefadroxil hemihydrate *first-generation cephalosporin antibiotic* 250, 500 mg/5 mL oral

Cefadyl powder for IV or IM injection (discontinued 2004) ℞ *first-generation cephalosporin antibiotic* [cephapirin sodium] 1 g

cefalexin INN, JAN *first-generation cephalosporin antibiotic* [also: cephalexin]

cefaloglycin INN *antibacterial* [also: cephaloglycin]

cefalonium INN [also: cephalonium]

cefaloram INN [also: cephaloram]

cefaloridine INN *antibacterial* [also: cephaloridine]

cefalotin INN *first-generation cephalosporin antibiotic* [also: cephalothin sodium; cephalothin]

cefalotin sodium [see: cephalothin sodium]

cefamandole USAN, INN *second-generation cephalosporin antibiotic* [also: cephamandole]

cefamandole nafate USAN, USP *second-generation cephalosporin antibiotic* [also: cephamandole nafate]

cefamandole sodium USP *second-generation cephalosporin antibiotic*

cefaparole USAN, INN *antibacterial*

cefapirin INN, BAN *first-generation cephalosporin antibiotic* [also: cephapirin sodium]

cefapirin sodium [see: cephapirin sodium]

cefatrizine USAN, INN, BAN *antibacterial*

cefazaflur INN *antibacterial* [also: cefazaflur sodium]

cefazaflur sodium USAN *antibacterial* [also: cefazaflur]

cefazedone INN, BAN

cefazolin USP, INN *first-generation cephalosporin antibiotic* [also: cephazolin]

cefazolin sodium USAN, USP *first-generation cephalosporin antibiotic* [also: cephazolin sodium] 0.5, 1, 5, 10, 20 g injection

cefbuperazone USAN, INN *antibacterial*

cefcanel INN

cefcanel daloxate INN

cefdinir USAN, INN *third-generation cephalosporin antibiotic* 300 mg oral; 125, 250 mg/5 mL oral

cefditoren pivoxil *broad-spectrum cephalosporin antibiotic*

cefedrolor INN

cefempidone INN, BAN

cefepime USAN, INN *fourth-generation cephalosporin antibiotic*

cefepime HCl USAN *fourth-generation cephalosporin antibiotic* 0.5, 1, 2 g injection

cefetamet USAN, INN *veterinary antibacterial*

cefetecol USAN, INN, BAN *antibacterial*

cefetrizole INN

cefivitril INN

cefixime USAN, USP, INN, BAN *third-generation cephalosporin antibiotic* ⑨ Zyvoxam

Cefizox powder or frozen premix for IV or IM injection ℞ *third-generation cephalosporin antibiotic* [ceftizoxime sodium] 0.5, 1, 2, 10 g

ceflatonin *investigational (orphan) anti-angiogenesis antineoplastic for chronic myeloid leukemia*

cefmenoxime INN *antibacterial* [also: cefmenoxime HCl]

cefmenoxime HCl USAN, USP *antibacterial* [also: cefmenoxime]

cefmepidium chloride INN

cefmetazole USAN, INN *second-generation cephalosporin antibiotic*

cefmetazole sodium USAN, USP, JAN *second-generation cephalosporin antibiotic*

cefminox INN

Cefobid powder or frozen premix for IV or IM injection (discontinued 2007) ℞ *third-generation cephalosporin antibiotic* [cefoperazone sodium] 1, 2, 10 g ☑ Cevi-Bid

cefodizime INN *cephalosporin antibiotic*

Cefol Filmtabs (film-coated tablets) ℞ *vitamin supplement* [multiple vitamins; folic acid] ± •0.5 mg ☑ Zyflo

cefonicid INN, BAN *second-generation cephalosporin antibiotic* [also: cefonicid monosodium]

cefonicid monosodium USAN *second-generation cephalosporin antibiotic* [also: cefonicid]

cefonicid sodium USAN, USP *second-generation cephalosporin antibiotic*

cefoperazone INN, BAN *third-generation cephalosporin antibiotic* [also: cefoperazone sodium]

cefoperazone sodium USAN, USP *third-generation cephalosporin antibiotic* [also: cefoperazone]

ceforanide USAN, USP, INN, BAN *cephalosporin antibiotic* ☑ Zofran ODT

Cefotan frozen premix for IV or IM injection (discontinued 2006) ℞ *cephamycin antibiotic* [cefotetan disodium] 1, 2, 10 g

Cefotan powder for IV or IM injection ℞ *cephamycin antibiotic* [cefotetan disodium] 1, 2, 10 g

cefotaxime INN, BAN *third-generation cephalosporin antibiotic* [also: cefotaxime sodium]

cefotaxime sodium USAN, USP *third-generation cephalosporin antibiotic* [also: cefotaxime] 0.5, 1, 2, 10 g injection

cefotetan USAN, INN, BAN *cephamycin antibiotic*

cefotetan disodium USAN, USP *cephamycin antibiotic* 1, 2, 10 g/vial injection

cefotiam INN, BAN *antibacterial* [also: cefotiam HCl]

cefotiam HCl USAN *antibacterial* [also: cefotiam]

cefoxazole INN [also: cephoxazole]

cefoxitin USAN, INN, BAN *cephamycin antibiotic*

cefoxitin sodium USAN, USP, BAN *cephamycin antibiotic* 1, 2, 10 g/vial injection

cefpimizole USAN, INN *antibacterial*

cefpimizole sodium USAN, JAN *antibacterial*

cefpiramide USAN, USP, INN *antibacterial* ☑ sevopramide

cefpiramide sodium USAN, JAN *antibacterial*

cefpirome INN, BAN *antibacterial* [also: cefpirome sulfate]

cefpirome sulfate USAN, JAN *antibacterial* [also: cefpirome]

cefpodoxime INN, BAN *broad-spectrum third-generation cephalosporin antibiotic* [also: cefpodoxime proxetil]

cefpodoxime proxetil USAN, JAN *broad-spectrum third-generation cephalosporin antibiotic* [also: cefpodoxime] 100, 200 mg oral; 50, 100 mg/5 mL oral

cefprozil USAN, INN *second-generation cephalosporin antibiotic* 250, 500 mg oral; 125, 250 mg/5 mL oral

cefquinome INN, BAN *veterinary antibacterial*

cefquinome sulfate USAN *veterinary antibacterial*

cefradine INN *first-generation cephalosporin antibiotic* [also: cephradine]

cefrotil INN

cefroxadine USAN, INN *antibacterial*

cefsulodin INN, BAN *antibacterial* [also: cefsulodin sodium]

cefsulodin sodium USAN *antibacterial* [also: cefsulodin]

cefsumide INN

ceftaroline *investigational (Phase III) broad-spectrum cephalosporin antibiotic for complicated skin and skin structure infections (SSSIs)*

ceftazidime USAN, USP, INN, BAN, JAN *third-generation cephalosporin antibiotic* 1, 2, 6 g injection

cefteram INN

ceftezole INN

ceftibuten USAN, INN, BAN *third-generation cephalosporin antibiotic*

Ceftin film-coated tablets, oral suspension ℞ *second-generation cephalosporin antibiotic* [cefuroxime axetil] 125, 250, 500 mg; 125, 250 mg/5 mL

ceftiofur INN, BAN *veterinary antibacterial* [also: ceftiofur HCl]

ceftiofur HCl USAN *veterinary antibacterial* [also: ceftiofur]

ceftiofur sodium USAN *veterinary antibacterial*

ceftiolene INN

ceftioxide INN

ceftizoxime INN, BAN *third-generation cephalosporin antibiotic* [also: ceftizoxime sodium]

ceftizoxime sodium USAN, USP *third-generation cephalosporin antibiotic* [also: ceftizoxime]

ceftobiprole *investigational (NDA filed) broad-spectrum cephalosporin antibiotic for complicated skin and skin structure infections (SSSIs) and community-acquired pneumonia (CAP)*

ceftriaxone INN, BAN *third-generation cephalosporin antibiotic* [also: ceftriaxone sodium]

ceftriaxone sodium USAN, USP *third-generation cephalosporin antibiotic* [also: ceftriaxone] 0.25, 0.5, 1, 2, 10 g injection

cefuracetime INN, BAN

cefuroxime USAN, INN, BAN *second-generation cephalosporin antibiotic*

cefuroxime axetil USAN, USP, BAN *second-generation cephalosporin antibiotic* 125, 250, 500 mg oral; 125, 250 mg/5 mL oral

cefuroxime pivoxetil USAN *second-generation cephalosporin antibiotic*

cefuroxime sodium USP, BAN *second-generation cephalosporin antibiotic* 0.75, 1.5, 7.5 g injection

cefuzonam INN

Cefzil film-coated tablets, powder for oral suspension ℞ *second-generation cephalosporin antibiotic* [cefprozil] 250, 500 mg; 125, 250 mg/5 mL

Cefzon (foreign name for U.S. product **Omnicef**) ⧈ Zefazone

celandine (Chelidonium majus) root and plant *medicinal herb used as an analgesic, antispasmodic, caustic, diaphoretic, diuretic, narcotic, and purgative*

Celebrex capsules ℞ *COX-2 inhibitor; nonsteroidal anti-inflammatory drug (NSAID) for osteoarthritis, rheumatoid arthritis, ankylosing spondylitis, and primary dysmenorrhea; reduces polyp growth in familial adenomatous polyposis; investigational (Phase III) for bladder cancer* [celecoxib] 50, 100, 200, 400 mg

celecoxib USAN *COX-2 inhibitor; nonsteroidal anti-inflammatory drug (NSAID) for osteoarthritis, rheumatoid arthritis, ankylosing spondylitis, and primary dysmenorrhea; reduces polyp growth in familial adenomatous polyposis; investigational (Phase III) for bladder cancer*

celery (Apium graveolens) root, stem, and seeds *medicinal herb for aiding digestion, arthritis, cancer, diuresis, gas, headache, hysteria, inducing menstruation, lumbago, nervousness, rheumatism, and terminating lactation* ⧈ Sular; Xolair

Celestone syrup, oral solution *corticosteroidal anti-inflammatory* [betamethasone] 0.6 mg/5 mL ⧈ sulisatin

Celestone tablets (discontinued 2005) *corticosteroidal anti-inflammatory* [betamethasone] 0.6 mg ⧈ sulisatin

Celestone Phosphate IV or IM injection (discontinued 2006) ℞ *corticosteroidal anti-inflammatory* [betamethasone sodium phosphate] 4 mg/mL

Celestone Soluspan intrabursal, intra-articular, intralesional injection ℞ *corticosteroidal anti-inflammatory* [betamethasone sodium phosphate; betamethasone acetate] 3•3 mg/mL

Celexa film-coated tablets, oral solution ℞ *selective serotonin reuptake inhibitor (SSRI) for major depression; also used*

for *obsessive-compulsive disorder (OCD),
post-traumatic stress disorder (PTSD),
generalized anxiety disorder (GAD),
and premenstrual dysphoric disorder
(PMDD)* [citalopram hydrobromide]
10, 20, 40 mg; 10 mg/5 mL ⧉ Cylex;
Salex

celgosivir HCl USAN *antiviral; α-glu-
cosidase I inhibitor for HIV*

celiprolol INN, BAN *antihypertensive;
antianginal; β-blocker* [also: celiprolol
HCl]

celiprolol HCl USAN *antihypertensive;
antianginal; β-blocker* [also: celiprolol]

cellacefate INN *tablet-coating agent*
[also: cellulose acetate phthalate;
cellacephate]

cellacephate BAN *tablet-coating agent*
[also: cellulose acetate phthalate;
cellacefate]

CellCept capsules, film-coated caplets,
powder for oral suspension ℞ *immunosuppressant for allogenic renal,
hepatic, or cardiac transplants (orphan)*
[mycophenolate mofetil] 250 mg;
500 mg; 200 mg/mL

CellCept powder for IV infusion ℞
*immunosuppressant for allogenic renal,
hepatic, or cardiac transplants*
[mycophenolate mofetil HCl] 500 mg

Cellegesic ointment *investigational
(NDA filed) treatment for anal fissures*
[nitroglycerin]

cellulase USAN *digestive enzyme*

cellulolytic enzyme [see: cellulase]

cellulose *bulk laxative*

cellulose, absorbable [see: cellulose,
oxidized]

cellulose, ethyl ester [see: ethylcellu-
lose]

**cellulose, hydroxypropyl methyl
ether** [see: hydroxypropyl methyl-
cellulose]

cellulose, microcrystalline NF *tablet
and capsule diluent* [also: dispersible
cellulose]

cellulose, oxidized USP *topical hemostat*

cellulose, oxidized regenerated USP
local hemostatic

cellulose, sodium carboxymethyl
[see: carboxymethylcellulose sodium]

cellulose acetate NF *tablet-coating
agent; insoluble polymer membrane*

cellulose acetate butyrate [see: cabufocon A; cabufocon B]

cellulose acetate dibutyrate [see:
porofocon A; porofocon B]

cellulose acetate phthalate (CAP)
NF *tablet-coating agent* [also: cellacefate; cellacephate]

**cellulose carboxymethyl ether,
sodium salt** [see: carboxymethylcellulose sodium]

cellulose diacetate [see: cellulose ace-
tate]

**cellulose dihydrogen phosphate,
disodium salt** [see: cellulose sodium
phosphate]

cellulose disodium phosphate [see:
cellulose sodium phosphate]

cellulose ethyl ether [see: ethylcellu-
lose]

cellulose gum, modified [now: croscarmellose sodium]

cellulose methyl ether [see: methyl-
cellulose]

cellulose nitrate [see: pyroxylin]

cellulose sodium phosphate (CSP)
USAN, USP *antiurolithic to prevent stone
formation in absorptive hypercalciuria
Type I*

cellulosic acid [see: cellulose, oxidized]

Celluvisc solution OTC *ophthalmic
moisturizer/lubricant* [carboxymethyl-
cellulose] 1%

celmoleukin INN *immunostimulant*

Celontin Kapseals (capsules) ℞ *succinimide anticonvulsant for petit mal
(absence) seizures* [methsuximide]
150, 300 mg

celucloral INN, BAN

**CEM (cytosine arabinoside, etopo-
side, methotrexate)** *chemotherapy
protocol*

Cenafed tablets, syrup OTC *nasal
decongestant* [pseudoephedrine HCl]
60 mg; 30 mg/5 mL

Cenafed Plus tablets (discontinued
2007) OTC *decongestant; antihistamine*

[pseudoephedrine HCl; triprolidine HCl] 60•2.5 mg

Cena-K oral liquid ℞ *potassium supplement* [potassium chloride] 20, 40 mEq K/15 mL ☒ senega; zinc

Cenestin film-coated tablets ℞ *synthetic estrogen for the treatment of postmenopausal symptoms* [synthetic conjugated estrogens, A] 0.3, 0.45, 0.625, 0.9, 1.25 mg

Cenogen Ultra capsules ℞ *vitamin/mineral/iron supplement* [multiple vitamins & minerals; iron; folic acid] ± •106•1 mg

Cenogen-OB capsules (discontinued 2004) ℞ *vitamin/mineral/iron supplement* [multiple vitamins & minerals; iron; folic acid] ± •106•1 mg

Cenolate IV, IM, or subcu injection ℞ *vitamin therapy; antiscorbutic* [vitamin C (as sodium ascorbate)] 500 mg/mL (562.5 mg/mL)

Centany ointment, kit (ointment + gauze pads) ℞ *antibiotic for impetigo due to* S. aureus *or* S. pyogenes [mupirocin] 2%

Centaurea cyanus medicinal herb [see: cornflower]

centaury (*Erythraea centaurium*) plant *medicinal herb for aiding digestion, blood cleansing, fever, and promoting menstruation*

Centella asiatica medicinal herb [see: gotu kola]

Center-Al subcu or IM injection ℞ *allergenic sensitivity testing (subcu); allergenic desensitization therapy (IM)* [allergenic extracts, alum-precipitated] ☒ zinterol

Centovir investigational (orphan) treatment and prophylaxis of CMV infections in allogenic bone marrow transplants [monoclonal antibody IgM (C-58) to cytomegalovirus (CMV)]

Centoxin investigational (orphan) for gram-negative bacteremia in endotoxin shock [nebacumab]

centrazene [see: simtrazene]

centrophenoxine [see: meclofenoxate]

Centrum, Advanced Formula oral liquid OTC *vitamin/mineral/iron supplement* [multiple vitamins & minerals; ferrous fumarate; biotin; alcohol 6.7%] ± •9•0.3 mg/15 mL

Centrum, Advanced Formula tablets OTC *vitamin/mineral/iron supplement* [multiple vitamins & minerals; ferrous fumarate; folic acid; biotin] ± •18 mg•0.4 mg•30 mcg

Centrum Jr. + Extra C; Centrum Jr. + Extra Calcium chewable tablets (discontinued 2008) OTC *vitamin/mineral/calcium/iron supplement* [multiple vitamins & minerals; calcium; iron; folic acid; biotin] ± •108•18• 0.4•0.045 mg; ± •160•18•0.4• 0.045 mg

Centrum Jr. with Iron tablets (discontinued 2008) OTC *vitamin/mineral/iron supplement* [multiple vitamins & minerals; iron; folic acid; biotin] ± •18 mg•0.4 mg•45 mcg

Centrum Performance tablets OTC *vitamin/mineral/calcium/iron supplement* [multiple vitamins & minerals; calcium; iron; folic acid; biotin] ± • 100•18 mg•0.4 mg•40 mcg

Centrum Silver tablets OTC *geriatric vitamin/mineral supplement* [multiple vitamins & minerals; folic acid; biotin] ± •400•30 mcg

centruroides immune F(ab)2 investigational (orphan) antitoxin for scorpion stings

Ceo-Two suppository OTC CO_2-releasing laxative [sodium bicarbonate; potassium bitartrate]

CEP (CCNU, etoposide, prednimustine) chemotherapy protocol

Cēpacol mouthwash/gargle OTC *oral antiseptic* [cetylpyridinium chloride] 0.05%

Cēpacol Anesthetic troches OTC *mucous membrane anesthetic; antiseptic* [benzocaine; cetylpyridinium chloride] 10 mg•0.07%

Cēpacol Dual Relief Sore Throat spray OTC *mucous membrane anes-*

thetic; emollient [benzocaine; glycerin] 5%•33%

Cēpacol Maximum Strength lozenges OTC *mucous membrane anesthetic* [benzocaine] 10 mg

Cēpacol Sore Throat lozenges OTC *mucous membrane anesthetic; antipruritic; counterirritant* [benzocaine; menthol] 10•2, 10•2.1, 10•2.6, 10•3.6, 10•4.5 mg

Cēpacol Sore Throat oral liquid OTC *decongestant; analgesic; antipyretic* [pseudoephedrine HCl; acetaminophen] 60•640 mg/30 mL

Cēpacol Sore Throat spray OTC *mucous membrane anesthetic; emollient* [dyclonine HCl; glycerin] 0.1%•33%

Cēpacol Sore Throat Postnasal Drip lozenges OTC *mild anesthetic; antipruritic; counterirritant* [menthol] 3, 5.4 mg

Cēpacol Throat lozenges OTC *antiseptic* [cetylpyridinium chloride] 0.07%

Cēpacol Ultra Sore Throat Plus Cough lozenges OTC *antitussive; mucous membrane anesthetic* [dextromethorphan hydrobromide; benzocaine] 5•7.5 mg

Cēpacol Viractin oral cream, oral gel (discontinued 2007) OTC *mucous membrane anesthetic for cold sores and fever blisters* [tetracaine HCl] 2%

Cēpastat Sore Throat lozenges OTC *mild anesthetic; antipruritic; counterirritant* [phenol] 14.5, 29 mg

cephacetrile sodium USAN, USP *antibacterial* [also: cefacetrile]

cephalexin USAN, USP, BAN *first-generation cephalosporin antibiotic* [also: cefalexin] 250, 500 mg oral; 125, 250 mg/5 mL oral

cephalexin HCl USAN, USP *first-generation cephalosporin antibiotic*

cephaloglycin USAN, USP, BAN *antibacterial* [also: cefaloglicin]

cephalonium BAN [also: cefalonium]

cephaloram BAN [also: cefaloram]

cephaloridine USAN, USP, BAN *antibacterial* [also: cefaloridine]

cephalosporin N [see: adicillin]

cephalosporins *a class of bactericidal antibiotics, divided into first-, second-, and third-generation; higher generations have increasing efficacy against gram-negative and decreasing efficacy against gram-positive bacteria*

cephalothin BAN *first-generation cephalosporin antibiotic* [also: cephalothin sodium; cefalotin]

cephalothin sodium USAN, USP *first-generation cephalosporin antibiotic* [also: cefalotin; cephalothin]

cephamandole BAN *second-generation cephalosporin antibiotic* [also: cefamandole]

cephamandole nafate BAN *second-generation cephalosporin antibiotic* [also: cefamandole nafate]

cephamycins *a class of bactericidal antibiotics similar to second-generation cephalosporins (q.v.)*

cephapirin sodium USAN, USP *first-generation cephalosporin antibiotic* [also: cefapirin]

cephazolin BAN *first-generation cephalosporin antibiotic* [also: cefazolin]

cephazolin sodium BAN *first-generation cephalosporin antibiotic* [also: cefazolin sodium]

cephoxazole BAN [also: cefoxazole]

cephradine USAN, USP, BAN *first-generation cephalosporin antibiotic* [also: cefradine]

Cephulac oral/rectal solution R *synthetic disaccharide used to prevent and treat portal-systemic encephalopathy* [lactulose] 10 g/15 mL

Ceplene *investigational (Phase III) histamine H_2 receptor agonist for malignant melanoma and acute myeloid leukemia (AML); investigational (Phase II) for hepatitis C and renal cell carcinoma* [histamine dihydrochloride]

CEPP (cyclophosphamide, etoposide, prednisone) *chemotherapy protocol for non-Hodgkin lymphoma*

CEPPB (cyclophosphamide, etoposide, prednisone, bleomycin) *che-*

motherapy protocol for non-Hodgkin lymphoma

Ceprotin powder for IV injection ℞ replacement therapy for severe congenital protein C deficiency in children and adults to prevent or treat thrombosis, pulmonary emboli, and purpura fulminans (orphan) [protein C concentrate (human)] 500, 1000 U ⊡ sparteine

Ceptaz powder for IV or IM injection ℞ third-generation cephalosporin antibiotic [ceftazidime pentahydrate] 1, 2 g

CERA (continuous erythropoietin receptor activator) [q.v.]

CeraLyte powder for oral liquid, ready-to-use oral liquid OTC supplementary feeding to maintain hydration and electrolyte balance in infants with diarrhea or vomiting [rice-based formula]

ceramide trihexosidase (CTH) & agalsidase beta investigational (orphan) enzyme replacement therapy for Fabry disease

Cerebyx IV or IM injection ℞ hydantoin anticonvulsant for grand mal status epilepticus (orphan) [fosphenytoin sodium (phenytoin sodium equivalent)] 75 (50) mg/mL ⊡ Surbex

Ceredase IV infusion ℞ glucocerebrosidase enzyme replacement for Gaucher disease type I (orphan); investigational (orphan) for types II and III [alglucerase] 80 U/mL

Cerefolin tablets ℞ vitamin B supplement for homocystinemia [vitamins B₂, B₆, and B₁₂; L-methylfolate] 5•50• 1•5.635 mg

cerelose [see: glucose]

Cereport investigational (Phase III) blood-brain barrier permeability-enhancing agent for carrying carboplatin to brain tumors [lobradimil]

Ceresine investigational (orphan) for severe head trauma, lactic acidosis, homozygous familial hypercholesterolemia, and monochloroacetic acid poisoning [sodium dichloroacetate]

Cerezyme powder for IV infusion ℞ glucocerebrosidase enzyme replacement for type 1 Gaucher disease (orphan);

investigational (orphan) for types 2 and 3 Gaucher disease [imiglucerase] 40 U/mL

cerium element (Ce) ⊡ Xyrem

cerium nitrate & silver sulfadiazine investigational (orphan) for life-threatening burns

cerium oxalate USP

cerivastatin sodium USAN HMG-CoA reductase inhibitor for hyperlipidemia and hypertriglyceridemia (discontinued 2001 due to safety concerns)

Cernevit-12 powder for IV injection ℞ parenteral vitamin therapy [multiple vitamins; folic acid; biotin] ≛•414• 60 mcg

Ceron syrup, oral drops ℞ decongestant; antihistamine; drops for children 6–24 months [phenylephrine HCl; chlorpheniramine maleate] 12.5•4 mg/5 mL; 3.5•1 mg/mL ⊡ Sereine

ceronapril USAN, INN antihypertensive

Ceron-DM oral drops ℞ antitussive; antihistamine; decongestant; for children 6–24 months [dextromethorphan hydrobromide; chlorpheniramine maleate; phenylephrine HCl] 3•1•3.5 mg/mL

Ceron-DM syrup ℞ antitussive; antihistamine; decongestant [dextromethorphan hydrobromide; chlorpheniramine maleate; phenylephrine HCl] 15•4•12.5 mg/5 mL

Cerovite; Cerovite Advanced Formula tablets OTC vitamin/mineral/iron supplement [multiple vitamins & minerals; ferrous fumarate; folic acid; biotin] ≛•18 mg•0.4 mg•30 mcg ⊡ Syrvite

Cerovite Jr. tablets OTC vitamin/mineral/iron supplement [multiple vitamins & minerals; ferrous fumarate; folic acid; biotin] ≛•18 mg•0.4 mg•45 mcg

Cerovite Senior tablets OTC geriatric vitamin/mineral supplement [multiple vitamins & minerals; folic acid; biotin] ≛•200•30 mcg

Cerovive investigational (Phase III) neuroprotectant for acute ischemic *stroke (AIS)* [NXY-059 (code name —generic name not yet assigned)]

Certagen film-coated tablets OTC *vitamin/mineral/iron supplement* [multiple vitamins & minerals; ferrous fumarate; folic acid; biotin] ±•18 mg• 0.4 mg•30 mcg

Certagen oral liquid OTC *vitamin/mineral/iron supplement* [multiple vitamins & minerals; iron; biotin; alcohol 6.6%] ±•9•0.3 mg

Certagen Senior tablets (discontinued 2008) OTC *geriatric vitamin/mineral supplement* [multiple vitamins & minerals; folic acid; biotin] ±•200•30 mcg

CertaVite tablets OTC *vitamin/mineral/iron supplement* [multiple vitamins & minerals; ferrous fumarate; folic acid; biotin] ±•18 mg•0.4 mg•30 mcg

Certa-Vite Golden tablets OTC *geriatric vitamin/mineral supplement* [multiple vitamins & minerals; biotin] ± •30 mcg

Certican ⓔⓤⓡ (European name for investigational U.S. product **Afinitor**)

certolizumab pegol *pegylated Fab fragment anti-TNF (tumor necrosis factor) anti-inflammatory for moderate to severe Crohn disease*

Cerubidine powder for IV injection ℞ *antibiotic antineoplastic for multiple nonlymphocytic leukemias* [daunorubicin HCl] 20 mg

ceruletide USAN, INN, BAN *gastric secretory stimulant*

ceruletide diethylamine USAN *gastric secretory stimulant*

Cerumenex ear drops (discontinued 2006) ℞ *cerumenolytic to emulsify and disperse ear wax* [trolamine polypeptide oleate-condensate] 10%

Cervarix ⓔⓤⓡ (available in Europe) *investigational (NDA filed) vaccine for cervical cancer and precancerous lesions caused by HPV infections* [human papillomavirus (HPV) recombinant vaccine, bivalent (types 16 and 18)]

Cervidil vaginal insert ℞ *prostaglandin for cervical ripening at term* [dinoprostone] 10 mg

Cesamet capsules ℞ *antiemetic for nausea and vomiting associated with cancer chemotherapy; restricted use due to the high possibility of disturbing psychomimetic reactions and psychological dependence* [nabilone] 1 mg

Cesia tablets (in packs of 28) ℞ *triphasic oral contraceptive* [desogestrel; ethinyl estradiol]
Phase 1 (7 days): 0.1 mg•25 mcg;
Phase 2 (7 days): 0,125 mg•25 mcg;
Phase 3 (7 days): 0.15 mg•25 mcg

cesium *element* (Cs)

cesium (^{131}Cs) **chloride** INN *radioactive agent* [also: cesium chloride Cs 131]

cesium chloride Cs 131 USAN *radioactive agent* [also: cesium (^{131}Cs) chloride]

Ceta topical liquid OTC *soap-free therapeutic skin cleanser*

Ceta Plus capsules ℞ *narcotic analgesic; antipyretic* [hydrocodone bitartrate; acetaminophen] 5•500 mg

cetaben INN *antihyperlipoproteinemic* [also: cetaben sodium] ② zotepine

cetaben sodium USAN *antihyperlipoproteinemic* [also: cetaben]

Cetacaine topical liquid, gel, ointment, aerosol ℞ *anesthetic; antiseptic* [benzocaine; tetracaine HCl; butamben; benzalkonium chloride] 14%• 2%•2%•0.5%

Cetacort lotion ℞ *corticosteroidal anti-inflammatory* [hydrocortisone] 0.25%, 0.5% ② S-T Cort

Cetafen; Cetafen Extra film-coated tablets OTC *analgesic; antipyretic* [acetaminophen] 325 mg; 500 mg ② Cytovene

Cetaklenz topical liquid OTC *soap-free skin cleanser* [cetyl alcohol; propylene glycol; sodium lauryl sulfate; stearyl alcohol]

cetalkonium *antiseptic*

cetalkonium chloride USAN, INN, BAN *topical anti-infective*

Cetamide ophthalmic ointment ℞ *antibiotic* [sulfacetamide sodium] 10%

cetamolol INN *antiadrenergic (β-receptor)* [also: cetamolol HCl]

cetamolol HCl USAN *antiadrenergic (β-receptor)* [also: cetamolol]

Cetaphil cream, lotion, cleansing bar, cleansing solution OTC *soap-free therapeutic skin cleanser*

cethexonium chloride INN

cetiedil INN *peripheral vasodilator* [also: cetiedil citrate] ⊡ Stadol

cetiedil citrate USAN *peripheral vasodilator; investigational (orphan) for sickle cell disease crisis* [also: cetiedil]

cetirizine INN, BAN *second-generation peripherally selective piperazine antihistamine for allergic rhinitis and chronic idiopathic urticaria* [also: cetirizine HCl] ⊡ Storzine 2

cetirizine HCl USAN *second-generation peripherally selective piperazine antihistamine for allergic rhinitis and chronic idiopathic urticaria* [also: cetirizine] 5, 10 mg oral; 5 mg/5 mL oral

Cetirizine Hydrochloride Allergy, Children's; Children's Cetirizine Chloride Hives Relief syrup OTC *nonsedating antihistamine for allergy and hives* [cetirizine HCl] 5 mg/5 mL

cetobemidone [see: ketobemidone]

cetocycline INN *antibacterial* [also: cetocycline HCl]

cetocycline HCl USAN *antibacterial* [also: cetocycline]

cetofenicol INN *antibacterial* [also: cetophenicol]

cetohexazine INN

cetomacrogol 1000 INN, BAN

cetophenicol USAN *antibacterial* [also: cetofenicol]

cetophenylbutazone [see: kebuzone]

cetostearyl alcohol NF *emulsifying agent*

cetotetrine HCl [now: cetocycline HCl]

cetotiamine INN

cetoxime INN, BAN

cetoxime HCl [see: cetoxime]

Cetraria islandica medicinal herb [see: Iceland moss]

cetraxate INN *GI antiulcerative* [also: cetraxate HCl]

cetraxate HCl USAN *GI antiulcerative* [also: cetraxate]

cetrimide INN, BAN *topical antiseptic*

cetrimonium bromide INN *topical antiseptic* [also: cetrimonium chloride]

cetrimonium chloride BAN *topical antiseptic* [also: cetrimonium bromide]

cetrorelix acetate USAN *gonadotropin-releasing hormone (GnRH) antagonist for infertility*

Cetrotide subcu injection ℞ *gonadotropin-releasing hormone (GnRH) antagonist for infertility* [cetrorelix acetate] 0.25, 3 mg

cetuximab USAN *monoclonal antibody to epidermal growth factor receptor (EGFR); antineoplastic for metastatic colorectal cancer and squamous cell carcinoma (SCC) of the head and neck (orphan); investigational (Phase III) for numerous other cancers*

cetyl alcohol NF *emulsifying and stiffening agent*

cetyl esters wax NF *stiffening agent*

cetyldimethylbenzyl ammonium chloride [see: cetalkonium chloride]

cetylpyridinium chloride USP, INN, BAN *topical antiseptic; preservative*

cetyltrimethyl ammonium bromide

CEV (cyclophosphamide, etoposide, vincristine) *chemotherapy protocol for small cell lung cancer (SCLC)*

Cevi-Bid tablets OTC *vitamin C supplement* [ascorbic acid] 500 mg ⊡ Cefobid

Cevi-Fer timed-release capsules (discontinued 2005) ℞ *hematinic; vitamin/iron supplement* [ferrous fumarate (source of iron); ascorbic acid; folic acid] 63 (20)•300•1 mg

cevimeline HCl USAN *cholinergic and muscarinic receptor agonist for dry mouth due to Sjögren syndrome*

cevitamic acid [see: ascorbic acid]

cevitan [see: ascorbic acid]

ceylon gelatin [see: agar]

Cezin-S capsules ℞ *geriatric vitamin/mineral supplement* [multiple vitamins & minerals; folic acid] ≟•0.5 mg

CF (carboplatin, fluorouracil) *chemotherapy protocol for head and neck cancer*

CF (cisplatin, fluorouracil) *chemotherapy protocol for adenocarcinoma and head and neck cancer*

CFC (chlorofluorocarbons) *the type of propellant used in older aerosol and pressurized metered-dose inhaler (pMDI) delivery systems; these are being replaced with products that use HFA-134a propellant (q.v.)*

CFL (cisplatin, fluorouracil, leucovorin [rescue]) *chemotherapy protocol*

CFM (cyclophosphamide, fluorouracil, mitoxantrone) *chemotherapy protocol for breast cancer* [also: CNF; FNC]

CFP (cyclophosphamide, fluorouracil, prednisone) *chemotherapy protocol*

CFPT (cyclophosphamide, fluorouracil, prednisone, tamoxifen) *chemotherapy protocol*

CFTR (cystic fibrosis transmembrane conductance regulator) [q.v.]

CG (Cardio-Green) [q.v.]

CG (chorionic gonadotropin) [see: gonadotropin, chorionic]

CGF (*Chlorella* growth factor) [q.v.]

CGF (Control Gel Formula) dressing [see: DuoDERM CGF]

CGU WC oral liquid ℞ *narcotic antitussive; expectorant* [codeine phosphate; guaifenesin] 6.3•100 mg/5 mL

CH1VPP; Ch1VPP (chlorambucil, vinblastine, procarbazine, prednisone) *chemotherapy protocol* Ⓓ CAFP; CAV/EP; CCVPP; CFP; CHVP; CVB; CVEB; CVP

CHAD (cyclophosphamide, hexamethylmelamine, Adriamycin, DDP) *chemotherapy protocol*

chalk, precipitated [see: calcium carbonate, precipitated]

Chamaelirium luteum *medicinal herb* [see: false unicorn]

CHAMOCA (cyclophosphamide, hydroxyurea, actinomycin D, methotrexate, Oncovin, calcium folinate, Adriamycin) *chemotherapy protocol for gestational trophoblastic neoplasm* [also known as: modified Bagshawe protocol]

chamomile (*Anthemis nobilis*; *Matricaria chamomilla*) flowers *medicinal herb for appetite stimulation, bronchitis, excessive menstruation with cramps, fever, gastrointestinal cramps, hysteria, inflammation, insomnia, nervousness, rheumatic disorders, and parasites*

Champix Ⓔ (European name for U.S. product **Chantix**)

channa; canna *medicinal herb* [see: kanna]

Chantix film-coated caplets ℞ *nicotine receptor agonist/antagonist; a non-nicotine smoking cessation aid; also used to reduce alcohol cravings* [varenicline tartrate] 0.5, 1 mg

CHAP (cyclophosphamide, Hexalen, Adriamycin, Platinol) *chemotherapy protocol for ovarian cancer*

CHAP (cyclophosphamide, hexamethylmelamine, Adriamycin, Platinol) *chemotherapy protocol*

Chap Stick Medicated Lip Balm stick, jar, squeezable tube OTC *mild anesthetic; antipruritic; counterirritant; moisturizer; protectant; emollient* [camphor; menthol; phenol] 1%•0.6%•0.5%

chaparral (*Larrea divaricata*; *L. glutinosa*; *L. tridentata*) leaves and stems *medicinal herb for arthritis, blood cleansing, bronchitis, cancer, chickenpox, colds, leukemia, rheumatic pain, stomach pain, and tumors; not generally regarded as safe and effective due to liver toxicity and the stimulation of some tumors*

CharcoAid oral suspension OTC *adsorbent antidote for poisoning* [activated charcoal] 15 g/120 mL, 30 g/150 mL

CharcoAid 2000 oral liquid, granules OTC *adsorbent antidote for poisoning* [activated charcoal] 15 g/120 mL, 50 g/240 mL; 15 g

charcoal *gastric adsorbent/detoxicant; antiflatulent* 260 mg oral

charcoal, activated USP *general purpose antidote/adsorbent* 15, 30, 40, 120, 240 g, 208 mg/mL oral

Charcoal Plus enteric-coated tablets OTC *adsorbent; detoxicant* [activated charcoal] 250 mg

CharcoCaps capsules OTC *adsorbent; detoxicant; antiflatulent* [charcoal] 260 mg

Chardonna-2 tablets (discontinued 2008) ℞ *GI/GU anticholinergic/antispasmodic; sedative* [belladonna extract; phenobarbital] 15•15 mg

chaste tree (Vitex agnus-castus) dried ripe fruit *medicinal herb for acne, balancing progesterone and estrogen production, increasing lactation, ovarian insufficiency, premenstrual breast pain, regulating menstrual cycle, and uterine bleeding*

chaulmosulfone INN

checkerberry *medicinal herb* [see: squaw vine; wintergreen]

cheese plant; cheeseflower *medicinal herb* [see: mallow]

cheese rennet *medicinal herb* [see: bedstraw]

Cheetah oral suspension ℞ *radiopaque contrast medium for gastrointestinal imaging* [barium sulfate] 2.2%

chelafrin [see: epinephrine]

Chelated Manganese tablets OTC *manganese supplement* [manganese] 20, 50 mg

chelating agents *a class of agents that prevent bodily absorption of and cause the excretion of substances such as heavy metals*

chelen [see: ethyl chloride]

Chelidonium majus *medicinal herb* [see: celandine]

Chelone glabra *medicinal herb* [see: turtlebloom]

Chemet capsules ℞ *heavy metal chelating agent for lead poisoning (orphan); investigational (orphan) for mercury poisoning and cysteine kidney stones* [succimer] 100 mg

Chemo-Pin (trademarked delivery form) *chemical-dispensing pin*

Chemstrip 2 GP; Chemstrip 2 LN; Chemstrip 4 the OB; Chemstrip 6; Chemstrip 7; Chemstrip 8; Chemstrip 9; Chemstrip 10 with SG; Chemstrip uGK reagent strips *in vitro diagnostic aid for multiple urine products*

Chemstrip bG reagent strips for home use OTC *in vitro diagnostic aid for blood glucose*

Chemstrip K reagent strips for professional use ℞ *in vitro diagnostic aid for acetone (ketones) in the urine*

Chemstrip Micral reagent strips for professional use ℞ *in vitro diagnostic aid for albumin (protein) in the urine*

Chemstrip uG reagent strips for home use OTC *in vitro diagnostic aid for urine glucose*

chenic acid [now: chenodiol]

Chenix tablets ℞ *anticholelithogenic for radiolucent gallstones (orphan)* [chenodiol] 250 mg

chenodeoxycholic acid INN, BAN *anticholelithogenic* [also: chenodiol]

chenodiol USAN *anticholelithogenic for radiolucent gallstones (orphan); investigational (orphan) for cerebrotendinous xanthomatosis* [also: chenodeoxycholic acid]

Chenofalk *investigational (orphan) agent for cerebrotendinous xanthomatosis* [chenodiol]

Cheracol Cough syrup (discontinued 2007) ℞ *narcotic antitussive; expectorant* [codeine phosphate; guaifenesin; alcohol 4.75%] 20•200 mg/10 mL

Cheracol D Cough Formula; Cheracol Plus syrup OTC *antitussive; expectorant* [dextromethorphan hydrobromide; guaifenesin; alcohol 4.75%] 10•100 mg/5 mL

Cheracol Sore Throat spray OTC *mild mucous membrane anesthetic; antipruritic; counterirritant* [phenol] 1.4%

Cheratussin AC syrup ℞ *narcotic antitussive; expectorant* [codeine phosphate; guaifenesin; alcohol 3.5%] 10•100 mg/5 mL

cherry, black; choke cherry; rum cherry *medicinal herb* [see: wild black cherry]

cherry, black; poison black cherry *medicinal herb* [see: belladonna]

cherry birch *medicinal herb* [see: birch]

cherry juice NF

chervil (Anthriscus cerefolium) *flowering plant medicinal herb used as a digestive, diuretic, expectorant, and stimulant*

chervil, sweet *medicinal herb* [see: sweet cicely]

chestnut *medicinal herb* [see: horse chestnut]

Chewable Multivitamins with Fluoride *pediatric tablets* ℞ *vitamin supplement; dental caries preventative* [multiple vitamins; fluoride; folic acid] ±•1•0.3 mg

Chewable Triple Vitamins with Fluoride *pediatric tablets* ℞ *vitamin supplement; dental caries preventative* [vitamins A, C, and D; fluoride] 2500 IU•60 mg•400 IU•1 mg

Chewable Vitamin C *chewable tablets* OTC *vitamin C supplement* [ascorbic acid and sodium ascorbate] 250, 500 mg

Chew-C *chewable tablets* OTC *vitamin C supplement* [ascorbic acid and sodium ascorbate] 500 mg

ChexUP; Chex-Up; CHEX-UP (cyclophosphamide, hexamethylmelamine, fluorouracil, Platinol) *chemotherapy protocol*

CHF (cyclophosphamide, hexamethylmelamine, fluorouracil) *chemotherapy protocol*

chicken's toes *medicinal herb* [see: coral root]

chickweed (Stellaria media) *plant medicinal herb for appetite suppression, bleeding, blood cleansing, convulsions, obesity, skin rashes, and ulcers; also used as a homeopathic remedy for psoriasis and rheumatic pain*

chicory (Chicorium intybus) *plant and root medicinal herb for blood cleansing, cardiac disease, jaundice,* *liver disorders, promoting expectoration, and removal of calcium deposits*

Chiggerex *ointment* OTC *anesthetic; antipruritic; counterirritant* [benzocaine; camphor; menthol]

Chigger-Tox *topical liquid* OTC *anesthetic* [benzocaine]

Chikusetsu ginseng (Panax pseudoginseng) *medicinal herb* [see: ginseng]

Children's Elixir DM Cough & Cold (discontinued 2007) OTC *antitussive; antihistamine; decongestant* [dextromethorphan hydrobromide; brompheniramine maleate; pseudoephedrine HCl] 5•1•15 mg/5 mL

Children's Ibuprofen Cold *oral suspension* (discontinued 2007) OTC *analgesic; antipyretic; nonsteroidal anti-inflammatory drug; nasal decongestant* [ibuprofen; pseudoephedrine] 100•15 mg/5 mL

Children's Loratadine *syrup* OTC *nonsedating antihistamine for allergic rhinitis* [loratadine] 5 mg/5 mL

chili pepper; chilies *medicinal herb* [see: cayenne]

chillifolinum [see: quillifoline]

Chimaphila umbellata *medicinal herb* [see: pipsissewa]

chimeric monoclonal antibodies *antibodies cloned from a single cell genetically engineered to combine the antigen-binding part of a murine (mouse/rat) antibody with the effector part of a human antibody, to prevent rejection by the human immune system* [see: monoclonal antibodies]

chinchona *medicinal herb* [see: quinine]

Chinese cucumber (Trichosanthes kirilowii) *gourd and root medicinal herb for abscesses, amenorrhea, cough, diabetes, edema, fever, inducing abortion, invasive moles, jaundice, polyuria, and tumors*

Chinese gelatin [see: agar]

Chinese isinglass [see: chiniofon]

Chinese rhubarb *medicinal herb* [see: rhubarb]

chinethazone [see: quinethazone]

chiniofon NF, INN

Chionanthus virginica medicinal herb [see: fringe tree]

ChiRhoStim powder for IV injection ℞ *diagnostic aid for pancreatic function* [secretin, human] 16, 40 mcg/vial

Chirocaine local or epidural injection (discontinued 2006) ℞ *long-acting local anesthetic* [levobupivacaine HCl] 2.5, 5, 7.5 mg/mL

chitosamine [see: glucosamine]

chitosan *natural cellulose-like biopolymer extracted from marine animal exoskeletons and used as a treatment for hypercholesterolemia, hyperlipidemia, and obesity; also used topically as an antimicrobial and vulnerary*

chittem bark *medicinal herb* [see: buckthorn; cascara sagrada]

CHL + PRED (chlorambucil, prednisone) *chemotherapy protocol* ☑ glyburide

Chlamydiazyme reagent kit for professional use ℞ *in vitro diagnostic aid for Chlamydia trachomatis* [solid phase enzyme immunoassay]

Chlo-Amine chewable tablets OTC *antihistamine* [chlorpheniramine maleate] 2 mg ☑ calamine; gallamine

chlophedianol BAN *antitussive* [also: chlophedianol HCl; clofedanol]

chlophedianol HCl USAN *antitussive* [also: clofedanol; chlophedianol]

chlophenadione [see: clorindione]

chloquinate [see: cloquinate]

chloracyzine INN

chloral betaine USAN, NF, BAN *sedative* [also: cloral betaine]

chloral hydrate USP, BAN *nonbarbiturate sedative and hypnotic; also abused as a street drug* 500 mg oral; 250, 500 mg/5 mL oral

chloral hydrate betaine [see: chloral betaine]

chloralformamide USP

chloralodol INN [also: chlorhexadol]

chloralose (α-chloralose) INN

chloralurethane [see: carbocloral]

chlorambucil USP, INN, BAN *nitrogen mustard-type alkylating antineoplastic for multiple leukemias and lymphomas*

chloramidobenzol [see: clofenamide]

chloramine [now: chloramine-T]

chloramine-T NF [also: tosylchloramide sodium]

chloramiphene [see: clomiphene citrate]

chloramphenicol USP, INN, BAN, JAN *bacteriostatic antibiotic; antirickettsial* 5 mg/mL eye drops; 10 mg/g ophthalmic ☑ cloramfenicol pantotenate complex

chloramphenicol palmitate USP, JAN *antibacterial; antirickettsial* 150 mg/5 mL oral ☑ cloramfenicol pantotenate complex

chloramphenicol pantothenate complex USAN *antibacterial; antirickettsial* [also: cloramfenicol pantotenate complex]

chloramphenicol sodium succinate USP, JAN *antibacterial; antirickettsial* 100 mg/mL injection ☑ cloramfenicol pantotenate complex

chloranautine [see: dimenhydrinate]

ChloraPrep One-Step swabs OTC *antiseptic* [chlorhexidine gluconate; isopropyl alcohol] 2% • 70%

chlorarsen [see: dichlorophenarsine HCl]

Chlorascrub Swab; Chlorascrub Swabstick; Chlorascrub Maxi swabs OTC *antiseptic* [chlorhexidine gluconate; isopropyl alcohol] 3.15% • 70% (1 mL; 1.6 mL; 5.1 mL)

Chloraseptic mouthwash/gargle OTC *oral antiseptic; antipruritic/counterirritant; mild local anesthetic* [phenol] 1.4%

Chloraseptic, Children's lozenges OTC *mucous membrane anesthetic* [benzocaine] 5 mg

Chloraseptic, Children's throat spray (name changed to **Chloraseptic Kids' Sore Throat** in 2005)

Chloraseptic Defense Daily Health Strips orally disintegrating film OTC *vitamin/mineral supplement* [vitamin C; zinc]

Chloraseptic Kids' Sore Throat orally disintegrating film OTC *mucous mem-*

brane anesthetic; antipruritic; counterirritant [benzocaine; menthol] 2•2 mg

Chloraseptic Sore Throat lozenges, orally disintegrating film OTC *mucous membrane anesthetic; antipruritic; counterirritant* [benzocaine; menthol] 6•10 mg; 3•3 mg

Chloraseptic Sore Throat oral liquid (discontinued 2008) OTC *analgesic; antipyretic* [acetaminophen] 166.6 mg/5 mL

Chloraseptic Sore Throat; Chloraseptic Kids' Sore Throat spray OTC *antipruritic/counterirritant; mild local anesthetic* [phenol] 1.4%; 0.5%

Chloraseptic Sugar Free Sore Throat lozenges OTC *mucous membrane anesthetic; antipruritic; counterirritant; (some flavors contain an antitussive)* [benzocaine; menthol; (dextromethorphan)]

chlorazanil INN

chlorazanil HCl [see: chlorazanil]

chlorazodin INN [also: chloroazodin]

chlorazone [see: chloramine-T]

chlorbenzoxamine INN

chlorbenzoxamine HCl [see: chlorbenzoxamine]

chlorbetamide INN, BAN

chlorbutanol [see: chlorobutanol]

chlorbutin [see: chlorambucil]

chlorbutol BAN *antimicrobial agent* [also: chlorobutanol]

chlorcinnazine [see: clocinizine]

chlorcyclizine INN, BAN *topical antihistamine* [also: chlorcyclizine HCl]

chlorcyclizine HCl USP *topical antihistamine* [also: chlorcyclizine]

chlordantoin USAN, BAN *antifungal* [also: clodantoin]

Chlordex GP syrup ℞ *antitussive; decongestant; antihistamine; expectorant* [dextromethorphan hydrobromide; phenylephrine HCl; chlorpheniramine maleate; guaifenesin] 7.5•10•2•100 mg/5 mL

chlordiazepoxide USP, INN, BAN, JAN *benzodiazepine anxiolytic; sedative; alcohol withdrawal aid*

chlordiazepoxide HCl USAN, USP, BAN, JAN *benzodiazepine anxiolytic; sedative; alcohol withdrawal aid; sometimes abused as a street drug* 5, 10, 25 mg oral

chlordiazepoxide HCl & clidinium bromide *anxiolytic; GI anticholinergic* 5•2.5 mg

chlordimorine INN

Chlorella a genus of single-cell algae used as a source of multiple vitamins and minerals, protein, chlorellin, chlorophyll and Chlorella growth factor (q.v.); immune enhancer and chelator of heavy metals

Chlorella growth factor (CGF) *natural extract of the nucleus of Chlorella algae (q.v.) that is widely used in wound healing and skin disorders*

Chloresium ointment, solution OTC *vulnerary and deodorant for wounds, burns, and ulcers* [chlorophyllin copper complex] 0.5%; 0.2%

Chloresium tablets OTC *systemic deodorant for ostomy, breath, and body odors* [chlorophyllin copper complex] 14 mg

chlorethate [see: clorethate]

chlorethyl [see: ethyl chloride]

Chlorex-A caplets ℞ *decongestant; antihistamine; sleep aid* [phenylephrine HCl; chlorpheniramine maleate; phenyltoloxamine citrate] 20•4•40 mg

Chlorex-A 12 oral suspension ℞ *decongestant; antihistamine; sleep aid* [phenylephrine tannate; chlorpheniramine tannate; pyrilamine tannate] 5•2•12.5 mg/5 mL

chlorfenisate [see: clofibrate]

chlorfenvinphos BAN [also: clofenvinfos]

chlorguanide HCl [see: chloroguanide HCl]

chlorhexadol BAN [also: chloralodol]

chlorhexidine INN, BAN *broad-spectrum antimicrobial* [also: chlorhexidine gluconate]

chlorhexidine gluconate USAN *broad-spectrum antimicrobial; investi-*

gational (orphan) for oral mucositis in bone marrow transplant patients [also: chlorhexidine] 0.12% oral rinse

chlorhexidine HCl USAN, BAN *broad-spectrum antimicrobial*

chlorhexidine phosphanilate USAN *broad-spectrum antimicrobial*

chlorimiphenin [see: imiclopazine]

chlorimpiphenine [see: imiclopazine]

chlorinated & iodized peanut oil [see: chloriodized oil]

chlorindanol USAN *spermaticide* [also: clorindanol]

chlorine *element (Cl)* ⑨ Klaron 10%

chloriodized oil USP

chlorisondamine chloride INN, BAN

chlorisondamone chloride [see: chlorisondamine chloride]

chlormadinone INN, BAN *progestin* [also: chlormadinone acetate]

chlormadinone acetate USAN, NF *progestin* [also: chlormadinone]

chlormerodrin NF, INN, BAN

chlormerodrin (¹⁹⁷Hg) INN *renal function test; radioactive agent* [also: chlormerodrin Hg 197]

chlormerodrin Hg 197 USAN, USP *renal function test; radioactive agent* [also: chlormerodrin (¹⁹⁷Hg)]

chlormerodrin Hg 203 USAN, USP *renal function test; radioactive agent*

chlormeroprin [see: chlormerodrin]

chlormethazanone [see: chlormezanone]

chlormethiazole BAN [also: clomethiazole]

chlormethine INN *nitrogen mustard-type alkylating antineoplastic* [also: mechlorethamine HCl; mustine; nitrogen mustard N-oxide HCl]

chlormethylencycline [see: clomocycline]

chlormezanone INN, BAN *mild anxiolytic*

chlormidazole INN, BAN

chlornaphazine INN

chloroacetic acid [see: monochloroacetic, dichloroacetic, or trichloroacetic acid]

8-chloroadenosine monophosphate, cyclic (8-Cl cAMP) [see: tocladesine]

chloroazodin USP [also: chlorazodin]

5-chlorobenzoxazolinone [see: chlorzoxazone]

chlorobutanol NF, INN *antimicrobial agent; preservative* [also: chlorbutol]

chlorochine [see: chloroquine]

chlorocresol USAN, NF, INN *antiseptic; disinfectant*

2-chloro-2'-deoxyadenosine (CdA) [now: cladribine]

chlorodeoxylincomycin [see: clindamycin]

chloroethane [see: ethyl chloride]

2-chloroethyl-3-sarcosinamide-1-nitrosourea *investigational (orphan) for malignant glioma*

chloroform NF *solvent*

chloroguanide HCl USP *antimalarial; dihydrofolate reductase inhibitor* [also: proguanil]

chloroguanide triazine pamoate [see: cycloguanil pamoate]

chloro-iodohydroxyquinoline [see: clioquinol]

chlorolincomycin [see: clindamycin]

Chloromag injection ℞ *magnesium replacement therapy* [magnesium chloride hexahydrate] 200 mg/mL

chloromethapyrilene citrate [see: chlorothen citrate]

Chloromycetin ophthalmic ointment (discontinued 2005) ℞ *antibiotic* [chloramphenicol] 10 mg/g

Chloromycetin powder for eye drops ℞ *antibiotic* [chloramphenicol] 25 mg/15 mL

Chloromycetin Sodium Succinate powder for IV injection ℞ *broad-spectrum bacteriostatic antibiotic* [chloramphenicol sodium succinate] 100 mg/mL

***p*-chlorophenol** [see: parachlorophenol]

chlorophenothane NF [also: clofenotane; dicophane]

chlorophenoxamide [see: clefamide]

chlorophenylmercury [see: phenylmercuric chloride]

chlorophyll, water soluble [see: chlorophyllin]

chlorophyllin *vulnerary; oral deodorant for ostomy, breath, and body odors; topical deodorant for wounds and ulcers* 20 mg oral

chlorophyllin copper complex USAN *oral deodorant for ostomy, breath, and body odors; topical deodorant for wounds and ulcers*

chloroprednisone INN

chloroprednisone acetate [see: chloroprednisone]

chloroprocaine INN *injectable local anesthetic* [also: chloroprocaine HCl]

chloroprocaine HCl USP *injectable local anesthetic; central or peripheral nerve block, including lumbar and epidural block* [also: chloroprocaine] 2%, 3% injection

Chloroptic eye drops (discontinued 2005) ℞ *antibiotic* [chloramphenicol] 5 mg/mL

Chloroptic S.O.P. ophthalmic ointment (discontinued 2005) ℞ *antibiotic* [chloramphenicol] 10 mg/g

chloropyramine INN [also: halopyramine]

chloropyrilene INN, BAN [also: chlorothen citrate]

chloroquine USP, INN, BAN *amebicide; antimalarial* ⚕ Klor-Con

chloroquine diphosphate [see: chloroquine phosphate]

chloroquine HCl USP *amebicide; antimalarial* [also: chloroquine]

chloroquine phosphate USP, BAN *amebicide; antimalarial; lupus erythematosus suppressant* 250, 500 mg oral

chloroserpidine INN

N-chlorosuccinimide [see: succinchlorimide]

chlorothen citrate NF [also: chloropyrilene]

chlorothenium citrate [see: chlorothen citrate]

chlorothenylpyramine [see: chlorothen]

chlorothiazide USP, INN, BAN *diuretic; antihypertensive* 250, 500 mg oral

chlorothiazide sodium USAN, USP *diuretic; antihypertensive*

chlorothymol NF

chlorotoxin *investigational (orphan) antineoplastic for malignant glioma*

chlorotrianisene USP, INN, BAN *estrogen for hormone replacement therapy or inoperable prostatic cancer*

chloroxine USAN *antibacterial and antifungal for seborrheic dermatitis of the scalp*

chloroxylenol USP, INN, BAN *antiseptic*

chlorozone [see: chloramine-T]

chlorpenthixol [see: clopenthixol]

chlorphenamine INN *antihistamine* [also: chlorpheniramine maleate; chlorpheniramine]

chlorphenamine maleate [see: chlorpheniramine maleate]

chlorphenecyclane [see: clofenciclan]

chlorphenesin INN, BAN *skeletal muscle relaxant* [also: chlorphenesin carbamate]

chlorphenesin carbamate USAN, JAN *skeletal muscle relaxant* [also: chlorphenesin]

chlorphenindione [see: clorindione]

chlorpheniramine BAN *alkylamine antihistamine* [also: chlorpheniramine maleate; chlorphenamine]

chlorpheniramine maleate USP *alkylamine antihistamine* [also: chlorphenamine; chlorpheniramine] 4, 8, 12 mg oral

chlorpheniramine maleate & phenylephrine HCl *antihistamine; decongestant* 4•20 mg oral; 4•12.5 mg/5 mL oral; 1•3.5 mg/mL oral

chlorpheniramine maleate & pseudoephedrine HCl *antihistamine; decongestant* 8•120, 12•100, 12•120 mg oral

chlorpheniramine polistirex USAN *alkylamine antihistamine*

chlorpheniramine tannate *alkylamine antihistamine*

chlorpheniramine tannate & pseudoephedrine tannate *antihistamine; decongestant*

chlorpheniramine tannate & pyrilamine tannate & phenylephrine tannate *antihistamine; decongestant* 2•12.5•5 mg/5 mL oral

chlorphenoctium amsonate INN, BAN

chlorphenotane [see: chlorophenothane]

chlorphenoxamine INN, BAN [also: chlorphenoxamine HCl]

chlorphenoxamine HCl USP [also: chlorphenoxamine]

chlorphentermine INN, BAN *anorectic* [also: chlorphentermine HCl]

chlorphentermine HCl USAN *anorectic* [also: chlorphentermine]

chlorphenylindandione [see: clorindione]

chlorphthalidone [see: chlorthalidone]

chlorprocaine chloride [see: chloroprocaine HCl]

chlorproethazine INN [also: chlorproethazine HCl]

chlorproethazine HCl [also: chlorproethazine]

chlorproguanil INN, BAN

chlorproguanil HCl [see: chlorproguanil]

chlorpromazine USP, INN, BAN *conventional (typical) phenothiazine antipsychotic for schizophrenia and manic episodes of a bipolar disorder; antiemetic for nausea and vomiting*

chlorpromazine HCl USP, BAN, JAN *phenothiazine antipsychotic for schizophrenia, manic episodes of a bipolar disorder, pediatric hyperactivity, and severe pediatric behavioral problems; treatment for acute intermittent porphyria, nausea/vomiting, and intractable hiccoughs* 10, 25, 50, 100, 200 mg oral; 100 mg/mL oral; 25 mg/mL injection

chlorpromazine hibenzate JAN *conventional (typical) phenothiazine antipsychotic for schizophrenia and manic episodes of a bipolar disorder; antiemetic for nausea and vomiting*

chlorpromazine phenolphthalinate JAN *conventional (typical) phenothiazine antipsychotic for schizophrenia and manic episodes of a bipolar disorder; antiemetic for nausea and vomiting*

chlorpromazine tannate USP, INN, BAN *conventional (typical) phenothiazine antipsychotic for schizophrenia and manic episodes of a bipolar disorder; antiemetic for nausea and vomiting*

chlorpropamide USP, INN, BAN, JAN *sulfonylurea antidiabetic that stimulates insulin secretion in the pancreas* 100, 250 mg oral

chlorprophenpyridamine maleate [see: chlorpheniramine maleate]

chlorprothixene USAN, USP, INN, BAN *thioxanthene antipsychotic*

chlorpyrifos BAN

chlorquinaldol INN, BAN

chlortalidone INN *antihypertensive; diuretic* [also: chlorthalidone]

chlortetracycline INN, BAN *antibiotic; antiprotozoal* [also: chlortetracycline bisulfate]

chlortetracycline bisulfate USP *antibiotic; antiprotozoal* [also: chlortetracycline]

chlortetracycline calcium *antibiotic; antiprotozoal*

chlortetracycline HCl USP, BAN *antibiotic; antiprotozoal*

chlorthalidone USAN, USP, BAN *antihypertensive; diuretic* [also: chlortalidone] 25, 50, 100 mg oral

chlorthalidone & atenolol *antihypertensive; diuretic; antiadrenergic (β-receptor)* 25•50, 25•100 mg oral

chlorthenoxazin BAN [also: chlorthenoxazine]

chlorthenoxazine INN [also: chlorthenoxazin]

chlorthiazide [see: chlorothiazide]

chlortrianisestrol [see: chlorotrianisene]

Chlor-Trimeton Allergy 8 Hour; Chlor-Trimeton Allergy 12 Hour timed-release tablets OTC *antihistamine* [chlorpheniramine maleate] 8 mg; 12 mg

Chlor-Trimeton Allergy-D 4 Hour tablets (discontinued 2007) OTC *decongestant; antihistamine* [pseudoephedrine sulfate; chlorpheniramine maleate] 60•4 mg

Chlor-Trimeton Allergy-D 12 Hour sustained-release tablets (discontinued 2007) OTC *decongestant; antihistamine* [pseudoephedrine sulfate; chlorpheniramine maleate] 120•8 mg

chlorzoxazone USP, INN, BAN, JAN *skeletal muscle relaxant* 250, 500 mg oral

chlosudimeprimylum [see: clopamide]

ChlVPP (chlorambucil, vinblastine, procarbazine, prednisone/prednisolone) *chemotherapy protocol for Hodgkin lymphoma* [note: prednisone is preferred in the U.S.; prednisolone is preferred in England]

ChlVPP/EVA (chlorambucil, vinblastine, procarbazine, prednisone/prednisolone, etoposide, vincristine, Adriamycin) *chemotherapy protocol for Hodgkin lymphoma* [note: prednisone is preferred in the U.S.; prednisolone is preferred in England]

CHO (cyclophosphamide, hydroxydaunomycin, Oncovin) *chemotherapy protocol*

CHO cells, recombinant [see: CD4, human truncated]

CHOB (cyclophosphamide, hydroxydaunomycin, Oncovin, bleomycin) *chemotherapy protocol*

CHOD (cyclophosphamide, hydroxydaunomycin, Oncovin, dexamethasone) *chemotherapy protocol*

choice dielytra *medicinal herb* [see: turkey corn]

Choice DM fingerstick test kit for home use OTC *in vitro diagnostic aid for glycosylated hemoglobin levels*

Choice DM; Choice DM Sugar-Free oral liquid OTC *enteral nutritional therapy for abnormal glucose tolerance* [lactose-free formula] 237 mL; 325 mL

Choice DM Daily Moisurizing lotion OTC *moisturizer; emollient*

Choice DM Gentle Care mouthwash

choke cherry; black choke *medicinal herb* [see: wild black cherry]

Cholac oral/rectal solution ℞ *synthetic disaccharide used to prevent and treat portal-systemic encephalopathy* [lactulose] 10 g/15 mL ⑨ shellac

cholagogues *a class of agents that stimulate the flow of bile into the duodenum*

cholalic acid [see: dehydrocholic acid]

cholecalciferol (vitamin D₃) USP, BAN, JAN *fat-soluble vitamin* (1 mcg= 400 IU) [also: colecalciferol] 1000 IU oral

Choledyl SA sustained-action tablets (discontinued 2004) ℞ *antiasthmatic; bronchodilator* [oxtriphylline] 400, 600 mg

cholera vaccine USP *active bacterin for cholera* (Vibrio cholerae)

cholesterin [see: cholesterol]

cholesterol NF *emulsifying agent*

cholestrin [see: cholesterol]

cholestyramine BAN *bile salts ion-exchange resin; cholesterol-lowering antihyperlipidemic* [also: cholestyramine resin; colestyramine]

Cholestyramine Light powder for oral suspension ℞ *cholesterol-lowering antihyperlipidemic; treatment for pruritus due to partial biliary obstruction; also used as an antidote to* Clostridium difficile *and digitalis toxicity* [cholestyramine resin] 4 g/dose

cholestyramine resin USP *bile salts ion-exchange resin; cholesterol-lowering antihyperlipidemic; treatment for pruritus due to partial biliary obstruction; also used as an antidote to* Clostridium difficile *and digitalis toxicity* [also: colestyramine; cholestyramine] 4 g powder for oral solution

Choletec IV injection ℞ *radioactive hepatobiliary imaging agent for cholescintigraphy* [technetium Tc 99m mebrofenin] 100 mCi in 45 mg

cholic acid [see: dehydrocholic acid]

Cholidase tablets OTC *dietary lipotropic with vitamin supplementation* [choline; inositol; vitamins B₆, B₁₂, and E] 185•150•2.5•0.005•7.5 mg

choline *dietary lipotropic supplement* 250, 300, 500, 650 mg oral

choline alfoscerate INN

choline bitartrate NF 250 mg oral

choline bromide hexamethylenedi-carbamate [see: hexacarbacholine bromide]

choline chloride INN *investigational (orphan) for choline deficiency of long-term parenteral nutrition*

choline chloride acetate [see: acetylcholine chloride]

choline chloride carbamate [see: carbachol]

choline chloride succinate [see: succinylcholine chloride]

choline dihydrogen citrate NF 650 mg oral

choline gluconate INN

choline glycerophosphate [see: choline alfoscerate]

choline perchlorate, nitrate ester [see: nitricholine perchlorate]

choline salicylate USAN, INN, BAN *analgesic; antipyretic; anti-inflammatory; antirheumatic*

choline theophyllinate INN, BAN *bronchodilator* [also: oxtriphylline]

cholinergic agonists *a class of agents that produce effects similar to those of the parasympathetic nervous system* [also called: parasympathomimetics]

cholinesterase inhibitors *a class of drugs which increase acetylcholine neurotransmitters, used as a cognition adjuvant in Alzheimer dementia* [also called: acetylcholinesterase (AChE) inhibitors]

Cholinoid capsules OTC *dietary lipotropic with vitamin supplementation* [choline; inositol; multiple B vitamins; vitamin C; lemon bioflavonoids] 111•111• ± •100•100 mg

Cholografin Meglumine injection R *radiopaque contrast medium for cholecystography and cholangiography* [iodipamide meglumine (49.2% iodine)] 520 mg/mL (257 mg/mL)

chondodendron tomentosum [see: tubocurarine chloride]

chondrocyte-alginate *investigational (orphan) gel suspension for vesicoureteral reflux in children*

chondroitin 4-sulfate [see: danaparoid sodium]

chondroitin 6-sulfate [see: danaparoid sodium]

chondroitin sulfate *natural remedy for arthritis, blood clots, and extravasation from needle sticks after certain chemotherapy treatments*

chondroitin sulfate sodium JAN

chondroitin sulfuric acid *natural remedy* [see: chondroitin sulfate]

chondroitinase *investigational (orphan) agent for vitrectomy*

Chondrox capsules OTC *dietary supplement for osteoarthritis; protects and rebuilds cartilage in joints* [N-acetyl-D-glucosamine; glucosamine sulfate; chondroitin sulfate; manganese (from manganese aspartate)] 500•500•800•0.17 mg

Chondrus crispus medicinal herb [see: Irish moss]

chonsurid *natural remedy* [see: chondroitin sulfate]

Chooz chewable tablets OTC *antacid* [calcium carbonate] 500 mg

CHOP (cyclophosphamide, hydroxydaunomycin, Oncovin, prednisone) *chemotherapy protocol for non-Hodgkin lymphoma*

CHOP-BLEO (cyclophosphamide, hydroxydaunomycin, Oncovin, prednisone, bleomycin) *chemotherapy protocol for non-Hodgkin lymphoma*

CHOPE (cyclophosphamide, hydroxydaunomycin, Oncovin, prednisone, etoposide) *chemotherapy protocol*

CHOR (cyclophosphamide, hydroxydaunomycin, Oncovin, radiation therapy) *chemotherapy protocol*

Chorex-5 powder for IM injection (discontinued 2006) R *gonad-stimulating hormone for prepubertal cryptorchidism or hypogonadism; ovulation*

stimulant [chorionic gonadotropin] 500 U/mL

Chorex-10 powder for IM injection (discontinued 2005) ℞ *gonad-stimulating hormone for prepubertal cryptorchidism or hypogonadism; ovulation stimulant* [chorionic gonadotropin] 1000 U/mL

choriogonadotropin alfa USAN, INN *recombinant human chorionic gonadotropin (rhCG); fertility stimulant for anovulatory women; adjuvant therapy for cryptorchidism*

chorionic gonadotrophin [see: gonadotropin, chorionic]

chorionic gonadotropin (CG) [see: gonadotropin, chorionic]

Choron-10 powder for IM injection ℞ *a human-derived hormone used for prepubertal cryptorchidism or hypogonadism and to induce ovulation in anovulatory women* [chorionic gonadotropin] 1000 U/mL ⊠ Creon 5; guarana

CHP (chlorhexidine phosphanilate) [q.v.]

Christmas factor [see: factor IX complex]

Chromagen film-coated caplets ℞ *hematinic* [iron; vitamins B_{12} and C; intrinsic factor concentrate; succinic acid] 70•0.01•152•50•75 mg

Chromagen capsules ℞ *hematinic* [ferrous fumarate; cyanocobalamin; ascorbic acid; intrinsic factor concentrate] 70•0.01•150•100 mg

Chromagen FA; Chromagen Forte capsules ℞ *hematinic* [iron; vitamins B_{12} & C; folic acid] 150•0.01•70•1 mg; 151•0.01•60•1 mg

Chromagen FA; Chromagen Forte film-coated caplets ℞ *hematinic* [iron; vitamins B_{12} & C; folic acid; succinic acid] 70•0.01•152•1•75 mg; 151•0.01•60.8•1•50 mg

Chromagen OB capsules OTC *prenatal vitamin/mineral/iron supplement* [multiple vitamins & minerals; iron; folic acid] ≛•28•1 mg

Chroma-Pak IV injection ℞ *chromium supplement* [chromic chloride

hexahydrate (20% elemental chromium)] 20.5, 102.5 mcg/mL (4, 20 mcg Cr/mL)

chromargyre [see: merbromin]

chromated albumin [see: albumin, chromated Cr 51 serum]

Chromelin Complexion Blender topical suspension OTC *skin darkening agent for vitiligo and hypopigmented areas* [dihydroxyacetone] 5%

chromic acid, disodium salt [see: sodium chromate Cr 51]

chromic chloride USP *dietary chromium supplement (20% elemental chromium)* 20.5, 102.5 mcg/mL (4, 20 mcg Cr/mL) injection

chromic chloride Cr 51 USAN *radioactive agent*

chromic chloride hexahydrate [see: chromic chloride]

chromic phosphate Cr 51 USAN *radioactive agent*

chromic phosphate P 32 USAN, USP *antineoplastic; radioactive agent*

chromium *element (Cr); trace mineral important in glucose metabolism*

Chromium Chloride IV injection ℞ *intravenous nutritional therapy* [chromic chloride hexahydrate] 4 mcg/mL

chromium chloride [see: chromic chloride Cr 51]

chromium chloride hexahydrate [see: chromic chloride]

chromium picolinate *dietary chromium supplement*

chromium polynicotinate *dietary chromium supplement*

chromocarb INN

chromonar HCl USAN *coronary vasodilator* [also: carbocromen]

Chronoforte capsules OTC *anti-aging supplement; glycation inhibitor; antioxidant* [acetyl-L-carnitine; alpha lipoic acid; carnosine; nettle leaf; quercetin; biotin] 333.3•50•166.7•166.7•12.5•0.5 mg

Chronogesic investigational (Phase III) *narcotic analgesic for cancer-related pain* [sufentanil]

Chronosule (trademarked dosage form) *sustained-action capsule* ⑨ Granisol

Chronotab (trademarked dosage form) *sustained-action tablet*

Chronulac oral/rectal solution ℞ *hyperosmotic laxative* [lactulose] 10 g/15 mL

Chrysanthemum parthenium medicinal herb [see: feverfew]

Chrysanthemum vulgare medicinal herb [see: tansy]

chrysazin *(withdrawn from the market by the FDA)* [see: danthron]

chrysin *natural aromatase inhibitor used to block the conversion of testosterone to estrogen* ⑨ Carrasyn; garcinia

CHVP (cyclophosphamide, hydroxydaunomycin, VM-26, prednisone) *chemotherapy protocol* ⑨ CAFP; CAV/EP; CCVPP; CFP; CH1VPP; CVB; CVEB; CVP

chymopapain USAN, INN, BAN *proteolytic enzyme for herniated lumbar discs*

chymotrypsin USP, INN, BAN *proteolytic enzyme; zonulolytic for intracapsular lens extraction*

C.I. acid orange 24 monosodium salt (color index) [see: resorcin brown]

C.I. basic violet 3 (color index) [see: gentian violet]

C.I. basic violet 14 monohydrochloride (color index) [see: fuchsin, basic]

C.I. direct blue 53 tetrasodium salt (color index) [see: Evans blue]

C.I. mordant yellow 5, disodium salt (color index) [see: olsalazine sodium]

ciadox INN ⑨ Cedax; Cidex; Sudex

Cialis film-coated tablets ℞ *phosphodiesterase type 5 (PDE5) inhibitor; selective vasodilator for erectile dysfunction (ED); approved for p.r.n. or q.d. dosing* [tadalafil] 2.5, 5, 10, 20 mg ⑨ Silace; xylose

ciamexon INN, BAN

cianergoline INN

cianidanol INN

cianidol [see: cianidanol]

cianopramine INN

ciapilome INN

Ciba Vision Cleaner for Sensitive Eyes solution OTC *surfactant cleaning solution for soft contact lenses*

Ciba Vision Saline aerosol solution OTC *rinsing/storage solution for soft contact lenses* [sodium chloride (saline solution)]

Cibacalcin subcu or IM injection ℞ *calcium regulator for Paget disease (osteitis deformans) (orphan)* [calcitonin (human)] 0.5 mg/vial

cibenzoline INN, BAN *antiarrhythmic* [also: cifenline]

cibenzoline succinate JAN *antiarrhythmic* [also: cifenline succinate]

cicaprost INN *prostacyclin analogue*

cicarperone INN

cicely, sweet *medicinal herb* [see: sweet cicely]

Cichorium intybus medicinal herb [see: chicory]

ciclacillin INN, BAN *antibacterial* [also: cyclacillin]

ciclactate INN

ciclafrine INN *antihypotensive* [also: ciclafrine HCl]

ciclafrine HCl USAN *antihypotensive* [also: ciclafrine]

ciclazindol USAN, INN, BAN *antidepressant*

ciclesonide *intranasal corticosteroidal anti-inflammatory for seasonal or perennial allergic rhinitis; once-daily treatment for persistent asthma*

cicletanine USAN, INN, BAN *antihypertensive*

ciclindole INN *antidepressant* [also: cyclindole]

cicliomenol INN ⑨ cyclomenol

ciclobendazole INN, BAN *anthelmintic* [also: cyclobendazole]

ciclofenazine INN *antipsychotic* [also: cyclophenazine HCl]

ciclofenazine HCl [see: cyclophenazine HCl]

cicloheximide INN *antipsoriatic* [also: cycloheximide]

ciclonicate INN

ciclonium bromide INN

ciclopirox USAN, INN, BAN *topical antifungal for tinea pedis, tinea cruris, tinea corporis, tinea versicolor, candidiasis, seborrheic dermatitis, and onychomycosis 0.77% topical; 8% nail lacquer*

ciclopirox olamine USAN, USP, JAN *topical antifungal for tinea pedis, tinea cruris, tinea corporis, tinea versicolor, candidiasis, seborrheic dermatitis, and onychomycosis 1% topical*

ciclopramine INN

cicloprofen USAN, INN, BAN *anti-inflammatory*

cicloprolol INN *antiadrenergic (β-receptor)* [also: cicloprolol HCl; cycloprolol]

cicloprolol HCl USAN *antiadrenergic (β-receptor)* [also: cicloprolol; cycloprolol]

ciclosidomine INN, BAN

ciclosporin INN *immunosuppressive* [also: cyclosporine; cyclosporin]

ciclotate INN *combining name for radicals or groups*

ciclotizolam INN, BAN

ciclotropium bromide INN

cicloxilic acid INN

cicloxolone INN, BAN

cicortonide INN

cicrotoic acid INN

cideferron INN ⊞ Pseudofrin

Cidex; Cidex-7; Cidex Plus 28 solution OTC *broad-spectrum antimicrobial* [glutaral] 2%; 2%; 3.2% ⊞ Cedax; ciadox; Sudex

cidofovir USAN, INN *nucleoside antiviral for AIDS-related cytomegalovirus (CMV) retinitis; investigational (Phase I/II) gel for AIDS-related genital herpes and Kaposi sarcoma*

cidoxepin INN *antidepressant* [also: cidoxepin HCl]

cidoxepin HCl USAN *antidepressant* [also: cidoxepin]

cifenline USAN *antiarrhythmic* [also: cibenzoline]

cifenline succinate USAN *antiarrhythmic* [also: cibenzoline succinate]

cifostodine INN

ciglitazone USAN, INN *antidiabetic*

cignolin [see: anthralin]

ciheptolane INN

ciladopa INN, BAN *antiparkinsonian; dopaminergic agent* [also: ciladopa HCl]

ciladopa HCl USAN *antiparkinsonian; dopaminergic agent* [also: ciladopa]

cilansetron INN *treatment for irritable bowel syndrome*

cilastatin INN, BAN *enzyme inhibitor* [also: cilastatin sodium]

cilastatin sodium USAN, JAN *enzyme inhibitor* [also: cilastatin]

cilazapril USAN, INN, BAN, JAN *antihypertensive; ACE inhibitor*

cilazaprilat INN, BAN

cilexetil USAN *combining name for radicals or groups*

ciliary neurotrophic factor *investigational (orphan) agent for amyotrophic lateral sclerosis*

ciliary neurotrophic factor, recombinant human *investigational (orphan) agent for amyotrophic lateral sclerosis and other muscular atrophies*

"cillins" *brief term for a class of antibiotics derived from various strains of the fungus* Penicillium, *or their semi-synthetic analogues, whose generic names end in "cillin," such as ampicillin* [properly called: penicillins] ⊞ Zolinza

cilmostim USAN *hematopoietic; macrophage colony-stimulating factor*

cilobamine INN *antidepressant* [also: cilobamine mesylate]

cilobamine mesylate USAN *antidepressant* [also: cilobamine]

cilofungin USAN, INN *antifungal*

ciloprost [see: iloprost]

cilostamide INN ⊞ salacetamide

cilostazol USAN, INN *antithrombotic; phosphodiesterase (PDE) III platelet aggregation inhibitor and vasodilator for intermittent claudication 50, 100 mg oral*

Ciloxan Drop-Tainers (eye drops), ointment ℞ *broad-spectrum fluoroquinolone antibiotic* [ciprofloxacin HCl] 3.5 mg/mL (3 mg/mL base); 3.33 mg/mL (3 mg/mL base)

ciltoprazine INN

cilutazoline INN

cimaterol USAN, INN *repartitioning agent* ⑨ Symmetrel; xamoterol
cimemoxin INN
cimepanol INN
cimetidine USAN, USP, INN, BAN, JAN *histamine H_2 antagonist for gastric and duodenal ulcers and gastric hypersecretory conditions* 200, 300, 400, 800 mg oral
cimetidine HCl USAN *histamine H_2 antagonist for gastric and duodenal ulcers and gastric hypersecretory conditions* 300 mg/5 mL oral; 300 mg/2 mL injection
Cimetidine in 0.9% Sodium Chloride IV infusion ℞ *histamine H_2 antagonist for gastric and duodenal ulcers and gastric hypersecretory conditions* [cimetidine HCl] 300 mg/50 mL bag
cimetropium bromide INN
Cimicifuga racemosa medicinal herb [see: black cohosh]
cimoxatone INN
Cimzia powder for subcu injection (discontinued 2008) ℞ *anti-inflammatory for moderate to severe Crohn disease* [certolizumab pegol] 200 mg
cinacalcet HCl *oral calcimimetic agent for hypercalcemia due to parathyroid carcinoma (orphan) and secondary hyperparathyroidism (SHPT) due to chronic kidney disease* (base=91%)
cinalukast USAN, INN *antiasthmatic*
cinametic acid INN
cinamolol INN
cinanserin INN *serotonin inhibitor* [also: cinanserin HCl]
cinanserin HCl USAN *serotonin inhibitor* [also: cinanserin]
cinaproxen INN
cincaine chloride [see: dibucaine HCl]
cinchocaine INN, BAN *local anesthetic* [also: dibucaine]
cinchocaine HCl BAN *local anesthetic* [also: dibucaine HCl]
Cinchona succirubra; C. ledgeriana; C. calisaya medicinal herb [see: quinine]
cinchonidine sulfate NF
cinchonine sulfate NF

cinchophen NF, INN, BAN
cinecromen INN
cinepaxadil INN
cinepazet INN, BAN *antianginal* [also: cinepazet maleate]
cinepazet maleate USAN *antianginal* [also: cinepazet]
cinepazic acid INN
cinepazide INN, BAN
cinfenine INN
cinfenoac INN, BAN
cinflumide USAN, INN *muscle relaxant*
cingestol USAN, INN *progestin*
cinitapride INN
cinmetacin INN
cinnamaldehyde NF
cinnamaverine INN
cinnamedrine USAN, INN *smooth muscle relaxant*
cinnamedrine HCl *smooth muscle relaxant*
cinnamic aldehyde [now: cinnamaldehyde]
cinnamon NF
cinnamon oil NF
cinnamon (Cinnamonum zeylanicum) bark and oil *medicinal herb for diarrhea, dysmenorrhea, gastrointestinal upset, microbial and fungal infections, and gas pain; also used as an aromatic, astringent, and stimulant*
cinnamon wood *medicinal herb* [see: sassafras]
cinnarizine USAN, INN, BAN *antihistamine*
cinnarizine clofibrate INN
cinnofuradione INN
cinnofuron [see: cinnofuradione]
cinnopentazone INN *anti-inflammatory* [also: cintazone]
cinnopropazone [see: apazone]
Cinobac capsules ℞ *urinary antibacterial* [cinoxacin] 250 mg ⑨ Sani-Pak
cinoctramide INN
cinodine HCl USAN *veterinary antibacterial*
cinolazepam INN
cinoquidox INN
cinoxacin USAN, USP, INN, BAN *urinary antibacterial*

cinoxate USAN, USP, INN *ultraviolet screen*

cinoxolone INN, BAN

cinoxopazide INN

cinperene USAN, INN *antipsychotic*

cinprazole INN

cinpropazide INN

cinquefoil (*Potentilla anserina; P. canadensis; P. reptans*) plant *medicinal herb used as an antispasmodic and astringent*

cinromide USAN, INN *anticonvulsant*

cintazone USAN *anti-inflammatory* [also: cinnopentazone]

cintramide INN *antipsychotic* [also: cintriamide]

cintredekin besudotox *investigational antineoplastic for brain tumors*

cintriamide USAN *antipsychotic* [also: cintramide]

cinuperone INN

cioteronel USAN, INN *antiandrogen* ☑ citronella; soterenol; SteriNail

cipamfylline USAN *antiviral agent; tumor necrosis factor alpha inhibitor*

cipemastat USAN, INN *matrix metalloproteinase inhibitor*

cipionate INN *combining name for radicals or groups* [also: cypionate]

ciprafamide INN

ciprazafone INN

ciprefadol INN *analgesic* [also: ciprefadol succinate]

ciprefadol succinate USAN *analgesic* [also: ciprefadol]

Cipro Cystitis Pack (6 film-coated tablets) ℞ *broad-spectrum fluoroquinolone antibiotic* [ciprofloxacin] 100 mg

Cipro film-coated tablets ℞ *broad-spectrum fluoroquinolone antibiotic* [ciprofloxacin HCl] 250, 500, 750 mg

Cipro powder for oral suspension ℞ *broad-spectrum fluoroquinolone antibiotic* [ciprofloxacin] 250, 500 mg/5 mL

Cipro HC Otic ear drop suspension ℞ *broad-spectrum fluoroquinolone antibiotic; corticosteroidal anti-inflammatory* [ciprofloxacin; hydrocortisone] 0.2%•1% (2•10 mg/mL)

Cipro I.V. ℞ *broad-spectrum fluoroquinolone antibiotic* [ciprofloxacin] 200, 400 mg/vial ☑ Spiriva

Cipro XR film-coated extended-release tablets ℞ *broad-spectrum fluoroquinolone antibiotic* [ciprofloxacin HCl] 500, 1000 mg

ciprocinonide USAN, INN *adrenocortical steroid*

Ciprodex ear drop suspension ℞ *broad-spectrum fluoroquinolone antibiotic; corticosteroidal anti-inflammatory* [ciprofloxacin HCl; dexamethasone] 0.3%•0.1%

ciprofibrate USAN, INN, BAN *antihyperlipoproteinemic*

ciprofloxacin USAN, INN, BAN *broad-spectrum fluoroquinolone antibiotic* 200, 400 mg injection ☑ sparfloxacin

ciprofloxacin HCl USAN, USP, JAN *broad-spectrum fluoroquinolone antibiotic* [3.5 mg/mL] 100, 250, 500, 750, 1000 mg oral; 3.5 mg/mL eye drops ☑ sparfloxacin

Ciprofloxacin in 5% Dextrose injection ℞ *broad-spectrum fluoroquinolone antibiotic* [ciprofloxacin] 200, 400 mg ☑ sparfloxacin

ciprofloxacin liposomal *broad-spectrum bactericidal antibiotic; investigational (orphan) aerosolized formulation for the treatment of cystic fibrosis*

cipropride INN

ciproquazone INN

ciproquinate INN *coccidiostat for poultry* [also: cyproquinate]

ciprostene INN *platelet antiaggregatory agent* [also: ciprostene calcium]

ciprostene calcium USAN *platelet anti-aggregatory agent* [also: ciprostene]

ciproximide INN *antipsychotic; antidepressant* [also: cyproximide]

ciramadol USAN, INN *analgesic*

ciramadol HCl USAN *analgesic*

cirazoline INN

Circadin *natural sleep aid; investigational (orphan) for circadian rhythm sleep disorders in blind people with no light perception* [melatonin]

Circavite-T tablets OTC *vitamin/mineral/iron supplement* [multiple vitamins & minerals; iron] $\pm$ • 12 mg

cirolemycin USAN, INN *antineoplastic; antibacterial*

cisapride USAN, INN, BAN, JAN *peristaltic stimulant; treatment for nocturnal heartburn due to gastroesophageal reflux disease; (withdrawn from the U.S. market in 2000 due to increased cardiac arrhythmias)*

cisatracurium besylate USAN *nondepolarizing neuromuscular blocker*

CISCA; CisCA (cisplatin, cyclophosphamide, Adriamycin) *chemotherapy protocol for bladder cancer*

CISCA$_{II}$/VB$_{IV}$ (cisplatin, cyclophosphamide, Adriamycin, vinblastine, bleomycin) *chemotherapy protocol for germ cell tumors*

cisclomiphene [now: enclomiphene]

cisconazole USAN, INN *antifungal*

cis-**DDP (diamminedichloroplatinum)** [see: cisplatin]

cis-**diamminedichloroplatinum (DDP)** [see: cisplatin]

cismadinone INN

cisplatin USAN, USP, INN, BAN *alkylating antineoplastic for metastatic testicular tumors, metastatic ovarian tumors, and advanced bladder cancer* 1 mg/mL injection

cisplatin & docetaxel *chemotherapy protocol for bladder cancer and non–small cell lung cancer (NSCLC)*

cisplatin & epinephrine *investigational (NDA filed, orphan) injectable gel for squamous cell carcinoma of the head and neck; investigational (orphan) for metastatic malignant melanoma*

cisplatin & fluorouracil *chemotherapy protocol for cervical cancer, used in conjunction with radiation therapy*

cisplatin & gemcitabine *chemotherapy protocol for metastatic bladder cancer*

cisplatin & vinorelbine *chemotherapy protocol for cervical cancer and non–small cell lung cancer (NSCLC)*

cis-**platinum** [now: cisplatin]

cis-**platinum II** [now: cisplatin]

9-*cis*-retinoic acid [see: alitretinoin]

13-*cis*-retinoic acid [see: isotretinoin]

cistinexine INN

citalopram INN, BAN *selective serotonin reuptake inhibitor (SSRI) for major depression*

citalopram hydrobromide USAN *selective serotonin reuptake inhibitor (SSRI) for major depression; also used for obsessive-compulsive disorder (OCD), post-traumatic stress disorder (PTSD), generalized anxiety disorder (GAD), and premenstrual dysphoric disorder (PMDD)* 10, 20, 40 mg oral; 10 mg/5 mL oral

Citanest Forte injection $\mathbb{R}$ *local anesthetic for dental procedures* [prilocaine HCl; epinephrine] 4% • 1:200 000

Citanest Plain injection $\mathbb{R}$ *local anesthetic for dental procedures* [prilocaine HCl] 4%

citatepine INN

citenamide USAN, INN *anticonvulsant*

citenazone INN

citicoline INN, JAN *neuroprotectant* [also: citicoline sodium]

citicoline sodium USAN *neuroprotectant* [also: citicoline]

citiolone INN

Citra pH oral solution OTC *antacid* [sodium citrate] 450 mg/5 mL

Citracal tablets OTC *calcium supplement* [calcium citrate] 200 mg Ca

Citracal Caplets + D OTC *dietary supplement* [calcium citrate; vitamin D] 315 mg • 200 IU

Citracal Creamy Bites chewable tablets (discontinued 2008) OTC *dietary supplement* [calcium citrate; vitamin D] 500 mg • 200 IU

Citracal Liquitab effervescent tablets OTC *calcium supplement* [calcium citrate] 500 mg Ca

Citracal Plus with Magnesium tablets OTC *dietary supplement* [calcium citrate; vitamin D; multiple minerals] 250 mg Ca • 125 IU • $\pm$

Citracal Prenatal 90 + DHA tablets + capsules $\mathbb{R}$ *calcium/iron supplement + omega-3 fatty acid supplement* [multiple vitamins & minerals; calcium citrate; carbonyl iron; folic acid; docusate sodium + docosahexaenoic acid (DHA)] ± • 200 • 90 • 1 • 50 mg (tablets) + 250 mg (capsules)

Citracal Prenatal + DHA tablets + capsules ℞ *calcium/iron supplement + omega-3 fatty acid supplement* [multiple vitamins & minerals; calcium citrate; iron; folic acid; docusate sodium + docosahexaenoic acid (DHA)] ± • 125 • 27 • 1 • 50 mg (tablets) + 250 mg (capsules)

Citracal Prenatal Rx tablets ℞ *calcium/iron supplement* [multiple vitamins & minerals; calcium citrate; iron; folic acid; docusate sodium] ± • 125 • 27 • 1 • 50 mg

Citralax effervescent granules OTC *saline laxative* [magnesium citrate; magnesium sulfate] ② Starlix

citrate dextrose [see: ACD solution]

citrate of magnesia [see: magnesium citrate]

citrate phosphate dextrose [see: anticoagulant citrate phosphate dextrose solution]

citrate phosphate dextrose adenine [see: anticoagulant citrate phosphate dextrose adenine solution]

citrated caffeine NF [see: caffeine citrate]

citric acid USP *pH adjusting agent; urinary acidifier* ② stearic acid

citric acid, magnesium oxide & sodium carbonate [see: Suby G solution]

citric acid & D-gluconic acid lactone & magnesium hydroxycarbonate *bladder and catheter irrigant for apatite or struvite calculi (orphan)*

citric acid & sodium citrate *urinary alkalinizing agent* 334 • 500 mg/5 mL oral

citrin [see: bioflavonoids]

Citrocarbonate effervescent granules OTC *antacid* [sodium bicarbonate; sodium citrate] 780 • 1820 mg/dose

Citrolith tablets ℞ *urinary alkalinizing agent* [potassium citrate; sodium citrate] 50 • 950 mg

citronella *(Cymbopogon nardus; C. winterianus)* oil *medicinal herb for gastrointestinal spasms, promoting diuresis, and worms; also used as an antibacterial; not generally regarded as safe and effective for internal use as it is highly toxic* ② cioteronel; soterenol; SteriNail

Citrotein oral liquid, powder for oral liquid OTC *enteral nutritional therapy* [lactose-free formula]

citrovorum factor [see: leucovorin calcium]

Citrucel powder, tablets OTC *bulk laxative* [methylcellulose] 2 g/tbsp. or scoop; 500 mg

Citrucel Fiber Shake; Citrucel Sugar Free powder for oral solution OTC *bulk laxative* [methylcellulose] 2 g/tbsp.

Citrus bergamia; C. aurantium medicinal herb [see: bergamot oil]

citrus bioflavonoids [see: bioflavonoids]

Citrus Calcium coated tablets OTC *calcium supplement* [calcium citrate] 200 mg Ca

Citrus limon medicinal herb [see: lemon]

Citrus paradisi medicinal herb [see: grapefruit]

civamide *investigational (orphan) agent for postherpetic neuralgia of the trigeminal nerve*

CIVPP (chlorambucil, vinblastine, procarbazine, prednisone) *chemotherapy protocol*

8-Cl cAMP (8-chloroadenosine monophosphate, cyclic) [see: tocladesine]

CLA (conjugated linoleic acid) [q.v.]

cladribine *antimetabolite antineoplastic for hairy-cell leukemia (orphan); investigational (Phase III, orphan) for relapsing multiple sclerosis; investigational (orphan) for chronic lymphocytic leukemia, myeloid leukemia, and non-Hodgkin lymphoma* 1 mg/mL injection

Claforan powder or frozen premix for IV or IM injection ℞ *third-generation cephalosporin antibiotic* [cefotaxime sodium] 0.5, 1, 2, 10 g ② Calphron; Kolephrin

clamidoxic acid INN, BAN

clamoxyquin BAN *antiamebic* [also: clamoxyquin HCl; clamoxyquine]

clamoxyquin HCl USAN *antiamebic* [also: clamoxyquine; clamoxyquin]

clamoxyquine INN *antiamebic* [also: clamoxyquin HCl; clamoxyquin]

clanfenur INN

clanobutin INN

clantifen INN

clara cell 10kDa protein, recombinant human *investigational (orphan) for prevention of bronchopulmonary dysplasia in neonates with respiratory distress syndrome (RDS)*

Claravis capsules ℞ *keratolytic for severe recalcitrant cystic acne* [isotretinoin] 10, 20, 30, 40 mg ② Klorvess

claretin-12 [see: cyanocobalamin]

Clarinex film-coated tablets, syrup ℞ *nonsedating antihistamine for allergic rhinitis and chronic idiopathic urticaria* [desloratadine] 5 mg; 2.5 mg/5 mL

Clarinex RediTabs (rapidly disintegrating tablets) ℞ *nonsedating antihistamine for allergic rhinitis and chronic idiopathic urticaria* [desloratadine] 2.5, 5 mg

Clarinex-D 12 Hour extended-release tablets (discontinued 2007) ℞ *nonsedating antihistamine and decongestant for allergic rhinitis* [desloratadine; pseudoephedrine sulfate] 2.5•120 mg

Clarinex-D 24 Hour extended-release tablets ℞ *nonsedating antihistamine and decongestant for allergic rhinitis* [desloratadine; pseudoephedrine sulfate] 5•240 mg

Claripel cream ℞ *hyperpigmentation bleaching agent* [hydroquinone] 4%

clarithromycin USAN, INN, BAN, JAN *macrolide antibiotic* 250, 500, 1000 mg oral; 125, 250 mg/5 mL oral

Claritin capsules, syrup OTC *nonsedating antihistamine for allergic rhinitis* [loratadine] 10 mg; 5 mg/5 mL

Claritin 24-Hour Allergy tablets OTC *nonsedating antihistamine for allergic rhinitis; also used for chronic idiopathic urticaria* [loratadine] 10 mg

Claritin Children's Allergy chewable tablets, oral solution OTC *nonsedating antihistamine for allergic rhinitis* [loratadine] 5 mg; 5 mg/5 mL

Claritin Hives Relief tablets OTC *nonsedating antihistamine for hives* [loratadine] 10 mg

Claritin RediTabs (orally disintegrating tablets) OTC *nonsedating antihistamine for allergic rhinitis* [loratadine] 5, 10 mg

Claritin-D 12 Hour; Claritin-D 24 Hour extended-release tablets OTC *nonsedating antihistamine; decongestant* [loratadine; pseudoephedrine sulfate] 5•120 mg; 10•240 mg

Clarityne (Mexican name for the U.S. product **Claritin**)

Claviceps purpurea medicinal herb [see: ergot]

clavulanate potassium USAN, USP *β-lactamase inhibitor; penicillin synergist*

clavulanic acid INN, BAN *β-lactamase inhibitor; penicillin synergist*

claw, scaly dragon's; turkey claw *medicinal herb* [see: coral root]

clay, kaolin *natural material* [see: kaolin]

clazolam USAN, INN *minor tranquilizer*

clazolimine USAN, INN *diuretic*

clazuril USAN, INN, BAN *coccidiostat for pigeons* ② Clozaril; glycerol

CLD-BOMP *chemotherapy protocol for cervical cancer* [see: BOMP]

Clean-N-Soak solution OTC *cleaning/soaking solution for hard contact lenses*

Clear Eyes ACR eye drops (name changed to **Clear Eyes Seasonal Relief** in 2006)

Clear Eyes Contact Lens Relief eye drops OTC *antiseptic; emollient* [sorbic acid; hypromellose; glycerin] 0.25%•②•②

Clear Eyes for Dry Eyes eye drops OTC *moisturizer; emollient* [carboxymethylcellulose sodium; glycerin] 1%•0.25%

Clear Eyes for Dry Eyes Plus Redness Relief eye drops OTC *decongestant; vasoconstrictor; moisturizer/lubricant* [naphazoline HCl; hypromellose; glycerin] 0.012%•0.8%•0.25%

Clear Eyes for Redness Relief eye drops OTC *decongestant; vasoconstrictor; moisturizer/lubricant* [naphazoline HCl; glycerin] 0.012%•0.2%

Clear Eyes Seasonal Relief eye drops OTC *decongestant; astringent* [naphazoline HCl; zinc sulfate] 0.012%•0.25%

Clearasil Acne Treatment cream OTC *keratolytic for acne* [benzoyl peroxide] 10%

Clearasil Acne-Fighting Pads OTC *keratolytic for acne* [salicylic acid; alcohol $\geq$ %] 2%

Clearasil Adult Care cream OTC *antiseptic, antifungal, and keratolytic for acne* [sulfur; resorcinol; alcohol 10%]

Clearasil Antibacterial Soap bar OTC *medicated cleanser for acne* [triclosan]

Clearasil Clearstick topical liquid OTC *keratolytic for acne* [salicylic acid; alcohol 39%] 1.25%, 2%

Clearasil Daily Face Wash topical liquid OTC *medicated cleanser for acne* [triclosan] 0.3%

Clearasil Double Clear; Clearasil Double Textured medicated pads OTC *keratolytic for acne* [salicylic acid; alcohol 40%] 1.25%, 2%; 2%

Clearasil Medicated Deep Cleanser topical liquid OTC *keratolytic cleanser for acne* [salicylic acid; alcohol 42%] 0.5%

Clear-Atadine tablets OTC *nonsedating antihistamine for allergic rhinitis; also used for chronic idiopathic urticaria* [loratadine] 10 mg

Clear-Atadine Children's oral liquid OTC *nonsedating antihistamine for allergic rhinitis* [loratadine] 5 mg/5 mL

Clear-Atadine D extended-release tablets OTC *nonsedating antihistamine; decongestant* [loratadine; pseudoephedrine sulfate] 10•240 mg

Clearblue Easy Digital Pregnancy Test test stick plus digital readout for home use OTC *in vitro diagnostic aid; urine pregnancy test*

Clearblue Easy Ovulation Test test sticks for home use (7 sticks per package) OTC *in vitro diagnostic aid; urine ovulation test*

Clearblue Easy Pregnancy Test test stick for home use OTC *in vitro diagnostic aid; urine pregnancy test*

Clearly Cala-gel OTC *topical antihistamine* [diphenhydramine HCl]

Clearplan Easy test kit for home use (discontinued 2004) OTC *in vitro diagnostic aid to predict ovulation time*

Clearview Chlamydia test for professional use ℞ *in vitro diagnostic aid for Chlamydia trachomatis* [color-label immunoassay]

cleavers; cleaverwort *medicinal herb* [see: bedstraw]

clebopride USAN, INN *antiemetic*

Cleeravue-M film-coated tablets ℞ *tetracycline antibiotic for gram-negative and gram-positive bacteria; antirickettsial* [minocycline] 50 mg

clefamide INN, BAN

clemastine USAN, BAN *ethanolamine antihistamine* ☒ galamustine

clemastine fumarate USAN, USP, BAN *ethanolamine antihistamine;* (base= 75%) 1.34, 2.68 mg oral; 0.67 mg/5 mL

Clematis cirrhosa; C. virginiana medicinal herb [see: woodbine]

clemeprol INN, BAN

clemizole INN, BAN

clemizole penicillin INN, BAN

clenbuterol INN, BAN

Clenia cream, foaming wash ℞ *antibiotic and keratolytic for acne, rosacea, and seborrheic dermatitis* [sulfacetamide sodium; sulfur] 10%•5% ☒ Calan; kaolin; khellin

clenoliximab *investigational (Phase I/II) anti-CD4 antibody for the treatment of rheumatoid arthritis*

clenpirin INN [also: clenpyrin]

clenpyrin BAN [also: clenpirin]

clentiazem INN *calcium channel antagonist* [also: clentiazem maleate]

clentiazem maleate USAN *calcium channel antagonist* [also: clentiazem]

Cleocin capsules ℞ *antibiotic; investigational (orphan) for AIDS-related* Pneumocystis *pneumonia (PCP)* [clindamycin (as HCl)] 75, 150, 300 mg

Cleocin vaginal cream in prefilled applicator, vaginal ovules (suppositories) ℞ *antibiotic for bacterial vaginosis* [clindamycin phosphate] 2%; 100 mg ☒ Galzin; glycine; Quelicin

Cleocin Pediatric granules for oral solution ℞ *antibiotic* [clindamycin (as palmitate HCl)] 75 mg/5 mL

Cleocin Phosphate IM injection ℞ *antibiotic; investigational (orphan) for AIDS-related* Pneumocystis *pneumonia (PCP)* [clindamycin (as phosphate)] 150 mg/mL

Cleocin Phosphate IV infusion ℞ *antibiotic; investigational (orphan) for AIDS-related* Pneumocystis *pneumonia (PCP)* [clindamycin (as phosphate)] 300, 600, 900 mg

Cleocin T gel, lotion, topical solution, pledgets ℞ *antibiotic for acne; also used for rosacea* [clindamycin phosphate] 1% ☒ Calcionate

Clerz 2; Clerz Plus solution OTC *rewetting solution for hard or soft contact lenses*

cletoquine INN, BAN

clevidipine butyrate *calcium channel blocker for the rapid control of hypertension*

Cleviprex emulsion for IV injection ℞ *calcium channel blocker for the rapid control of hypertension* [clevidipine butyrate] 50, 100 mL

Clexane (Eur) (European name for U.S. product **Lovenox**)

clibucaine INN

click.easy (trademarked device) *reconstitution device used with the* **one.click** *prefilled auto-injector* ☒ Caelyx; glucose

clidafidine INN

clidanac INN

clidinium bromide USAN, USP, INN, BAN *GI/GU anticholinergic/antispasmodic; peptic ulcer adjunct*

clidinium bromide & chlordiazepoxide HCl *GI/GU anticholinergic/antispasmodic; anxiolytic* 2.5•5 mg

Climara transdermal patch ℞ *estrogen replacement therapy for the treatment of postmenopausal symptoms and prevention of postmenopausal osteoporosis* [estradiol] 25, 37.5, 50, 60, 75, 100 mcg/day

ClimaraPro transdermal patch ℞ *hormone replacement therapy for the treatment of postmenopausal symptoms and prevention of postmenopausal osteoporosis* [levonorgestrel; estradiol] 15•45 mcg/day

climazolam INN

climbazole INN, BAN

climiqualine INN

Clinac BPO gel ℞ *keratolytic for acne* [benzoyl peroxide] 7%

clinafloxacin HCl USAN *quinolone antibacterial*

Clindagel gel ℞ *antibiotic for acne; also used for rosacea* [clindamycin phosphate] 1%

ClindaMax gel, lotion ℞ *antibiotic for acne; also used for rosacea* [clindamycin phosphate] 1%

ClindaMax vaginal cream in prefilled applicators ℞ *antibiotic for bacterial vaginosis* [clindamycin phosphate] 2%

clindamycin USAN, INN, BAN *lincosamide antibiotic; investigational (orphan) for AIDS-related* Pneumocystis *pneumonia (PCP)*

clindamycin HCl USP, BAN *lincosamide antibiotic; investigational (orphan) for AIDS-related* Pneumocystis *pneumonia (PCP)* 150, 300 mg oral

clindamycin palmitate HCl USAN, USP *lincosamide antibiotic*

clindamycin phosphate USAN, USP *lincosamide antibiotic* 1%, 2% topical; 150 mg/mL injection

Clindesse vaginal cream in prefilled applicators ℞ *antibiotic for bacterial vaginosis* [clindamycin phosphate] 2%

Clindets topical solution, pledgets ℞ *antibiotic for acne; also used for rosacea* [clindamycin; alcohol 52%] 1%

Clinipak (trademarked packaging form) *unit dose package*

Clinistix reagent strips for home use OTC *in vitro diagnostic aid for urine glucose*

Clinitest reagent tablets for home use OTC *in vitro diagnostic aid for urine glucose*

clinocaine HCl [see: procaine HCl]

clinofibrate INN

clinolamide INN

Clinoril tablets ℞ *nonsteroidal anti-inflammatory drug (NSAID) for osteoarthritis, rheumatoid arthritis, ankylosing spondylitis, acute bursitis/tendinitis, and other inflammatory conditions* [sulindac] 150, 200 mg

clioquinol USP, INN, BAN *topical antibacterial/antifungal* 3% topical

clioxanide USAN, INN, BAN *anthelmintic*

clipoxamine [see: cliropamine]

cliprofen USAN, INN *anti-inflammatory*

cliropamine INN

Clivarine *investigational (orphan) for deep vein thrombosis (DVT) in pediatric or pregnant patients* [reviparin sodium]

clobamine mesylate [now: cilobamine mesylate]

clobazam USAN, INN, BAN *minor benzodiazepine tranquilizer; anxiolytic*

clobedolum [see: clonitazene]

clobenoside INN

clobenzepam INN

clobenzorex INN

clobenztropine INN

clobetasol INN, BAN *topical corticosteroidal anti-inflammatory* [also: clobetasol propionate]

clobetasol propionate USAN *topical corticosteroidal anti-inflammatory for scalp dermatoses and plaque psoriasis* [also: clobetasol] 0.05% topical

clobetasone INN, BAN *topical corticosteroidal anti-inflammatory* [also: clobetasone butyrate]

clobetasone butyrate USAN *topical corticosteroidal anti-inflammatory* [also: clobetasone]

Clobex topical spray, lotion, shampoo ℞ *corticosteroidal anti-inflammatory* [clobetasol propionate] 0.05%

clobutinol INN

clobuzarit INN, BAN

clocanfamide INN

clocapramine INN

clociguanil INN, BAN

clocinizine INN

clocortolone INN *topical corticosteroid* [also: clocortolone acetate]

clocortolone acetate USAN *topical corticosteroid* [also: clocortolone]

clocortolone pivalate USAN, USP *topical corticosteroid*

clocoumarol INN

Clocream cream OTC *moisturizer; emollient* [cod liver oil (vitamins A and E); cholecalciferol; vitamin A palmitate]

clodacaine INN

clodanolene USAN, INN *skeletal muscle relaxant*

clodantoin INN *antifungal* [also: chlordantoin]

clodazon INN *antidepressant* [also: clodazon HCl] ② Caldesene

clodazon HCl USAN *antidepressant* [also: clodazon]

Cloderm cream ℞ *corticosteroidal anti-inflammatory* [clocortolone pivalate] 0.1%

clodoxopone INN

clodronate disodium *bisphosphonate bone resorption inhibitor for hypercalcemia of malignancy* [also: disodium clodronate]

clodronic acid USAN, INN, BAN *calcium regulator*

clofarabine *purine nucleoside antimetabolite antineoplastic for children with acute lymphoblastic leukemia (orphan); investigational (Phase III, orphan) for acute myelogenous leukemia*

Clofarex (name changed to **Clolar** upon marketing release in 2004)

clofazimine USAN, INN, BAN *bactericidal; tuberculostatic; leprostatic (orphan);*

*available only to physicians enrolled in
the National Hansen Disease Program
through the FDA*

clofedanol INN *antitussive* [also: chlophedianol HCl; chlophedianol]

clofedanol HCl [see: chlophedianol
HCl]

clofenamic acid INN

clofenamide INN

clofenciclan INN

clofenetamine INN

clofenetamine HCl [see: clofeneta-
mine]

clofenotane INN [also: chlorophenothane; dicophane]

clofenoxyde INN

clofenpyride [see: nicofibrate]

clofenvinfos INN [also: chlorfenvin-
phos]

clofeverine INN

clofexamide INN

clofezone INN ☑ Calphosan

clofibrate USAN, USP, INN, BAN *triglyceride-lowering antihyperlipidemic for
primary dysbetalipoproteinemia (type
III hyperlipidemia) and hypertriglyceridemia (types IV and V hyperlipidemia)*

clofibric acid INN

clofibride INN

clofilium phosphate USAN, INN *antiarrhythmic*

clofinol [see: nicofibrate]

cloflucarban USAN *disinfectant* [also:
halocarban]

clofluperol INN, BAN *antipsychotic*
[also: seperidol HCl]

clofluperol HCl [see: seperidol HCl]

clofoctol INN

cloforex INN

clofurac INN

clogestone INN, BAN *progestin* [also:
clogestone acetate]

clogestone acetate USAN *progestin*
[also: clogestone]

cloguanamil INN, BAN [also: clogua-
namile]

cloguanamile BAN [also: cloguanamil]

Clolar IV infusion ℞ *purine nucleoside
antimetabolite antineoplastic for children with acute lymphoblastic leukemia*

*(orphan); investigational (Phase III,
orphan) for acute myelogenous leukemia* [clofarabine] 1 mg/mL

clomacran INN, BAN *antipsychotic*
[also: clomacran phosphate]

clomacran phosphate USAN *antipsychotic* [also: clomacran]

clomegestone INN *progestin* [also: clomegestone acetate]

clomegestone acetate USAN *progestin*
[also: clomegestone]

clometacin INN

clometerone INN *antiestrogen* [also:
clometherone]

clometherone USAN *antiestrogen* [also:
clometerone]

clomethiazole INN [also: chlormethia-
zole]

clomethiazole edisylate USAN *GABA
(A) receptor modulator for acute
ischemic stroke*

clometocillin INN

Clomid tablets ℞ *ovulation stimulant*
[clomiphene citrate] 50 mg

clomide [see: aklomide]

clomifene INN *gonad-stimulating principle; ovulation stimulant* [also: clomiphene citrate; clomiphene]

clomifenoxide INN

clominorex USAN, INN *anorectic*

clomiphene BAN *gonad-stimulating
principle; ovulation stimulant* [also:
clomiphene citrate; clomifene]

clomiphene citrate USAN, USP *gonad-
stimulating principle; ovulation stimulant* [also: clomifene; clomiphene] 50
mg oral

clomipramine INN, BAN *tricyclic antidepressant for obsessive-compulsive disorders* [also: clomipramine HCl]

clomipramine HCl USAN *tricyclic
antidepressant for obsessive-compulsive
disorders* [also: clomipramine] 25, 50,
75 mg oral

clomocycline INN, BAN ☑ colimecycline

clomoxir INN

clonazepam USAN, USP, INN, BAN
*anticonvulsant; anxiolytic for panic dis-
order; also used for parkinsonian dysar-*

thria, neuralgias, multifocal tics, and
manic episodes of a bipolar disorder;
investigational (orphan) for hyperexplexia (startle disease) 0.125, 0.25,
0.5, 1, 2 mg oral
clonazoline INN
CloniBID sustained release *investigational (NDA filed) antihypertensive*
[clonidine HCl]
clonidine USAN, INN, BAN *centrally
acting antiadrenergic antihypertensive;
adjunct to epidural opioid analgesics for
severe cancer pain (orphan)*
clonidine HCl USAN, USP, BAN *centrally acting antiadrenergic antihypertensive; adjunct to epidural opioid analgesics for severe cancer pain (orphan)*
0.1, 0.2, 0.3 mg oral
clonitazene INN, BAN
clonitrate USAN, INN *coronary vasodilator*
clonixeril USAN, INN *analgesic*
clonixin USAN, INN *analgesic*
clopamide USAN, INN, BAN *antihypertensive; diuretic*
clopenthixol USAN, INN, BAN *antipsychotic*
cloperastine INN
cloperidone INN *sedative* [also: cloperidone HCl]
cloperidone HCl USAN *sedative* [also:
cloperidone]
clophenoxate [see: meclofenoxate]
clopidogrel INN, BAN *platelet aggregation inhibitor for stroke, myocardial
infarction, peripheral artery disease, and
acute coronary syndrome*
clopidogrel bisulfate USAN *platelet
aggregation inhibitor for stroke, myocardial infarction, peripheral artery disease, and acute coronary syndrome*
(base=76.6%) 75 mg oral
clopidol USAN, INN, BAN *coccidiostat
for poultry*
clopimozide USAN, INN *antipsychotic*
clopipazan INN *antipsychotic* [also: clopipazan mesylate]
clopipazan mesylate USAN *antipsychotic* [also: clopipazan]

clopirac USAN, INN, BAN *anti-inflammatory*
cloponone INN, BAN
clopoxide [see: chlordiazepoxide]
clopoxide chloride [see: chlordiazepoxide HCl]
Clopra tablets (discontinued 2005) ℞
*antidopaminergic; antiemetic for che-
motherapy; peristaltic* [metoclopra-
mide HCl] 10 mg
cloprednol USAN, INN, BAN *corticosteroid; anti-inflammatory*
cloprostenol INN, BAN *prostaglandin*
[also: cloprostenol sodium]
cloprostenol sodium USAN *prostaglandin* [also: cloprostenol]
cloprothiazole INN ② glyprothiazol
cloquinate INN, BAN
cloquinozine INN
cloracetadol INN
cloral betaine INN *sedative* [also: chloral betaine]
cloramfenicol pantotenate complex
INN *antibacterial; antirickettsial* [also:
chloramphenicol pantothenate com-
plex] ② chloramphenicol palmitate
cloranolol INN
clorarsen [see: dichlorophenarsine HCl]
clorazepate dipotassium USAN, USP
*benzodiazepine anxiolytic; minor tran-
quilizer; alcohol withdrawal aid; anticonvulsant adjunct* [also: dipotassium
clorazepate] 3.75, 7.5, 15 mg oral
clorazepate monopotassium USAN
minor tranquilizer
clorazepic acid BAN
cloretate INN *sedative; hypnotic* [also:
clorethate]
Cloretazine *investigational (orphan) for
acute myelogenous leukemia*
clorethate USAN *sedative; hypnotic*
[also: cloretate]
clorexolone USAN, INN, BAN *diuretic*
Clorfed extended-release tablets (discontinued 2006) ℞ *decongestant;
antihistamine* [pseudoephedrine HCl;
chlorpheniramine maleate] 60•4 mg
clorgiline INN [also: clorgyline]
clorgyline BAN [also: clorgiline]
cloricromen INN

cloridarol INN

clorindanic acid INN

clorindanol INN *spermaticide* [also: chlorindanol]

clorindione INN, BAN

clormecaine INN

clorofene INN *disinfectant* [also: clorophene]

cloroperone INN *antipsychotic* [also: cloroperone HCl]

cloroperone HCl USAN *antipsychotic* [also: cloroperone]

clorophene USAN *disinfectant* [also: clorofene]

cloroqualone INN

clorotepine INN

Clorpactin WCS-90 powder for topical solution OTC *antimicrobial* [oxychlorosene sodium] 2 g

clorprenaline INN, BAN *adrenergic; bronchodilator* [also: clorprenaline HCl]

clorprenaline HCl USAN *adrenergic; bronchodilator* [also: clorprenaline]

Clorpres tablets ℞ *antihypertensive; central antiadrenergic; diuretic* [clonidine HCl; chlorthalidone] 0.1•15 mg; 0.2•15 mg; 0.3•15 mg

clorquinaldol [see: chlorquinaldol]

clorsulon USAN, INN *antiparasitic; fasciolicide*

clortermine INN *anorectic* [also: clortermine HCl]

clortermine HCl USAN *anorectic* [also: clortermine]

closantel USAN, INN, BAN *anthelmintic*

closilate INN *combining name for radicals or groups* [also: closylate]

closiramine INN *antihistamine* [also: closiramine aceturate]

closiramine aceturate USAN *antihistamine* [also: closiramine]

clostebol INN [also: clostebol acetate] ⑨ colestipol

clostebol acetate BAN [also: clostebol]

clostridial collagenase *investigational (Phase II, orphan) for advanced Dupuytren disease*

Clostridium botulinum **toxin** [see: botulinum toxin]

closylate USAN, BAN *combining name for radicals or groups* [also: closilate]

clotbur *medicinal herb* [see: burdock]

clothiapine USAN, BAN *antipsychotic* [also: clotiapine]

clothixamide maleate USAN *antipsychotic* [also: clotixamide]

clotiapine INN *antipsychotic* [also: clothiapine]

clotiazepam INN

cloticasone INN, BAN *anti-inflammatory* [also: cloticasone propionate]

cloticasone propionate USAN *anti-inflammatory* [also: cloticasone]

clotioxone INN

clotixamide INN *antipsychotic* [also: clothixamide maleate]

clotixamide maleate [see: clothixamide maleate]

clotrimazole (CLT) USAN, USP, INN, BAN, JAN *broad-spectrum antifungal; investigational (orphan) for sickle cell disease* 1% topical; 100 mg vaginal; 10 mg troches

clotrimazole & betamethasone dipropionate *broad-spectrum antifungal; corticosteroidal anti-inflammatory* 1%•0.05% topical

cloudberry *medicinal herb* [see: blackberry]

clove oil NF ⑨ Calafol

clover, king's; sweet clover *medicinal herb* [see: melilot]

clover, marsh *medicinal herb* [see: buckbean]

clover, purple; wild clover *medicinal herb* [see: red clover]

clover, winter *medicinal herb* [see: squaw vine]

cloves (*Caryophyllus aromaticus; Eugenia caryophyllata; Syzygium aromaticum*) seed and oil *medicinal herb for bad breath, bronchial secretions, dizziness, earache, fever, nausea, platelet aggregation inhibition, poor circulation, and thrombosis; also used topically as an analgesic and antiseptic*

clovoxamine INN

cloxacepride INN

cloxacillin INN, BAN *penicillinase-resistant penicillin antibiotic* [also: cloxacillin benzathine]

cloxacillin benzathine USP *penicillinase-resistant penicillin antibiotic* [also: cloxacillin]

cloxacillin sodium USAN, USP *penicillinase-resistant penicillin antibiotic*

cloxazolam INN

cloxestradiol INN

cloxifenol [see: triclosan]

cloximate INN

cloxiquine INN *antibacterial* [also: cloxyquin]

cloxotestosterone INN

cloxphendyl [see: cloxypendyl]

cloxypendyl INN

cloxyquin USAN *antibacterial* [also: cloxiquine]

clozapine USAN, INN, BAN *novel (atypical) dibenzapine antipsychotic for severe schizophrenia and recurrent suicidal behavior; sedative; also used for agitation and psychosis due to Alzheimer and other dementias* 12.5, 25, 50, 100, 200 mg oral

Clozaril tablets ℞ *novel (atypical) dibenzapine antipsychotic for severe schizophrenia and recurrent suicidal behavior; sedative; also used for agitation and psychosis due to Alzheimer and other dementias* [clozapine] 25, 100 mg ⊘ clazuril; glycerol

CLT (clotrimazole) [q.v.]

club, shepherd's *medicinal herb* [see: mullein]

club moss (Lycopodium clavatum) spores *medicinal herb used as a hemostatic and vulnerary*

cluster, wax *medicinal herb* [see: wintergreen]

C-Max gradual-release tablets (discontinued 2007) OTC *vitamin/mineral supplement* [vitamin C; multiple minerals] 1•± g

CMC (carboxymethylcellulose) gum [see: carboxymethylcellulose sodium]

CMC (cyclophosphamide, methotrexate, CCNU) *chemotherapy protocol*

CMC-VAP (cyclophosphamide, methotrexate, CCNU, vincristine, Adriamycin, procarbazine) *chemotherapy protocol*

CMF; CMF-IV (cyclophosphamide, methotrexate, fluorouracil) *chemotherapy protocol for breast cancer*

CMF/AV (cyclophosphamide, methotrexate, fluorouracil, Adriamycin, Oncovin) *chemotherapy protocol*

CMFAVP (cyclophosphamide, methotrexate, fluorouracil, Adriamycin, vincristine, prednisone) *chemotherapy protocol*

CMFP; CMF-P (cyclophosphamide, methotrexate, fluorouracil, prednisone) *chemotherapy protocol for breast cancer*

CMFPT (cyclophosphamide, methotrexate, fluorouracil, prednisone, tamoxifen) *chemotherapy protocol*

CMFPTH (cyclophosphamide, methotrexate, fluorouracil, prednisone, tamoxifen, Halotestin) *chemotherapy protocol*

CMFT (cyclophosphamide, methotrexate, fluorouracil, tamoxifen) *chemotherapy protocol*

CMFVaT (cyclophosphamide, methotrexate, fluorouracil, vincristine, Adriamycin, testosterone) *chemotherapy protocol*

CMFVP (cyclophosphamide, methotrexate, fluorouracil, vincristine, prednisone) *chemotherapy protocol for breast cancer* [two dosing protocols: Cooper protocol and SWOG protocol]

CMH (cyclophosphamide, m-AMSA, hydroxyurea) *chemotherapy protocol*

C-MOPP (cyclophosphamide, mechlorethamine, Oncovin, procarbazine, prednisone) *chemotherapy protocol for Hodgkin or non-Hodgkin lymphoma* ⊘ CAMB; COMB

CMV (cisplatin, methotrexate, vinblastine) *chemotherapy protocol for bladder cancer*

CMV-IGIV (cytomegalovirus immune globulin intravenous) [see: cytomegalovirus immune globulin, human]

CN2 HCl [see: mechlorethamine HCl]

CNF (cyclophosphamide, Novantrone, fluorouracil) *chemotherapy protocol for breast cancer* [also: CFM; FNC]

Cnicus benedictus *medicinal herb* [see: blessed thistle]

CNOP (cyclophosphamide, Novantrone, Oncovin, prednisone) *chemotherapy protocol for non-Hodgkin lymphoma*

CNTO 148 *investigational (Phase III) injectable anti-inflammatory for rheumatoid and psoriatic arthritis and ankylosing spondylitis*

CNTO 1275 *investigational (Phase III) injectable anti-inflammatory for psoriasis*

Co I (coenzyme I) [see: nadide]

CO$_2$ (carbon dioxide) [q.v.]

^{57}Co [see: cobaltous chloride Co 57]

^{57}Co [see: cyanocobalamin Co 57]

^{58}Co [see: cyanocobalamin (^{58}Co)]

^{60}Co [see: cobaltous chloride Co 60]

^{60}Co [see: cyanocobalamin Co 60]

coachweed *medicinal herb* [see: bedstraw]

CoaguChek PT test strips for home use OTC *in vitro diagnostic aid for the management of anticoagulation therapy*

coagulants *a class of agents that promote or accelerate clotting of the blood*

coagulation factor VIIa [see: factor VIIa, recombinant]

coagulation factor IX (human) [see: factor IX complex; nonacog alfa]

Coagulin-B *investigational (orphan) agent for moderate to severe hemophilia* [adeno-associated viral vector containing the gene for human coagulation Factor IX]

coakum *medicinal herb* [see: pokeweed]

coal tar USP *topical antieczematic; antiseborrheic* ▣ Caltro; Kaletra

co-amoxiclav (amoxicillin & potassium clavulanate) [q.v.]

COAP (cyclophosphamide, Oncovin, ara-C, prednisone) *chemotherapy protocol*

COAP-BLEO (cyclophosphamide, Oncovin, ara-C, prednisone, bleomycin) *chemotherapy protocol* ▣ COP-BLEO

COB (cisplatin, Oncovin, bleomycin) *chemotherapy protocol for head and neck cancer*

cobalamin concentrate USP *vitamin B$_{12}$; hematopoietic*

cobalt *element (Co)* ▣ caplet

cobalt-labeled vitamin B$_{12}$ [see: cyanocobalamin Co 57 & Co 60]

cobaltous chloride Co 57 USAN *radioactive agent*

cobaltous chloride Co 60 USAN *radioactive agent*

cobamamide INN

COBARTin *investigational (orphan) for steatorrhea in short bowel syndrome* [conjugated bile acids]

cocaine USP, BAN *topical anesthetic for mucous membranes; widely abused as a street drug, derived from coca leaves* 4%, 10% topical

cocaine, crack *street drug made by converting cocaine HCl into a form that can be smoked, which causes a faster, more intense effect*

cocaine HCl USP *topical anesthetic for mucous membranes; widely abused as a street drug, derived from coca leaves* 135 mg oral; 4%, 10% topical

Cocaine Viscous topical solution ℞ *mucous membrane anesthetic* [cocaine] 4%, 10%

cocarboxylase INN [also: co-carboxylase]

co-carboxylase BAN [also: cocarboxylase]

cocashweed *medicinal herb* [see: life root]

coccidioidin USP *dermal coccidioidomycosis test*

cocculin [see: picrotoxin]

Cocculus lacunosus; C. suberosus *medicinal herb* [see: levant berry]

Cocculus palmatus *medicinal herb* [see: colombo]

Cochlearia armoracia *medicinal herb* [see: horseradish]

cocklebur *medicinal herb* [see: agrimony; burdock]

cockspur pepper *medicinal herb* [see: cayenne]

cockspur rye *medicinal herb* [see: ergot]

cocoa NF

cocoa (Theobromo cacao) *bean medicinal herb used as a cardiac stimulant, diuretic, and vasodilator*

cocoa butter NF *suppository base; emollient/protectant* ☒ cacao butter

cocowort *medicinal herb* [see: shepherd's purse]

cod liver oil USP, BAN *vitamins A and D source; emollient/protectant*

cod liver oil, nondestearinated NF

codactide INN, BAN

Codal-DH *syrup* ℞ *narcotic antitussive; antihistamine; sleep aid; decongestant* [hydrocodone bitartrate; pyrilamine maleate; phenylephrine HCl] 1.66•8.33•5 mg/5 mL

Codal-DM *syrup* OTC *antitussive; antihistamine; sleep aid; decongestant* [dextromethorphan hydrobromide; pyrilamine maleate; phenylephrine HCl] 10•8.33•5 mg/5 mL

CODE (cisplatin, Oncovin, doxorubicin, etoposide) *chemotherapy protocol for small cell lung cancer (SCLC)*

codehydrogenase I [see: nadide]

codeine USP, BAN *narcotic analgesic used as an antitussive; sometimes abused as a street drug* ☒ Kadian; Quad Tann

codeine & acetaminophen *narcotic analgesic* 15•300, 30•300, 60•300 mg oral; 12•30 mg/5 mL oral

codeine phosphate USP, BAN *narcotic analgesic used as an antitussive* 15 mg/5 mL oral; 15, 30 mg/mL injection

codeine phosphate & aspirin *narcotic antitussive; analgesic; antipyretic* 325•15 mg oral

codeine phosphate & aspirin & carisoprodol *narcotic analgesic; skeletal muscle relaxant* 16•325•200 mg oral

codeine phosphate & butalbital & acetaminophen & caffeine *narcotic antitussive; barbiturate sedative; analgesic* 30•50•325•40 mg oral

codeine phosphate & guaifenesin *antitussive; narcotic analgesic; expectorant* 10•300 mg oral

codeine phosphate & promethazine HCl *narcotic antitussive; antihistamine* 10•6.25 mg/5 mL oral

codeine phosphate & promethazine HCl & phenylephrine HCl *narcotic antitussive; antihistamine; decongestant* 10•6.25•5 mg/5 mL oral

codeine polistirex USAN *narcotic analgesic used as an antitussive*

codeine sulfate USP *narcotic analgesic used as an antitussive* 15, 30, 60 mg oral

codelcortone [see: prednisolone]

Codeprex *extended-release oral suspension (discontinued 2007)* ℞ *narcotic antitussive; antihistamine* [codeine polistirex; chlorpheniramine polistirex] 40•8 mg/10 mL

co-dergocrine mesylate BAN *cognition adjuvant* [also: ergoloid mesylates]

Codiclear DH *syrup* ℞ *narcotic antitussive; expectorant* [hydrocodone bitartrate; guaifenesin] 3.5•300 mg/5 mL

Codimal DH *syrup* ℞ *narcotic antitussive; antihistamine; decongestant* [hydrocodone bitartrate; dexchlorpheniramine maleate; phenylephrine HCl] 2•1•5 mg/5 mL

Codimal DM *syrup* OTC *antitussive; antihistamine; sleep aid; decongestant* [dextromethorphan hydrobromide; pyrilamine maleate; phenylephrine HCl] 10•8.33•5 mg/5 mL

Codimal PH *syrup* ℞ *narcotic antitussive; antihistamine; sleep aid; decongestant* [codeine phosphate; pyrilamine maleate; phenylephrine HCl] 20•16.7•10 mg/10 mL

codorphone [now: conorphone HCl]

codoxime USAN, INN *antitussive*

Coease *intraocular injection* ℞ *viscoelastic agent for ophthalmic surgery* [hyaluronate sodium] 12 mg/mL

coenzyme Q10 *natural enzyme cofactor used as a cardiac protectant, free radical scavenger, and membrane stabilizer; investigational (orphan) for Huntington disease, pediatric CHF, and mitochondrial cytopathies* [also: ubiquinol; ubiquinone]

CoFactor *investigational (Phase III) chemotherapy rescue agent for fluorouracil toxicity*

COF/COM (cyclophosphamide, Oncovin, fluorouracil + cyclophosphamide, Oncovin, methotrexate) *chemotherapy protocol*

coffeine [see: caffeine]

cofisatin INN

cofisatine [see: cofisatin]

cogazocine INN

Cogentin tablets, IV or IM injection ℞ *anticholinergic; antiparkinsonian* [benztropine mesylate] 0.5, 1, 2 mg; 1 mg/mL

Co-Gesic tablets ℞ *narcotic analgesic; antipyretic* [hydrocodone bitartrate; acetaminophen] 5•500 mg

Cognex capsules ℞ *reversible cholinesterase inhibitor; cognition adjuvant for Alzheimer dementia* [tacrine HCl] 10, 20, 30, 40 mg ⊇ Kionex

Cognitex; Cognitex with Pregnenolone softgels OTC *anti-aging supplement for improving mental function* [glyceryl phosphorylcholine; choline dihydrogen citrate; choline bitartrate; phosphatidylserine; vinpocetine; pantothenic acid; RNA/DNA; (pregnenolone)] 100•250•200•16.7•2.5•83.3•70.8(•8.3) mg

cohosh *medicinal herb* [see: black cohosh; blue cohosh; white cohosh]

Cola acuminata *medicinal herb* [see: kola nut]

Colace capsules, syrup, oral liquid OTC *laxative; stool softener* [docusate sodium] 50, 100 mg; 60 mg/15 mL; 150 mg/15 mL ⊇ Cal-Cee; K-Lease

Colace; Colace Infant/Child suppositories OTC *hyperosmolar laxative* [glycerin] ⊇ Cal-Cee; K-Lease

colaspase BAN *antineoplastic for acute lymphocytic leukemia (ALL)* [also: asparaginase]

Colazal capsules ℞ *gastrointestinal anti-inflammatory for ulcerative colitis* [balsalazide disodium] 750 mg ⊇ Gelseal

Colazide ⓔ (European name for U.S. product **Colazal**) ⊇ khelloside

colchamine [see: demecolcine]

colchicine USP, JAN *gout suppressant; investigational (orphan) to stop the progression of multiple sclerosis* 0.6 mg oral; 1 mg injection

Colchicum autumnale; C. speciosum; C. vernum *medicinal herb* [see: autumn crocus]

Cold & Cough Tussin softgels (discontinued 2007) OTC *antitussive; decongestant; expectorant* [dextromethorphan hydrobromide; pseudoephedrine HCl; guaifenesin] 10•30•200 mg

cold cream USP

Cold Symptoms Relief tablets (discontinued 2007) OTC *antitussive; antihistamine; decongestant; analgesic; antipyretic* [dextromethorphan hydrobromide; chlorpheniramine maleate; pseudoephedrine HCl; acetaminophen] 10•2•30•325 mg

Coldcough PD syrup (discontinued 2005) ℞ *narcotic antitussive; decongestant; antihistamine* [dihydrocodeine bitartrate; phenylephrine HCl; chlorpheniramine maleate] 3•7.5•2 mg/5 mL

Coldec D extended-release caplets (discontinued 2007) ℞ *decongestant; antihistamine* [pseudoephedrine HCl; carbinoxamine maleate] 80•8 mg

Coldec DM oral liquid (discontinued 2007) ℞ *antitussive; antihistamine; decongestant* [dextromethorphan hydrobromide; brompheniramine maleate; pseudoephedrine HCl] 15•4•60 mg/5 mL

Coldmist JR sustained-release tablets ℞ *decongestant; expectorant* [pseudoephedrine HCl; guaifenesin] 48•595 mg

Coldmist LA extended-release caplets ℞ *decongestant; expectorant* [pseudoephedrine HCl; guaifenesin] 85•795 mg

Coldonyl tablets OTC *decongestant; expectorant; analgesic; antipyretic* [phenylephrine HCl; guaifenesin; acetaminophen] 5•100•325 mg

colecalciferol (vitamin D₃) INN *fat-soluble vitamin* [also: cholecalciferol]

colesevelam HCl USAN *bile acid sequestrant; nonabsorbable cholesterol-lowering polymer for hyperlipidemia and to improve glycemic control in type 2 diabetes*

Colestid tablets, granules for oral suspension ℞ *cholesterol-lowering antihyperlipidemic* [colestipol HCl] 1 g; 5 g/dose

colestipol INN, BAN *bile acid sequestrant; cholesterol-lowering antihyperlipidemic* [also: colestipol HCl] ⊡ clostebol

colestipol HCl USAN, USP *bile acid sequestrant; cholesterol-lowering antihyperlipidemic* [also: colestipol] 1, 5 g oral

colestolone USAN, INN *hypolipidemic*

colestyramine INN *bile salt ion-exchange resin; antihyperlipoproteinemic* [also: cholestyramine resin; cholestyramine]

colestyramine resin [see: cholestyramine]

colextran INN

Colfed-A sustained-release capsules ℞ *decongestant; antihistamine* [pseudoephedrine HCl; chlorpheniramine maleate] 120•8 mg

colfenamate INN

colforsin USAN, INN *antiglaucoma agent*

colfosceril palmitate USAN, INN, BAN *pulmonary surfactant for hyaline membrane disease and neonatal respiratory distress syndrome (orphan); investigational (orphan) for adult respiratory distress syndrome (ARDS)*

colic root *medicinal herb* [see: blazing star; star grass; wild yam]

Colic Tablets OTC *natural product to relieve colic, stomach cramps, hiccups, and gas in infants* [wild yam; chamomile; bitter apple]

Colic-Ease Gripe Water oral liquid OTC *natural product to relieve colic, stomach cramps, hiccups, and gas in infants* [dill weed seed oil; caraway seed oil; cinnamon bark oil; clove bud oil; cardamom seed oil]

colimecycline INN ⊡ clomocycline

colistimethate sodium USAN, USP, INN *bactericidal antibiotic* [also: colistin sulphomethate] 150 mg/vial injection

colistin INN, BAN *bactericidal antibiotic* [also: colistin sulfate] ⊡ glycitein

colistin methanesulfonate [see: colistimethate sodium]

colistin sulfate USP *bactericidal antibiotic* [also: colistin]

colistin sulphomethate BAN *bactericidal antibiotic* [also: colistimethate sodium]

collagen *ophthalmic implant to block the puncta and retain moisture; urethral injection for stress urinary incontinence; dermal filler for moderate to deep facial wrinkles and folds* ⊡ Cala-gen; Glaucon; Glyquin; Qualaquin

collagen, purified bovine *injectable dermal filler for scars, wrinkles, and facial folds*

collagen, purified human *injectable dermal filler for scars, wrinkles, and facial folds*

collagen, purified type II *investigational (Phase III, orphan) oral treatment for juvenile rheumatoid arthritis*

collagen sponge, absorbable *topical hemostat for surgery*

collagenase *topical proteolytic enzymes for necrotic tissue debridement; investigational (orphan) for Peyronie disease*

collagenase, clostridial [see: clostridial collagenase]

Collagenase Santyl ointment ℞ *proteolytic enzymes for debriding dermal ulcers and severely burned areas* [collagenase] 250 U/g

collard *medicinal herb* [see: skunk cabbage]

Collinsonia canadensis medicinal herb
[see: stone root]

collodion USP *topical protectant*

colloidal aluminum hydroxide [see:
aluminum hydroxide gel]

colloidal oatmeal *demulcent*

colloidal silicon dioxide [see: silicon
dioxide, colloidal]

Colloral *investigational (Phase III,
orphan) treatment of juvenile rheumatoid arthritis* [purified type II collagen]

Collyrium for Fresh Eyes *ophthalmic solution* OTC *extraocular irrigating
solution* [sterile isotonic solution]

Collyrium Fresh *eye drops* (discontinued 2006) OTC *decongestant; vasoconstrictor* [tetrahydrozoline HCl] 0.05%

ColoCare *test kit for home use* OTC *in
vitro diagnostic aid for fecal occult blood*

Colocort *rectal suspension* ℞ *corticosteroidal anti-inflammatory* [hydrocor-
tisone] 100 mg/60 mL

colombo *(Cocculus palmatus)* root
*medicinal herb used as an antiemetic
and febrifuge*

Colomed *enema investigational (orphan)
for left-sided ulcerative colitis and
chronic radiation proctitis* [short chain
fatty acids]

colony-stimulating factors *a class of
glycoproteins that stimulate the production of granulocytes and macrophages*

**Color Allergy Screening Test
(CAST)** *reagent assay tubes in vitro
diagnostic aid for immunoglobulin E in
serum*

Color Ovulation Test *kit for home
use* (discontinued 2004) OTC *in vitro
diagnostic aid to predict ovulation time*

ColoScreen *slide test for professional
use* ℞ *in vitro diagnostic aid for fecal
occult blood*

colterol INN *bronchodilator* [also: colterol mesylate] ◎ glutaral

colterol mesylate USAN *bronchodilator*
[also: colterol]

colt's tail *medicinal herb* [see: fleabane;
horseweed]

coltsfoot *(Tussilago farfara)* buds,
flowers, and leaves *medicinal herb for*

*asthma, bronchitis, dry cough, hay
fever, lung disorders, excess mucus,
and throat irritation*

Columbia Antiseptic *powder* OTC
emollient; astringent; antiseptic [zinc
oxide; talc; carbolic acid; boric acid]

columbine *(Aquilegia vulgaris)* plant
*medicinal herb used as an astringent,
diaphoretic, and diuretic*

Coly-Mycin M *powder for IV or IM
injection* ℞ *bactericidal antibiotic*
[colistimethate sodium] 150 mg

Coly-Mycin S Otic *suspension* ℞ *corticosteroidal anti-inflammatory; antibiotic* [hydrocortisone acetate; neomycin sulfate; colistin sulfate] 1%•4.71
mg•3 mg per mL

CoLyte *powder for oral solution* ℞
pre-procedure bowel evacuant [poly-
ethylene glycol–electrolyte solution
(PEG 3350)] 60 g/L ◎ Klout; K-Lyte

**COM (cyclophosphamide, Oncovin,
MeCCNU)** *chemotherapy protocol*

**COM (cyclophosphamide, Onco-
vin, methotrexate)** *chemotherapy
protocol*

**COMA-A (cyclophosphamide,
Oncovin, methotrexate/citrovo-
rum factor, Adriamycin, ara-C)**
chemotherapy protocol

**COMB (cyclophosphamide, Onco-
vin, MeCCNU, bleomycin)** *chemotherapy protocol* ◎ CAMB; C-MOPP

**COMB (Cytoxin, Oncovin, metho-
trexate, bleomycin)** *chemotherapy
protocol* ◎ CAMB; C-MOPP

ComBgen *tablets* ℞ *vitamin B supplement* [vitamins B_6 and B_{12}; folic acid]
25•0.5•2.2 mg

Combiflex *capsules* ℞ *antihistamine;
sleep aid; analgesic; antipyretic* [phen-
yltoloxamine citrate; acetaminophen; salicylamide; caffeine] 20•
325•250•50 mg

Combiflex ES *caplets* ℞ *antihistamine;
sleep aid; analgesic; antipyretic* [phenyl-
toloxamine citrate; acetaminophen;
magnesium salicylate; caffeine] 20•
500•500•50 mg

Combigan eye drops ℞ *combination* α_2 *agonist and β-blocker for glaucoma and ocular hypertension* [brimonidine tartrate; timolol maleate] 0.2%•0.5%

CombiPatch transdermal patch ℞ *hormone replacement therapy for postmenopausal symptoms, hypogonadism, castration, and primary ovarian failure* [estradiol; norethindrone acetate] 5•14, 5•25 mcg/day

Combipres 0.1; Combipres 0.2; Combipres 0.3 tablets (discontinued 2007) ℞ *antihypertensive; diuretic* [clonidine HCl; chlorthalidone] 0.1•15 mg; 0.2•15 mg; 0.3•15 mg

Combistix reagent strips *in vitro diagnostic aid for multiple urine products*

Combivent oral inhalation aerosol ℞ *anticholinergic bronchodilator for chronic bronchospasm with COPD* [ipratropium bromide; albuterol sulfate] 18•103 mcg/dose

Combivir film-coated caplets ℞ *nucleoside reverse transcriptase inhibitor combination for HIV* [lamivudine; zidovudine] 150•300 mg

combretastatin A4 phosphate *investigational (orphan) agent for anaplastic, medullary, papillary, or follicular thyroid cancer*

Combunox film-coated caplets ℞ *narcotic analgesic; antipyretic* [oxycodone HCl; ibuprofen] 5•400 mg

COMe (Cytoxin, Oncovin, methotrexate) *chemotherapy protocol*

COMF (cyclophosphamide, Oncovin, methotrexate, fluorouracil) *chemotherapy protocol* ② CAMF; CMF; CMV

Comfort eye drops (discontinued 2006) OTC *decongestant; vasoconstrictor* [naphazoline HCl] 0.03%

Comfort Tears eye drops OTC *moisturizer/lubricant* [hydroxyethylcellulose]

ComfortCare GP Wetting & Soaking solution OTC *disinfecting/wetting/soaking solution for rigid gas permeable contact lenses*

Comfortine ointment (discontinued 2004) OTC *moisturizer; emollient;* *astringent; antiseptic* [vitamins A and D; lanolin; zinc oxide]

comfrey (Symphytum officinale; S. tuberosum) leaves and roots *medicinal herb for anemia, arthritis, blood cleansing, boils and sores, bruises, burns, edema, emphysema, fractures, gastric ulcers, hemorrhoids, and sprains; not generally regarded as safe and effective as it may be carcinogenic and hepatotoxic* ② camphor

comfrey, spotted *medicinal herb* [see: lungwort]

COMLA (cyclophosphamide, Oncovin, methotrexate, leucovorin [rescue], ara-C) *chemotherapy protocol for non-Hodgkin lymphoma* ② Cameo Oil

Commiphora abssynica; C. molmol; C. myrrha *medicinal herb* [see: myrrh]

Commiphora mukul *medicinal herb* [see: guggul]

Commit lozenges OTC *smoking cessation aid for the relief of nicotine withdrawal symptoms* [nicotine polacrilex] 2, 4 mg

common bugloss *medicinal herb* [see: borage]

common elder *medicinal herb* [see: elderberry]

common flax *medicinal herb* [see: flaxseed]

comosain *investigational (orphan) proteolytic enzymes for debridement of severe burns*

COMP (CCNU, Oncovin, methotrexate, procarbazine) *chemotherapy protocol* ② CAMB; C-MOPP

COMP (cyclophosphamide, Oncovin, methotrexate, prednisone) *chemotherapy protocol for pediatric Hodgkin lymphoma* ② CAMB; C-MOPP

Compack (trademarked packaging form) *patient compliance package for oral contraceptives*

Compazine suppositories ℞ *conventional (typical) phenothiazine antipsychotic for schizophrenia; anxiolytic; antiemetic for nausea and vomiting; also used for acute treatment of migraine*

headaches [prochlorperazine] 2.5, 5, 25 mg

Compazine syrup, IV or IM injection ℞ *conventional (typical) phenothiazine antipsychotic for schizophrenia; anxiolytic; antiemetic for nausea and vomiting; also used for acute treatment of migraine headaches* [prochlorperazine edisylate] 5 mg/5 mL; 5 mg/mL

Compazine tablets, Spansules (sustained-release capsules) ℞ *conventional (typical) phenothiazine antipsychotic for schizophrenia; anxiolytic; antiemetic for nausea and vomiting; also used for acute treatment of migraine headaches* [prochlorperazine maleate] 5, 10, 25 mg; 30 mg

Compete tablets OTC *vitamin/iron supplement* [multiple vitamins; ferrous gluconate; folic acid] ≛•27•0.4 mg

Compleat Modified Formula closed system containers OTC *enteral nutritional therapy* [lactose-free formula]

Compleat Modified Formula ready-to-use oral liquid OTC *enteral nutritional therapy* [lactose-free formula]

Compleat Regular Formula ready-to-use oral liquid OTC *enteral nutritional therapy* [milk-based formula]

complement receptor type I, myristoylated recombinant *investigational (orphan) to prevent delayed graft function following solid organ transplant*

complement receptor type I, soluble recombinant human *investigational (orphan) for adult respiratory distress syndrome and to prevent postcardiopulmonary bypass syndrome in children undergoing cardiopulmonary bypass*

Complete solution OTC *rewetting solution for soft contact lenses*

Complete All-in-One solution OTC *cleaning/disinfecting/rinsing/storage solution for soft contact lenses* [polyhexamethylene biguanide] 0.0001%

Complete Weekly Enzymatic Cleaner effervescent tablets OTC *enzymatic cleaner for soft contact lenses* [subtilisin A]

Complex 15 Face cream OTC *moisturizer; emollient*

Complex 15 Hand & Body cream, lotion OTC *moisturizer; emollient*

Comply oral liquid OTC *enteral nutritional therapy* [lactose-free formula]

component pertussis vaccine (alternate name for acellular pertussis vaccine) [see: diphtheria & tetanus toxoids & acellular pertussis (DTaP) vaccine, adsorbed]

Compound 347 liquid for vaporization ℞ *inhalation general anesthetic* [enflurane]

compound 42 [see: warfarin]

compound CB3025 [see: melphalan]

compound E [see: cortisone acetate]

compound F [see: hydrocortisone]

compound orange spirit [see: orange spirit, compound]

compound S [see: zidovudine]

compound solution of sodium chloride INN *fluid and electrolyte replenisher* [also: Ringer injection]

compound solution of sodium lactate INN *electrolyte and fluid replenisher; systemic alkalizer* [also: Ringer injection, lactated]

Compound W topical liquid, gel OTC *keratolytic* [salicylic acid in collodion] 17%

Compound W Freeze Off aerosol spray OTC *cryoablation of common and plantar warts* [dimethyl ether; propane; isobutane]

Compound W One Step Wart Remover for Kids pad OTC *keratolytic* [salicylic acid] 40%

Compoz gelcaps OTC *antihistamine; sleep aid* [diphenhydramine HCl] 25 mg

Compoz Nighttime Sleep Aid tablets OTC *antihistamine; sleep aid* [diphenhydramine HCl] 50 mg

compressible sugar [see: sugar, compressible]

Compro suppositories ℞ *conventional (typical) phenothiazine antipsychotic for schizophrenia; anxiolytic; antiemetic for nausea and vomiting; also used for* *acute treatment of migraine headaches* [prochlorperazine] 25 mg

Computer Eye Drops (discontinued 2008) OTC *ophthalmic moisturizer and emollient* [glycerin] 1%

COMT (catechol-O-methyltransferase) inhibitors *a class of antiparkinson agents that stabilize serum levodopa levels by inhibiting an enzyme that breaks down the levodopa before it reaches the brain*

Comtan film-coated tablets ℞ COMT *(catechol-O-methyltransferase) inhibitor for Parkinson disease* [entacapone] 200 mg

Comtrex Acute Head Cold caplets (discontinued 2007) OTC *decongestant; antihistamine; analgesic; antipyretic* [pseudoephedrine HCl; brompheniramine maleate; acetaminophen] 30•2•500 mg

Comtrex Allergy-Sinus Treatment caplets, tablets (discontinued 2006) OTC *decongestant; antihistamine; analgesic; antipyretic* [pseudoephedrine HCl; chlorpheniramine maleate; acetaminophen] 30•2•500 mg

Comtrex Cold & Cough Relief, Multi-Symptom caplets (discontinued 2007) OTC *antitussive; antihistamine; decongestant; analgesic; antipyretic* [dextromethorphan hydrobromide; chlorpheniramine maleate; pseudoephedrine HCl; acetaminophen] 15•2•30•500 mg

Comtrex Day and Night Flu Therapy; Comtrex Day and Night Severe Cold and Sinus caplets OTC *decongestant; analgesic; antipyretic; antihistamine added* PM [phenylephrine HCl; acetaminophen; chlorpheniramine maleate (PM)] 5•325 mg AM; 5•325•2 mg PM

Comtrex Day & Night Cold & Cough caplets OTC *antitussive; decongestant; analgesic; antipyretic; antihistamine added* PM [dextromethorphan hydrobromide; phenylephrine HCl; acetaminophen; chlor-

pheniramine maleate (PM)] 10•5• 325 mg AM; 10•5•325•2 mg PM

Comtrex Multi-Symptom Deep Chest Cold caplets OTC *expectorant; analgesic; antipyretic* [guaifenesin; acetaminophen] 200•325 mg

Comtrex Multi-Symptom Deep Chest Cold softgels (discontinued 2007) OTC *antitussive; decongestant; expectorant; analgesic; antipyretic* [dextromethorphan hydrobromide; pseudoephedrine HCl; guaifenesin; acetaminophen] 10•30•100•250 mg

Comtrex Multi-Symptom Non-Drowsy Cold & Cough Relief caplets (discontinued 2007) OTC *antitussive; decongestant; analgesic; antipyretic* [dextromethorphan hydrobromide; pseudoephedrine HCl; acetaminophen] 15•30•500 mg

Comtrex Nighttime Acute Head Cold oral liquid (discontinued 2007) OTC *decongestant; antihistamine; analgesic; antipyretic* [pseudoephedrine HCl; brompheniramine maleate; acetaminophen] 60•4• 1000 mg/30 mL

Comtrex Nighttime Cold & Cough caplets OTC *antitussive; antihistamine; decongestant; analgesic; antipyretic* [dextromethorphan hydrobromide; chlorpheniramine maleate; phenylphrine HCl; acetaminophen] 10•2•5•325 mg

Comtrex Nighttime Cold & Cough oral liquid (discontinued 2007) OTC *antitussive; antihistamine; decongestant; analgesic; antipyretic* [dextromethorphan hydrobromide; chlorpheniramine maleate; pseudoephedrine HCl; acetaminophen] 30•4•60• 1000 mg/30 mL

Comtrex Nighttime Flu Therapy oral liquid (discontinued 2007) OTC *decongestant; antihistamine; analgesic; antipyretic* [pseudoephedrine HCl; chlorpheniramine maleate; acetaminophen] 60•4•1000 mg/30 mL

**Comtrex Non-Drowsy Cold &
Cough** caplets OTC *antitussive;
decongestant; analgesic; antipyretic*
[dextromethorphan hydrobromide;
phenylephrine HCl; acetamino-
phen] 10•5•325 mg

**Comtrex Sinus & Nasal Deconges-
tant** caplets (discontinued 2007)
OTC *decongestant; antihistamine; analgesic; antipyretic* [pseudoephedrine
HCl; chlorpheniramine maleate;
acetaminophen] 30•2•500 mg

Comtrex Sore Throat oral liquid
(discontinued 2008) OTC *analgesic;
antipyretic* [acetaminophen] 166.6
mg/5 mL

Comtussin HC syrup (discontinued
2007) ℞ *narcotic antitussive; antihistamine; decongestant* [hydrocodone
bitartrate; chlorpheniramine maleate; phenylephrine HCl] 5•4•10
mg/10 mL

Comvax IM injection ℞ *vaccine for* H.
*influenzae and hepatitis B infections in
children 1½–15 months* [Haemophilus
b purified capsular polysaccharide;
Neisseria meningitidis OMPC; hepatitis B virus vaccine] 7.5•125•5 mcg/
0.5 mL

Conal oral suspension ℞ *decongestant;
antihistamine; sleep aid* [phenyleph-
rine tannate; chlorpheniramine tannate; pyrilamine tannate] 15•8•
12.5 mg/5 mL

Conceive Ovulation Predictor 5-day
test kit for professional use (discontinued 2004) ℞ *in vitro diagnostic aid
to predict ovulation time*

Conceive Pregnancy test kit for
home use OTC *in vitro diagnostic aid;
urine pregnancy test*

Concentrated Cleaner solution OTC
*cleaning solution for rigid gas permeable
contact lenses*

**Conceptrol Disposable Contracep-
tive** vaginal gel OTC *spermicidal contraceptive* [nonoxynol 9] 4%

Concerta OROS dual-release tablets
(22% immediate release, 78%
extended release) ℞ *CNS stimulant;*
*once-daily treatment for attention-defi-
cit/hyperactivity disorder (ADHD)*
[methylphenidate HCl] 18, 27, 36,
54, 72 mg

Condylox solution, gel ℞ *antimitotic
for external genital and perianal warts*
[podofilox] 0.5%

cone flower, purple *medicinal herb*
[see: echinacea]

conessine INN

conessine hydrobromide [see: cones-
sine]

confectioner's sugar [see: sugar, confectioner's]

Confide test kit for home use OTC *in
vitro diagnostic aid for HIV in the blood*

congazone sodium [see: Congo red]

Congestac caplets OTC *decongestant;
expectorant* [pseudoephedrine HCl;
guaifenesin] 60•400 mg

Congestaid tablets OTC *nasal decongestant* [pseudoephedrine HCl] 30 mg

Congo red USP

conivaptan HCl *arginine vasopressin
antagonist; diuretic for euvolemic and
hypervolemic hyponatremia in hospitalized patients; treatment for syndrome
of inappropriate antidiuretic hormone
(SIADH)*

conjugated bile acids [see: bile acids,
conjugated]

conjugated equine estrogen (CEE)
[see: estrogens, conjugated]

conjugated estrogens [see: estrogens,
conjugated]

conjugated linoleic acid (CLA) *natural omega-6 essential fatty acid shown
to be effective in weight management
and cancer prevention*

conorfone INN *analgesic* [also: conorphone HCl]

conorfone HCl [see: conorphone HCl]

conorphone HCl USAN *analgesic* [also:
conorfone]

**CONPADRI; CONPADRI-I (cyclo-
phosphamide, Oncovin, L-phenylalanine mustard, Adriamycin)**
chemotherapy protocol

Conray; Conray 30; Conray 43
injection ℞ *radiopaque contrast*

medium [iothalamate meglumine (47% iodine)] 600 mg/mL (282 mg/mL); 300 mg/mL (141 mg/mL); 430 mg/mL (202 mg/mL)

Constilac oral/rectal solution ℞ *hyperosmotic laxative* [lactulose] 10 g/15 mL

Constulose oral/rectal solution ℞ *hyperosmotic laxative* [lactulose] 10 g/ 15 mL

consumptive's weed *medicinal herb* [see: yerba santa]

Contac Cold + Flu caplets OTC *decongestant; antihistamine; analgesic; antipyretic* [phenylephrine HCl; chlorpheniramine maleate; acetaminophen] 5•7•500 mg

Contac Cold + Flu Day & Night caplets OTC *decongestant; analgesic; antipyretic; antihistamine added* PM [phenylephrine HCl; acetaminophen; chlorpheniramine maleate (PM)] 5•500 mg AM; 5•500•2 mg PM

Contac Day & Night Allergy/Sinus Relief caplets (discontinued 2007) OTC *decongestant; analgesic; antipyretic; antihistamine/sleep aid added* PM [pseudoephedrine HCl; acetaminophen; diphenhydramine HCl (PM)] 60•650 mg AM; 60•650•50 mg PM

Contac Day & Night Cold & Flu caplets (discontinued 2007) OTC *decongestant; analgesic; antipyretic; antitussive added* AM; *antihistamine/ sleep aid added* PM [pseudoephedrine HCl; acetaminophen; dextromethorphan hydrobromide (AM); diphenhydramine HCl (PM)] 60•650•30 mg AM; 60•650•50 mg PM

Contac Severe Cold & Flu caplets (discontinued 2007) OTC *antitussive; antihistamine; decongestant; analgesic; antipyretic* [dextromethorphan hydrobromide; chlorpheniramine maleate; pseudoephedrine HCl; acetaminophen] 15•2•30•500 mg

conteben [see: thioacetazone; thiacetazone]

continuous erythropoietin receptor activator (CERA) *investigational*

(Phase III) hematopoietic for anemia in patients with chronic kidney disease

ContolRx toothpaste ℞ *dental caries preventative* [sodium fluoride] 1.1%

Contrin capsules ℞ *hematinic* [ferrous fumarate; cyanocobalamin; ascorbic acid; intrinsic factor concentrate; folic acid] 110 mg•15 mcg•75 mg•240 mg•0.5 mg

ControlPak (trademarked packaging form) *tamper-resistant unit-dose package*

conval lily *medicinal herb* [see: lily of the valley]

Convallaria majalis *medicinal herb* [see: lily of the valley]

conventional (typical) antipsychotics *a class of dopamine receptor antagonists with a higher affinity to the D_2 than D_1 receptors and little affinity to the nondopaminergic receptors; high incidence of extrapyramidal side effects (EPS)* [compare to: novel (atypical) antipsychotics]

Convolvulus sepium *medicinal herb* [see: hedge bindweed]

convulsion root; convulsion weed *medicinal herb* [see: fit root]

Conyza canadensis *medicinal herb* [see: horseweed]

cool.click (trademarked delivery device) *needle-free subcutaneous injector*

Cooper regimen *chemotherapy protocol for breast cancer* [see: CMFVP]

COP [see: creatinolfosfate]

COP (cyclophosphamide, Oncovin, prednisone) *chemotherapy protocol for non-Hodgkin lymphoma*

COP 1 (copolymer 1) [see: glatiramer acetate]

COPA (Cytoxin, Oncovin, prednisone, Adriamycin) *chemotherapy protocol*

COPA-BLEO (cyclophosphamide, Oncovin, prednisone, Adriamycin, bleomycin) *chemotherapy protocol*

COPAC (CCNU, Oncovin, prednisone, Adriamycin, cyclophosphamide) *chemotherapy protocol* 🖭 CPB WC; CPC; Gy-Pak; K-Pek

Copaxone subcu injection in **Auto-ject2** (prefilled glass syringe) ℞ *immunomodulator for relapsing-remitting multiple sclerosis (orphan)* [glatiramer acetate] 20 mg

COPB (cyclophosphamide, Oncovin, prednisone, bleomycin) *chemotherapy protocol*

COP-BLAM (cyclophosphamide, Oncovin, prednisone, bleomycin, Adriamycin, Matulane) *chemotherapy protocol*

COP-BLEO (cyclophosphamide, Oncovin, prednisone, bleomycin) *chemotherapy protocol* ⊉ COAP-BLEO

Cope tablets OTC *analgesic; antipyretic; anti-inflammatory; antacid* [aspirin; caffeine; magnesium hydroxide; aluminum hydroxide] 421•32•50•25 mg

COPE (cyclophosphamide, Oncovin, Platinol, etoposide) *chemotherapy protocol for small cell lung cancer (SCLC) and pediatric brain tumors*

Copegus film-coated tablets ℞ *nucleoside antiviral for chronic hepatitis C infections (orphan) and clinically stable HIV disease; also used for viral hemorrhagic fevers* [ribavirin] 200 mg ⊉ Capex

copolymer 1 (COP 1) [see: glatiramer acetate]

copovithane BAN

COPP (CCNU, Oncovin, procarbazine, prednisone) *chemotherapy protocol*

COPP (cyclophosphamide, Oncovin, procarbazine, prednisone) *chemotherapy protocol for Hodgkin or non-Hodgkin lymphoma*

copper *element (Cu)* ⊉ CAPPr; Keppra

copper chloride dihydrate [see: cupric chloride]

copper gluconate (copper D-gluconate) USP *dietary copper supplement*

copper sulfate pentahydrate [see: cupric sulfate]

copper 10-undecenoate [see: copper undecylenate]

copper undecylenate USAN

copperhead snake antivenin [see: antivenin (Crotalidae) polyvalent]

Coptis trifolia *medicinal herb* [see: gold thread]

CoQ10 [see: coenzyme Q10]

coral (Goniopora spp.; Porite spp.) *natural material used as a substrate for bone grafts and fractures and in reconstructive surgery* ⊉ caraway oil; Kerol

coral root (Corallorhiza odontorhiza) *medicinal herb for diaphoresis, fever, insomnia, and sedation*

coral snake antivenin [see: antivenin (Micrurus fulvius)]

corbadrine INN *adrenergic; vasoconstrictor* [also: levonordefrin]

Cordaptive extended-release tablets (available in the European Union as **Tredaptive**) *investigational (Phase III) antihyperlipidemic for hypertriglyceridemia plus prostaglandin inhibitor to prevent flushing* [niacin; laropiprant] 1000•20 mg

Cordarone tablets, IV infusion ℞ *antiarrhythmic for acute ventricular tachycardia and fibrillation (orphan)* [amiodarone HCl] 200 mg; 50 mg/mL

Cordox *investigational (Phase III, orphan) cytoprotective agent for vaso-occlusive episodes of sickle cell disease* [fructose-1,6-diphosphate]

Cordran ointment, lotion, tape ℞ *corticosteroidal anti-inflammatory* [flurandrenolide] 0.05%; 0.05%; 4 mcg/cm^2

Cordran SP cream ℞ *corticosteroidal anti-inflammatory* [flurandrenolide] 0.05%

Cordron-D; Cordron-D NR oral liquid ℞ *decongestant; antihistamine* [pseudoephedrine HCl; carbinoxamine maleate] 17.5•2 mg/5 mL; 12.5•2 mg/5 mL

Cordron-DM NR oral liquid ℞ *antitussive; antihistamine; decongestant* [dextromethorphan hydrobromide; carbinoxamine maleate; pseudoephedrine HCl] 15•3•12.5 mg/5 mL

Cordron-HC oral liquid ℞ *narcotic antitussive; antihistamine; decongestant* [hydrocodone bitartrate; chlorpheniramine maleate; phenylephrine HCl] 1.67•2.5•20 mg/5 mL

Cordron-HC NR syrup Ŗ *narcotic antitussive; antihistamine; decongestant* [hydrocodone bitartrate; chlorpheniramine maleate; pseudoephedrine HCl] 1.67•2.5•17.5 mg/5 mL

Coreg Tiltab (film-coated tablets) Ŗ *α- and β-blocker for hypertension, congestive heart failure (CHF), and left ventricular dysfunction (LVD) following myocardial infarction (MI); also used for chronic angina pectoris and idiopathic cardiomyopathy* [carvedilol] 3.125, 6.25, 12.5, 25 mg ⊡ Carac; Kuric

Coreg CR extended-release capsules Ŗ *α- and β-blocker for hypertension, congestive heart failure (CHF), and left ventricular dysfunction (LVD) following myocardial infarction (MI)* [carvedilol phosphate] 10, 20, 40, 80 mg

Corgard tablets Ŗ *antianginal; antihypertensive; antiadrenergic (β-blocker)* [nadolol] 20, 120, 160 mg

coriander *(Coriandrum sativum)* seed *medicinal herb used as antispasmodic, appetizer, carminative, and stomachic*

coriander oil NF

Coricidin D Cold, Flu, & Sinus tablets OTC *decongestant; antihistamine; analgesic; antipyretic* [phenylephrine HCl; chlorpheniramine maleate; acetaminophen] 5•2•325 mg

Coricidin HBP Chest Congestion & Cough softgels OTC *antitussive; expectorant* [dextromethorphan hydrobromide; guaifenesin] 10•200 mg

Coricidin HBP Cold & Flu tablets OTC *antihistamine; analgesic; antipyretic* [chlorpheniramine maleate; acetaminophen] 2•325 mg

Coricidin HBP Cough & Cold tablets OTC *antitussive; antihistamine* [dextromethorphan hydrobromide; chlorpheniramine maleate] 30•4 mg

Coricidin HBP Flu tablets OTC *antitussive; antihistamine; analgesic; antipyretic* [dextromethorphan hydrobromide; chlorpheniramine maleate; acetaminophen] 15•2•500 mg

corkwood tree *(Duboisia myoporoides)* leaves *medicinal herb used as a central nervous system stimulant and in homeopathic therapy for eye disorders; not generally regarded as safe and effective as it contains scopolamine and related alkaloids, which may be fatal in high doses*

Corlopam IV infusion Ŗ *rapid-acting vasodilator for in-hospital management of hypertensive emergencies* [fenoldopam mesylate] 10 mg/mL

Corlux *investigational (Phase III) GR-II antagonist to reduce abnormal cortisol release in psychotic major depression* [mifepristone]

Cormax cream, ointment Ŗ *corticosteroidal anti-inflammatory* [clobetasol propionate] 0.05%

cormed [see: nikethamide]

cormetasone INN *topical anti-inflammatory* [also: cormethasone acetate]

cormetasone acetate [see: cormethasone acetate]

cormethasone acetate USAN *topical anti-inflammatory* [also: cormetasone]

corn, turkey *medicinal herb* [see: turkey corn]

corn cockle *(Agrostemma githago)* seeds and root *medicinal herb for cancer, edema, exanthema, hemorrhoids, jaundice, and worms; also used as an emmenagogue and expectorant, and in homeopathic remedies for gastritis and paralysis; not generally regarded as safe and effective as it is extremely poisonous*

Corn Huskers lotion OTC *moisturizer; emollient*

corn oil NF *solvent; caloric replacement*

corn silk *(stigmata maidis)* *medicinal herb* [see: Indian corn]

cornflower *(Centaurea cyanus)* plant *medicinal herb for conjunctivitis, corneal ulcers and other eye disorders and for nervous disorders and poisonous bites and stings*

corpse plant *medicinal herb* [see: fit root]

corpus luteum extract [see: progesterone]

Corque cream ℞ *corticosteroidal anti-inflammatory; antifungal; antibacterial* [hydrocortisone; clioquinol] 1%•3% ⊘ Carac; Kuric

Correctol enteric-coated tablets OTC *stimulant laxative* [bisacodyl] 5 mg

CortaGel OTC *corticosteroidal anti-inflammatory* [hydrocortisone] 1%

Cortaid cream, ointment OTC *corticosteroidal anti-inflammatory* [hydrocortisone acetate] 1%

Cortaid pump spray OTC *corticosteroidal anti-inflammatory* [hydrocortisone] 1%

Cortaid Faststick roll-on stick OTC *corticosteroidal anti-inflammatory* [hydrocortisone; alcohol 55%] 1%

Cortaid Intensive Therapy cream (discontinued 2004) OTC *corticosteroidal anti-inflammatory* [hydrocortisone] 1%

Cortaid with Aloe cream, ointment OTC *corticosteroidal anti-inflammatory* [hydrocortisone acetate] 0.5%

Cortane-B lotion ℞ *corticosteroidal anti-inflammatory; local anesthetic; antiseptic* [hydrocortisone acetate; pramoxine HCl; chloroxylenol] 1%•1%•0.1%

Cortane-B Aqueous; Cortane-B Otic ear drops ℞ *corticosteroidal anti-inflammatory; local anesthetic; antiseptic* [hydrocortisone; pramoxine HCl; chloroxylenol] 1%•1%•0.1%

Cortatrigen ear drop solution, ear drop suspension (discontinued 2006) ℞ *corticosteroidal anti-inflammatory; antibiotic* [hydrocortisone; neomycin sulfate; polymyxin B sulfate] 1%•5 mg•10 000 U per mL

Cort-Dome cream ℞ *corticosteroidal anti-inflammatory* [hydrocortisone] 0.5%, 1%

Cort-Dome High Potency rectal suppositories ℞ *corticosteroidal anti-inflammatory* [hydrocortisone acetate] 25 mg

Cortef tablets, oral suspension ℞ *corticosteroid; anti-inflammatory* [hydrocortisone] 5, 10, 20 mg; 10 mg/5 mL

Cortef Feminine Itch cream OTC *corticosteroidal anti-inflammatory* [hydrocortisone acetate] 0.5%

Cortenema retention enema (discontinued 2004) ℞ *corticosteroidal anti-inflammatory for ulcerative colitis* [hydrocortisone] 100 mg/60 mL

cortenil [see: desoxycorticosterone acetate]

cortexolone [see: cortodoxone]

Cortic; Cortic-ND ear drops ℞ *corticosteroidal anti-inflammatory; local anesthetic; antiseptic* [hydrocortisone; pramoxine HCl; chloroxylenol] 1%•1%•0.1%

Corticaine cream OTC *corticosteroidal anti-inflammatory* [hydrocortisone acetate] 0.5% ⊘ carticaine

corticorelin ovine triflutate USAN, INN *corticotropin-releasing hormone; diagnostic aid for Cushing syndrome and adrenocortical insufficiency* (orphan)

corticosteroids *a class of anti-inflammatory drugs*

corticotrophin INN, BAN *adrenocorticotropic hormone; corticosteroid; anti-inflammatory; diagnostic aid* [also: corticotropin]

corticotrophin-zinc hydroxide INN *adrenocorticotropic hormone; corticosteroid; anti-inflammatory; diagnostic aid* [also: corticotropin zinc hydroxide]

corticotropin USP *adrenocorticotropic hormone; corticosteroid; anti-inflammatory; diagnostic aid* [also: corticotrophin]

corticotropin, repository USP *adrenocorticotropic hormone; corticosteroid; anti-inflammatory; diagnostic aid for testing adrenocortical function; investigational* (orphan) *for infantile spasms*

corticotropin tetracosapeptide [see: cosyntropin]

corticotropin zinc hydroxide USP *adrenocorticotropic hormone; corticosteroid; anti-inflammatory; diagnostic aid* [also: corticotrophin-zinc hydroxide]

corticotropin-releasing factor *investigational (Phase I/II, orphan) for peritumoral brain edema*

Cortifoam intrarectal foam aerosol (discontinued 2004) ℞ *corticosteroidal anti-inflammatory for ulcerative proctitis* [hydrocortisone acetate] 90 mg/dose

cortisol [see: hydrocortisone]

cortisol 21-acetate [see: hydrocortisone acetate]

cortisol 21-butyrate [see: hydrocortisone butyrate]

cortisol 21-cyclopentanepropionate [see: hydrocortisone cypionate]

cortisol cyclopentylpropionate [see: hydrocortisone cypionate]

cortisol 21-valerate [see: hydrocortisone valerate]

cortisone INN, BAN *corticosteroid; anti-inflammatory* [also: cortisone acetate]

cortisone acetate USP *corticosteroid; anti-inflammatory* [also: cortisone] 25 mg oral

Cortisporin cream ℞ *corticosteroidal anti-inflammatory; antibiotic* [hydrocortisone acetate; neomycin sulfate; polymyxin B sulfate] 0.5%•3.5 mg•10 000 U per g

Cortisporin eye drop suspension ℞ *corticosteroidal anti-inflammatory; antibiotic* [hydrocortisone; neomycin sulfate; polymyxin B sulfate] 1%•0.35%•10 000 U per mL

Cortisporin ointment (discontinued 2006) ℞ *corticosteroidal anti-inflammatory; antibiotic* [hydrocortisone; neomycin sulfate; bacitracin zinc; polymyxin B sulfate] 1%•3.5 mg•400 U•5000 U per g

Cortisporin ophthalmic ointment (discontinued 2006) ℞ *ophthalmic corticosteroidal anti-inflammatory; antibiotic* [hydrocortisone; neomycin sulfate; bacitracin zinc; polymyxin B sulfate] 1%•0.35%•400 U/g•10 000 U/g

Cortisporin Otic ear drop solution, ear drop suspension ℞ *corticosteroidal anti-inflammatory; antibiotic* [hydrocortisone; neomycin sulfate; polymyxin B sulfate] 1%•5 mg•10 000 U per mL

Cortisporin-TC Otic ear drop suspension ℞ *corticosteroidal anti-inflammatory; antibiotic; surface-active synergist* [hydrocortisone acetate; neomycin sulfate; colistin sulfate; thonzonium bromide] 10•3.3•3•0.5 mg/mL

cortisuzol INN

cortivazol USAN, INN *corticosteroid; anti-inflammatory*

Cortizone for Kids cream OTC *corticosteroidal anti-inflammatory* [hydrocortisone] 0.5%

Cortizone-5 cream (discontinued 2005) OTC *corticosteroidal anti-inflammatory* [hydrocortisone] 1%

Cortizone-5 ointment OTC *corticosteroidal anti-inflammatory* [hydrocortisone] 0.5%

Cortizone-10 cream, ointment OTC *corticosteroidal anti-inflammatory* [hydrocortisone] 1%

Cortizone-10 External Anal Itch cream OTC *corticosteroidal anti-inflammatory* [hydrocortisone] 1%

Cortizone-10 Plus cream OTC *corticosteroidal anti-inflammatory* [hydrocortisone] 1%

Cortizone-10 Quickshot spray OTC *corticosteroidal anti-inflammatory* [hydrocortisone] 1%

cortodoxone USAN, INN, BAN *anti-inflammatory*

Cortone Acetate intra-articular or intralesional injection ℞ *corticosteroidal anti-inflammatory* [cortisone acetate] 50 mg/mL

Cortrosyn powder for IM or IV injection ℞ *diagnostic aid for testing adrenocortical function* [cosyntropin] 0.25 mg

Corvert IV infusion ℞ *antiarrhythmic for atrial fibrillation/flutter* [ibutilide fumarate] 0.1 mg/mL

corydalis (Corydalis cava) root *medicinal herb used as an antispasmodic, hypnotic, and antiparkinsonian*

Corydalis formosa medicinal herb [see: turkey corn]

Corynanthe johimbe medicinal herb [see: yohimbe]

Corzide 40/5; Corzide 80/5 tablets ℞ *antihypertensive; β-blocker; diuretic* [nadolol; bendroflumethiazide] 40•5 mg; 80•5 mg

Cosmegen powder for IV injection ℞ *antibiotic antineoplastic for various tumors, carcinomas, and sarcomas; potentiator for radiation therapy* [dactinomycin] 0.5 mg/vial

CosmoDerm gel for subcu injection ℞ *dermal filler for shallow scars and fine wrinkles* [collagen, purified human] 35 mg/mL

cosmoline [see: petrolatum]

CosmoPlast gel for subcu injection ℞ *dermal filler for scars, deep wrinkles, and facial folds* [collagen, purified human, cross-linked] 35 mg/mL

Cosopt eye drops ℞ *combination carbonic anhydrase inhibitor and beta-blocker for glaucoma* [dorzolamide HCl; timolol maleate] 2%•0.5%

cosyntropin USAN *adrenocorticotropic hormone; diagnostic aid for testing adrenocortical function* [also: tetracosactide; tetracosactrin] 0.25 mg/mL injection

Cotara *investigational (Phase III) agent for glioblastoma multiforme* [chimeric monoclonal antibody labeled with iodine-131]

cotarnine chloride NF

cotarnine HCl [see: cotarnine chloride]

cotinine INN *antidepressant* [also: cotinine fumarate]

cotinine fumarate USAN *antidepressant* [also: cotinine]

Cotrim; Cotrim D.S. tablets ℞ *anti-infective; antibacterial* [trimethoprim; sulfamethoxazole] 80•400 mg; 160•800 mg

Cotrim Pediatric oral suspension ℞ *anti-infective; antibacterial* [trimethoprim; sulfamethoxazole] 40•200 mg/5 mL

co-trimoxazole BAN [also: trimethoprim + sulfamethoxazole]

cotriptyline INN

cotton, purified USP *surgical aid*

cottonseed oil NF *solvent*

cottonweed *medicinal herb* [see: milkweed]

Cotuss EX syrup (discontinued 2007) ℞ *narcotic antitussive; expectorant* [hydrocodone bitartrate; potassium guaiacolsulfonate] 2.5•120 mg/5 mL

Cotuss HD; Cotuss MS syrup (discontinued 2007) ℞ *narcotic antitussive; antihistamine; decongestant* [hydrocodone bitartrate; chlorpheniramine maleate; phenylephrine HCl] 5•8•20 mg/10 mL; 10•4•20 mg/10 mL

couch grass (Agropyron repens) rhizomes, roots, and stems *medicinal herb for blood cleansing, cystitis, diabetes, jaundice, kidney problems, upper respiratory tract inflammation with mucous discharge, rheumatism, and urinary infections*

coughroot *medicinal herb* [see: birthroot]

Coughtuss oral liquid ℞ *narcotic antitussive; antihistamine; decongestant* [hydrocodone bitartrate; chlorpheniramine maleate; phenylephrine HCl] 5•2•5 mg/5 mL

coughweed *medicinal herb* [see: life root]

coughwort *medicinal herb* [see: coltsfoot]

Cough-X lozenges OTC *antitussive; mucous membrane anesthetic* [dextromethorphan hydrobromide; benzocaine] 5•2 mg

Coumadin tablets, powder for IV injection ℞ *coumarin-derivative anticoagulant* [warfarin sodium] 1, 2, 2.5, 3, 4, 5, 6, 7.5, 10 mg; 2 mg/mL

coumafos INN [also: coumaphos]

coumamycin INN *antibacterial* [also: coumermycin]

coumaphos BAN [also: coumafos]

coumarin NF *anticoagulant; investigational (orphan) for renal cell carcinoma*

coumarins *a class of anticoagulants that interfere with vitamin K-dependent clotting factors*

coumazoline INN

coumermycin USAN *antibacterial* [also: coumamycin]

coumermycin sodium USAN *antibacterial*

coumetarol INN [also: cumetharol]

counterirritants *a class of agents that produce superficial irritation in one part of the body to relieve irritation in another part*

Covaryx; Covaryx H.S. film-coated caplets ℞ *combination equine estrogen and synthetic androgen; hormone replacement therapy for postmenopausal symptoms* [esterified estrogens; methyltestosterone] 1.25•2.5 mg; 0.625•1.25 mg

covatin HCl [see: captodiame HCl]

Covera-HS extended-release film-coated tablets ℞ *antihypertensive; antianginal; antiarrhythmic; calcium channel blocker* [verapamil HCl] 180, 240 mg

cow cabbage *medicinal herb* [see: masterwort; white pond lily]

cow parsnip *medicinal herb* [see: masterwort]

cowslip *(Caltha palustris)* plant *medicinal herb used as an analgesic, antispasmodic, diaphoretic, diuretic, expectorant, and rubefacient*

cowslip, Jerusalem *medicinal herb* [see: lungwort]

COX-2 (cyclooxygenase-2) inhibitors *a class of nonsteroidal anti-inflammatory drugs (NSAIDs) for osteoarthritis, rheumatoid arthritis, acute pain, and primary dysmenorrhea; these agents also have antipyretic activity*

Cozaar film-coated tablets ℞ *angiotensin II receptor antagonist for hypertension; treatment to delay the progression of diabetic nephropathy* [losartan potassium] 25, 50, 100 mg

CP (chlorambucil, prednisone) *chemotherapy protocol for chronic lymphocytic leukemia (CLL)*

CP (cyclophosphamide, Platinol) *chemotherapy protocol for ovarian cancer*

CP (cyclophosphamide, prednisone) *chemotherapy protocol*

CP DEC syrup, oral drops ℞ *decongestant; antihistamine; drops for children 6–24 months* [phenylephrine HCl; chlorpheniramine maleate] 12.5•4 mg/5 mL; 3.5•1 mg/mL

CP DEC-DM oral drops ℞ *antitussive; antihistamine; decongestant; for children 6–24 months* [dextromethorphan hydrobromide; chlorpheniramine maleate; phenylephrine HCl] 3•1•3.5 mg/mL

CP DEC-DM syrup ℞ *antitussive; antihistamine; decongestant* [dextromethorphan hydrobromide; chlorpheniramine maleate; phenylephrine HCl] 15•4•12.5 mg/5 mL

CPB (cyclophosphamide, Platinol, BCNU) *chemotherapy protocol*

CPB WC oral liquid ℞ *narcotic antitussive; antihistamine; decongestant* [codeine phosphate; brompheniramine maleate; pseudoephedrine HCl] 6.3•1.3•10 mg/5 mL ☑ COPAC; CPC; Gy-Pak; K-Pek

CPC (cyclophosphamide, Platinol, carboplatin) *chemotherapy protocol*

C.P.-DM oral drops (discontinued 2007) ℞ *antitussive; antihistamine; decongestant; for children 1–24 months* [dextromethorphan hydrobromide; carbinoxamine maleate; pseudoephedrine HCl] 4•1•15 mg/mL

C-Phed Tannate oral suspension (discontinued 2007) ℞ *decongestant; antihistamine* [pseudoephedrine tannate; chlorpheniramine tannate] 150•9 mg/10 mL

C-Phen syrup, oral drops ℞ *decongestant; antihistamine; drops for children 6–24 months* [phenylephrine HCl; chlorpheniramine maleate] 12.5•4 mg/5 mL; 3.5•1 mg/mL ☑ caffeine; Kuvan

C-Phen DM oral drops ℞ *antitussive; antihistamine; decongestant; for children 6–24 months* [dextromethorphan hydrobromide; chlorpheniramine maleate; phenylephrine HCl] 3•1•3.5 mg/mL ☑ G Phen DM; GFN 1000/DM 50; Guaifen DM

C-Phen DM syrup ℞ *antitussive; antihistamine; decongestant* [dextromethorphan hydrobromide; chlorpheniramine maleate; phenylephrine HCl] 15•4•12.5 mg/5 mL ☑ G Phen DM; GFN 1000/DM 50; Guaifen DM

CPM (CCNU, procarbazine, methotrexate) *chemotherapy protocol*

CPM 8/PE 20/MSC 1.25 caplets ℞ *antihistamine; decongestant; anticholinergic to dry mucosal secretions* [chorpheniramine maleate; phenylephrine HCl; methscopolamine nitrate] 8•20•1.25 mg

CPM 8/PSE 90/MSC 2.5 sustained-release tablets ℞ *antihistamine; decongestant; anticholinergic to dry mucosal secretions* [chorpheniramine maleate; pseudoephedrine HCl; methscopolamine nitrate] 8•90•2.5 mg

CPOB (cyclophosphamide, prednisone, Oncovin, bleomycin) *chemotherapy protocol* ⦸ CABOP; CAP-BOP; cubeb; Q-Pap

CPT-11 (camptothecin-11) [see: irinotecan]

CP-Tannic oral suspension (discontinued 2007) ℞ *decongestant; antihistamine* [pseudoephedrine tannate; chlorpheniramine tannate] 150•9 mg/10 mL

CR1 (complement receptor 1) [see: complement receptor type I]

⁵¹Cr [see: albumin, chromated Cr 51 serum]

⁵¹Cr [see: chromic chloride Cr 51]

⁵¹Cr [see: chromic phosphate Cr 51]

⁵¹Cr [see: sodium chromate Cr 51]

cramp bark (*Viburnum opulus*) bark and berries *medicinal herb for asthma, convulsions, cramps, heart palpitations, hypertension, hysteria, leg cramps, nervousness, spasm, and urinary disorders*

crampweed *medicinal herb* [see: cinquefoil]

cranberry (*Vaccinium edule; V. erythrocarpum; V. macrocarpon; V. oxycoccos; V. vitis*) fruit *medicinal herb for bladder, kidney, and urinary tract infections; also used to decrease the rate of urine degradation and odor formation in incontinent patients*

cranesbill; spotted cranesbill *medicinal herb* [see: alum root]

Crantex oral liquid ℞ *decongestant; expectorant* [phenylephrine HCl; guaifenesin] 7.5•100 mg/5 mL

Crantex ER extended-release capsules (discontinued 2007) ℞ *decongestant; expectorant* [phenylephrine HCl; guaifenesin] 10•300 mg

Crataegus laevigata; C. monogyna; C. oxyacantha *medicinal herb* [see: hawthorn]

crawley; crawley root *medicinal herb* [see: coral root]

Creamy Tar shampoo OTC *antiseborrheic; antipsoriatic; antipruritic; antibacterial* [coal tar] 8.65%

Creapure *investigational (orphan) agent for amyotrophic lateral sclerosis (ALS)* [creatine]

creatine *investigational (orphan) agent for amyotrophic lateral sclerosis (ALS)*

creatinolfosfate INN

Creomulsion Adult Formula syrup OTC *antitussive* [dextromethorphan hydrobromide] 20 mg/15 mL

Creomulsion for Children syrup OTC *antitussive* [dextromethorphan hydrobromide] 5 mg/5 mL

Creon 5; Creon 10: Creon 20 delayed-release capsules containing enteric-coated microspheres ℞ (available OTC in Canada) *porcine-derived digestive enzymes* [lipase; protease; amylase] 5000•18 750•16 600 USP units; 10 000•37 500•33 200 USP units; 20 000•75 000•66 400 USP units ⦸ Choron-10; guarana

creosote carbonate USP

Creo-Terpin oral liquid OTC *antitussive* [dextromethorphan hydrobromide; alcohol 25%] 10 mg/15 mL

cresol NF *disinfectant* ⦸ Cryselle; Kerasal

cresotamide INN

cresoxydiol [see: mephenesin]

crestomycin sulfate [see: paromomycin sulfate]

Crestor tablets ℞ *HMG-CoA reductase inhibitor for hypercholesterolemia, mixed dyslipidemia, and hypertriglyceridemia; reduces atheroma (plaque build-*

up) in coronary arteries [rosuvastatin (as calcium)] 5, 10, 20, 40 mg

Cresylate ear drops ℞ *antiseptic; antibacterial; antifungal* [m-cresyl acetate; chlorobutanol; alcohol] 25%•25%•1%

cresylic acid [see: cresol]

crilanomer INN

crilvastatin USAN, INN *antihyperlipidemic*

Crinone vaginal gel in prefilled applicators ℞ *natural progestin; hormone replacement or supplementation for assisted reproductive technology (ART) treatments* [progesterone] 8% (90 mg)

crisnatol INN *antineoplastic* [also: crisnatol mesylate]

crisnatol mesylate USAN *antineoplastic* [also: crisnatol]

Criticare HN ready-to-use oral liquid OTC *enteral nutritional therapy* [lactose-free formula]

Crixivan capsules ℞ *antiretroviral protease inhibitor for HIV infection* [indinavir sulfate] 125, 250, 416.3, 500 mg (100, 200, 333, 400 mg base)

crobefate INN *combining name for radicals or groups*

croconazole INN

crocus, autumn *medicinal herb* [see: autumn crocus]

Crocus sativus medicinal herb [see: saffron]

CroFab injection ℞ *treatment of pit viper (rattlesnake, copperhead, and cottonmouth moccasin) snake bites (orphan)* [antivenin (Crotalidae) polyvalent immune Fab (ovine)]

crofelemer USAN *investigational (Phase III) treatment for AIDS-related diarrhea; investigational (Phase II) antiviral for AIDS-related genital herpes*

crofilcon A USAN *hydrophilic contact lens material*

Crolom eye drops ℞ *mast cell stabilizer; antiallergic and antiviral for vernal keratoconjunctivitis* [cromolyn sodium] 4%

cromacate INN *combining name for radicals or groups*

cromakalim INN, BAN

Cro-Man-Zin tablets OTC *mineral supplement* [chromium; manganese; zinc] 0.2•5•25 mg

cromesilate INN *combining name for radicals or groups*

cromitrile INN *antiasthmatic* [also: cromitrile sodium]

cromitrile sodium USAN *antiasthmatic* [also: cromitrile]

cromoglicic acid INN *prophylactic antiasthmatic* [also: cromolyn sodium; cromoglycic acid]

cromoglycic acid BAN *prophylactic antiasthmatic* [also: cromolyn sodium; cromoglicic acid]

cromolyn sodium USAN, USP *antiinflammatory; mast cell stabilizer for prophylactic treatment of allergy, asthma, and bronchospasm; treatment for mastocytosis and vernal keratoconjunctivitis (orphan)* [also: cromoglicic acid; cromoglycic acid] 20 mg/2 mL inhalation

Cronassial *investigational (orphan) agent for retinitis pigmentosa* [gangliosides, sodium salts]

cronetal [see: disulfiram]

cronidipine INN

cropropamide INN, BAN

croscarmellose INN *tablet disintegrant* [also: croscarmellose sodium]

croscarmellose sodium USAN, NF *tablet disintegrant* [also: croscarmellose]

crosfumaril [see: hemoglobin crosfumaril]

crospovidone NF *tablet excipient*

cross-linked carboxymethylcellulose sodium [now: croscarmellose sodium]

cross-linked carmellose sodium [see: croscarmellose sodium]

crotaline antivenin [see: antivenin (Crotalidae) polyvalent]

crotamiton USP, INN, BAN *scabicide; antipruritic*

crotetamide INN [also: crotethamide]

crotethamide BAN [also: crotetamide]

crotoniazide INN

crotonylidenisoniazid [see: crotoniazide]

crotoxyfos BAN

crowfoot *medicinal herb* [see: alum root; buttercup]

crowfoot buttercup; acrid crowfoot; cursed crowfoot; marsh crowfoot; meadow crowfoot; tall crowfoot; water crowfoot *medicinal herb* [see: buttercup]

crown, priest's *medicinal herb* [see: dandelion]

crude tuberculin [see: tuberculin, old]

Cruex cream OTC *antifungal* [clotrimazole] 1%

Cruex cream, aerosol powder OTC *antifungal* [undecylenic acid; zinc undecylenate] 20% total; 19% total

Cruex topical powder OTC *antifungal* [calcium undecylenate] 10%

crufomate USAN, INN, BAN *veterinary anthelmintic* ⊘ carfimate

cryofluorane INN *aerosol propellant* [also: dichlorotetrafluoroethane]

Cryptaz *antiprotozoal; investigational (orphan) for intestinal amebiasis* [nitazoxanide]

cryptenamine acetates

Crypto-LA slide test for professional use ℞ *in vitro diagnostic aid for Cryptococcus neoformans antigens*

Cryptosporidium parvum bovine colostrum IgG concentrate *investigational (orphan) treatment of cryptosporidiosis-induced diarrhea in immunocompromised patients*

Cryselle tablets (in packs of 21 and 28) ℞ *monophasic oral contraceptive; emergency postcoital contraceptive* [norgestrel; ethinyl estradiol] 0.3 mg•30 mcg ⊘ cresol; Kerasal

crystal violet [see: gentian violet]

crystallized trypsin [see: trypsin, crystallized]

Crystamine IM or subcu injection ℞ *hematinic; vitamin B_{12} supplement* [cyanocobalamin] 1000 mcg/mL

Crysti 1000 IM or subcu injection ℞ *hematinic; vitamin B_{12} supplement* [cyanocobalamin] 1000 mcg/mL

crystografin [see: meglumine diatriazole]

^{131}Cs [see: cesium chloride Cs 131]

CS-92 *investigational (Phase I/II) nucleoside reverse transcriptase inhibitor (NRTI) for HIV infection*

C-Solve OTC *lotion base*

CSP (cellulose sodium phosphate) [q.v.]

CT (cisplatin, Taxol) *chemotherapy protocol for ovarian cancer*

CT (cytarabine, thioguanine) *chemotherapy protocol*

CT-2584 mesylate *investigational (Phase II, orphan) antineoplastic for soft tissue sarcomas and malignant mesothelioma*

CTAB (cetyltrimethyl ammonium bromide) ⊘ K-Tab; Q-Tapp

C-Tan D oral suspension ℞ *decongestant; antihistamine* [phenylephrine tannate; brompheniramine tannate] 5•4 mg/5 mL

C-Tanna 12D oral suspension ℞ *antitussive; antihistamine; sleep aid; decongestant* [carbetapentane tannate; pyrilamine tannate; phenylephrine tannate] 30•30•5 mg/5 mL

C-Tanna 12D tablets (discontinued 2006) ℞ *antitussive; antihistamine; sleep aid; decongestant* [carbetapentane tannate; pyrilamine tannate; phenylephrine tannate] 60•40•10 mg

CTCb (cyclophosphamide, thiotepa, carboplatin) *chemotherapy protocol*

CTH (ceramide trihexosidase) [q.v.]

CTP-37 *investigational (Phase III) theraccine for cervical and pancreatic cancer; investigational (Phase II) for prostate and advanced colorectal cancers*

CTX (cyclophosphamide) [q.v.]

Ctx-Plat (cyclophosphamide, Platinol) *chemotherapy protocol*

^{64}Cu [see: cupric acetate Cu 64]

cubeb (Piper cubeba) unripe berries *medicinal herb used as an antiseptic, antisyphilitic, carminative, diuretic, expectorant, stimulant, and stomachic* ⊘ CABOP; CAP-BOP; CPOB; Q-Pap

Cubicin powder for IV infusion ℞ *cyclic lipopeptide antibiotic for skin and skin structure infections (SSSIs), Staph-*

ylococcus aureus *bloodstream infections, and right-sided endocarditis* [daptomycin] 500 mg/vial ⑨ Capsin; kebuzone; quipazine

cucurbita (*Cucurbita maxima; C. moschata; C. pepa*) seeds *medicinal herb for prophylaxis, immobilizing, and aiding in the expulsion of intestinal worms and parasites; also used in prostate gland disorders*

Culturette 10 Minute Group A Strep ID slide test for professional use ℞ *in vitro diagnostic test for Group A streptococcal antigens in throat swabs* [latex agglutination test]

Culver physic *medicinal herb* [see: Culver root]

Culver root (*Varonicastrum virginicum*) *medicinal herb for blood cleansing, diarrhea, and liver and stomach disorders*

cumetharol BAN [also: coumetarol]

cumin (*Cuminum cyminum; C. odorum*) seeds and oil *medicinal herb for gastric cancer; also used as an antioxidant*

cupric acetate Cu 64 USAN *radioactive agent*

cupric chloride USP *dietary copper supplement*

cupric sulfate USP *antidote to phosphorus overload; dietary copper supplement* (40% elemental copper) 0.4, 2 mg/mL injection

Cuprimine capsules ℞ *metal chelating agent for rheumatoid arthritis, Wilson disease, and cystinuria* [penicillamine] 125, 250 mg

cuprimyxin USAN, INN *veterinary antibacterial; antifungal*

cuproxoline INN, BAN

Curaçao aloe *medicinal herb* [see: aloe]

curare [see: metocurine iodide; tubocurarine chloride]

Curcuma domestica; C. longa *medicinal herb* [see: turmeric]

cure-all *medicinal herb* [see: lemon balm]

CureLight BroadBand Model 01 (device) *red-light illuminator; used with* **Metvixia** (methyl aminolevuli-

nate HCl) *for photodynamic therapy of precancerous actinic keratoses of the face and scalp*

curium *element* (Cm)

curled dock; curly dock *medicinal herb* [see: yellow dock]

curled mint *medicinal herb* [see: peppermint]

curls, blue *medicinal herb* [see: woundwort]

Curosurf intratracheal suspension ℞ *porcine lung extract for respiratory distress syndrome (RDS) in premature infants* (orphan); *also used for severe meconium aspiration in term infants* [poractant alfa] 1.5, 3 mL (120, 240 mg phospholipids)

curral [see: diallybarbituric acid]

currant (*Ribes nigrum; R. rubrum*) leaves and fruit *medicinal herb used as a diaphoretic and diuretic* ⑨ green tea

Curretab tablets (discontinued 2004) ℞ *synthetic progestin for secondary amenorrhea, abnormal uterine bleeding, and endometrial hyperplasia* [medroxyprogesterone acetate] 10 mg

custard apple *medicinal herb* [see: pawpaw]

custirsen sodium *investigational antineoplastic for progressive metastatic prostate cancer*

Cūtar Bath Oil Emulsion OTC *antipsoriatic; antiseborrheic; antipruritic; emollient* [coal tar] 7.5%

Cūtemol cream OTC *moisturizer; emollient* [allantoin]

Cuticura Medicated Soap bar OTC *therapeutic skin cleanser; antiseptic* [triclocarban] 1%

Cutivate cream, lotion, ointment ℞ *corticosteroidal anti-inflammatory* [fluticasone propionate] 0.05%; 0.05%; 0.005%

CV (cisplatin, VePesid) *chemotherapy protocol*

CVA (cyclophosphamide, vincristine, Adriamycin) *chemotherapy protocol*

CVA-BMP; CVA + BMP (cyclophosphamide, vincristine, Adria-

mycin, BCNU, methotrexate, procarbazine) *chemotherapy protocol*

CVAD; C-VAD (cyclophosphamide, vincristine, Adriamycin, dexamethasone) *chemotherapy protocol* ⑨ CVD; Guaifed

CVB (CCNU, vinblastine, bleomycin) *chemotherapy protocol*

CVBD (CCNU, bleomycin, vinblastine, dexamethasone) *chemotherapy protocol*

CVD (cisplatin, vinblastine, dacarbazine) *chemotherapy protocol for malignant melanoma*

CVD+IL-2I (cisplatin, vinblastine, dacarbazine, interleukin-2, interferon alfa) *chemotherapy protocol for malignant melanoma*

CVEB (cisplatin, vinblastine, etoposide, bleomycin) *chemotherapy protocol* ⑨ CAFP; CAV/EP; CCVPP; CFP; CH1VPP; CHVP; CVB; CVP

CVI (carboplatin, VePesid, ifosfamide [with mesna rescue]) *chemotherapy protocol for non–small cell lung cancer (NSCLC)* [also: VIC]

CVM (cyclophosphamide, vincristine, methotrexate) *chemotherapy protocol*

CVP (cyclophosphamide, vincristine, prednisone) *chemotherapy protocol for non-Hodgkin lymphoma and chronic lymphocytic leukemia (CLL)*

CVPP (CCNU, vinblastine, procarbazine, prednisone) *chemotherapy protocol for Hodgkin lymphoma* ⑨ CAFP; CAV/EP; CCVPP; CFP; CH1VPP; CHVP; CVB; CVEB

CVPP (cyclophosphamide, Velban, procarbazine, prednisone) *chemotherapy protocol* ⑨ CAFP; CAV/EP; CCVPP; CFP; CH1VPP; CHVP; CVB; CVEB

CVPP-CCNU (cyclophosphamide, vinblastine, procarbazine, prednisone, CCNU) *chemotherapy protocol*

CY-1503 *investigational (Phase III, orphan) adjunct to surgery for congenital heart defects in newborns; investiga-* *tional (orphan) for postischemic pulmonary reperfusion edema*

CY-1899 *investigational (orphan) agent for chronic active hepatitis B*

cyacetacide INN [also: cyacetazide]

cyacetazide BAN [also: cyacetacide]

CyADIC (cyclophosphamide, Adriamycin, DIC) *chemotherapy protocol* ⑨ Cydec; Xedec; Zodeac-100

cyamemazine INN

cyamepromazine [see: cyamemazine]

cyanamide JAN [also: calcium carbimide]

cyani *medicinal herb* [see: cornflower]

Cyanide Antidote Package ℞ *emergency treatment of cyanide poisoning* [sodium nitrite; sodium thiosulfate; amyl nitrite inhalant] 300 mg•12.5 g•0.3 mL

cyanoacetohydrazide [see: cyacetazide]

cyanoacrylate *topical skin adhesive for closing surgical incisions and traumatic lacerations; topical mucous membrane sealant and protectant for canker and mouth sores*

cyanocobalamin (vitamin B$_{12}$) USP, INN, BAN, JAN *water-soluble vitamin; hematopoietic* 50, 100, 250, 500, 1000, 5000 mcg oral; 100, 1000 mcg/mL injection

cyanocobalamin (^{57}Co) INN *pernicious anemia test; radioactive agent* [also: cyanocobalamin Co 57]

cyanocobalamin (^{58}Co) INN

cyanocobalamin (^{60}Co) INN *pernicious anemia test; radioactive agent* [also: cyanocobalamin Co 60]

cyanocobalamin Co 57 USAN, USP *pernicious anemia test; radioactive agent* [also: cyanocobalamin (^{57}Co)]

cyanocobalamin Co 60 USAN, USP *pernicious anemia test; radioactive agent* [also: cyanocobalamin (^{60}Co)]

Cyanoject IM or subcu injection ℞ *hematinic; vitamin B$_{12}$ supplement* [cyanocobalamin] 1000 mcg/mL

Cyanokit *powder for IV infusion* ℞ *antidote to acute cyanide poisoning*

194   cyclacillin

(orphan) [hydroxocobalamin] 25
mg/mL (5 g/dose) ⊡ Senokot; Zincate
cyclacillin USAN, USP *antibacterial*
[also: ciclacillin]
cyclamate calcium NF
cyclamic acid USAN, BAN *non-nutritive
sweetener (banned in the U.S.)*
cyclamide [see: glycyclamide]
cyclandelate INN, BAN, JAN *peripheral
vasodilator; vascular smooth muscle
relaxant*
cyclarbamate INN, BAN
cyclazocine USAN, INN *analgesic*
cyclazodone INN
Cyclessa tablets (in packs of 28) ℞
*triphasic oral contraceptive; emergency
postcoital contraceptive* [desogestrel;
ethinyl estradiol] ⊡ Sequels
Phase 1 (7 days): 0.1 mg•25 mcg;
Phase 2 (7 days): 0.125 mg•25 mcg;
Phase 3 (7 days): 0.15 mg•25 mcg
cyclexanone INN
**cyclic adenosine monophosphate
(cAMP)** [see: adenosine phosphate]
cyclic lipopeptides *a class of antibiotics that binds to bacterial membranes
and causes a rapid depolarization of
membrane potential, which inhibits
RNA/DNA synthesis, leading to bacterial cell death*
cyclic propylene carbonate [see:
propylene carbonate]
cyclindole USAN *antidepressant* [also:
ciclindole]
Cyclinex-1 powder OTC *formula for
infants with urea cycle disorders or
gyrate atrophy*
Cyclinex-2 powder OTC *enteral nutritional therapy for urea cycle disorders
or gyrate atrophy* [multiple essential
amino acids]
cycliramine INN *antihistamine* [also:
cycliramine maleate]
cycliramine maleate USAN *antihistamine* [also: cycliramine]
cyclizine USP, INN, BAN *anticholinergic;
antihistamine; antiemetic; motion sickness relief* ⊡ seclazone

cyclizine HCl USP, BAN *anticholinergic;
antihistamine; antiemetic; motion sickness relief*
cyclizine lactate USP, BAN *antinauseant*
cyclobarbital NF, INN [also: cyclobar-
bitone]
cyclobarbital calcium NF
cyclobarbitone BAN [also: cyclobarbi-
tal]
cyclobendazole USAN *anthelmintic*
[also: ciclobendazole]
cyclobenzaprine INN *skeletal muscle
relaxant* [also: cyclobenzaprine HCl]
cyclobenzaprine HCl USAN, USP
skeletal muscle relaxant [also: cyclo-
benzaprine] 5, 7.5, 10 mg oral
cyclobutoic acid INN
cyclobutyrol INN
cyclocarbothiamine [see: cycotiamine]
Cyclocort ointment, cream, lotion ℞
corticosteroidal anti-inflammatory
[amcinonide] 0.1%
cyclocoumarol BAN
cyclocumarol [see: cyclocoumarol]
α-cyclodextrin [see: alfadex]
Cyclofed Pediatric syrup (discontinued
2005) ℞ *narcotic antitussive; decongestant; expectorant* [codeine phosphate;
pseudoephedrine HCl; guaifenesin;
alcohol 6%] 10•30•100 mg/5 mL
cyclofenil INN, BAN
cyclofilcon A USAN *hydrophilic contact
lens material*
cycloguanil embonate INN, BAN *antimalarial* [also: cycloguanil pamoate]
cycloguanil pamoate USAN *antimalarial* [also: cycloguanil embonate]
Cyclogyl Drop-Tainers (eye drops) ℞
cycloplegic; mydriatic [cyclopentolate
HCl] 0.5%, 1%, 2%
cyclohexanehexol [see: inositol]
cyclohexanesulfamate dihydrate
[see: sodium cyclamate]
cyclohexanesulfamic acid *(banned in
the U.S.)* [see: cyclamic acid]
cycloheximide USAN *antipsoriatic*
[also: cicloheximide]
p-cyclohexylhydratropic acid [see:
hexaprofen]

N-cyclohexyllinoleamide [see: clinolamide]

4-cyclohexyloxybenzoate [see: cyclomethycaine]

1-cyclohexylpropyl carbamate [see: procymate]

N-cyclohexylsulfamic acid *(banned in the U.S.)* [see: cyclamic acid]

cyclomenol INN ⊡ cicliomenol

cyclomethicone NF *wetting agent*

cyclomethycaine INN, BAN *local anesthetic* [also: cyclomethycaine sulfate]

cyclomethycaine sulfate USP *local anesthetic* [also: cyclomethycaine]

Cyclomydril Drop-Tainers (eye drops) ℞ *cycloplegic; mydriatic* [cyclopentolate HCl; phenylephrine HCl] 0.2% •1%

cyclonium iodide [see: oxapium iodide]

cyclooxygenase-2 (COX-2) inhibitors *a class of nonsteroidal anti-inflammatory drugs (NSAIDs) for osteoarthritis, rheumatoid arthritis, acute pain, and primary dysmenorrhea; these agents also have antipyretic activity*

cyclopentamine INN, BAN [also: cyclopentamine HCl]

cyclopentamine HCl USP [also: cyclopentamine]

cyclopentaphene [see: cyclarbamate]

cyclopenthiazide USAN, INN, BAN *antihypertensive*

cyclopentolate INN, BAN *ophthalmic anticholinergic* [also: cyclopentolate HCl]

cyclopentolate HCl USP *ophthalmic anticholinergic; mydriatic; cycloplegic* [also: cyclopentolate] 1% eye drops

8-cyclopentyl 1,3-dipropylxanthine *investigational (orphan) for cystic fibrosis*

cyclophenazine HCl USAN *antipsychotic* [also: ciclofenazine]

cyclophosphamide USP, INN, BAN, JAN *nitrogen mustard–type alkylating antineoplastic; immunosuppressive* 25, 50 mg oral; 0.5, 1, 2 g injection

cycloplegics *a class of drugs that paralyze the ciliary muscles of the eye*

cyclopolydimethylsiloxane [see: cyclomethicone]

cyclopregnol INN

cycloprolol BAN *antiadrenergic (β-receptor)* [also: cicloprolol HCl; cicloprolol]

cyclopropane USP, INN *inhalation general anesthetic*

Cycloprostin *investigational (orphan) heparin replacement for hemodialysis* [epoprostenol]

cyclopyrronium bromide INN

cycloserine (D-cycloserine) *investigational treatment for phobias and other severe anxiety disorders*

cycloserine (L-cycloserine) USP, INN, BAN, JAN *bacteriostatic; tuberculosis retreatment; investigational (orphan) for Gaucher disease*

Cyclospire *oral aerosol investigational (orphan) to prevent and treat lung allograft and other pulmonary rejection associated with bone marrow transplantation* [cyclosporine, liposomal]

cyclosporin BAN *immunosuppressant* [also: cyclosporine; ciclosporin]

cyclosporin A [now: cyclosporine]

cyclosporine USAN, USP *immunosuppressant for transplants (orphan), rheumatoid arthritis, and psoriasis; tear stimulant for Sjögren keratoconjunctivitis sicca (orphan); investigational (orphan) for corneal melting syndrome* [also: ciclosporin; cyclosporin] 25, 50, 100 mg oral; 100 mg/mL oral; 50 mg/mL injection

cyclosporine, liposomal *investigational (orphan) oral aerosol to prevent and treat lung allograft and other pulmonary rejection associated with bone marrow transplantation*

cyclosporine & ketoconazole *investigational (orphan) to diminish nephrotoxicity from organ transplantation*

CycloTech *(trademarked delivery device) provides premeasured doses of oral liquids and records dosing times*

cyclothiazide USAN, USP, INN, BAN *diuretic; antihypertensive*

cyclovalone INN

cycobemin [see: cyanocobalamin]

Cycofed syrup (discontinued 2007) ℞ *narcotic antitussive; decongestant* [codeine phosphate; pseudoephedrine HCl] 20•60 mg/5 mL

cycotiamine INN

cycrimine INN, BAN [also: cycrimine HCl]

cycrimine HCl USP [also: cycrimine]

Cycrin tablets (discontinued 2004) ℞ *synthetic progestin for secondary amenorrhea, abnormal uterine bleeding, and endometrial hyperplasia* [medroxyprogesterone acetate] 2.5, 5, 10 mg ⊡ Secran

Cydec oral drops (discontinued 2007) ℞ *decongestant; antihistamine* [pseudoephedrine HCl; carbinoxamine maleate] 25•2 mg/mL ⊡ CyADIC; Xedec; Zodeac-100

Cydec-DM syrup, pediatric oral drops (discontinued 2007) ℞ *antitussive; antihistamine; decongestant* [dextromethorphan hydrobromide; carbinoxamine maleate; pseudoephedrine HCl] 15•4•60 mg/5 mL; 4•2•25 mg/mL

cyfluthrin BAN

cyhalothrin BAN

cyheptamide USAN, INN *anticonvulsant*

cyheptropine INN

CyHOP (cyclophosphamide, Halotestin, Oncovin, prednisone) *chemotherapy protocol*

Cyklokapron tablets, IV injection ℞ *systemic hemostatic; surgical adjunct for patients with congenital coagulopathies (orphan); investigational (orphan) for hereditary angioneurotic edema* [tranexamic acid] 500 mg; 100 mg/mL

Cylert tablets, chewable tablets (withdrawn from the market in 2005 due to safety concerns) ℞ *CNS stimulant for attention-deficit/hyperactivity disorder (ADHD)* [pemoline] 18.75, 37.5, 75 mg; 37.5 mg

Cylex; Cylex Sugar-Free lozenges OTC *mucous membrane anesthetic; antiseptic* [benzocaine; cetylpyridinium chloride] 15•5 mg ⊡ Celexa; Salex

Cylexin *investigational (Phase III, orphan) adjunct to surgery for congenital heart defects in newborns; investigational (orphan) for postischemic pulmonary reperfusion edema* [CY-1503 (code name—generic name not yet assigned)]

Cymbalta enteric-coated pellets in capsules ℞ *selective serotonin and norepinephrine reuptake inhibitor (SSNRI) for major depressive disorder (MDD) and generalized anxiety disorder (GAD); analgesic for diabetic peripheral neuropathy (DPN) and fibromyalgia* [duloxetine HCl] 20, 30, 60 mg ⊡ Simplet

Cymbopogon citratus *medicinal herb* [see: lemongrass]

Cymbopogon nardus; C. winterianus *medicinal herb* [see: citronella]

cymemoxine [see: cimemoxin]

Cymevene (foreign name for the U.S. product **Cytovene**)

Cynara scolymus *medicinal herb* [see: artichoke]

cynarine INN

Cyomin IM or subcu injection ℞ *hematinic; vitamin B_{12} supplement* [cyanocobalamin] 1000 mcg/mL ⊡ Zymine

cypenamine INN, BAN *antidepressant* [also: cypenamine HCl]

cypenamine HCl USAN *antidepressant* [also: cypenamine]

cypionate USAN, BAN *combining name for radicals or groups* [also: cipionate]

cypothrin USAN *veterinary insecticide*

cyprazepam USAN, INN *sedative*

cyprenorphine INN, BAN

cyprenorphine HCl [see: cyprenorphine]

Cypripedium pubescens *medicinal herb* [see: lady's slipper]

cyprodemanol [see: cyprodenate]

cyprodenate INN

cyproheptadine INN, BAN *nonselective piperidine antihistamine for hypersensitivity reactions; antipruritic* [also: cyproheptadine HCl]

cyproheptadine HCl USP, JAN *nonselective piperidine antihistamine for allergic rhinitis and type I hypersensitiv-*

ity reactions; antipruritic; adjunctive anaphylactic therapy; also used for post-traumatic stress disorder (PTSD) [also: cyproheptadine] 4 mg oral; 2 mg/5 mL oral

cyprolidol INN *antidepressant* [also: cyprolidol HCl]

cyprolidol HCl USAN *antidepressant* [also: cyprolidol]

cyproquinate USAN *coccidiostat for poultry* [also: ciproquinate]

cyproterone INN, BAN *antiandrogen* [also: cyproterone acetate]

cyproterone acetate USAN *antiandrogen; investigational (orphan) for severe hirsutism* [also: cyproterone]

cyproximide USAN *antipsychotic; antidepressant* [also: ciproximide]

cyren A [see: diethylstilbestrol]

cyren B [see: diethylstilbestrol dipropionate]

cyromazine INN, BAN ② Seromycin

Cystadane powder for oral solution ℞ *electrolyte replenisher for homocystinuria (orphan)* [betaine HCl] 1 g

Cystagon capsules ℞ *antiurolithic for nephropathic cystinosis (orphan)* [cysteamine bitartrate] 50, 150 mg

cystamin [see: methenamine]

cysteamine USAN, BAN *antiurolithic for nephropathic cystinosis (orphan)* [also: mercaptamine]

cysteamine bitartrate *antiurolithic for nephropathic cystinosis (orphan)*

cysteamine HCl USAN *antiurolithic; investigational (orphan) for corneal cystine crystal accumulation in cystinosis patients*

cysteine (L-cysteine) INN *nonessential amino acid; symbols: Cys, C; investigational (orphan) for erythropoietic protoporphyria photosensitivity* [also: cysteine HCl]

cysteine HCl (L-cysteine HCl) USP *nonessential amino acid* [also: cysteine] 50 mg/mL injection

L-cysteine HCl monohydrate [see: cysteine HCl]

Cystex tablets ℞ *urinary antibiotic; analgesic; acidifier* [methenamine;

sodium salicylate; benzoic acid] 162•162.5•32 mg

cystic fibrosis gene therapy *investigational (orphan) for cystic fibrosis*

cystic fibrosis transmembrane conductance regulator (CFTR) *investigational (orphan) for cystic fibrosis*

cystic fibrosis transmembrane conductance regulator, recombinant adenovirus (AdGV-CFTR) *investigational (orphan) for cystic fibrosis*

cystine (L-cystine) USAN *amino acid* ② Sustain; Systane

Cysto-Conray; Cysto-Conray II intracavitary instillation (discontinued 2005) ℞ *radiopaque contrast medium for urological imaging* [iothalamate meglumine (47% iodine)] 430 mg/mL (202 mg/mL); 172 mg/mL (81 mg/mL)

cystogen [see: methenamine]

Cystografin; Cystografin Dilute intracavitary instillation ℞ *radiopaque contrast medium for urological imaging* [diatrizoate meglumine (46.67% iodine)] 300 mg/mL (141 mg/mL); 180 mg/mL (85 mg/mL)

Cystospaz tablets ℞ *GI/GU antispasmodic; antiparkinsonian; anticholinergic "drying agent" for allergic rhinitis and hyperhidrosis* [hyoscyamine sulfate] 0.15 mg

Cystospaz-M timed-release capsules (discontinued 2004) ℞ *GI/GU antispasmodic; antiparkinsonian; anticholinergic "drying agent" for allergic rhinitis and hyperhidrosis* [hyoscyamine sulfate] 0.375 mg

CYTABOM (cytarabine, bleomycin, Oncovin, mechlorethamine) *chemotherapy protocol*

Cytadren tablets (discontinued 2008) ℞ *adrenal steroid inhibitor; antisteroidal antineoplastic for corticotropin-producing tumors* [aminoglutethimide] 250 mg

cytarabine USAN, USP, INN, BAN *antimetabolite antineoplastic for various leukemias* 100, 500, 1000, 2000 mg injection

cytarabine, liposomal *antimetabolite antineoplastic for lymphomatous neoplastic meningitis (NM) arising from solid tumors or non-Hodgkin lymphoma (orphan)*

cytarabine HCl USAN *antiviral*

Cytisus scoparius medicinal herb [see: broom]

CytoGam IV infusion ℞ *prevention of primary cytomegalovirus in bone marrow and organ transplants from a CMV seropositive donor to an immunocompromised CMV seronegative recipient (orphan)* [cytomegalovirus immune globulin, solvent/detergent treated] 50 mg/mL

CytoImplant *investigational (orphan) agent for pancreatic cancer* [blood mononuclear cells, allogenic peripheral]

Cytoimplant *investigational (orphan) treatment for pancreatic cancer* [peripheral blood mononuclear cells]

cytolin *investigational (Phase I/II) monoclonal antibody for AIDS*

cytomegalovirus immune globulin (CMV-IG), human *prevention of primary cytomegalovirus in bone marrow and organ transplants from a CMV seropositive donor to an immunocompromised CMV seronegative recipient (orphan)*

cytomegalovirus immune globulin intravenous (CMV-IGIV) & ganciclovir sodium *investigational (orphan) for cytomegalovirus pneumonia in bone marrow transplant patients*

Cytomel tablets ℞ *synthetic thyroid hormone (T$_3$ fraction only)* [liothyronine sodium] 5, 25, 50 mcg

cytoprotective agents *a class of drugs that provide prophylaxis against the side effects of antineoplastic agents*

Cytosar-U powder for subcu, intrathecal or IV injection (discontinued 2005) ℞ *antimetabolite antineoplastic for various leukemias* [cytarabine] 100, 500, 1000, 2000 mg/vial

cytosine arabinoside (ara-C) [see: cytarabine]

cytosine arabinoside HCl [now: cytarabine HCl]

Cytosol topical liquid ℞ *for general irrigating, washing, and rinsing* [physiological irrigating solution]

Cytotec tablets ℞ *prevents NSAID-induced gastric ulcers; has been used for cervical ripening and induction of labor; use by pregnant women can cause abortion, premature birth, or birth defects* [misoprostol] 100, 200 mcg

cytotoxic lymphocyte maturation factor [see: edodekin alfa]

Cytovene capsules ℞ *antiviral for AIDS-related cytomegalovirus (CMV) infections (orphan) and CMV retinitis (orphan)* [ganciclovir] 250, 500 mg ⊡ Cetafen

Cytovene powder for IV infusion ℞ *antiviral for AIDS-related cytomegalovirus (CMV) infections (orphan)* [ganciclovir sodium] 500 mg/vial ⊡ Cetafen

Cytoxan tablets, powder for IV injection (discontinued 2008) ℞ *nitrogen mustard-type alkylating antineoplastic for multiple leukemias, lymphomas, blastomas, sarcomas and organ cancers* [cyclophosphamide] 25, 50 mg; 100 mg

Cytra-2 solution ℞ *urinary alkalizing agent* [sodium citrate; citric acid] 500•334 mg/5 mL ⊡ Zetar

Cytra-3 syrup ℞ *urinary alkalinizing agent* [potassium citrate; sodium citrate; citric acid] 550•500•334 mg/5 mL ⊡ Zetar

Cytra-K oral solution ℞ *urinary alkalizing agent* [potassium citrate; citric acid] 1100•334 mg/5 mL

Cytra-LC solution ℞ *urinary alkalizer* [potassium citrate; sodium citrate; citric acid] 550•500•334 mg/5 mL

Cytuss HC; Cytuss HC NR oral liquid ℞ *narcotic antitussive; antihistamine; decongestant* [hydrocodone bitartrate; chlorpheniramine maleate; phenylephrine HCl] 2.5•2•5 mg/5 mL; 2.5•1•5 mg/5 mL

CY-VA-DACT (Cytoxin, vincristine, Adriamycin, dactinomycin) *chemotherapy protocol*
CYVADIC; CY-VA-DIC; CyVADIC (cyclophosphamide, vincristine, **Adriamycin, DIC)** *chemotherapy protocol for bone and soft tissue sarcomas*
CYVMAD (cyclophosphamide, vincristine, methotrexate, Adriamycin, DTIC) *chemotherapy protocol*

D (vitamin D) [q.v.]
D-2.5-W; D-5-W; D-10-W; D-20-W; D-25-W; D-30-W; D-40-W; D-50-W; D-60-W; D-70-W ℞ *intravenous nutritional therapy* [dextrose]
D₂ (vitamin D₂) [see: ergocalciferol]
D₃ (vitamin D₃) [see: cholecalciferol]
d4T [see: stavudine]
D.A. chewable tablets ℞ *decongestant; antihistamine; anticholinergic to dry mucosal secretions* [phenylephrine HCl; chlorpheniramine maleate; methscopolamine nitrate] 10•2•1.25 mg
DA (daunorubicin, ara-C) *chemotherapy protocol for acute myelocytic leukemia (AML)*
D.A. II tablets (discontinued 2006) ℞ *decongestant; antihistamine; anticholinergic to dry mucosal secretions* [phenylephrine HCl; chlorpheniramine maleate; methscopolamine nitrate] 10•4•1.25 mg
DAA (dihydroxyaluminum aminoacetate) [q.v.]
dabigatran etexilate *direct thrombin inhibitor; investigational (Phase III) oral anticoagulant for the prevention of deep vein thrombosis (DVT) or other venous thromboembolism (VTE) following total hip or total knee replacement surgery*
dacarbazine USAN, USP, INN, BAN *alkylating antineoplastic for metastatic malignant melanoma and Hodgkin disease* 100, 200 mg injection
dacemazine INN ⊉ duazomycin
Dacex-A oral drops (discontinued 2007) ℞ *antitussive; antihistamine;* *decongestant; for children 3–24 months* [dextromethorphan hydrobromide; carbinoxamine maleate; phenylephrine HCl] 4•1•2 mg/mL ⊉ Desoxi; Diskus
Dacex-DM syrup ℞ *antitussive; decongestant; expectorant* [dextromethorphan hydrobromide; phenylephrine HCl; guaifenesin] 25•12.5•175 mg/5 mL
Dacex-PE extended-release caplets ℞ *antitussive; decongestant; expectorant* [dextromethorphan hydrobromide; phenylephrine HCl; guaifenesin] 30•10•600 mg
dacisteine INN
dacliximab [now: daclizumab]
daclizumab USAN, INN, BAN *immunosuppressant; monoclonal antibody (MAb) to prevent acute rejection of organ and bone marrow transplants (orphan)*
Dacogen IV infusion ℞ *antineoplastic for myelodysplastic syndromes (MDS; orphan); investigational (NDA filed, orphan) for chronic myelogenous leukemia and sickle cell anemia; investigational (Phase III) for multiple myeloma* [decitabine] 50 mg
Dacriose ophthalmic solution OTC *extraocular irrigating solution* [sterile isotonic solution]
dactinomycin USAN, USP, BAN *antibiotic antineoplastic for various tumors, carcinomas, and sarcomas; potentiator for radiation therapy* [also: actinomycin D]
dacuronium bromide INN, BAN
DADDS (diacetyl diaminodiphenylsulfone) [see: acedapsone]

dagapamil INN

daidzein *one of several soy isoflavones that provide cell-protective effects*

daidzin *isoform precursor to daidzein* [q.v.]

Daily Vitamins oral liquid OTC *vitamin supplement* [multiple vitamins]

Daily-Vite with Iron & Minerals tablets OTC *vitamin/mineral/iron supplement* [multiple vitamins & minerals; iron; folic acid; biotin] ±•18•0.4•± mg

Dairy Ease chewable tablets OTC *digestive aid for lactose intolerance* [lactase enzyme] 3000 U ☒ Diurese; Dry Eyes; DUROS

daisy, wild *medicinal herb* [see: wild daisy]

Dakin solution [see: sodium hypochlorite]

Dalalone intra-articular, intralesional, soft tissue, or IM injection ℞ *corticosteroid; anti-inflammatory* [dexamethasone sodium phosphate] 4 mg/mL

Dalalone D.P. intra-articular, soft tissue, or IM injection ℞ *corticosteroid; anti-inflammatory* [dexamethasone acetate] 16 mg/mL

Dalalone L.A. intralesional, intra-articular, soft tissue, or IM injection ℞ *corticosteroid; anti-inflammatory* [dexamethasone acetate] 8 mg/mL

dalanated insulin [see: insulin, dalanated]

dalbavancin *glycopeptide antibiotic for anaerobic and gram-positive aerobic bacteria; investigational (NDA filed) once-weekly treatment for methicillin-resistant* Staphylococcus aureus *(MRSA) and methicillin-resistant* S. epidermidis *(MRSE)*

dalbraminol INN

daledalin INN *antidepressant* [also: daledalin tosylate]

daledalin tosylate USAN *antidepressant* [also: daledalin]

dalfopristin USAN, INN *streptogramin antibacterial antibiotic for life-threatening infections*

dalfopristin & quinupristin *two streptogramin antibiotics that are syner-gistically bactericidal to gram-positive infections; investigational (NDA filed) for pneumonia*

Dallergy oral drops ℞ *decongestant; antihistamine; for children 1–24 months* [phenylephrine HCl; chlorpheniramine maleate] 2•1 mg/mL ☒ Dolorac

Dallergy sustained-release caplets (discontinued 2007) ℞ *decongestant; antihistamine; anticholinergic to dry mucosal secretions* [phenylephrine HCl; chlorpheniramine maleate; methscopolamine nitrate] 20•12•2.5 mg ☒ Dolorac

Dallergy tablets, syrup ℞ *decongestant; antihistamine; anticholinergic to dry mucosal secretions* [phenylephrine HCl; chlorpheniramine maleate; methscopolamine nitrate] 10•4•1.25 mg; 8•2•0.75 mg/5 mL ☒ Dolorac

Dallergy DM syrup ℞ *antitussive; decongestant; antihistamine* [dextromethorphan hydrobromide; pseudoephedrine HCl; brompheniramine maleate] 15•30•3 mg/5 mL

Dallergy-JR extended-release capsules, oral suspension ℞ *decongestant; antihistamine* [phenylephrine HCl; chlorpheniramine maleate] 20•4 mg; 20•4 mg/5 mL

Dalmane capsules ℞ *benzodiazepine sedative and hypnotic; anticonvulsant; muscle relaxant; also abused as a street drug* [flurazepam HCl] 15, 30 mg ☒ Dilomine; diolamine

d′Alpha E 400 softgels (discontinued 2004) OTC *vitamin supplement* [vitamin E (as d-alpha tocopherol)] 400 IU

d′Alpha E 1000 softgels OTC *vitamin supplement* [vitamin E (as d-alpha tocopherol)] 1000 IU

dalteparin sodium USAN, INN, BAN *a low molecular weight heparin–type anticoagulant and antithrombotic for prevention of deep vein thrombosis (DVT), venous thromboembolism (VTE), unstable angina, and myocardial infarction*

daltroban USAN, INN *immunosuppressive*

Damason-P tablets ℞ *narcotic analgesic; antipyretic* [hydrocodone bitartrate; aspirin] 5•500 mg

dambose [see: inositol]

dametralast INN

damiana *(Turnera aphrodisiaca; T. diffusa; T. microphylla)* leaves *medicinal herb for bed-wetting, bronchitis, emphysema, headache, hormonal imbalance, hot flashes, menopause, and Parkinson disease; also used as an aphrodisiac*

damotepine INN

danaparoid sodium USAN, BAN *glycosaminoglycan anticoagulant and antithrombotic for prevention of deep vein thrombosis (DVT)*

danazol USAN, USP, INN, BAN *anterior pituitary suppressant; gonadotropin inhibitor for endometriosis, fibrocystic breast disease, and hereditary angioedema* 50, 100, 200 mg oral

dandelion *(Leontodon taraxacum; Taraxacum officinale)* leaves and root *medicinal herb for anemia, analgesia, blisters, blood cleansing, blood glucose regulation, constipation, diaphoresis, dyspepsia, edema, endurance, gallbladder disease, hypertension, and liver disorders*

daniplestim USAN *treatment for chemotherapy-induced bone marrow suppression*

daniquidone BAN

danitamon [see: menadione]

danitracen INN

Danocrine capsules (discontinued 2005) ℞ *gonadotropin inhibitor for endometriosis, fibrocystic breast disease, and hereditary angioedema* [danazol] 50, 100, 200 mg

danofloxacin INN *veterinary antibacterial* [also: danofloxacin mesylate]

danofloxacin mesylate USAN *veterinary antibacterial* [also: danofloxacin]

danosteine INN

danshen *(Salvia miltiorrhiza)* medicinal herb for abdominal pain, bruises, circulatory problems, insomnia, menstrual irregularity, and stroke; also used as an aid in granulation of wounds

danthron USP, BAN *(withdrawn from market by FDA)* [also: dantron]

Dantrium capsules, powder for IV injection ℞ *skeletal muscle relaxant; investigational (orphan) for neuroleptic malignant syndrome* [dantrolene sodium] 25, 50, 100 mg; 20 mg/vial (0.32 mg/mL)

dantrolene USAN, INN, BAN *skeletal muscle relaxant*

dantrolene sodium USAN, BAN *skeletal muscle relaxant; investigational (orphan) for neuroleptic malignant syndrome* 25, 50, 100 mg oral; 20 mg injection

dantron INN *(withdrawn from market by FDA)* [also: danthron]

dapagliflozin *investigational (Phase III) sodium glucose uptake transporter 2 (SGLT-2) inhibitor for diabetes*

Daphne mezereum *medicinal herb* [see: mezereon]

dapiprazole INN *α-adrenergic blocker; miotic; neuroleptic* [also: dapiprazole HCl]

dapoxetine *investigational (NDA filed) selective serotonin reuptake inhibitor (SSRI) for various urogenital indications, including moderate to severe premature ejaculation (PE)*

dapsone USAN, USP, BAN *antibacterial for acne vulgaris; leprostatic; herpetiform dermatitis suppressant; investigational (Phase III, orphan) for Pneumocystis pneumonia (PCP) and toxoplasmosis* 25, 100 mg oral

dapsone & trimethoprim *investigational (Phase III) for Pneumocystis pneumonia (PCP)*

Daptacel IM injection ℞ *active immunizing agent for diphtheria, tetanus, and pertussis; Dtap (diphtheria predominant) vaccine used in the initial immunization series of infants and children 6 weeks to 6 years* [diphtheria toxoid; tetanus toxoid; acellular pertussis toxoid (DTaP vaccine)] 15 Lf• 5 Lf•10 mcg per 0.5 mL dose

daptazole [see: amiphenazole]

daptomycin USAN, INN, BAN *cyclic lipopeptide antibiotic for complicated skin and skin structure infections (cSSSIs),* Staphylococcus aureus *bloodstream infections, and right-sided endocarditis*

Daranide tablets (discontinued 2004) ℞ *carbonic anhydrase inhibitor; diuretic* [dichlorphenamide] 50 mg

Daraprim tablets ℞ *antimalarial; toxoplasmosis treatment adjunct* [pyrimethamine] 25 mg

darbepoetin alfa USAN *erythropoiesis-stimulating agent (ESA); recombinant human erythropoietin for anemia associated with chronic renal failure or chemotherapy for nonmyeloid malignancies*

darbufelone mesylate USAN *anti-inflammatory; antiarthritic; cyclooxygenase inhibitor; 5-lipoxygenase inhibitor*

darenzepine INN

darglitazone sodium USAN *oral hypoglycemic*

darifenacin hydrobromide *selective muscarinic M₃ receptor antagonist for urinary frequency, urgency, and incontinence*

darodipine USAN, INN *antihypertensive; bronchodilator; vasodilator*

darunavir ethanolate *antiretroviral protease inhibitor for HIV-1 infections*

Darvocet A500 film-coated tablets ℞ *narcotic analgesic; antipyretic* [propoxyphene napsylate; acetaminophen] 100•500 mg

Darvocet-N 50; Darvocet-N 100 tablets ℞ *narcotic analgesic; antipyretic* [propoxyphene napsylate; acetaminophen] 50•325 mg; 100•650 mg

Darvon Pulvules (capsules) ℞ *narcotic analgesic for mild to moderate pain* [propoxyphene HCl] 65 mg ② Duraphen II

Darvon Compound 32 Pulvules (capsules) (discontinued 2007) ℞ *narcotic analgesic; antipyretic* [propoxyphene HCl; aspirin; caffeine] 32•389•32.4 mg

Darvon Compound 65 Pulvules (capsules) ℞ *narcotic analgesic; antipyretic* [propoxyphene HCl; aspirin; caffeine] 65•389•32.4 mg

Darvon-N film-coated tablets ℞ *narcotic analgesic for mild to moderate pain* [propoxyphene napsylate] 100 mg ② Duraphen II

dasatinib *multiple tyrosine kinase inhibitor; antineoplastic for chronic myeloid leukemia (CML) and Philadelphia chromosome–positive acute lymphoblastic leukemia (Ph+ ALL)*

DaT (daunorubicin, ara-C, thioguanine) *chemotherapy protocol for acute myelocytic leukemia (AML)* [also: DCT; TAD]

datelliptium chloride INN

Datura stramonium medicinal herb [see: jimsonweed]

daturine hydrobromide [see: hyoscyamine hydrobromide]

DaTVP (daunorubicin, ara-C, thioguanine, vincristine, prednisone) *chemotherapy protocol*

Daucus carota medicinal herb [see: carrot]

daunomycin [see: daunorubicin HCl]

daunorubicin (DNR) INN, BAN *anthracycline antibiotic antineoplastic for various leukemias* [also: daunorubicin HCl]

daunorubicin citrate, liposomal *anthracycline antibiotic antineoplastic for advanced HIV-related Kaposi sarcoma (orphan)*

daunorubicin HCl USAN, USP, JAN *anthracycline antibiotic antineoplastic for various leukemias* [also: daunorubicin] 20, 50 mg injection

DaunoXome IV infusion ℞ *antibiotic antineoplastic for advanced AIDS-related Kaposi sarcoma (orphan)* [daunorubicin citrate, liposomal] 2 mg/mL (50 mg/dose)

DAV (daunorubicin, ara-C, VePesid) *chemotherapy protocol for acute myelocytic leukemia (AML)*

DAVA (desacetyl vinblastine amide) [see: vindesine]

DAVH (dibromodulcitol, Adriamycin, vincristine, Halotestin) *chemotherapy protocol*

davitamon [see: menadione]

Daxas *investigational (Phase III) agent for chronic obstructive pulmonary disease (COPD) and asthma* [roflumilast]

Dayalets Filmtabs (film-coated tablets) OTC *vitamin supplement* [multiple vitamins; folic acid] ± •0.4 mg

Dayalets + Iron Filmtabs (film-coated tablets) OTC *vitamin/iron supplement* [multiple vitamins; ferrous sulfate; folic acid] ± •18•0.4 mg

Dayhist-1 tablets OTC *antihistamine for allergic rhinitis and urticaria* [clemastine fumarate] 1.34 mg ⊠ Duohist DH

Daypro film-coated caplets ℞ *analgesic; nonsteroidal anti-inflammatory drug (NSAID) for osteoarthritis and rheumatoid arthritis* [oxaprozin] 600 mg ⊠ Dopar

Daypro Alta film-coated caplets ℞ *analgesic; nonsteroidal anti-inflammatory drug (NSAID) for osteoarthritis and rheumatoid arthritis* [oxaprozin potassium] 678 mg (600 mg base)

DayQuil Multi-Symptom Cold/Flu Relief LiquiCaps (liquid-filled gelcaps), oral liquid OTC *antitussive; decongestant; analgesic; antipyretic* [dextromethorphan hydrobromide; phenylephrine HCl; acetaminophen] 10•5•325 mg; 10•5•325 mg/15 mL

DayQuil Sinus Liqui-caps (liquid-filled gelcaps) OTC *decongestant; analgesic; antipyretic* [phenylephrine HCl; acetaminophen] 5•325 mg

Daytime Sinus Relief Non-Drowsy caplets (discontinued 2007) OTC *decongestant; analgesic; antipyretic* [pseudoephedrine HCl; acetaminophen] 30•500 mg

Daytrana transdermal patch ℞ *CNS stimulant for attention-deficit/hyperactivity disorder (ADHD)* [methylphenidate] 10, 15, 20, 30 mg/day

dazadrol INN *antidepressant* [also: dazadrol maleate]

dazadrol maleate USAN *antidepressant* [also: dazadrol]

Dazamide tablets (discontinued 2005) ℞ *carbonic anhydrase inhibitor diuretic; treatment for acute mountain sickness* [acetazolamide] 250 mg

dazepinil INN *antidepressant* [also: dazepinil HCl]

dazepinil HCl USAN *antidepressant* [also: dazepinil]

dazidamine INN

dazmegrel USAN, INN, BAN *thromboxane synthetase inhibitor*

dazolicine INN

dazopride INN *peristaltic stimulant* [also: dazopride fumarate]

dazopride fumarate USAN *peristaltic stimulant* [also: dazopride]

dazoquinast INN

dazoxiben INN, BAN *antithrombotic* [also: dazoxiben HCl]

dazoxiben HCl USAN *antithrombotic* [also: dazoxiben]

DBED (dibenzylethylenediamine dipenicillin G) [see: penicillin G benzathine]

DBM (dibromomannitol) [see: mitobronitol]

DC softgels OTC *laxative; stool softener* [docusate calcium] 240 mg

DC (daunorubicin, cytarabine) *chemotherapy protocol*

D&C Brown No. 1 (drugs & cosmetics) [see: resorcin brown]

DCA (desoxycorticosterone acetate) [q.v.]

DCA (dichloroacetate) [see: sodium dichloroacetate]

DCF (2'-deoxycoformycin) [see: pentostatin]

DCL (descarboethoxyloratadine) [q.v.]

DCMP (daunorubicin, cytarabine, mercaptopurine, prednisone) *chemotherapy protocol*

DCPM (daunorubicin, cytarabine, prednisone, mercaptopurine) *chemotherapy protocol*

DCT (daunorubicin, cytarabine, thioguanine) *chemotherapy protocol*

for acute myelocytic leukemia (AML) [also: DaT; TAD]

DCV (DTIC, CCNU, vincristine) *chemotherapy protocol*

DCVax-Brain *investigational (Phase II, orphan) vaccine for glioblastoma multiforme* [dendritic cells pulsed with glioblastoma multiforme acid-eluted tumor antigens]

DCVax-Prostate *investigational (Phase II, orphan) vaccine for prostate cancer*

DDAVP tablets, nasal spray, rhinal tube, subcu or IV injection ℞ *posterior pituitary hormone for hemophilia A (orphan), von Willebrand disease (orphan), central diabetes insipidus, and nocturnal enuresis* [desmopressin acetate] 0.1, 0.2 mg; 10 mcg/dose; 0.1 mg/mL; 15 mcg/mL ☑ DVB; DVP

DDAVP (1-deamino-8-D-arginine-vasopressin) [see: desmopressin acetate]

DDC; ddC (dideoxycytidine) [see: zalcitabine]

*o,p'-***DDD** [now: mitotane]

DDI; ddI (dideoxyinosine) [see: didanosine]

DDP; *cis*-DDP (diamminedichloroplatinum) [see: cisplatin]

DDS (diaminodiphenylsulfone) [now: dapsone]

DDT (dichlorodiphenyltrichloroethane) [see: chlorophenothane]

DDVP (dichlorovinyl dimethyl phosphate) [see: dichlorvos]

DEA (diethanolamine) [q.v.]

deacetyllanatoside C [see: deslanoside]

17-deacylnorgestimate [see: norelgestromin]

deadly nightshade *medicinal herb* [see: belladonna]

deadly nightshade leaf [see: belladonna extract]

DEAE-rebeccamycin *investigational (orphan) for bile duct tumors*

deal pine *medicinal herb* [see: white pine]

1-deamino-8-D-arginine-vasopressin (DDAVP) [see: desmopressin acetate]

deanil INN *combining name for radicals or groups*

deanol BAN [also: deanol aceglumate]

deanol aceglumate INN [also: deanol]

deanol acetamidobenzoate

deba [see: barbital]

Debacterol oral solution with swab applicator ℞ *antiseptic and analgesic for ulcerating mouth and gum lesions such as aphthous ulcers (canker sores) and necrotizing ulcerative gingivitis (pyorrhea)* [sulfuric acid; sulfonated phenolics] 30%•50%

deboxamet INN

debrase *investigational (orphan) agent for debridement of acute, deep dermal burns*

Debridase *investigational (orphan) agent for debridement of acute, deep dermal burns* [debrase]

Debrisan beads, paste ℞ *debrider and cleanser for wet wounds* [dextranomer] ☑ Diprosone

debrisoquin sulfate USAN *antihypertensive* [also: debrisoquine]

debrisoquine INN, BAN *antihypertensive* [also: debrisoquin sulfate]

Debrox ear drops OTC *cerumenolytic to emulsify and disperse ear wax* [carbamide peroxide] 6.5%

Decadron tablets ℞ *corticosteroidal anti-inflammatory* [dexamethasone] 0.5, 0.75 mg

Decadron Phosphate intra-articular, intralesional, soft tissue or IM injection ℞ *corticosteroidal anti-inflammatory* [dexamethasone sodium phosphate] 4 mg/mL

Decadron Phosphate IV injection ℞ *corticosteroidal anti-inflammatory* [dexamethasone sodium phosphate] 24 mg/mL

Decadron Phosphate Ocumeter (eye drops) (discontinued 2006) ℞ *corticosteroidal anti-inflammatory* [dexamethasone sodium phosphate] 0.1%

Decadron with Xylocaine soft tissue injection ℞ *corticosteroidal anti-inflammatory; anesthetic* [dexamethasone sodium phosphate; lidocaine HCl] 4•10 mg/mL

Decadron-LA intralesional, intra-articular, soft tissue, or IM injection (discontinued 2004) ℞ *corticosteroidal anti-inflammatory* [dexamethasone acetate] 8 mg/mL

Deca-Durabolin IM injection (discontinued 2005) ℞ *anabolic steroid for anemia of renal insufficiency; sometimes abused as a street drug* [nandrolone decanoate (in oil)] 100, 200 mg/mL

Decagen tablets OTC *vitamin/mineral/iron supplement* [multiple vitamins & minerals; iron; folic acid; biotin] ± • 18 mg•0.4 mg•30 mcg

Decaject intra-articular, intralesional, soft tissue, or IM injection ℞ *corticosteroidal anti-inflammatory* [dexamethasone sodium phosphate] 4 mg/mL

Decaject-L.A. intralesional, intra-articular, soft tissue, or IM injection ℞ *corticosteroidal anti-inflammatory* [dexamethasone acetate] 8 mg/mL

DECAL (dexamethasone, etoposide, cisplatin, ara-C, L-asparaginase) *chemotherapy protocol* ② Dical

decamethonium bromide USP, INN [also: decamethonium iodide]

decamethonium iodide BAN [also: decamethonium bromide]

Decapinol oral rinse ℞ *gingivitis treatment*

decapinol [see: delmopinol]

Decavac IM injection ℞ *active immunizing agent for diphtheria and tetanus* [diphtheria & tetanus toxoids, adsorbed] 2•5 LfU per 0.5 mL dose

decavitamin USP

De-Chlor HC; De-Chlor HD oral liquid ℞ *narcotic antitussive; antihistamine; decongestant* [hydrocodone bitartrate; chlorpheniramine maleate; phenylephrine HCl] 2.5•2•10 mg/5 mL; 2.5•4•10 mg/5 mL

De-Chlor NX oral liquid ℞ *narcotic antitussive; expectorant* [hydrocodone bitartrate; potassium guaiacolsulfonate] 3•150 mg/5 mL

Decholin tablets OTC *laxative; hydrocholeretic* [dehydrocholic acid] 250 mg ② Dyclone

decicain [see: tetracaine HCl]

decil INN *combining name for radicals or groups* ② Dicel

decimemide INN

decitabine USAN, INN, BAN *DNA synthesis inhibitor; antineoplastic for myelodysplastic syndromes (MDS; orphan); investigational (NDA filed, orphan) for chronic myelogenous leukemia and sickle cell anemia; investigational (Phase III) for multiple myeloma*

decitropine INN

declaben [now: lodelaben]

declenperone USAN, INN *veterinary sedative*

Declomycin film-coated tablets ℞ *broad-spectrum antibiotic* [demeclocycline HCl] 150, 300 mg

decloxizine INN

Decodult tablets (discontinued 2007) OTC *decongestant; antihistamine; analgesic; antipyretic* [phenylephrine HCl; chlorpheniramine maleate; acetaminophen] 5•2•300 mg

Decofed syrup OTC *nasal decongestant* [pseudoephedrine HCl] 30 mg/5 mL

Decohistine DH oral liquid (discontinued 2007) ℞ *narcotic antitussive; antihistamine; decongestant* [codeine phosphate; chlorpheniramine maleate; pseudoephedrine HCl; alcohol 5.8%] 10•2•30 mg/5 mL

Decolate tablets (discontinued 2007) ℞ *decongestant; antihistamine; expectorant* [phenylephrine HCl; chlorpheniramine maleate; guaifenesin] 5•4•100 mg

decominol INN

Deconamine tablets (discontinued 2007) ℞ *decongestant; antihistamine* [pseudoephedrine HCl; chlorpheniramine maleate] 60•4 mg

Deconamine syrup ℞ *decongestant; antihistamine* [pseudoephedrine HCl; chlorpheniramine maleate] 30•2 mg/5 mL

Deconamine SR sustained-release capsules ℞ *decongestant; antihistamine* [pseudoephedrine HCl; chlorpheniramine maleate] 120•8 mg

Deconex DM extended-release tablets ℞ *antitussive; decongestant; expectorant* [dextromethorphan hydrobromide; phenylephrine HCl; guaifenesin] 30•30•900 mg

Deconomed SR sustained-release capsules ℞ *decongestant; antihistamine* [pseudoephedrine HCl; chlorpheniramine maleate] 120•8 mg

Deconsal II extended-release capsules (discontinued 2007) ℞ *decongestant; expectorant* [phenylephrine HCl; guaifenesin] 20•375 mg ⓢ doconazole

Deconsal II extended-release tablets ℞ *decongestant; expectorant* [phenylephrine HCl; guaifenesin] 25•275 mg ⓢ doconazole

decoquinate USAN, INN, BAN *coccidiostat for poultry*

dectaflur USAN, INN *dental caries prophylactic*

Decylenes ointment OTC *antifungal* [undecylenic acid; zinc undecylenate]

deditonium bromide INN

Deep-Down Rub OTC *analgesic; mild anesthetic; antipruritic; counterirritant* [methyl salicylate; menthol; camphor] 15%•5%•0.5%

deer musk *(Moschus moschiferus) natural remedy in ancient Chinese medicine; reported to have antianginal, antibacterial, antihistaminic, antiinflammatory, CNS-depressant, and stimulant activity in clinical studies*

deerberry *medicinal herb* [see: holly; squaw vine; wintergreen]

DEET (diethyltoluamide) [q.v.]

Defen-LA sustained-release tablets (discontinued 2004) ℞ *decongestant; expectorant* [pseudoephedrine HCl; guaifenesin] 60•600 mg

deferasirox *oral iron chelating agent for chronic iron overload due to blood transfusions (orphan)*

deferiprone *investigational (orphan) agent for chronic iron overload due to transfusion-dependent anemias*

deferitrin *investigational (orphan) for iron overload*

deferoxamine USAN, INN *chelating agent for acute or chronic iron poisoning* [also: desferrioxamine]

deferoxamine HCl USAN *chelating agent for acute or chronic iron poisoning*

deferoxamine mesylate USAN, USP *chelating agent for acute or chronic iron poisoning* [also: desferrioxamine mesylate] 500, 2000 mg injection

defibrotide BAN *investigational (orphan) agent for thrombotic thrombocytopenic purpura and hepatic veno-occlusive disease*

Definity injection ℞ *radiopaque contrast medium to enhance echocardiography* [perflutren] 6.52 mg/mL

deflazacort USAN, INN, BAN *antiinflammatory*

defosfamide INN

defungit sodium salt [see: bensuldazic acid]

Defy eye drops ℞ *aminoglycoside antibiotic* [tobramycin] 0.3%

degarelix *investigational (Phase III) gonadotropin-releasing hormone (GnRH) blocker for prostate cancer*

Degas chewable tablets OTC *antiflatulent* [simethicone] 80 mg ⓢ Doxy 100

Degest 2 eye drops (discontinued 2006) OTC *decongestant; vasoconstrictor* [naphazoline HCl] 0.012%

Dehistine syrup ℞ *decongestant; antihistamine; anticholinergic to dry mucosal secretions* [phenylephrine HCl; chlorpheniramine maleate; methscopolamine nitrate] 10•2•1.25 mg/5 mL

dehydrated alcohol [see: alcohol, dehydrated]

Dehydrex drops *investigational (orphan) treatment for recurrent corneal erosion* [dextran 70]

dehydroacetic acid NF *preservative*

dehydroandrosterone [see: prasterone]

dehydrocholate sodium USP [also: sodium dehydrocholate]

7-dehydrocholesterol, activated [now: cholecalciferol]

dehydrocholic acid USP, INN, BAN, JAN *choleretic; laxative; investigational (orphan) agent for congenital errors of* *cholesterol and bile acid synthesis* 250 mg oral

dehydrocholin [see: dehydrocholic acid]

dehydroemetine INN, BAN *anti-infective for amebiasis and amebic dysentery*

dehydroepiandrosterone (DHEA) *natural hormone precursor; investigational (NDA filed, orphan) for systemic lupus erythematosus (SLE); investigational (orphan) replacement therapy for adrenal insufficiency*

dehydroepiandrosterone sulfate (DHEAS)

dehydroepiandrosterone sulfate sodium *investigational (orphan) agent for re-epithelialization of serious burns and skin graft donor sites*

Deka oral liquid (discontinued 2007) ℞ *antitussive; antihistamine; decongestant; expectorant* [dextromethorphan hydrobromide; dexbrompheniramine maleate; pseudoephrine HCl; guaifenesin] 30•1•30•200 mg/10 mL

Deka Pediatric oral drops (discontinued 2007) ℞ *antitussive; decongestant; antihistamine; expectorant; for children 1–24 months* [dextromethorphan hydrobromide; pseudoephedrine HCl; dexbrompheniramine maleate; guaifenesin] 4•12.5•0.5•40 mg/mL

delanterone INN

delapril INN *antihypertensive; angiotensin-converting enzyme (ACE) inhibitor* [also: delapril HCl]

delapril HCl USAN *antihypertensive; angiotensin-converting enzyme (ACE) inhibitor* [also: delapril]

Delatestryl IM injection ℞ *androgen replacement for hypogonadism or testosterone deficiency in men, delayed puberty in boys, and metastatic breast cancer in women; hormone replacement therapy (HRT) for postandropausal symptoms; sometimes abused as a street drug* [testosterone enanthate (in oil)] 200 mg/mL

delavirdine INN *antiviral; non-nucleoside reverse transcriptase inhibitor (NNRTI) for HIV and AIDS* [also: delavirdine mesylate]

delavirdine mesylate USAN *antiviral; non-nucleoside reverse transcriptase inhibitor (NNRTI) for HIV-1 infection* [also: delavirdine]

delayed-release aspirin [see: aspirin]

Delcap (trademarked device) *unit dispensing cap*

Delcort cream OTC *corticosteroidal anti-inflammatory* [hydrocortisone] 0.5%, 1%

delequamine INN α_2 *adrenoreceptor antagonist for sexual dysfunction* [also: delequamine HCl]

delequamine HCl USAN α_2 *adrenoreceptor antagonist for sexual dysfunction* [also: delequamine]

delergotrile INN

Delestrogen IM injection ℞ *synthetic estrogen for the treatment of postmenopausal symptoms and prevention of postmenopausal osteoporosis; hormonal antineoplastic for prostate and metastatic breast cancers* [estradiol valerate in oil] 10, 20, 40 mg/mL

delfantrine INN

delfaprazine INN

Delfen Contraceptive vaginal foam OTC *spermicidal contraceptive* [nonoxynol 9] 12.5%

delmadinone INN, BAN *progestin; antiandrogen; antiestrogen* [also: delmadinone acetate]

delmadinone acetate USAN *progestin; antiandrogen; antiestrogen* [also: delmadinone]

delmetacin INN

delmopinol INN

delnav [see: dioxathion]

delorazepam INN

deloxolone INN

m-delphene [see: diethyltoluamide]

delprostenate INN, BAN

Delsym extended-release oral suspension OTC *antitussive* [dextromethorphan polistirex] 30 mg/5 mL

Delta-Cortef tablets (discontinued 2005) ℞ *corticosteroid; anti-inflammatory* [prednisolone] 5 mg

deltacortone [see: prednisone]

Delta-D tablets OTC *vitamin supplement* [cholecalciferol (vitamin D₃)] 400 IU

deltafilcon A USAN *hydrophilic contact lens material*

deltafilcon B USAN *hydrophilic contact lens material*

delta-1-hydrocortisone [see: prednisolone]

Deltasone tablets (discontinued 2008) ℞ *corticosteroid; anti-inflammatory* [prednisone] 2.5, 5, 10, 20 mg

delta-9-tetrahydrocannabinol (THC) [see: dronabinol]

delta-9-THC (tetrahydrocannabinol) [see: dronabinol]

Delta-Tritex cream, ointment ℞ *corticosteroidal anti-inflammatory* [triamcinolone acetonide] 0.1%

Deltavac vaginal cream ℞ *broad-spectrum antibiotic; antiseptic; moisturizer/lubricant* [sulfanilamide; aminacrine HCl; allantoin] 15%•0.2%•2%

deltibant USAN *bradykinin antagonist for treatment of systemic inflammatory response syndrome*

deltra-stab [see: prednisolone]

delucemine HCl USAN *NMDA receptor antagonist; neuroprotectant*

Demadex tablets, IV injection ℞ *antihypertensive; loop diuretic* [torsemide] 5, 10, 20, 100 mg; 10 mg/mL

dembrexine INN, BAN

dembroxol [see: dembrexine]

demecarium bromide USP, INN, BAN *antiglaucoma agent; reversible cholinesterase inhibitor miotic*

demeclocycline USP, BAN *tetracycline antibiotic*

demeclocycline HCl USP, BAN *tetracycline antibiotic; antirickettsial* 150, 300 mg oral

demecolcine INN, BAN

demecycline USAN, INN *antibacterial*

demegestone INN

demekastigmine bromide [see: demecarium bromide]

demelverine INN

Demerol tablets, syrup, IV or IM injection ℞ *narcotic analgesic; also*

abused as a street drug [meperidine HCl] 50, 100 mg; 50 mg/5 mL; 25, 50, 75, 100 mg/mL

demetacin [see: delmetacin]

11-demethoxyreserpine [see: deserpidine]

demethylchlortetracycline (DMCT) [now: demeclocycline]

demethylchlortetracycline HCl [see: demeclocycline HCl]

N-demethylcodeine [see: norcodeine]

demexiptiline INN

Demi-Regroton tablets (discontinued 2007) ℞ *antihypertensive; diuretic* [chlorthalidone; reserpine] 25•0.125 mg

democonazole INN

demoxepam USAN, INN *minor tranquilizer*

demoxytocin INN

Demser capsules ℞ *antihypertensive for pheochromocytoma* [metyrosine] 250 mg

demulcents *a class of agents that soothe irritated or abraded tissues, particularly mucous membranes*

Demulen 1/35; Demulen 1/50 tablets (in Compacks of 21 or 28) (discontinued 2008) ℞ *monophasic oral contraceptive* [ethynodiol diacetate; ethinyl estradiol] 1 mg•35 mcg; 1 mg•50 mcg

denatonium benzoate USAN, NF, INN, BAN *alcohol denaturant; flavoring agent*

denaverine INN

Denavir cream ℞ *antiviral for recurrent herpes labialis* [penciclovir] 1%

Denaze oral liquid ℞ *decongestant; antihistamine; anticholinergic to dry mucosal secretions* [phenylephrine HCl; chlorpheniramine maleate; methscopolamine nitrate] 10•4•1.25 mg/5 mL ② Doan's

denbufylline INN, BAN

Dendracin Neurodendtraxcin lotion OTC *anesthetic; analgesic; antipruritic; counterirritant* [benzocaine; methyl salicylate; menthol] 15%•30%•5%

dendritic cells pulsed with glioblastoma multiforme acid-eluted

tumor antigens *investigational (orphan) agent for glioblastoma multiforme*

denileukin diftitox USAN, INN *antineoplastic for cutaneous T-cell lymphoma (orphan)*

denipride INN

denofungin USAN *antifungal; antibacterial*

denopamine INN

Denorex Everyday Dandruff shampoo OTC *antiseborrheic; antibacterial; antifungal* [pyrithione zinc] 2%

denosumab *investigational (Phase III) twice-yearly subcu injection to increase bone density, prevent postmenopausal osteoporosis, and prevent bone metastasis; investigational (Phase II) for rheumatoid arthritis*

denpidazone INN

Denquel toothpaste OTC *tooth desensitizer* [potassium nitrate] 5%

DENSPM (diethylnorspermine) [q.v.]

Denta 5000 Plus dental cream Ṛ *caries preventative* [sodium fluoride] 1.1%

DentaGel Ṛ *dental caries preventative* [sodium fluoride] 1.1%

dental antiformin [see: antiformin, dental]

dental-type silica [see: silica, dental-type]

Dentipatch transmucosal patch Ṛ *mucous membrane anesthetic* [lidocaine HCl] 23, 46.1 mg

Dent-O-Kain/20 topical liquid OTC *mucous membrane anesthetic* [benzocaine] 20%

Dent's Lotion-Jel OTC *mucous membrane anesthetic* [benzocaine]

Dent's Toothache Gum; Dent's Toothache Drops OTC *mucous membrane anesthetic* [benzocaine] 20%

denufosol tetrasodium *P2Y₂ uridine 5'-triphosphate (UTP) agonist to increase mucosal hydration and enhance mucus clearance from the lungs; investigational (Phase III, orphan) inhalation solution for cystic fibrosis*

denyl sodium [see: phenytoin sodium]

denzimol INN

deodorants *a class of agents that mask undesirable or offensive odors* [also called: antibromics]

2'-deoxycoformycin (DCF) [see: pentostatin]

deoxycorticosterone acetate [see: desoxycorticosterone acetate]

deoxycorticosterone pivalate [see: desoxycorticosterone pivalate]

deoxycortolone pivalate BAN *salt-regulating adrenocortical steroid* [also: desoxycorticosterone pivalate]

deoxycortone BAN *salt-regulating adrenocortical steroid* [also: desoxycorticosterone acetate; desoxycortone]

2'-deoxycytidine *investigational (orphan) host-protective agent in acute myelogenous leukemia*

deoxyephedrine HCl [see: methamphetamine HCl]

12-deoxyerythromycin [see: berythromycin]

1-deoxygalactonojirimycin *investigational (orphan) for Fabry disease*

deoxyribonuclease, recombinant human (rhDNase) [see: dornase alfa]

deoxyribonucleic acid (DNA)

15-deoxyspergualin trihydrochloride [now: gusperimus trihydrochloride]

Depacin capsules (discontinued 2008) OTC *analgesic; antipyretic* [acetaminophen] 325 mg

Depacon IV infusion Ṛ *anticonvulsant for complex partial seizures and simple or complex absence seizures* [valproate sodium] 500 mg/vial ② dibucaine

Depade tablets (discontinued 2004) Ṛ *narcotic antagonist for opiate dependence or overdose (orphan) and alcoholism* [naltrexone HCl] 50 mg

Depakene capsules Ṛ *anticonvulsant for complex partial seizures and simple or complex absence seizures* [valproic acid] 250 mg ② dibucaine

Depakene syrup Ṛ *anticonvulsant for complex partial seizures and simple or complex absence seizures* [valproic acid] 250 mg/5 mL ② dibucaine

Depakote delayed-release enteric-coated tablets ℞ *anticonvulsant for complex partial seizures and simple or complex absence seizures; treatment for manic episodes of a bipolar disorder; migraine headache prophylaxis* [divalproex sodium] 125, 250, 500 mg

Depakote sprinkle capsules ℞ *anticonvulsant for complex partial seizures and simple or complex absence seizures* [divalproex sodium] 125 mg

Depakote ER extended-release tablets ℞ *anticonvulsant for complex partial seizures and simple or complex absence seizures; treatment for manic episodes of a bipolar disorder; migraine headache prophylaxis* [divalproex sodium] 250, 500 mg

Depen titratable tablets ℞ *metal chelating agent for rheumatoid arthritis, Wilson disease, and cystinuria* [penicillamine] 250 mg

depepsen [see: sodium amylosulfate]

Deplin tablets ℞ *hematinic* [folic acid] 7.5 mg

depMedalone 40; depMedalone 80 intralesional, soft tissue, and IM injection (discontinued 2008) ℞ *corticosteroid; anti-inflammatory; immunosuppressant* [methylprednisolone acetate] 40 mg/mL; 80 mg/mL

DepoCyt sustained-release intrathecal injection ℞ *antineoplastic for lymphomatous neoplastic meningitis (NM) arising from solid tumors or non-Hodgkin lymphoma (orphan)* [cytarabine, liposomal] 10 mg/mL

DepoDur extended-release liposomal suspension for epidural injection ℞ *narcotic analgesic* [morphine sulfate] 10 mg/mL

Depo-Estradiol IM injection ℞ *synthetic estrogen; hormone replacement therapy for the treatment of postmenopausal symptoms* [estradiol cypionate in oil] 5 mg/mL

Depoject intralesional, soft tissue, and IM injection (discontinued 2008) ℞ *corticosteroid; anti-inflammatory; immunosuppressant* [methylprednisolone acetate] 40, 80 mg/mL

Depo-Medrol intralesional, soft tissue, and IM injection ℞ *corticosteroid; anti-inflammatory; immunosuppressant* [methylprednisolone acetate] 20, 40, 80 mg/mL

Deponit transdermal patch (discontinued 2005) ℞ *coronary vasodilator; antianginal* [nitroglycerin] 0.2, 0.4 mg/hr. (16, 32 mg total) ⊘ Dibent

Depopred-40; Depopred-80 intralesional, soft tissue, and IM injection (discontinued 2006) ℞ *corticosteroid; anti-inflammatory; immunosuppressant* [methylprednisolone acetate] 40 mg/mL; 80 mg/mL ⊘ dobupride

Depo-Provera IM injection ℞ *hormonal antineoplastic adjunct for metastatic endometrial and renal carcinoma; long-term injectable contraceptive* [medroxyprogesterone acetate] 150, 400 mg/mL

Depo-Sub Q Provera 104 subcu injection in prefilled syringes ℞ *hormonal antineoplastic adjunct for metastatic endometrial and renal carcinoma; long-term injectable contraceptive* [medroxyprogesterone acetate] 104 mg

Depo-Testadiol IM injection (discontinued 2004) ℞ *estrogen/androgen combination for hormone replacement therapy for postmenopausal symptoms* [estradiol cypionate; testosterone cypionate] 2•50 mg/mL

Depo-Testosterone IM injection ℞ *androgen for hypogonadism or testosterone deficiency in men; hormone replacement therapy for postandropausal symptoms; sometimes abused as a street drug* [testosterone cypionate (in oil)] 100, 200 mg/mL

depramine INN [also: balipramine]

deprenyl (L-deprenyl) [see: selegiline HCl]

depreotide USAN *radiopharmaceutical imaging agent*

depressants *a class of agents that reduce functional activity and vital energy in* *general by producing muscular relaxation and diaphoresis*

deprodone INN, BAN ② diperodon

deprostil USAN, INN *gastric antisecretory* ② dipyrocetyl

depsipeptide *investigational (orphan) for cutaneous T-cell lymphoma*

deptropine INN, BAN

deptropine citrate [see: deptropine]

depurants; depuratives *a class of agents that purify or cleanse the system, particularly the blood* [also called: pellants]

dequalinium chloride INN, BAN

Dequasine tablets OTC *dietary supplement* [multiple minerals & amino acids; vitamin C] ≛•200 mg

deracoxib USAN *COX-2 inhibitor anti-inflammatory and analgesic for osteoarthritis and rheumatoid arthritis*

deramciclane *serotonin 5-HT₂ receptor antagonist; antidepressant; anxiolytic*

Derifil tablets OTC *systemic deodorant for ostomy, breath, and body odors* [chlorophyllin] 100 mg ② Duraflu

Derma Viva lotion (discontinued 2004) OTC *moisturizer; emollient*

Dermabase OTC *cream base*

Dermabond topical liquid OTC *skin adhesive for closing surgical incisions and traumatic lacerations*

Dermacoat aerosol (discontinued 2007) OTC *anesthetic* [benzocaine] 4.5%

Dermacort cream, lotion ℞ *corticosteroidal anti-inflammatory* [hydrocortisone] 1%

Dermadrox ointment OTC *astringent; skin protectant; emollient* [aluminum hydroxide gel; zinc chloride; lanolin]

DermaFlex gel OTC *anesthetic* [lidocaine; alcohol 79%] 2.5%

Dermal-Rub balm OTC *analgesic; counterirritant* [methyl salicylate; camphor; racemic manthol; cajuput oil]

Dermamycin cream, spray OTC *antihistamine* [diphenhydramine HCl] 2%

Derma-Pax lotion OTC *antihistamine; antiseptic; antipruritic* [pyrilamine maleate; chlorpheniramine maleate; alcohol 35%] 0.44%•0.06%

Dermarest gel OTC *antihistamine; antifungal* [diphenhydramine HCl; resorcinol] 2%•2%

Dermarest Dricort Creme OTC *corticosteroidal anti-inflammatory* [hydrocortisone acetate] 1%

Dermarest Plus gel, spray OTC *antihistamine; mild anesthetic; antipruritic; counterirritant* [diphenhydramine HCl; menthol] 2%•1%

Dermasept Antifungal spray liquid OTC *antifungal; antiseptic; anesthetic; astringent* [tolnaftate; tannic acid; zinc chloride; benzocaine; methylbenzethonium HCl; undecylenic acid; alcohol 58.54%] 1.017%•6.098%•5.081%•2.032%•3.049%•5.081%

Dermasil lotion OTC *bath emollient*

Derma-Smoothe/FS oil ℞ *corticosteroidal anti-inflammatory; emollient* [fluocinolone acetonide] 0.01%

dermatan sulfate [see: danaparoid sodium]

dermatol [see: bismuth subgallate]

Dermatop E cream, ointment ℞ *corticosteroidal anti-inflammatory* [prednicarbate] 0.1%

DermaVite tablets OTC *vitamin/mineral supplement* [multiple vitamins & minerals; folic acid; biotin] ≛•400•600 mcg

Dermazinc shampoo OTC *antiseborrheic; antibacterial; antifungal* [pyrithione zinc] 0.25%

Derm-Cleanse topical liquid OTC *soap-free therapeutic skin cleanser*

Dermol HC anorectal cream, anorectal ointment ℞ *corticosteroidal anti-inflammatory* [hydrocortisone] 1%, 2.5%; 1%

Dermolate Anti-Itch cream OTC *corticosteroidal anti-inflammatory* [hydrocortisone] 0.5%

Dermolin liniment OTC *analgesic; mild anesthetic; antipruritic; counterirritant; antiseptic* [methyl salicylate; camphor; racemic menthol; mustard oil; alcohol 8%] ② Dramilin

Dermoplast aerosol spray, lotion OTC *anesthetic; antipruritic; counterirritant* [benzocaine; menthol] 20%•0.5%; 8%•0.5%

Dermoplast Antibacterial aerosol spray OTC *anesthetic; antiseptic* [benzocaine; benzethonium chloride] 20%•0.2%

DermOtic Oil ear drops ℞ *corticosteroidal anti-inflammatory* [fluocinolone acetonide in oil] 0.01%

Dermovan OTC *cream base*

Dermprotective Factor (DPF) (trademarked ingredient) *aromatic syrup* [eriodictyon]

Dermtex HC with Aloe cream OTC *corticosteroidal anti-inflammatory* [hydrocortisone] 0.5%

Dermuspray aerosol spray ℞ *proteolytic enzyme for debridement of necrotic tissue; vulnerary* [trypsin; Peruvian balsam] 0.1•72.5 mg/0.82 mL

derpanicate INN

DES (diethylstilbestrol) [q.v.]

desacetyl vinblastine amide (DAVA) [see: vindesine]

desacetyl-lanatoside C [see: deslanoside]

desaglybuzole [see: glybuzole]

desamino-oxytocin [see: demoxytocin]

desaspidin INN

desciclovir USAN, INN *antiviral*

descinolone INN *corticosteroid; anti-inflammatory* [also: descinolone acetonide]

descinolone acetonide USAN *corticosteroid; anti-inflammatory* [also: descinolone]

Desenex cream OTC *antifungal* [clotrimazole] 1%

Desenex foam, soap OTC *antifungal* [undecylenic acid] 10%

Desenex powder OTC *antifungal* [miconazole nitrate] 2%

Desenex powder, aerosol powder, ointment, cream OTC *antifungal* [undecylenic acid; zinc undecylenate] 25% total

Desenex, Prescription Strength spray liquid, spray powder OTC *antifungal for tinea pedis, tinea cruris, and tinea corporis* [miconazole nitrate] 2%

Desenex Antifungal cream (discontinued 2007) OTC *antifungal for tinea pedis, tinea cruris, and tinea corporis* [miconazole nitrate] 2%

DesenexMax cream OTC *allylamine antifungal* [terbinafine HCl] 1%

deserpidine INN, BAN *antihypertensive; peripheral antiadrenergic; rauwolfia derivative*

desert herb; desert tea *medicinal herb* [see: ephedra]

Desert Pure Calcium film-coated tablets OTC *calcium supplement* [calcium carbonate; vitamin D] 500 mg•125 IU

Desferal powder for IM, IV, or subcu injection ℞ *chelating agent for acute or chronic iron poisoning* [deferoxamine mesylate] 500, 2000 mg

desferrioxamine BAN *chelating agent for acute or chronic iron poisoning* [also: deferoxamine]

desferrioxamine mesylate BAN *chelating agent for acute or chronic iron poisoning* [also: deferoxamine mesylate]

desflurane USAN, INN *inhalation general anesthetic*

desglugastrin INN

desipramine INN, BAN *tricyclic antidepressant* [also: desipramine HCl] ⊡ diisopromine

desipramine HCl USAN, USP *tricyclic antidepressant* [also: desipramine] 10, 25, 50, 75, 100, 150 mg oral

desirudin USAN *anticoagulant; thrombin inhibitor for the prevention of deep vein thrombosis (DVT) in elective hip replacement surgery*

Desitin ointment OTC *moisturizer; emollient; astringent* [cod liver oil; zinc oxide]

Desitin Clear ointment OTC *diaper rash treatment* [white petrolatum] 60%

Desitin Creamy ointment OTC *diaper rash treatment* [zinc oxide] 10%

Desitin with Zinc Oxide powder OTC *diaper rash treatment* [zinc oxide; cornstarch] 10%•88.2%

deslanoside USP, INN, BAN *cardiotonic; cardiac glycoside*

desloratadine USAN *second-generation peripherally selective piperidine antihistamine for allergic rhinitis and chronic idiopathic urticaria; active metabolite of loratadine*

deslorelin USAN, INN *LHRH agonist*

desmethylmoramide INN

desmoglein 3 synthetic peptide *investigational (orphan) for pemphigus vulgaris*

desmophosphamide [see: defosfamide]

desmopressin INN, BAN *posterior pituitary antidiuretic hormone (ADH)* [also: desmopressin acetate]

desmopressin acetate USAN *antidiuretic; posterior pituitary antidiuretic hormone for hemophilia A (orphan), von Willebrand disease (orphan), and nocturnal enuresis* [also: desmopressin] 0.1, 0.2 mg oral; 4 mcg/mL injection; 10 mcg nasal spray

desmoteplase *investigational antiplatelet drug for ischemic stroke; synthetic analogue of vampire bat saliva*

desocriptine INN

Desogen tablets (in packs of 28) ℞ *monophasic oral contraceptive* [desogestrel; ethinyl estradiol] 0.15 mg• 30 mcg × 21 days; counters × 7 days ☑ Diascan

desogestrel USAN, INN, BAN *progestin*

desolone [see: deprodone]

desomorphine INN, BAN

Desonate gel ℞ *corticosteroidal anti-inflammatory* [desonide] 0.05%

desonide USAN, INN, BAN *topical corticosteroidal anti-inflammatory* 0.05% topical

DesOwen ointment, cream, lotion ℞ *corticosteroidal anti-inflammatory* [desonide] 0.05%

desoximetasone USAN, USP, INN *topical corticosteroidal anti-inflammatory* [also: desoxymethasone] 0.05%, 0.25% topical

desoxycholic acid *increases secretion of bile acids*

desoxycorticosterone acetate (DCA; DOCA) USP *salt-regulating adrenocortical steroid* [also: desoxycortone; deoxycortone]

desoxycorticosterone pivalate USP *salt-regulating adrenocortical steroid* [also: deoxycortolone pivalate]

desoxycorticosterone trimethylacetate USP

desoxycortone INN *salt-regulating adrenocortical steroid* [also: desoxycorticosterone acetate; deoxycortone]

l-**desoxyephedrine** [see: levmetamfetamine]

desoxyephedrine HCl [see: methamphetamine HCl]

desoxymethasone BAN *topical corticosteroidal anti-inflammatory* [also: desoximetasone]

Desoxyn tablets ℞ *CNS stimulant; sometimes abused as a street drug* [methamphetamine HCl] 5 mg

desoxyribonuclease [see: fibrinolysin & desoxyribonuclease]

Despec oral drops ℞ *antitussive; decongestant; expectorant; for children 1–24 months* [dextromethorphan hydrobromide; pseudoephedrine HCl; guaifenesin] 4•20•10 mg/mL ☑ Dosepak

Despec oral liquid ℞ *decongestant; expectorant* [phenylephrine HCl; guaifenesin] 10•200 mg/10 mL ☑ Dosepak

Despec DM extended-release tablets (discontinued 2007) ℞ *antitussive; decongestant; expectorant* [dextromethorphan hydrobromide; pseudoephedrine HCl; guaifenesin] 60• 120•800 mg

Despec DM oral liquid (discontinued 2007) ℞ *antitussive; decongestant; expectorant* [dextromethorphan hydrobromide; phenylephrine HCl; guaifenesin] 30•10•200 mg/10 mL

Despec NR oral drops ℞ *antitussive; decongestant; expectorant; for children 1–24 months* [dextromethorphan hydrobromide; phenylephrine HCl; guaifenesin] 4•1.5•20 mg/mL

Desquam-E 5; Desquam-E 10 gel ℞ *keratolytic for acne* [benzoyl peroxide] 5%; 10%

Desquam-X cleansing bar ℞ *keratolytic for acne* [benzoyl peroxide] 10%

Desquam-X 5; Desquam-X 10 gel ℞ *keratolytic for acne* [benzoyl peroxide] 5%; 10%

de-Stat 3; de-Stat 4 solution OTC *cleaning/disinfecting/soaking solution for rigid gas permeable contact lenses* ⚕ Diastat

destradiol [see: estradiol]

desulfated heparin [see: heparin, 2-0-desulfated]

63-desulfohirudin [see: desirudin]

desvenlafaxine succinate *selective serotonin and norepinephrine reuptake inhibitor (SSNRI) for major depressive disorder (MDD); investigational (NDA filed) for postmenopausal vasomotor symptoms; investigational (Phase III) for fibromyalgia and diabetic peripheral neuropathy; single isomer of venlafaxine*

Desyrel film-coated tablets, Dividose (multiple-scored tablets) ℞ *antidepressant; also used for aggressive behavior, alcoholism, panic disorder, agoraphobia, and cocaine withdrawal* [trazodone HCl] 50, 100 mg; 150, 300 mg

DET (diethyltryptamine) [q.v.]

Detachol topical liquid OTC *adhesive remover for the skin*

detajmium bitartrate INN

Detane gel OTC *anesthetic* [benzocaine] 7.5% ⚕ Dytan

detanosal INN

Detect-A-Strep slide tests for professional use ℞ *in vitro diagnostic aid for streptococcal antigens in throat swabs*

Detecto-Seal (trademarked packaging form) *tamper-resistant parenteral package*

deterenol INN *ophthalmic adrenergic* [also: deterenol HCl]

deterenol HCl USAN *ophthalmic adrenergic* [also: deterenol]

detergents *a class of agents that cleanse wounds and sores*

detigon HCl [see: chlophedianol HCl]

detirelix INN *luteinizing hormone-releasing hormone (LHRH) antagonist* [also: detirelix acetate]

detirelix acetate USAN *luteinizing hormone-releasing hormone (LHRH) antagonist* [also: detirelix]

detomidine INN, BAN *veterinary analgesic; sedative* [also: detomidine HCl]

detomidine HCl USAN *veterinary analgesic; sedative* [also: detomidine]

detorubicin INN

detralfate INN

Detrol film-coated tablets ℞ *muscarinic receptor antagonist for urinary frequency, urgency, and incontinence* [tolterodine tartrate] 1, 2 mg

Detrol LA extended-release capsules ℞ *muscarinic receptor antagonist for urinary frequency, urgency, and incontinence* [tolterodine tartrate] 2, 4 mg

detrothyronine INN

Detrusitol Ⓔ (European name for U.S. product **Detrol**)

Detussin oral liquid (discontinued 2007) ℞ *narcotic antitussive; decongestant* [hydrocodone bitartrate; pseudoephedrine HCl; alcohol 5%] 5•60 mg/5 mL

deuterium oxide USAN *radioactive agent*

devapamil INN

devazepide USAN *cholecystokinin antagonist*

devil's bones *medicinal herb* [see: wild yam]

devil's claw (Harpagophytum procumbens) root *medicinal herb for arrhythmias, arteriosclerosis, arthritis, blood cleansing, diabetes, hypertension, liver disease, lowering cholesterol, rheumatism, stomach disorders, and strengthening bladder and kidneys*

devil's club (Echinopanax horridum; Fatsia horrida; Oplopanax horridus; Panax horridum) cambium and stem *medicinal herb for arthritis, burns and cuts, colds, cough, fever, inducing vomiting and bowel evacuation, pneumonia, and tuberculosis*

devil's dung *medicinal herb* [see: asafetida]

devil's eye *medicinal herb* [see: henbane]

devil's fuge *medicinal herb* [see: mistletoe]

devil's shrub *medicinal herb* [see: eleuthero]

Devrom chewable tablets OTC *systemic deodorizer for ostomy and incontinence odors* [bismuth subgallate] 200 mg

dewberry *medicinal herb* [see: blackberry]

Dex GG TR timed-release tablets (discontinued 2007) ℞ *antitussive; expectorant* [dextromethorphan hydrobromide; guaifenesin] 60•1000 mg

Dex4 Glucose chewable tablets OTC *blood glucose elevating agent for hypoglycemia* [glucose]

dexa [see: dexamethasone]

Dexacidin eye drop suspension ℞ *corticosteroidal anti-inflammatory; antibiotic* [dexamethasone; neomycin sulfate; polymyxin B sulfate] 0.1%• 0.35%•10 000 U/mL

Dexacine ophthalmic ointment (discontinued 2004) ℞ *corticosteroidal anti-inflammatory; antibiotic* [dexamethasone; neomycin sulfate; polymyxin B sulfate] 0.1%•0.35%• 10 000 U/g

Dexacort Phosphate Respihaler (oral inhalation aerosol) ℞ *corticosteroid for bronchial asthma* [dexamethasone sodium phosphate] 84 mcg/dose

Dexacort Phosphate Turbinaire (nasal inhalation aerosol) ℞ *intranasal corticosteroidal anti-inflammatory* [dexamethasone sodium phosphate; alcohol 2%] 84 mcg/dose

DexAlone liquid-filled gelcaps OTC *antitussive* [dextromethorphan hydrobromide] 30 mg

Dexameth tablets (discontinued 2004) ℞ *corticosteroidal anti-inflammatory* [dexamethasone] 0.5, 0.75, 1.5, 4 mg ⑨ dioxamate

dexamethasone USP, INN, BAN *corticosteroidal anti-inflammatory; investigational (orphan) for idiopathic intermediate uveitis* 0.25, 0.5, 0.75, 1, 1.5, 2, 4, 6 mg oral; 0.5 mg/5 mL oral

dexamethasone acefurate USAN, INN *corticosteroidal anti-inflammatory*

dexamethasone acetate USAN, USP, BAN *corticosteroidal anti-inflammatory* 8 mg/mL injection

dexamethasone dipropionate USAN *corticosteroidal anti-inflammatory*

Dexamethasone Intensol oral drops ℞ *corticosteroidal anti-inflammatory* [dexamethasone] 1 mg/mL

dexamethasone & neomycin sulfate & polymyxin B sulfate *topical ophthalmic corticosteroidal anti-inflammatory and antibiotic* 0.1%•0.35%• 10 000 U/mL eye drops

dexamethasone sodium phosphate USP, BAN *corticosteroid; anti-inflammatory* 0.1% eye drops; 4, 10 mg/mL injection

dexamfetamine INN *CNS stimulant* [also: dextroamphetamine; dexamphetamine]

dexamisole USAN, INN *antidepressant*

dexamphetamine BAN *CNS stimulant* [also: dextroamphetamine; dexamfetamine]

dexanabinol *nonpsychotropic synthetic analogue of marijuana; investigational (Phase II, orphan) for the attenuation or amelioration of long-term neurological sequelae of severe head trauma*

Dexasol eye drops/ear drops ℞ *corticosteroidal anti-inflammatory for corneal injury, ophthalmic inflammation, and otic inflammation* [dexamethasone sodium phosphate] 0.1%

Dexasone intra-articular, intralesional, soft tissue, or IM injection ℞ *corticosteroid; anti-inflammatory* [dexamethasone sodium phosphate] 4 mg/mL

Dexasone L.A. intralesional, intra-articular, soft tissue, or IM injection ℞ *corticosteroid; anti-inflammatory* [dexamethasone acetate] 8 mg/mL

Dexasporin ophthalmic ointment ℞ *corticosteroidal anti-inflammatory; antibiotic* [dexamethasone; neomycin sulfate; polymyxin B sulfate] 0.1%• 0.35%•10 000 U/g

dexbrompheniramine INN, BAN *alkylamine antihistamine* [also: dexbrompheniramine maleate]

dexbrompheniramine maleate USP *alkylamine antihistamine* [also: dexbrompheniramine]

dexchlorpheniramine INN *alkylamine antihistamine* [also: dexchlorpheniramine maleate]

dexchlorpheniramine maleate USP *alkylamine antihistamine* [also: dexchlorpheniramine] 4, 6 mg oral; 2 mg/5 mL oral

dexchlorpheniramine tannate *alkylamine antihistamine*

dexclamol INN *sedative* [also: dexclamol HCl]

dexclamol HCl USAN *sedative* [also: dexclamol]

Dexcon-DM syrup (discontinued 2007) R̶ *antitussive; decongestant; expectorant* [dextromethorphan hydrobromide; phenylephrine HCl; guaifenesin] 20•10•100 mg/5 mL

Dexedrine Spansules (sustained-release capsules) R̶ *amphetamine; CNS stimulant; widely abused as a street drug* [dextroamphetamine sulfate] 5, 10, 15 mg

Dexedrine tablets (discontinued 2008) R̶ *amphetamine; CNS stimulant; widely abused as a street drug* [dextroamphetamine sulfate] 5 mg

dexetimide USAN, INN, BAN *anticholinergic*

dexetozoline INN

dexfenfluramine INN, BAN *anorexiant; appetite suppressant; serotonin reuptake inhibitor* [also: dexfenfluramine HCl]

dexfenfluramine HCl USAN *anorexiant; appetite suppressant; serotonin reuptake inhibitor* [also: dexfenfluramine]

DexFerrum IV or IM injection R̶ *hematinic* [iron dextran] 50, 100 mg/dose

DexFol tablets R̶ *vitamin B supplement* [vitamins B_1, B_2, B_3, B_5, B_6, B_{12}, and C; folic acid; biotin] 1.5•1.5•20•10•50•1•60•5•0.3 mg

dexibuprofen USAN, INN *analgesic; cyclooxygenase inhibitor; anti-inflammatory*

dexibuprofen lysine USAN *analgesic; cyclooxygenase inhibitor; anti-inflammatory* [also: dexibuprofen]

deximafen USAN, INN *antidepressant*

dexindoprofen INN

dexivacaine USAN, INN *anesthetic*

dexlofexidine INN

dexmedetomidine USAN, INN, BAN *sedative*

dexmedetomidine HCl *sedative for intubated and ventilated patients in an intensive care setting; premedication to anesthesia*

dexmethylphenidate HCl *CNS stimulant for attention-deficit/hyperactivity disorder (ADHD) and narcolepsy; active isomer of methylphenidate HCl* 2.5, 5, 10 mg oral

dexnorgestrel acetime [now: norgestimate]

Dexodryl chewable caplets, oral suspension R̶ *antihistamine; anticholinergic to dry mucosal secretions* [chlorpheniramine maleate; methscopolamine nitrate] 2•1.5 mg; 2•1.5 mg/5 mL ☒ dioxadrol

Dexone intra-articular, intralesional, soft tissue, or IM injection (discontinued 2004) R̶ *corticosteroidal anti-inflammatory* [dexamethasone sodium phosphate] 4 mg/mL ☒ Dequasine

Dexone tablets (discontinued 2004) R̶ *corticosteroidal anti-inflammatory* [dexamethasone] 0.5, 0.75, 1.5, 4 mg ☒ Dequasine

Dexone LA intralesional, intra-articular, soft tissue, or IM injection R̶ *corticosteroidal anti-inflammatory* [dexamethasone acetate] 8 mg/mL ☒ docosanol

dexormaplatin USAN, INN *antineoplastic*

dexoxadrol INN *CNS stimulant; analgesic* [also: dexoxadrol HCl]

dexoxadrol HCl USAN *CNS stimulant; analgesic* [also: dexoxadrol]

DexPak; DexPak 13 Day; DexPak Jr. 10 Day Taperpak (tablets) R̶ *corticosteroidal anti-inflammatory* [dexamethasone] 1.5 mg

dexpanthenol USAN, USP, INN, BAN *cholinergic; antipruritic; emollient; postoperative prophylaxis for paralytic ileus* 250 mg/mL injection

dexpemedolac USAN *analgesic*

Dexphen M oral solution ℞ *antihistamine; decongestant; anticholinergic to dry mucosal secretions* [dexchlorpheniramine maleate; phenylephrine HCl; methscopolamine nitrate] 1•10• 1.25 mg/5 mL

dexpropranolol HCl USAN *antiarrhythmic; antiadrenergic (β-receptor)* [also: dexpropranolol]

dexproxibutene INN

dexrazoxane USAN, INN, BAN *cardioprotectant for doxorubicin-induced cardiomyopathy (orphan) and anthracycline extravasation; chelates intracellular iron*

dexrazoxane HCl *cardioprotectant for doxorubicin-induced cardiomyopathy (orphan) and anthracycline extravasation; chelates intracellular iron* (base= 85%) 294, 589 mg injection (250, 500 mg base)

dexsecoverine INN

dexsotalol HCl USAN *class III antiarrhythmic*

dextilidine INN

dextran INN, BAN *blood flow adjuvant; plasma volume extender* [also: dextran 40]

dextran, high molecular weight [see: dextran 70]

dextran, low molecular weight [see: dextran 40]

dextran 1 *monovalent hapten for prevention of dextran-induced anaphylactic reactions; investigational (orphan) for cystic fibrosis*

dextran 40 USAN *blood flow adjuvant; plasma volume extender* [also: dextran] 10% injection

dextran 70 USAN *plasma volume extender; viscosity-increasing agent; investigational (orphan) for recurrent corneal erosion* 6% injection

dextran 75 USAN *plasma volume extender; viscosity-increasing agent* 6% injection

dextran sulfate *investigational (orphan) inhalant for cystic fibrosis*

dextran sulfate, sodium salt, aluminum complex [see: detralfate]

dextran sulfate sodium *investigational (orphan) for AIDS*

dextranomer INN, BAN *wound cleanser and debrider*

dextrates USAN, NF *tablet binder and diluent*

dextriferron NF, INN, BAN

dextrin NF, BAN *suspending agent; tablet binder and diluent*

dextroamphetamine USAN *CNS stimulant; widely abused as a street drug, which causes strong psychic dependence* [also: dexamfetamine; dexamphetamine]

dextroamphetamine phosphate USP *CNS stimulant*

dextroamphetamine saccharate *CNS stimulant*

dextroamphetamine sulfate USP *CNS stimulant; widely abused as a street drug, which causes psychic dependence* 5, 10, 15 mg oral; 5 mg/5 mL oral

dextrobrompheniramine maleate [see: dexbrompheniramine maleate]

dextrochlorpheniramine maleate [see: dexchlorpheniramine maleate]

dextrofemine INN

dextromethorphan USP, INN, BAN *antitussive*

dextromethorphan hydrobromide USP, BAN *antitussive*

dextromethorphan hydrobromide & guaifenesin *antitussive; expectorant* 30•500 mg oral

dextromethorphan hydrobromide & pseudoephedrine HCl & guaifenesin *antitussive; decongestant; expectorant* 60•90•800 mg oral

dextromethorphan polistirex USAN *antitussive*

dextromethorphan & quinidine *investigational (NDA filed) dual-action* *glutamate inhibitor to treat involuntary emotional expression disorder (IEED)*

dextromethorphan tannate *antitussive*

dextromoramide INN, BAN

dextromoramide tartrate [see: dextromoramide]

dextro-pantothenyl alcohol [see: dexpanthenol]

dextropropoxiphene chloride [see: propoxyphene HCl]

dextropropoxyphene INN, BAN *narcotic analgesic* [also: propoxyphene HCl]

dextropropoxyphene HCl BAN [also: propoxyphene HCl]

dextrorphan INN, BAN *adjunct to vasospastic therapy* [also: dextrorphan HCl]

dextrorphan HCl USAN *adjunct to vasospastic therapy* [also: dextrorphan]

dextrose USP *fluid and nutrient replenisher; parenteral antihypoglycemic*

5% Dextrose and Electrolyte #48; 5% Dextrose and Electrolyte #75; 10% Dextrose and Electrolyte #48 IV infusion ℞ *intravenous nutritional/electrolyte therapy* [combined electrolyte solution; dextrose]

dextrose excipient NF *tablet excipient*

Dextrose Thermoject System IV injection ℞ *diagnostic aid for the measurement of cardiac output by the thermodilution method* [dextrose] 0.9%, 5%

DextroStat tablets ℞ *amphetamine; CNS stimulant* [dextroamphetamine sulfate] 5, 10 mg

Dextrostix reagent strips for home use (discontinued 2004) OTC *in vitro diagnostic aid for blood glucose*

dextrothyronine [see: detrothyronine]

dextrothyroxine BAN *antihyperlipidemic* [also: dextrothyroxine sodium]

dextrothyroxine sodium USAN, USP, INN *antihyperlipidemic* [also: dextrothyroxine]

Dex-Tuss oral liquid ℞ *narcotic antitussive; expectorant* [codeine phosphate; guaifenesin] 10•300 mg/5 mL

Dex-Tuss DM oral liquid ℞ *antitussive; expectorant* [dextromethorphan

hydrobromide; guaifenesin] 10•100 mg/5 mL ⓐ docusate sodium

dexverapamil INN *adjunct to chemotherapy*

Dey-Dose (delivery device) *nebulizer*

Dey-Lute (trademarked delivery device) *nebulizer*

Dey-Pak Sodium Chloride 3% & 10% solution ℞ *for inducing sputum production for specimen collection* [sodium chloride] 3%; 10%

dezaguanine USAN, INN *antineoplastic*

dezaguanine mesylate USAN *antineoplastic*

dezinamide USAN, INN *anticonvulsant*

dezocine USAN, INN *narcotic analgesic*

DFMO (difluoromethylornithine) [see: eflornithine]

DFMO (difluoromethylornithine) HCl [see: eflornithine HCl]

DFMO-MGBG (eflornithine, mitoguazone) *chemotherapy protocol* [see also: DFMO; MGBG]

DFP (diisopropyl flurophosphate) [see: isoflurophate]

DFV (DDP, fluorouracil, VePesid) *chemotherapy protocol*

DHA (docosahexaenoic acid) [q.v.; also: doconexent]

DHAP (dexamethasone, high-dose ara-C, Platinol) *chemotherapy protocol for non-Hodgkin lymphoma*

DHC Plus capsules ℞ *narcotic analgesic; antipyretic* [dihydrocodeine bitartrate; acetaminophen; caffeine] 16•356.4•30 mg ⓐ DOK-Plus

DHE (dihydroergotamine) [see: dihydroergotamine mesylate]

D.H.E. 45 IV or IM injection ℞ *ergot alkaloid for the rapid control of migraine and cluster headaches* [dihydroergotamine mesylate] 1 mg/mL

DHEA (dehydroepiandrosterone) [q.v.]

D-Hist D extended-release caplets ℞ *decongestant; antihistamine; anticholinergic to dry mucosal secretions* [pseudoephedrine HCl; dexchlorpheniramine maleate; methscopolamine bromide] 45•3.5•1 mg ⓐ Dosette; Duocet

DHPG (dihydroxy propoxymethyl guanine) [see: ganciclovir]

DHS Tar liquid shampoo, gel shampoo OTC *antiseborrheic; antipsoriatic; antipruritic; antibacterial* [coal tar] 0.5%

DHS Zinc shampoo OTC *antiseborrheic; antibacterial; antifungal* [pyrithione zinc] 2%

DHT tablets, Intensol (concentrated oral solution) ℞ *vitamin D therapy for tetany and hypoparathyroidism* [dihydrotachysterol] 0.125, 0.2, 0.4 mg; 0.2 mg/mL

DHT (dihydrotachysterol) [q.v.]

DHT (dihydrotestosterone) [see: androstanolone; stanolone]

DI (doxorubicin, ifosfamide [with mesna rescue]) *chemotherapy protocol for soft tissue sarcoma*

Diaβeta (or DiaBeta) tablets ℞ *sulfonylurea antidiabetic that stimulates insulin secretion in the pancreas* [glyburide] 1.25, 2.5, 5 mg

Diabetic Tussin oral liquid OTC *expectorant* [guaifenesin] 100 mg/5 mL

Diabetic Tussin DM oral liquid OTC *antitussive; expectorant* [dextromethorphan hydrobromide; guaifenesin] 10•100, 10•200 mg/5 mL

Diabinese tablets ℞ *sulfonylurea antidiabetic that stimulates insulin secretion in the pancreas* [chlorpropamide] 100, 250 mg

diacerein INN

diacetamate INN, BAN

diacetolol INN, BAN *antiadrenergic (β-receptor)* [also: diacetolol HCl]

diacetolol HCl USAN *antiadrenergic (β-receptor)* [also: diacetolol]

diacetoxyphenylisatin [see: oxyphenisatin acetate]

diacetoxyphenyloxindol [see: oxyphenisatin acetate]

diacetrizoate sodium [see: diatrizoate sodium]

diacetyl diaminodiphenylsulfone (DADDS) [see: acedapsone]

diacetylated monoglycerides NF *plasticizer*

diacetylcholine chloride [see: succinylcholine chloride]

diacetyl-dihydroxydiphenylisatin [see: oxyphenisatin acetate]

diacetyldioxphenylisatin [see: oxyphenisatin acetate]

diacetylmorphine HCl USP *(heroin; banned in USA)* [also: diamorphine]

diacetylmorphine salts *(heroin; banned in USA)*

diacetylsalicylic acid [see: dipyrocetyl]

diacetyltannic acid [see: acetyltannic acid]

diacetylthiamine [see: acetiamine]

diagniol [see: sodium acetrizoate]

diallylbarbituric acid [see: allobarbital]

diallylbarbituric acid [now: allobarbital]

diallylnortoxiferene dichloride [see: alcuronium chloride]

diallymal [see: allobarbital]

Dialpak (trademarked packaging form) *reusable patient compliance package for oral contraceptives*

Dialume capsules ℞ *antacid* [aluminum hydroxide gel] 500 mg

Dialyte Pattern LM solution ℞ *peritoneal dialysis solution* [multiple electrolytes; dextrose] 1.5%•⚕, 2.5%•⚕, 4.5%•⚕

Dialyvite 3000 tablets OTC *vitamin/mineral supplement* [multiple vitamins & minerals; folic acid; biotin] ⚕•3•0.3 mg

Dialyvite Multi-Vitamins for Dialysis Patients tablets ℞ *vitamin/mineral supplement* [multiple vitamins; folic acid; biotin] ⚕•1•0.3 mg

Dialyvite with Zinc tablets ℞ *vitamin/mineral supplement* [multiple vitamins & minerals; folic acid; biotin] ⚕•1•0.3 mg

dia-mer-sulfonamides (sulfadiazine & sulfamerazine) [q.v.]

diamethine [see: dimethyltubocurarinium chloride; dimethyltubocurarine]

diamfenetide INN [also: diamphenethide]

diaminedipenicillin G [see: penicillin G benzathine]

diaminodiphenylsulfone (DDS)
[now: dapsone]

3,4-diaminopyridine *investigational
(orphan) for Lambert-Eaton myasthenic
syndrome*

***cis*-diamminedichloroplatinum
(DDP)** [see: cisplatin]

diammonium phosphate [see: ammonium phosphate]

diamocaine INN, BAN *local anesthetic*
[also: diamocaine cyclamate]

diamocaine cyclamate USAN *local
anesthetic* [also: diamocaine]

diamorphine BAN *(heroin; banned in the
U.S.)* [also: diacetylmorphine HCl]

Diamox powder for IV injection (discontinued 2005) ℞ *carbonic anhydrase inhibitor diuretic; antiglaucoma;
anticonvulsant* [acetazolamide sodium]
500 mg ☑ DMax

Diamox tablets, Sequels (sustained-release capsules) ℞ *carbonic anhydrase inhibitor diuretic; antiglaucoma;
anticonvulsant; treatment for acute
mountain sickness* [acetazolamide]
125, 250 mg; 500 mg ☑ DMax

diamphenethide BAN [also: diamfenetide]

diampromide INN, BAN

diampron [see: amicarbalide]

diamthazole BAN [also: dimazole]

diamthazole dihydrochloride [see:
diamthazole]

Dianabol tablets (discontinued 1982)
℞ *anabolic steroid; discontinued for
human use, but the veterinary product
is still available and sometimes abused
as a street drug* [methandrostenolone]
2.5, 5 mg

Dianeal *investigational (orphan) nutritional supplement for continuous
ambulatory peritoneal dialysis patients*
[peritoneal dialysis solution with
1.1% amino acids]

diapamide USAN *diuretic; antihypertensive* [also: tiamizide]

Diaparene Baby cream OTC *diaper
rash treatment*

Diaparene Cornstarch Baby powder
OTC *diaper rash treatment* [cornstarch;
aloe]

Diaparene Diaper Rash ointment
OTC *diaper rash treatment* [zinc oxide]

Diaper Guard ointment OTC *diaper
rash treatment* [dimethicone; vitamins
A, D, and E; zinc oxide] 1%•⸏•⸎

Diaper Rash ointment OTC *diaper rash
treatment* [zinc oxide]

diaphene [see: dibromsalan]

diaphenylsulfone [see: dapsone]

diaphoretics *a class of agents that promote profuse perspiration* [also called:
sudorifics]

Diar-Aid tablets OTC *antidiarrheal; GI
adsorbent* [loperamide HCl] 2 mg

diarbarone INN

Diascan reagent strips for home use OTC
in vitro diagnostic aid for blood glucose

DiaScreen reagent strips for professional use ℞ *in vitro diagnostic aid for
multiple disease markers in the urine*

Diasorb tablets, oral liquid OTC *antidiarrheal; GI adsorbent* [activated attapulgite] 750 mg; 750 mg/5 mL

Diastat rectal gel in a disposable applicator ("pediatric" and "adult" refer
to the length of the applicator tip)
(discontinued 2006) ℞ *benzodiazepine anticonvulsant for acute repetitive
seizures (orphan)* [diazepam] 2.5, 5,
10 mg (pediatric); 10, 15, 20 mg
(adult) ☑ de-Stat 3

Diastat AcuDial rectal gel in prefilled
disposable applicators ℞ *benzodiazepine anticonvulsant for acute repetitive
seizures (orphan)* [diazepam; alcohol
10%] 2.5, 5, 7.5, 10, 12.5, 15, 17.5, 20
mg/dose (2.5, 10, 20 mg/applicator)

Diastix reagent strips for home use OTC
in vitro diagnostic aid for urine glucose

diathymosulfone INN

diatrizoate meglumine USP *oral/
parenteral radiopaque contrast medium
(46.67% iodine)* [also: meglumine
diatrizoate]

diatrizoate methylglucamine [see:
diatrizoate meglumine]

diatrizoate sodium USP *oral/rectal/ parenteral radiopaque contrast medium (59.87% iodine)* [also: sodium amidotrizoate; sodium diatrizoate]

diatrizoate sodium I 125 USAN *radioactive agent*

diatrizoate sodium I 131 USAN *radioactive agent*

diatrizoic acid USAN, USP, BAN *radiopaque contrast medium* [also: amidotrizoic acid]

Diatx tablets ℞ *hematinic* [multiple B vitamins; folic acid; biotin] ≐•5•0.3 mg

Diatx Fe tablets ℞ *vitamin/mineral supplement for anemia* [multiple B vitamins; folic acid; biotin; ferrous fumarate] ≐•5•0.3•100 mg

diaveridine USAN, INN, BAN *antibacterial*

diazacholesterol dihydrochloride [see: azacosterol HCl]

diazepam USAN, USP, INN, BAN, JAN *benzodiazepine anxiolytic; sedative; skeletal muscle relaxant; anticonvulsant for acute repetitive seizures (orphan); alcohol withdrawal aid; also abused as a street drug* 2, 5, 10 mg oral; 5 mg/5 mL oral; 5 mg/mL injection

Diazepam Intensol oral drops ℞ *benzodiazepine sedative; anxiolytic; skeletal muscle relaxant; anticonvulsant; also abused as a street drug* [diazepam; alcohol 19%] 5 mg/mL

diazinon BAN [also: dimpylate]

diaziquone USAN, INN *antineoplastic; investigational (orphan) for primary brain malignancies (astrocytomas)*

diazoxide USAN, USP, INN, BAN *emergency antihypertensive; vasodilator; glucose-elevating agent for hyperinsulinemia due to pancreatic cancer*

dibasic calcium phosphate [see: calcium phosphate, dibasic]

dibasic potassium phosphate [see: potassium phosphate, dibasic]

dibasic sodium phosphate [see: sodium phosphate, dibasic]

dibasol [see: bendazol]

dibazol [see: bendazol]

dibekacin INN, BAN

dibemethine INN

dibencil [see: penicillin G benzathine]

dibencozide [see: cobamamide]

Dibent IM injection ℞ *gastrointestinal anticholinergic/antispasmodic for irritable bowel syndrome (IBS)* [dicyclomine HCl] 10 mg/mL ⊘ Deponit

dibenthiamine [see: bentiamine]

dibenzathione [see: sulbentine]

dibenzepin INN, BAN *antidepressant* [also: dibenzepin HCl]

dibenzepin HCl USAN *antidepressant* [also: dibenzepin]

dibenzodiazepines *a class of novel (atypical) antipsychotic agents*

dibenzothiazepines *a class of novel (atypical) antipsychotic agents*

dibenzothiazine [see: phenothiazine]

dibenzothiophene USAN *keratolytic*

dibenzoxazepines *a class of dopamine receptor antagonists with antipsychotic, hypotensive, antiemetic, antispasmodic, and antihistaminic activity*

dibenzoyl peroxide [see: benzoyl peroxide]

dibenzoylthiamin [see: bentiamine]

dibenzthion [see: sulbentine]

dibenzylethylenediamine dipenicillin G (DBED) [see: penicillin G benzathine]

Dibenzyline capsules ℞ *antihypertensive for pheochromocytoma* [phenoxybenzamine HCl] 10 mg

N,N-dibenzylmethylamine [see: dibemethine]

dibromodulcitol [see: mitolactol]

dibromohydroxyquinoline [see: broxyquinoline]

dibromomannitol (DBM) [see: mitobronitol]

dibromopropamidine BAN [also: dibrompropamidine]

4,5-dibromorhodamine 123 *investigational (orphan) for chronic myelogenous leukemia*

dibrompropamidine INN [also: dibromopropamidine]

dibromsalan USAN, INN *disinfectant*

dibrospidium chloride INN

dibucaine USP *topical anesthetic* [also: cinchocaine] 1% topical ⊘ Depacon

dibucaine HCl USP *local anesthetic* [also: cinchocaine HCl]

dibudinate INN *combining name for radicals or groups*

dibunate INN *combining name for radicals or groups* ⊘ Deponit

dibuprol INN

dibupyrone INN, BAN

dibusadol INN

dibutoline sulfate

DIC (dimethyl imidazole carboxamide) [see: dacarbazine]

Dical CapTabs (capsule-shaped tablets) OTC *dietary supplement* [dibasic calcium phosphate; vitamin D] 117 mg (Ca)•90 mg (P)•133 IU ⊘ DECAL

dicalcium phosphate [see: calcium phosphate, dibasic]

Dical-D chewable wafers (discontinued 2005) OTC *dietary supplement* [dibasic calcium phosphate; vitamin D] 232 mg (Ca)•180 mg (P)•200 IU

Dical-D tablets OTC *dietary supplement* [dibasic calcium phosphate; vitamin D] 105 mg (Ca)•81 mg (P)•120 IU

dicarbine INN

dicarfen INN

Dicel oral suspension ℞ *decongestant; antihistamine* [pseudoephedrine tannate; chlorpheniramine tannate] 75•5 mg/5 mL ⊘ decil

Dicel DM oral suspension ℞ *antitussive; antihistamine; decongestant* [dextromethorphan tannate; chlorpheniramine tannate; pseudoephedrine tannate] 25•5•75 mg/5 mL

dichlofenthion BAN

dichloralantipyrine [see: dichloralphenazone]

dichloralphenazone (chloral hydrate & phenazone) BAN *mild sedative*

dichloralphenazone & acetaminophen & isometheptane mucate *cerebral vasoconstrictor and analgesic for vascular and tension headaches; "possibly effective" for migraine headaches* 100•325•65 mg oral

dichloralpyrine [see: dichloralphenazone]

dichloramine-T NF

dichloranilino imidazolin [see: clonidine HCl]

dichloren [see: mechlorethamine HCl]

dichlorisone INN

dichlorisone acetate [see: dichlorisone]

dichlormethazanone [see: dichlormezanone]

dichlormezanone INN

dichloroacetic acid *strong keratolytic/ cauterant*

dichlorodifluoromethane NF *aerosol propellant; topical refrigerant anesthetic*

dichlorodiphenyl trichloroethane (DDT) [see: chlorophenothane]

dichlorometaxylenol [see: dichloroxylenol]

dichloromethane [see: methylene chloride]

dichlorophen INN, BAN

dichlorophenarsine INN, BAN [also: dichlorophenarsine HCl]

dichlorophenarsine HCl USP [also: dichlorophenarsine]

dichlorotetrafluoroethane NF *aerosol propellant; topical refrigerant anesthetic* [also: cryofluorane]

dichlorovinyl dimethyl phosphate (DDVP) [see: dichlorvos]

dichloroxylenol INN, BAN

dichlorphenamide USP, BAN *carbonic anhydrase inhibitor; diuretic* [also: diclofenamide]

dichlorvos USAN, INN, BAN *anthelmintic*

dichysterol [see: dihydrotachysterol]

diciferron INN

dicirenone USAN, INN *hypotensive; aldosterone antagonist*

Dick test (scarlet fever streptococcus toxin)

diclazuril USAN, INN, BAN *coccidiostat for poultry*

diclofenac INN, BAN *analgesic; antiarthritic; nonsteroidal anti-inflammatory drug (NSAID) for ankylosing spondylitis* [also: diclofenac potassium]

diclofenac epolamine *transdermal analgesic; nonsteroidal anti-inflamma-*

tory drug (NSAID) for acute pain due to strains, sprains, and contusions

diclofenac potassium USAN *analgesic; nonsteroidal anti-inflammatory drug (NSAID) for osteoarthritis, rheumatoid arthritis, ankylosing spondylitis, and dysmenorrhea; topical treatment for actinic keratoses* [also: diclofenac] 50 mg oral

diclofenac sodium USAN, JAN *analgesic; nonsteroidal anti-inflammatory drug (NSAID) for osteoarthritis, rheumatoid arthritis, and ankylosing spondylitis; ocular treatment for cataract extraction and corneal refractive surgery; topical treatment for actinic keratoses* 25, 50, 75, 100 mg oral; 0.1% eye drops

diclofenamide INN *carbonic anhydrase inhibitor* [also: dichlorphenamide]

diclofensine INN

diclofibrate [see: simfibrate]

diclofurime INN

diclometide INN

diclonixin INN

dicloralurea USAN, INN *veterinary food additive*

dicloxacillin USAN, INN, BAN *penicillinase-resistant penicillin antibiotic*

dicloxacillin sodium USAN, USP, BAN *penicillinase-resistant penicillin antibiotic* 250, 500 mg oral

dicobalt edetate INN, BAN

dicolinium iodide INN

Dicomal-DH syrup (discontinued 2007) R *narcotic antitussive; antihistamine; sleep aid; decongestant* [hydrocodone bitartrate; pyrilamine maleate; phenylephrine HCl] 1.66•8.33• 5 mg/5 mL

Dicomal-DM syrup (discontinued 2007) OTC *antitussive; antihistamine; sleep aid; decongestant* [dextromethorphan hydrobromide; pyrilamine maleate; phenylephrine HCl] 20•16.7• 10 mg/10 mL

dicophane BAN [also: chlorophenothane; clofenotane]

dicoumarin [see: dicumarol]

dicoumarol INN *coumarin-derivative anticoagulant* [also: dicumarol]

dicresulene INN

Dictamnus albus *medicinal herb* [see: fraxinella]

dicumarol USAN, USP *coumarin-derivative anticoagulant* [also: dicoumarol]

dicyclomine BAN *gastrointestinal anticholinergic/antispasmodic* [also: dicyclomine HCl; dicycloverine]

dicyclomine HCl USP *gastrointestinal anticholinergic/antispasmodic for irritable bowel syndrome (IBS)* [also: dicycloverine; dicyclomine] 10, 20 mg oral; 10 mg/5 mL oral; 10 mg/mL injection

dicycloverine INN *anticholinergic* [also: dicyclomine HCl; dicyclomine]

dicycloverine HCl [see: dicyclomine HCl]

dicysteine [see: cystine]

didanosine USAN, INN, BAN *antiviral nucleoside reverse transcriptase inhibitor for HIV-1 infections (orphan)* 200, 250, 400 mg oral

didehydrodideoxythymidine [see: stavudine]

Di-Delamine gel, spray OTC *antihistamine* [diphenhydramine HCl; tripelennamine HCl] 1%•0.5%•

2′,3′-dideoxyadenosine (ddA) *investigational (orphan) treatment for AIDS*

dideoxycytidine (DDC; ddC) [see: zalcitabine]

dideoxyinosine (DDI; ddI) [see: didanosine]

Didrex tablets R *anorexiant* [benzphetamine HCl] 50 mg

Didro-Kit (Italian name for U.S. product **Didronel**)

Didronel caplets R *bisphosphonate bone resorption inhibitor for Paget disease, heterotopic ossification, and hypercalcemia of malignancy (orphan); also used for corticosteroid-induced osteoporosis* [etidronate disodium] 200, 400 mg

Didronel IV infusion (discontinued 2004) R *bisphosphonate bone resorption inhibitor for hypercalcemia of malignancy (orphan); investigational*

(orphan) for metabolic bone disease [etidronate disodium] 300 mg/ampule

didrovaltrate INN

didroxane [see: dichlorophen]

dieldrin INN, BAN

dielytra; choice dielytra *medicinal herb* [see: turkey corn]

diemal [see: barbital]

dienestrol USP, INN *estrogen* [also: dienoestrol]

dienoestrol BAN *estrogen* [also: dienestrol]

dienogest INN

dietamiphylline [see: etamiphyllin]

dietamiverine HCl [see: bietamiverine HCl]

diethadione INN, BAN

diethanolamine NF *alkalizing agent*

diethazine INN, BAN ⑨ Detussin

diethazine HCl [see: diethazine]

diethyl phthalate NF *plasticizer*

diethylamine *p*-aminobenzenestibonate [see: stibosamine]

3-diethylaminobutyranilide [see: octacaine]

diethylbarbiturate monosodium [see: barbital sodium]

diethylbarbituric acid [see: barbital]

diethylcarbamazine INN, BAN *anthelmintic for Bancroft filariasis, onchocerciasis, tropical eosinophilia, and loiasis* [also: diethylcarbamazine citrate]

diethylcarbamazine citrate USP *anthelmintic for Bancroft filariasis, onchocerciasis, tropical eosinophilia, and loiasis* [also: diethylcarbamazine]

diethylcarbamazine dihydrogen citrate [see: diethylcarbamazine citrate]

diethyldithiocarbamate *investigational (Phase II/III, orphan) immunomodulator for HIV and AIDS*

diethyldixanthogen [see: dixanthogen]

diethylenediamine citrate [see: piperazine citrate]

diethylenetriaminepentaacetic acid (DTPA) [see: pentetic acid]

N,N-diethyllysergamide [see: lysergide]

diethylmalonylurea [see: barbital]

diethylmalonylurea sodium [see: barbital sodium]

N,N-diethylnicotinamide [see: nikethamide]

diethylnorspermine *investigational (orphan) for hepatocellular carcinoma*

diethylpropion BAN *anorexiant; CNS stimulant* [also: diethylpropion HCl; amfepramone] 75 mg oral

diethylpropion HCl USP *anorexiant; CNS stimulant* [also: amfepramone; diethylpropion] 25 mg oral

diethylstilbestrol (DES) USP, INN *hormonal antineoplastic for inoperable prostatic and breast cancer* [also: stilboestrol]

diethylstilbestrol diphosphate USP *hormonal antineoplastic* [also: fosfestrol]

diethylstilbestrol dipropionate NF

***p*-diethylsulfamoylbenzoic acid** [see: etebenecid; ethebenecid]

diethylthiambutene INN, BAN

diethyltoluamide (DEET) USP, BAN *arthropod repellent*

diethyltryptamine (DET) *a hallucinogenic street drug closely related to dimethyltryptamine (DMT), but prepared synthetically*

N,N-diethylvanillamide [see: ethamivan]

dietifen INN

dietroxine [see: diethadione]

diexanthogen [see: dixanthogen]

difebarbamate INN

difemerine INN [also: difemerine HCl]

difemerine HCl [also: difemerine]

difemetorex INN

difenamizole INN

difencloxazine INN

difencloxazine HCl [see: difencloxazine]

difenidol INN *antiemetic; antivertigo* [also: diphenidol]

difenoximide INN *antiperistaltic* [also: difenoximide HCl]

difenoximide HCl USAN *antiperistaltic* [also: difenoximide]

difenoxin USAN, INN, BAN *antiperistaltic*

difenoxin HCl *antiperistaltic*

diferuloylmethane *investigational (orphan) agent for cystic fibrosis*

difetarsone INN, BAN

difeterol INN

Differin gel ℞ *synthetic retinoid analogue for acne* [adapalene] 0.1%, 0.3%

Differin solution, cream, single-use pledgets ℞ *synthetic retinoid analogue for acne* [adapalene] 0.1%

Difil-G caplets ℞ *antiasthmatic; bronchodilator; expectorant* [dyphylline; guaifenesin] 200•300 mg ⊘ Duphalac

Difil-G Forte oral liquid ℞ *antiasthmatic; bronchodilator; expectorant* [dyphylline; guaifenesin] 100•100 mg/5 mL

diflorasone INN, BAN *topical corticosteroidal anti-inflammatory* [also: diflorasone diacetate]

diflorasone diacetate USAN, USP *topical corticosteroidal anti-inflammatory* [also: diflorasone] 0.05% topical

difloxacin INN *anti-infective; DNA gyrase inhibitor* [also: difloxacin HCl]

difloxacin HCl USAN *anti-infective; DNA gyrase inhibitor* [also: difloxacin]

difluanazine INN *CNS stimulant* [also: difluanine HCl]

difluanazine HCl [see: difluanine HCl]

difluanine HCl USAN *CNS stimulant* [also: difluanazine]

Diflucan tablets, powder for oral suspension, IV infusion ℞ *systemic triazole antifungal* [fluconazole] 50, 100, 150, 200 mg; 10, 40 mg/mL; 2 mg/mL

diflucortolone USAN, INN, BAN *corticosteroid; anti-inflammatory*

diflucortolone pivalate USAN *corticosteroid; anti-inflammatory*

diflumidone INN, BAN *anti-inflammatory* [also: diflumidone sodium]

diflumidone sodium USAN *anti-inflammatory* [also: diflumidone]

diflunisal USAN, USP, INN, BAN *anti-inflammatory; analgesic; antipyretic; antiarthritic; antirheumatic* 500 mg oral

difluoromethylornithine (DFMO) [see: eflornithine]

difluoromethylornithine HCl [see: eflornithine HCl]

difluprednate USAN, INN *topical corticosteroidal anti-inflammatory*

difolliculin [see: estradiol benzoate]

diftalone USAN, INN *anti-inflammatory*

digalloyl trioleate USAN

Di-Gel oral liquid OTC *antacid; antiflatulent* [aluminum hydroxide; magnesium hydroxide; simethicone] 200•200•20 mg/5 mL ⊘ DECAL; Dical

Di-Gel, Advanced Formula chewable tablets OTC *antacid; antiflatulent* [magnesium hydroxide; calcium carbonate; simethicone] 128•280•20 mg

digestants; digestives *a class of agents that promote or aid in digestion*

digestive enzymes (amylase; lipase; protease) [q.v.]

Digibind powder for IV injection ℞ *antidote to digoxin/digitoxin overdose (orphan)* [digoxin immune Fab (ovine)] 38 mg/vial

Digidote *investigational (orphan) antidote to cardiac glycoside intoxication* [digoxin immune Fab (ovine)]

DigiFab powder for IV injection ℞ *antidote to digoxin/digitoxin overdose (orphan)* [digoxin immune Fab (ovine)] 40 mg/vial

digitalis USP *cardiotonic*

Digitalis ambigua; D. ferriginea; D. grandiflora; D. lanata; D. lutea; D. purpurea medicinal herb [see: foxglove]

digitalis glycosides *a class of cardiovascular drugs that increase the force of cardiac contractions* [also called: cardiac glycosides]

Digitek tablets ℞ *cardiac glycoside to increase cardiac output; antiarrhythmic* [digoxin] 0.125, 0.25 mg

digitoxin USP, INN, BAN *cardiotonic; cardiac glycoside; investigational (orphan) for soft tissue sarcomas and ovarian cancer*

digitoxin, acetyl [see: acetyldigitoxin]

α-digitoxin monoacetate [see: acetyldigitoxin]

digitoxoside [see: digitoxin]

digolil INN *combining name for radicals or groups*

digoxin USP, INN, BAN *cardiotonic; cardiac glycoside antiarrhythmic* 0.125, 0.25 mg oral, 0.05 mg/mL oral, 0.1, 0.25 mg/mL injection

digoxin antibody [see: digoxin immune Fab]

digoxin immune Fab (ovine) *antidote to digoxin/digitoxin intoxication (orphan); investigational (orphan) for other cardiac glycoside intoxication*

dihexyverine INN *anticholinergic* [also: dihexyverine HCl]

dihexyverine HCl USAN *anticholinergic* [also: dihexyverine]

Dihistine DH elixir (discontinued 2006) ℞ *narcotic antitussive; antihistamine; decongestant* [codeine phosphate; chlorpheniramine maleate; pseudoephedrine HCl] 20•4•60 mg/10 mL

Dihistine Expectorant oral liquid (discontinued 2007) ℞ *narcotic antitussive; decongestant; expectorant* [codeine phosphate; pseudoephedrine HCl; guaifenesin; alcohol 7.5%] 10•30•100 mg/5 mL

dihydan soluble [see: phenytoin sodium]

dihydralazine INN, BAN

dihydralazine sulfate [see: dihydralazine]

5,6-dihydro-5-azacytidine *investigational (orphan) for malignant mesothelioma*

dihydrobenzthiazide [see: hydrobentizide]

dihydrocodeine INN, BAN *narcotic analgesic and antitussive* [also: dihydrocodeine bitartrate]

dihydrocodeine bitartrate USP *narcotic analgesic and antitussive* [also: dihydrocodeine]

dihydrocodeine bitartrate & acetaminophen & caffeine *narcotic antitussive; analgesic* 32•712.8•60 mg

dihydrocodeinone bitartrate [see: hydrocodone bitartrate]

dihydroergocornine [see: ergoloid mesylates]

dihydroergocristine [see: ergoloid mesylates]

dihydroergocryptine [see: ergoloid mesylates]

dihydroergotamine (DHE) INN, BAN *antiadrenergic; anticoagulant; ergot alkaloid for rapid control of migraines* [also: dihydroergotamine mesylate; dihydroergotamine mesilate]

dihydroergotamine mesilate JAN *antiadrenergic; anticoagulant; ergot alkaloid for rapid control of migraines* [also: dihydroergotamine mesylate; dihydroergotamine]

dihydroergotamine mesylate USAN, USP *antiadrenergic; anticoagulant; ergot alkaloid for the rapid control of migraine and cluster headaches* [also: dihydroergotamine; dihydroergotamine mesilate] 1 mg/mL injection

dihydroergotamine methanesulfonate [see: dihydroergotamine mesylate]

dihydroergotoxine mesylate [now: ergoloid mesylates]

dihydroergotoxine methanesulfonate [now: ergoloid mesylates]

dihydroethaverine [see: drotaverine]

dihydrofollicular hormone [see: estradiol]

dihydrofolliculine [see: estradiol]

dihydrogenated ergot alkaloids [now: ergoloid mesylates]

dihydrohydroxycodeinone [see: oxycodone]

dihydrohydroxycodeinone HCl [see: oxycodone HCl]

6-dihydro-6-iminopurine [see: adenine]

dihydroindolones *a class of dopamine receptor antagonists with conventional (typical) antipsychotic activity* [also called: indolones]

dihydroisoperparine [see: drotaverine]

dihydromorphinone HCl [now: hydromorphone HCl]

dihydroneopine [see: dihydrocodeine bitartrate]

dihydropyridines *a class of calcium channel blockers*

dihydrostreptomycin (DST) INN *antibacterial* [also: dihydrostreptomycin sulfate]

dihydrostreptomycin sulfate USP *antibacterial* [also: dihydrostreptomycin]

dihydrostreptomycin-streptomycin [see: streptoduocin]

dihydrotachysterol (DHT) USP, INN, BAN, JAN *fat-soluble vitamin; synthetic reduction product of tachysterol, a vitamin D isomer; calcium regulator for tetany and hypoparathyroidism* 0.125, 0.2, 0.4 mg oral; 0.2 mg/mL oral

dihydrotestosterone (DHT) *anabolic steroid; investigational (Phase II, orphan) for AIDS-wasting syndrome* [also: androstanolone; stanolone]

dihydrotheelin [see: estradiol]

dihydroxy(stearato)aluminum [see: aluminum monostearate]

dihydroxy propoxymethyl guanine (DHPG) [see: gancyclovir]

dihydroxyacetone *skin darkener for vitiligo and hypopigmented areas*

dihydroxyaluminum aminoacetate (DAA) USP *antacid*

dihydroxyaluminum sodium carbonate USP *antacid*

dihydroxyanthranol [see: anthralin]

dihydroxyanthraquinone *(withdrawn from market)* [see: danthron]

1α,25-dihydroxycholecalciferol [see: calcitriol]

24,25-dihydroxycholecalciferol *investigational (orphan) for uremic osteodystrophy*

dihydroxyestrin [see: estradiol]

5,7-dihydroxyflavone [see: chrysin]

dihydroxyfluorane [see: fluorescein]

dihydroxyphenylalanine (DOPA) [see: levodopa]

dihydroxyphenylisatin [see: oxyphenisatin acetate]

dihydroxyphenyloxindol [see: oxyphenisatin acetate]

dihydroxyprogesterone acetophenide [see: algestone acetophenide]

dihydroxypropyl theophylline [see: dyphylline]

diiodobuphenine [see: bufeniode]

diiodohydroxyquin [now: iodoquinol]

diiodohydroxyquinoline INN, BAN *antiamebic* [also: iodoquinol]

diisopromine INN ② desipramine

diisopromine HCl [see: diisopromine]

diisopropanolamine NF *alkalizing agent*

diisopropyl flurophosphate (DFP) [see: isoflurophate]

diisopropyl flurophosphonate [see: isoflurophate]

diisopropyl phosphorofluoridate [see: isoflurophate]

2,6-diisopropylphenol [see: propofol]

Dilacor XR sustained-release capsules ℞ *antihypertensive; antianginal; antiarrhythmic; calcium channel blocker* [diltiazem HCl] 120, 180, 240 mg

Dilantin Infatabs (chewable tablets) ℞ *hydantoin anticonvulsant* [phenytoin] 50 mg

Dilantin Kapseals (capsules) ℞ *hydantoin anticonvulsant* [phenytoin sodium] 30, 100 mg

Dilantin-125 oral suspension ℞ *hydantoin anticonvulsant* [phenytoin] 125 mg/5 mL

Dilatrate-SR sustained-release capsules ℞ *coronary vasodilator; antianginal* [isosorbide dinitrate] 40 mg

Dilaudid tablets, oral liquid, subcu or IM injection, suppositories ℞ *narcotic analgesic; widely abused as a street drug* [hydromorphone HCl] 2, 4, 8 mg; 1 mg/mL; 1, 2, 4 mg/mL; 3 mg

Dilaudid Cough syrup (discontinued 2007) ℞ *narcotic antitussive; expectorant* [hydromorphone HCl; guaifenesin; alcohol 5%] 1•100 mg/5 mL

Dilaudid-HP subcu or IM injection; powder for subcu or IM injection ℞ *narcotic analgesic* [hydromorphone HCl] 10 mg/mL; 250 mg

dilazep INN

dilevalol INN, BAN *antihypertensive; antiadrenergic (β-receptor)* [also: dilevalol HCl]

dilevalol HCl USAN, JAN *antihypertensive; antiadrenergic (β-receptor)* [also: dilevalol]

Dilex-G; Dilex-G 200 syrup ℞ *antiasthmatic; bronchodilator; expectorant* [dyphylline; guaifenesin] 100•100 mg/5 mL; 100•200 mg/5 mL

Dilex-G 400 tablets ℞ *antiasthmatic; bronchodilator; expectorant* [dyphylline; guaifenesin] 200•400 mg

dilithium carbonate [see: lithium carbonate]

dill *(Anethum graveolens)* fruit and seed *medicinal herb used as an aromatic, carminative, diaphoretic, stimulant, and stomachic*

dilmefone

Dilomine IM injection ℞ *gastrointestinal anticholinergic/antispasmodic for irritable bowel syndrome (IBS)* [dicyclomine HCl] 10 mg/mL ⃞ Dalmane; diolamine

Dilor elixir, IM injection (discontinued 2005) ℞ *antiasthmatic; bronchodilator* [dyphylline] 160 mg/15 mL; 250 mg/mL

Dilor tablets (discontinued 2006) ℞ *antiasthmatic; bronchodilator* [dyphylline] 200 mg

Dilor 400 tablets (discontinued 2006) ℞ *antiasthmatic; bronchodilator* [dyphylline] 400 mg

Dilotab tablets (discontinued 2007) OTC *decongestant; analgesic; antipyretic* [pseudoephedrine HCl; acetaminophen] 30•500 mg

Dilotab II tablets OTC *decongestant; analgesic; antipyretic* [phenylephrine HCl; acetaminophen] 5•325 mg

diloxanide INN, BAN

diloxanide furoate *investigational anti-infective for amebiasis* (available only from the Centers for Disease Control and Prevention)

Dilt-CD extended-release capsules ℞ *antihypertensive; calcium channel blocker* [diltiazem HCl] 120, 180, 240, 300 mg

Diltia XT sustained-release capsules ℞ *antihypertensive; calcium channel blocker* [diltiazem HCl] 120, 180, 240 mg

diltiazem INN, BAN *coronary vasodilator; calcium channel blocker; antianginal; antihypertensive* [also: diltiazem HCl]

diltiazem HCl USAN, USP, JAN *coronary vasodilator; calcium channel blocker; antianginal; antihypertensive; antiarrhythmic* [also: diltiazem] 30, 60, 90, 120, 180, 240, 300, 360, 420 mg oral; 5 mg/mL injection

diltiazem malate USAN *coronary vasodilator; calcium channel blocker; antianginal; antihypertensive; antiarrhythmic*

Dilt-XR extended-release capsules ℞ *antihypertensive; calcium channel blocker* [diltiazem HCl] 120, 180, 240 mg

diluted acetic acid [see: acetic acid, diluted]

diluted alcohol [see: alcohol, diluted]

diluted hydrochloric acid [see: hydrochloric acid, diluted]

diluted sodium hypochlorite [see: sodium hypochlorite, diluted]

dimabefylline INN

dimantine INN *anthelmintic* [also: dymanthine HCl]

dimantine HCl INN [also: dymanthine HCl]

Dimaphen elixir OTC *decongestant; antihistamine* [pseudoephedrine HCl; brompheniramine maleate] 30•2 mg/10 mL

Dimaphen DM Cold & Cough elixir OTC *antitussive; antihistamine; decongestant* [dextromethorphan hydrobromide; brompheniramine maleate; pseudoephedrine HCl] 10•2•30 mg/10 mL

dimazole INN [also: diamthazole]

dimazole dihydrochloride [see: dimazole; diamthazole]

dimebolin HCl *investigational (Phase III) treatment for Alzheimer disease*

Dimebon *investigational (Phase III) treatment for Alzheimer disease* [dimebolin HCl]

dimecamine INN

dimecolonium iodide INN

dimecrotic acid INN

dimedrol [see: diphenhydramine HCl]

dimefadane USAN, INN *analgesic*

dimefilcon A USAN *hydrophilic contact lens material*

dimefline INN, BAN *respiratory stimulant* [also: dimefline HCl]

dimefline HCl USAN *respiratory stimulant* [also: dimefline]

dimefocon A USAN *hydrophobic contact lens material*

dimekolin [see: dimecolonium iodide]

dimelazine INN

dimelin [see: dimecolonium iodide]

dimemorfan INN

dimenhydrinate USP, INN, BAN *antiemetic; anticholinergic; antivertigo; motion sickness prophylaxis* 50 mg oral; 12.5 mg/4 mL oral; 50 mg/mL injection

dimenoxadol INN [also: dimenoxadole]

dimenoxadole BAN [also: dimenoxadol]

dimepheptanol INN, BAN

dimepranol INN *immunomodulator* [also: dimepranol acedoben]

dimepranol acedoben USAN *immunomodulator* [also: dimepranol]

dimepregnen INN, BAN

dimepropion BAN [also: metamfepramone]

dimeprozan INN

dimeprozinum [see: dimeprozan]

dimercaprol USP, INN *chelating agent for arsenic, gold, and mercury poisoning; adjunct to lead poisoning*

dimercaptopropanol [see: dimercaprol]

2,3-dimercaptosuccinic acid (DMSA) [see: succimer]

dimesna INN

dimesone INN, BAN

Dimetabs tablets ℞ *anticholinergic; antiemetic; antivertigo agent; motion sickness preventative* [dimenhydrinate] 50 mg

dimetacrine INN

dimetamfetamine INN

Dimetane-DX Cough syrup (discontinued 2004) ℞ *antitussive; decongestant; antihistamine* [dextromethorphan hydrobromide; pseudoephedrine HCl; brompheniramine maleate; alcohol 1%] 20•60•4 mg/10 mL

Dimetapp 12-Hour Non-Drowsy Extentabs (extended-release tablets) OTC *decongestant* [pseudoephedrine HCl] 120 mg

Dimetapp Children's Cold & Allergy elixir OTC *decongestant; antihistamine* [phenylephrine HCl; brompheniramine maleate] 2.5•1 mg/10 mL

Dimetapp Children's Cold & Fever oral suspension (discontinued 2007) OTC *decongestant; analgesic; antipyretic* [pseudoephedrine HCl; ibuprofen] 15•100 mg

Dimetapp Children's ND Non-Drowsy Allergy orally disintegrating tablets, syrup OTC *nonsedating antihistamine for allergic rhinitis* [loratadine] 10 mg; 5 mg/5 mL

Dimetapp Children's Nighttime Flu syrup (discontinued 2007) OTC *antitussive; antihistamine; decongestant; analgesic; antipyretic* [dextromethorphan hydrobromide; brompheniramine maleate; pseudoephedrine HCl; acetaminophen] 5•1•15•160 mg/5 mL

Dimetapp Children's Non-Drowsy Flu syrup (discontinued 2007) OTC *antitussive; decongestant; analgesic; antipyretic; for children 2–11 years* [dextromethorphan hydrobromide; pseudoephedrine HCl; acetaminophen] 5•15•160 mg/5 mL

Dimetapp Decongestant Pediatric oral drops OTC *nasal decongestant* [pseudoephedrine HCl] 7.5 mg/0.8 mL

Dimetapp DM Children's Cold & Cough elixir (discontinued 2007) OTC *antitussive; antihistamine; decongestant* [dextromethorphan hydrobromide; brompheniramine maleate; pseudoephedrine HCl] 5•1•15 mg/5 mL

Dimetapp Long Acting Cough Plus Cold syrup OTC *antitussive; antihistamine* [dextromethorphan hydrobromide; chlorpheniramine maleate] 15•2 mg/10 mL

Dimetapp Non-Drowsy Liqui-Gels (liquid-filled softgels) OTC *decongestant* [pseudoephedrine HCl] 30 mg

Dimetapp Sinus caplets OTC *decongestant; analgesic; antipyretic* [pseudoephedrine HCl; ibuprofen] 30•200 mg

Dimetapp Toddler's Decongestant Plus Cough oral drops OTC *antitussive; decongestant; for children 2–5 years* [dextromethorphan hydrobromide; pseudoephedrine HCl] 5•2.5 mg/1.6 mL

dimethadione USAN, INN *anticonvulsant*

dimethazan ② duometacin

dimethazine [see: mebolazine]

dimethicone USAN, NF, BAN *lubricant and hydrophobing agent; soft tissue prosthetic aid* [also: dimeticone]

dimethicone 350 USAN *soft tissue prosthetic aid*

dimethindene BAN *antihistamine* [also: dimethindene maleate; dimetindene]

dimethindene maleate USP *antihistamine* [also: dimetindene; dimethindene]

dimethiodal sodium INN

dimethisoquin BAN [also: dimethisoquin HCl; quinisocaine]

dimethisoquin HCl USAN [also: quinisocaine; dimethisoquin]

dimethisterone USAN, NF, INN, BAN *progestin*

dimetholizine INN

dimethothiazine BAN *serotonin inhibitor* [also: fonazine mesylate; dimetotiazine]

dimethoxanate INN, BAN

dimethoxanate HCl [see: dimethoxanate]

2,5-dimethoxy-4-methylamphetamine (DOM) *a hallucinogenic street drug derived from amphetamine, popularly called STP*

dimethoxyphenyl penicillin sodium [see: methicillin sodium]

dimethpyridene maleate [see: dimethindene maleate]

dimethyl ketone [see: acetone]

dimethyl phthalate USP

dimethyl polysiloxane [see: dimethicone]

dimethyl sulfoxide (DMSO) USAN, USP, INN *solvent; anti-inflammatory for symptomatic relief of interstitial cystitis; investigational (orphan) for traumatic brain coma; investigational (orphan) topical treatment for scleroderma and extravasation of cytotoxic drugs* [also: dimethyl sulphoxide] 50% solution

dimethyl sulphoxide BAN *topical anti-inflammatory; solvent* [also: dimethyl sulfoxide]

dimethyl triazeno imidazole carboxamide (DIC; DTIC) [see: dacarbazine]

3-(3,5-dimethyl-1H-methylene)-1,3-dihydro-indole-2-one *investigational (orphan) for Kaposi sarcoma and von Hippel-Lindau disease*

dimethylaminoethanol (DMAE) *natural precursor to the neurotransmitter acetylcholine; readily crosses the blood-brain barrier to enhance memory and cognitive function*

dimethylaminoethanol bitartrate *natural precursor to the neurotransmitter acetylcholine; readily crosses the blood-brain barrier to enhance memory and cognitive function* (base=37%)

dimethylaminophenazone [see: aminopyrine]

dimethylcysteine [see: penicillamine]

dimethylglycine HCl (DMG) *amino acid; natural immune system booster*

dimethylhexestrol [see: methestrol]

1,5-dimethylhexylamine [see: octodrine]

5,5-dimethyl-2,4-oxazolidinedione (DMO) [see: dimethadione]

dimethyloxyquinazine [see: antipyrine]

o,α-dimethylphenethylamine [see: ortetamine]

dimethylsiloxane polymers [see: dimethicone]

dimethylthiambutene INN, BAN

dimethyltryptamine (DMT) *hallucinogenic street drug derived from a plant*

native to South America and the West Indies

dimethyltubocurarine BAN [also: dimethyltubocurarinium chloride]

dimethyltubocurarine iodide [see: metocurine iodide]

dimethyltubocurarinium chloride INN [also: dimethyltubocurarine]

dimethylxanthine [see: theophylline]

dimeticone INN *lubricant and hydrophobing agent; soft tissue prosthetic aid* [also: dimethicone]

dimetindene INN *antihistamine* [also: dimethindene maleate; dimethindene]

dimetindene maleate [see: dimethindene maleate]

dimetipirium bromide INN

dimetofrine INN

dimetotiazine INN *serotonin inhibitor* [also: fonazine mesylate; dimethothiazine]

dimetridazole INN, BAN

dimevamide INN

dimevamide sulfate [see: dimevamide]

diminazene INN, BAN

dimoxamine HCl USAN *memory adjuvant*

dimoxaprost INN

dimoxyline INN

dimpylate INN [also: diazinon]

dinaline INN

Dinate IV or IM injection ℞ *anticholinergic; antiemetic; antivertigo agent; motion sickness preventative* [dimenhydrinate] 50 mg/mL ② D-Tann aT; Duonate-12

dinazafone INN

diniprofylline INN

dinitolmide INN, BAN

dinitrotoluamide [see: dinitolmide]

dinoprost USAN, INN, BAN *oxytocic for induction of labor; prostaglandin-type abortifacient; cervical ripening agent*

dinoprost trometamol BAN *oxytocic for induction of labor; prostaglandin-type abortifacient; cervical ripening agent* [also: dinoprost tromethamine]

dinoprost tromethamine USAN *oxytocic for induction of labor; prostaglandin-type abortifacient; treatment for postpartum uterine bleeding* [also: dinoprost trometamol]

dinoprostone USAN, INN, BAN *oxytocic for induction of labor; prostaglandin-type abortifacient; cervical ripening agent*

dinsed USAN, INN *coccidiostat for poultry* ② Donna-Sed

Diocto oral liquid, syrup (discontinued 2004) OTC *laxative; stool softener* [docusate sodium] 150 mg/15 mL; 60 mg/15 mL ② DCT

dioctyl calcium sulfosuccinate [now: docusate calcium]

dioctyl potassium sulfosuccinate [now: docusate potassium]

dioctyl sodium sulfosuccinate (DSS) [now: docusate sodium]

Dioctyn softgels OTC *laxative; stool softener* [docusate sodium] 100 mg

diodone INN [also: iodopyracet]

diohippuric acid I 125 USAN *radioactive agent*

diohippuric acid I 131 USAN *radioactive agent*

diolamine USAN, INN *combining name for radicals or groups* ② Dalmane; Dilomine

diolostene [see: methandriol]

dionin [see: ethylmorphine HCl]

diophyllin [see: aminophylline]

Dioscorea villosa medicinal herb [see: wild yam]

diosmin INN

Diostate D tablets OTC *dietary supplement* [calcium; phosphorus; vitamin D] 114 mg•88 mg•133 IU

diotyrosine I 125 USAN *radioactive agent* ② dotarizine

diotyrosine I 131 USAN *radioactive agent* ② dotarizine

Diovan tablets ℞ *angiotensin II receptor antagonist for hypertension, heart failure, or myocardial infarction* [valsartan] 40, 80, 160, 320 mg ② D-Phen 1000

Diovan HCT tablets ℞ *antihypertensive; angiotensin II receptor antagonist; diuretic* [valsartan; hydrochlorothiazide] 80•12.5, 160•12.5, 160•25, 320•12.5, 320•25 mg

dioxadilol INN

dioxadrol INN *antidepressant* [also: dioxadrol HCl] 🔲 Dexodryl

dioxadrol HCl USAN *antidepressant* [also: dioxadrol]

***d*-dioxadrol HCl** [see: dexoxadrol HCl]

dioxamate INN, BAN

dioxaphetyl butyrate INN, BAN

dioxathion BAN [also: dioxation]

dioxation INN [also: dioxathion]

dioxethedrin INN

dioxethedrin HCl [see: dioxethedrin]

dioxifedrine INN

dioxindol [see: oxyphenisatin acetate]

dioxyanthranol [see: anthralin]

dioxyanthraquinone *(withdrawn from market)* [see: danthron]

dioxybenzone USAN, USP, INN *ultraviolet screen*

dipalmitoylphosphatidylcholine (DPPC) [see: colfosceril palmitate]

diparcol HCl [see: diethazine HCl]

dipegyl [see: niacinamide]

dipenicillin G [see: penicillin G benzathine]

dipenine bromide BAN [also: diponium bromide]

Dipentum capsules ℞ *anti-inflammatory for ulcerative colitis* [olsalazine sodium] 250 mg

dipeptidyl peptidase-4 (DPP-4) inhibitors *a class of oral antidiabetic agents that enhance the function of the body's incretin system to increase insulin production in the pancreas and reduce glucose production in the liver*

diperodon USP, INN, BAN *topical anesthetic* 🔲 deprodone

diperodon HCl *topical anesthetic*

diphemanil methylsulfate USP *anticholinergic* [also: diphemanil metilsulfate; diphemanil methylsulphate]

diphemanil methylsulphate BAN *anticholinergic* [also: diphemanil methylsulfate; diphemanil metilsulfate]

diphemanil metilsulfate INN *anticholinergic* [also: diphemanil methylsulfate; diphemanil methylsulphate]

Diphen AF oral liquid OTC *antihistamine; sleep aid* [diphenhydramine HCl] 12.5 mg/5 mL

Diphen Tann 25 mg/PE Tann 10 mg/CT Tann 30 mg chewable tablets ℞ *antitussive; antihistamine; sleep aid; decongestant* [carbetapentane tannate; diphenhydramine tannate; phenylephrine tannate] 30•25•10 mg

diphenadione USP, INN, BAN

diphenan INN

diphenatil [see: diphemanil methylsulfate]

diphenchloxazine HCl [see: difencloxazine HCl]

diphenesenic acid [see: xenyhexenic acid]

Diphenhist caplets, capsules, oral liquid OTC *antihistamine; sleep aid* [diphenhydramine HCl] 25 mg; 25 mg; 12.5 mg/5 mL

diphenhydramine INN, BAN *ethanolamine antihistamine; antitussive; motion sickness preventative; sleep aid* [also: diphenhydramine citrate]

diphenhydramine citrate USP *ethanolamine antihistamine; antitussive; motion sickness preventative; sleep aid* [also: diphenhydramine]

diphenhydramine HCl USP, BAN *ethanolamine antihistamine; antitussive; motion sickness preventative; sleep aid* 25, 50 mg oral; 50 mg/mL injection

diphenhydramine tannate *ethanolamine antihistamine; antitussive; motion sickness preventative; sleep aid*

diphenhydramine theoclate [see: dimenhydrinate]

diphenidol USAN, BAN *antiemetic; antivertigo* [also: difenidol]

diphenidol HCl USAN *antiemetic*

diphenidol pamoate USAN *antiemetic*

DiphenMax D chewable tablets ℞ *decongestant; antihistamine; sleep aid* [phenylephrine tannate; diphenhydramine tannate] 10•25 mg

diphenmethanil methylsulfate [see: diphemanil methylsulfate]

diphenoxylate INN, BAN *antiperistaltic* [also: diphenoxylate HCl]

diphenoxylate HCl USP *antiperistaltic* [also: diphenoxylate]

diphenylacetylindandione [see: diphenadione]

diphenylalkylamines *a class of calcium channel blockers*

Diphenylan Sodium capsules ℞ *anticonvulsant* [phenytoin sodium] 30, 100 mg

diphenylbutazone [see: phenylbutazone]

diphenylbutylpiperidines [see: phenylbutylpiperidines]

diphenylcyclopenone *investigational (orphan) agent for severe alopecia areata, alopecia totalis, and alopecia universalis*

diphenylhydantoin [now: phenytoin]

diphenylhydantoin sodium [now: phenytoin sodium]

diphenylisatin [see: oxyphenisatin]

diphenylpyraline INN, BAN *antihistamine* [also: diphenylpyraline HCl]

diphenylpyraline HCl USP *antihistamine* [also: diphenylpyraline]

diphetarsone [see: difetarsone]

diphexamide iodomethylate [see: buzepide metiodide]

diphosphonic acid [see: etidronic acid]

diphosphopyridine nucleotide (DPN) [now: nadide]

diphosphoric acid, tetrasodium salt [see: sodium pyrophosphate]

diphosphothiamin [see: co-carboxylase]

diphoxazide INN

diphtheria antitoxin USP *passive immunizing agent for diphtheria* [also: diphtheria toxoid] 500 U/mL injection

diphtheria CRM₁₀₇ conjugate *investigational (orphan) carrier for human transferrin to treat malignant tumors of the central nervous system*

diphtheria CRM₁₉₇ conjugate *carrier protein for hemophilus b and pneumococcal vaccines*

diphtheria equine antitoxin *investigational passive immunizing agent*

(available only from the Centers for Disease Control and Prevention)

diphtheria & tetanus toxoids, adsorbed (DT; Td) USP *active immunizing agent for diphtheria and tetanus* 2•2, 2•5, 2•10, 6.6•5, 7.5• 7.5, 10•5, 12.5•5, 15•10 LfU/0.5 mL injection

diphtheria & tetanus toxoids & acellular pertussis (DTaP; Dtap; Tdap) vaccine *active immunizing agent for diphtheria, tetanus, and pertussis* [compare variants: Tdap; Dtap]

diphtheria & tetanus toxoids & pertussis vaccine (DTP) USP *active immunizing agent for diphtheria, tetanus, and pertussis*

diphtheria & tetanus toxoids & whole-cell pertussis vaccine (DTwP) *active immunizing agent for diphtheria, tetanus, and pertussis* 6.5• 5•4, 10•5.5•4 LfU/0.5 mL injection

diphtheria toxin, diagnostic [now: diphtheria toxin for Schick test]

diphtheria toxin, inactivated diagnostic [now: Schick test control]

diphtheria toxin for Schick test USP *dermal diphtheria immunity test*

diphtheria toxoid USP *active immunizing agent for diphtheria* [also: diphtheria antitoxin]

diphtheria toxoid, adsorbed USP *active immunizing agent for diphtheria* 15 LfU/0.5 mL injection

dipipanone INN, BAN

dipipanone HCl [see: dipipanone]

dipiproverine INN

dipiproverine HCl [see: dipiproverine]

dipivalyl epinephrine (DPE) [now: dipivefrin]

dipivefrin USAN *ophthalmic adrenergic* [also: dipivefrine]

dipivefrin HCl USP *topical antiglaucoma agent* 0.1% eye drops

dipivefrine INN, BAN *ophthalmic adrenergic* [also: dipivefrin]

diponium bromide INN [also: dipenine bromide]

dipotassium carbonate [see: potassium carbonate]

dipotassium clorazepate INN *benzodi-azepine anxiolytic; minor tranquilizer; anticonvulsant adjunct; alcohol withdrawal aid* [also: clorazepate dipotassium]

dipotassium hydrogen phosphate [see: potassium phosphate, dibasic]

dipotassium phosphate [see: potassium phosphate, dibasic]

dipotassium pyrosulfite [see: potassium metabisulfite]

diprafenone INN

diprenorphine INN, BAN

Diprivan emulsion for IV R *general anesthetic* [propofol] 10 mg/mL

diprobutine INN, BAN

diprofene INN

diprogulic acid INN

diproleandomycin INN

Diprolene ointment, gel, lotion R *corticosteroidal anti-inflammatory* [betamethasone dipropionate, augmented] 0.05%

Diprolene AF cream R *corticosteroidal anti-inflammatory* [betamethasone dipropionate, augmented] 0.05%

diprophylline INN, BAN *bronchodilator* [also: dyphylline]

dipropylacetic acid [see: valproic acid]

2-dipropylaminoethyl diphenylthioacetate [see: diprofene]

1,1-dipropylbutylamine [see: diprobutine]

diproqualone INN

Diprosone ointment, cream, lotion, aerosol R *corticosteroidal anti-inflammatory* [betamethasone dipropionate] 0.05%; 0.05%; 0.05%; 0.1% ⑨ Debrisan

diproteverine INN, BAN

diprothazine [see: dimelazine]

diprotrizoate sodium USP [also: sodium diprotrizoate]

diproxadol INN

Dipteryx odorata; D. oppositifolia medicinal herb [see: tonka bean]

dipyridamole USAN, USP, INN, BAN *coronary vasodilator; platelet aggregation inhibitor to prevent postoperative thromboembolic complications of cardiac valve* replacement; diagnostic aid for coronary artery function 25, 50, 75 mg oral

dipyrithione USAN, INN *antibacterial; antifungal*

dipyrocetyl INN ⑨ deprostil

dipyrone USAN, BAN *analgesic; antipyretic* [also: metamizole sodium] ⑨ duoperone

diquafosol tetrasodium *investigational (NDA filed) treatment for dry eye*

dirithromycin USAN, INN, BAN *macrolide antibiotic*

disaccharide tripeptide glycerol dipalmitoyl *investigational (orphan) immunostimulant for pulmonary and hepatic metastases of colorectal adenocarcinoma, Ewing sarcoma, and osteosarcoma*

Disalcid film-coated tablets, capsules R *analgesic; antipyretic; anti-inflammatory; antirheumatic* [salsalate] 500, 750 mg; 500 mg

disalicylic acid [see: salsalate]

Dis-Co Pack (trademarked packaging form) *unit-dose package*

DisCoVisc prefilled syringes R *viscoelastic agent for ophthalmic surgery* [hyaluronate sodium; chondroitin sulfate sodium] 17•40 mg/mL

discutients *a class of agents that cause a dispersal or disappearance of a pathological condition, such as a tumor*

disease-modifying antirheumatic drugs (DMARDs) *a class of agents that slow the progression of rheumatic arthritis (RA) by modifying immune system response; this is in contrast to NSAIDs, which treat only the symptoms of the disease*

disinfectants *a class of agents that inhibit the growth and development of microorganisms, usually on an inanimate surface, without necessarily killing them* [see also: antiseptics; germicides]

Disinfecting Solution OTC *chemical disinfecting solution for soft contact lenses* [chlorhexidine; EDTA; thimerosal] 0.005%•0.1%•0.00%

disiquonium chloride USAN, INN *antiseptic*

Diskets (trademarked dosage form) *dispersible tablets*

Diskets dispersible tablets ℞ *narcotic analgesic; narcotic addiction detoxicant; often abused as a street drug* [methadone HCl] 40 mg

Diskhaler (trademarked delivery device) *inhalation powder dispenser for use with a* **Rotadisk**

Diskus (trademarked delivery device) *breath-activated inhalation powder dispenser* ☒ Dacex-A; Desoxi

disobutamide USAN, INN *antiarrhythmic*

disodium carbenicillin [see: carbenicillin disodium]

disodium carbonate [see: sodium carbonate]

disodium cefotetan [see: cefotetan disodium]

disodium chromate [see: sodium chromate]

disodium clodronate tetrahydrate [available in Canada; investigational (orphan) in the U.S.] *bisphosphonate bone resorption inhibitor for hypercalcemia and osteolysis of malignancy*

disodium cromoglycate (DSC; DSCG) [see: cromolyn sodium]

disodium dihydrogen methylenediphosphonate [see: medronate disodium]

disodium edathamil [see: edathamil disodium]

disodium edetate BAN *metal-chelating agent* [also: edetate disodium]

disodium ethylenediamine tetraacetate [see: edetate disodium]

disodium hydrogen phosphate [see: sodium phosphate]

disodium hydrogen phosphate heptahydrate [see: sodium phosphate, dibasic]

disodium hydrogen phosphate hydrate [see: sodium phosphate, dibasic]

(disodium) methylene diphosphonate (MDP) [now: medronate disodium]

disodium phosphate [see: sodium phosphate, dibasic]

disodium phosphate heptahydrate [see: sodium phosphate]

disodium phosphonoacetate monohydrate [see: fosfonet sodium]

disodium phosphorofluoridate [see: sodium monofluorophosphate]

disodium pyrosulfite [see: sodium metabisulfite]

disodium silibinin dihemisuccinate *investigational (orphan) antitoxin for* Amanita phalloides *(mushroom) intoxication*

disodium sulfate decahydrate [see: sodium sulfate]

disodium thiosulfate pentahydrate [see: sodium thiosulfate]

disofenin USAN, INN, BAN *carrier agent in diagnostic tests*

disogluside INN

disoprofol [see: propofol]

disopromine HCl [see: diisopromine HCl]

disoproxil *combining name for radicals or groups* [also: soproxil]

disopyramide USAN, INN, BAN *antiarrhythmic for severe ventricular arrhythmias*

disopyramide phosphate USAN, USP, BAN *antiarrhythmic for severe ventricular arrhythmias* 100, 150 mg oral

disoxaril USAN, INN *antiviral*

Di-Spaz capsules, IM injection ℞ *gastrointestinal anticholinergic/antispasmodic for irritable bowel syndrome (IBS)* [dicyclomine HCl] 10 mg; 10 mg/mL

Dispenserpak (trademarked packaging form) *unit-of-use package*

DisperMox tablets for oral suspension ℞ *aminopenicillin antibiotic* [amoxicillin] 200, 400 mg

dispersible cellulose BAN *tablet and capsule diluent* [also: cellulose, microcrystalline]

Dispertab (trademarked dosage form) *delayed-release tablet*

Dispette (trademarked delivery device) *disposable pipette*

Dispos-a-Med (trademarked dosage form) *solution for inhalation*

distaquaine [see: penicillin V]

distigmine bromide INN, BAN

disulergine INN

disulfamide INN [also: disulphamide]

disulfiram USP, INN, BAN *deterrent to alcohol consumption*

disulfurous acid, dipotassium salt [see: potassium metabisulfite]

disulfurous acid, disodium salt [see: sodium metabisulfite]

disulphamide BAN [also: disulfamide]

disuprazole INN

ditazole INN

ditekiren USAN *antihypertensive; renin inhibitor*

ditercalinium chloride INN

dithiazanine BAN [also: dithiazanine iodide]

dithiazanine iodide USP, INN [also: dithiazanine]

dithranol INN, BAN *topical antipsoriatic* [also: anthralin] ☒ deterenol

D.I.T.I.-2 vaginal cream ℞ *broad-spectrum antibiotic; antiseptic; moisturizer/lubricant* [sulfanilamide; aminacrine HCl; allantoin] 15%•0.2%•2%

ditiocarb sodium INN

ditiomustine INN

ditolamide INN

ditophal INN, BAN

Ditropan tablets, syrup ℞ *urinary antispasmodic for urge urinary incontinence and frequency* [oxybutynin chloride] 5 mg; 5 mg/5 mL

Ditropan XL extended-release tablets ℞ *urinary antispasmodic for urge urinary incontinence and frequency* [oxybutynin chloride] 5, 10, 15 mg

Diurese tablets (discontinued 2006) ℞ *diuretic; antihypertensive* [trichlormethiazide] 4 mg ☒ Dairy Ease; Dry Eyes; DUROS

diuretics *a class of agents that stimulate increased excretion of urine* ☒ Drytex

Diurigen tablets (discontinued 2008) ℞ *diuretic* [chlorothiazide] 500 mg ☒ DuraGen

Diuril oral suspension ℞ *diuretic* [chlorothiazide] 250 mg/5 mL ☒ Doral

Diuril powder for IV injection ℞ *diuretic* [chlorothiazide sodium] 500 mg ☒ Doral

Diuril tablets (discontinued 2008) ℞ *diuretic* [chlorothiazide] 250, 500 mg ☒ Doral

Diutensen-R tablets (discontinued 2007) ℞ *antihypertensive* [methyclothiazide; reserpine] 2.5•0.1 mg

divabuterol INN

divalproex sodium USAN *anticonvulsant for complex partial seizures and simple or complex absence seizures; treatment for manic episodes of a bipolar disorder; migraine headache prophylaxis; valproic acid derivative* [also: valproate semisodium; semisodium valproate] 125, 250, 500 mg oral

divanilliden cyclohexanone [see: cyclovalone]

divaplon INN

Divide-Tab (trademarked dosage form) *scored tablet*

Dividose (trademarked dosage form) *multiple-scored tablets*

Divigel gel ℞ *estrogen-replacement therapy for moderate-to-severe hot flashes associated with menopause* [estradiol] 0.1% (0.25, 0.5, 1.0 g/pkt.)

diviminol [see: viminol]

divinyl ether [see: vinyl ether]

divinyl oxide [see: vinyl ether]

dixamone bromide [see: methantheline bromide]

dixanthogen INN

dixarit [see: clonidine]

dizatrifone INN

dizocilpine INN *neuroprotective; NMDA (N-methyl-D-aspartate) antagonist* [also: dizocilpine maleate]

dizocilpine maleate USAN *neuroprotective; NMDA (N-methyl-D-aspartate) antagonist* [also: dizocilpine]

D-Lay (trademarked dosage form) *timed-release tablet*

DMAE (dimethylaminoethanol) [q.v.]

DMARDs (disease-modifying antirheumatic drugs) *a class of agents that slow the progression of rheumatic* arthritis (RA) by modifying immune system response; this is in contrast to NSAIDs, which treat only the symptoms of the disease

DMax syrup (discontinued 2007) ℞ antitussive; antihistamine; decongestant [dextromethorphan hydrobromide; carbinoxamine maleate; phenylephrine HCl] 30•8•16 mg/10 mL ☒ Diamox

DMax Pediatric oral drops (discontinued 2007) ℞ antitussive; antihistamine; decongestant; for children 1–24 months [dextromethorphan hydrobromide; carbinoxamine maleate; phenylephrine HCl] 4•2•2 mg/mL

DMC (dactinomycin, methotrexate, cyclophosphamide) chemotherapy protocol

DMCT (demethylchlortetracycline) [see: demeclocycline]

DMG (dimethylglycine) [q.v.]

DML lotion OTC moisturizer; emollient

DML Forte cream OTC moisturizer; emollient

DMO (dimethyl oxazolidinedione) [see: dimethadione]

DMP 777 investigational (orphan) for the management of cystic fibrosis lung disease

DMSA (dimercaptosuccinic acid) [see: succimer]

DMSO (dimethyl sulfoxide) [q.v.]

DMT (dimethyltryptamine) street drug [q.v.]

DNA (deoxyribonucleic acid)

DNA polymerase [see: reverse transcriptase inhibitors; non-nucleoside reverse transcriptase inhibitors]

DNase (recombinant human deoxyribonuclease I) [see: dornase alfa]

DNP-conjugated tumor vaccine investigational (Phase III, orphan) theraccine for postsurgical stage III malignant melanoma

DNR (daunorubicin) [q.v.]

Doak Tar shampoo OTC antiseborrheic; antipsoriatic; antipruritic; antibacterial [coal tar] 1.2%

Doak Tar Oil topical liquid OTC antiseborrheic; antipsoriatic; antipruritic; antibacterial [coal tar] 0.8%, 2%

Doan's caplets OTC analgesic; antirheumatic [magnesium salicylate] 325, 377, 500 mg ☒ Denaze

Doan's P.M. caplets OTC analgesic; antirheumatic; antihistamine; sleep aid [magnesium salicylate; diphenhydramine HCl] 500•25 mg

DOAP (daunorubicin, Oncovin, ara-C, prednisone) chemotherapy protocol

dobupride INN ☒ Depored-40

dobutamine USAN, INN, BAN vasopressor for cardiac shock

dobutamine HCl USAN, USP, BAN vasopressor for cardiac shock 12.5 mg/mL injection

dobutamine lactobionate USAN cardiotonic

dobutamine tartrate USAN cardiotonic

Dobutrex IV infusion (discontinued 2006) ℞ vasopressor for cardiac shock [dobutamine HCl] 12.5 mg/mL

DOCA (desoxycorticosterone acetate) [q.v.]

docarpamine INN

docebenone USAN, INN 5-lipoxygenase inhibitor

docetaxel USAN, INN antineoplastic for advanced or metastatic breast, prostate, stomach, head, neck, and non–small cell lung cancer (NSCLC); also used for ovarian, esophageal, and other cancers; analogue to paclitaxel 10 mg/mL injection

docetaxel & cisplatin chemotherapy protocol for bladder cancer and non–small cell lung cancer (NSCLC)

dock, curled; curly dock; narrow dock; sour dock medicinal herb [see: yellow dock]

dock, patience; sweet dock medicinal herb [see: bistort]

doconazole USAN, INN antifungal ☒ Deconsal II

doconexent INN omega-3 marine triglyceride [also: docosahexaenoic acid (DHA)]

docosahexaenoic acid (DHA) *natural omega-3 fatty acid used to prevent a wide range of degenerative diseases; high concentrations are found in the brain, where supplementation may increase brain function; effective in treating depression and other brain disorders* [also: doconexent]

docosanol (n-docosanol) USAN *antiviral for herpes simplex labialis; topical treatment of oral herpes simplex type 1* ⑨ Dexone LA

docosil INN *combining name for radicals or groups*

Docu oral liquid; syrup OTC *laxative; stool softener* [docusate sodium] 150 mg/15 mL; 20 mg/5 mL

docusate calcium USAN, USP *laxative; stool softener* 240 mg oral

docusate potassium USAN, USP *laxative; stool softener*

docusate sodium USAN, USP, BAN *stool softener; surfactant/wetting agent* [also: sodium dioctyl sulfosuccinate] 50, 100, 250 mg oral; 50 mg/15 mL oral ⑨ Dex-Tuss DM

Docusate with Casanthranol capsules OTC *stool softener; stimulant laxative* [docusate sodium; casanthranol] 100•30 mg

dodecafluoropentane [see: perflenapent]

dodeclonium bromide INN

2-dodecylisoquinolinium bromide [see: lauryl isoquinolinium bromide]

dofamium chloride INN, BAN

dofetilide USAN, INN, BAN *antiarrhythmic; potassium channel blocker*

dofosfate INN *combining name for radicals or groups*

dog grass *medicinal herb* [see: couch grass]

dog poison (Aethusa cynapium) plant *medicinal herb used as an antispasmodic and emetic in homeopathic remedies; not generally regarded as safe and effective as ingestion may be fatal*

dogbane (Apocynum androsaemifolium) root *medicinal herb used as a cathartic, diuretic, emetic, expectorant, stimulant, and sudorific*

dogwood, black; black alder dogwood *medicinal herb* [see: buckthorn; cascara sagrada]

DOK-Plus syrup OTC *stimulant laxative; stool softener* [casanthranol; docusate sodium; alcohol 10%] 30•60 mg/15 mL ⑨ DHC Plus

Dolacet capsules ℞ *narcotic analgesic; antipyretic* [hydrocodone bitartrate; acetaminophen] 5•500 mg ⑨ Dulcet

dolantal [see: meperidine HCl]

dolantin [see: meperidine HCl]

dolasetron INN *serotonin 5-HT₃ receptor antagonist; antiemetic to prevent nausea and vomiting following chemotherapy or surgery; also used to prevent radiation-induced nausea and vomiting* [also: dolasetron mesylate]

dolasetron mesylate USAN *serotonin 5-HT₃ receptor antagonist; antiemetic to prevent nausea and vomiting following chemotherapy or surgery; also used to prevent radiation-induced nausea and vomiting* [also: dolasetron]

Dolgic caplets ℞ *barbiturate sedative; analgesic; antipyretic* [butalbital; acetaminophen] 50•650 mg

Dolgic LQ oral solution ℞ *barbiturate sedative; analgesic; antipyretic* [butalbital; acetaminophen; caffeine; alcohol 7.4%] 50•325•40 mg/15 mL

Dolgic Plus oral liquid ℞ *barbiturate sedative; analgesic; antipyretic* [butalbital; acetaminophen; caffeine] 50•750•40 mg

doliracetam INN

Dolobid film-coated tablets (discontinued 2007) ℞ *analgesic; antiarthritic; antirheumatic; anti-inflammatory; antipyretic* [diflunisal] 250, 500 mg

dolomite *nutritional supplement; source of calcium and magnesium*

Dolomite tablets OTC *mineral supplement* [calcium; magnesium] 130•78 mg

Dolono elixir (discontinued 2008) OTC *analgesic; antipyretic* [acetaminophen] 160 mg/5 mL

Dolophine HCl subcu or IM injection (discontinued 2004) ℞ *narcotic analgesic; narcotic addiction detoxicant; often abused as a street drug* [methadone HCl] 10 mg/mL

Dolophine HCl tablets ℞ *narcotic analgesic; narcotic addiction detoxicant; often abused as a street drug* [methadone HCl] 5, 10 mg

Dolorac cream OTC *analgesic; counterirritant* [capsaicin] 0.025%

dolosal [see: meperidine HCl]

Dolsed sugar-coated tablets (discontinued 2008) ℞ *urinary antibiotic; analgesic; antispasmodic; acidifier* [methenamine; phenyl salicylate; atropine sulfate; methylene blue; hyoscyamine sulfate; benzoic acid] 40.8•18.1•0.03•5.4•0.03•4.5 mg

dolvanol [see: meperidine HCl]

DOM (2,5-dimethoxy-4-methylamphetamine) *a hallucinogenic street drug derived from amphetamine, popularly called STP*

domazoline INN *anticholinergic* [also: domazoline fumarate]

domazoline fumarate USAN *anticholinergic* [also: domazoline]

Domeboro powder packets, effervescent tablets OTC *astringent wet dressing (modified Burow solution)* [aluminum sulfate; calcium acetate]

Domeboro Otic [see: Otic Domeboro]

Dome-Paste medicated gauze bandage OTC *protection and support of extremities* [zinc oxide; calamine; gelatin]

domestrol [see: diethylstilbestrol]

domibrom [see: domiphen bromide]

domiodol USAN, INN *mucolytic*

domiphen bromide USAN, BAN *topical anti-infective*

domipizone INN

Domol Bath and Shower Oil OTC *bath emollient*

domoprednate INN

domoxin INN

domperidone USAN, INN, BAN, JAN *antiemetic for diabetic gastroparesis and chronic gastritis*

domperidone maleate INN, BAN *antiemetic for diabetic gastroparesis and chronic gastritis* (base=78.6%)

Donatussin oral drops ℞ *decongestant; expectorant; for children 1–24 months* [phenylephrine HCl; guaifenesin] 1.5•20 mg/mL

Donatussin syrup ℞ *antitussive; decongestant; antihistamine; expectorant* [dextromethorphan hydrobromide; phenylephrine HCl; chlorpheniramine maleate; guaifenesin] 15•10•2•100 mg/5 mL

Donatussin DC syrup ℞ *narcotic antitussive; decongestant; expectorant* [hydrocodone bitartrate; phenylephrine HCl; guaifenesin] 2.5•6•120 mg/5 mL

Donatussin DM oral drops ℞ *antitussive; antihistamine; decongestant; for children 3–24 months* [dextromethorphan hydrobromide; chlorpheniramine maleate; phenylephrine HCl] 3•1•1.5 mg/mL

Donatussin DM syrup OTC *antitussive; decongestant; expectorant* [dextromethorphan hydrobromide; pseudoephedrine HCl; guaifenesin] 15•30•150 mg/5 mL

donepezil HCl USAN *reversible acetylcholinesterase (AChE) inhibitor; cognition adjuvant for Alzheimer dementia; also used for vascular dementia, poststroke aphasia, and memory improvement in multiple sclerosis patients* 5, 10 mg oral

donetidine USAN, INN, BAN *antagonist to histamine H_2 receptors*

dong quai (Angelica polymorpha; A. sinensis; A. dahurica) *root medicinal herb for allergies, anemia, blood cleansing, constipation, female hormonal problems, hypertension, internal bleeding, menopausal symptoms, nourishing brain, and ulcers; not generally regarded as safe and effective as it contains coumarins and safrole*

Donnagel chewable tablets, oral liquid (discontinued 2004) OTC *antidi-*

arrheal; GI adsorbent [attapulgite] 600 mg; 600 mg/15 mL ⊡ Denquel

Donnamar tablets (discontinued 2004) ℞ *GI/GU antispasmodic; antiparkinsonian; anticholinergic "drying agent" for allergic rhinitis and hyperhidrosis* [hyoscyamine sulfate] 0.125 mg

Donna-Sed elixir ℞ *GI antispasmodic; anticholinergic; sedative* [atropine sulfate; scopolamine hydrobromide; hyoscyamine hydrobromide; phenobarbital] 0.0194•0.0065•0.1037• 16.2 mg/5 mL ⊡ dinsed

Donnatal capsules (discontinued 2004) ℞ *GI/GU anticholinergic/antispasmodic; sedative* [atropine sulfate; scopolamine hydrobromide; hyoscyamine sulfate; phenobarbital] 0.0194• 0.0065•0.1037•16.2 mg

Donnatal Extentabs (extended-release tablets), tablets, elixir ℞ *GI/GU anticholinergic/antispasmodic; sedative* [atropine sulfate; scopolamine hydrobromide; hyoscyamine sulfate; phenobarbital] 0.0582•0.0195• 0.3111•48.6 mg; 0.0194•0.0065• 0.1037•16.2 mg; 0.0194•0.0065• 0.1037•16.2 mg/5 mL

Donnatal No. 2 tablets (discontinued 2004) ℞ *GI antispasmodic; anticholinergic; sedative* [atropine sulfate; scopolamine hydrobromide; hyoscyamine sulfate; phenobarbital] 0.0194•0.0065•0.1037•32.4 mg

DOPA (dihydroxyphenylalanine) [see: levodopa]

L-dopa [see: levodopa]

dopamantine USAN, INN *antiparkinsonian*

dopamine INN, BAN *vasopressor for cardiac, pulmonary, traumatic, septic, or renal shock* [also: dopamine HCl]

dopamine HCl USAN, USP *vasopressor for cardiac, pulmonary, traumatic, septic, or renal shock; also used for chronic obstructive pulmonary disease (COPD), congestive heart failure (CHF), and respiratory distress syndrome (RDS) in infants* [also: dopamine] 40, 80, 160 mg/mL injection

Dopamine HCl in 5% Dextrose IV injection ℞ *vasopressor for cardiac, pulmonary, traumatic, septic, or renal shock; also used for chronic obstructive pulmonary disease (COPD), congestive heart failure (CHF), and respiratory distress syndrome (RDS) in infants* [dopamine HCl; dextrose] 80, 160, 320 mg/100 mL

dopaminergics *a class of antiparkinsonian agents that affect the dopamine neurotransmitters in the brain*

Dopar capsules ℞ *dopamine precursor for Parkinson disease* [levodopa] 100, 250, 500 mg ⊡ Daypro

dopexamine USAN, INN, BAN *cardiovascular agent*

dopexamine HCl USAN, BAN *cardiovascular agent*

Dopram IV injection or infusion ℞ *CNS stimulant; analeptic; adjunct to postanesthesia "stir-up"; respiratory stimulant for chronic obstructive pulmonary disease (COPD); also used for apnea of prematurity* [doxapram HCl] 20 mg/mL

dopropidil INN

doqualast INN

Doral caplets ℞ *benzodiazepine sedative and hypnotic* [quazepam] 7.5, 15 mg ⊡ Diuril

dorastine INN *antihistamine* [also: dorastine HCl]

dorastine HCl USAN *antihistamine* [also: dorastine]

doreptide INN

doretinel USAN, INN *antikeratinizing agent*

Doribax IV infusion ℞ *broad-spectrum carbapenem antibiotic for complicated urinary tract infections (cUTI), including pyelonephritis, and complicated intra-abdominal infections (cIAI); investigational (Phase III, orphan) for nosocomial pneumonia* [doripenem] 500 mg

doripenem *broad-spectrum carbapenem antibiotic for complicated urinary tract infections (cUTI), including pyelonephritis, and complicated intra-abdominal* infections (cIAI); investigational (Phase III, orphan) for nosocomial pneumonia

Dormarex 2 tablets OTC antihistamine; sleep aid; motion sickness preventative [diphenhydramine HCl] 50 mg

dormethan [see: dextromethorphan hydrobromide]

Dormin caplets, capsules OTC antihistamine; sleep aid [diphenhydramine HCl] 25 mg

dormiral [see: phenobarbital]

dormonal [see: barbital]

dornase alfa USAN, INN reduces respiratory viscoelasticity of sputum in cystic fibrosis (orphan)

Doryx coated pellets in capsules, delayed-release tablets ℞ tetracycline antibiotic [doxycycline hyclate] 75, 100, 150 mg ⊡ Droxia

dorzolamide HCl USAN topical carbonic anhydrase inhibitor for glaucoma

D.O.S. softgels OTC laxative; stool softener [docusate sodium] 100, 250 mg

Dosa-Trol Pack (trademarked packaging form) unit-of-use package

Dosepak (trademarked packaging form) unit-of-use package ⊡ Despec

dosergoside INN

Dosette (trademarked packaging form) injectable unit-of-use system (vials, ampules, syringes, etc.) ⊡ Duocet

Dospan (trademarked dosage form) controlled-release tablets

Dostinex tablets (discontinued 2008) ℞ dopamine agonist for hyperprolactinemia [cabergoline] 0.5 mg

dosulepin INN antidepressant [also: dothiepin HCl; dothiepin; dosulepin HCl]

dosulepin HCl JAN antidepressant [also: dothiepin HCl; dosulepin; dothiepin]

dotarizine INN ⊡ diotyrosine I 125

dotefonium bromide INN

dothiepin BAN antidepressant [also: dothiepin HCl; dosulepin; dosulepin HCl]

dothiepin HCl USAN antidepressant [also: dosulepin; dothiepin; dosulepin HCl]

Double Antibiotic ointment OTC antibiotic [polymyxin B sulfate; bacitracin zinc] 10 000•500 U/g

Double Ice ArthriCare [see: ArthriCare, Double Ice]

Double-Action Toothache Kit tablets + topical liquid OTC analgesic; antipyretic + mucous membrane anesthetic [acetaminophen + benzocaine; alcohol 74%] 325 mg + ²

Dovobet (foreign name for U.S. product **Taclonex**)

Dovonex cream, ointment, scalp solution ℞ antipsoriatic [calcipotriene] 0.005%

DOX → CMF, sequential (doxorubicin; cyclophosphamide, methotrexate, fluorouracil) chemotherapy protocol for breast cancer

doxacurium chloride USAN, INN, BAN nondepolarizing neuromuscular blocker; muscle relaxant; adjunct to anesthesia

doxaminol INN

doxapram INN, BAN respiratory stimulant; analeptic [also: doxapram HCl]

doxapram HCl USAN, USP CNS stimulant; analeptic; adjunct to postanesthesia "stir-up"; respiratory stimulant for chronic obstructive pulmonary disease (COPD); also used for apnea of prematurity [also: doxapram] 20 mg/mL injection

doxaprost USAN, INN bronchodilator

doxate [see: docusate sodium]

doxazosin INN, BAN alpha$_1$-adrenergic blocker for hypertension and benign prostatic hyperplasia (BPH) [also: doxazosin mesylate]

doxazosin mesylate USAN alpha$_1$-adrenergic blocker for hypertension and benign prostatic hyperplasia (BPH) [also: doxazosin] 1, 2, 4, 8 mg oral

doxefazepam INN

doxenitoin INN

doxepin INN, BAN tricyclic antidepressant; anxiolytic; topical antihistamine [also: doxepin HCl]

doxepin HCl USAN, USP tricyclic antidepressant; anxiolytic; topical antihistamine; investigational (NDA filed) for *chronic insomnia* [also: doxepin] 10, 25, 50, 75, 100, 150 mg oral; 10 mg/mL oral

doxercalciferol USAN *synthetic vitamin D analogue; serum calcium regulator for hyperparathyroidism due to chronic kidney disease*

doxibetasol INN [also: doxybetasol]

Doxidan delayed-release tablets OTC *stimulant laxative* [bisacodyl] 5 mg

doxifluridine INN, JAN *antineoplastic*

Doxil IV injection suspension ℞ *antineoplastic for Kaposi sarcoma, ovarian cancer (orphan), and multiple myeloma (orphan); investigational (Phase III) for breast cancer* [doxorubicin HCl, liposome-encapsulated] 20, 60 mg/vial

doxofylline USAN, INN *bronchodilator*

doxorubicin USAN, INN, BAN *anthracycline antibiotic antineoplastic*

doxorubicin HCl USP *anthracycline antibiotic antineoplastic* 10, 20, 50 mg, 2 mg/mL injection

doxorubicin HCl, liposome-encapsulated (LED) *anthracycline antibiotic antineoplastic for Kaposi sarcoma, ovarian cancer (orphan), and multiple myeloma (orphan); investigational (Phase III) for breast cancer*

doxorubicin & vinorelbine *chemotherapy protocol for breast cancer*

doxpicodin HCl [now: doxpicomine HCl]

doxpicomine INN *analgesic* [also: doxpicomine HCl]

doxpicomine HCl USAN *analgesic* [also: doxpicomine]

Doxy 100; Doxy 200 powder for IV infusion ℞ *tetracycline antibiotic* [doxycycline hyclate] 100 mg/vial; 200 mg/vial ② Degas

doxybetasol BAN [also: doxibetasol]

doxycycline USAN, USP, INN, BAN *tetracycline antibiotic for the treatment of rosacea; antirickettsial; malaria prophylaxis* 25 mg/5 mL oral

doxycycline calcium USP *tetracycline antibiotic; antiprotozoal*

doxycycline fosfatex USAN, BAN *tetracycline antibiotic*

doxycycline hyclate USP *tetracycline antibiotic; periodontitis treatment* 20, 50, 75, 100 mg oral; 100 mg/vial injection

doxycycline monohydrate *tetracycline antibiotic* 50, 75, 100, 150 mg oral

doxylamine INN, BAN *antihistamine; sleep aid* [also: doxylamine succinate]

doxylamine succinate USP *antihistamine; sleep aid* [also: doxylamine]

DPE (dipivalyl epinephrine) [now: dipivefrin]

DPF [see: Dermprotective Factor]

D-Phen 1000 extended-release caplets ℞ *decongestant; expectorant* [phenylephrine HCl; guaifenesin] 30•1000 mg ② Diovan

DPN (diphosphopyridine nucleotide) [now: nadide]

DPP-4 (dipeptidyl peptidase-4) inhibitors *a class of oral antidiabetic agents that enhance the function of the body's incretin system to increase insulin production in the pancreas and reduce glucose production in the liver*

DPPC (dipalmitoylphosphatidylcholine) [see: colfosceril palmitate]

DPPE (diethyl-phenylmethyl-phenoxy ethenamine) HCl [see: tesmilifene HCl]

Dr. Brown's Home Drug Testing System *in vitro diagnostic aid for detection of multiple illicit drugs in the urine*

Dr. Dermi-Heal ointment OTC *vulnerary; antipruritic; astringent* [allantoin; zinc oxide; Peruvian balsam] 1%•?•?

Dr. Edwards' Olive tablets OTC *stimulant laxative* [sennosides] 8.6 mg

Dr. Scholl's Advanced Pain Relief Corn Removers; Dr. Scholl's Callus Removers; Dr Scholl's Clear Away; Dr. Scholl's Corn Removers medicated discs OTC *keratolytic* [salicylic acid in a rubber-based vehicle] 40%

Dr. Scholl's Athlete's Foot powder, spray powder, spray liquid OTC *antifungal* [tolnaftate] 1%

Dr. Scholl's Clear Away OneStep; Dr. Scholl's OneStep Corn Removers medicated strips OTC *keratolytic* [salicylic acid in a rubber-based vehicle] 40%

Dr. Scholl's Corn/Callus Remover topical liquid OTC *keratolytic* [salicylic acid in flexible collodion] 17%

Dr. Scholl's Cracked Heel Relief cream OTC *anesthetic; antiseptic* [lidocaine HCl; benzalkonium chloride] 2%•0.13%

Dr. Scholl's Moisturizing Corn Remover Kit medicated discs + cushions + moisturizing cream OTC *keratolytic* [salicylic acid in a rubber-based vehicle] 40%

Dr. Scholl's Tritin powder, spray powder OTC *antifungal* [tolnaftate] 1%

Dr. Scholl's Wart Remover Kit topical liquid + adhesive pads OTC *keratolytic* [salicylic acid in flexible collodion] 17%

Dr. Smith's Adult Care; Dr. Smith's Diaper ointment OTC *astringent; moisturizer; emollient* [zinc oxide] 10%

draflazine USAN *cardioprotectant*

dragée (French for "sugar plum") *a sugar-coated pill or medicated confection* [pronounced "drah zhá"]

dragon's claw, scaly *medicinal herb* [see: coral root]

dragonwort *medicinal herb* [see: bistort]

Dramamine oral liquid ℞ *antinauseant; antiemetic; antivertigo agent; motion sickness preventative* [dimenhydrinate] 15.62 mg/5 mL

Dramamine tablets, chewable tablets, oral liquid OTC *antinauseant; antiemetic; antivertigo agent; motion sickness preventative* [dimenhydrinate] 50 mg; 50 mg; 12.5 mg/4 mL

Dramamine, Children's oral liquid OTC *antinauseant; antiemetic; antivertigo agent; motion sickness preventative* [dimenhydrinate; alcohol 5%] 12.5 mg/5 mL

Dramamine Less Drowsy Formula tablets OTC *anticholinergic; antihista-mine; antivertigo agent; motion sickness preventative* [meclizine HCl] 25 mg

Dramanate IV or IM injection ℞ *antinauseant; antiemetic; antivertigo agent; motion sickness preventative* [dimenhydrinate] 50 mg/mL

dramarin [see: dimenhydrate]

dramedilol INN

Dramilin IV or IM injection ℞ *antinauseant; antiemetic; antivertigo agent; motion sickness preventative* [dimenhydrinate] 50 mg/mL ☒ Dermolin

dramyl [see: dimenhydrate]

draquinolol INN

drazidox INN

Drepanol *investigational (orphan) for prophylactic treatment of sickle cell disease* [OM 401 (code name—generic name not yet assigned)]

dribendazole USAN, INN *anthelmintic*

dricol [see: amidephrine]

Dri/Ear ear drops OTC *antiseptic; emollient* [isopropyl alcohol; glycerin] 95%•5%

dried aluminum hydroxide gel [see: aluminum hydroxide gel, dried]

dried basic aluminum carbonate [see: aluminum carbonate, basic]

dried ferrous sulfate [see: ferrous sulfate, dried]

dried yeast [see: yeast, dried]

DriHist SR sustained-release caplets ℞ *decongestant; antihistamine; anticholinergic to dry mucosal secretions* [phenylephrine HCl; chlorpheniramine maleate; methscopolamine nitrate] 20•8•2.5 mg

drinidene USAN, INN *analgesic*

Drisdol capsules ℞ *vitamin deficiency therapy for refractory rickets, familial hypophosphatemia, and hypoparathyroidism* [ergocalciferol (vitamin D_2)] 50 000 IU

Drisdol Drops for oral or IM administration OTC *vitamin supplement; vitamin deficiency therapy for refractory rickets, familial hypophosphatemia, and hypoparathyroidism* [ergocalciferol (vitamin D_2)] 8000 IU/mL

Dristan 12-Hr. nasal spray OTC *nasal decongestant* [oxymetazoline HCl] 0.05%

Dristan Cold, Maximum Strength caplets OTC *decongestant; antihistamine; analgesic; antipyretic* [pseudoephedrine HCl; brompheniramine maleate; acetaminophen] 30•2•500 mg

Dristan Cold Multi-Symptom Formula tablets OTC *decongestant; antihistamine; analgesic; antipyretic* [phenylephrine HCl; chlorpheniramine maleate; acetaminophen] 5•2•325 mg

Dristan Cold Non-Drowsy caplets (discontinued 2007) OTC *decongestant; analgesic; antipyretic* [pseudoephedrine HCl; acetaminophen] 30•500 mg

Dristan Fast Acting Formula nasal spray OTC *nasal decongestant; antihistamine* [phenylephrine HCl; pheniramine maleate] 0.5%•0.2%

Dristan Sinus caplets (discontinued 2007) OTC *decongestant; analgesic; antipyretic* [pseudoephedrine HCl; ibuprofen] 30•200 mg

Drithocreme; Drithocreme HP 1% cream (discontinued 2006) ℞ *antipsoriatic* [anthralin] 0.1%, 0.25%, 0.5%; 1%

Dritho-Scalp cream ℞ *antipsoriatic for the scalp* [anthralin] 0.5%

Drixomed sustained-release tablets ℞ *decongestant; antihistamine* [pseudoephedrine sulfate; dexbrompheniramine maleate] 120•6 mg

Drixoral 12 hour Non-Drowsy Formula extended-release tablets OTC *nasal decongestant* [pseudoephedrine sulfate] 120 mg

Drixoral Allergy Sinus extended-release tablets (discontinued 2007) OTC *decongestant; antihistamine; analgesic; antipyretic* [pseudoephedrine sulfate; dexbrompheniramine maleate; acetaminophen] 60•3•500 mg

Drixoral Cold & Allergy extended-release tablets OTC *decongestant; antihistamine* [pseudoephedrine sulfate; dexbrompheniramine maleate] 120•6 mg

drobuline USAN, INN *antiarrhythmic*

drocarbil NF

drocinonide USAN, INN *anti-inflammatory*

droclidinium bromide INN

drocode [see: dihydrocodeine]

drofenine INN

droloxifene INN *antiestrogen antineoplastic*

droloxifene citrate USAN *antineoplastic; antiestrogen*

drometrizole USAN, INN *ultraviolet screen*

dromostanolone propionate USAN, USP *antineoplastic* [also: drostanolone]

dronabinol USAN, USP, INN *cannabinoid; antiemetic for chemotherapy; appetite stimulant for AIDS patients (orphan)* 2.5, 5, 10 mg oral

dronedarone *investigational (Phase III) multi-channel antiarrhythmic that affects the calcium, potassium, and sodium channels*

drop chalk [see: calcium carbonate]

dropberry *medicinal herb* [see: Solomon's seal]

Drop-Dose (trademarked delivery form) *prefilled eye drop dispenser*

dropempine INN

droperidol USAN, USP, INN, BAN *general anesthetic; antiemetic; antipsychotic*

Dropperettes (delivery form) *prefilled droppers*

droprenilamine USAN, INN *coronary vasodilator*

dropropizine INN, BAN

Drop-Tainers (trademarked delivery form) *prefilled eye drop dispenser*

drospirenone USAN *progestin; spironolactone analogue; aldosterone antagonist; androgen and mineralocorticoid blocker*

drostanolone INN, BAN *antineoplastic* [also: dromostanolone propionate]

drotaverine INN

drotebanol INN, BAN

Drotic ear drops (discontinued 2006) ℞ *corticosteroidal anti-inflammatory; antibiotic* [hydrocortisone; neomycin sulfate; polymyxin B sulfate] 1%•5 mg•10 000 U per mL

drotrecogin alfa *recombinant human activated protein C (rhAPC); thrombolytic/fibrinolytic for severe sepsis*

DroTuss *oral liquid* ℞ *narcotic antitussive; decongestant; antihistamine; expectorant* [hydrocodone bitartrate; pseudoephedrine HCl; chlorpheniramine maleate; guaifenesin] 2.5•15•2•100 mg/5 mL ☑ Duratuss

droxacin INN *antibacterial* [also: droxacin sodium]

droxacin sodium USAN *antibacterial* [also: droxacin]

Droxia *capsules* ℞ *sickle cell anemia treatment (orphan)* [hydroxyurea] 200, 300, 400 mg ☑ Doryx

droxicainide INN

droxicam INN

droxidopa INN *synthetic precursor of norepinephrine; investigational (orphan) for neurogenic orthostatic hypotension*

droxifilcon A USAN *hydrophilic contact lens material*

droxinavir HCl USAN *antiviral; HIV-1 protease inhibitor*

droxypropine INN, BAN

Dry E 400 *tablets (discontinued 2004)* OTC *vitamin supplement* [vitamin E (as d-alpha tocopheryl acid succinate)] 400 IU

Dry Eyes *eye drops* OTC *moisturizer/lubricant* [polyvinyl alcohol] 1.4% ☑ Dairy Ease; Diurese; DUROS

Dry Eyes *ophthalmic ointment* OTC *ocular moisturizer/lubricant* [white petrolatum; mineral oil] ☑ Dairy Ease; Diurese; DUROS

Dryopteris filix-mas medicinal herb [see: aspidium]

Dryphen Multi-Symptom Formula *tablets* OTC *decongestant; antihistamine; analgesic; antipyretic* [phenylephrine HCl; chlorpheniramine maleate; acetaminophen] 5•2•325 mg

Drysec *sustained-release tablets* ℞ *decongestant; antihistamine; anticholinergic to dry mucosal secretions* [phenylephrine HCl; chlorpheniramine

maleate; methscopolamine nitrate] 20•8•2.5 mg

Drysol *solution* ℞ *astringent for hyperhidrosis* [aluminum chloride (hexahydrate)] 20% ☑ Durasal II

Drytergent *topical liquid* OTC *soap-free therapeutic skin cleanser*

Drytex *lotion* OTC *keratolytic cleanser for acne* [salicylic acid; acetone; isopropyl alcohol] ≗•10%•40% ☑ diuretics

Dryvax *powder for reconstitution* ℞ *active immunization against smallpox using the multiple-puncture technique (scarification); licensed for restricted use and available only from the CDC* [smallpox vaccine] 100 million infectious vaccinia viruses/mL

DSC; DSCG (disodium cromoglycate) [see: cromolyn sodium]

D-S-S *capsules* OTC *laxative; stool softener* [docusate sodium] 100 mg

DSS (dioctyl sodium sulfosuccinate) [now: docusate sodium]

DST (dihydrostreptomycin) [q.v.]

DT; Td (diphtheria & tetanus [toxoids]) *the designation DT (or TD) denotes the pediatric vaccine; Td denotes the adult vaccine* [see: diphtheria & tetanus toxoids, adsorbed]

D-Tab *film-coated extended-release caplets* ℞ *decongestant; expectorant* [phenylephrine HCl; guaifenesin] 40•1200 mg

D-Tann *chewable tablets, oral suspension* ℞ *decongestant; antihistamine; sleep aid* [phenylephrine tannate; diphenhydramine tannate] 10•25 mg; 7.5•25 mg/5 mL

D-Tann aT *oral suspension* ℞ *antitussive; antihistamine; sleep aid* [carbetapentane tannate; diphenhydramine tannate] 30•25 mg/5 mL ☑ Dinate; Duonate-12

D-Tann CT *tablets, oral suspension* ℞ *antitussive; antihistamine; sleep aid; decongestant* [carbetapentane tannate; diphenhydramine tannate; phenylephrine tannate] 30•25•10 mg; 30•25•7.5 mg/5 mL

D-Tann DM oral suspension ℞ *antitus-sive; antihistamine; sleep aid; deconges-tant* [dextromethorphan tannate; diphenhydramine tannate; phenyl-ephrine tannate] 75•25•7.5 mg/5 mL

Dtap (diphtheria, tetanus, & acel-lular pertussis) vaccine Dtap (diphtheria predominant) is the vac-cine used in the initial immuniza-tion series of infants and children 6 weeks to 6 years; compare to Tdap [see: diphtheria & tetanus toxoids & acellular pertussis (DTaP; Dtap; Tdap) vaccine]

DTaP (diphtheria & tetanus [tox-oids] & acellular pertussis [vac-cine]) [q.v.]

DTIC (dimethyl triazeno imidazole carboxamide) [see: dacarbazine]

DTIC & tamoxifen *chemotherapy pro-tocol for malignant melanoma*

DTIC-ACTD; DTIC-ACT-D (DTIC, actinomycin D) *chemotherapy proto-col*

DTIC-Dome IV injection ℞ *antineo-plastic for metastatic malignant mela-noma and Hodgkin disease* [dacarba-zine] 100, 200 mg

DTP (diphtheria & tetanus [tox-oids] & pertussis [vaccine]) [q.v.]

DTPA (diethylenetriaminepenta-acetic acid) [see: pentetic acid]

DTPA (diethylenetriaminepenta-acetic acid) technetium (^{99m}Tc), human serum albumin [see: tech-netium Tc 99m pentetate]

DTwP (diphtheria & tetanus [tox-oids] & whole-cell pertussis [vac-cine]) [q.v.]

Duac gel ℞ *antibiotic and keratolytic for acne* [clindamycin; benzoyl peroxide] 1%•5%

Duadacin Cold & Flu caplets (dis-continued 2004) OTC *decongestant; antihistamine; analgesic; antipyretic* [pseudoephedrine HCl; chlorphenir-amine maleate; acetaminophen] 30•2•500 mg

duazomycin USAN, INN *antineoplastic* ⏚ dacemazine

duazomycin A [see: duazomycin]

duazomycin B [see: azotomycin]

duazomycin C [see: ambomycin]

Duboisia myoporoides medicinal herb [see: corkwood]

duck's foot *medicinal herb* [see: man-drake]

ducodal [see: oxycodone]

Duet chewable tablets ℞ *prenatal vita-min/mineral/calcium/iron supplement* [multiple vitamins & minerals; cal-cium; iron; folic acid] ≚•100•29•1 mg

Duet tablets ℞ *vitamin/mineral/calcium/iron supplement* [multiple vitamins & minerals; calcium; iron] ≚•200•29 mg

Duet DHA tablets + capsules ℞ *pre-natal vitamin/mineral/calcium/iron/omega-3 supplement* [multiple vita-mins & minerals; calcium; iron; folic acid + docosahexaenoic acid (DHA)] ≚•200•29•1 mg + 200 mg

Duet DHA^{EC} tablets + enteric-coated capsules ℞ *prenatal vitamin/mineral/calcium/iron/omega-3 supplement* [mul-tiple vitamins & minerals; calcium; iron; folic acid + docosahexaenoic acid (DHA)] ≚•200•29•1 mg + 200 mg

Duetact tablets ℞ *antidiabetic combina-tion for type 2 diabetes that increases cellular response to insulin and stimu-lates insulin secretion in the pancreas* [pioglitazone HCl; glimepiride] 30•2, 30•4 mg

Dulcet (trademarked dosage form) *chewable tablet* ⏚ Dolacet

Dulcolax enteric-coated tablets, sup-positories OTC *stimulant laxative* [bis-acodyl] 5 mg; 10 mg

Dulcolax oral liquid OTC *saline laxa-tive; antacid* [magnesium hydroxide] 400 mg/5 mL

Dulcolax Bowel Prep Kit 4 enteric-coated tablets + 1 suppository OTC *pre-procedure bowel evacuant* [bisaco-dyl] 5 mg; 10 mg

Dulcolax Stool Softener softgels OTC *laxative; stool softener* [docusate sodium] 100 mg

Dull-C powder for oral liquid OTC *vitamin C supplement* [ascorbic acid] 4.24 g/tsp.

dulofibrate INN

duloxetine INN *selective serotonin and norepinephrine reuptake inhibitor (SSNRI) for depression* [also: duloxetine HCl]

duloxetine HCl USAN *selective serotonin and norepinephrine reuptake inhibitor (SSNRI) for major depressive disorder (MDD) and generalized anxiety disorder (GAD); analgesic for diabetic peripheral neuropathy (DPN) and fibromyalgia* [also: duloxetine]

dulozafone INN

dumorelin INN

duneryl [see: phenobarbital]

Duocaine injection ℞ *local anesthetic; peripheral nerve block for ophthalmic surgery* [bupivacaine HCl; lidocaine HCl] 3.75•10 mg/mL

Duocet tablets ℞ *narcotic analgesic; antipyretic* [hydrocodone bitartrate; acetaminophen] 5•500 mg ⧉ D-Hist D; Dosette

DuoDerm CGF; DuoDerm Extra Thin; DuoDerm Hydroactive adhesive dressings OTC *occlusive wound dressing* [hydrocolloid gel]

DuoDerm Hydroactive paste, granules OTC *wound dressing* [hydrocolloid gel] 30 g; 5 g

Duodopa investigational (orphan) *dopamine precursor plus potentiator for late-stage Parkinson disease* [levodopa; carbidopa]

DuoDote prefilled IM auto-injectors ℞ *antidote to organophosphate nerve agents and organophosphate insecticide poisoning* [atropine; pralidoxime chloride] 2.1•600 mg

DuoFilm patch OTC *keratolytic* [salicylic acid in a rubber-based vehicle] 40%

DuoFilm topical liquid OTC *keratolytic* [salicylic acid in flexible collodion] 17%

Duohist DH oral liquid ℞ *narcotic antitussive; antihistamine; decongestant* [dihydrocodeine bitartrate; chlorpheniramine maleate; phenylephrine HCl] 7.25•2•5 mg/5 mL ⧉ Dayhist-1

duometacin INN

duomycin [see: chlortetracycline HCl]

Duonate-12 oral suspension (discontinued 2007) ℞ *decongestant; antihistamine; sleep aid* [phenylephrine tannate; pyrilamine tannate] 5•30 mg/5 mL ⧉ Dinate; D-Tann aT

DuoNeb oral inhalation aerosol ℞ *anticholinergic bronchodilator for chronic obstructive pulmonary disease (COPD)* [ipratropium bromide; albuterol sulfate] 0.5•3 mg/dose

duoperone INN *neuroleptic* [also: duoperone fumarate] ⧉ dipyrone

duoperone fumarate USAN *neuroleptic* [also: duoperone]

DuoPlant gel ℞ *keratolytic* [salicylic acid in flexible collodion] 17%

duotal [see: guaiacol carbonate]

Duotan PD pediatric oral suspension (discontinued 2007) ℞ *decongestant; antihistamine* [pseudoephedrine tannate; dexchlorpheniramine tannate] 75•2.5 mg/5 mL

DuoVisc prefilled syringes ℞ *dispersive/cohesive viscoelastic agent for ophthalmic surgery* [Viscoat (q.v.); ProVisc (q.v.)] 0.35•0.4, 0.5•0.55 mL

Duphalac oral/rectal solution ℞ *hyperosmotic laxative* [lactulose] 10 g/15 mL ⧉ Difil-G

Duplex topical liquid (discontinued 2004) OTC *soap-free therapeutic skin cleanser* [sodium lauryl sulfate] 15%

duponol [see: sodium lauryl sulfate]

dupracetam INN

Durabac Forte tablets ℞ *analgesic; antipyretic; antihistamine* [acetaminophen; magnesium salicylate; phenyltoloxamine citrate; caffeine] 500•500•20•50 mg

Duracaps (dosage form) *sustained-release capsules*

DURAcare II solution OTC *surfactant cleaning solution for soft contact lenses*

Duraclon continuous epidural infusion ℞ *central analgesic; adjunct to opioid analgesics for severe cancer pain (orphan)* [clonidine HCl] 500 mcg/mL

DuraDEX extended-release tablets (discontinued 2007) ℞ *antitussive; expectorant* [dextromethorphan hydrobromide; guaifenesin] 20•1200 mg

Duradrin capsules (discontinued 2008) ℞ *cerebral vasoconstrictor and analgesic for vascular and tension headaches; "possibly effective" for migraine headaches* [isometheptene mucate; dichloralphenazone; acetaminophen] 65•100•325 mg

Duradryl syrup ℞ *decongestant; antihistamine; anticholinergic to dry mucosal secretions* [phenylephrine HCl; chlorpheniramine maleate; methscopolamine nitrate] 10•2•1.25 mg/5 mL

Duradryl JR pediatric capsules (discontinued 2004) ℞ *decongestant; antihistamine; anticholinergic to dry mucosal secretions* [phenylephrine HCl; chlorpheniramine maleate; methscopolamine nitrate] 10•4•1.25 mg

Duraflu tablets ℞ *antitussive; decongestant; expectorant; analgesic; antipyretic* [dextromethorphan hydrobromide; pseudoephedrine HCl; guaifenesin; acetaminophen] 20•60•200•500 mg ☑ Derifil

DuraGen ℞ *resorbable graft matrix to repair the dura mater following brain surgery or traumatic injury* ☑ Diurigen

Duragesic-12; Duragesic-25; Duragesic-50; Duragesic-75; Duragesic-100 transdermal patch ℞ *narcotic analgesic* [fentanyl] 12.5 mcg/hr.; 25 mcg/hr.; 50 mcg/hr.; 75 mcg/hr.; 100 mcg/hr.

Durahist sustained-release tablets ℞ *decongestant; antihistamine; anticholinergic to dry mucosal secretions* [pseudoephedrine HCl; chlorpheniramine maleate; methscopolamine bromide] 60•8•1.25 mg

Durahist D extended-release caplets ℞ *decongestant; antihistamine; anticholinergic to dry mucosal secretions* [pseudoephedrine HCl; dexchlorpheniramine maleate; methscopolamine bromide] 45•3.5•1 mg

Duralone-40; Duralone-80 intralesional, soft tissue, and IM injection (discontinued 2004) ℞ *corticosteroid; anti-inflammatory; immunosuppressant* [methylprednisolone acetate] 40 mg/mL; 80 mg/mL

Duramist Plus 12-Hour Decongestant nasal spray OTC *nasal decongestant* [oxymetazoline HCl] 0.05%

Duramorph IV, IM, or subcu injection ℞ *narcotic analgesic* [morphine sulfate] 0.5, 1 mg/mL

duramycin *investigational (orphan) agent for cystic fibrosis*

durapatite USAN *prosthetic aid* [also: calcium phosphate, tribasic; hydroxyapatite]

Duraphen II; Duraphen 1000 extended-release tablets (discontinued 2008) ℞ *decongestant; expectorant* [phenylephrine HCl; guaifenesin] 25•800 mg; 30•1000 mg ☑ Darvon

Duraphen II DM extended-release tablets (discontinued 2007) ℞ *antitussive; decongestant; expectorant* [dextromethorphan hydrobromide; phenylephrine HCl; guaifenesin] 20•20•800 mg

Duraphen Forte extended-release tablets (discontinued 2007) ℞ *antitussive; decongestant; expectorant* [dextromethorphan hydrobromide; phenylephrine HCl; guaifenesin] 30•30•1200 mg

DuraPrep Surgical Solution self-contained applicator OTC *broad-spectrum antimicrobial prep for surgical procedures* [iodine; isopropyl alcohol] 0.7%•74%

Durasal II sustained-release tablets (discontinued 2007) ℞ *decongestant; expectorant* [pseudoephedrine HCl; guaifenesin] 60•600 mg ☑ Drysol

DuraSite (trademarked dosage form) *polymer-based eye drops*

DuraSolv (trademarked dosage form) *orally disintegrating tablets*

Durasphere injection ℞ *tissue-bulking agent for female stress urinary incontinence* [carbon-coated beads]

Dura-Tab (trademarked dosage form) *sustained-release tablet*

DuraTan DM oral suspension ℞ *antitussive; antihistamine; decongestant* [dextromethorphan tannate; brompheniramine tannate; phenylephrine tannate] 20•8•20 mg/5 mL

DuraTan Forte oral suspension ℞ *antitussive; antihistamine; decongestant* [dextromethorphan tannate; dexchlorpheniramine tannate; pseudoephedrine tannate] 30•3.5•45 mg/5 mL

DuraTan PE oral suspension ℞ *decongestant; antihistamine; anticholinergic to dry mucosal secretions* [phenylephrine HCl; chlorpheniramine maleate; methscopolamine nitrate] 10•2•1.5 mg/5 mL

Duratears Naturale ophthalmic ointment OTC *moisturizer/lubricant* [white petrolatum; mineral oil; lanolin]

Duration nasal spray OTC *nasal decongestant* [oxymetazoline HCl] 0.05%

Duratuss; Duratuss GP extended-release tablets ℞ *decongestant; expectorant* [phenylephrine HCl; guaifenesin] 25•900 mg; 25•1200 mg ▣ DroTuss

Duratuss A extended-release tablets ℞ *decongestant; expectorant; analgesic; antipyretic* [phenylephrine HCl; guaifenesin; acetaminophen] 20•600•650 mg ▣ DroTuss

Duratuss AC 12 Tannate oral suspension ℞ *antitussive; antihistamine; sleep aid; decongestant* [dextromethorphan tannate; diphenhydramine tannate; phenylephrine tannate] 30•25•30 mg/5 mL

Duratuss CS extended-release caplets ℞ *antitussive; expectorant* [carbetapentane citrate; guaifenesin] 60•900 mg

Duratuss DM elixir ℞ *antitussive; expectorant* [dextromethorphan hydrobromide; guaifenesin] 25•225 mg/5 mL

Duratuss HD elixir ℞ *narcotic antitussive; decongestant; expectorant* [hydrocodone bitartrate; phenylephrine HCl; guaifenesin] 2.5•10•225 mg/5 mL

Duratuss PE extended-release tablets ℞ *decongestant; expectorant* [phenylephrine HCl; guaifenesin] 30•1050 mg

Dura-Vent/DA sustained-release tablets ℞ *decongestant; antihistamine; anticholinergic to dry mucosal secretions* [phenylephrine HCl; chlorpheniramine maleate; methscopolamine nitrate] 20•8•2.5 mg

Duraxin capsules (discontinued 2007) ℞ *antihistamine; sleep aid; analgesic; antipyretic* [phenyltoloxamine citrate; acetaminophen; salicylamide] 25•325•200 mg

Durezol eye drop emulsion ℞ *corticosteroidal anti-inflammatory* [difluprednate] 0.05% ▣ Drysol

Duricef capsules, tablets, powder for oral suspension (discontinued 2008) ℞ *first-generation cephalosporin antibiotic* [cefadroxil] 500 mg; 1000 mg; 125, 250, 500 mg/5 mL

DUROS (trademarked delivery device) *implantable drug carrier, osmotically driven to provide a daily dose of several micrograms for up to one year; it is not biodegradable and must be removed or replaced when exhausted* ▣ Dairy Ease; Diurese; Dry Eyes

Dur-Tann DM oral suspension ℞ *antitussive; antihistamine; decongestant* [dextromethorphan tannate; brompheniramine tannate; phenylephrine tannate] 20•8•20 mg/5 mL

Dur-Tann Forte oral suspension ℞ *antitussive; antihistamine; decongestant* [dextromethorphan tannate; dexchlorpheniramine tannate; pseudoephedrine tannate] 30•3.5•45 mg/5 mL

dusting powder, absorbable USP *surgical glove lubricant*

dutasteride USAN *5α-reductase blocker; inhibits the conversion of testosterone to dihydrotestosterone (DHT); treatment for benign prostatic hyperplasia (BPH); investigational (Phase III) for prostate cancer*

Dutonin ⓔⓤⓡ (British name for U.S. product **Serzone**)

DVB (DDP, vindesine, bleomycin) *chemotherapy protocol*

DVP (daunorubicin, vincristine, prednisone) *chemotherapy protocol for acute lymphocytic leukemia (ALL)*

DVPL-ASP (daunorubicin, vincristine, prednisone, L-asparaginase) *chemotherapy protocol*

dwarf ginseng (Panax trifolius) *medicinal herb* [see: ginseng]

dwarf palm; dwarf palmetto *medicinal herb* [see: saw palmetto]

dwarf sumach *medicinal herb* [see: sumach]

Dyazide capsules R̸ *antihypertensive; diuretic* [triamterene; hydrochlorothiazide] 37.5•25 mg

dyclocaine BAN *topical anesthetic* [also: dyclonine HCl; dyclonine]

Dyclone solution (discontinued 2004) R̸ *anesthetic prior to upper GI and respiratory endoscopies* [dyclonine HCl] 0.5%, 1%

dyclonine INN *mucous membrane anesthetic* [also: dyclonine HCl; dyclocaine]

dyclonine HCl USP *mucous membrane anesthetic* [also: dyclonine; dyclocaine]

dydrogesterone USAN, USP, INN, BAN *progestin*

dyer's broom (Genista tinctoria) flowering twigs *medicinal herb used as an aperient, diuretic, stimulant, and vasoconstrictor*

dyer's bugloss *medicinal herb* [see: henna (Alkanna)]

dyer's saffron *medicinal herb* [see: safflower]

dyer's weed *medicinal herb* [see: goldenrod]

Dyflex-G tablets R̸ *antiasthmatic; bronchodilator; expectorant* [dyphylline; guaifenesin] 200•200 mg

dyflos BAN *antiglaucoma agent; irreversible cholinesterase inhibitor miotic* [also: isoflurophate]

Dy-G oral liquid R̸ *antiasthmatic; bronchodilator; expectorant* [dyphylline; guaifenesin] 100•100 mg/5 mL

dylate [see: clonitrate]

Dyline-GG tablets, oral liquid (discontinued 2005) R̸ *antiasthmatic; bronchodilator; expectorant* [dyphylline; guaifenesin] 200•200 mg; 300•300 mg/15 mL

Dylix elixir R̸ *antiasthmatic; bronchodilator* [dyphylline] 100 mg/15 mL

dymanthine HCl USAN *anthelmintic* [also: dimantine HCl]

Dymelor tablets (discontinued 2006) R̸ *sulfonylurea antidiabetic that stimulates insulin secretion in the pancreas* [acetohexamide] 250, 500 mg

Dymenate IV or IM injection R̸ *antinauseant; antiemetic; antivertigo; motion sickness preventative* [dimenhydrinate] 50 mg/mL

Dynabac enteric-coated delayed-release tablets (discontinued 2008) R̸ *once-daily macrolide antibiotic for respiratory and dermatological infections* [dirithromycin] 250 mg

Dynacin capsules, film-coated tablets R̸ *tetracycline antibiotic for gram-negative and gram-positive bacteria; antirickettsial* [minocycline HCl] 50, 75, 100 mg

DynaCirc capsules R̸ *antihypertensive; dihydropyridine calcium channel blocker* [isradipine] 2.5, 5 mg

DynaCirc CR controlled-release tablets R̸ *once-daily antihypertensive; dihydropyridine calcium channel blocker* [isradipine] 5, 10 mg

dynacoryl [see: nikethamide]

Dynafed Asthma Relief tablets OTC *bronchodilator; decongestant; expectorant* [ephedrine HCl; guaifenesin] 25•200 mg

Dynafed E.X. tablets (discontinued 2008) OTC *analgesic; antipyretic* [acetaminophen] 500 mg

Dynafed Jr., Children's chewable tablets (discontinued 2008) OTC *analgesic; antipyretic* [acetaminophen] 80 mg

Dyna-Hex Skin Cleanser; Dyna-Hex 2 Skin Cleanser topical liquid OTC *broad-spectrum antimicrobial; germicidal* [chlorhexidine gluconate; alcohol 4%] 4%; 2%

dynamine *investigational (orphan) agent for Lambert-Eaton myasthenic syndrome and Charcot-Marie-Tooth disease*

dynarsan [see: acetarsone]

Dynatuss DF syrup (discontinued 2007) ℞ *narcotic antitussive; expectorant* [hydrocodone bitartrate; guaifenesin] 5•200 mg/10 mL

Dynatuss EX syrup ℞ *antitussive; decongestant; expectorant* [dextromethorphan hydrobromide; phenylephrine HCl; guaifenesin] 30•10•200 mg/5 mL

Dynex sustained-release caplets (discontinued 2007) ℞ *decongestant; expectorant* [pseudoephedrine HCl; guaifenesin] 90•1200 mg

Dynex LA dual-release caplets ℞ *decongestant; expectorant* [phenylephrine HCl; guaifenesin (50% immediate release; 50% extended release)] 30•800 mg

Dynex VR dual-release capsules ℞ *antitussive; expectorant* [carbetapentane citrate (sustained release); guaifenesin (immediate release)] 30•400 mg

dyphylline USP *antiasthmatic; bronchodilator* [also: diprophylline]

dyphylline & guaifenesin *antiasthmatic; bronchodilator; expectorant* 200•200 mg oral

Dyphylline-GG elixir OTC *antiasthmatic; bronchodilator; expectorant* [dyphylline; guaifenesin] 100•100 mg/15 mL

Dyprotex pads OTC *diaper rash treatment* [zinc oxide; dimethicone] 40%•2.5%

Dyrenium capsules ℞ *antihypertensive; potassium-sparing diuretic* [triamterene] 50, 100 mg

Dysport *investigational (orphan) agent for blepharospasm and strabismus of dystonia, pediatric cerebral palsy, and cervical dystonia* [botulinum toxin, type A]

dysprosium *element (Dy)*

Dytan chewable tablets, oral suspension ℞ *antihistamine; sleep aid* [diphenhydramine tannate] 25 mg; 25 mg/5 mL ⑨ Detane

Dytan-CD oral suspension ℞ *antitussive; antihistamine; sleep aid; decongestant* [carbetapentane tannate; diphenhydramine tannate; phenylephrine tannate] 30•25•15 mg/5 mL

Dytan-CS tablets, oral suspension ℞ *antitussive; antihistamine; sleep aid; decongestant* [carbetapentane tannate; diphenhydramine tannate; phenylephrine tannate] 30•25•10 mg; 30•25•7.5 mg/5 mL

Dytan-D chewable tablets, oral suspension ℞ *decongestant; antihistamine; sleep aid* [phenylephrine tannate; diphenhydramine tannate] 10•25 mg; 7.5•25 mg/5 mL

DZAPO (daunorubicin, azacitidine, ara-C, prednisone, Oncovin) *chemotherapy protocol*

E

E₂C (estradiol cypionate) [q.v.]

EACA (epsilon-aminocaproic acid) [see: aminocaproic acid]

EAP (etoposide, Adriamycin, Platinol) *chemotherapy protocol for gastric and small bowel cancer*

ear, lion's *medicinal herb* [see: motherwort]

Ear-Dry *ear drops* OTC *antiseptic; astringent* [boric acid] 2.75% Auro-Dri

Ear-Eze *ear drops* ℞ *corticosteroidal anti-inflammatory; antibiotic* [hydrocortisone; neomycin sulfate; polymyxin B sulfate] 1%•5 mg•10 000 U per mL Aerius; Oracea; OROS; Urso 250

EarSol-HC *ear drops* OTC *corticosteroidal anti-inflammatory; antiseptic* [hydrocortisone; alcohol 44%] 1%

earthnut oil [see: peanut oil]

Easprin *delayed-release enteric-coated tablets* ℞ *analgesic; antipyretic; anti-inflammatory; antirheumatic* [aspirin] 975 mg aceperone; azaperone; esuprone

Easter giant *medicinal herb* [see: bistort]

Easy A1C *fingerstick test kit for home use* OTC *in vitro diagnostic aid for glycosylated hemoglobin levels*

EasyInjector (trademarked delivery device) *self-injector*

E-Base *enteric-coated delayed-release caplets and tablets* (discontinued 2005) ℞ *macrolide antibiotic* [erythromycin] 333, 500 mg

ebastine USAN, INN *antihistamine* epostane

ebiratide INN

ebrotidine INN

ebselen INN epicillin

EC (epicatechin); ECG, ECg (epicatechin gallate) [q.v.]

EC (etoposide, carboplatin) *chemotherapy protocol for lung cancer*

ecadotril USAN, INN *antihypertensive*

ecalcidene USAN *antipsoriatic*

ecallantide *investigational (Phase III, orphan) kallikrein inhibitor for angioedema*

ecamsule USAN *UVA sunscreen*

ecarazine [see: todralazine]

EC-ASA (enteric-coated aspirin) [see: aspirin]

ecastolol INN

Ecee Plus *tablets* OTC *vitamin/mineral supplement* [vitamins C and E; zinc sulfate; magnesium sulfate] 100•165•80•70 mg

echinacea (Echinacea angustifolia; E. purpurea; E. pallida) *root medicinal herb for anemia, blood diseases, blood poisoning, boils, dizziness, immune system stimulation, lymph disorders, promoting wound healing, prostate disorders, skin infections, and snake bites*

echinocandins *a class of antifungals* [also: glucan synthesis inhibitors]

Echinopanax horridum *medicinal herb* [see: devil's club]

ECHO (etoposide, cyclophosphamide, hydroxydaunomycin, Oncovin) *chemotherapy protocol*

echothiophate iodide USP *antiglaucoma agent; irreversible cholinesterase inhibitor miotic* [also: ecothiopate iodide]

ecipramidil INN

eclanamine INN *antidepressant* [also: eclanamine maleate]

eclanamine maleate USAN *antidepressant* [also: eclanamine]

eclazolast USAN, INN *antiallergic; mediator release inhibitor*

EC-Naprosyn *enteric-coated delayed-release caplets* ℞ *analgesic; nonsteroidal anti-inflammatory drug (NSAID) for osteoarthritis, rheumatoid arthritis, juvenile arthritis, ankylosing spondylitis, primary dysmenorrhea, bursitis/tendinitis, and other mild to moderate pain* [naproxen] 375, 500 mg

ecogramostim BAN

ecomustine INN

econazole USAN, INN, BAN *topical antifungal*

econazole nitrate USAN, USP, BAN *topical antifungal* 1% topical

Econo B & C caplets OTC *vitamin supplement* [multiple B vitamins; vitamin C] ≛•300 mg

Econopred Drop-Tainers (eye drop suspension) (discontinued 2006) ℞ *corticosteroidal anti-inflammatory* [prednisolone acetate] 0.125%

Econopred Plus Drop-Tainers (eye drop suspension) ℞ *corticosteroidal anti-inflammatory* [prednisolone acetate] 1%

ecopipam HCl USAN *selective dopamine receptor antagonist for addiction*

ecostigmine iodide [see: echothiophate iodide]

ecothiopate iodide INN, BAN *antiglaucoma agent; irreversible cholinesterase inhibitor miotic* [also: echothiophate iodide]

Ecotrin enteric-coated tablets, enteric-coated caplets OTC *analgesic; antipyretic; anti-inflammatory; antiarthritic* [aspirin] 325, 500 mg

Ecotrin Adult Low Strength enteric-coated tablets OTC *analgesic; antipyretic; anti-inflammatory; antiarthritic* [aspirin] 81 mg

Ecovia *investigational (orphan) for Huntington disease* [remacemide HCl]

ecraprost USAN *treatment of peripheral occlusive disease*

ecteinascidin *investigational (Phase III, orphan) tetrahydroisoquinoline alkaloid for soft tissue sarcoma and relapsed ovarian cancer*

ectylurea BAN

eculizumab *monoclonal antibody; antihemolytic for paroxysmal nocturnal hemoglobinuria (PNH; orphan); investigational (orphan) for idiopathic membranous glomerular nephropathy*

Ed-A-Hist sustained-release tablets, oral liquid ℞ *decongestant; antihistamine* [phenylephrine HCl; chlorpheniramine maleate] 20•8 mg; 10•4 mg/5 mL

Ed-A-Hist DM oral liquid ℞ *antitussive; antihistamine; decongestant* [dextromethorphan hydrobromide; chlorpheniramine maleate; phenylephrine HCl] 15•4•10 mg/5 mL

Ed-Apap, Children's oral liquid OTC *analgesic; antipyretic* [acetaminophen] 160 mg/5 mL

Ed-Bron G oral liquid ℞ *antiasthmatic; bronchodilator; expectorant* [dyphylline; guaifenesin] 150•100 mg/15 mL

Ed Chlor-PED D oral drops ℞ *decongestant; antihistamine* [phenylephrine tannate; chlorpheniramine tannate] 6•2 mg/mL

Ed Chlor-Tan caplets ℞ *antihistamine* [chlorpheniramine tannate] 8 mg

ED Tuss HC syrup (discontinued 2007) ℞ *narcotic antitussive; antihistamine; decongestant* [hydrocodone bitartrate; chlorpheniramine maleate; phenylephrine HCl] 2.5•4•10 mg/5 mL

edamine [see: ethylenediamine]

EDAP (etoposide, dexamethasone, ara-C, Platinol) *chemotherapy protocol* ▨ ADOAP; UDIP

edathamil [now: edetate calcium disodium]

edathamil calcium disodium [now: edetate calcium disodium]

edathamil disodium [now: edetate disodium]

edatrexate USAN, INN *antineoplastic; methotrexate analogue*

Edecrin tablets ℞ *antihypertensive; loop diuretic* [ethacrynic acid] 25, 50 mg

Edecrin Sodium powder for IV injection ℞ *antihypertensive; loop diuretic* [ethacrynate sodium] 50 mg

edelfosine INN

edetate calcium disodium USAN, USP *heavy metal chelating agent for acute or chronic lead poisoning and lead encephalopathy* [also: sodium calcium edetate; sodium calciumedetate; calcium disodium edetate]

edetate dipotassium USAN *chelating agent*

edetate disodium USP *chelating agent; preservative; antioxidant* [also: disodium edetate] 150 mg/mL injection

edetate magnesium disodium *chelating agent for atherosclerosis*

edetate sodium USAN *chelating agent*

edetate trisodium USAN *chelating agent*

edetic acid NF, INN, BAN *chelating agent*

edetol USAN, INN *alkalizing agent*

Edex injection, pre-filled syringes ℞ *vasodilator for erectile dysfunction* [alprostadil] 10, 20, 40 mcg/mL 🔊 ADEKs; Adoxa; Iodex

Ed-Flex capsules (discontinued 2007) ℞ *antihistamine; sleep aid; analgesic; antipyretic* [phenyltoloxamine citrate; acetaminophen; salicylamide] 20•300•200 mg (note: one of two products with the same name)

Ed-Flex capsules (discontinued 2007) ℞ *antihistamine; sleep aid; analgesic; antipyretic* [phenyltoloxamine citrate; acetaminophen; magnesium salicylate] 20•500•500 mg (note: one of two products with the same name)

edifolone INN *antiarrhythmic* [also: edifolone acetate]

edifolone acetate USAN *antiarrhythmic* [also: edifolone]

Ed-In-Sol drops (discontinued 2005) OTC *hematinic; iron supplement* [ferrous sulfate (source of iron)] 75 mg/0.6 mL (15 mg/0.6 mL)

edisilate INN *combining name for radicals or groups* [also: edisylate]

edisylate USAN, BAN *combining name for radicals or groups* [also: edisilate]

edithamil [see: edetate ...]

edobacomab USAN *monoclonal antibody to endotoxin for gram-negative sepsis*

edodekin alfa USAN *antiasthmatic; immunomodulator; investigational (orphan) for renal cell carcinoma*

edogestrone INN, BAN

edonentan USAN *endothelin A (ETA) inhibitor for heart failure*

edoxudine USAN, INN *antiviral*

edrecolomab USAN *investigational (orphan) antineoplastic adjunct for pancreatic cancer*

edrofuradene [see: nifurdazil]

edrophone chloride [see: edrophonium chloride]

edrophonium chloride USP, INN, BAN *cholinergic/anticholinesterase muscle stimulant; antidote to curare; myasthenia gravis diagnostic aid*

Ed-Spaz tablets ℞ *GI/GU antispasmodic; antiparkinsonian; anticholinergic "drying agent" for allergic rhinitis and hyperhidrosis* [hyoscyamine sulfate] 0.125 mg

EDTA (ethylenediaminetetraacetic acid) [see: edetate disodium]

EDTA calcium [see: edetate calcium disodium]

ED-TLC; ED-Tuss HC oral liquid ℞ *narcotic antitussive; antihistamine; decongestant* [hydrocodone bitartrate; chlorpheniramine maleate; phenylephrine HCl] 1.67•2•5 mg/5 mL; 3.5•4•10 mg/5 mL

E.E.S. granules for oral suspension ℞ *macrolide antibiotic* [erythromycin ethylsuccinate] 200 mg/5 mL

EES (erythromycin ethylsuccinate) [q.v.]

E.E.S. 200 oral suspension ℞ *macrolide antibiotic* [erythromycin ethylsuccinate] 200 mg/5 mL

E.E.S. 400 film-coated tablets, oral suspension ℞ *macrolide antibiotic* [erythromycin ethylsuccinate] 400 mg; 400 mg/5 mL

efalizumab *recombinant humanized monoclonal antibody (rhuMAb) to leukocyte function–associated antigen-1 (LFA-1); immunosuppressant for moderate to severe plaque psoriasis*

efaproxiral *investigational (NDA filed, orphan) radiosensitizer for brain tumors; investigational (NDA filed) for breast and lung cancer*

Efaproxyn *investigational (NDA filed) radiosensitizer for breast, lung, and brain tumors* [efaproxiral]

efaroxan INN, BAN

efavirenz *antiviral non-nucleoside reverse transcriptase inhibitor (NNRTI) for HIV infection*

efegatran sulfate USAN *antithrombotic*

efetozole INN

effector molecules *a class of cytotoxic or radioactive drugs delivered to specific tissue—usually a cancerous tumor— by targeted monoclonal antibody vehicles (T-MAVs; q.v.)*

Effer-K effervescent tablets ℞ *potassium supplement* [potassium bicarbonate; potassium citrate] 10, 20, 25 mEq K

Effervescent Potassium effervescent tablets (discontinued 2007) ℞ *potassium supplement* [potassium bicarbonate; potassium citrate] 25 mEq K

Effervescent Potassium Chloride effervescent tablets for oral solution ℞ *potassium supplement* [potassium chloride] 25 mEq K

Effexor tablets ℞ *antidepressant; anxiolytic; selective serotonin and norepinephrine reuptake inhibitor (SSNRI) for major depressive disorder (MDD)* [venlafaxine HCl] 25, 37.5, 50, 75, 100 mg

Effexor XR extended-release capsules ℞ *antidepressant; anxiolytic; selective serotonin and norepinephrine reuptake inhibitor (SSNRI) for major depressive disorder (MDD), generalized anxiety disorder (GAD), social anxiety disorder (SAD), and panic disorder* [venlafaxine HCl] 37.5, 75, 150 mg

Effient *investigational (NDA filed) oral adenosine phosphate inhibitor to block platelet aggregation in patients with acute coronary syndrome (ACS)* [prasugrel]

Efidac 24 dual-release tablets OTC *antihistamine* [chlorpheniramine maleate] 16 mg (4 mg immediate release, 12 mg extended release)

Efidac 24 Pseudoephedrine dual-release tablets OTC *nasal decongestant* [pseudoephedrine HCl] 240 mg (60 mg immediate release, 180 mg extended release)

efletirizine *investigational second-generation peripherally selective piperazine antihistamine*

eflornithine INN, BAN *antineoplastic; antiprotozoal; topical hair growth inhibitor* [also: eflornithine HCl]

eflornithine HCl USAN *antiprotozoal for* Trypanosoma brucei *gambiense (sleeping sickness) infection (orphan); topical hair growth inhibitor; investigational (Phase III) for bladder cancer; investigational (orphan) for AIDS-related* Pneumocystis pneumonia *(PCP)* [also: eflornithine]

efloxate INN

eflumast INN

Efodine ointment OTC *broad-spectrum antimicrobial* [povidone-iodine] 1%

eformoterol fumarate BAN *long-acting β₂ agonist; sympathomimetic bronchodilator for asthma* [also: formoterol; formoterol fumarate]

EFP (etoposide, fluorouracil, Platinol) *chemotherapy protocol for gastric and small bowel cancer*

efrotomycin USAN, INN, BAN *veterinary growth stimulant*

Efudex cream, topical solution ℞ *antineoplastic for actinic keratoses (AK) and basal cell carcinomas (BCC)* [fluorouracil] 5%; 2%, 5%

Efudex Occlusion Pack cream + bandages ℞ *antineoplastic for actinic keratoses (AK) and basal cell carcinomas (BCC)* [fluorouracil] 5%

efungumab *investigational (Phase III, orphan) for invasive candidiasis and other severe fungal infections*

EGC (epigallocatechin); EGCG, EGCg (epigallocatechin gallate) [q.v.]

EGFR (epidermal growth factor receptor) inhibitors [q.v.]

egtazic acid USAN, INN *pharmaceutic aid*

Egyptian privet *medicinal herb* [see: henna (Lawsonia)]

Egyptian thorn *medicinal herb* [see: acacia]

EHDP (ethane hydroxydiphosphonate) [see: etidronate disodium]

Ehrlich 594 [see: acetarsone]

Ehrlich 606 [see: arsphenamine]

eicosapentaenoic acid (EPA) *natural omega-3 fatty acid used to prevent a wide range of degenerative diseases; precursor to the anti-inflammatory and* *anticoagulant series 3 prostaglandins; effective in treating depression and other mental disorders* [also: icosapent]

8 in 1 (methylprednisolone, vincristine, lomustine, procarbazine, hydroxyurea, cisplatin, cytarabine, cyclophosphamide) *chemotherapy protocol* ⊡ Attain

8 in 1 (methylprednisolone, vincristine, lomustine, procarbazine, hydroxyurea, cisplatin, cytarabine, dacarbazine) *chemotherapy protocol for pediatric brain tumors* ⊡ Attain

8-MOP capsules ℞ *systemic psoralens for psoriasis, repigmentation of idiopathic vitiligo, and cutaneous T-cell lymphoma (CTCL); used to increase tolerance to sunlight and enhance pigmentation* [methoxsalen] 10 mg

einsteinium *element (Es)*

eIPV (enhanced, inactivated polio vaccine) [see: poliovirus vaccine, enhanced inactivated]

elacridar HCl USAN *chemotherapy potentiator; multi–drug-resistance inhibitor*

elantrine USAN, INN *anticholinergic*

elanzepine INN ⊡ olanzapine

Elaprase injection ℞ *iduronate-2-sulfatase enzyme to improve walking capacity in patients with Hunter syndrome (mucopolysaccharidosis II; MPS II; orphan)* [idursulfase] 2 mg/mL

elastofilcon A USAN *hydrophilic contact lens material*

Elavil film-coated tablets (discontinued 2004) ℞ *tricyclic antidepressant* [amitriptyline HCl] 10, 25, 50, 75, 100, 150 mg ⊡ olive oil

elbanizine INN

elcatonin INN, JAN *investigational (orphan) intrathecal treatment of intractable pain*

eldacimibe USAN *antihyperlipidemic; antiatherosclerotic; AcylCoA transferase (ACaT) inhibitor*

Eldepryl capsules ℞ *monoamine oxidase inhibitor (MAOI); dopaminergic for Parkinson disease (orphan)* [selegiline HCl] 5 mg

elder flower; elderberry (Sambucus canadensis; S. ebulus; S. nigra; S. racemosa) *berries and flowers medicinal herb for allergies, asthma, bronchitis, colds, constipation, edema, fever, hay fever, pneumonia, and sinus congestion; also used topically as an astringent*

Eldercaps capsules ℞ *vitamin/mineral supplement* [multiple vitamins & minerals; folic acid] ≛•1 mg

Eldertonic oral liquid OTC *vitamin/mineral supplement* [multiple B vitamins & minerals; alcohol 13.5%]

eldexomer INN

Eldisine *investigational (NDA filed) synthetic vinca alkaloid antineoplastic for leukemia, melanoma, breast and lung cancers* [vindesine sulfate]

Eldopaque; Eldopaque-Forte cream OTC *hyperpigmentation bleaching agent; sunscreen* [hydroquinone in a sunblock base] 2%; 4%

Eldoquin-Forte cream OTC *hyperpigmentation bleaching agent* [hydroquinone] 4%

elecampane (Inula helenium) *root medicinal herb for chronic bronchitis and cough*

electrocortin [see: aldosterone]

eledoisin INN

Elestat eye drops ℞ *antihistamine; mast cell stabilizer* [epinastine HCl] ⊡ AlaSTaT

Elestrin transdermal gel in a metered-dose pump ℞ *estrogen replacement therapy for postmenopausal symptoms* [estradiol] 0.06% (0.52 mg/dose) ⊡ alosetron

eletriptan hydrobromide USAN *vascular serotonin 5-HT$_{1B/1D/1F}$-receptor agonist for the acute treatment of migraine (base=82.5%)*

eleuthero (Eleutherococcus senticosus) *root medicinal herb for age spots, blood diseases, depression, hemorrhage, immune system stimulation, increasing endurance and longevity, normalizing blood pressure, platelet aggregation inhibition, sexual stimulation, and* *stress* [previously called: Siberian ginseng]

Elevess subcu injection ℞ *dermal filler for facial wrinkles and scar remediation* [cross-linked hyaluronic acid; lidocaine]

ELF (etoposide, leucovorin [rescue], fluorouracil) *chemotherapy protocol for gastric cancer*

elfazepam USAN, INN *veterinary appetite stimulant*

elfdock; elfwort *medicinal herb* [see: elecampane]

elgodipine INN

Elidel cream ℞ *immunomodulator for atopic dermatitis* [pimecrolimus] 1%

Eligard sustained-release subcu injection ℞ *antihormonal antineoplastic for advanced prostate cancer* [leuprolide acetate] 7.5 mg (1-month depot), 22.5 mg (3-month depot), 30 mg (4-month depot), 45 mg (6-month depot) ☑ Allegra ODT

Elimite cream ℞ (available OTC in Canada as **Kwellada-P** lotion) *pediculicide for lice; scabicide* [permethrin] 5% ☑ Alimta

eliprodil INN *treatment for ischemic stroke*

Elitek powder for IV infusion ℞ *antimetabolite antineoplastic for leukemia, lymphoma, and solid tumor malignancies (orphan)* [rasburicase] 1.5, 7.5 mg/vial

Elixomin elixir (discontinued 2008) ℞ *antiasthmatic; bronchodilator* [theophylline] 80 mg/15 mL

Elixophyllin capsules (discontinued 2008) ℞ *antiasthmatic; bronchodilator* [theophylline] 100, 200 mg

Elixophyllin elixir ℞ *antiasthmatic; bronchodilator* [theophylline] 80 mg/ 15 mL

Elixophyllin GG oral liquid (discontinued 2007) ℞ *antiasthmatic; bronchodilator; expectorant* [theophylline; guaifenesin] 100•100 mg/15 mL

Elixophyllin-KI elixir (discontinued 2007) ℞ *antiasthmatic; bronchodilator; expectorant* [theophylline; potassium iodide] 80•130 mg/15 mL

ElixSure Children's Cough syrup OTC *antitussive* [dextromethorphan hydrobromide] 7.5 mg/5 mL

ElixSure Congestion; ElixSure Children's Congestion syrup OTC *decongestant* [pseudoephedrine HCl] 15 mg/5 mL

ElixSure Fever Reducer/Pain Reliever oral solution OTC *analgesic; antipyretic* [acetaminophen] 160 mg/ 5 mL

ElixSure IB oral suspension OTC *analgesic; antipyretic; nonsteroidal anti-inflammatory drug (NSAID) for minor aches and pains* [ibuprofen] 100 mg/5 mL

ellagic acid INN

Ellence IV infusion ℞ *anthracycline antibiotic antineoplastic for breast cancer (orphan)* [epirubicin HCl] 50, 200 mg/vial

Elliott's B solution *investigational (orphan) intrathecal chemotherapy diluent*

elliptinium acetate INN, BAN

elm, American; Indian elm; moose elm; red elm; rock elm; sweet elm; winged elm *medicinal herb* [see: slippery elm]

Elmiron capsules ℞ *urinary tract anti-inflammatory and analgesic for interstitial cystitis (orphan)* [pentosan polysulfate sodium] 100 mg

elmustine INN

elnadipine INN

Elocon ointment, cream, lotion ℞ *corticosteroidal anti-inflammatory* [mometasone furoate] 0.1% ☑ AlaQuin; Alcaine; elucaine

Elon Barrier Protectant liquid OTC *skin protectant* [paraffin based]

Elon Dual Defense Antifungal Formula topical liquid OTC *antifungal* [undecylenic acid] 25%

Eloxatin IV infusion ℞ *alkylating antineoplastic for advanced or metastatic colorectal cancers; also used for non-Hodgkin lymphoma and advanced ovarian cancer (orphan); investigational (Phase III) for pancreatic cancer* [oxaliplatin] 50, 100, 200 mg

elsamitrucin USAN, INN *antineoplastic*

Elspar powder for IV or IM injection
℞ *antineoplastic adjunct for acute lymphocytic leukemia* [asparaginase]
10 000 IU

eltanolone INN *IV anesthetic*

eltenac INN ② Altinac

eltoprazine INN

eltrombopag *investigational (NDA filed) oral thrombopoietin (TPO) receptor agonist to increase platelet production in idiopathic thrombocytopenia purpura (ITP)*

elucaine USAN, INN *gastric anticholinergic* ② Ala-Quin; Alcaine; Elocon

Elymus repens medicinal herb [see: couch grass]

elziverine INN

EMA (estramustine L-alanine) [q.v.]

EMA 86 (etoposide, mitoxantrone, ara-C) *chemotherapy protocol for acute myelocytic leukemia (AML)*

EMACO (etoposide, methotrexate, actinomycin D, cyclophosphamide, Oncovin) *chemotherapy protocol*

Emadine eye drops ℞ *antihistamine for allergic conjunctivitis* [emedastine difumarate] 0.05%

Embeline ointment, gel, cream, scalp application ℞ *corticosteroidal anti-inflammatory* [clobetasol propionate] 0.05%

embinal [see: barbital sodium]

embonate INN, BAN *combining name for radicals or groups* [also: pamoate]

embramine INN, BAN ② ampyrimine; imipramine

embramine HCl [see: embramine]

Embrex 600 chewable tablets ℞ *vitamin/mineral/calcium/iron supplement* [multiple vitamins & minerals; calcium; iron; folic acid] ± • 240 • 90 • 1 mg

embutramide USAN, INN, BAN *veterinary anesthetic; veterinary euthanasia*

Emcyt capsules ℞ *nitrogen mustard-type alkylating antineoplastic for metastatic or progressive prostatic carcinoma* [estramustine phosphate sodium] 140 mg

emedastine INN *ophthalmic antihistamine* [also: emedastine difumarate]

emedastine difumarate USAN, JAN *ophthalmic antihistamine* [also: emedastine]

Emend capsules ℞ *antiemetic for chemotherapy-induced and postoperative nausea and vomiting* [aprepitant] 40, 80, 125 mg ② Immun-Aid

Emend IV infusion ℞ *antiemetic for chemotherapy-induced nausea and vomiting* [fosaprepitant dimeglumine] 188 mg (115 mg base)

emepronium bromide INN, BAN

emepronium carrageenate BAN

Emersal topical emulsion (discontinued 2004) ℞ *antipsoriatic; antiseborrheic* [ammoniated mercury; salicylic acid] 5% • 2.5%

emetic herb; emetic weed *medicinal herb* [see: lobelia]

emetics *a class of agents that induce vomiting*

emetine BAN *antiamebic* [also: emetine HCl] ② Amitone; iometin

emetine bismuth iodide [see: emetine HCl]

emetine HCl USP *amebicide* [also: emetine]

Emetrol oral solution OTC *antiemetic for nausea associated with influenza, morning sickness, motion sickness, inhalation anesthesia, or food and drink indiscretions* [phosphorated carbohydrate solution (fructose, dextrose, and phosphoric acid)] 1.87 g • 1.87 g • 21.5 mg ② amiterol

EMF oral liquid OTC *protein supplement* [multiple amino acids] 15 g protein

Emgel gel ℞ *antibiotic for acne* [erythromycin; alcohol 77%] 2%

emiglitate INN, BAN

emilium tosilate INN *antiarrhythmic* [also: emilium tosylate]

emilium tosylate USAN *antiarrhythmic* [also: emilium tosilate]

emitefur USAN *antineoplastic for stomach, colorectal, breast, pancreatic, and non–small cell lung cancers (NSCLC)* ② amitivir

EMLA (eutectic mixture of local anesthetics) cream, adhesive disc ℞ *anesthetic* [lidocaine; prilocaine] 2.5%•2.5% ⧈ Emollia; emu oil

emmenagogues *a class of agents that induce or increase menstruation*

Emollia lotion OTC *moisturizer; emollient* ⧈ EMLA; emu oil

emollient laxatives *a subclass of laxatives that work by retarding colonic absorption of fecal water to soften the stool and ease its movement through the intestines* [see also: laxatives]

emollients *a class of dermatological agents that soften and soothe the skin*

emonapride INN

emopamil INN

emorfazone INN

Empirin tablets OTC *analgesic; antipyretic; anti-inflammatory; antirheumatic* [aspirin] 325 mg ⧈ amiperone

Empirin with Codeine No. 3 & No. 4 tablets ℞ *narcotic antitussive; analgesic; antipyretic; sometimes abused as a street drug* [codeine phosphate; aspirin] 30•325 mg; 60•325 mg

Emsam transdermal patch ℞ *monoamine oxidase inhibitor (MAOI); once-daily treatment for major depressive disorder (MDD)* [selegiline HCl] 6, 9, 12 mg/day

Emselex ⓔ (European name for U.S. product **Enablex**)

emtricitabine USAN *synthetic cytosine analogue; antiviral nucleoside analogue reverse transcriptase inhibitor for HIV-1 infection; also used for hepatitis B virus (HBV) infection*

Emtriva capsules, oral solution ℞ *antiviral nucleoside analogue reverse transcriptase inhibitor for HIV-1 infection; also used for hepatitis B virus (HBV) infection* [emtricitabine] 200 mg; 10 mg/mL

emtryl [see: dimetridazole]

emu oil *natural remedy for arthritis pain, hair loss prevention, and chronic skin disorders* ⧈ EMLA; Emollia

emulsifying wax [see: wax, emulsifying]

Emulsoil oral emulsion OTC *stimulant laxative* [castor oil] 95%

E-Mycin enteric-coated tablets (discontinued 2005) ℞ *macrolide antibiotic* [erythromycin] 250, 333 mg ⧈ Amosan

emylcamate INN, BAN

Enablex extended-release tablets ℞ *selective muscarinic receptor antagonist for urinary frequency, urgency, and incontinence* [darifenacin hydrobromide] 7.5, 15 mg

enadoline INN *analgesic* [also: enadoline HCl]

enadoline HCl USAN *analgesic; investigational (orphan) for severe head injury* [also: enadoline]

enalapril INN, BAN *antihypertensive; angiotensin-converting enzyme (ACE) inhibitor; treatment for congestive heart failure (CHF)* [also: enalapril maleate]

enalapril maleate USAN, USP *antihypertensive; angiotensin-converting enzyme (ACE) inhibitor; treatment for congestive heart failure (CHF)* [also: enalapril] 2.5, 5, 10, 20 mg oral

enalapril maleate & hydrochlorothiazide *antihypertensive; angiotensin-converting enzyme (ACE) inhibitor; diuretic* 5•12.5, 10•25 mg oral

enalaprilat USAN, USP, INN, BAN *antihypertensive; angiotensin-converting enzyme (ACE) inhibitor* 1.25 mg/mL injection

enalkiren USAN, INN *antihypertensive; renin inhibitor*

enallynymal sodium [see: methohexital sodium]

enantate INN *combining name for radicals or groups* [also: enanthate]

enanthate USAN, USP, BAN *combining name for radicals or groups* [also: enantate]

enantiomer [def.] *One of a pair of chemical compounds having the same molecular formula, but with the atoms arranged in mirror image. Subdivided into (+) (formerly d- or dextro-) and (−) (formerly l- or levo-).* [see also: isomer; racemic]

Enbrel powder for subcu injection, pre-filled syringes ℞ *soluble tumor necrosis factor receptor (sTNFR) inhibitor for rheumatoid arthritis, juvenile rheumatoid arthritis (orphan), psoriatic arthritis, and ankylosing spondylitis; investigational (NDA filed) for congestive heart failure; investigational (orphan) for Wegener granulomatosis* [etanercept] 25 mg/vial; 25, 50 mg

enbucrilate INN, BAN

encainide INN, BAN *antiarrhythmic* [also: encainide HCl]

encainide HCl USAN *antiarrhythmic* [also: encainide]

Encare vaginal suppositories OTC *spermicidal contraceptive* [nonoxynol 9] 2.27%

enciprazine INN, BAN *minor tranquilizer* [also: enciprazine HCl]

enciprazine HCl USAN *minor tranquilizer* [also: enciprazine]

enclomifene INN [also: enclomiphene]

enclomiphene USAN [also: enclomifene]

encyprate USAN, INN *antidepressant*

EndaCof caplets (discontinued 2007) ℞ *narcotic antitussive; expectorant* [hydrocodone bitartrate; guaifenesin] 2.5•300 mg

EndaCof DM syrup ℞ *antitussive; antihistamine; decongestant* [dextromethorphan hydrobromide; brompheniramine maleate; pseudoephedrine HCl] 30•4•60 mg/5 mL

EndaCof-PD oral drops OTC *antitussive; antihistamine; decongestant; for children 1–24 months* [dextromethorphan hydrobromide; brompheniramine maleate; pseudoephedrine HCl] 3•1•12.5 mg/mL

EndaCof-XP oral liquid (discontinued 2007) ℞ *narcotic antitussive; expectorant* [hydrocodone bitartrate; guaifenesin] 5•400 mg/10 mL

Endagen-HD oral liquid (discontinued 2007) ℞ *narcotic antitussive; antihistamine; decongestant* [hydrocodone bitartrate; chlorpheniramine maleate; phenylephrine HCl] 3.4•4•10 mg/10 mL ☑ indecainide

Endal Expectorant syrup (discontinued 2005) ℞ *narcotic antitussive; decongestant; expectorant* [codeine phosphate; phenylephrine HCl; guaifenesin; alcohol 5%] 12.5•4•125 mg/5 mL

Endal HD syrup (discontinued 2007) ℞ *narcotic antitussive; antihistamine; sleep aid; decongestant* [hydrocodone bitartrate; diphenhydramine HCl; phenylephrine HCl] 4•25•15 mg/10 mL

Endal HD Plus syrup ℞ *narcotic antitussive; antihistamine; decongestant* [hydrocodone bitartrate; chlorpheniramine maleate; phenylephrine HCl] 3.5•2•7.5 mg/5 mL

Endal Nasal Decongestant timed-release caplets (discontinued 2006) ℞ *decongestant; expectorant* [phenylephrine HCl; guaifenesin] 20•300 mg

endiemal [see: metharbital]

endive *medicinal herb* [see: chicory]

endive, white; wild endive *medicinal herb* [see: dandelion]

endixaprine INN

endobenzyline bromide

endocaine [see: pyrrocaine]

Endocet tablets ℞ *narcotic analgesic; antipyretic* [oxycodone HCl; acetaminophen] 5•325, 7.5•325, 7.5•500, 10•325, 10•650 mg

Endocodone tablets (discontinued 2005) ℞ *narcotic analgesic* [oxycodone HCl] 5 mg

endolate [see: meperidine HCl]

Endometrin vaginal inserts ℞ *natural progestin; hormone replacement or supplementation for assisted reproductive technology (ART) treatments* [progesterone, micronized] 100 mg

endomide INN

endomycin

endostatin protein, recombinant human *investigational (orphan) for neuroendocrine tumors and metastatic melanoma*

endothelin-1 receptor antagonists *a class of vasodilator antihypertensives* *that block the action of endothelin-1 (ET-1), a vascular vasoconstrictor more potent than angiotensin II*

endothelin-A (EtA; ETA; ET$_A$) receptor antagonists *a class of antineoplastic agents that mediate the action of endothelin-1 (ET-1) to retard the proliferation of cancerous cells*

endralazine INN, BAN *antihypertensive* [also: endralazine mesylate]

endralazine mesylate USAN *antihypertensive* [also: endralazine]

Endrate IV infusion (discontinued 2008) ℞ *chelating agent for hypercalcemia and ventricular arrhythmias due to digitalis toxicity* [edetate disodium] 150 mg/mL ⊡ woundwort

endrisone INN *topical ophthalmic anti-inflammatory* [also: endrysone]

endrysone USAN *topical ophthalmic anti-inflammatory* [also: endrisone]

Enduret (trademarked dosage form) *prolonged-action tablet* ⊡ woundwort

Enduron tablets ℞ *antihypertensive; diuretic* [methyclothiazide] 5 mg

Enecat CT concentrated rectal suspension ℞ *radiopaque contrast medium for gastrointestinal imaging* [barium sulfate] 5%

enefexine INN

Enerjets lozenges OTC *CNS stimulant; analeptic* [caffeine] 75 mg

enestebol INN

EnfaCare [see: Enfamil EnfaCare]

Enfalyte ready-to-use oral liquid OTC *supplementary feeding to maintain hydration and electrolyte balance in infants with diarrhea or vomiting* 33.8 oz bottles ⊡ Infalyte

Enfamil oral liquid, powder for oral liquid OTC *total or supplementary infant feeding*

Enfamil EnfaCare oral liquid, powder for oral liquid OTC *enriched formula for premature infants* [milk-based formula] 3 oz bottles; 14 oz cans

Enfamil Human Milk Fortifier powder OTC *supplement to breast milk*

Enfamil LactoFree oral liquid, concentrate for oral liquid, powder for

oral liquid OTC *hypoallergenic infant formula* [milk-based formula, lactose free] 946 mL; 384 mL; 397 g

Enfamil LIPIL with Iron Nursette bottles, ready-to-use oral liquid, concentrate for oral liquid, powder for oral liquid OTC *infant formula fortified with omega-3 fatty acids* 3, 6 oz. bottles; 32 oz. cans; 13 oz. cans; 12.9, 25.9 oz. cans

Enfamil Next Step oral liquid, powder for oral liquid OTC *total or supplementary infant feeding*

Enfamil Premature Formula oral liquid OTC *total or supplementary infant feeding*

Enfamil with Iron oral liquid, powder for oral liquid OTC *total or supplementary infant feeding*

enfenamic acid INN

enflurane USAN, USP, INN, BAN *inhalation general anesthetic* 125, 250 mL

enfuvirtide *fusion inhibitor that prevents HIV from binding to T-cells, thus preventing viral entry into healthy cells*

Engerix-B IM injection ℞ *active immunizing agent for hepatitis B and D in adults* [hepatitis B virus vaccine, inactivated, recombinant] 20 mcg/mL

English elm (Ulmus campestris) *medicinal herb* [see: slippery elm]

English hawthorn *medicinal herb* [see: hawthorn]

English ivy (Hedera helix) leaves *medicinal herb used as an antispasmodic and antiexanthematous agent*

English oak (Quercus robur) *medicinal herb* [see: white oak]

English valerian *medicinal herb* [see: valerian]

English walnut (Juglans regia) leaves *medicinal herb used as an astringent*

englitazone INN *antidiabetic* [also: englitazone sodium]

englitazone sodium USAN *antidiabetic* [also: englitazone]

enhanced, inactivated polio vaccine (eIPV) [see: poliovirus vaccine, enhanced inactivated]

Enhancer powder for oral suspension ℞ *radiopaque contrast medium for gastrointestinal imaging* [barium sulfate] 98%

enhexymal [see: hexobarbital]

eniclobrate INN

enilconazole USAN, INN, BAN *antifungal*

enilospirone INN

eniluracil USAN *antineoplastic potentiator for fluorouracil; uracil reductase inhibitor*

enisoprost USAN, INN *antiulcerative; investigational (orphan) to reduce cyclosporine nephrotoxicity and acute rejection following organ transplants*

Enisyl tablets OTC *dietary amino acid supplement* [L-lysine] 334, 500 mg ⊇ anise oil; Anusol; Enseal; Unisol

Enjuvia film-coated tablets ℞ *hormone replacement therapy for severe postmenopausal vasomotor symptoms* [synthetic conjugated estrogens, B] 0.3, 0.45, 0.625, 0.9, 1.25 mg

Enlive! ready-to-use oral liquid OTC *enteral nutritional therapy* 240 mL ⊇ One-Alpha

Enlon IV or IM injection (discontinued 2008) ℞ *myasthenia gravis treatment; antidote to curare overdose* [edrophonium chloride] 10 mg/mL ⊇ inulin

Enlon Plus IV or IM injection (discontinued 2008) ℞ *muscle stimulant; neuromuscular blocker antagonist* [edrophonium chloride; atropine sulfate] 10•0.14 mg

enloplatin USAN, INN *antineoplastic*

enocitabine INN ⊇ ancitabine

enofelast USAN, INN *antiasthmatic*

enolicam INN *anti-inflammatory; antirheumatic* [also: enolicam sodium]

enolicam sodium USAN *anti-inflammatory; antirheumatic* [also: enolicam]

enoxacin USAN, INN, BAN, JAN *broad-spectrum fluoroquinolone antibiotic*

enoxamast INN

enoxaparin BAN *a low molecular weight heparin–type anticoagulant and antithrombotic for the prevention of deep vein thrombosis (DVT), unstable angina, and myocardial infarction* [also: enoxaparin sodium]

enoxaparin sodium USAN, INN *a low molecular weight heparin–type anticoagulant and antithrombotic for the prevention of deep vein thrombosis (DVT), unstable angina, and myocardial infarction* [also: enoxaparin]

enoximone USAN, INN, BAN *cardiotonic*

enoxolone INN, BAN

enphenemal [see: mephobarbital]

enpiprazole INN, BAN

enpiroline INN *antimalarial* [also: enpiroline phosphate]

enpiroline phosphate USAN *antimalarial* [also: enpiroline]

enprazepine INN

Enpresse tablets (in packs of 28) ℞ *triphasic oral contraceptive; emergency postcoital contraceptive* [levonorgestrel; ethinyl estradiol]
Phase 1 (6 days): 0.5 mg•30 mcg;
Phase 2 (5 days): 0.75 mg•40 mcg;
Phase 3 (10 days): 0.125 mg•30 mcg

enprofen [now: furaprofen]

enprofylline USAN, INN *bronchodilator*

enpromate USAN, INN *antineoplastic*

enprostil USAN, INN, BAN *antisecretory; antiulcerative*

enramycin INN

enrofloxacin USAN, INN, BAN *veterinary antibacterial*

Enseal (trademarked dosage form) *enteric-coated tablet* ⊇ anise oil; Anusol; Enisyl; Unisol

Ensure oral liquid, powder for oral liquid OTC *enteral nutritional therapy* [lactose-free formula]

Ensure pudding OTC *enteral nutritional therapy* [milk-based formula] 150 g

Ensure Glucerna beverage, bars OTC *diabetic nutritional supplements/snacks*

Ensure High Calcium ready-to-use oral liquid OTC *enteral nutritional therapy for postmenopausal women*

Ensure High Protein ready-to-use oral liquid OTC *enteral nutritional therapy* [lactose-free formula] 237 mL

Ensure HN; Ensure with Fiber ready-to-use oral liquid OTC *enteral nutritional therapy* [lactose-free formula]

Ensure Plus; Ensure Plus HN oral liquid OTC *enteral nutritional therapy* [lactose-free formula]

EN-tab (trademarked dosage form) *enteric-coated tablet*

entacapone USAN COMT *(catechol-O-methyltransferase) inhibitor for Parkinson disease*

entecavir USAN *nucleoside reverse transcriptase inhibitor (NRTI); antiviral for chronic hepatitis B virus (HBV) infection*

enteramine [see: serotonin]

Entereg capsules ℞ *peripherally acting opioid receptor antagonist for postoperative ileus (POI); restores normal bowel function after surgery* [alvimopan] 12 mg

Entero Vu oral suspension ℞ *radiopaque contrast agent for small bowel imaging* [barium sulfate] 13%, 24% in 600 mL

Entero Vu powder for oral liquid ℞ *radiopaque contrast agent for small bowel imaging* [barium sulfate] 100 g packets

Entero-Test; Entero-Test Pediatric string capsules for professional use ℞ *in vitro diagnostic aid for GI disorders*

Entertainer's Secret throat spray OTC *saliva substitute*

Entex oral liquid ℞ *decongestant; expectorant* [phenylephrine HCl; guaifenesin] 7.5•100 mg/5 mL ▣ Antiox

Entex ER extended-release capsules (discontinued 2007) ℞ *decongestant; expectorant* [phenylephrine HCl; guaifenesin] 10•300 mg ▣ Uni-Tex ER

Entex HC oral liquid ℞ *narcotic antitussive; decongestant; expectorant* [hydrocodone bitartrate; pseudoephedrine HCl; guaifenesin] 3.75•22.5•50 mg/5 mL

Entex LA dual-release capsules ℞ *decongestant; expectorant* [phenylephrine HCl (extended release); guaifenesin (immediate release)] 30•400 mg

Entex LA dual-release tablets ℞ *decongestant; expectorant (50% immediate release; 50% extended release)* [phenylephrine HCl; guaifenesin] 30•800 mg

Entex PSE dual-release capsules ℞ *decongestant; expectorant* [pseudoephedrine HCl (extended release); guaifenesin (immediate release)] 120•400 mg

Entex PSE sustained-release caplets ℞ *decongestant; expectorant* [pseudoephedrine HCl; guaifenesin] 50•525 mg

Entocort EC oral capsules for ileal release ℞ *corticosteroidal anti-inflammatory for Crohn disease* [budesonide (micronized)] 3 mg

Entri-Pak (delivery form) *liquid-filled pouch*

Entrition 0.5 oral liquid OTC *enteral nutritional therapy* [lactose-free formula]

Entrition HN Entri-Pak (liquid-filled pouch) OTC *enteral nutritional therapy* [lactose-free formula]

Entrobar oral suspension ℞ *radiopaque contrast medium for gastrointestinal imaging* [barium sulfate] 50% ▣ winterberry

EntroEase oral suspension (discontinued 2008) ℞ *radiopaque contrast medium for gastrointestinal imaging* [barium sulfate] 13%

EntroEase Dry powder for oral suspension (discontinued 2008) ℞ *radiopaque contrast medium for gastrointestinal imaging* [barium sulfate] 92%

entsufon INN *detergent* [also: entsufon sodium]

entsufon sodium USAN *detergent* [also: entsufon]

Entuss oral liquid (discontinued 2007) ℞ *narcotic antitussive; expectorant* [hydrocodone bitartrate; potassium guaiacolsulfonate] 5•300 mg/5 mL

Enuclene eye drops OTC *cleaning, wetting and lubricating agent for artificial eyes* [tyloxapol] 0.25%

Enulose oral/rectal solution ℞ *synthetic disaccharide used to prevent and treat portal-systemic encephalopathy* [lactulose] 10 g/15 mL

enviomycin INN

enviradene USAN, INN *antiviral*

Enviro-Stress slow-release tablets OTC *vitamin/mineral supplement* [multiple vitamins & minerals; folic acid] ≛• 0.4 mg

enviroxime USAN, INN *antiviral*

enzacamene USAN *ultraviolet sunscreen*

enzastaurin *serine-threonine kinase inhibitor; investigational (Phase III) tumor growth suppressor for non-Hodgkin lymphoma*

Enzone cream ℞ *corticosteroidal anti-inflammatory; anesthetic* [hydrocortisone acetate; pramoxine HCl] 1%• 1% ⊘ Anacin; inosine; Unasyn

Enzymatic Cleaner for Extended Wear tablets OTC *enzymatic cleaner for soft contact lenses* [pork pancreatin]

Eovist IV injection ℞ *MRI contrast agent for liver imaging* [gadoxetate disodium] 181.43 mg/mL in 10 mL vials ⊘ Evista

EP (etoposide, Platinol) *chemotherapy protocol for adenocarcinoma, lung cancer, and testicular cancer*

EPA capsules OTC *dietary supplement* [omega-3 fatty acids] 1000 mg

EPA (eicosapentaenoic acid) [q.v.; also: icosapent]

epalrestat INN *treatment for diabetic neuropathy*

epanolol USAN, INN, BAN

eperezolid USAN *antibacterial*

eperisone INN ⊘ euprocin

epervudine INN

ephedra (*Ephedra* spp.) plant *medicinal herb for asthma, blood cleansing, bronchitis, bursitis, chills, colds, edema, fever, flu, headache, kidney disorders, nasal congestion, and venereal disease* ⊘ Ivy-Dry

ephedrine USP, BAN *sympathomimetic bronchodilator; nasal decongestant; vasopressor for shock*

ephedrine HCl USP, BAN *sympathomimetic bronchodilator; nasal decongestant; vasopressor for shock*

ephedrine sulfate USP *sympathomimetic bronchodilator; nasal decongestant; vasopressor for acute hypotensive shock* [also: ephedrine sulphate] 25 mg oral; 50 mg/mL injection

ephedrine sulphate BAN *sympathomimetic bronchodilator; nasal decongestant* [also: ephedrine sulfate]

ephedrine tannate *sympathomimetic bronchodilator; nasal decongestant*

Epi-C concentrated oral suspension ℞ *radiopaque contrast medium for gastrointestinal imaging* [barium sulfate] 150% ⊘ ABC; APC; Apo-K; EPOCH

epicainide INN

epicatechin (EC); epicatechin gallate (ECG; ECg) *natural polyphenolic antioxidants found in green tea, believed to be primarily responsible for its anticarcinogenic property* [see also: epicatechins; epigallocatechin]

epicatechins *a class of natural polyphenolic antioxidants found in green tea and grape seed extract, used for their anticarcinogenic, anti-inflammatory, and antiatherosclerotic properties and to promote thermogenesis* [see also: catechins; kunecatechins]

epicillin USAN, INN, BAN *antibacterial* ⊘ ebselen

epicriptine INN

epidermal growth factor (EGF), human *investigational (orphan) for acceleration of corneal regeneration and the healing of severe burns*

epidermal growth factor receptor (EGFR) inhibitors *a class of antineoplastics, predominantly monoclonal antibodies, that suppress the growth of breast, colorectal, head, and neck cancers; includes HER1 (q.v.), HER2 (q.v.), HER3, and HER4* [also known as: human epidermal growth factor receptor (HER) inhibitors]

epiestriol INN [also: epioestriol]

Epifoam aerosol foam ℞ *corticosteroidal anti-inflammatory; anesthetic* [hydrocortisone acetate; pramoxine] 1%•1%

Epifrin eye drops (discontinued 2004) ℞ *antiglaucoma agent* [epinephrine HCl] 0.5%, 1%, 2% ⊘ ibuverine

epigallocatechin (EGC); epigallo-catechin gallate (EGCG; EGCg) *natural polyphenolic antioxidants found in green tea, believed to be primarily responsible for its anticarcinogenic property* [see also: epicatechins]

epilin [see: dietifen]

E-Pilo-1; E-Pilo-2; E-Pilo-4; E-Pilo-6 eye drops (discontinued 2004) ℞ *antiglaucoma agent* [pilocarpine HCl; epinephrine bitartrate] 1%•1%; 2%•1%; 4%•1%; 6%•1% ⊡ A.P.L.; apple; IPOL; OPAL

Epilyt lotion concentrate OTC *moisturizer; emollient*

epimestrol USAN, INN, BAN *anterior pituitary activator*

Epinal eye drops ℞ *antiglaucoma agent* [epinephryl borate] 0.5%, 1% ⊡ Abenol

epinastine INN *ophthalmic antihistamine* [also: epinastine HCl]

epinastine HCl *ophthalmic antihistamine* [also: epinastine]

epinephran [see: epinephrine]

epinephrine USP, INN *vasoconstrictor; sympathomimetic bronchodilator; topical antiglaucoma agent; vasopressor for shock* [also: adrenaline] 1:1000, 1:10 000 (1, 0.1 mg/mL) injection

epinephrine bitartrate USP *sympathomimetic bronchodilator; ophthalmic adrenergic; topical antiglaucoma agent*

epinephrine borate *topical antiglaucoma agent*

epinephrine & cisplatin *investigational (NDA filed, orphan) injectable gel for squamous cell carcinoma of the head and neck; investigational (orphan) for metastatic malignant melanoma*

epinephrine HCl *sympathomimetic bronchodilator; nasal decongestant; topical antiglaucoma agent; vasopressor for shock* 0.1% eye drops; 1:1000 (1 mg/mL) injection

Epinephrine Mist inhalation aerosol OTC *sympathomimetic bronchodilator; vasopressor for shock* [epinephrine] 0.22 mg/spray

epinephryl borate USAN, USP *adrenergic; topical antiglaucoma agent*

epioestriol BAN [also: epiestriol]

EpiPen; EpiPen Jr. auto-injector (automatic IM injection device) ℞ *emergency treatment of anaphylaxis; vasopressor for shock* [epinephrine] 1:1000 (1 mg/mL); 1:2000 (0.5 mg/mL)

epipropidine USAN, INN *antineoplastic*

EpiQuin Micro cream ℞ *hyperpigmentation bleaching agent* [hydroquinone (in a base containing vitamins A, C, and E)] 4%

epirizole USAN, INN *analgesic; antiinflammatory*

epiroprim INN

epirubicin INN, BAN *anthracycline antibiotic antineoplastic* [also: epirubicin HCl]

epirubicin HCl USAN, JAN *anthracycline antibiotic antineoplastic for breast cancer (orphan)* [also: epirubicin] 50, 200 mg/vial injection

epirubicin & tamoxifen *chemotherapy protocol for breast cancer*

epitetracycline HCl USP *antibacterial*

epithiazide USAN, BAN *antihypertensive; diuretic* [also: epitizide]

epithioandrostanol [see: epitiostanol]

epitiostanol INN

epitizide INN *antihypertensive; diuretic* [also: epithiazide]

Epitol tablets ℞ *iminostilbene anticonvulsant; analgesic for trigeminal neuralgia; also used for restless legs syndrome (RLS), alcohol withdrawal, and postherpetic neuralgia* [carbamazepine] 200 mg ⊡ Apetil

Epivir film-coated tablets, oral solution ℞ *antiviral for HIV infection* [lamivudine] 150, 300 mg; 10 mg/mL

Epivir-HBV film-coated caplets, oral solution ℞ *antiviral for hepatitis B virus (HBV) infection* [lamivudine] 100 mg; 5 mg/mL

eplerenone USAN *aldosterone receptor antagonist for hypertension and congestive heart failure (CHF); improves survival after a cardiovascular event* 25, 50 mg oral

EPO (epoetin alfa) [q.v.]

EPO (evening primrose oil) [see: evening primrose]

EPOCH (etoposide, prednisone, Oncovin, cyclophosphamide, Halotestin) chemotherapy protocol ② ABC; APC; Apo-K; Epi-C; iboga

epoetin alfa (EPO) USAN, INN, BAN, JAN hematopoietic to stimulate RBC production for anemia of chronic renal failure, HIV, and chemotherapy (orphan) and to reduce the need for blood transfusions in surgery; investigational (orphan) for myelodysplastic syndrome

epoetin beta USAN, INN, BAN, JAN erythropoiesis-stimulating agent (ESA) for the treatment of anemia due to chronic renal failure (orphan)

Epogen IV or subcu injection ℞ hematopoietic to stimulate RBC production for anemia of chronic renal failure, HIV, and chemotherapy (orphan) and to reduce the need for blood transfusions in surgery [epoetin alfa] 2000, 3000, 4000, 10 000, 20 000, 40 000 U/mL ② Apokyn; Opcon-A

epoprostenol USAN, INN platelet aggregation inhibitor and vasodilator for pulmonary hypertension (orphan); investigational (orphan) heparin replacement for hemodialysis

epoprostenol sodium USAN, BAN platelet aggregation inhibitor and vasodilator for pulmonary hypertension (orphan); investigational (orphan) heparin replacement for hemodialysis 0.5, 1.5 mg injection

epostane USAN, INN, BAN interceptive ② ebastine

epoxytropine tropate methylbromide [see: methscopolamine bromide]

epratuzumab investigational (Phase III, orphan) monoclonal antibody to CD22, radiolabeled with yttrium Y 90 for AIDS-related non-Hodgkin lymphoma; investigational (Phase III) for systemic lupus erythematosus (SLE)

eprazinone INN

eprinomectin USAN veterinary antiparasitic

epristeride USAN, INN, BAN alpha reductase inhibitor

eprodisate investigational (NDA filed, orphan) amyloid fibrinogen inhibitor for AA (secondary) amyloidosis

eprosartan USAN antihypertensive; angiotensin II receptor antagonist

eprosartan mesylate USAN antihypertensive; angiotensin II receptor antagonist

eprovafen INN

eproxindine INN

eprozinol INN

epsikapron [see: aminocaproic acid]

epsilon-aminocaproic acid (EACA) [see: aminocaproic acid]

epsiprantel INN, BAN

Epsom salt granules OTC saline laxative [magnesium sulfate]

Epsom salt [see: magnesium sulfate]

e.p.t. Quick Stick test stick for home use OTC in vitro diagnostic aid; urine pregnancy test

eptacog alfa (activated) activated recombinant human blood coagulation Factor VII (rFVIIa) for hemophilia A and B

eptaloprost INN

eptamestrol [see: etamestrol]

eptaprost [see: eptaloprost]

eptastatin sodium [see: pravastatin sodium]

eptastigmine INN treatment for Alzheimer disease

eptazocine INN

eptifibatide glycoprotein (GP) IIb/IIIa receptor antagonist; platelet aggregation inhibitor for acute coronary syndrome, unstable angina, myocardial infarction, and cardiac surgery

Epulor oral liquid OTC enteral nutritional therapy [milk-based formula]

Epzicom film-coated tablets ℞ once-daily nucleoside reverse transcriptase inhibitor (NRTI) antiviral combination for HIV infections [abacavir sulfate; lamivudine] 600•300 mg

Equagesic tablets ℞ *analgesic; antipyretic; anti-inflammatory; anxiolytic; sedative* [aspirin; meprobamate] 325•200 mg

Equalactin chewable tablets OTC *bulk laxative; antidiarrheal* [calcium polycarbophil] 625 mg

Equanil tablets (discontinued 2004) ℞ *anxiolytic* [meprobamate] 200, 400 mg ☒ Aquanil

Equetro extended-release capsules ℞ *iminostilbene antipsychotic for manic episodes of a bipolar disorder; also used for restless legs syndrome (RLS), alcohol withdrawal, and postherpetic neuralgia* [carbamazepine] 100, 200, 300 mg

Equilet chewable tablets OTC *antacid* [calcium carbonate] 500 mg ☒ Accolate

equilin USP *estrogen*

Equipoise *brand name for boldenone undecylenate, a veterinary anabolic steroid abused as a street drug* ☒ Aquabase; ICaps

Equisetum arvens medicinal herb [see: horsetail]

Eraxis powder for IV infusion ℞ *antifungal for candidemia of the internal organs, esophageal candidiasis, and other serious fungal infections* [anidulafungin] 50, 100 mg/vial

Erbitux IV infusion ℞ *antineoplastic for metastatic colorectal cancer and squamous cell carcinoma (SCC) of the head and neck (orphan); investigational (Phase III) for brain, breast, bladder, gastric, lung, prostate, and pancreatic cancers* [cetuximab] 100, 200 mg/vial

erbium *element (Er)* ☒ europium

erbulozole USAN, INN *antineoplastic adjunct*

erbumine USAN, INN, BAN *combining name for radicals or groups*

Ercaf tablets ℞ *migraine-specific vasoconstrictor* [ergotamine tartrate; caffeine] 1•100 mg

erdosteine INN

Erechtites hieracfolia medicinal herb [see: pilewort]

Ergamisol tablets (discontinued 2006) ℞ *biological response modifier; antineoplastic adjunct for colon cancer* [levamisole HCl] 50 mg

ergocalciferol (vitamin D₂) USP, INN, BAN, JAN *fat-soluble vitamin for refractory rickets, familial hypophosphatemia, and hypoparathyroidism* (1 mg=40 000 IU) 50 000 U oral

ergoloid mesylates USAN, USP *cognition adjuvant for age-related mental capacity decline* [also: co-dergocrine mesylate] 0.5, 1 mg oral

Ergomar sublingual tablets ℞ *prophylaxis or treatment of migraine and other vascular headaches* [ergotamine tartrate] 2 mg

ergometrine INN, BAN *oxytocic for induction of labor* [also: ergonovine maleate]

ergonovine maleate USP *oxytocic for the induction of labor and prevention of postpartum and postabortal hemorrhage* [also: ergometrine]

ergosterol, activated [see: ergocalciferol]

ergot (Claviceps purpurea) *dried sclerotia medicinal herb used as an abortifacient, emmenagogue, hemostatic, oxytocic, and vasoconstrictor; source of ergotamine and LSD* ☒ Irrigate

ergot alkaloids [see: ergoloid mesylates]

ergotamine INN, BAN *migraine-specific analgesic* [also: ergotamine tartrate]

ergotamine tartrate USP *prophylaxis or treatment of migraine and other vascular headaches* [also: ergotamine]

ergotamine tartrate & caffeine *prophylaxis or treatment of migraine and other vascular headaches* 1•100 mg oral

Ergotrate Maleate IM or IV injection (discontinued 2004) ℞ *oxytocic for the induction of labor and prevention of postpartum and postabortal hemorrhage* [ergonovine maleate] 0.2 mg/mL

Ergotrate Maleate tablets ℞ *oxytocic for the induction of labor and prevention of postpartum and postabortal hemorrhage* [ergonovine maleate] 0.2 mg

ericolol INN

Erigeron canadensis *medicinal herb* [see: fleabane; horseweed]

eriodictyon NF

Eriodictyon californicum *medicinal herb* [see: yerba santa]

eritrityl tetranitrate INN *coronary vasodilator* [also: erythrityl tetranitrate]

erizepine INN ⊡ AeroSpan

erlizumab USAN *monoclonal antibody to treat reperfusion injury following acute myocardial infarction*

erlotinib HCl *human epidermal growth factor receptor type 1 (HER1) inhibitor; tyrosine kinase inhibitor; antineoplastic for advanced or metastatic non–small cell lung and pancreatic cancer; investigational (Phase III) for breast cancer; investigational (orphan) for malignant gliomas*

E·R·O Ear Drops OTC *cerumenolytic to emulsify and disperse ear wax* [carbamide peroxide] 6.5% ⊡ Auro Ear Drops

erocainide INN

errhines *a class of agents that promote nasal discharge or secretion* ⊡ Orencia; Orinase

Errin tablets (in packs of 28) ℞ *oral contraceptive (progestin only)* [norethindrone] 0.35 mg ⊡ iron

ersofermin USAN, INN *wound healing agent; transglutaminase inhibitor for the treatment of scar tissue*

Ertaczo cream ℞ *antifungal* [sertaconazole nitrate] 2% ⊡ AeroTuss; Artiss

ertapenem sodium USAN *broad-spectrum carbapenem antibiotic*

Erwinase *investigational (orphan) antineoplastic for acute lymphocytic leukemia* [erwinia L-asparaginase]

erwinia L-asparaginase *investigational (orphan) antineoplastic for acute lymphocytic leukemia*

Ery Pads pledgets ℞ *antibiotic for acne* [erythromycin; alcohol 60.5%] 2%

ERYC delayed-release capsules containing enteric-coated pellets ℞ *macrolide antibiotic* [erythromycin] 250 mg ⊡ ara-C

EryDerm 2% topical solution ℞ *antibiotic for acne* [erythromycin; alcohol 77%] 2%

Erygel gel ℞ *antibiotic for acne* [erythromycin; alcohol 92%] 2% ⊡ Orajel

Eryngium aquaticum *medicinal herb* [see: water eryngo]

EryPed oral drops ℞ *macrolide antibiotic* [erythromycin ethylsuccinate] 100 mg/2.5 mL ⊡ AeroBid

EryPed 200; EryPed 400 oral suspension ℞ *macrolide antibiotic* [erythromycin ethylsuccinate] 200 mg/5 mL; 400 mg/5 mL ⊡ AeroBid

Ery-Tab enteric-coated delayed-release tablets ℞ *macrolide antibiotic* [erythromycin] 250, 333, 500 mg

erythorbic acid

Erythraea centaurium *medicinal herb* [see: centaury]

erythrityl tetranitrate USAN, USP *coronary vasodilator; antianginal* [also: eritrityl tetranitrate]

Erythrocin Lactobionate powder for IV injection ℞ *macrolide antibiotic* [erythromycin lactobionate] 500, 1000 mg/vial

Erythrocin Stearate Filmtabs (film-coated tablets) ℞ *macrolide antibiotic* [erythromycin stearate] 250, 500 mg

erythrol tetranitrate [now: erythrityl tetranitrate]

erythromycin USP, INN, BAN *macrolide antibiotic* 250, 500 mg oral; 2% topical; 0.5% ophthalmic

erythromycin 2'-acetate octadecanoate [see: erythromycin acistrate]

erythromycin 2'-acetate stearate [see: erythromycin acistrate]

erythromycin acistrate USAN, INN *macrolide antibiotic*

erythromycin B [see: berythromycin]

erythromycin & benzoyl peroxide *antibiotic and keratolytic for acne* 3%•5% topical

erythromycin estolate USAN, USP, BAN *macrolide antibiotic*

erythromycin ethyl succinate BAN *macrolide antibiotic* [also: erythromycin ethylsuccinate]

erythromycin ethylcarbonate USP
macrolide antibiotic

erythromycin ethylsuccinate (EES)
USP *macrolide antibiotic* [also: erythromycin ethyl succinate] 400 mg oral;
200, 400 mg/5 mL oral

erythromycin gluceptate USP *macrolide antibiotic*

erythromycin glucoheptonate [see:
erythromycin gluceptate]

erythromycin lactobionate USP *macrolide antibiotic*

**erythromycin lauryl sulfate, propi-
onyl** [now: erythromycin estolate]

**erythromycin monoglucohepto-
nate** [see: erythromycin gluceptate]

erythromycin octadecanoate [see:
erythromycin stearate]

erythromycin 2′-propanoate [see:
erythromycin propionate]

erythromycin propionate USAN *macrolide antibiotic*

**erythromycin 2′-propionate dodecyl
sulfate** [see: erythromycin estolate]

**erythromycin propionate lauryl
sulfate** [now: erythromycin estolate]

erythromycin salnacedin USAN *macrolide antibiotic for acne vulgaris*

erythromycin stearate USP, BAN *macrolide antibiotic* 250, 500 mg oral

erythromycin stinoprate INN *macrolide antibiotic*

Erythronium americanum medicinal
herb [see: adder's tongue]

**erythropoietin, recombinant human
(rEPO)** [see: epoetin alfa; epoetin
beta]

erythrosine sodium USP *dental disclosing agent*

Eryzole granules for oral suspension ℞
antibiotic [erythromycin ethylsuccinate; sulfisoxazole acetyl] 200•600
mg/5 mL ⊘ Orasol; uracil

esafloxacin INN

esaprazole INN

escitalopram oxalate USAN *selective
serotonin reuptake inhibitor (SSRI) for
major depressive disorder (MDD) and
generalized anxiety disorder (GAD);*
*also used for panic disorder; isomer of
citalopram* 5, 10, 20 mg oral

Esclim transdermal patch ℞ *estrogen
replacement therapy for the treatment
of postmenopausal symptoms* [estra-
diol] 25, 37.5 mcg/day ⊘ Oesclim

esculamine INN

eseridine INN

eserine [see: physostigmine]

esflurbiprofen INN, BAN

Esgic caplets, capsules ℞ *barbiturate
sedative; analgesic; antipyretic* [butal-
bital; acetaminophen; caffeine] 50•
325•40 mg

Esgic-Plus caplets, capsules ℞ *barbiturate sedative; analgesic; antipyretic*
[butalbital; acetaminophen; caffeine]
50•500•40 mg

**ESHAP (etoposide, Solu-Medrol,
high-dose ara-C, Platinol)** *chemotherapy protocol for non-Hodgkin lymphoma* ⊘ ASHAP

**ESHAP-MINE (alternating cycles
of ESHAP and MINE)** *chemotherapy protocol*

Esidrix tablets (discontinued 2006) ℞
antihypertensive; diuretic [hydrochlo-
rothiazide] 25, 50, 100 mg

esilate INN *combining name for radicals
or groups* [also: esylate] ⊘ Isolyte E

Esimil tablets (discontinued 2007) ℞
antihypertensive; diuretic [hydrochlo-
rothiazide; guanethidine monosul-
fate] 25•10 mg ⊘ Isomil

Eskalith capsules ℞ *antipsychotic for
manic episodes* [lithium carbonate]
300 mg

Eskalith tablets (discontinued 2005)
℞ *antipsychotic for manic episodes*
[lithium carbonate] 300 mg

Eskalith CR controlled-release tablets
℞ *antipsychotic for manic episodes*
[lithium carbonate] 450 mg

esmolol INN, BAN *antihypertensive;
antiadrenergic (β-receptor)* [also:
esmolol HCl]

esmolol HCl USAN *antihypertensive;
antiarrhythmic; antiadrenergic (β-
receptor)* [also: esmolol] 10 mg/mL
injection

E-Solve OTC *lotion base*

esomeprazole magnesium USAN *oral proton pump inhibitor for gastric and duodenal ulcers, erosive esophagitis, gastroesophageal reflux disease (GERD), and other gastroesophageal disorders; isomer of omeprazole*

esomeprazole sodium *injectable proton pump inhibitor for the short-term treatment of GERD in patients who cannot take the drug orally; isomer of omeprazole*

esorubicin INN *antineoplastic* [also: esorubicin HCl]

esorubicin HCl USAN *antineoplastic* [also: esorubicin]

Esotérica Dry Skin Treatment lotion OTC *moisturizer; emollient*

Esotérica Facial; Esotérica Regular cream OTC *hyperpigmentation bleaching agent* [hydroquinone] 2%

Esotérica Soap OTC *bath emollient*

Esotérica Sunscreen cream OTC *hyperpigmentation bleaching agent; sunscreen* [hydroquinone; padimate O; oxybenzone] 2%•3.3%•2.5%

esproquin HCl USAN *adrenergic* [also: esproquine]

esproquine INN *adrenergic* [also: esproquin HCl]

Essential ProPlus powder for oral solution OTC *oral protein supplement with vitamins and minerals* [soy protein; multiple vitamins and minerals]

Essential Protein powder OTC *oral protein supplement* [soy protein]

Estar gel (discontinued 2004) OTC *antipsoriatic; antiseborrheic* [coal tar] 5%

estazolam USAN, INN *benzodiazepine sedative and hypnotic* 1, 2 mg oral

Ester-C Plus Multi-Mineral capsules OTC *vitamin C/mineral supplement with multiple bioflavonoids* [vitamin C; multiple minerals; citrus bioflavonoids; acerola; rose hips; rutin] 425• ≛•50•12.5•12.5•5 mg

Ester-C Plus Vitamin C capsules OTC *vitamin C/calcium supplement with multiple bioflavonoids* [vitamin C; calcium; citrus bioflavonoids; acerola; rose hips; rutin] 500•62•25•10•10• 5 mg; 1000•125•200•25•25•25 mg

esterified estrogens [see: estrogens, esterified]

esterifilcon A USAN *hydrophilic contact lens material*

estilben [see: diethylstilbestrol dipropionate]

estolate INN *combining name for radicals or groups*

estomycin sulfate [see: paromomycin sulfate]

Estorra tablets (name changed to **Lunesta** in 2004)

Estrace tablets ℞ *estrogen replacement therapy for the treatment of postmenopausal symptoms and prevention of postmenopausal osteoporosis; palliative therapy for prostate and metastatic breast cancers* [estradiol, soy-derived] 0.5, 1, 2 mg

Estrace Vaginal cream ℞ *estrogen replacement for postmenopausal atrophic vaginitis* [estradiol] 0.1 mg/g

Estraderm transdermal patch ℞ *estrogen replacement therapy for the treatment of postmenopausal symptoms and prevention of postmenopausal osteoporosis* [estradiol] 50, 100 mcg/day

estradiol USP, INN *estrogen replacement therapy for the treatment of postmenopausal disorders and the prevention of postmenopausal osteoporosis; palliative therapy for breast and prostate cancers; may be naturally derived or a synthetic analogue* [also: oestradiol] 0.5, 1, 2 mg oral

estradiol acetate *synthetic estrogen; hormone replacement therapy for the treatment of postmenopausal symptoms*

estradiol-17β *estrogen replacement therapy for postmenopausal disorders*

estradiol benzoate USP, INN, JAN [also: oestradiol benzoate]

estradiol 17-cyclopentanepropionate [see: estradiol cypionate]

estradiol cypionate USP *synthetic estrogen; hormone replacement therapy for the treatment of postmenopausal symptoms*

estradiol dipropionate NF, JAN

estradiol enanthate USAN *estrogen*

estradiol hemihydrate *synthetic estrogen; topical hormone therapy for atrophic vaginitis*

estradiol 17-heptanoate [see: estradiol enanthate]

estradiol monobenzoate [see: estradiol benzoate]

estradiol 17-nicotinate 3-propionate [see: estrapronicate]

estradiol & norethindrone acetate *a mixture of natural and synthetic hormones; hormone replacement therapy for postmenopausal symptoms* 1•0.5 mg oral

estradiol phosphate polymer [see: polyestradiol phosphate]

Estradiol Transdermal System patch ℞ *estrogen replacement therapy for the treatment of postmenopausal symptoms and prevention of postmenopausal osteoporosis* [estradiol] 25, 37.5, 50, 60, 75, 100 mcg/day

estradiol 17-undecanoate [see: estradiol undecylate]

estradiol undecylate USAN, INN *estrogen*

estradiol valerate USP, INN, JAN *synthetic estrogen; hormone replacement therapy for the treatment of postmenopausal symptoms and the prevention of postmenopausal osteoporosis; hormonal antineoplastic for breast and prostate cancers* [also: oestradiol valerate] 10, 20, 40 mg/mL injection

Estra-L 40 IM injection ℞ *estrogen replacement therapy for postmenopausal symptoms; antineoplastic for prostatic cancer* [estradiol valerate in oil] 40 mg/mL ☑ Ezetrol

estramustine USAN, INN, BAN *nitrogen mustard-type alkylating antineoplastic*

estramustine phosphate sodium USAN, BAN, JAN *nitrogen mustard-type alkylating antineoplastic for prostate cancer*

estramustine & vinblastine sulfate *chemotherapy protocol for prostate cancer*

estrapronicate INN

Estrasorb topical emulsion (discontinued 2007) ℞ *estrogen replacement therapy for postmenopausal symptoms* [estradiol hemihydrate] 2.5 mg/g (4.35 mg/pouch; base=25 mcg/pouch)

Estratest; Estratest H.S. sugar-coated tablets ℞ *combination equine estrogen and synthetic androgen; hormone replacement therapy for postmenopausal symptoms* [esterified estrogens; methyltestosterone] 1.25•2.5 mg; 0.625•1.25 mg

estrazinol INN *estrogen* [also: estrazinol hydrobromide]

estrazinol hydrobromide USAN *estrogen* [also: estrazinol]

Estring vaginal ring ℞ *three-month estrogen replacement for postmenopausal atrophic vaginitis* [estradiol] 2 mg (7.5 mcg/day) ☑ Oestring

estriol USP *estrogen* [also: estriol succinate; oestriol succinate] ☑ Ezetrol

estriol succinate INN *estrogen* [also: estriol; oestriol succinate]

estrobene [see: diethylstilbestrol]

estrobene DP [see: diethylstilbestrol dipropionate]

estrofurate USAN, INN *estrogen*

Estrogel transdermal gel ℞ *estrogen replacement therapy for postmenopausal symptoms* [estradiol] 0.06%

estrogenic substances, conjugated [see: estrogens, conjugated]

estrogenine [see: diethylstilbestrol]

estrogens *a class of sex hormones that includes estradiol, estrone, and estriol, also used as an antineoplastic*

estrogens, conjugated USP, JAN *a mixture of equine estrogens; hormone replacement therapy for the treatment of postmenopausal symptoms and prevention of postmenopausal osteoporosis; palliative therapy for breast and prostate cancers*

estrogens, esterified USP *a mixture of equine estrogens; hormone replacement therapy for the treatment of postmenopausal disorders; palliative therapy for breast and prostate cancers*

estrogens, esterified & methyltestosterone *combination equine estrogen and synthetic androgen; hormone replacement therapy for postmenopausal symptoms* 0.625•1.25, 1.25•2.5 mg oral

estrogens, synthetic conjugated, A *a mixture of 9 synthetic estrogenic substances; hormone replacement therapy for postmenopausal symptoms*

estrogens, synthetic conjugated, B *a mixture of 10 synthetic estrogenic substances; hormone replacement therapy for severe postmenopausal vasomotor symptoms*

estromenin [see: diethylstilbestrol]

estrone USP, INN *bioidentical human estrogen; natural hormone replacement therapy for postmenopausal disorders; palliative therapy for breast and prostate cancers* [also: oestrone] ② isoetarine

estrone hydrogen sulfate [see: estrone sodium sulfate]

estrone sodium sulfate *synthetic estrogen*

Estrophasic (trademarked/patented dosing regimen) *gradual estrogen intake with steady progestin intake*

estropipate USP *natural estrogen replacement therapy for the treatment of postmenopausal symptoms and prevention of postmenopausal osteoporosis; a stabilized form of estrone, the bioidentical human estrogen* 0.75, 1.5, 3, 6 mg oral

Estrostep 21 tablets (in packs of 21) (discontinued 2008) ℞ *triphasic oral contraceptive; treatment for acne vulgaris in females* [norethindrone acetate; ethinyl estradiol]
Phase 1 (5 days): 1 mg•20 mcg;
Phase 2 (7 days): 1 mg•30 mcg;
Phase 3 (9 days): 1 mg•35 mcg

Estrostep Fe tablets (in packs of 28) ℞ *triphasic oral contraceptive; iron supplement* [norethindrone acetate; ethinyl estradiol; ferrous fumarate]
Phase 1 (5 days): 1•0.02•75 mg;
Phase 2 (7 days): 1•0.03•75 mg;
Phase 3 (9 days): 1•0.035•75 mg;
Counters (7 days): 0•0•75 mg

esuprone INN ② aceperone; aspirin; azaperone; Easprin

esylate USAN, BAN *combining name for radicals or groups* [also: esilate] ② Isolyte E

eszopiclone *nonbarbiturate sedative and hypnotic for chronic insomnia; isomer of zopiclone*

etabenzarone INN

etabonate USAN, INN *combining name for radicals or groups*

etacepride INN

etacrynic acid INN, JAN *antihypertensive; loop diuretic* [also: ethacrynic acid]

etafedrine INN, BAN *adrenergic* [also: etafedrine HCl]

etafedrine HCl USAN *adrenergic* [also: etafedrine]

etafenone INN ② etifenin

etafilcon A USAN *hydrophilic contact lens material*

etamestrol INN

etaminile INN

etamiphyllin INN [also: etamiphylline]

etamiphyllin methesculetol [see: metescufylline]

etamiphylline BAN [also: etamiphyllin]

etamivan INN *central and respiratory stimulant* [also: ethamivan]

etamocycline INN

etamsylate INN *hemostatic* [also: ethamsylate]

etanercept USAN *soluble tumor necrosis factor receptor (sTNFR) inhibitor for rheumatoid arthritis, juvenile rheumatoid arthritis (orphan), psoriatic arthritis, and ankylosing spondylitis; investigational (orphan) for Wegener granulomatosis*

etanidazole USAN, INN *antineoplastic; hypoxic cell radiosensitizer*

etanterol INN

etaperazine [see: perphenazine]

etaqualone INN

etarotene USAN, INN *keratolytic*

etasuline INN ② etozolin

etazepine INN ② atosiban

etazolate INN *antipsychotic* [also: etazolate HCl]

etazolate HCl USAN *antipsychotic* [also: etazolate]

etebenecid INN [also: ethebenecid]

etenzamide BAN [also: ethenzamide]

eterobarb USAN, INN, BAN *anticonvulsant*

etersalate INN

ethacridine INN [also: ethacridine lactate; acrinol]

ethacridine lactate [also: ethacridine; acrinol]

ethacrynate sodium USAN, USP *antihypertensive; loop diuretic*

ethacrynic acid USAN, USP, BAN *antihypertensive; loop diuretic* [also: etacrynic acid]

ethambutol INN, BAN *bacteriostatic; primary tuberculostatic* [also: ethambutol HCl]

ethambutol HCl USAN, USP *bacteriostatic; primary tuberculostatic* [also: ethambutol] 100, 400 mg oral

ethamivan USAN, USP, BAN *central and respiratory stimulant* [also: etamivan]

Ethamolin IV injection ℞ *sclerosing agent for bleeding esophageal varices (orphan)* [ethanolamine oleate] 5%

ethamsylate USAN, BAN *hemostatic* [also: etamsylate]

ethanol JAN *topical anti-infective/antiseptic; astringent; solvent; a widely abused "legal street drug" used to produce euphoria* [also: alcohol]

ethanol, dehydrated JAN *antidote* [also: alcohol, dehydrated]

ethanolamine oleate USAN *sclerosing agent for bleeding esophageal varices (orphan)* [also: monoethanolamine oleate]

ethanolamines *a class of antihistamines that includes diphenhydramine HCl and clemastine fumarate*

ethaverine INN *peripheral vasodilator*

ethaverine HCl *peripheral vasodilator for peripheral and vascular insufficiency due to arterial spasm* [also: ethaverine]

ethchlorvynol USP, INN, BAN *sedative; hypnotic*

ethebenecid BAN [also: etebenecid]

EtheDent chewable tablets ℞ *dental caries preventative* [sodium fluoride] 0.25, 0.5, 1 mg

EtheDent dental cream ℞ *caries preventative* [sodium fluoride] 1.1%

ethenzamide INN, JAN [also: etenzamide]

ether USP *inhalation anesthetic* ② water O 15

Ethezyme; Ethezyme 830 ointment ℞ *proteolytic enzyme for debridement of necrotic tissue; vulnerary* [papain; urea] 1 100 000 U•100 mg per gram; 830 000 IU•100 mg per gram

ethiazide INN, BAN ② Atuss HD

ethidium bromide [see: homidium bromide]

ethinamate USP, INN, BAN *sedative; hypnotic*

ethinyl estradiol USP *estrogen replacement therapy for the treatment of postmenopausal disorders; palliative therapy for prostate and breast cancers; investigational (orphan) for Turner syndrome* [also: ethinylestradiol; ethinyloestradiol]

ethinylestradiol INN *estrogen replacement therapy for the treatment of postmenopausal disorders; palliative therapy for prostate and breast cancers* [also: ethinyl estradiol; ethinyloestradiol]

ethinyloestradiol BAN *estrogen replacement therapy for the treatment of postmenopausal disorders; palliative therapy for prostate and breast cancers* [also: ethinyl estradiol; ethinylestradiol]

ethiodized oil USP *parenteral radiopaque contrast medium (37% iodine)*

ethiodized oil (¹³¹I) INN *antineoplastic; radioactive agent* [also: ethiodized oil I 131]

ethiodized oil I 131 USAN *antineoplastic; radioactive agent* [also: ethiodized oil (¹³¹I)]

Ethiodol intracavitary instillation ℞ *radiopaque contrast medium for lymphography and gynecological imaging* [ethiodized oil (37% iodine)] 1284 mg/mL (475 mg/mL)

ethiofos [now: amifostine]

ethionamide USAN, USP, INN, BAN *bacteriostatic; tuberculosis retreatment*

ethisterone NF, INN, BAN ☒ itasetron

Ethmozine film-coated tablets (discontinued 2008) ℞ *antiarrhythmic for severe ventricular arrhythmias* [moricizine HCl] 200, 250, 300 mg

ethodryl [see: diethylcarbamazine citrate]

ethoglucid BAN [also: etoglucid]

ethoheptazine BAN [also: ethoheptazine citrate]

ethoheptazine citrate NF, INN [also: ethoheptazine]

ethohexadiol USP

ethomoxane INN, BAN

ethomoxane HCl [see: ethomoxane]

ethonam nitrate USAN *antifungal* [also: etonam]

ethopabate BAN

ethopropazine BAN *anticholinergic; antiparkinsonian* [also: ethopropazine HCl; profenamine]

ethopropazine HCl USP *anticholinergic; antiparkinsonian* [also: profenamine; ethopropazine]

ethosalamide BAN [also: etosalamide]

ethosuximide USAN, USP, INN, BAN *anticonvulsant* 250 mg oral; 250 mg/ 5 mL oral

ethotoin USP, INN, BAN *hydantoin anticonvulsant*

ethoxarutine [see: ethoxazorutoside]

ethoxazene HCl USAN *analgesic* [also: etoxazene]

ethoxazorutoside INN

ethoxyacetanilide *(withdrawn from the market)* [see: phenacetin]

o-**ethoxybenzamide** [see: ethenzamide; etenzamide]

ETH-Oxydose oral drops ℞ *narcotic analgesic* [oxycodone HCl] 20 mg/mL

ethoxzolamide USP

Ethrane liquid for vaporization ℞ *inhalation general anesthetic* [enflurane]

ethybenztropine USAN, BAN *anticholinergic* [also: etybenzatropine]

ethyl acetate NF *solvent*

ethyl alcohol (EtOH; ETOH) [now: alcohol; ethanol]

ethyl aminobenzoate (ethyl *p*-aminobenzoate) JAN *topical anesthetic; nonprescription diet aid* [also: benzocaine]

ethyl 2-benzimidazolecarbamate [see: lobendazole]

ethyl N-benzylcyclopropanecarbamate [see: encyprate]

ethyl biscoumacetate NF, INN, BAN

ethyl biscumacetate [see: ethyl biscoumacetate]

ethyl carbamate [now: urethane]

ethyl carfluzepate INN

ethyl cartrizoate INN

ethyl chloride USP *topical refrigerant anesthetic*

ethyl dibunate USAN, INN, BAN *antitussive*

ethyl dirazepate INN

ethyl eicosapentaenoate *investigational (orphan) agent for Huntington disease*

ethyl ether [see: ether]

ethyl *p*-fluorophenyl sulfone [see: fluoresone]

ethyl *p*-hydroxybenzoate [see: ethylparaben]

ethyl loflazepate INN

ethyl nitrite NF

ethyl oleate NF *vehicle*

ethyl oxide [see: ether]

ethyl vanillin NF *flavoring agent*

ethylcellulose NF *tablet binder*

ethylchlordiphene [see: etofamide]

ethyldicoumarol [see: ethyl biscoumacetate]

ethylene NF *inhalation general anesthesia* ☒ Atolone

ethylene distearate [see: glycol distearate]

ethylenediamine USP, JAN

ethylenediaminetetraacetate [see: edetate disodium]

ethylenediaminetetraacetic acid (EDTA) [see: edetate disodium]

N,N-ethylenediarsanilic acid [see: difetarsone]

ethylenedinitrilotetraacetate disodium [see: edetate disodium]

ethylenetriaminepentaacetate
(pentetate trisodim) [see: pentetic
acid, sodium salts]

ethylestrenol USAN, INN *anabolic steroid; also abused as a street drug* [also: ethyloestrenol; ethylnandrol]

ethylhexanediol [see: ethohexadiol]

2-ethylhexyl diphenyl phosphate
[see: octicizer]

2-ethylhexyl p-methoxycinnamate
[see: octinoxate]

2-ethylhexyl salicylate [see: octisalate]

ethylhydrocupreine HCl NF

ethylmethylthiambutene INN, BAN

ethylmorphine BAN [also: ethylmorphine HCl]

ethylmorphine HCl NF [also: ethylmorphine]

ethylnandrol JAN *anabolic steroid; also abused as a street drug* [also: ethylestrenol; ethyloestrenol]

ethylnorepinephrine HCl USP *sympathomimetic bronchodilator*

ethyloestradiol BAN *estrogen* [also: ethinyl estradiol]

ethyloestrenol BAN *anabolic steroid; also abused as a street drug* [also: ethylestrenol; ethylnandrol]

ethylpapaverine HCl [see: ethaverine HCl]

ethylparaben NF *antifungal agent*

ethylphenacemide [see: pheneturide]

ethylstibamine [see: stibosamine]

2-ethylthioisonicotinamide [see: ethionamide]

ethynerone USAN, INN *progestin*

ethynodiol BAN *progestin* [also: ethynodiol diacetate; etynodiol]

ethynodiol diacetate USAN, USP *progestin* [also: etynodiol; ethynodiol]

(–)-5-ethynylnicotine [see: altinicline]

5-ethynyluracil [see: eniluracil]

Ethyol powder for IV infusion ℞ *chemoprotective agent for cisplatin and paclitaxel chemotherapy (orphan); treatment for moderate to severe xerostomia following postoperative radiation therapy (orphan); investigational (orphan) for cyclophosphamide-induced granulocytopenia* [amifostine] 500 mg/vial

ethypicone INN

ethypropymal sodium [see: probarbital sodium]

etibendazole USAN, INN *anthelmintic*

eticlopride INN

eticyclidine INN

etidocaine USAN, INN, BAN *injectable local anesthetic*

etidocaine HCl *injectable local anesthetic*

etidronate disodium USAN, USP *bisphosphonate bone resorption inhibitor for Paget disease, heterotopic ossification, and hypercalcemia of malignancy (orphan); also used for corticosteroid-induced osteoporosis; investigational (orphan) for metabolic bone disease* 200, 400 mg oral

etidronate monosodium

etidronate sodium (*this term is used only when the form of sodium cannot be more accurately identified*)

etidronate tetrasodium

etidronate trisodium

etidronic acid USAN, INN, BAN *calcium regulator*

etifelmine INN

etifenin USAN, INN, BAN *diagnostic aid*
 🔊 etafenone

etifoxin BAN [also: etifoxine]

etifoxine INN [also: etifoxin]

etilamfetamine INN

etilefrine INN

etilefrine pivalate INN

etintidine INN *antagonist to histamine H_2 receptors* [also: etintidine HCl]

etintidine HCl USAN *antagonist to histamine H_2 receptors* [also: etintidine]

etiocholanedione *investigational (orphan) for aplastic anemia and Prader-Willi syndrome*

etipirium iodide INN

etiproston INN

etiracetam INN

etiroxate INN

etisazole INN, BAN

etisomicin INN, BAN

etisulergine INN

etizolam INN

etobedolum [see: etonitazene]

etocarlide INN

etocrilene INN *ultraviolet screen* [also: etocrylene]

etocrylene USAN *ultraviolet screen* [also: etocrilene]

etodolac USAN, INN, BAN *analgesic; nonsteroidal anti-inflammatory drug (NSAID) for osteoarthritis, rheumatoid arthritis, juvenile rheumatoid arthritis, and other chronic pain* [also: etodolic acid] 200, 300, 400, 500, 600 mg oral

R-etodolac *investigational (orphan) treatment for chronic lymphocytic leukemia*

etodolic acid INN *analgesic; antiarthritic; nonsteroidal anti-inflammatory drug (NSAID)* [also: etodolac]

etodroxizine INN

etofamide INN

etofenamate USAN, INN, BAN *analgesic; anti-inflammatory*

etofenprox INN

etofibrate INN

etoformin INN *antidiabetic* [also: etoformin HCl]

etoformin HCl USAN *antidiabetic* [also: etoformin]

etofuradine INN ⊘ atevirdine

etofylline INN

etofylline clofibrate INN *antihyperlipoproteinemic* [also: theofibrate]

etoglucid INN [also: ethoglucid]

EtOH; ETOH (ethyl alcohol) [now: alcohol]

etolorex INN

etolotifen INN

etoloxamine INN

etomidate USAN, INN, BAN *rapid-acting nonbarbiturate general anesthetic; hypnotic* 2 mg/mL injection

etomidoline INN

etomoxir INN

etonam INN *antifungal* [also: ethonam nitrate]

etonam nitrate [see: ethonam nitrate]

etonitazene INN, BAN

etonogestrel USAN, INN *progestin for vaginal (1 month) and parenteral (3 years) contraception*

etoperidone INN *antidepressant* [also: etoperidone HCl]

etoperidone HCl USAN *antidepressant* [also: etoperidone]

etophylate [see: acepifylline]

Etopophos powder for IV injection ℞ *antineoplastic for testicular and small cell lung cancers (SCLC)* [etoposide phosphate diethanolate] 119.3 mg/vial

etoposide USAN, INN, BAN *antineoplastic* 50 mg oral; 20, 30 mg/mL injection

etoposide & paclitaxel & carboplatin *chemotherapy protocol for primary adenocarcinoma and small cell lung cancer (SCLC)*

etoposide phosphate USAN *antineoplastic*

etoprindole INN

etoprine USAN *antineoplastic*

etoricoxib USAN *antiarthritic; antipyretic; COX-2 inhibitor; nonsteroidal anti-inflammatory drug (NSAID); investigational (NDA filed) for osteoarthritis, rheumatoid arthritis, musculoskeletal pain, and gout*

etorphine INN, BAN ⊘ Etrafon; Otrivin

etosalamide INN [also: ethosalamide]

etoxadrol INN *anesthetic* [also: etoxadrol HCl]

etoxadrol HCl USAN *anesthetic* [also: etoxadrol]

etoxazene INN *analgesic* [also: ethoxazene HCl]

etoxazene HCl [see: ethoxazene HCl]

etoxeridine INN, BAN

etozolin USAN, INN *diuretic* ⊘ etasuline

etrabamine INN

Etrafon; Etrafon 2–10; Etrafon-A; Etrafon-Forte tablets ℞ *conventional (typical) phenothiazine antipsychotic for schizophrenia and psychotic disorders; antidepressant* [perphenazine; amitriptyline HCl] 2•25 mg; 2•10 mg; 4•10 mg; 4•25 mg ⊘ etorphine; Otrivin

etravirine *non-nucleoside reverse transcriptase inhibitor (NNRTI) for drug-resistant HIV-1 infections*

etretin [see: acitretin]

etretinate USAN, INN, BAN, JAN *systemic antipsoriatic; retinoic acid analogue*

etryptamine INN, BAN *CNS stimulant* [also: etryptamine acetate]

etryptamine acetate USAN *CNS stimulant* [also: etryptamine]

etybenzatropine INN *anticholinergic* [also: ethybenztropine]

etymemazine INN

etymemazine HCl [see: etymemazine]

etynodiol INN *progestin* [also: ethynodiol diacetate; ethynodiol]

etyprenaline [see: isoetharine]

eucaine HCl NF

Eucalyptamint ointment, gel OTC *mild anesthetic; antipruritic; counterirritant; antiseptic* [menthol; eucalyptus oil] 16%• ⨪; 8%• ⨪

eucalyptol USAN *antiseptic/germicide*

eucalyptus (Eucalyptus globulus) oil *medicinal herb for bronchitis, lung disorders, neuralgia, and skin sores; source of bioflavonoids*

eucalyptus oil NF *topical antiseptic*

eucatropine INN, BAN *ophthalmic anticholinergic* [also: eucatropine HCl]

eucatropine HCl USP *ophthalmic anticholinergic* [also: eucatropine]

Eucerin cream, lotion OTC *moisturizer; emollient*

Eucerin OTC *cream base*

Eucerin Itch-Relief Moisturizing spray OTC *mild anesthetic; antipruritic; counterirritant* [menthol] 0.15%

Eucerin Plus lotion OTC *moisturizer; emollient* [sodium lactate; urea] 5%• 5%

eucodal [see: oxycodone]

euflavine [see: acriflavine]

Euflexxa intra-articular injection in prefilled syringes ℞ *viscoelastic lubricant and "shock absorber" for osteoarthritis and temporomandibular joint syndrome* [hyaluronate sodium] 20 mg/2 mL syringe ② Avelox; I-Valex

Eugenia caryophyllata *medicinal herb* [see: cloves]

Eugenia pimenta *medicinal herb* [see: allspice]

eugenol USP *dental analgesic* ② Aquanil; Equanil

eukadol [see: oxycodone]

Eulexin capsules ℞ *antiandrogen antineoplastic adjunct to metastatic prostate cancer* [flutamide] 125 mg

Euonymus atropurpureus *medicinal herb* [see: wahoo]

Eupatorium cannabinum *medicinal herb* [see: hemp agrimony]

Eupatorium perfoliatum *medicinal herb* [see: boneset]

Eupatorium purpureum *medicinal herb* [see: queen of the meadow]

Euphorbia poinsettia; E. pulcherrima *medicinal herb* [see: poinsettia]

euphoretics; euphoriants; euphoragens *a class of agents that produce euphoria*

Euphrasia officinalis; E. rostkoviana; E. strica *medicinal herb* [see: eyebright]

euprocin INN *topical anesthetic* [also: euprocin HCl] ② eperisone

euprocin HCl USAN *topical anesthetic* [also: euprocin]

euquinine [see: quinine ethylcarbonate]

Eurax cream, lotion ℞ *scabicide; antipruritic* [crotamiton] 10% ② Urex

European alder; European black alder; European buckthorn *medicinal herb* [see: buckthorn]

European aspen *medicinal herb* [see: black poplar]

europium *element (Eu)* ② erbium

EVA (etoposide, vinblastine, Adriamycin) *chemotherapy protocol for Hodgkin lymphoma*

Evac-Q-Mag carbonated oral solution OTC *saline laxative* [magnesium citrate; citric acid; potassium citrate]

Evac-Q-Tabs tablets OTC *stimulant laxative* [bisacodyl] 5 mg

Evac-U-Gen chewable tablets OTC *stimulant laxative* [sennosides] 10 mg

EvaMist metered-dose transdermal spray ℞ *hormone replacement for postmenopausal vasomotor symptoms* [estradiol] 1.53 mg/spray

evandamine INN

Evans blue USP *diagnostic aid for blood volume* [also: azovan blue] 5 mL injection

evening primrose *(Oenothera biennis)* bark, leaves, oil *medicinal herb for cardiovascular health, hypertension, mastalgia, multiple sclerosis, nerves, obesity, premenstrual syndrome, prostate disorders, rheumatoid arthritis, and skin disorders*

everlasting *(Anaphalis margaritacea; Gnaphalium polycephalum; G. uliginosum)* plant *medicinal herb used as an astringent, diaphoretic, febrifuge, pectoral, vermifuge, and vulnerary*

evernimicin USAN *antibiotic*

everolimus *investigational (NDA filed) once-daily oral antineoplastic for kidney and neuroendocrine cancer*

Evista film-coated tablets ℞ *selective estrogen receptor modulator (SERM) for the prevention and treatment of postmenopausal osteoporosis; hormone antagonist for breast cancer (orphan)* [raloxifene HCl] 60 mg ⍰ Eovist

E-Vitamin ointment OTC *emollient* [vitamin E] 30 mg/g ⍰ iofetamine

Evithrom topical solution *hemostatic to minimize blood loss during surgery* [thrombin, human] 800–1200 IU/mL

E-VMAC (escalated methotrexate, vinblastine, Adriamycin, cis-platin) *chemotherapy protocol*

E-VMAC (escalated methotrexate, vinblastine, Adriamycin, cyclophosphamide) *chemotherapy protocol*

Evoclin topical foam ℞ *antibiotic for acne; also used for rosacea* [clindamycin phosphate] 1% ⍰ ivoqualine

Evolence subcu injection in prefilled syringes ℞ *dermal filler for moderate to deep facial wrinkles and folds* [collagen, purified porcine] 3.5%

Evoxac capsules ℞ *cholinergic and muscarinic receptor agonist for treatment of dry mouth due to Sjögren syndrome* [cevimeline HCl] 30 mg

Evra [see: Ortho Evra]

Exact vanishing cream OTC *keratolytic for acne* [benzoyl peroxide] 5%

exalamide INN

exametazime USAN, INN, BAN *regional cerebral perfusion imaging aid*

Exanta Ⓔ tablets (available in 14 European countries; U.S trials discontinued 2006 due to safety concerns) *investigational (NDA filed) oral anticoagulant and direct thrombin inhibitor for the prevention of stroke due to atrial fibrillation and the prevention and treatment of a venous thromboembolic event (VTE)* [ximelagatran]

exaprolol INN *antiadrenergic (β-receptor)* [also: exaprolol HCl]

exaprolol HCl USAN *antiadrenergic (β-receptor)* [also: exaprolol]

exatecan mesylate USAN *antineoplastic; topoisomerase I inhibitor for skin cancer*

Excedrin Aspirin Free caplets, geltabs OTC *analgesic; antipyretic; anti-inflammatory* [acetaminophen; caffeine] 500•65 mg

Excedrin Back & Body caplets OTC *analgesic; antipyretic; anti-inflammatory* [acetaminophen; buffered aspirin] 250•250 mg

Excedrin Extra Strength caplets, tablets, geltabs OTC *analgesic; antipyretic; anti-inflammatory* [acetaminophen; aspirin; caffeine] 250•250•65 mg ⍰ oxidronic acid

Excedrin Migraine tablets OTC *analgesic for relief of migraine headache syndrome, including prodrome, pain, and associated symptoms* [acetaminophen; aspirin; caffeine] 250•250•65 mg

Excedrin P.M. oral liquid, liquigels OTC *antihistamine; sleep aid; analgesic; antipyretic* [diphenhydramine HCl; acetaminophen] 50•1000 mg/30 mL; 25•500 mg

Excedrin P.M. tablets, caplets, geltabs OTC *antihistamine; sleep aid; analgesic; antipyretic* [diphenhydramine citrate; acetaminophen] 38•500 mg

Excedrin QuickTabs (orally dissolving tablets) (discontinued 2008) OTC *analgesic; antipyretic; anti-inflammatory* [acetaminophen; caffeine] 500•65 mg

Excedrin Sinus Headache film-coated tablets OTC *decongestant; analgesic; antipyretic* [phenylephrine HCl; acetaminophen] 5•325 mg

Excedrin Tension Headache caplets, geltabs OTC *analgesic; antipyretic; anti-inflammatory* [acetaminophen; caffeine] 500•65 mg

Excita Extra premedicated condom OTC *spermicidal/barrier contraceptive* [nonoxynol 9] 8%

ExeCof extended-release tablets ℞ *antitussive; decongestant; expectorant* [dextromethorphan hydrobromide; phenylephrine HCl; guaifenesin] 60•40•1000 mg

ExeFen-PD extended-release caplets ℞ *decongestant; expectorant* [phenylephrine HCl; guaifenesin] 10•600 mg

Exelderm solution ℞ *antifungal* [sulconazole nitrate] 1%

Exelon capsules, oral solution ℞ *acetylcholinesterase inhibitor to increase cognition in Alzheimer and Parkinson disease* [rivastigmine tartrate] 1.5, 3, 4.5, 6 mg; 2 mg/mL ☒ ioxilan

Exelon Patch ℞ *acetylcholinesterase inhibitor to increase cognition in Alzheimer and Parkinson disease* [rivastigmine] 4.6, 9.5 mg/day

exemestane INN *aromatase inhibitor; antihormonal antineoplastic for advanced breast cancer in postmenopausal women (orphan)*

exenatide *synthetic exendin-4 analogue; incretin mimetic antidiabetic for type 2 diabetes that improves the body's normal glucose-sensing mechanisms and slows gastric emptying; synthetic analogue of Gila monster saliva*

exepanol INN

ExeTuss; ExeTuss GP extended-release caplets ℞ *decongestant; expectorant* [phenylephrine HCl; guaifenesin] 25•900 mg; 25•1200 mg

Exforge film-coated tablets ℞ *combination calcium channel blocker and angiotensin II receptor antagonist for hypertension* [amlodipine besylate; valsartan] 5•160, 5•320, 10•160, 10•320 mg

Ex-Histine syrup (discontinued 2007) ℞ *decongestant; antihistamine; anticholinergic to dry mucosal secretions*

[phenylephrine HCl; chlorpheniramine maleate; methscopolamine bromide] 20•4•2.5 mg/10 mL

Exidine Skin Cleanser; Exidine-2 Scrub; Exidine-4 Scrub topical liquid OTC *broad-spectrum antimicrobial; germicidal* [chlorhexidine gluconate; alcohol 4%] 4%; 2%; 4%

exifone INN

exiproben INN

exisulind *investigational (NDA filed, orphan) antineoplastic for familial adenomatous polyposis (FAP; also known as adenomatous polyposis coli, or APC); investigational (Phase III) for lung cancer*

Exjade tablets ℞ *once-daily iron chelating agent for chronic iron overload due to blood transfusions (orphan)* [deferasirox] 125, 250, 500 mg

Ex-Lax tablets, chocolated chewable tablets OTC *stimulant laxative* [sennosides] 15 mg

Ex-Lax Gentle Strength caplets OTC *stimulant laxative; stool softener* [sennosides; docusate sodium] 10•65 mg

Ex-Lax Maximum Relief tablets OTC *stimulant laxative* [sennosides] 25 mg

Ex-Lax Stool Softener caplets OTC *laxative; stool softener* [docusate sodium] 100 mg

Ex-Lax Ultra enteric-coated tablets OTC *stimulant laxative* [bisacodyl] 5 mg

Exocaine Medicated Rub; Exocaine Plus Rub OTC *analgesic; counterirritant* [methyl salicylate] 25%; 30%

Exosurf *investigational (orphan) pulmonary surfactant for adult respiratory distress syndrome (ARDS)* [colfosceril palmitate]

Exosurf Neonatal intratracheal suspension ℞ *pulmonary surfactant for hyaline membrane disease and respiratory distress syndrome (orphan)* [colfosceril palmitate] 108 mg

expectorants *a class of drugs that promote the ejection of mucus from the respiratory tract*

Expidet (trademarked dosage form) *fast-dissolving dose*

Exratuss oral suspension (discontinued 2007) ℞ *antitussive; antihistamine; decongestant* [carbetapentane tannate; chlorpheniramine tannate; phenylephrine tannate] 30•4•12.5 mg

Exsel lotion/shampoo (discontinued 2004) ℞ *antiseborrheic; dandruff treatment* [selenium sulfide] 2.5% ▣ Oxizole; Oxycel

exsiccated sodium arsenate [see: sodium arsenate, exsiccated]

Extavia ⓔᵁᴿ (European name for U.S. product **Betaseron**)

Extencap (trademarked dosage form) *extended-release capsule*

extended insulin zinc [see: insulin zinc, extended]

Extendryl chewable tablets ℞ *decongestant; antihistamine; anticholinergic to dry mucosal secretions* [phenylephrine HCl; chlorpheniramine maleate; methscopolamine nitrate] 10•2•1.25 mg

Extendryl syrup ℞ *decongestant; antihistamine; anticholinergic to dry mucosal secretions* [phenylephrine HCl; dexchlorpheniramine maleate; methscopolamine nitrate] 10•1•1.25 mg/5 mL

Extendryl DM extended-release tablets ℞ *antitussive; antihistamine; anticholinergic to dry mucosal secretions* [dextromethorphan hydrobromide; chlorpheniramine maleate; methscopolamine nitrate] 30•8•2.5 mg

Extendryl G extended-release tablets ℞ *decongestant; expectorant* [phenylephrine HCl; guaifenesin] 30•1000 mg

Extendryl GCP oral solution ℞ *antitussive; decongestant; expectorant* [carbetapentane citrate; phenylephrine HCl; guaifenesin] 15•5•100 mg/5 mL

Extendryl JR sustained-release pediatric capsules (discontinued 2007) ℞ *decongestant; antihistamine; anticholinergic to dry mucosal secretions* [phenylephrine HCl; chlorpheniramine maleate; methscopolamine nitrate] 10•4•1.25 mg

Extendryl PEM extended-release tablets ℞ *decongestant; anticholinergic to dry mucosal secretions* [phenylephrine HCl; methscopolamine nitrate] 30•1.25 mg

Extendryl SR sustained-release capsules (discontinued 2007) ℞ *decongestant; antihistamine; anticholinergic to dry mucosal secretions* [phenylephrine HCl; chlorpheniramine maleate; methscopolamine nitrate] 20•8•2.5 mg

Extentab (trademarked dosage form) *extended-release tablet*

Extina topical foam ℞ *antifungal for seborrheic dermatitis* [ketoconazole] 2%

Extra Action Cough syrup (discontinued 2007) OTC *antitussive; expectorant* [dextromethorphan hydrobromide; guaifenesin] 20•200 mg/10 mL

"Extra Strength" products [see under product name]

Extra Strength Pain Reliever PM caplets OTC *antihistaminic sleep aid; analgesic; antipyretic* [diphenhydramine HCl; acetaminophen] 25•500 mg

Extraneal IV infusion (supplied in Ultrabag and Ambu-Flex) ℞ *peritoneal dialysis solution for end-stage renal disease (orphan)* [icodextrin] 75 g

Extratuss oral suspension (discontinued 2007) ℞ *antitussive; antihistamine; decongestant* [carbetapentane tannate; brompheniramine tannate; phenylephrine tannate] 30•4•12.5 mg/5 mL

Exubera powder for oral inhalation in unit dose blisters, for use with an **Exubera Release Unit** (inhalation device) (discontinued 2007) ℞ *antidiabetic; each milligram of inhaled powder is approximately equivalent to 3 units of injected insulin* [insulin, human (rDNA)] 1, 3 mg/blister ▣ AK-Spore

Exubera Release Unit (trademarked delivery device) (discontinued 2007) *inhalation powder dispenser for use with* **Exubera**

eye balm; eye root *medicinal herb*
[see: goldenseal]

Eye Drops OTC *decongestant; vasocon-strictor* [tetrahydrozoline HCl] 0.05%

Eye Irrigating Solution OTC *extraocular irrigating solution* [sterile isotonic solution]

Eye Irrigating Wash (discontinued 2006) OTC *extraocular irrigating solution* [sterile isotonic solution]

Eye Scrub solution OTC *eyelid cleanser for blepharitis or contact lenses*

Eye Stream ophthalmic solution OTC *extraocular irrigating solution* [sterile isotonic solution]

Eye Wash ophthalmic solution OTC *extraocular irrigating solution* [sterile isotonic solution]

eyebright (*Euphrasia officinalis; E. rostkoviana; E. strica*) *plant medicinal herb for blood cleansing, cataracts, colds, conjunctivitis, eye disorders and infections, and stimulating liver function;* *not generally regarded as safe and effective for topical ophthalmic use* 🅐 Iberet

Eye-Lube-A eye drops OTC *moisturizer/lubricant* [glycerin] 0.25% 🅐 Albay

EZ Detect test kit for home use OTC *in vitro diagnostic aid for fecal occult blood*

ezetimibe USAN *antihyperlipidemic for primary hypercholesterolemia and mixed hyperlipidemia; intestinal cholesterol absorption inhibitor*

Ezetrol 🄲🄴 caplets (foreign name for U.S. product **Zetia**) 🅐 Estra-L

EZFE 200 capsules OTC *hematinic; iron supplement* [iron] 200 mg 🅐 Isovue

Ezide tablets ℞ *antihypertensive; diuretic* [hydrochlorothiazide] 50 mg

ezlopitant USAN *substance P receptor antagonist for emesis, pain, and inflammation*

E-Z-Paque oral suspension ℞ *radiopaque contrast agent* [barium sulfate] 6.2, 10, 12 oz.

F

1+1-F Creme ℞ *corticosteroidal anti-inflammatory; antifungal; antibacterial; anesthetic* [hydrocortisone; clioquinol; pramoxine] 1%•3%•1%

¹⁸F [see: fludeoxyglucose F 18]

¹⁸F [see: sodium fluoride F 18]

Fab (fragment, antigen-binding) [def.] *one side of an immunoglobulin that contains an antigen binding site*

FAB (French-American-British) [def.] *a classification system for acute leukemia*

Fablyn *second-generation selective estrogen receptor modulator (SERM); investigational (NDA filed) for osteoporosis and the reduction of LDL cholesterol; investigational (Phase III) for breast cancer* [lasofoxifene tartrate]

FABRase *investigational (orphan) enzyme replacement therapy for Fabry disease* [agalsidase alfa]

Fabrazyme powder for IV infusion ℞ *enzyme replacement therapy for Fabry disease (orphan)* [agalsidase beta] 5.5, 37 mg/dose

FAC (fluorouracil, Adriamycin, cyclophosphamide) *chemotherapy protocol for breast cancer*

FAC-LEV (fluorouracil, Adriamycin, Cytoxin, levamisole) *chemotherapy protocol*

FAC-M (fluorouracil, Adriamycin, cyclophosphamide, methotrexate) *chemotherapy protocol* 🅐 Vicam

Fact Plus test kit for home use OTC *in vitro diagnostic aid; urine pregnancy test*

Factive film-coated tablets ℞ *broad-spectrum fluoroquinolone antibiotic for respiratory tract infections* [gemifloxacin mesylate] 320 mg 🅐 Viactiv

factor II (prothrombin)

factor III [see: thromboplastin]

factor VIIa, recombinant *coagulant for hemophilia A and B (orphan); investigational (orphan) for Glanzmann thrombasthenia*

factor VIII [see: antihemophilic factor]

factor VIII (rDNA) BAN *blood coagulating factor*

factor VIII fraction BAN *blood coagulating factor*

factor IX complex USP *systemic hemostatic; antihemophilic for factor IX deficiency (hemophilia B; Christmas disease) (orphan)* [also: factor IX fraction; nonacog alfa]

factor IX fraction BAN *systemic hemostatic; antihemophilic* [also: factor IX complex; nonacog alfa]

factor XIII, human plasma–derived *investigational (orphan) hemostatic for congenital factor XIII deficiency*

factor XIII [A2] homodimer, recombinant *investigational (orphan) hemostatic for congenital factor XIII deficiency*

Factrel *powder for subcu or IV injection* ℞ *gonadotropin releasing hormone; diagnostic aid for anterior pituitary function* [gonadorelin HCl] 100, 500 mcg

fadrozole INN *antineoplastic; aromatase inhibitor* [also: fadrozole HCl]

fadrozole HCl USAN *antineoplastic; aromatase inhibitor* [also: fadrozole]

falintolol INN

falipamil INN

Falkochol *investigational (orphan) agent for congenital errors of cholesterol and bile acid synthesis* [dehydrocholic acid]

false foxglove *medicinal herb* [see: feverweed]

false unicorn (Chamaelirium luteum) *root medicinal herb used for amenorrhea, morning sickness, and preventing miscarriages; also used for colic, cough, and digestive, kidney, and prostate problems; emetic in high doses*

false valerian *medicinal herb* [see: life root]

false vervain *medicinal herb* [see: blue vervain]

FAM (fluorouracil, Adriamycin, mitomycin) *chemotherapy protocol for adenocarcinoma and gastric cancer*

FAM-CF (fluorouracil, Adriamycin, mitomycin, citrovorum factor) *chemotherapy protocol*

famciclovir USAN, INN, BAN *oral antiviral for herpes labialis (cold sores), herpes simplex type 2 (genital herpes), and herpes zoster (shingles) infections; suppressive therapy for recurrent outbreaks* 125, 250, 500 mg oral

FAME; FAMe (fluorouracil, Adriamycin, MeCCNU) *chemotherapy protocol*

famiraprinium chloride INN

FAMMe (fluorouracil, Adriamycin, mitomycin, MeCCNU) *chemotherapy protocol*

famotidine USAN, USP, INN, BAN *histamine H_2 antagonist for gastric and duodenal ulcers, gastroesophageal reflux disease (GERD), and gastric hypersecretory conditions* 10, 20, 40 mg oral; 10 mg/mL injection; 20 mg/50 mL infusion

famotine INN *antiviral* [also: famotine HCl]

famotine HCl USAN *antiviral* [also: famotine]

fampridine USAN, INN *investigational (Phase III, orphan) agent for multiple sclerosis and spinal cord injury*

famprofazone INN, BAN

FAM-S (fluorouracil, Adriamycin, mitomycin, streptozocin) *chemotherapy protocol* ② FMS

FAMTX (fluorouracil, Adriamycin, methotrexate [with leucovorin rescue]) *chemotherapy protocol for gastric cancer*

Famvir *film-coated tablets* ℞ *antiviral for herpes labialis (cold sores), herpes simplex type 2 (HSV-2, genital herpes) and herpes zoster (shingles) infections; suppressive therapy for recurrent outbreaks* [famciclovir] 125, 250, 500, 1000 mg

fananserin USAN *antipsychotic; anti-schizophrenic; dopamine D*$_2$ *and serotonin 5-HT*$_2$ *receptor antagonist*

fanetizole INN, BAN *immunoregulator* [also: fanetizole mesylate]

fanetizole mesylate USAN *immunoregulator* [also: fanetizole]

Fansidar tablets ℞ *antimalarial* [sulfadoxine; pyrimethamine] 500•25 mg

fanthridone BAN *antidepressant* [also: fantridone HCl; fantridone]

fantridone INN *antidepressant* [also: fantridone HCl; fanthridone]

fantridone HCl USAN *antidepressant* [also: fantridone; fanthridone]

FAP (fluorouracil, Adriamycin, Platinol) *chemotherapy protocol for gastric cancer*

Farbee with Vitamin C caplets OTC *vitamin supplement* [multiple B vitamins; vitamin C] ±•300 mg

Fareston tablets ℞ *antiestrogen antineoplastic for metastatic breast cancer in postmenopausal women (orphan); investigational (orphan) for desmoid tumors* [toremifene citrate] 60 mg

farglitazar USAN *thiazolidinedione (TZD) antidiabetic that increases cellular response to insulin without increasing insulin secretion*

farnesil INN *combining name for radicals or groups* 🔲 Fer-In-Sol

faropenem [see: fropenem]

fasiplon INN

Faslodex prefilled syringe for IM injection ℞ *once monthly antiestrogen antineoplastic for metastatic breast cancer in postmenopausal women* [fulvestrant] 50 mg/mL

Faspak (trademarked packaging form) *flexible plastic bag* 🔲 Visipak

Fastic (Japanese name for U.S. product **Starlix**) 🔲 Vasotec

Fast-Trak (trademarked delivery device) *quick-loading syringe*

fat, hard NF *suppository base*

fat emulsion, intravenous *parenteral essential fatty acid replacement*

Father John's Medicine Plus oral liquid (discontinued 2007) OTC *anti-*

tussive; antihistamine; decongestant [dextromethorphan hydrobromide; chlorpheniramine maleate; phenylephrine HCl] 10•4•10 mg/30 mL

Fatsia horrida *medicinal herb* [see: devil's club]

FazaClo orally disintegrating tablets ℞ *novel (atypical) dibenzapine antipsychotic for severe schizophrenia and recurrent suicidal behavior; sedative; also used for agitation and psychosis due to Alzheimer disease* [clozapine] 12.5, 25, 50, 100 mg 🔲 Visicol

fazadinium bromide INN, BAN

fazarabine USAN, INN *antineoplastic*

5-FC (5-fluorocytosine) [see: flucytosine]

FCAP (fluorouracil, cyclophosphamide, Adriamycin, Platinol) *chemotherapy protocol* 🔲 FCP; VACP; VCAP; VCP; VOCAP

FCE (fluorouracil, cisplatin, etoposide) *chemotherapy protocol*

F-CL (fluorouracil, leucovorin calcium [rescue]) *chemotherapy protocol for colorectal cancer* [also: FU/LV]

FCP (fluorouracil, cyclophosphamide, prednisone) *chemotherapy protocol*

FD&C Red No. 2 (Food, Drug & Cosmetic [Act]) [see: amaranth]

FD&C Red No. 3 (Food, Drug & Cosmetic [Act]) [see: erythrosine sodium]

F-ddA (fluorodideoxyadenosine) [see: lodenosine]

FDDNP ([^{18}F] fluoroethyl [methyl] amino-2-naphthyl ethylidene malononitrile) *PET scan contrast medium for detection of β-amyloid senile plaques and neurofibrillary tangles for early detection of Alzheimer disease*

^{18}FDG (fludeoxyglucose) [see: fludeoxyglucose F 18]

FDh (2(3H) furanone di-hydro) *a precursor to gamma hydroxybutyrate (GHB); a formerly legal alternative to GHB, now also illegal (Schedule I); also known as gamma butyrolactone (GBL)* [see: gamma hydroxybutyrate (GHB)]

FDP (fructose-1,6-diphosphate) [q.v.]

FE Aspartate tablets OTC *hematinic; iron supplement* [ferrous aspartate] 112 mg (18 mg Fe)

Fe⁵⁰ (or Fe50) extended-release caplets (discontinued 2005) OTC *hematinic; iron supplement* [ferrous sulfate, dried (source of iron)] 160 mg (50 mg)

⁵⁹Fe [see: ferric chloride Fe 59]

⁵⁹Fe [see: ferric citrate (⁵⁹Fe)]

⁵⁹Fe [see: ferrous citrate Fe 59]

⁵⁹Fe [see: ferrous sulfate Fe 59]

febantel USAN, INN, BAN *veterinary anthelmintic*

febarbamate INN

febricides *a class of agents that relieve or reduce fever* [also called: antifebriles; antipyretics; antithermics; febrifuges]

febrifuges *a class of agents that relieve or reduce fever* [also called: antifebriles; antipyretics; antithermics; febricides]

febuprol INN

febuverine INN

febuxostat *investigational (NDA filed) selective xanthine oxidase inhibitor for gout*

FEC (fluorouracil, epirubicin, cyclophosphamide) *chemotherapy protocol for breast cancer*

feclemine INN

feclobuzone INN

FED (fluorouracil, etoposide, DDP) *chemotherapy protocol for non–small cell lung cancer (NSCLC)*

fedotozine INN *kappa selective opioid agonist for irritable bowel syndrome*

fedrilate INN

Feen-A-Mint enteric-coated tablets OTC *stimulant laxative* [bisacodyl] 5 mg

Feiba VH Immuno IV injection or drip ℞ *antihemophilic to correct factor VIII deficiency and coagulation deficiency* [anti-inhibitor coagulant complex, vapor heated and freeze-dried] (each bottle is labeled with dosage)

felbamate USAN, INN *anticonvulsant; adjunctive therapy for Lennox-Gastaut syndrome (orphan)*

Felbatol tablets, oral suspension (the FDA and the manufacturer strongly caution against its use due to adverse side effects) ℞ *anticonvulsant; adjunctive therapy for Lennox-Gastaut syndrome (orphan)* [felbamate] 400, 600 mg; 600 mg/5 mL

felbinac USAN, INN, BAN *anti-inflammatory*

Feldene capsules ℞ *analgesic; nonsteroidal anti-inflammatory drug (NSAID) for osteoarthritis and rheumatoid arthritis* [piroxicam] 10, 20 mg

felipyrine INN

felodipine USAN, INN, BAN *vasodilator; antihypertensive; calcium channel blocker* 2.5, 5, 10 mg oral

felonwood; felonwort *medicinal herb* [see: bittersweet nightshade]

felvizumab USAN *monoclonal antibody for prophylaxis and treatment of respiratory syncytial virus (RSV)*

felypressin USAN, INN, BAN *vasoconstrictor* ⃞ fluprazine

Fem pH vaginal jelly OTC *acidity modifier; antiseptic* [acetic acid, glacial; oxyquinoline sulfate] 0.9%•0.025% ⃞ FMV

Fem-1 tablets OTC *analgesic; antipyretic; diuretic* [acetaminophen; pamabrom] 500•25 mg

female fern (Polypodium vulgare) root *medicinal herb used as an anthelmintic, cholagogue, demulcent, and purgative*

female regulator *medicinal herb* [see: life root]

Femara film-coated tablets ℞ *aromatase inhibitor; estrogen antagonist; antineoplastic for early, advanced, or metastatic breast cancer in postmenopausal women* [letrozole] 2.5 mg

FemBack caplets OTC *analgesic; antipyretic; antihistamine; sleep aid* [acetaminophen; salicylamide; phenyltoloxamine citrate] 150•150•44 mg

Femcon Fe chewable tablets (in packs of 28) ℞ *monophasic oral contraceptive; iron supplement* [norethindrone; ethinyl estradiol; ferrous fumarate]

0.4 mg•35 mcg•75 mg × 21 days; 0•0•75 mg × 7 days

femhrt 1/5 tablets (in packs of 28) ℞ *a mixture of synthetic and equine hormones; hormone replacement therapy for postmenopausal symptoms* [norethindrone acetate; ethinyl estradiol] 1 mg•5 mcg

femhrtLo tablets (in packs of 28) ℞ *a mixture of synthetic and equine hormones; hormone replacement therapy for postmenopausal symptoms* [norethindrone acetate; ethinyl estradiol] 0.5 mg•2.5 mcg

Feminique Disposable Douche vaginal solution OTC *acidity modifier; cleanser and deodorizer* [vinegar (acetic acid)]

Femiron tablets (discontinued 2005) OTC *hematinic; iron supplement* [ferrous fumarate (source of iron)] 63 mg (20 mg)

Femiron Multi-Vitamins and Iron tablets (discontinued 2005) OTC *vitamin/iron supplement* [multiple vitamins; ferrous fumarate; folic acid] ± •20•0.4 mg

Femizol-M vaginal cream OTC *antifungal* [miconazole nitrate] 2%

femoxetine INN

Femring vaginal ring ℞ *synthetic estrogen; three-month hormone replacement for postmenopausal atrophic vaginitis* [estradiol acetate] 12.4 mg (50 mcg/day), 24.8 mg (100 mcg day)

FemSoft urethral insert *treatment for stress urinary incontinence* [silicone plug]

Femstat 3 vaginal cream in prefilled applicator (discontinued 2004) OTC *antifungal* [butoconazole nitrate] 2%

Femtrace tablets ℞ *synthetic estrogen; hormone replacement for postmenopausal symptoms* [estradiol acetate] 0.45, 0.9, 1.8 mg

Fem-V kit for home use OTC *in vitro diagnostic aid for vaginal infections* ☒ FMV

fenabutene INN

fenacetinol INN

fenaclon INN

fenadiazole INN ☒ Vandazole

fenaftic acid INN

fenalamide USAN, INN *smooth muscle relaxant*

fenalcomine INN

fenamifuril INN

fenamisal INN *antibacterial; tuberculostatic* [also: phenyl aminosalicylate]

fenamole USAN, INN *anti-inflammatory* ☒ Venomil

fenaperone INN

fenarsone [see: carbarsone]

fenasprate [see: benorilate]

fenbendazole USAN, INN, BAN *anthelmintic*

fenbenicillin INN [also: phenbenicillin]

fenbufen USAN, INN, BAN *anti-inflammatory*

fenbutrazate INN [also: phenbutrazate]

fencamfamin INN, BAN

fencamfamin HCl [see: fencamfamin]

fencarbamide INN *anticholinergic* [also: phencarbamide]

fenchlorphos BAN *systemic insecticide* [also: ronnel; fenclofos]

fencilbutirol USAN, INN *choleretic*

fenclexonium metilsulfate INN

fenclofenac USAN, INN, BAN *anti-inflammatory*

fenclofos INN *systemic insecticide* [also: ronnel; fenchlorphos]

fenclonine USAN, INN *serotonin inhibitor*

fenclorac USAN, INN *anti-inflammatory*

fenclozic acid INN, BAN

fendiline INN

fendizoate INN *combining name for radicals or groups*

fendosal USAN, INN, BAN *anti-inflammatory* ☒ Vandazole

feneritrol INN

Fenesin sustained-release tablets (discontinued 2004) ℞ *expectorant* [guaifenesin] 600 mg ☒ phenazone; Vanocin

Fenesin DM tablets (discontinued 2005) ℞ *antitussive; expectorant* [dextromethorphan hydrobromide; guaifenesin] 30•600 mg

Fenesin DM IR tablets OTC *antitussive; expectorant* [dextromethorphan hydrobromide; guaifenesin] 15•400 mg

fenestrel USAN, INN *estrogen*

fenethazine INN ⚕ *phenothiazine*

fenethylline BAN *CNS stimulant* [also: fenethylline HCl; fenetylline] ⚕ phenythilone; Ventolin

fenethylline HCl USAN *CNS stimulant* [also: fenetylline; fenethylline]

fenetradil INN

fenetylline INN *CNS stimulant* [also: fenethylline HCl; fenethylline] ⚕ Ventolin

fenflumizole INN

fenfluramine INN, BAN *anorexiant; CNS depressant* [also: fenfluramine HCl]

fenfluramine HCl USAN *anorexiant; CNS depressant* [also: fenfluramine]

fenfluthrin INN, BAN

fengabine USAN, INN, BAN *mood regulator*

fenharmane INN ⚕ *pheniramine*

fenimide USAN, INN, BAN *antipsychotic* ⚕ Vanamide

feniodium chloride INN

fenipentol INN

fenirofibrate INN

fenisorex USAN, INN, BAN *anorectic*

fenleuton USAN *5-lipoxygenase inhibitor for asthma*

fenmetozole INN *antidepressant; narcotic antagonist* [also: fenmetozole HCl]

fenmetozole HCl USAN *antidepressant; narcotic antagonist* [also: fenmetozole]

fenmetramide USAN, INN, BAN *antidepressant*

fennel (*Anethum foeniculum; Foeniculum officinale; F. vulgare*) seeds *medicinal herb for colic, gas, intestinal problems, promoting expectoration, stimulating lactation and menses, and sedation in children* ⚕ phenol; vanilla

fennel oil NF

fenobam USAN, INN *sedative*

fenocinol INN

fenoctimine INN *gastric antisecretory* [also: fenoctimine sulfate]

fenoctimine sulfate USAN *gastric antisecretory* [also: fenoctimine]

fenofibrate INN, BAN *PPARα agonist for primary hypercholesterolemia, hypertriglyceridemia, and mixed dyslipidemia; also used for hyperuricemia* 40, 54, 67, 107, 134, 160, 200 mg oral

fenoldopam INN, BAN *dopamine agonist; vasodilator for hypertensive emergencies* [also: fenoldopam mesylate]

fenoldopam mesylate USAN *dopamine agonist; rapid-acting vasodilator for in-hospital management of hypertensive emergencies* [also: fenoldopam] 10 mg/mL injection

fenoprofen USAN, INN, BAN *analgesic; nonsteroidal anti-inflammatory drug (NSAID) for osteoarthritis, rheumatoid arthritis, and other mild to moderate pain; also used for juvenile rheumatoid arthritis, migraine headaches, and sunburn pain*

fenoprofen calcium USAN, USP, BAN *analgesic; nonsteroidal anti-inflammatory drug (NSAID) for osteoarthritis, rheumatoid arthritis, and other mild to moderate pain; also used for juvenile rheumatoid arthritis, migraine headaches, and sunburn pain* 200, 300, 600 mg oral

fenoterol USAN, INN, BAN *bronchodilator; β-blocker* [also: fenoterol hydrobromide] ⚕ Phentrol 2

fenoterol hydrobromide JAN *bronchodilator; antiasthmatic; β-blocker* [also: fenoterol]

fenoverine INN

fenoxazol [see: pemoline]

fenoxazoline INN

fenoxazoline HCl [see: fenoxazoline]

fenoxedil INN

fenoxypropazine INN [also: phenoxypropazine]

fenozolone INN

fenpentadiol INN

fenperate INN

fenpipalone USAN, INN *anti-inflammatory*

fenpipramide INN, BAN

fenpiprane INN, BAN

fenpiprane HCl [see: fenpiprane]

fenpiverinium bromide INN

fenprinast INN *bronchodilator; antiallergic* [also: fenprinast HCl]

fenprinast HCl USAN *bronchodilator; antiallergic* [also: fenprinast]

fenproporex INN

fenprostalene USAN, INN, BAN *luteolysin*

fenquizone USAN, INN *diuretic* ② Vancocin

fenretinide USAN, INN *synthetic retinoid; investigational (Phase III) chemopreventative for bladder, oral, and skin cancers*

fenspiride INN *bronchodilator; antiadrenergic (α-receptor)* [also: fenspiride HCl]

fenspiride HCl USAN *bronchodilator; antiadrenergic (α-receptor)* [also: fenspiride]

fentanyl INN, BAN *narcotic analgesic; also abused as a street drug* [also: fentanyl citrate] 12.5, 25, 50, 75, 100 mcg/hr. transdermal

fentanyl citrate USAN, USP, JAN *narcotic analgesic for breakthrough pain in cancer patients; adjunct to anesthesia; also abused as a street drug* [also: fentanyl] 50 mcg/mL injection; 200, 400, 600, 800, 1200, 1600 mcg oral transmucosal

Fentanyl Citrate Transmucosal lozenge on a stick ℞ *narcotic analgesic for anesthesia premedication* [fentanyl citrate] 200, 400, 600, 800, 1200, 1600 mcg

fentanyl HCl *transdermal narcotic analgesic for short-term management of postoperative pain*

Fentanyl Oralet lozenges (discontinued 2005) ℞ *transmucosal narcotic analgesic for anesthesia premedication* [fentanyl citrate] 100, 200, 300, 400 mcg

fenthion BAN ② phenytoin; Vantin

fentiazac USAN, INN, BAN *anti-inflammatory*

fenticlor USAN, INN, BAN *topical anti-infective*

fenticonazole INN, BAN *antifungal* [also: fenticonazole nitrate]

fenticonazole nitrate USAN *antifungal* [also: fenticonazole]

fentonium bromide INN

Fentora buccal tablets ℞ *transmucosal narcotic analgesic for chronic pain in opioid-tolerant cancer patients* [fentanyl citrate] 100, 200, 400, 600, 800 mcg

fenugreek (Trigonella foenum-graecum) seeds *medicinal herb for boils, bronchial secretions, cellulitis, diabetes, hypercholesterolemia, kidney stones, lung infections, promoting expectoration, stomach irritation, and tuberculosis*

fenyramidol INN *analgesic; skeletal muscle relaxant* [also: phenyramidol HCl]

fenyripol INN *skeletal muscle relaxant* [also: fenyripol HCl]

fenyripol HCl USAN *skeletal muscle relaxant* [also: fenyripol]

Feocyte prolonged-action tablets ℞ *hematinic* [iron (as ferrous fumarate, ferrous gluconate, and ferrous sulfate); desiccated liver; vitamins B_6, B_{12}, and C; folic acid] 110•15•2•0.05•100•0.8 mg

FeoGen capsules ℞ *hematinic* [ferrous fumarate; cyanocobalamin; ascorbic acid; intrinsic factor concentrate] 66•0.01•250•100 mg ② Phicon

FeoGen FA; FeoGen Forte gelcaps ℞ *hematinic* [iron; vitamins B_{12} & C; folic acid] 66•0.01•250•1 mg; 151•0.01•60•1 mg ② Phicon F

Feosol elixir (discontinued 2005) OTC *hematinic; iron supplement* [ferrous sulfate (source of iron)] 220 mg/5 mL (44 mg/5 mL) ② PhosLo; VaZol

Feosol tablets OTC *hematinic; iron supplement* [carbonyl iron] 45 mg (note: one of three different products with the same name) ② PhosLo; VaZol

Feosol tablets OTC *hematinic; iron supplement* [ferrous sulfate (source of iron)] 325 mg (65 mg) (note: one of three different products with the same name) ② PhosLo; VaZol

Feosol tablets OTC *hematinic; iron supplement* [ferrous sulfate, dried (source of iron)] 200 mg (65 mg) (note: one of three different products with the same name) ⍰ PhosLo; VaZol

Feostat chewable tablets (discontinued 2006) OTC *hematinic; iron supplement* [ferrous fumarate (source of iron)] 100 mg (33 mg)

Feostat suspension, drops (discontinued 2005) OTC *hematinic; iron supplement* [ferrous fumarate (source of iron)] 100 mg/5 mL (33 mg/5 mL); 45 mg/0.6 mL (15 mg/0.6 mL)

fepentolic acid INN

fepitrizol INN

fepradinol INN

feprazone INN, BAN

fepromide INN

feprosidnine INN

Feratab tablets OTC *hematinic; iron supplement* [ferrous sulfate, dried (source of iron)] 187 mg (60 mg)

Fer-Gen-Sol drops OTC *hematinic; iron supplement* [ferrous sulfate (source of iron)] 75 mg/0.6 mL (15 mg/0.6 mL) ⍰ voriconazole

Fergon tablets OTC *hematinic; iron supplement* [ferrous gluconate (source of iron)] 225 mg (27 mg) ⍰ Vergon

Feridex I.V. injection ℞ *radiopaque contrast medium to enhance MRIs of the liver* [ferumoxides] 11.2 mg iron

Fer-In-Sol drops OTC *hematinic; iron supplement* [ferrous sulfate (source of iron)] 75 mg/0.6 mL (15 mg/0.6 mL) ⍰ farnesil

Fer-In-Sol syrup (discontinued 2005) OTC *hematinic; iron supplement* [ferrous sulfate (source of iron)] 90 mg/5 mL (18 mg/5 mL) ⍰ farnesil

Fer-Iron drops (discontinued 2005) OTC *hematinic; iron supplement* [ferrous sulfate (source of iron)] 75 mg/0.6 mL (15 mg/0.6 mL)

fermium *element (Fm)*

fern; fern brake *medicinal herb* [see: buckhorn brake; female fern]

fern, flowering; king's fern; water fern *medicinal herb* [see: buckhorn brake]

fern-leaved foxglove *medicinal herb* [see: feverweed]

Fero-Folic-500 controlled-release Filmtabs (film-coated tablets) ℞ *hematinic* [ferrous sulfate; ascorbic acid; folic acid] 105•500•0.8 mg

Fero-Grad-500 controlled-release tablets OTC *hematinic; vitamin/iron supplement* [ferrous sulfate; sodium ascorbate] 105 mg Fe•500 mg

FeroSul tablets OTC *hematinic; iron supplement* [ferrous sulfate (source of iron)] 325 mg (65 mg) ⍰ vorozole

Ferotrinsic capsules ℞ *hematinic* [ferrous fumarate; cyanocobalamin; ascorbic acid; intrinsic factor concentrate; folic acid] 110 mg•15 mcg•75 mg•240 mg•0.5 mg

Ferralet 90 film-coated tablets ℞ *hematinic* [carbonyl iron] 90 mg

Ferralet Plus tablets OTC *hematinic; vitamin/iron supplement* [ferrous gluconate; cyanocobalamin; ascorbic acid; folic acid] 46 mg•25 mcg•400 mg•0.8 mg

Ferretts film-coated caplets OTC *hematinic; iron supplement* [ferrous fumarate (source of iron)] 325 mg (106 mg) ⍰ Fortaz

Ferrex 150 capsules OTC *hematinic; iron supplement* [polysaccharide-iron complex] 150 mg Fe

Ferrex 150 Forte capsules ℞ *hematinic* [polysaccharide-iron complex; vitamin B_{12}; folic acid] 150 mg iron•25 mcg•1 mg

Ferrex 150 Forte Plus capsules ℞ *hematinic* [polysaccharide-iron complex; vitamins B_{12} and C; folic acid] 150•0.025•60•1 mg

Ferrex 150 Plus capsules OTC *hematinic; vitamin/iron supplement* [polysaccharide-iron complex; vitamin C] 150 mg Fe•50 mg

Ferrex PC; Ferrex PC Forte film-coated tablets ℞ *vitamin/mineral/iron supplement for pregnancy and lactation* [multiple vitamins & minerals; polysaccharide-iron complex; folic acid] ±•60 mg Fe•1 mg

ferric ammonium citrate NF

ferric ammonium sulfate

ferric cacodylate NF

ferric chloride (FeCl₃)

ferric chloride Fe 59 (⁵⁹FeCl₃) USAN *radioactive agent*

ferric citrate (⁵⁹Fe) INN

ferric citrochloride NF

ferric fructose USAN, INN *hematinic*

ferric glycerophosphate NF

ferric hexacyanoferrate (insoluble Prussian blue) *chelating agent for internal contamination with radioactive or nonradioactive cesium and/or thallium (orphan)*

ferric hyaluronate *adhesion barrier for open gynecological and lower GI surgery*

ferric hydroxide sucrose complex [see: iron sucrose; saccharated ferric oxide]

ferric hypophosphite NF

ferric oxide NF *coloring agent*

ferric oxide, red NF

ferric oxide, yellow NF

ferric pyrophosphate, soluble NF

ferric subsulfate NF *hemostatic used in a solution or paste to control superficial bleeding from skin biopsies, cervical biopsies, colposcopy, etc.*

ferricholinate [see: ferrocholinate]

ferriclate calcium sodium USAN *hematinic* [also: calcium sodium ferriclate]

Ferriprox *investigational (orphan) agent for chronic iron overload due to transfusion-dependent anemias* [deferiprone]

ferristene USAN *paramagnetic imaging agent for MRI*

Ferrlecit IV infusion ℞ *hematinic for iron deficiency due to chronic hemodialysis with erythropoietin therapy* [sodium ferric gluconate (source of iron)] 62.5 mg Fe/5 mL

ferrocholate [see: ferrocholinate]

ferrocholinate INN

Ferromar *sustained-release caplets* OTC *hematinic; vitamin/iron supplement* [ferrous fumarate; vitamin C] 201.5 • 200 mg

ferropolimaler INN

Ferro-Sequels *timed-release tablets* OTC *hematinic; iron supplement* [ferrous fumarate (source of iron); docusate sodium] 150 (50) • 100 mg

ferrotrenine INN

ferrous aspartate *hematinic; iron supplement (16% elemental iron)*

ferrous citrate Fe 59 USAN, USP *radioactive agent*

ferrous fumarate USP *hematinic; iron supplement (33% elemental iron)* 90, 324 mg oral

ferrous gluconate USP *hematinic; iron supplement (11.6% elemental iron)* 225, 300, 324, 325 mg oral

ferrous lactate NF

ferrous orotate JAN

ferrous sulfate (FeSO₄ · 7H₂O) USP, JAN *hematinic; iron supplement (20% elemental iron)* 325 mg oral; 220, 300 mg/5 mL oral; 75 mg/0.6 mL oral

ferrous sulfate, dried (FeSO₄ · xH₂O) USP *hematinic; iron supplement (30% elemental iron)* 160 mg oral

ferrous sulfate, exsiccated [see: ferrous sulfate, dried]

ferrous sulfate Fe 59 (⁵⁹FeSO₄) USAN *radioactive agent*

fertirelin INN, BAN *veterinary gonadotropin-releasing hormone* [also: fertirelin acetate]

fertirelin acetate USAN *veterinary gonadotropin-releasing hormone* [also: fertirelin]

ferucarbotran USAN *superparamagnetic diagnostic aid*

Ferula assafoetida; F. foetida; F. rubricaulis *medicinal herb* [see: asafetida; asafoetida]

ferumoxides USAN *parenteral radiopaque contrast medium to enhance MRIs of the liver*

ferumoxsil USAN *oral MRI contrast medium for upper GI tract imaging*

ferumoxtran-10 USAN *superparamagnetic diagnostic aid*

ferumoxytol *investigational (NDA filed) iron replacement for iron deficiency in patients with chronic kidney disease*

FeSO₄ (ferrous sulfate) [q.v.]

fesosterodine *muscarinic receptor antagonist for overactive bladder* (available in Europe; investigational (NDA filed) in the U.S.)

Fetal Fibronectin Test kit for professional use ℞ *in vitro diagnostic aid for fetal fibronectin in vaginal secretions at 24–34 weeks, a predictor of preterm delivery*

fetal neural cells [see: neural cells, porcine fetal]

fetid helebore (*Helleborus foetidus*) [see: helebore]

Fe-Tinic 150 capsules ℞ *hematinic* [polysaccharide-iron complex] 150 mg Fe

Fe-Tinic 150 Forte capsules ℞ *hematinic* [polysaccharide-iron complex; vitamin B_{12}; folic acid] 150 mg Fe• 25 mcg•1 mg

fetoxilate INN *smooth muscle relaxant* [also: fetoxylate HCl; fetoxylate]

fetoxylate BAN *smooth muscle relaxant* [also: fetoxylate HCl; fetoxilate]

fetoxylate HCl USAN *smooth muscle relaxant* [also: fetoxilate; fetoxylate]

fever root *medicinal herb* [see: coral root]

fever twig *medicinal herb* [see: bittersweet nightshade]

FeverAll; Children's FeverAll; Infant's FeverAll; Junior FeverAll suppositories OTC *analgesic; antipyretic* [acetaminophen] 650 mg; 120 mg; 80 mg; 325 mg

FeverAll, Children's; Junior FeverAll Sprinkle Caps (powder) (discontinued 2008) OTC *analgesic; antipyretic* [acetaminophen] 80 mg; 160 mg

feverbush *medicinal herb* [see: winterberry]

feverfew (*Chrysanthemum parthenium; Leucanthemum parthenium; Pyrethrum parthenium; Tanacetum parthenium*) leaves and flowers *medicinal herb used as an aspirin substitute for chills, colds, fever, inflammation, and migraine and sinus headache*

feverweed (*Gerardia pedicularia*) plant *medicinal herb used as an antiseptic, diaphoretic, febrifuge, and sedative*

fexicaine INN

fexinidazole INN

Fexmid film-coated tablets ℞ *skeletal muscle relaxant* [cyclobenzaprine HCl] 7.5 mg

fexofenadine HCl USAN *second-generation peripherally selective piperidine antihistamine for allergic rhinitis and chronic idiopathic urticaria* 30, 60, 180 mg oral

fezatione INN

fezolamine INN *antidepressant* [also: fezolamine fumarate]

fezolamine fumarate USAN *antidepressant* [also: fezolamine]

FGF-20 (fibroblast growth factor-20) [q.v.]

FGN-1 [now: exisulind]

fiacitabine (FIAC) USAN, INN *antiviral*

fialuridine (FIAU) USAN, INN *investigational (orphan) antiviral for chronic active hepatitis B*

Fiberall powder OTC *bulk laxative* [psyllium hydrophilic mucilloid] 3.5 g/ tsp. ⑨ Vaporole

FiberCon tablets OTC *bulk laxative; antidiarrheal* [calcium polycarbophil] 500 mg

Fiberlan oral liquid OTC *enteral nutritional therapy* [lactose-free formula]

Fiber-Lax tablets OTC *bulk laxative; antidiarrheal* [calcium polycarbophil] 625 mg

FiberNorm tablets OTC *bulk laxative; antidiarrheal* [calcium polycarbophil] 625 mg

Fibersure powder for oral solution OTC *bulk laxative; antidiarrheal; dietary fiber supplement* [inulin]

fibracillin INN

fibrin INN

fibrin sealant, human *topical agent to adhere autologous skin grafts to wounds due to burns*

fibrinase [see: factor XIII]

fibrinogen (^{125}I) INN [also: fibrinogen I 125]

fibrinogen, human USP *investigational (orphan) agent to control bleeding in fibrinogen-deficient patients*

fibrinogen I 125 USAN *vascular patency test; radioactive agent* [also: fibrinogen (^{125}I)]

fibrinoligase [see: factor XIII]

fibrinolysin, human INN [also: plasmin]

fibrin-stabilizing factor (FSF) [see: factor XIII]

fibroblast growth factor, basic (bFGF) [see: ersofermin]

fibroblast growth factor-20, recombinant human (rhFGF-20) *investigational (orphan) for radiation-induced oral mucositis*

fibroblast interferon [now: interferon beta]

Fibrogammin P *investigational (orphan) hemostatic for congenital factor XIII deficiency* [factor XIII, human plasma–derived]

fibronectin *investigational (orphan) for nonhealing corneal ulcers or epithelial defects*

Ficus carica medicinal herb [see: fig]

Fidelin *natural hormone precursor; investigational (NDA filed, orphan) for systemic lupus erythematosus (SLE); investigational (orphan) replacement therapy for adrenal insufficiency* [dehydroepiandrosterone (DHEA)]

fiduxosin HCl USAN α_{1a}-*adrenoceptor antagonist for benign prostatic hyperplasia (BPH)*

fig (*Ficus carica*) *fruit medicinal herb used as a demulcent, emollient, and laxative*

figwort (*Scrophularia nodosa*) *leaves, stems, and roots medicinal herb for abrasions, athlete's foot, cradle cap, fever, impetigo, restlessness, skin diseases, and skin tumors*

filaminast USAN *selective phosphodiesterase IV inhibitor for asthma*

filenadol INN

filgrastim USAN, INN, BAN *hematopoietic stimulant for severe chronic neutropenia (orphan); investigational (Phase III, orphan) cytokine for AIDS-related cytomegalovirus retinitis; investigational (orphan) for myelodysplastic syndrome*

Filipendula ulmaria medicinal herb [see: meadowsweet]

filipin USAN, INN *antifungal* ② *fleabane; Velban*

Filmix *investigational (orphan) neurosonographic contrast medium for intracranial tumors* [microbubble contrast agent]

Filmlok (trademarked dosage form) *film-coated tablet*

Filmseal (trademarked dosage form) *film-coated tablet* ② *flumizole*

Filmtabs (trademarked dosage form) *film-coated tablets*

FIME (fluorouracil, ICRF-159, MeCCNU) *chemotherapy protocol*

Finac *lotion* OTC *keratolytic for acne* [salicylic acid; isopropyl alcohol] 2%•22.5% ② *FNC; Fung-O; Vaniqa*

Finacea *gel* ℞ *antimicrobial and keratolytic for mild to moderate rosacea* [azelaic acid] 15% ② *Phenazo; Vanos*

Finajet; Finaplix *brand names for trenbolone acetate, a European veterinary anabolic steroid abused as a street drug*

finasteride USAN, INN, BAN α-*reductase inhibitor; androgen hormone inhibitor for benign prostatic hyperplasia (BPH) and androgenic alopecia in men; investigational for aggressive prostate tumors* 5 mg oral

Finevin *cream* ℞ *antimicrobial and keratolytic for inflammatory acne vulgaris* [azelaic acid] 20%

finger leaf *medicinal herb* [see: cinquefoil]

Fioricet *tablets* ℞ *barbiturate sedative; analgesic; antipyretic* [butalbital; acetaminophen; caffeine] 50•325•40 mg

Fioricet with Codeine *capsules* ℞ *narcotic antitussive; barbiturate sedative; analgesic* [codeine phosphate; butalbital; acetaminophen; caffeine] 30•50•325•40 mg

Fiorinal *capsules* ℞ *barbiturate sedative; analgesic; antipyretic* [butalbital; aspirin; caffeine] 50•325•40 mg

Fiorinal with Codeine *capsules* ℞ *barbiturate sedative; narcotic antitussive; analgesic; antipyretic* [butalbital; codeine phosphate; aspirin; caffeine] 50•30•325•40 mg

Fiortal capsules (discontinued 2004) ℞ *barbiturate sedative; analgesic; antipyretic* [butalbital; aspirin; caffeine] 50•325•40 mg

fipexide INN

fire ant venom allergenic extract *investigational (orphan) skin test and immunotherapy for fire ant anaphylactic reactions*

fireweed *medicinal herb* [see: pilewort]

First Choice reagent strips for home use OTC *in vitro diagnostic aid for blood glucose*

First Response; First Response Early Result test stick for home use OTC *in vitro diagnostic aid; urine pregnancy test*

First Response Ovulation Predictor test kit for home use OTC *in vitro diagnostic aid to predict ovulation time*

fisalamine [see: mesalamine]

fit root (*Monotropa uniflora*) *medicinal herb used as an antispasmodic, febrifuge, nervine, and sedative*

FIV-ASA suppositories ℞ *anti-inflammatory for active ulcerative colitis, proctosigmoiditis, and proctitis* [mesalamine (5-aminosalicylic acid)] 500 mg

5 + 2 protocol (cytarabine, daunorubicin) *chemotherapy protocol for acute myelocytic leukemia (AML)*

5 + 2 protocol (cytarabine, mitoxantrone) *chemotherapy protocol for acute myelocytic leukemia (AML)*

5-ALA HCl; ALA [see: aminolevulinic acid HCl]

5% Alcohol and 5% Dextrose in Water; 10% Alcohol and 5% Dextrose in Water IV infusion ℞ *for caloric replacement and rehydration* [dextrose; alcohol] 5%•5%; 10%•5%

5 Benzagel; 10 Benzagel gel ℞ *keratolytic for acne* [benzoyl peroxide] 5%; 10%

5% Travert and Electrolyte No. 2; 10% Travert and Electrolyte No. 2 IV infusion ℞ *intravenous nutritional/electrolyte therapy* [combined electrolyte solution; invert sugar (50% dextrose + 50% fructose)]

506U78 *investigational (orphan) for chronic lymphocytic leukemia*

5-FC (5-fluorocytosine) [see: flucytosine]

five-finger grass; five fingers *medicinal herb* [see: cinquefoil]

five-fingers root *medicinal herb* [see: ginseng]

5-HT (5-hydroxytryptamine) [see: serotonin]

5-HT₃ (hydroxytryptamine) receptor antagonists *a class of antiemetic and antinauseant agents used primarily after emetogenic cancer chemotherapy* [also called: selective serotonin 5-HT₃ blockers]

5-HTP (5-hydroxytryptophan) [see: L-5 hydroxytryptophan]

FL (flutamide, leuprolide acetate) *chemotherapy protocol for prostate cancer*

FLAC (fluorouracil, leucovorin [rescue], Adriamycin, cyclophosphamide) *chemotherapy protocol* ⊞ Velac

flag, sweet; myrtle flag *medicinal herb* [see: calamus]

flag lily; poison flag; water flag *medicinal herb* [see: blue flag]

Flagyl film-coated tablets, capsules ℞ *antibiotic; antiprotozoal; amebicide* [metronidazole] 250, 500 mg; 375 mg ⊞ Ful-Glo

Flagyl topical *investigational (orphan) treatment for advanced decubitus ulcers* [metronidazole]

Flagyl ER film-coated extended-release tablets ℞ *once-daily antibiotic for bacterial vaginosis* [metronidazole] 750 mg

Flagyl IV powder for injection ℞ *antibiotic; antiprotozoal; amebicide* [metronidazole HCl] 500 mg

Flagyl IV RTU (ready-to-use) injection (discontinued 2006) ℞ *antibiotic; antiprotozoal; amebicide* [metronidazole] 500 mg/100 mL

flamenol INN

Flammacerium *investigational (orphan) for life-threatening burns* [silver sulfadiazine; cerium nitrate]

Flanders Buttocks ointment OTC *diaper rash treatment* [zinc oxide; Peruvian balsam]

flannel flower *medicinal herb* [see: mullein]

FLAP (fluorouracil, leucovorin [rescue], Adriamycin, Platinol) *chemotherapy protocol* ▣ FLEP; VLP

Flarex Drop-Tainers (eye drop suspension) ℞ *corticosteroidal anti-inflammatory* [fluorometholone acetate] 0.1% ▣ Fluarix

FlashDose (trademarked dosage form) *orally disintegrating tablets*

Flatulex drops OTC *antiflatulent* [simethicone] 40 mg/0.6 mL

Flatulex tablets OTC *adsorbent; detoxicant; antiflatulent* [activated charcoal; simethicone] 250•80 mg

flavamine INN

flavine [see: acriflavine HCl]

flavocoxid *natural flavonoids and flavins; natural COX-2 inhibitor; analgesic and anti-inflammatory for the dietary management of osteoarthritis*

flavodic acid INN

flavodilol INN *antihypertensive* [also: flavodilol maleate]

flavodilol maleate USAN *antihypertensive* [also: flavodilol]

flavonoid [see: troxerutin]

Flavons tablets OTC *dietary supplement* [mixed bioflavonoids] 500 mg

Flavons-500 tablets OTC *dietary supplement* [citrus bioflavonoids] 500 mg

flavopiridol *investigational (Phase III) kinase inhibitor for lung cancer*

flavoxate INN, BAN *smooth muscle relaxant; urinary antispasmodic* [also: flavoxate HCl]

flavoxate HCl USAN *anticholinergic; smooth muscle relaxant; urinary antispasmodic* [also: flavoxate] 100 mg oral

flaxseed (Linum usitatissimum) *medicinal herb for arthritis, autoimmune diseases, colds, constipation, cough, heart disease, lowering cholesterol levels, skin disorders, and urinary tract infections*

flazalone USAN, INN, BAN *anti-inflammatory* ▣ flusalan

FLe (fluorouracil, levamisole) *chemotherapy protocol for colorectal cancer*

flea seed; fleawort *medicinal herb* [see: plantain]

fleabane; horseweed (Erigeron canadensis) *plant medicinal herb used as an astringent, diuretic, and hemostatic* ▣ filipin; Velban

fleawort; flea seed *medicinal herb* [see: plantain]

Flebogamma 5% IV infusion ℞ *passive immunizing agent for primary (inherited) immunodeficiency disorders* [immune globulin (IGIV)] 5% (0.5, 2.5, 5, 10 g/dose))

flecainide INN, BAN *antiarrhythmic* [also: flecainide acetate]

flecainide acetate USAN *antiarrhythmic* [also: flecainide] 50, 100, 150 mg oral

Flector transdermal patch ℞ *analgesic; nonsteroidal anti-inflammatory drug (NSAID) for acute pain due to strains, sprains, and contusions* [diclofenac epolamine] 180 mg

Fleet disposable enema OTC *saline laxative* [sodium phosphate, monobasic; sodium phosphate, dibasic] 7•19 g/118 mL dose ▣ violet

Fleet Babylax rectal liquid OTC *hyperosmolar laxative* [glycerin] 4 mL/dose

Fleet Bisacodyl disposable enema OTC *stimulant laxative* [bisacodyl] 10 mg/30 mL dose

Fleet Laxative enteric-coated tablets, suppositories OTC *stimulant laxative* [bisacodyl] 5 mg; 10 mg

Fleet Medicated Wipes cleansing pads OTC *moisturizer and cleanser for external rectal/vaginal areas; astringent; antiseptic; antifungal* [hamamelis water (witch hazel); glycerin; alcohol] 50%•10%•7%

Fleet Mineral Oil disposable enema OTC *emollient laxative* [mineral oil] 118 mL dose

Fleet Pain Relief anorectal wipes OTC *local anesthetic* [pramoxine HCl; glycerin] 1%•12%

Fleet Phospho-soda oral solution OTC *saline laxative* [sodium phosphate, monobasic; sodium phosphate, dibasic] 7.2•2.7 g/15 mL

Fleet Phospho-soda EZ-Prep two-dose kit OTC *pre-procedure bowel evacuant* [sodium phosphate, monobasic; sodium phosphate, dibasic]
First dose: 21.6•5.4 g/45 mL;
Second dose: 14.4•3.6 g/30 mL

Fleet Prep Kits No. 1 to No. 3 OTC *pre-procedure bowel evacuant* [other Fleet products in combination kits]

FLEP (fluorouracil, leucovorin, etoposide, Platinol) *chemotherapy protocol* ② FLAP; VLP

flerobuterol INN

fleroxacin USAN, INN *antibacterial*

flesinoxan INN *antidepressant; anxiolytic*

flestolol INN *antiadrenergic (β-receptor)* [also: flestolol sulfate]

flestolol sulfate USAN *antiadrenergic (β-receptor)* [also: flestolol]

fletazepam USAN, INN, BAN *skeletal muscle relaxant*

Fletcher's Castoria oral liquid OTC *stimulant laxative* [senna concentrate] 33.3 mg/mL

fleur-de-lis *medicinal herb* [see: blue flag]

Flex-all 454 gel OTC *analgesic; mild anesthetic; antipruritic; counterirritant* [methyl salicylate; menthol] ≟•16%

Flexaphen capsules ℞ *skeletal muscle relaxant; analgesic; antipyretic* [chlorzoxazone; acetaminophen] 250•300 mg

Flex-Care Especially for Sensitive Eyes solution OTC *chemical disinfecting solution for soft contact lenses* [note: the soft contact indication is different from RGP contact indication for the same product]

Flex-Care Especially for Sensitive Eyes solution OTC *disinfecting/wetting/soaking solution for rigid gas permeable contact lenses* [note: the RGP contact indication is different from soft contact indication for the same product]

Flexderm sheets *absorbent wound dressing* [hydrogel polymer]

Flexeril film-coated tablets ℞ *skeletal muscle relaxant* [cyclobenzaprine HCl] 5, 10 mg

FlexiGel Strands wound dressing OTC *absorbent dressing*

Flexoject IV or IM injection (discontinued 2005) ℞ *skeletal muscle relaxant; analgesic; anticholinergic* [orphenadrine citrate] 30 mg/mL

Flexon IV or IM injection ℞ *skeletal muscle relaxant; analgesic; anticholinergic* [orphenadrine citrate] 30 mg/mL ② Floxin; fluquazone

FlexPack HP test for professional use ℞ *diagnostic aid for serum IgG antibodies to H. pylori (for peptic ulcers)*

FlexPen (trademarked delivery form) *disposable prefilled self-injector for insulin*

Flex-Power Performance Sports cream OTC *analgesic* [trolamine salicylate] 10%

Flextra-DS tablets ℞ *analgesic; antipyretic; antihistamine; sleep aid* [acetaminophen; phenyltoloxamine citrate] 500•50 mg

Flexzan; Flexzan Extra adhesive sheets *absorbent, semi-occlusive wound dressing* [polyurethane foam] ② viloxazine

flibanserin USAN *rapid-acting antidepressant; investigational agent to increase sexual desire and arousal in women*

Flintstones Children's; Flintstones Plus Calcium; Flintstones Plus Extra C Children's chewable tablets OTC *vitamin supplement* [multiple vitamins; folic acid] ≟•0.3 mg

Flintstones Complete chewable tablets OTC *vitamin/mineral/iron supplement* [multiple vitamins & minerals; iron; folic acid; biotin] ≟•18 mg•0.4 mg•40 mcg

Flintstones Plus Iron chewable tablets OTC *vitamin/iron supplement* [multiple vitamins; iron; folic acid] ≟•15•0.3 mg

Flixotide (foreign name for U.S. product **Flovent**)

Flo-Coat rectal suspension ℞ *radi-opaque contrast medium for gastrointestinal imaging* [barium sulfate] 100%

Flocor *investigational (Phase III, orphan) coagulation inhibitor for treatment of sickle cell vaso-occlusive crisis; investigational (orphan) for severe burns and for vasospasm following cerebral aneurysm repair* [poloxamer 188]

floctafenine USAN, INN, BAN *analgesic*

Flolan IV infusion ℞ *platelet aggregation inhibitor and vasodilator for pulmonary hypertension (orphan); investigational (orphan) heparin replacement for hemodialysis* [epoprostenol sodium] 0.5, 1.5 mg

Flomax capsules ℞ *alpha₁-adrenergic blocker for benign prostatic hyperplasia (BPH); also used as adjunctive therapy for ureteral stones* [tamsulosin HCl] 0.4 mg 🔁 Volmax

flomoxef INN

Flonase nasal spray in a metered-dose pump ℞ *corticosteroidal anti-inflammatory for seasonal or perennial allergic rhinitis* [fluticasone propionate] 50 mcg/dose

Flo-Pack (trademarked delivery form) *vial for IV drip*

Flo-Pred oral suspension ℞ *corticosteroid; anti-inflammatory* [prednisolone acetate] 5, 15 mg/5 mL

flopropione INN

Floranex chewable tablets OTC *natural intestinal bacteria; probiotic; dietary supplement* [Lactobacillus acidophilus; L. bulgaricus] 1 million CFU mixed culture

florantyrone INN, BAN

Flora-Q capsules ℞ *digestive enzymes* [Lactobacillus acidophilus; L. paracasei; Bifidobacterium; Streptococcus thermophilus] 8 million CFU

Florastor capsules OTC *natural intestinal bacteria; probiotic; dietary supplement* [Saccharomyces boulardii lyo] 250 mg

Florastor Kids oral powder OTC *natural intestinal bacteria; probiotic; dietary supplement* [Saccharomyces boulardii lyo] 250 mg

flordipine USAN, INN *antihypertensive*

floredil INN

Florentine iris *medicinal herb* [see: orris root]

floretione [see: fluoresone]

florfenicol USAN, INN, BAN *veterinary antibacterial*

Florical capsules, tablets OTC *calcium/fluoride supplement* [calcium carbonate; sodium fluoride] 364•8.3 mg

Florida Sunburn Relief lotion OTC *mild anesthetic; antipruritic; counterirritant; antiseptic* [phenol; camphor; menthol; benzyl alcohol] 0.4%•0.2%•0.15%•3%

florifenine INN

Florinef Acetate tablets ℞ *replacement therapy for adrenocortical insufficiency in Addison disease* [fludrocortisone acetate] 0.1 mg

Florone cream, ointment ℞ *corticosteroidal anti-inflammatory* [diflorasone diacetate] 0.05% 🔁 fluorine; valerian

Florone E cream ℞ *corticosteroidal anti-inflammatory; emollient* [diflorasone diacetate] 0.05% 🔁 fluorine; valerian

floropipamide [now: pipamperone]

floropipeton [see: propyperone]

Florvite pediatric oral drops ℞ *vitamin supplement; dental caries preventative* [multiple vitamins; sodium fluoride] ≞•0.25, ≞•0.5 mg/mL

Florvite; Florvite Half Strength pediatric chewable tablets ℞ *vitamin supplement; dental caries preventative* [multiple vitamins; sodium fluoride; folic acid] ≞•1•0.3 mg; ≞•0.5•0.3 mg

Florvite + Iron pediatric oral drops ℞ *vitamin/iron supplement; dental caries preventative* [multiple vitamins & minerals; sodium fluoride; ferrous sulfate] ≞•0.25•10, ≞•0.5•10 mg/mL

Florvite + Iron; Half Strength Florvite + Iron pediatric chewable tablets ℞ *vitamin/iron supplement; dental caries preventative* [multiple vitamins & minerals; sodium fluo-

ride; ferrous sulfate; folic acid] ± •
1 • 12 • 0.3 mg; ± • 0.5 • 12 • 0.3 mg

flosequinan USAN, INN, BAN *antihypertensive; vasodilator; treatment for congestive heart failure*

flotrenizine INN

Flovent Diskus (prefilled inhalation powder device) (discontinued 2007) ℞ *corticosteroidal anti-inflammatory for chronic asthma; not indicated for acute attacks* [fluticasone propionate] 50, 100, 250 mcg/dose

Flovent Rotadisk (inhalation powder) (discontinued 2007) ℞ *corticosteroidal anti-inflammatory for chronic asthma; not indicated for acute attacks* [fluticasone propionate] 50, 100, 250 mcg/dose

Flovent HFA inhalation aerosol in a metered-dose inhaler ℞ *corticosteroidal anti-inflammatory for chronic asthma; not indicated for acute attacks* [fluticasone propionate] 44, 110, 220 mcg/dose

floverine INN ⊡ Fluvirin

flower velure *medicinal herb* [see: coltsfoot]

flower-de-luce *medicinal herb* [see: blue flag]

floxacillin USAN *antibacterial* [also: flucloxacillin]

floxacrine INN

Floxin film-coated tablets, UroPak (3-day supply) ℞ *broad-spectrum fluoroquinolone antibiotic* [ofloxacin] 200, 300, 400 mg; 6 tablets × 200 mg ⊡ Flexon; fluquazone

Floxin IV injection (discontinued 2004) ℞ *broad-spectrum fluoroquinolone antibiotic* [ofloxacin] 200, 400 mg/vial ⊡ Flexon; fluquazone

Floxin Otic ear drops ℞ *broad-spectrum fluoroquinolone antibiotic* [ofloxacin] 0.3%

Floxin Otic Singles (premeasured containers) ℞ *broad-spectrum fluoroquinolone antibiotic* [ofloxacin] 0.3% (0.75 mg per 0.25 mL container)

floxuridine USAN, USP, INN *antimetabolic antineoplastic for GI adenocarci-*
noma metastatic to the liver; investigational (orphan) for intraperitoneal treatment of gastric cancer; also used for ovarian and kidney cancer 500 mg injection

Flu OIA (Optical ImmunoAssay) test for professional use ℞ *rapid (less than 20 minutes) diagnostic aid for influenza A and B in sputum, nasal aspirate, or nasopharyngeal swab*

fluacizine INN ⊡ volazocine

flualamide INN

fluanisone INN, BAN

Fluarix suspension for IM injection in prefilled syringes ℞ *vaccine for influenza virus types A and B for patients ≥ 18 years* [influenza split-virus vaccine (preservative free)] 0.5 mL/dose ⊡ Flarex

fluazacort USAN, INN *anti-inflammatory*

flubanilate INN *CNS stimulant* [also: flubanilate HCl]

flubanilate HCl USAN *CNS stimulant* [also: flubanilate]

flubendazole USAN, INN, BAN *antiprotozoal*

flubenisolone [see: betamethasone]

flubepride INN

flubuperone [see: melperone]

Flucaine eye drops ℞ *local anesthetic; corneal disclosing agent* [proparacaine HCl; fluorescein sodium] 0.5% • 0.25%

flucarbril INN

flucetorex INN

flucindole USAN, INN *antipsychotic*

fluciprazine INN

fluclorolone acetonide INN, BAN *corticosteroid; anti-inflammatory* [also: flucloronide]

flucloronide USAN *corticosteroid; anti-inflammatory* [also: fluclorolone acetonide]

flucloxacillin INN, BAN *antibacterial* [also: floxacillin]

fluconazole USAN, INN, BAN *systemic triazole antifungal* 50, 100, 150, 200 mg oral; 50, 200 mg/5 mL oral; 2 mg/mL injection ⊡ valconazole

flucrilate INN *tissue adhesive* [also: flu-crylate]

flucrylate USAN *tissue adhesive* [also: flucrilate]

flucytosine USAN, USP, INN, BAN *systemic antifungal*

fludalanine USAN, INN *antibacterial*

Fludara powder for IV injection Ŗ *antineoplastic for chronic lymphocytic leukemia (CLL) and non-Hodgkin lymphoma (orphan)* [fludarabine phosphate] 50 mg

fludarabine INN *antimetabolite antineoplastic* [also: fludarabine phosphate]

fludarabine phosphate USAN *antimetabolite antineoplastic for chronic lymphocytic leukemia (CLL) and non-Hodgkin lymphoma (orphan)* [also: fludarabine] 25, 50 mg injection

fludazonium chloride USAN, INN *topical anti-infective*

fludeoxyglucose (^{18}F) INN *diagnostic aid; radioactive agent* [also: fludeoxyglucose F 18]

fludeoxyglucose F 18 USAN, USP *diagnostic aid; radioactive agent* [also: fludeoxyglucose (^{18}F)]

fludiazepam INN

fludorex USAN, INN *anorectic; antiemetic*

fludoxopone INN

fludrocortisone INN, BAN *salt-regulating adrenocortical steroid; mineralocorticoid* [also: fludrocortisone acetate]

fludrocortisone acetate USP *salt-regulating adrenocortical steroid; mineralocorticoid; for adrenocortical insufficiency in Addison disease* [also: fludrocortisone] 0.1 mg oral

fludroxicortide [see: flurandrenolide]

fludroxycortide INN *topical corticosteroid* [also: flurandrenolide; flurandrenolone]

flufenamic acid USAN, INN, BAN *anti-inflammatory*

flufenisal USAN, INN *analgesic*

flufosal INN

flufylline INN

flugestone INN, BAN *progestin* [also: flurogestone acetate]

flugestone acetate [see: flurogestone acetate]

fluindarol INN

fluindione INN

FluLaval IM injection Ŗ *flu vaccine for influenza virus types A and B for patients ≥ 18 years* [influenza split-virus vaccine (with thimerosal preservative)] 0.5 mL/dose (mercury 25 mcg/dose)

Flumadine film-coated tablets Ŗ *antiviral; prophylaxis and treatment for influenza A virus* [rimantadine HCl] 100 mg

Flumadine syrup (discontinued 2008) Ŗ *antiviral; prophylaxis and treatment for influenza A virus* [rimantadine HCl] 50 mg/5 mL

flumazenil USAN, INN, BAN *benzodiazepine antagonist to reverse anesthesia or treat overdose* 0.1 mg/mL injection

flumazepil [see: flumazenil]

flumecinol INN *investigational (orphan) agent for neonatal hyperbilirubinemia*

flumedroxone INN, BAN

flumequine USAN, INN, BAN *antibacterial*

flumeridone USAN, INN, BAN *antiemetic*

flumetasone INN *corticosteroid; anti-inflammatory* [also: flumethasone]

flumethasone USAN, BAN *topical corticosteroidal anti-inflammatory* [also: flumetasone]

flumethasone pivalate USAN, USP, BAN *topical corticosteroidal anti-inflammatory*

flumethiazide INN, BAN

flumethrin BAN

flumetramide USAN, INN *skeletal muscle relaxant*

flumexadol INN

flumezapine USAN, INN, BAN *antipsychotic; neuroleptic*

fluminorex USAN, INN *anorectic*

FluMist prefilled single-use intranasal sprayers Ŗ *flu vaccine for influenza types A and B for patients 2–49 years* [influenza virus vaccine, live attenuated (preservative free)] 0.5 mL/dose

flumizole USAN, INN *anti-inflammatory* ⑨ Filmseal

flumoxonide USAN, INN *adrenocortical steroid*

flunamine INN

flunarizine INN, BAN *vasodilator* [also: flunarizine HCl]

flunarizine HCl USAN *investigational (orphan) vasodilator for alternating hemiplegia* [also: flunarizine]

flunidazole USAN, INN *antiprotozoal*

flunisolide USAN, USP, INN, BAN *corticosteroidal anti-inflammatory for chronic asthma and rhinitis* 0.025% (25, 29 mcg/dose) nasal spray

flunisolide acetate USAN *anti-inflammatory*

flunisolide hemihydrate [see: flunisolide]

flunitrazepam USAN, INN, BAN, JAN *benzodiazepine sedative and hypnotic; also abused as a "date rape" street drug*

flunixin USAN, INN, BAN *anti-inflammatory; analgesic*

flunixin meglumine USAN *anti-inflammatory; analgesic*

flunoprost INN

flunoxaprofen INN

fluocinolide [now: fluocinonide]

fluocinolone BAN *topical corticosteroidal anti-inflammatory* [also: fluocinolone acetonide]

fluocinolone acetonide USAN, USP, INN *topical corticosteroidal anti-inflammatory; ocular implant for uveitis (orphan)* [also: fluocinolone] 0.01%, 0.025% topical

fluocinonide USAN, USP, INN, BAN *topical corticosteroidal anti-inflammatory* 0.05% topical

fluocortin INN *anti-inflammatory* [also: fluocortin butyl]

fluocortin butyl USAN, BAN *anti-inflammatory* [also: fluocortin]

fluocortolone USAN, INN, BAN *corticosteroid; anti-inflammatory*

fluocortolone caproate USAN *corticosteroid; anti-inflammatory*

Fluonex cream ℞ *corticosteroidal anti-inflammatory* [fluocinonide] 0.05%

Fluonid topical solution ℞ *corticosteroidal anti-inflammatory* [fluocinolone acetonide] 0.01%

fluopromazine BAN *antipsychotic* [also: triflupromazine]

Fluoracaine eye drops ℞ *local anesthetic; corneal disclosing agent* [proparacaine HCl; fluorescein sodium] 0.5%•0.25%

fluoracizine [see: fluacizine]

fluorescein USP, BAN, JAN *ophthalmic diagnostic agent*

fluorescein, soluble [now: fluorescein sodium]

Fluorescein Injection Lite ℞ *ophthalmic diagnostic agent* [fluorescein sodium] 10%, 25%

fluorescein sodium USP, BAN, JAN *ophthalmic diagnostic agent* 2% eye drops

fluorescein sodium & proparacaine HCl *corneal disclosing agent; topical ophthalmic anesthetic* 0.25%•0.5% eye drops

Fluorescite antecubital venous injection ℞ *ophthalmic diagnostic agent* [fluorescein sodium] 10%, 25%

Fluoresoft eye drops ℞ *diagnostic aid in fitting contact lenses* [fluorexon] 0.35%

fluoresone INN

Fluorets ophthalmic strips OTC *corneal disclosing agent* [fluorescein sodium] 1 mg

fluorexon *diagnosis and fitting aid for contact lenses*

fluorhydrocortisone acetate [see: fludrocortisone acetate]

Fluoride tablets OTC *dental caries preventative* [sodium fluoride] 2.21 mg

Fluoride Loz lozenges ℞ *dental caries preventative* [sodium fluoride] 2.21 mg

Fluoridex Daily Defense Sensitivity Relief toothpaste OTC *tooth desensitizer; dental caries preventative* [potassium nitrate; sodium fluoride]

Fluorigard oral rinse OTC *dental caries preventative; antiseptic* [sodium fluoride; alcohol 6%] 0.05%

Fluori-Methane spray (discontinued 2005) ℞ *vapo-coolant anesthetic/anal-*

gesic [trichloromonofluoromethane; dichlorodifluoromethane] 85%•15%

fluorine *element (F)* ⊠ Florone; valerian

fluorine F 18 fluorodeoxyglucose [see: fludeoxyglucose F 18]

Fluorinse oral rinse ℞ *dental caries preventative* [sodium fluoride] 0.2%

Fluor-I-Strip; Fluor-I-Strip A.T. ophthalmic strips ℞ *corneal disclosing agent* [fluorescein sodium] 9 mg; 1 mg

Fluoritab chewable tablets, drops ℞ *dental caries preventative* [sodium fluoride] 1.1, 2.2 mg; 0.55 mg/drop

fluormethylprednisolone [see: dexamethasone]

5-fluorocytosine (5-FC) [see: flucytosine]

fluorodeoxyglucose F 18 [see: fludeoxyglucose F 18]

fluorodideoxyadenosine (F-ddA) [see: lodenosine]

fluorometholone USAN, INN, BAN *topical ophthalmic corticosteroidal anti-inflammatory* 0.1% eye drops

fluorometholone acetate USAN *topical ophthalmic corticosteroidal anti-inflammatory*

fluoromethylene deoxycytidine (FMdC) [now: tezacitabine]

Fluor-Op eye drop suspension (discontinued 2006) ℞ *corticosteroidal anti-inflammatory* [fluorometholone] 0.1%

Fluoroperm 32 ℞ *hydrophobic contact lens material* [paflufocon C]

Fluoroperm 62 ℞ *hydrophobic contact lens material* [paflufocon B]

Fluoroperm 92 ℞ *hydrophobic contact lens material* [paflufocon A]

Fluoroperm 151 ℞ *hydrophobic contact lens material* [paflufocon D]

Fluoroplex cream ℞ *antineoplastic for actinic keratoses (AK)* [fluorouracil] 1%

Fluoroplex topical solution (discontinued 2008) ℞ *antineoplastic for actinic keratoses (AK)* [fluorouracil] 1%

fluoroquinolones *a class of synthetic, broad-spectrum, antimicrobial, bactericidal antibiotics*

fluorosalan USAN *disinfectant* [also: flusalan]

fluorouracil (5-FU) USAN, USP, INN, BAN *antimetabolite antineoplastic for colorectal (orphan), esophageal (orphan), breast, stomach, and pancreatic cancers; topical treatment for actinic keratoses and basal cell carcinoma; investigational (orphan) for glioblastoma multiforme* 50 mg/mL injection; 2%, 5% topical

fluorouracil & cisplatin *chemotherapy protocol for cervical cancer, used in conjunction with radiation therapy*

fluorouracil & leucovorin *antineoplastic for metastatic colorectal cancer (orphan)*

fluoruridine deoxyribose [see: floxuridine]

fluostigmine [see: isoflurophate]

Fluothane liquid for vaporization ℞ *inhalation general anesthetic* [halothane]

fluotracen INN *antipsychotic; antidepressant* [also: fluotracen HCl]

fluotracen HCl USAN *antipsychotic; antidepressant* [also: fluotracen]

fluoxetine USAN, INN, BAN *selective serotonin reuptake inhibitor (SSRI) for depression, obsessive-compulsive disorder, bulimia nervosa, premenstrual dysphoric disorder, and panic disorder*

fluoxetine HCl USAN *selective serotonin reuptake inhibitor (SSRI) for major depressive disorder (MDD), obsessive-compulsive disorder (OCD), bulimia nervosa, premenstrual dysphoric disorder (PMDD), and panic disorder; investigational (orphan) for autism* 10, 20, 40 mg oral; 20 mg/5 mL oral

fluoximesterone [see: fluoxymesterone]

Flu-Oxinate eye drops (discontinued 2006) ℞ *topical anesthetic; corneal disclosing agent* [benoxinate HCl; fluorescein sodium] 0.4%•0.25%

fluoxiprednisolone [see: triamcinolone]

fluoxymesterone USP, INN, BAN *oral androgen for hypogonadism or testosterone deficiency in men, delayed puberty in boys, and metastatic breast cancer in women; hormone replacement therapy*

(HRT) for postandropausal symptoms 10 mg oral

fluparoxan INN, BAN *antidepressant* [also: fluparoxan HCl]

fluparoxan HCl USAN *antidepressant* [also: fluparoxan]

flupenthixol BAN *thioxanthene antipsychotic* [also: flupentixol]

flupentixol INN *thioxanthene antipsychotic* [also: flupenthixol]

fluperamide USAN, INN *antiperistaltic* ② valpromide

fluperlapine INN

fluperolone INN, BAN *corticosteroid; anti-inflammatory* [also: fluperolone acetate]

fluperolone acetate USAN *corticosteroid; anti-inflammatory* [also: fluperolone]

fluphenazine INN, BAN *conventional (typical) phenothiazine antipsychotic for schizophrenia and psychotic disorders* [also: fluphenazine enanthate]

fluphenazine decanoate *conventional (typical) phenothiazine antipsychotic for schizophrenia and psychotic disorders; used for prolonged parenteral neuroleptic therapy* 25 mg/mL injection

fluphenazine enanthate USP *conventional (typical) phenothiazine antipsychotic for schizophrenia and psychotic disorders* [also: fluphenazine]

fluphenazine HCl USP, BAN *conventional (typical) phenothiazine antipsychotic for schizophrenia and psychotic disorders* 1, 2.5, 5, 10 mg oral; 2.5 mg/ 5 mL oral; 5 mg/mL oral; 2.5 mg/L injection

flupimazine INN

flupirtine INN, BAN *non-narcotic analgesic* [also: flupirtine maleate]

flupirtine maleate USAN *non-narcotic analgesic* [also: flupirtine]

flupranone INN

fluprazine INN ② felypressin

fluprednidene INN, BAN

fluprednisolone USAN, NF, INN, BAN *corticosteroid; anti-inflammatory*

fluprednisolone valerate USAN *corticosteroid; anti-inflammatory*

fluprofen INN, BAN

fluprofylline INN

fluproquazone USAN, INN, BAN *analgesic*

fluprostenol INN, BAN *prostaglandin* [also: fluprostenol sodium]

fluprostenol sodium USAN *prostaglandin* [also: fluprostenol]

fluquazone USAN, INN *anti-inflammatory* ② Flexon; Floxin

Flura tablets ℞ *dental caries preventative* [sodium fluoride] 2.2 mg

fluracil [see: fluorouracil]

fluradoline INN *analgesic* [also: fluradoline HCl]

fluradoline HCl USAN *analgesic* [also: fluradoline]

Flura-Drops ℞ *dental caries preventative* [sodium fluoride] 0.55 mg/drop

Flura-Loz lozenges ℞ *dental caries preventative* [sodium fluoride] 2.2 mg

flurandrenolide USAN, USP *topical corticosteroid* [also: fludroxycortide; flurandrenolone] 0.05% topical

flurandrenolone BAN *topical corticosteroid* [also: flurandrenolide; fludroxycortide]

flurantel INN

Flurate eye drops ℞ *topical anesthetic; corneal disclosing agent* [benoxinate HCl; fluorescein sodium] 0.4%• 0.25%

flurazepam INN, BAN *benzodiazepine sedative and hypnotic; anticonvulsant; muscle relaxant; also abused as a street drug* [also: flurazepam HCl]

flurazepam HCl USAN, USP *benzodiazepine sedative and hypnotic; anticonvulsant; muscle relaxant; also abused as a street drug* [also: flurazepam] 15, 30 mg oral

flurbiprofen USAN, USP, INN, BAN *analgesic; nonsteroidal anti-inflammatory drug (NSAID) for osteoarthritis and rheumatoid arthritis* 50, 100 mg oral

flurbiprofen sodium USP *prostaglandin synthesis inhibitor; ophthalmic nonsteroidal anti-inflammatory drug (NSAID); intraoperative miosis inhibitor* 0.03% eye drops

Fluress eye drops ℞ *topical anesthetic; corneal disclosing agent* [benoxinate HCl; fluorescein sodium] 0.4%•0.25%

fluretofen USAN, INN *anti-inflammatory; antithrombotic*

flurfamide [now: flurofamide]

flurithromycin INN

flurocitabine USAN, INN *antineoplastic*

Fluro-Ethyl aerosol spray ℞ *refrigerant anesthetic* [ethyl chloride; dichlorotetrafluoroethane] 25%•75%

flurofamide USAN, INN *urease enzyme inhibitor*

flurogestone acetate USAN *progestin* [also: flugestone]

Flurosyn ointment, cream (discontinued 2006) ℞ *corticosteroidal anti-inflammatory* [fluocinolone acetonide] 0.025%; 0.01, 0.025%

flurothyl USAN, USP, BAN *CNS stimulant* [also: flurotyl]

flurotyl INN *CNS stimulant* [also: flurothyl]

Flurox eye drops ℞ *topical anesthetic; corneal disclosing agent* [benoxinate HCl; fluorescein sodium] 0.4%•0.25% ☒ Flarex

fluroxene USAN, NF, INN *inhalation anesthetic*

fluroxyspiramine [see: spiramide]

flusalan INN *disinfectant* [also: fluorosalan] ☒ flazalone

flusoxolol INN, BAN

fluspiperone USAN, INN *antipsychotic*

fluspirilene USAN, INN, BAN *diphenylbutylpiperidine antipsychotic*

Flutabs caplets ℞ *antitussive; decongestant; expectorant; analgesic; antipyretic* [dextromethorphan hydrobromide; pseudoephedrine HCl; guaifenesin; acetaminophen] 20•60•200•500 mg

flutamide USAN, INN, BAN *antiandrogen antineoplastic for prostatic carcinoma* 125 mg oral

flutazolam INN

flutemazepam INN

Flutex ointment, cream ℞ *corticosteroidal anti-inflammatory* [triamcinolone acetonide] 0.025%, 0.1%, 0.5% ☒ Foltx

flutiazin USAN, INN *veterinary anti-inflammatory*

fluticasone INN, BAN *corticosteroidal anti-inflammatory for chronic asthma or allergic rhinitis* [also: fluticasone propionate] ☒ Valtaxin

fluticasone furoate *corticosteroidal anti-inflammatory; nasal aerosol for seasonal or perennial allergic rhinitis*

fluticasone propionate USAN *topical corticosteroidal anti-inflammatory; oral inhalation aerosol for chronic asthma; nasal aerosol for allergic rhinitis* [also: fluticasone] 0.005%, 0.05% topical; 50 mcg nasal spray

Flutiform *investigational (Phase III) combination inhaled corticosteroidal anti-inflammatory and bronchodilator for mild-to-moderate asthma* [fluticasone; formoterol]

flutizenol INN

flutomidate INN

flutonidine INN

flutoprazepam INN

flutrimazole INN

flutroline USAN, INN *antipsychotic*

flutropium bromide INN

FluTuss HC oral liquid ℞ *narcotic antitussive; antihistamine; decongestant* [hydrocodone bitartrate; brompheniramine maleate; phenylephrine HCl] 2.5•4•7.5 mg/5 mL

fluvastatin INN, BAN *HMG-CoA reductase inhibitor for hypercholesterolemia and atherosclerosis* [also: fluvastatin sodium]

fluvastatin sodium USAN *HMG-CoA reductase inhibitor for hypercholesterolemia, hypertriglyceridemia, mixed dyslipidemia, atherosclerosis, and coronary heart disease (CHD)* [also: fluvastatin]

Fluvirin suspension for IM injection in prefilled syringes ℞ *flu vaccine for influenza virus types A and B for patients ≥ 4 years* [influenza split-virus vaccine (preservative free)] 0.5 mL/dose ☒ floverine

fluvoxamine INN, BAN *selective seroto-nin reuptake inhibitor (SSRI) for obses-sive-compulsive disorder (OCD)* [also: fluvoxamine maleate]

fluvoxamine maleate USAN *selective serotonin reuptake inhibitor (SSRI) for obsessive-compulsive disorder (OCD); also used for depression, bulimia ner-vosa, panic disorder, social phobia, and nocturnal enuresis* [also: fluvoxamine] 25, 50, 100 mg oral

flux root *medicinal herb* [see: pleurisy root]

fluzinamide USAN, INN *anticonvulsant*

Fluzone suspension for IM injection in multidose vials ℞ *flu vaccine for influenza virus types A and B for patients ≥ 6 months* [influenza split-virus vaccine (with thimerosal pre-servative)] 0.5 mL/dose (mercury 25 mcg/dose) ▣ Valisone

Fluzone suspension for IM injection in prefilled syringes ℞ *flu vaccine for influenza virus types A and B for patients ≥ 6 months* [influenza split-virus vaccine (preservative free)] 0.5 mL/dose ▣ Valisone

Fluzone Preservative-Free: Pedi-atric Dose prefilled syringes for IM injection ℞ *flu vaccine* [influenza split-virus or whole-virus vaccine] 0.25 mL/dose

fluzoperine INN

flytrap *medicinal herb* [see: dogbane]

FMdC (fluoromethylene deoxycy-tidine) [now: tezacitabine]

FML; FML Forte eye drop suspension ℞ *corticosteroidal anti-inflammatory* [fluorometholone] 0.1%; 0.25%

FML S.O.P. ophthalmic ointment ℞ *corticosteroidal anti-inflammatory* [flu-orometholone] 0.1%

FML-S eye drop suspension ℞ *cortico-steroidal anti-inflammatory; antibiotic* [fluorometholone; sulfacetamide sodium] 0.1%•10%

FMS (fluorouracil, mitomycin, streptozocin) *chemotherapy protocol*

FMV (fluorouracil, MeCCNU, vin-cristine) *chemotherapy protocol*

FNC (fluorouracil, Novantrone, cyclophosphamide) *chemotherapy protocol for breast cancer* [also: CFN; CNF]

FNM (fluorouracil, Novantrone, methotrexate) *chemotherapy protocol*

foal's foot *medicinal herb* [see: coltsfoot]

FOAM (fluorouracil, Oncovin, Adriamycin, mitomycin) *chemo-therapy protocol*

Foamicon chewable tablets OTC *antacid* [aluminum hydroxide; magnesium trisilicate] 80•20 mg ▣ fomocaine

Focalin tablets ℞ *CNS stimulant for attention-deficit/hyperactivity disorder (ADHD)* [dexmethylphenidate HCl] 2.5, 5, 10 mg ▣ viqualine

Focalin XR extended-release capsules ℞ *CNS stimulant for attention-deficit/hyperactivity disorder (ADHD)* [dex-methylphenidate HCl] 5, 10, 15, 20 mg

focofilcon A USAN *hydrophilic contact lens material*

fodipir USAN *excipient*

Foeniculum officinale; F. vulgare *medicinal herb* [see: fennel]

Foille spray OTC *anesthetic; antiseptic* [benzocaine; chloroxylenol] 5%•0.63%

Foille Medicated First Aid ointment, aerosol spray OTC *anesthetic; antisep-tic* [benzocaine; chloroxylenol] 5%•0.1%; 5%•0.6%

Foille Plus aerosol spray OTC *anes-thetic; antiseptic* [benzocaine; alcohol 57.33%] 5%

folacin [see: folic acid]

folate [see: folic acid]

folate sodium USP

Folergot-DF tablets (discontinued 2008) ℞ *GI/GU anticholinergic/anti-spasmodic; sedative; analgesic* [bella-donna alkaloids; phenobarbital; ergotamine tartrate] 0.2•40•0.6 mg

folescutol INN

Folgard tablets OTC *vitamin B supple-ment* [vitamins B_6 and B_{12}; folic acid] 10•0.115•0.8 mg

Folgard RX 2.2 film-coated tablets ℞ *vitamin B supplement* [vitamins B₆ and B₁₂; folic acid] 25•0.5•2.3 mg

folic acid USP, INN, BAN *vitamin B꜀; vitamin M; hematopoietic; birth defect preventative* 0.4, 0.8, 1 mg oral; 5 mg/mL injection

folinate-SF calcium [see: leucovorin calcium]

folinic acid [see: leucovorin calcium]

follicle-stimulating hormone (FSH) BAN [also: menotropins]

follidrin [see: estradiol benzoate]

Follistim powder for subcu or IM injection (name changed to **Follistim AQ** in 2006)

Follistim AQ subcu or IM injection ℞ *recombinant follicle-stimulating hormone (FSH) for the induction of ovulation in women and spermatogenesis in men; adjunct to assisted reproductive technologies (ART)* [follitropin beta] 75, 150 FSH units/vial

Follistim AQ Cartridge prefilled Follistim Pen cartridges for subcu or IM injection ℞ *recombinant follicle-stimulating hormone (FSH) for the induction of ovulation in women and spermatogenesis in men; adjunct to assisted reproductive technologies (ART)* [follitropin beta] 150, 300, 600, 600 FSH units/cartridge

follitropin alfa INN *recombinant follicle-stimulating hormone (FSH) for the induction of ovulation in women and spermatogenesis in men (orphan); adjunct to assisted reproductive technologies (ART)*

follitropin beta INN *recombinant follicle-stimulating hormone (FSH) for the induction of ovulation in women and spermatogenesis in men; adjunct to assisted reproductive technologies (ART)* [also: menotropins]

follotropin [see: menotropins]

Follow-Up [see: **Carnation Follow-Up**]

Folmor tablets ℞ *nutritional supplement for homocystinemia* [folic acid; vitamins B₆ and B₁₂; Primorine (q.v.)] 2.5•25•2•875 mg

Folpace tablets ℞ *vitamin/magnesium supplement* [vitamins B₆ and B₁₂; folic acid; vitamin E; magnesium] 25 mg•425 mcg•2.05 mg•100 IU•100 mg ℞ Phillips'

Foltrin capsules ℞ *hematinic* [ferrous fumarate; cyanocobalamin; ascorbic acid; intrinsic factor concentrate; folic acid] 110 mg•15 mcg•75 mg•240 mg•0.5 mg ℞ Voltaren

Foltx tablets ℞ *vitamin B therapy for arteriosclerosis, cardiovascular and peripheral vascular disease, and neurological disorders* [vitamins B₆ and B₁₂; folic acid] 25•2•2.5 mg ℞ Flutex

Folvite IM injection ℞ *hematinic* [folic acid] 5 mg/mL ℞ Velivet

fomepizole USAN, INN *antidote; alcohol dehydrogenase inhibitor for methanol or ethylene glycol poisoning (orphan)* 1 g/mL injection

FOMI; FOMi (fluorouracil, Oncovin, mitomycin) *chemotherapy protocol*

fomidacillin INN, BAN

fominoben INN [also: fominoben HCl]

fominoben HCl JAN [also: fominoben]

fomivirsen sodium *antisense drug for AIDS-related CMV retinitis*

fomocaine INN, BAN ℞ Foamicon

fonatol [see: diethylstilbestrol]

fonazine mesylate USAN *serotonin inhibitor* [also: dimetotiazine; dimethothiazine]

fondaparinux sodium *selective factor Xa inhibitor; antithrombotic for prevention of deep vein thrombosis (DVT) and acute pulmonary embolism (PE) following abdominal or orthopedic surgery*

fontarsol [see: dichlorophenarsine HCl]

fopirtoline INN

Foradil encapsulated powder for inhalation (used with an **Aerolizer** device) ℞ *twice-daily bronchodilator for asthma, COPD, and emphysema* [formoterol fumarate] 12 mcg/dose

Forane liquid for vaporization ℞ *inhalation general anesthetic* [isoflurane] ℞ Fourneau 309

forasartan USAN *antihypertensive; angiotensin II receptor antagonist; treatment for congestive heart failure (CHF)*

foreign colombo *medicinal herb* [see: colombo]

forfenimex INN

Formalaz topical liquid in a roll-on bottle ℞ *drying agent for pre- and postsurgical removal of warts* [formaldehyde] 10%

formaldehyde solution USP *disinfectant; anhidrotic for hyperhidrosis and bromhidrosis*

Formalyde-10 spray ℞ *anhidrotic for hyperhidrosis and bromhidrosis* [formaldehyde] 10%

formebolone INN, BAN

formetamide [see: formetorex]

formetorex INN

formidacillin [see: fomidacillin]

forminitrazole INN, BAN

formocortal USAN, INN, BAN *corticosteroid; anti-inflammatory*

formoterol INN *long-acting β₂ agonist; sympathomimetic bronchodilator for asthma and bronchospasm* [also: eformoterol; formoterol fumarate]

formoterol fumarate USAN, JAN *long-acting β₂ agonist; sympathomimetic bronchodilator for asthma and bronchospasm, and for the long-term treatment of COPD* [also: formoterol; eformoterol fumarate]

Formula 44 Cough Relief oral liquid OTC *antitussive* [dextromethorphan hydrobromide; alcohol 5%] 10 mg/5 mL

Formula 44D Cough & Head Congestion Relief oral liquid OTC *antitussive; decongestant* [dextromethorphan hydrobromide; phenylephrine HCl] 20•10 mg/15 mL

Formula 44E Cough & Chest Congestion Relief; Pediatric Formula 44e Cough & Chest Congestion Relief oral liquid OTC *antitussive; expectorant* [dextromethorphan hydrobromide; guaifenesin] 20•200 mg/15 mL; 10•100 mg/15 mL

Formula 44M Cough, Cold, & Flu Relief oral liquid OTC *antitussive; antihistamine; analgesic; antipyretic* [dextromethorphan hydrobromide; chlorpheniramine maleate; acetaminophen] 30•4•650 mg/20 mL

Formula 44M Pediatric Cough & Cold Relief oral liquid (discontinued 2007) OTC *antitussive; antihistamine; for adults and children ≥ 6 years* [dextromethorphan hydrobromide; chlorpheniramine maleate] 15•2 mg/15 mL

Formula 405 cleansing bar, cream OTC *therapeutic skin cleanser*

Formula B tablets ℞ *vitamin supplement* [multiple B vitamins; vitamin C; folic acid] ±•500•0.5 mg

Formula B Plus tablets ℞ *vitamin/mineral/iron supplement* [multiple vitamins & minerals; ferrous fumarate; folic acid; biotin] ±•27•0.8•0.15 mg

Formula EM oral solution OTC *antiemetic for nausea associated with influenza, morning sickness, motion sickness, inhalation anesthesia, or food and drink indiscretions* [phosphorated carbohydrate solution (fructose; dextrose; phosphoric acid)] 1.87 g•1.87 g•21.5 mg per 5 mL

Formula VM-2000 tablets OTC *dietary supplement* [multiple vitamins & minerals; multiple amino acids; iron; folic acid; biotin] ±•5 mg•0.2 mg•50 mcg

Formulation R anorectal cream, anorectal ointment OTC *temporary relief of hemorrhoidal symptoms* [phenylephrine HCl] 0.25%

4′-formylacetanilide thiosemicarbazone [see: thioacetazone; thiacetazone]

foropafant INN

forskolin [see: colforsin]

Forta Drink powder OTC *enteral nutritional therapy* [lactose-free formula]

Forta Shake powder OTC *enteral nutritional therapy* [milk-based formula]

Fortamet extended-release film-coated tablets ℞ *biguanide antidiabetic that decreases hepatic glucose production* and increases cellular response to insulin [metformin HCl] 500, 1000 mg

Fortaz powder or frozen premix for IV or IM injection ℞ *third-generation cephalosporin antibiotic* [ceftazidime] 0.5, 1, 2, 6 g ⑨ Ferretts

Fortel Midstream test stick for professional use ℞ *in vitro diagnostic aid; urine pregnancy test*

Fortel Plus test kit for home use OTC *in vitro diagnostic aid; urine pregnancy test*

Fortéo subcu injection via prefilled self-injector ℞ *parathyroid hormone (PTH) for postmenopausal osteoporosis in women and primary or hypogonadal osteoporosis in men* [teriparatide] 20 mcg/day (750 mcg/3 mL injector)

Fortical nasal spray in a metered-dose inhaler ℞ *calcium regulator for postmenopausal osteoporosis* [calcitonin (salmon)] 200 U/0.9 mL dose

fortimicin A [now: astromicin sulfate]

Fortovase softgels (discontinued 2005) ℞ *antiretroviral protease inhibitor for HIV* [saquinavir] 200 mg

40 winks capsules OTC *antihistamine; sleep aid* [diphenhydramine HCl] 50 mg

Forvade gel *investigational (Phase I/II) nucleoside antiviral for AIDS-related genital herpes and Kaposi sarcoma* [cidofovir]

Forzest (Indian name for U.S. product Cialis)

Fosamax tablets, oral solution ℞ *bisphosphonate bone resorption inhibitor for Paget disease and corticosteroid-induced or age-related osteoporosis in men and women; investigational (orphan) for bone manifestations of Gaucher disease and pediatric osteogenesis imperfecta* [alendronate sodium] 5, 10, 35, 40, 70 mg; 70 mg/bottle

Fosamax Plus D caplets ℞ *once-weekly bisphosphonate bone resorption inhibitor and vitamin D supplement for age-related osteoporosis in men and women* [alendronate sodium; cholecalciferol] 70 mg•70mcg (2800 IU), 70•140 mcg (5600 IU)

fosamprenavir calcium USAN *antiretroviral; HIV-1 protease inhibitor; prodrug of amprenavir* (amprenavir conversion=86%)

fosamprenavir sodium USAN *antiretroviral; HIV-1 protease inhibitor; prodrug of amprenavir*

fosaprepitant dimeglumine *antiemetic for chemotherapy-induced nausea and vomiting; prodrug of aprepitant* (aprepitant conversion=61%)

fosarilate USAN, INN *antiviral*

fosazepam USAN, INN, BAN *hypnotic*

Foscan *investigational (NDA filed, orphan) palliative treatment for head and neck cancer* [temoporfin]

foscarnet sodium USAN, INN, BAN *antiviral for cytomegalovirus (CMV) and various herpes viruses (HSV-1, HSV-2)* 24 mg/mL injection

Foscavir IV injection ℞ *antiviral for cytomegalovirus (CMV) retinitis and herpes simplex virus (HSV) infections in immunocompromised patients* [foscarnet sodium] 24 mg/mL

foscolic acid INN

fosenazide INN

fosenopril sodium [see: fosinopril sodium]

fosfestrol INN, BAN *antineoplastic; estrogen* [also: diethylstilbestrol diphosphate]

fosfocreatinine INN

fosfomycin USAN, INN, BAN *antibacterial* [also: fosfomycin calcium; fosfomycin sodium]

fosfomycin calcium JAN *antibacterial* [also: fosfomycin; fosfomycin sodium]

fosfomycin sodium JAN *antibacterial* [also: fosfomycin; fosfomycin calcium]

fosfomycin tromethamine USAN *broad-spectrum bactericidal antibiotic for urinary tract infections*

fosfonet sodium USAN, INN *antiviral*

fosfosal INN

Fosfree tablets OTC *vitamin/iron supplement* [multiple vitamins; iron] ≜ •29 mg

fosfructose trisodium USAN *cardioprotectant*

fosinopril INN, BAN *antihypertensive; angiotensin-converting enzyme (ACE) inhibitor; adjunctive treatment for congestive heart failure (CHF)* [also: fosinopril sodium]

fosinopril sodium USAN *antihypertensive; angiotensin-converting enzyme (ACE) inhibitor; adjunctive treatment for congestive heart failure (CHF)* [also: fosinopril] 10, 20, 40 mg oral

fosinopril sodium & hydrochlorothiazide *antihypertensive; angiotensin-converting enzyme (ACE) inhibitor; diuretic* 10•12.5, 20•12.5 mg

fosinoprilat USAN, INN *antihypertensive*

fosmenic acid INN

fosmidomycin INN

fosphenytoin INN *hydantoin anticonvulsant* [also: fosphenytoin sodium]

fosphenytoin sodium USAN *hydantoin anticonvulsant for grand mal status epilepticus (orphan)* [also: fosphenytoin] 50 mg/mL injection

fospirate USAN, INN *veterinary anthelmintic*

fospropofol disodium *investigational anesthetic; precursor to* **propofol**, *an injectable general anesthetic*

fosquidone USAN, INN, BAN *antineoplastic*

Fosrenol chewable tablets R *phosphate binder for hyperphosphatemia in end-stage renal disease (ESRD)* [lanthanum carbonate] 250, 500, 750, 1000 mg

fostedil USAN, INN *vasodilator; calcium channel blocker*

Fosteum capsule R *dietary supplement for the management of osteopenia and osteoporosis* [genistein; zinc chelazome; cholecalciferol (vitamin D₃)] 27 mg•20 mg•200 IU ℞ P-Hist DM

Fostex Acne Cleansing cream OTC *keratolytic for acne* [salicylic acid] 2%

Fostex Acne Medication Cleansing bar OTC *medicated cleanser for acne* [salicylic acid] 2%

Fostex Medicated Cleansing Shampoo OTC *antiseborrheic; keratolytic* [sulfur; salicylic acid] 2%•2%

fostriecin INN *antineoplastic* [also: fostriecin sodium]

fostriecin sodium USAN *antineoplastic* [also: fostriecin]

Fostril lotion (discontinued 2004) OTC *antiseptic and keratolytic for acne* [sulfur; zinc oxide] ℞ Vistaril

fosveset USAN *ligant excipient*

fotemustine INN, BAN

fo-ti; ho-shou-wu *(Polygonum multiflorum)* root *medicinal herb for atherosclerosis, blood cleansing, constipation, improving liver and kidney function, insomnia, malaria, muscle aches, TB, and weak bones; also used to increase fertility, prevent aging, and promote longevity*

Fototar cream OTC *antipsoriatic; antiseborrheic* [coal tar] 2%

fotretamine INN

Fouchet reagent (solution)

4 Hair softgel capsules OTC *vitamin/mineral/iron supplement* [multiple vitamins & minerals; iron; folic acid; biotin] ±•2.5•33.3•0.25 mg

4 Nails softgel capsules OTC *vitamin/mineral/calcium/iron supplement* [multiple vitamins & minerals; calcium; iron; folic acid; biotin] ±•167•3•0.333•0.0083 mg

4 Trace Elements IV injection R *intravenous nutritional therapy* [multiple trace elements (metals)]

4-Way Fast Acting nasal spray OTC *nasal decongestant* [phenylephrine HCl] 1%

4-Way Menthol nasal spray OTC *nasal decongestant; mild anesthetic* [phenylephrine HCl; menthol] 1%•⅔

4-Way Moisturizing Relief nasal spray OTC *nasal decongestant* [xylometazoline HCl] 0.1%

40DS02 *investigational (orphan) for chronic iron overload due to transfusional treatments*

480848 *lipoprotein-associated phospholipase A2 (Lp-PLA2) blocker; investigational (Phase III) gene-based antiatherosclerotic agent*

Fourneau 309 (available only from the Centers for Disease Control) ℞ *antiparasitic for African trypanosomiasis and onchocerciasis* [suramin sodium] ⑨ Forane

foxglove (*Digitalis ambigua; D. ferriginea; D. grandiflora; D. lanata; D. lutea; D. purpurea*) leaves *medicinal herb for asthma, burns, congestive heart failure, edema, promoting wound healing, and sedation; not generally regarded as safe and effective for children as ingestion can be fatal*

foxglove, American; false foxglove; fern-leaved foxglove *medicinal herb* [see: feverweed]

foxtail *medicinal herb* [see: club moss]

frabuprofen INN

Fractar (trademarked ingredient) *antipsoriatic; antiseborrheic* [crude coal tar]

Fragaria vesca *medicinal herb* [see: strawberry]

Fragmin deep subcu injection, prefilled syringes ℞ *anticoagulant/antithrombotic for prevention of deep vein thrombosis (DVT) and venous thromboembolism (VTE) after abdominal or hip replacement surgery, unstable angina, and myocardial infarction* [dalteparin sodium] 10 000, 25 000 IU (64, 160 mg)/mL; 2500, 5000, 7500, 10 000, 12 500, 15 000, 18 000 IU (16, 32, 48, 64, 80, 96, 115 mg)

framycetin INN, BAN *anti-infective wound dressing*

francium *element* (Fr)

Frangula purshiana *medicinal herb* [see: cascara sagrada]

frankincense (*Boswellia serrata*) leaves and bark *medicinal herb for anaphylaxis, arthritis, asthma, blood cleansing, bronchial disorders, dysentery, rheumatism, skin ailments, ulcers, and wound healing*

fraxinella (*Dictamnus albus*) root, plant, and seed *medicinal herb used as an anthelmintic, diuretic, emmenagogue, expectorant, and febrifuge*

FreAmine III 3% (8.5%) with Electrolytes IV infusion ℞ *total parenteral nutrition (8.5% only); peripheral parenteral nutrition (both)* [multiple essential and nonessential amino acids; electrolytes] ⑨ furomine; Viramune

FreAmine III 8.5%; FreAmine III 10% IV infusion ℞ *total parenteral nutrition; peripheral parenteral nutrition* [multiple essential and nonessential amino acids] ⑨ furomine; Viramune

FreAmine HBC 6.9% IV infusion ℞ *nutritional therapy for high metabolic stress* [multiple branched-chain essential and nonessential amino acids; electrolytes]

Free & Clear shampoo OTC *soap-free therapeutic cleanser*

Freedavite tablets OTC *vitamin/mineral/iron supplement* [multiple vitamins & minerals; ferrous fumarate] ≛•10 mg

Freezone topical liquid OTC *keratolytic* [salicylic acid in a collodion-like vehicle] 13.6% ⑨ Furacin

frentizole USAN, INN, BAN *immunoregulator*

Freshkote eye drops ℞ *moisturizer/lubricant for moderate to severe dry eye* [polyvinyl alcohol; polyvinyl pyrrolidone] 2.7%•2%

fringe tree (*Chionanthus virginica*) bark *medicinal herb used as an aperient, diuretic, febrifuge, and tonic*

fronepidil INN

fropenem INN *broad-spectrum carbapenem antibiotic*

frost plant; frost weed; frostwort *medicinal herb* [see: rock rose]

Frova film-coated tablets ℞ *vascular serotonin 5-HT$_{1B/1D}$ receptor agonist for the acute treatment of migraine* [frovatriptan succinate] 2.5 mg

frovatriptan succinate USAN *vascular serotonin 5-HT$_{1B/1D}$ receptor agonist for the acute treatment of migraine*

froxiprost INN

β-fructofuranosidase [see: sacrosidase]

fructose (D-fructose) USP *nutrient; caloric replacement* [also: levulose]

fructose-1,6-diphosphate (FDP) *investigational (Phase III, orphan)* *cytoprotective agent for vaso-occlusive episodes of sickle cell disease*

Fruit C 100; Fruit C 200; Fruit C 500 chewable tablets OTC *vitamin C supplement* [ascorbic acid and calcium ascorbate] 100 mg; 200 mg; 500 mg

Fruity Chews chewable tablets OTC *vitamin supplement* [multiple vitamins; folic acid] ± •0.3 mg

Fruity Chews with Iron chewable tablets OTC *vitamin/iron supplement* [multiple vitamins; iron; folic acid] ± •12•0.3 mg

frusemide BAN *antihypertensive; loop diuretic* [also: furosemide]

FSF (fibrin-stabilizing factor) [see: factor XIII]

FSH (follicle-stimulating hormone) [see: menotropins]

ftalofyne INN *veterinary anthelmintic* [also: phthalofyne]

ftaxilide INN

ftivazide INN

ftormetazine INN

ftorpropazine INN

5-FU (5-fluorouracil) [see: fluorouracil]

fubrogonium iodide INN

fuchsin, basic USP *topical antibacterial/ antifungal*

Fucus versiculosus medicinal herb [see: kelp]

FUDR powder for intra-arterial infusion R *antimetabolite antineoplastic for GI adenocarcinoma metastatic to the liver; investigational (orphan) for intraperitoneal treatment of gastric cancer; also used for ovarian and kidney cancer* [floxuridine] 500 mg

FUDR; FUdR (5-fluorouracil deoxyribonucleoside) [see: floxuridine]

fuge, devil's *medicinal herb* [see: mistletoe]

Ful-Glo ophthalmic strips OTC *corneal disclosing agent* [fluorescein sodium] 0.6 mg ⊠ Flagyl

Full Spectrum B tablets OTC *vitamin supplement* [multiple B vitamins]

Full Term test kit for professional use R *in vitro diagnostic aid for fetal*

fibronectin; an elevated level indicates an increased risk of preterm birth

fulmicoton [see: pyroxylin]

FU/LV (fluorouracil, leucovorin calcium [rescue]) *chemotherapy protocol for colorectal cancer* [also: F-CL]

FU/LV/CPT-11 (fluorouracil, leucovorin calcium [rescue], CPT-11) *chemotherapy protocol for metastatic colorectal cancer*

fulvestrant USAN *steroidal selective estrogen receptor down-regulator; antineoplastic for metastatic breast cancer in postmenopausal women*

FUM (fluorouracil, methotrexate) *chemotherapy protocol*

fumagillin INN, BAN

Fumaria officinalis medicinal herb [see: fumitory]

fumaric acid NF *acidifier*

Fumatinic sustained-release capsules R *hematinic* [ferrous fumarate; cyanocobalamin; ascorbic acid] 200 mg (66 mg Fe)•5 mcg•60 mg

fumitory (*Fumaria officinalis*) plant *medicinal herb for cardiovascular disorders, constipation, eczema, edema, and hepatobiliary disorders*

fumoxicillin USAN, INN *antibacterial*

Funduscein-10; Funduscein-25 antecubital venous injection R *ophthalmic diagnostic agent* [fluorescein sodium] 10%; 25% ⊠ vindesine

fungicidin [see: nystatin]

fungimycin USAN *antifungal* ⊠ vancomycin

Fungi-Nail topical liquid OTC *antifungal; keratolytic; anesthetic; antiseptic* [resorcinol; salicylic acid; chloroxylenol; benzocaine; alcohol 50%] 1%•2%•2%•0.5% ⊠ vincanol

Fungizone oral suspension (discontinued 2004) R *systemic polyene antifungal; "swish and swallow" treatment for oral candidiasis* [amphotericin B] 100 mg/mL ⊠ fenquizone; Vancocin

Fungizone powder for IV infusion R *systemic polyene antifungal* [amphotericin B deoxycholate] 50 mg/vial ⊠ fenquizone; Vancocin

Fung-O topical liquid OTC *keratolytic* [salicylic acid] 17% ☑ Finac; FNC

Fungoid tincture OTC *antifungal for tinea pedis, tinea cruris, and tinea corporis* [miconazole nitrate] 2%

Fungoid-HC cream ℞ *corticosteroidal anti-inflammatory; antipruritic; antifungal; antibacterial* [miconazole nitrate; hydrocortisone] 2%•1%

FUP (fluorouracil, Platinol) *chemotherapy protocol for gastric cancer*

fuprazole INN ☑ Vaprisol

furacilin [see: nitrofurazone]

Furacin topical solution, cream ℞ *broad-spectrum antibacterial; adjunct to burn therapy and skin grafting* [nitrofurazone] 0.2% ☑ Freezone

Furacin Soluble Dressing ointment ℞ *broad-spectrum antibacterial; adjunct to burn therapy and skin grafting* [nitrofurazone] 0.2%

furacrinic acid INN, BAN

Furadantin oral suspension ℞ *urinary antibiotic* [nitrofurantoin] 25 mg/5 mL

furafylline INN ☑ verofylline

Furalan tablets ℞ *urinary antibiotic* [nitrofurantoin] 50, 100 mg ☑ Verelan; Virilon

furalazine INN

furaltadone INN, BAN

Furamide (available only from the Centers for Disease Control and Prevention) *investigational anti-infective for amebiasis* [diloxanide furoate]

2(3H) furanone di-hydro (FDh) *a precursor to gamma hydroxybutyrate (GHB); a formerly legal alternative to GHB, now also illegal (Schedule I); also known as gamma butyrolactone (GBL)* [see: gamma hydroxybutyrate (GHB)]

furaprofen USAN, INN *anti-inflammatory*

furazabol INN

furazolidone USP, INN, BAN *bactericidal; antiprotozoal; treatment of diarrhea and enteritis due to bacterial or protozoal organisms*

furazolium chloride USAN, INN *antibacterial*

furazolium tartrate USAN *antibacterial*

furbucillin INN

furcloprofen INN

furegrelate INN *thromboxane synthetase inhibitor* [also: furegrelate sodium]

furegrelate sodium USAN *thromboxane synthetase inhibitor* [also: furegrelate]

furethidine INN, BAN

furfenorex INN

furfuryltrimethylammonium iodide [see: furtrethonium iodide]

furidarone INN

furmethoxadone INN

furobufen USAN, INN *anti-inflammatory*

furodazole USAN, INN *anthelmintic*

furofenac INN

furomazine INN

furomine USAN, INN, BAN *ligand* ☑ FreAmine; Viramune

furosemide USAN, USP, INN, JAN *antihypertensive; loop diuretic* [also: frusemide] 20, 40, 80 mg oral; 10 mg/mL oral; 40 mg/5 mL oral; 10 mg/mL injection

furostilbestrol INN

furoxicillin [see: fumoxicillin]

Furoxone oral liquid (discontinued 2005) ℞ *antibacterial* [furazolidone] 50 mg/15 mL ☑ Viroxyn

Furoxone tablets (discontinued 2008) ℞ *bactericidal; antiprotozoal; treatment of diarrhea and enteritis due to bacterial or protozoal organisms* [furazolidone] 100 mg ☑ Viroxyn

fursalan USAN, INN *disinfectant*

fursultiamine INN

furterene INN

furtrethonium iodide INN

furtrimethonium iodide [see: furtrethonium iodide]

fusafungine INN, BAN

fusidate sodium USAN *antibiotic for staphylococcal and other gram-positive infections*

fusidic acid USAN, INN, BAN *topical and systemic antibiotic for staphylococcal and other gram-positive infections*

fusidic acid, sodium salt [see: fusidate sodium]

FUVAC (5-FU, vinblastine, Adriamycin, cyclophosphamide) *chemotherapy protocol* ☑ VAFAC

Fuzeon powder for subcu injection ℞
fusion inhibitor for HIV infection
[enfuvirtide] 90 mg/mL (108 mg/
dose) ⑨ Visine; Vusion

fuzlocillin INN, BAN
fytic acid INN
FZ (flutamide, Zoladex) *chemother-*
apy protocol for prostate cancer

G Phen DM film-coated extended-
release tablets (discontinued 2007)
℞ *antitussive; decongestant; expecto-*
rant [dextromethorphan hydrobromide; phenylephrine HCl; guaifene-
sin] 60•40•600 mg ⑨ C-Phen DM;
GFN 1000/DM 50; Guaifen DM
G17DT immunogen *investigational*
(orphan) agent for gastric cancer and
adenocarcinoma of the pancreas
G-3139 *investigational (Phase I/II)*
adjunct used with docetaxel for AIDS-
related non-Hodgkin lymphoma
^{67}**Ga** [see: gallium citrate Ga 67]
GAA (glucosidase-alpha acid) [see:
alglucosidase alfa]
GABA (gamma-aminobutyric acid)
[see: γ-aminobutyric acid]
gabapentin USAN, INN *anticonvulsant;*
treatment for postherpetic neuralgia;
investigational (orphan) for amyotrophic
lateral sclerosis; investigational (Phase
II) for moderate to severe postmeno-
pausal hot flashes 100, 300, 400, 600,
800 mg oral
gabapentin enacarbil *investigational*
(NDA filed) treatment for moderate-
to-severe restless legs syndrome (RLS);
gabapentin prodrug
Gabapentin GR *investigational (Phase*
III) extended-release formulation for
the treatment of postherpetic neuralgia;
investigational (Phase II) for moderate
to severe postmenopausal hot flashes
[gabapentin]
Gabarone tablets ℞ *anticonvulsant for*
partial-onset seizures; treatment for post-
herpetic neuralgia [gabapentin] 100,
300, 400 mg ⑨ gepirone; Quibron

Gabbromicina *investigational (orphan)*
agent for tuberculosis and Mycobacterium avium *complex (MAC)* [amino-
sidine]
gabexate INN
Gabitril Filmtabs (film-coated tablets)
℞ *anticonvulsant; adjunctive treatment*
for partial seizures [tiagabine HCl] 2,
4, 12, 16 mg ⑨ Capitrol
gaboxadol INN *investigational (Phase*
III) GABA$_A$ *agonist for the treatment*
of insomnia
gadobenate dimeglumine USAN *paren-*
teral radiopaque contrast medium to
enhance MRIs of the brain, spine, and
other CNS tissue [also: gadobenic acid]
gadobenic acid INN *MRI diagnostic aid*
[also: gadobenate dimeglumine]
gadobutrol INN *adjunct to MRI*
gadodiamide USAN, INN, BAN *paren-*
teral radiopaque contrast medium for
thoracic, abdominal, pelvic, and retro-
peritoneal imaging and to enhance
MRIs of the brain, spine, and other
CNS tissue
gadofosveset trisodium USAN *contrast*
agent for vascular enhancement of
MRI scans
gadolinium *element (Gd)*
gadolinium texaphyrin (Gd-Tex)
[now: motexafin gadolinium]
gadopenamide INN
gadopentetate dimeglumine USAN
parenteral radiopaque contrast medium
for imaging of the head and neck, and
to enhance MRIs of the brain, spine,
and other CNS tissue [also: gadopentetic acid]

gadopentetic acid INN, BAN *parenteral MRI contrast medium* [also: gadopentetate dimeglumine]

gadoteric acid INN

gadoteridol USAN, INN, BAN *parenteral radiopaque contrast media for head and neck imaging and to enhance MRIs of the brain, spine, and other CNS tissue*

gadoversetamide USAN, INN *parenteral radiopaque contrast medium to enhance MRIs of the brain, head, and spine and liver structure and vascularity*

gadoxanum USAN *gadolinium-xanthan gum complex; diagnostic aid*

gadoxetate disodium *MRI contrast agent for liver imaging*

gadozelite USAN *gadolinium zeolite complex; diagnostic aid*

gaiactamine [see: guaiactamine]

gaietamine [see: guaiactamine]

galactagogues *a class of agents that promote or increase the flow of breast milk* [also called: lactagogues]

α-D-galactopyranose [see: galactose]

galactose USAN *ultrasound contrast medium*

α-galactosidase [see: agalsidase alfa]

galamustine INN ⊠ clemastine

galangal (*Alpinia galanga; A. officinarum*) *rhizomes medicinal herb for diuresis, fungal infections, gas, hypertension, tumors, ulcers, and worms; also used as an antiplatelet agent*

galantamine USAN, INN *acetylcholinesterase inhibitor to increase cognition in Alzheimer disease*

galantamine hydrobromide USAN *acetylcholinesterase inhibitor to increase cognition in Alzheimer disease; investigational to block the effects of nerve gas agents agents sarin and soman 4, 8, 12, 16, 24 mg oral*

galanthamine [see: galantamine]

Galardin *investigational (orphan) matrix metalloproteinase (MMP) inhibitor for corneal ulcers* [ilomastat]

galdansetron INN, BAN *antiemetic* [also: galdansetron HCl]

galdansetron HCl USAN *antiemetic* [also: galdansetron]

Galeopsis tetrahit *medicinal herb* [see: hemp nettle]

Galida *investigational (Phase III) peroxisome proliferator–activated receptor (PPAR) agonist for type 2 diabetes* [tesaglitazar]

Galium aparine; G. verum *medicinal herb* [see: bedstraw]

Galium odoratum *medicinal herb* [see: sweet woodruff]

gallamine BAN *neuromuscular blocker* [also: gallamine triethiodide] ⊠ calamine; Chlo-Amine

gallamine triethiodide USP, INN *neuromuscular blocker; muscle relaxant* [also: gallamine]

gallamone triethiodide [see: gallamine triethiodide]

gallic acid NF ⊠ Gly-Oxide

gallic acid, bismuth basic salt [see: bismuth subgallate]

gallium *element (Ga)* ⊠ Kolyum

gallium (^{67}Ga) citrate INN *radiopaque contrast medium; radioactive agent* [also: gallium citrate Ga 67] ⊠ Kolyum

gallium citrate Ga 67 USAN, USP *radiopaque contrast medium; radioactive agent* [also: gallium (^{67}Ga) citrate]

gallium nitrate USAN *bone resorption inhibitor for hypercalcemia of malignancy (orphan)*

gallium nitrate nonahydrate [see: gallium nitrate]

gallopamil INN, BAN

gallotannic acid [see: tannic acid]

gallstone solubilizing agents *a class of drugs that dissolve gallstones*

galosemide INN ⊠ Calcium 600 + D

galsulfase *recombinant human enzyme N-acetylgalactosamine 4-sulfatase; treatment for mucopolysaccharidosis VI (MPS VI; Maroteaux-Lamy syndrome) (orphan)*

galtifenin INN

Galvus Ⓔ *tablets (available in Europe) investigational (NDA filed) DPP-4 inhibitor for type 2 diabetes that enhances the function of the body's incretin system to increase insulin production in* the pancreas and reduce glucose production in the liver [vildagliptin] 50 mg

Galzin capsules ℞ copper blocking/complexing agent for Wilson disease (orphan) [zinc acetate] 25, 50 mg ☒ Cleocin; glycine; Quelicin

GamaSTAN S/D IM injection ℞ immunizing agent for hepatitis A, measles, varicella, and rubella; treatment for immunoglobulin G deficiency and acquired agammaglobulinemia [immune globulin, solvent/detergent treated] 2, 10 mL

gamfexine USAN, INN antidepressant

Gamimune N IV infusion (discontinued 2005) ℞ passive immunizing agent for HIV, ITP, and bone marrow transplantation; infection prophylaxis in pediatric HIV (orphan) [immune globulin, solvent/detergent treated] 5%, 10%

gamma benzene hexachloride [now: lindane]

gamma butyraldehyde (GHB-aldehyde) a precursor to gamma hydroxybutyrate (GHB) [see: gamma hydroxybutyrate (GHB)]

gamma butyrolactone (GBL) precursor to gamma hydroxybutyrate (GHB); a formerly legal alternative to GHB, now also illegal (Schedule I); also known as 2(3H) furanone di-hydro (FDh) [see: gamma hydroxybutyrate (GHB)]

gamma globulin [see: globulin, immune]

gamma hydroxybutyrate (GHB) a CNS depressant used as an anesthetic in some countries; sometimes abused as a "date rape" street drug; illegal in the U.S. (Schedule I) as GHB, but available (Schedule III) as sodium oxybate to treat cataplexy due to narcolepsy [also known as: sodium oxybate]

gamma hydroxybutyric (GHB) acid investigational (orphan) CNS depressant for narcolepsy, cataplexy, sleep paralysis, hypnagogic hallucinations, and automatic behavior

gamma oryzanol; gamma-oz medicinal herb [see: rice bran oil]

gamma-aminobutyric acid (GABA) [see: γ-aminobutyric acid]

gamma-c cDNA, retroviral vector investigational (orphan) for X-linked severe combined immunodeficiency disease (SCID)

Gammagard Liquid IV infusion ℞ passive immunizing agent for HIV, idiopathic thrombocytopenic purpura (ITP), B-cell chronic lymphocytic leukemia, and Kawasaki syndrome [immune globulin (IGIV)] 10% (1, 2.5, 5, 10, 20 g/dose)

Gammagard S/D freeze-dried powder for IV infusion (discontinued 2004) ℞ passive immunizing agent for HIV, idiopathic thrombocytopenic purpura (ITP), B-cell chronic lymphocytic leukemia, and Kawasaki syndrome [immune globulin (IGIV), solvent/detergent treated] 50 mg/mL

gamma-hydroxybutyrate sodium [see: sodium oxybate]

gamma-linolenic acid (GLA) natural omega-6 fatty acid; investigational (orphan) for juvenile rheumatoid arthritis

gammaphos [now: ethiofos]

Gammar-P I.V. (pasteurized) powder for IV infusion (discontinued 2007) ℞ passive immunizing agent and immunomodulator for HIV; pediatric treatment of primary immune deficiency (PID) [immune globulin, heat treated; human albumin] 5%●3%

gamma-vinyl GABA (gamma-aminobutyric acid) [see: vigabatrin]

gamolenic acid INN, BAN

Gamunex IV infusion ℞ passive immunizing agent for primary humoral immunodeficiency and idiopathic thrombocytopenic purpura; investigational (orphan) for chronic inflammatory demyelinating polyneuropathy [immune globulin (IGIV), chromatography purified] 10% (1, 2.5, 10, 20 g/dose)

ganaxolone USAN investigational (orphan) neuroactive steroid for infantile spasms

ganciclovir USAN, INN, BAN antiviral for AIDS-related cytomegalovirus

(CMV) infections (orphan) and CMV retinitis (orphan) [also: ganciclovir sodium] 250, 500 mg oral

ganciclovir sodium USAN antiviral for cytomegalovirus retinitis (orphan) [also: ganciclovir]

ganglefene INN

gangliosides, sodium salts investigational (orphan) agent for retinitis pigmentosa

Ganidin NR oral liquid ℞ expectorant [guaifenesin] 100 mg/5 mL

ganirelix INN gonadotropin-releasing hormone (GnRH) antagonist for infertility [also: ganirelix acetate]

ganirelix acetate USAN gonadotropin-releasing hormone (GnRH) antagonist for infertility [also: ganirelix] 250 mcg/0.5 mL injection

Ganite IV infusion ℞ bone resorption inhibitor for hypercalcemia of malignancy (orphan) [gallium nitrate] 25 mg/mL

Gani-Tuss NR oral liquid ℞ narcotic antitussive; expectorant [codeine phosphate; guaifenesin] 10•100 mg/5 mL

Gani-Tuss-DM NR oral liquid ℞ antitussive; expectorant [dextromethorphan hydrobromide; guaifenesin] 10•100 mg/5 mL

Gantrisin pediatric suspension ℞ broad-spectrum sulfonamide antibiotic [sulfisoxazole acetyl; alcohol 0.3%] 500 mg/5 mL

gapicomine INN

gapromidine INN

Garamicina (Mexican name for U.S. product Garamycin)

Garamycin eye drops, ophthalmic ointment ℞ aminoglycoside antibiotic [gentamicin sulfate] 3 mg/mL; 3 mg/g

Garamycin IV or IM injection (discontinued 2006) ℞ aminoglycoside antibiotic [gentamicin sulfate] 40 mg/mL

garcinia (Garcinia cambogia) fruit medicinal herb for appetite suppressant, thermogenesis, and weight control ⊡ Carrasyn; chrysin

Gardasil IM injection ℞ vaccine for genital warts (condylomata acuminata), cervical cancer, and precancerous or dysplastic vaginal, vulvar, or cervical intraepithelial neoplasia caused by HPV infections; currently approved for women 9–26 years [human papillomavirus (HPV) recombinant vaccine, quadrivalent (types 6, 11, 16, and 18)] 20•40•40•20 mcg/0.5 mL dose

garden nightshade medicinal herb [see: bittersweet nightshade]

garden patience medicinal herb [see: yellow dock]

Garfield; Garfield Plus Extra C chewable tablets OTC vitamin supplement [multiple vitamins; folic acid] ±•0.3 mg

Garfield Complete with Minerals chewable tablets OTC vitamin/mineral/iron supplement [multiple vitamins & minerals; iron; folic acid; biotin] ±•18•0.4•0.04 mg

Garfield Plus Iron chewable tablets OTC vitamin/iron supplement [multiple vitamins; iron; folic acid] ±•15•0.3 mg

garget medicinal herb [see: pokeweed]

garlic (Allium sativum) bulb medicinal herb for asthma, cancer immunity, diabetes, digestive disorders, ear infections, flatulence, hypercholesterolemia, hypertension, and infectious diseases ⊡ Keralac

Garlique enteric-coated caplets OTC herbal supplement for cardiovascular support [garlic bulb extract] ≥ 5000 mcg allicin ⊡ Keralac

Gas chewable tablets OTC antiflatulent [simethicone] 125 mg

gas gangrene antitoxin, pentavalent

gas gangrene antitoxin, polyvalent [see: gas gangrene antitoxin, pentavalent]

Gas Permeable Daily Cleaner solution OTC cleaning solution for rigid gas permeable contact lenses

Gas Relief chewable tablets, drops OTC antiflatulent [simethicone] 80, 125 mg; 40 mg/0.6 mL

Gas-Ban tablets OTC antacid; antiflatulent [calcium carbonate; simethicone] 300•40 mg ⊡ Kao-Spen

Gas-Ban DS oral liquid OTC *antacid; antiflatulent* [aluminum hydroxide; magnesium hydroxide; simethicone] 400•400•40 mg/5 mL

gastric acid inhibitors [see: proton pump inhibitors]

gastric mucin BAN

Gastroccult slide test for professional use ℞ *in vitro diagnostic aid for gastric occult blood*

Gastrocrom oral solution ℞ *mastocytosis treatment (orphan)* [cromolyn sodium] 100 mg/5 mL

Gastrografin oral solution ℞ *radiopaque contrast medium for gastrointestinal imaging* [diatrizoate meglumine; diatrizoate sodium (48.29% total iodine)] 660•100 mg/mL (367 mg/mL)

GastroMARK oral suspension (discontinued 2005) ℞ *MRI contrast medium for upper GI tract imaging* [ferumoxsil] 175 mcg iron/mL

Gastrosed drops, tablets (discontinued 2004) ℞ *GI/GU antispasmodic; antiparkinsonian; anticholinergic "drying agent" for allergic rhinitis and hyperhidrosis* [hyoscyamine sulfate] 0.125 mg/mL; 0.125 mg

Gastro-Test string capsules for professional use ℞ *in vitro diagnostic aid for GI disorders*

Gas-X chewable tablets, softgels OTC *antiflatulent* [simethicone] 80, 125 mg; 125 mg

Gas-X Infant Drops, Baby oral drops OTC *antiflatulent* [simethicone] 20 mg/0.3 mL

Gas-X Thin Strips (orally dissolving film) OTC *antiflatulent* [simethicone] 62.5 mg

Gas-X with Maalox chewable tablets OTC *antiflatulent; antacid* [simethicone; calcium carbonate] 125•500 mg

gatifloxacin USAN *broad-spectrum fluoroquinolone antibiotic*

Gattex *investigational (Phase III) glucagon-like peptide 2 (GLP-2) analogue for short bowel syndrome* [teduglutide]

gaulheria oil [see: methyl salicylate]

Gaultheria procumbens *medicinal herb* [see: wintergreen]

gauze, absorbent USP *surgical aid*

gauze, petrolatum USP *surgical aid*

gauze bandage [see: bandage, gauze]

gavestinel USAN *N-methyl-D-aspartate (NMDA) receptor antagonist for stroke*

gavilimomab *investigational (orphan) monoclonal antibody for acute graft vs. host disease*

Gaviscon chewable tablets OTC *antacid* [aluminum hydroxide; magnesium trisilicate] 80•20 mg

Gaviscon oral liquid OTC *antacid* [aluminum hydroxide; magnesium carbonate] 31.7•119.3 mg/5 mL

Gaviscon Antacid chewable tablets OTC *antacid* [aluminum hydroxide; magnesium carbonate] 160•105 mg

Gaviscon Relief Formula chewable tablets, oral liquid OTC *antacid* [aluminum hydroxide; magnesium carbonate] 160•105 mg; 254•237.5 mg/5 mL

Gaviscon-2 chewable tablets (name changed to **Gaviscon Antacid** in 2006)

GBH *a mistaken acronym for gamma hydroxybutyrate (GHB)* [see: gamma hydroxybutyrate (GHB)]

G-Bid DM TR extended-release tablets (discontinued 2007) ℞ *antitussive; expectorant* [dextromethorphan hydrobromide; guaifenesin] 60•1200 mg

GBL (gamma butyrolactone) *precursor to gamma hydroxybutyrate (GHB); a formerly legal alternative to GHB, now also illegal (Schedule I); also known as 2(3H) furanone di-hydro (FDh)* [see: gamma hydroxybutyrate (GHB)]

G-CSF (granulocyte colony-stimulating factor) [see: filgrastim]

Gd texaphyrin [see: motexafin gadolinum]

Gebauer's Spray and Stretch topical spray ℞ *refrigerant anesthetic* [tetrafluoroethane; pentafluoropropane]

gedocarnil INN *treatment of central nervous system disorders*

gefarnate INN, BAN

gefitinib *epidermal growth factor receptor-tyrosine kinase inhibitor (EGFR-TKI); antineoplastic for advanced or metastatic non–small cell lung cancer (NSCLC); investigational (Phase III) for head and neck cancers*

gelatin NF *encapsulating, suspending, binding and coating agent*

gelatin film, absorbable USP *topical hemostat for surgery*

gelatin powder, absorbable *topical hemostat for surgery*

gelatin solution, special intravenous [see: polygeline]

gelatin sponge, absorbable USP *topical hemostat for surgery*

gelcaps (dosage form) *soft gelatin capsules* ⊠ Cal-C-Caps

Gelclair *oral gel "swish and spit" treatment for oral mucositis or lesions; occlusive coating for exposed nerve endings* [povidone; hyaluronic acid] 15 mL/pkt.

Gelfilm; Gelfilm Ophthalmic ℞ *topical hemostat for surgery* [absorbable gelatin film]

Gelfoam powder ℞ *topical hemostat for surgery* [absorbable gelatin powder]

Gelfoam sponge, packs, dental packs, prostatectomy cones ℞ *topical hemostat for surgery* [absorbable gelatin sponge]

Gelhist pediatric oral suspension ℞ *decongestant; antihistamine; sleep aid* [phenylephrine tannate; chlorpheniramine tannate; pyrilamine tannate] 5•2•12.5 mg/5 mL ⊠ Calcet; Glyset

Gel-Kam Rinse dental gel OTC *caries preventative* [stannous fluoride] 0.63%

Gelseal (trademarked dosage form) *soft gelatin capsule* ⊠ Colazal

gelsemium *(Bignonia sempervirens; Gelsemium nitidum; G. sempervirens)* plant *medicinal herb for asthma, neuralgia, and respiratory disorders; not generally regarded as safe and effective as it is highly toxic*

gelsolin, recombinant human *investigational (orphan) for respiratory symptoms of cystic fibrosis and bronchiectasis*

Gel-Tin gel OTC *dental caries preventative* [stannous fluoride] 0.4%

Gelusil chewable tablets OTC *antacid; antiflatulent* [aluminum hydroxide; magnesium hydroxide; simethicone] 200•200•25 mg ⊠ Colazal

gemazocine INN

gemcadiol USAN, INN *antihyperlipoproteinemic*

gemcitabine USAN, INN, BAN *antimetabolite antineoplastic*

gemcitabine & carboplatin *chemotherapy protocol for non–small cell lung cancer (NSCLC)*

gemcitabine & cisplatin *chemotherapy protocol for metastatic bladder cancer*

gemcitabine HCl USAN *antimetabolite antineoplastic for advanced or metastatic breast, ovarian, pancreatic, and non–small cell lung cancers (NSCLC); investigational (Phase III) for cervical cancer; also used for biliary, bladder, and testicular cancer* 200, 1000 mg/dose injection

gemcitabine & vinorelbine *chemotherapy protocol for non–small cell lung cancer (NSCLC)*

gemcitabine-cis (gemcitabine, cisplatin) *chemotherapy protocol for non–small cell lung cancer (NSCLC)*

Gemcor film-coated tablets ℞ *antihyperlipidemic for hypercholesterolemia* [gemfibrozil] 600 mg

gemeprost USAN, INN, BAN *prostaglandin*

gemfibrozil USAN, USP, INN, BAN *triglyceride-lowering antihyperlipidemic for hypertriglyceridemia (types IV and V hyperlipidemia) and coronary heart disease* 600 mg oral

gemifloxacin mesylate USAN *broad-spectrum fluoroquinolone antibiotic for respiratory tract infections*

gemopatrilat USAN *antihypertensive; angiotensin-converting enzyme (ACE) inhibitor; vasopeptidase inhibitor (VPI); treatment for congestive heart failure (CHF)*

gemtuzumab ozogamicin USAN *monoclonal antibody–targeted chemo-*

therapy agent for acute myeloid leuke-mia (orphan)

Gemzar powder for IV infusion ℞ *anti-metabolite antineoplastic for advanced or metastatic breast, ovarian, pancre-atic, and non–small cell lung cancers (NSCLC); investigational (Phase III) for cervical cancer; also used for biliary, bladder, and testicular cancer* [gemcit-abine HCl] 200, 1000 mg/dose

Genac tablets OTC *decongestant; anti-histamine* [pseudoephedrine HCl; tri-prolidine HCl] 60•2.5 mg ℞ Gonak; Kank-a

Genacol Cold & Flu Relief tablets (discontinued 2007) OTC *antitussive; antihistamine; decongestant; analgesic; antipyretic* [dextromethorphan hydro-bromide; chlorpheniramine maleate; pseudoephedrine HCl; acetamino-phen] 15•2•30•500 mg

Genahist tablets, capsules, oral liquid OTC *antihistamine; sleep aid* [diphen-hydramine HCl] 25 mg; 25 mg; 12.5 mg/5 mL

Gen-Allerate tablets OTC *antihistamine* [chlorpheniramine maleate] 4 mg

Genantussidex oral liquid (discontin-ued 2007) ℞ *antitussive; deconges-tant; expectorant* [dextromethorphan hydrobromide; phenylephrine HCl; guaifenesin] 30•10•200 mg/5 mL

Genapap tablets, caplets, rapid-release gelcaps OTC *analgesic; antipyretic* [acetaminophen] 325, 500 mg; 500 mg; 500 mg

Genapap, Children's chewable tab-lets OTC *analgesic; antipyretic* [aceta-minophen] 80 mg

Genapap, Children's elixir (discon-tinued 2008) OTC *analgesic; antipy-retic* [acetaminophen] 160 mg/5 mL

Genapap, Infants' drops (discontin-ued 2008) OTC *analgesic; antipyretic* [acetaminophen] 100 mg/mL

Genaphed tablets OTC *nasal deconges-tant* [pseudoephedrine HCl] 30 mg ℞ Confide

Genaphed Plus tablets ℞ *deconges-tant; antihistamine* [pseudoephedrine HCl; chlorpheniramine maleate] 60•4 mg

Genasal nasal spray OTC *nasal decon-gestant* [oxymetazoline HCl] 0.05% ℞ Goniosol; Gynazole-1; Konsyl

Genasense *antisense antineoplastic; investigational (NDA filed, orphan) for malignant melanoma; investigational (Phase III, orphan) for multiple myeloma and chronic lymphocytic leu-kemia (CLL)* [oblimersen sodium]

Genasoft softgels OTC *laxative; stool softener* [docusate sodium] 100 mg

Genaspor cream OTC *antifungal* [tol-naftate] 1%

Genaton chewable tablets OTC *antacid* [aluminum hydroxide; magnesium trisilicate] 80•20 mg

Genaton oral liquid OTC *antacid* [alu-minum hydroxide; magnesium car-bonate] 31.7•137.3 mg/5 mL

Genaton, Extra Strength chewable tablets OTC *antacid* [aluminum hydroxide; magnesium carbonate] 160•105 mg

Genatuss DM syrup OTC *antitussive; expectorant* [dextromethorphan hydrobromide; guaifenesin] 10•100 mg/5 mL

Gen-bee with C caplets OTC *vitamin supplement* [multiple B vitamins; vitamin C] ±•300 mg

Gendex 75 IV infusion ℞ *plasma vol-ume expander for shock due to hemor-rhage, burns, or surgery* [dextran 75] 6% ℞ Quinidex

gene plasmid hVEGF165 [see: vascu-lar endothelial growth factor (VEGF)]

Genebrom-DM oral liquid (discon-tinued 2007) ℞ *antitussive; antihista-mine; decongestant* [dextromethor-phan hydrobromide; brompheniramine maleate; pseudo-ephedrine HCl] 20•4•60 mg/10 mL

Genebs tablets, caplets OTC *analgesic; antipyretic* [acetaminophen] 325, 500 mg; 500 mg

Genelan-NF oral liquid (discontinued 2007) ℞ *antitussive; antihistamine; decongestant; expectorant* [dextromethorphan hydrobromide; chlorpheniramine maleate; phenylephrine HCl; guaifenesin] 30•4•20•200 mg/10 mL

Generet-500 timed-release tablets OTC *hematinic* [ferrous sulfate; multiple B vitamins; sodium ascorbate] 105• ± •500 mg ② Kineret

Generix-T tablets OTC *vitamin/mineral/iron supplement* [multiple vitamins & minerals; iron] ± •15 mg

GenESA computer-controlled IV infusion device ("GenESA System") (discontinued 2007) Ŗ *cardiac stressor for diagnosis of coronary artery disease* [arbutamine HCl] 0.05 mg/mL ② Canasa

Gene-T-Press oral liquid (discontinued 2007) Ŗ *antitussive; decongestant; expectorant* [dextromethorphan hydrobromide; phenylephrine HCl; guaifenesin] 15•5•200 mg/5 mL

Genevax-HIV *investigational (Phase I/II) vaccine for HIV*

Geneye eye drops OTC *decongestant; vasoconstrictor* [tetrahydrozoline HCl] 0.05%

Geneye Extra eye drops (discontinued 2006) OTC *decongestant; vasoconstrictor; moisturizer/lubricant* [tetrahydrozoline HCl; polytheylene glycol 400] 0.05%•1%

Genfiber powder OTC *bulk laxative* [psyllium hydrophilic mucilloid] 3.4 g/tsp.

Gengraf capsules, oral drops Ŗ *immunosuppressant for allogenic kidney, liver, and heart transplants (orphan), rheumatoid arthritis (RA), and psoriasis* [cyclosporine] 25, 100 mg; 100 mg/mL

Genista tinctoria medicinal herb [see: dyer's broom]

genistein *one of several soy isoflavones that provide cell-protective effects*

genistin *isoform precursor to genistein* [q.v.]

Gen-K powder for oral solution Ŗ *potassium supplement* [potassium chloride] 20 mEq K/pkt. ② Gonak; Kank-a

genophyllin [see: aminophylline]

Genoptic eye drops Ŗ *aminoglycoside antibiotic* [gentamicin sulfate] 3 mg/mL

Genoptic S.O.P. ophthalmic ointment Ŗ *aminoglycoside antibiotic* [gentamicin sulfate] 3 mg/g

Genotropin MiniQuick (prefilled syringes in packs of 7) Ŗ *growth hormone for children and adults with congenital or endogenous growth hormone deficiency (GHD), short bowel syndrome, or AIDS-wasting syndrome; for children with Turner syndrome, Prader-Willi syndrome, or renal-induced growth failure* [somatropin] 0.2, 0.4, 0.6, 0.8, 1, 1.2, 1.4, 1.6, 1.8, 2 mg/syringe

Genotropin powder for subcu injection Ŗ *growth hormone for children and adults with congenital or endogenous growth hormone deficiency (GHD), short bowel syndrome, or AIDS-wasting syndrome; for children with Turner syndrome, Prader-Willi syndrome, or renal-induced growth failure* [somatropin] 5.8, 13.8 mg (17.4, 41.4 IU) per vial

Genpril film-coated tablets (discontinued 2006) OTC *analgesic; antiarthritic; antipyretic; nonsteroidal anti-inflammatory drug (NSAID) for mild to moderate pain, migraine headaches, and primary dysmenorrhea* [ibuprofen] 200 mg ② quinapril

Genprin tablets OTC *analgesic; antipyretic; anti-inflammatory; antirheumatic* [aspirin] 325 mg

Gentacidin eye drops Ŗ *aminoglycoside antibiotic* [gentamicin sulfate] 3 mg/mL

Gentak eye drops (discontinued 2005) Ŗ *aminoglycoside antibiotic* [gentamicin sulfate] 3 mg/mL

Gentak ophthalmic ointment Ŗ *aminoglycoside antibiotic* [gentamicin sulfate] 3 mg/g

gentamicin BAN *aminoglycoside antibiotic* [also: gentamicin sulfate]

gentamicin sulfate USAN, USP *aminoglycoside antibiotic* [also: gentamicin] 3 mg/mL eye drops; 3 mg/g ophthalmic; 0.1% topical; 10, 40 mg/mL injection

gentamicin sulfate, liposomal *investigational (orphan) agent for disseminated* Mycobacterium avium-intracellulare *infection*

Gentamicin Sulfate in 0.9% Sodium Chloride injection ℞ *aminoglycoside antibiotic* [gentamicin sulfate; sodium chloride] 0.8, 0.9, 1, 1.2, 1.4, 1.6 mg/mL (60, 70, 80, 90, 100 mg/dose)

gentamicin-impregnated polymethyl methacrylate (PMMA) beads *investigational (orphan) agent for chronic osteomyelitis*

GenTeal gel OTC *ophthalmic moisturizer/lubricant* [carboxymethylcellulose sodium; hypromellose] 0.25%•0.3% ⊉ Cantil

GenTeal; GenTeal Mild eye drops OTC *moisturizer/lubricant* [hydroxypropyl methylcellulose] ⊉ Cantil

Gentex HC oral liquid ℞ *narcotic antitussive; decongestant; expectorant* [hydrocodone bitartrate; phenylephrine HCl; guaifenesin] 2.5•7.5•100 mg/5 mL

Gentex LA extended-release caplets ℞ *decongestant; expectorant* [phenylephrine HCl; guaifenesin] 23.75•650 mg

gentian (*Gentiana lutea*) root *medicinal herb for aiding digestion, appetite stimulation, arthritis, hysteria, jaundice, liver disorders, and sore throat*

gentian violet USP *topical anti-infective/antifungal* [also: methylrosanilinium chloride] 1%, 2%

gentisic acid ethanolamide NF *complexing agent*

Gentlax tablets OTC *stimulant laxative* [bisacodyl] 5 mg

Gentle Cream OTC *moisturizer; emollient*

Gentran 40 IV injection ℞ *plasma volume expander for shock due to hemorrhage, burns, or surgery* [dextran 40] 10% ⊉ Contrin

Gentran 70 IV infusion ℞ *plasma volume expander for shock due to hemorrhage, burns, or surgery* [dextran 70] 6% ⊉ Contrin

Geocillin film-coated caplets (discontinued 2008) ℞ *extended-spectrum penicillin antibiotic* [carbenicillin indanyl sodium] 500 mg (382 mg base)

Geodon capsules ℞ *novel (atypical) benzisoxazole antipsychotic for schizophrenia and manic episodes of a bipolar disorder* [ziprasidone HCl] 20, 40, 60, 80 mg ⊉ codeine; Kadian; Quad Tann

Geodon powder for IM injection ℞ *novel (atypical) benzisoxazole antipsychotic for rapid control of acute agitation in schizophrenic patients* [ziprasidone mesylate] 20 mg ⊉ codeine; Kadian; Quad Tann

gepefrine INN

gepirone INN *azapirone tranquilizer; anxiolytic; antidepressant* [also: gepirone HCl] ⊉ Gabarone; Quibron

gepirone HCl USAN *investigational (NDA filed) azapirone tranquilizer; anxiolytic; antidepressant* [also: gepirone]

Geranium maculatum medicinal herb [see: alum root]

2-geranylhydroquinone [see: geroquinol]

Gerardia pedicularia medicinal herb [see: feverweed]

Geravim elixir OTC *vitamin/mineral supplement* [multiple B vitamins & minerals] ⊉ CarraFoam; Kerafoam

Geravite elixir OTC *geriatric vitamin supplement* [multiple B vitamins] ⊉ Carafate

Gerber Baby Low Iron Formula oral liquid, powder for oral liquid OTC *total or supplementary infant feeding*

Gerber Soy Formula powder OTC *hypoallergenic infant formula* [soy protein formula]

Geref powder for IV injection ℞ *diagnostic aid for pituitary function; treatment for growth hormone deficiency (orphan), anovulation (orphan), and AIDS-related weight loss (orphan)* [sermorelin acetate] 50 mcg ⊉ Kariva

Geri SS lotion OTC *moisturizer; emollient*

Geridium tablets ℞ *urinary tract analgesic for relief of pain, burning, urgency, and frequency due to mucosal irritation from surgery, catheterization, endoscopic procedures, or trauma; adjunct*

to antibacterial agents for urinary tract infections [phenazopyridine HCl] 100, 200 mg ⊡ Karidium

Geri-Hydrolac cream OTC *moisturizer; emollient* [ammonium lactate] 12%

Geri-Hydrolac 5% lotion OTC *moisturizer; emollient* [lactic acid, buffered] 5%

Gerimal sublingual tablets, tablets ℞ *cognition adjuvant for age-related mental capacity decline* [ergoloid mesylates] 0.5, 1 mg; 1 mg ⊡ caramel

Gerimed film-coated tablets OTC *geriatric vitamin/mineral supplement* [multiple vitamins & minerals]

Geriot film-coated tablets OTC *hematinic; vitamin/mineral supplement* [carbonyl iron; multiple vitamins & minerals; folic acid; biotin] 50 mg•±•0.4 mg•45 mcg ⊡ carrot

Geri-Silk bath oil OTC *moisturizer; emollient* [mineral oil]

Geri-Soft lotion OTC *moisturizer; emollient*

Geritol Complete tablets OTC *vitamin/mineral/iron supplement* [multiple vitamins & minerals; ferrous fumarate; folic acid; biotin] ±•18 mg•0.4 mg•45 mcg

Geritol Extend caplets OTC *vitamin/mineral/iron supplement* [multiple vitamins & minerals; ferrous fumarate; folic acid] ±•10•0.2 mg

Geritol Tonic oral liquid OTC *hematinic* [ferric pyrophosphate; multiple B vitamins; alcohol 12%] 18•± mg/15 mL

Geritonic oral liquid OTC *hematinic* [ferric ammonium citrate; liver fraction 1; multiple B vitamins & minerals; alcohol 20%] 105•375•± mg/15 mL

Gerivite oral liquid OTC *geriatric vitamin/mineral supplement* [multiple B vitamins & minerals; alcohol 18%] ⊡ Carafate

Gerivites tablets (discontinued 2004) OTC *hematinic; vitamin/mineral supplement* [ferrous sulfate; multiple vitamins & minerals; folic acid] 50•±•0.4 mg

German valerian *medicinal herb* [see: valerian]

Germanin (available only from the Centers for Disease Control) ℞ *antiparasitic for African trypanosomiasis and onchocerciasis* [suramin sodium]

germanium *element (Ge)* ⊡ carumonam

germicides *a class of agents that destroy micro-organisms* [see also: antiseptics; disinfectants]

geroquinol INN

Geroton Forte oral liquid OTC *geriatric vitamin/mineral supplement* [multiple B vitamins & minerals; alcohol 13.5%]

gesarol [see: chlorophenothane]

gestaclone USAN, INN *progestin*

gestadienol INN

gestanin [see: allyloestrenol]

Gestiva injection *investigational (NDA filed) long-acting progesterone to prevent preterm birth in women with a history of preterm delivery* [17 alpha-hydroxyprogesterone caproate (17P)]

gestodene USAN, INN, BAN *progestin*

gestonorone caproate USAN, INN *progestin* [also: gestronol]

gestrinone USAN, INN *progestin*

gestronol BAN *progestin* [also: gestonorone caproate]

Get Better Bear Sore Throat Pops OTC *throat emollient and protectant* [pectin] 19 mg

Gets-It topical liquid OTC *keratolytic* [salicylic acid; zinc chloride; alcohol 28%] ⊡ QTest

gevotroline INN *antipsychotic* [also: gevotroline HCl]

gevotroline HCl USAN *antipsychotic* [also: gevotroline]

Gevrabon oral liquid OTC *vitamin/mineral supplement* [multiple B vitamins & minerals; alcohol 18%]

Gevral tablets OTC *vitamin/mineral/iron supplement* [multiple vitamins & minerals; ferrous fumarate; folic acid] ±•18 mg•0.4 mg

Gevral Protein powder OTC *oral protein supplement* [calcium caseinate; sucrose]

G-F 20 [see: hylan G-F 20]

GFN (guaifenesin) [q.v.]

GFN 550/PSE 60/DM 30 sustained-release tablets (discontinued 2007) ℞ expectorant; decongestant; antitussive [guaifenesin; pseudoephedrine HCl; dextromethorphan hydrobromide] 550•60•30 mg

GFN 600/Phenylephrine 20 tablets ℞ expectorant; decongestant [guaifenesin; phenylephrine HCl] 600•20 mg

GFN 600/PSE 60/DM 30 sustained-release caplets ℞ expectorant; decongestant; antitussive [guaifenesin; pseudoephedrine HCl; dextromethorphan hydrobromide] 600•60•30 mg

GFN 1000/DM 50 sustained-release caplets (discontinued 2007) ℞ expectorant; antitussive [guaifenesin; dextromethorphan hydrobromide] 1000•50 mg ⊡ C-Phen DM; G Phen DM; Guaifen DM

GFN 1000/DM 60; GFN 1200/DM 60 sustained-release caplets ℞ expectorant; antitussive [guaifenesin; dextromethorphan hydrobromide] 1000•60 mg; 1200•60 mg ⊡ C-Phen DM; G Phen DM; Guaifen DM

GFN 1200/DM 20/PE 40 extended-release tablets ℞ expectorant; antitussive; decongestant [guaifenesin; dextromethorphan hydrobromide; phenylephrine HCl] 1200•20•40 mg

GFN 1200/DM 60/PSE 120 sustained-release caplets (discontinued 2007) ℞ expectorant; antitussive; decongestant [guaifenesin; dextromethorphan hydrobromide; pseudoephedrine HCl] 1200•60•120 mg

GFN/PSE sustained-release tablets ℞ expectorant; decongestant [guaifenesin; pseudoephedrine HCl] 1200•120 mg

GHB (gamma hydroxybutyrate) a CNS depressant used as an anesthetic in some countries, produced and abused as a "date rape" street drug in the U.S.; illegal in the U.S. (Schedule I) [the sodium salt is medically known as sodium oxybate]

GHB-aldehyde (gamma butyraldehyde) a precursor to gamma hydroxy-butyrate (GHB) [see: gamma hydroxybutyrate (GHB)]

GHRF; GH-RF (growth hormone-releasing factor) [q.v.]

Gilead, balm of medicinal herb [see: balm of Gilead]

Gilphex TR film-coated caplets ℞ decongestant; expectorant [phenylephrine HCl; guaifenesin] 10•388 mg

Giltuss oral liquid ℞ antitussive; decongestant; expectorant [dextromethorphan hydrobromide; phenylephrine HCl; guaifenesin] 15•10•300 mg/5 mL ⊡ Glutose

Giltuss Ped-C oral liquid ℞ narcotic antitussive; decongestant; expectorant; for children 2–12 years [codeine phosphate; phenylephrine HCl; guaifenesin] 3•2.5•50 mg/5 mL

Giltuss Pediatric oral liquid ℞ antitussive; decongestant; expectorant; for children 2–12 years [dextromethorphan hydrobromide; phenylephrine HCl; guaifenesin] 3•2.5•50 mg/5 mL

Giltuss TR capsules, tablets OTC antitussive; decongestant; expectorant [dextromethorphan hydrobromide; phenylephrine HCl; guaifenesin] 14•7•288 mg; 30•20•600 mg

ginger (Zingiber officinale) root medicinal herb for childhood diseases, colds, colic, dizziness, fever, flu, gas pains, headache, indigestion, morning sickness, nausea, poor circulation, toothache, and vestibular disorders ⊡ canaigre

ginger, wild medicinal herb [see: wild ginger]

ginkgo (Ginkgo biloba) leaves medicinal herb for Alzheimer disease, antioxidant, anxiety, asthma, attention-deficit disorder, chilblains, cerebral insufficiency, dementia, dizziness, memory loss, poor circulation, Raynaud disease, stroke, and tinnitus

ginseng (Panax spp.) root medicinal herb for age spots, blood diseases, depression, hemorrhage, increasing endurance and longevity, and stress; also used as an aphrodisiac

ginseng, blue; yellow ginseng *medicinal herb* [see: blue cohosh]

giparmen INN ⊡ Cuprimine

giractide INN

girisopam INN

gitalin NF [also: gitalin amorphous] ⊡ guaietolin

gitalin amorphous INN [also: gitalin]

gitaloxin INN

gitoformate INN

gitoxin 16-formate [see: gitaloxin]

gitoxin pentaacetate [see: pengitoxin]

GLA (gamma-linolenic acid) [q.v.]

glacial acetic acid [see: acetic acid, glacial]

Gladase ointment ℞ *proteolytic enzyme for debridement of necrotic tissue; vulnerary* [papain; urea] 830 000 U•100 mg per gram

Gladase-C ointment ℞ *proteolytic enzyme for debridement of necrotic tissue; vulnerary; topical wound deodorant* [papain; urea; chlorophyllin copper complex] 521 700 U/g•10%•0.5%

glafenine INN, JAN

glaphenine [see: glafenine]

glatiramer acetate USAN *immunomodulator for relapsing-remitting multiple sclerosis* (orphan)

Glauber salt [see: sodium sulfate]

glaucarubin

Glaucon Drop-Tainers (eye drops) (discontinued 2004) ℞ *antiglaucoma agent* [epinephrine HCl] 1%, 2% ⊡ Glyquin; Qualaquin

glaze, pharmaceutical NF *tablet-coating agent*

glaziovine INN

Gleevec film-coated tablets ℞ *antineoplastic for chronic myeloid leukemia* (orphan), *acute lymphoblastic leukemia, chronic eosinophilic leukemia, myelodysplastic diseases, gastrointestinal stromal tumors* (orphan), *systemic mastitis, and dermatofibrosarcoma protuberans* [imatinib mesylate] 100, 400 mg ⊡ Glivec

glemanserin USAN, INN *anxiolytic*

gleptoferron USAN, INN, BAN *veterinary hematinic*

Gliadel wafers ℞ *nitrosourea-type alkylating antineoplastic cerebral implants for excised brain tumors* [carmustine] 7.7 mg

gliamilide USAN, INN *antidiabetic*

glibenclamide INN, BAN *sulfonylurea antidiabetic that stimulates insulin secretion in the pancreas* [also: glyburide]

glibornuride USAN, INN, BAN *antidiabetic*

glibutimine INN

glicaramide INN

glicetanile INN *antidiabetic* [also: glicetanile sodium]

glicetanile sodium USAN *antidiabetic* [also: glicetanile]

gliclazide INN, BAN *sulfonylurea antidiabetic that stimulates insulin secretion in the pancreas*

glicondamide INN

glidazamide INN

gliflumide USAN, INN *antidiabetic*

glimepiride USAN, INN, BAN *sulfonylurea antidiabetic that stimulates insulin secretion in the pancreas* 1, 2, 4 mg oral

glipentide [see: glisentide]

glipizide USAN, INN, BAN *sulfonylurea antidiabetic for type 2 diabetes that stimulates insulin secretion in the pancreas* 5, 10 mg oral

Glipizide ER extended-release tablets ℞ *sulfonylurea antidiabetic that stimulates insulin secretion in the pancreas* [glipizide] 2.5, 5, 10 mg

glipizide & metformin HCl *antidiabetic combination for type 2 diabetes that stimulates insulin secretion in the pancreas, decreases hepatic glucose production, and increases cellular response to insulin* 2.5•250, 2.5•500, 5•500 mg

gliquidone INN, BAN

glisamuride INN

glisentide INN

glisindamide INN

glisolamide INN

glisoxepide INN, BAN

Glivec (foreign name for U.S. product Gleevec) ⊡ Gleevec

globin zinc insulin INN [also: insulin, globin zinc]

globulin, aerosolized pooled immune *investigational (orphan) agent for respiratory syncytial virus lower respiratory tract disease*

globulin, immune USP *passive immunizing agent for HIV, ITP, B-cell CLL, PID, and bone marrow transplantation; infection prophylaxis in pediatric HIV (orphan); investigational (orphan) for juvenile rheumatoid arthritis, GI disturbances due to autism, and idiopathic myopathies* [also see: Rh$_0$D immune globulin]

globulin, immune, with high titers of West Nile virus antibodies *investigational (orphan) passive immunizing agent for the West Nile virus*

globulin, immune human serum [now: globulin, immune]

Glossets (trademarked dosage form) *sublingual or rectal administration*

gloxazone USAN, INN, BAN *veterinary anaplasmodastat*

gloximonam USAN, INN *antibacterial*

GlucaGen Diagnostic Kit IV injection ℞ *agent to inhibit movement of the gastrointestinal tract during radiographic procedures* [glucagon, recombinant] 1 mg

GlucaGen Emergency Kit; GlucaGen HypoKit subcu, IV, or IM injection ℞ *emergency treatment of hypoglycemic crisis* [glucagon, recombinant] 1 mg

glucagon USP, INN, BAN *antidiabetic; glucose elevating agent; diagnostic aid for GI imaging*

Glucagon Diagnostic Kit IM or IV injection ℞ *to inhibit GI tract movement during radiographic procedures* [glucagon, recombinant] 1 mg (1 U)

Glucagon Emergency Kit subcu, IM, or IV injection ℞ *emergency treatment for hypoglycemic crisis* [glucagon, recombinant] 1 mg (1 U)

glucalox INN [also: glycalox] ② Glyco-Lax

glucametacin INN

glucan synthesis inhibitors *a class of antifungals* [also: echinocandins]

D-**glucaric acid, calcium salt tetrahydrate** [see: calcium saccharate]

gluceptate USAN, USP, INN, BAN *combining name for radicals or groups*

gluceptate sodium USAN *pharmaceutic aid*

Glucerna; Glucerna Select; Glucerna Weight Loss Shake ready-to-use oral liquid OTC *enteral nutritional therapy for abnormal glucose tolerance* ② glycerin

D-**glucitol** [see: sorbitol]

D-**glucitol hexanicotinate** [see: sorbinicate]

β-**glucocerebrosidase, macrophage-targeted** [see: alglucerase]

glucocerebrosidase, recombinant retroviral vector *investigational (orphan) enzyme replacement for types I, II, or III Gaucher disease*

glucocerebrosidase-β-glucosidase [see: alglucerase]

glucocorticoids *a class of adrenal cortical steroids that modify the body's immune response*

Glucofilm reagent strips for home use OTC *in vitro diagnostic aid for blood glucose*

glucoheptonic acid, calcium salt [see: calcium gluceptate]

glucomannan (*Amorphophallus konjac*) *root medicinal herb for constipation, diverticular disease, hemorrhoids, hypercholesterolemia, and obesity; it may produce altered insulin requirements or hypoglycemia in diabetics*

Glucometer Encore; Glucometer Elite reagent strips for home use OTC *in vitro diagnostic aid for blood glucose*

D-**gluconic acid, calcium salt** [see: calcium gluconate]

D-**gluconic acid, magnesium salt** [see: magnesium gluconate]

D-**gluconic acid, monopotassium salt** [see: potassium gluconate]

D-**gluconic acid, monosodium salt** [see: sodium gluconate]

Glucophage film-coated tablets ℞ *biguanide antidiabetic that decreases hepatic glucose production and* *increases cellular response to insulin* [metformin HCl] 500, 850, 1000 mg

Glucophage XR extended-release caplets ℞ *once-daily biguanide antidiabetic* [metformin HCl] 500, 750 mg

β-D-glucopyranuronamide [see: glucuronamide]

glucosamine USAN, INN *pharmaceutic aid; natural remedy for osteoarthritis*

glucosamine sulfate *natural remedy for osteoarthritis*

glucose NF *blood glucose elevating agent for hypoglycemia; diagnostic aid for diabetes; tablet binder and coating agent* ℞ Caelyx; click.easy

***d*-glucose** [see: dextrose]

***d*-glucose monohydrate** [see: dextrose]

glucose oxidase

glucose polymers *caloric replacement*

Glucostix reagent strips for home use OTC *in vitro diagnostic aid for blood glucose*

glucosulfamide INN

glucosulfone INN

glucosylceramidase [see: alglucerase]

Glucotrol tablets ℞ *sulfonylurea antidiabetic that stimulates insulin secretion in the pancreas* [glipizide] 5, 10 mg

Glucotrol XL extended-release tablets ℞ *sulfonylurea antidiabetic that stimulates insulin secretion in the pancreas* [glipizide] 2.5, 5, 10 mg

Glucovance film-coated caplets ℞ *antidiabetic combination for type 2 diabetes that stimulates insulin secretion in the pancreas, decreases hepatic glucose production, and increases cellular response to insulin* [glyburide; metformin HCl] 1.25•250, 2.5•500, 5•500 mg

glucurolactone INN

glucuronamide INN, BAN

Glumetza extended-release film-coated tablets ℞ *biguanide antidiabetic that decreases hepatic glucose production and increases cellular response to insulin* [metformin HCl] 500, 1000 mg

glunicate INN

gluside [see: saccharin]

gluside, soluble [see: saccharin sodium]

glusoferron INN

glutamic acid (L-glutamic acid) USAN, INN *nonessential amino acid; symbols: Glu, E 340,* 500 mg oral

glutamic acid HCl *gastric acidifier*

glutamine (L-glutamine) USAN, USP, JAN *nonessential amino acid that reduces fatigue, increases exercise endurance, and strengthens the GI tract; growth hormone secretagogue; investigational (NDA filed) for oral mucositis; investigational (orphan) for short bowel syndrome and sickle cell disease; symbol: Gln, Q*

L-glutamyl-L-tryptophan *investigational (orphan) agent for AIDS-related Kaposi sarcoma*

glutaral USAN, USP, INN *disinfectant* ℞ colterol

glutaraldehyde [see: glutaral]

Glutarex-1 powder OTC *formula for infants with glutaric aciduria type I* ℞ Klotrix

Glutarex-2 powder OTC *enteral nutritional therapy for glutaric aciduria type I* ℞ Klotrix

glutasin [see: glutamic acid HCl]

glutathione *endogenous antioxidant produced in the liver; unstable as an oral supplement; endogenous levels are increased by using transdermal preparations, by supplementing its precursors, MSM and NAC (q.v.), or by regenerating it with SAMe (q.v.)*

L-glutathione, reduced *investigational (orphan) for AIDS-related cachexia*

glutaurine INN

glutethimide USP, INN, BAN *sedative; sometimes abused as a street drug* 250, 500 mg oral

Glutofac tablets OTC *vitamin/mineral supplement* [multiple vitamins & minerals]

Glutofac-ZX caplets ℞ *vitamin/mineral supplement* [multiple vitamins & minerals; folic acid; biotin] ±•1•0.2 mg

Glutose oral gel OTC *blood glucose elevating agent for hypoglycemia* [glucose] 40% ℞ Giltuss

glyburide USAN *sulfonylurea antidiabetic for type 2 diabetes that stimulates* *insulin secretion in the pancreas* [also: glibenclamide] 1.25, 1.5, 2.5, 3, 4.5, 5, 6 mg oral ⧆ CHL + PRED

glyburide & metformin HCl *antidiabetic combination for type 2 diabetes that stimulates insulin secretion in the pancreas, decreases hepatic glucose production, and increases cellular response to insulin* 1.25•250, 2.5•500, 5•500 mg oral

glybutamide [see: carbutamide]

glybuthiazol INN ⧆ clobetasol

glybuthizol [see: glybuthiazol]

glybuzole INN

glycalox BAN [also: glucalox]

glyceol *investigational (orphan) agent for decreasing intracranial hypertension or cerebral edema*

glycerides oleiques polyoxyethylenes [see: peglicol 5 oleate]

glycerin USP *humectant; solvent; osmotic diuretic; hyperosmotic laxative; emollient/protectant; ophthalmic moisturizer* [also: glycerol] ⧆ Glucerna

glycerol INN *humectant; solvent; osmotic diuretic; hyperosmotic laxative; emollient/protectant; monoctanoin component D* [also: glycerin] ⧆ clazuril; Clozaril

glycerol, iodinated USAN, BAN *(disapproved for use as an expectorant in 1991)*

glycerol 1-decanoate *monoctanoin component B* [see: monoctanoin]

glycerol 1,2-dioctanoate *monoctanoin component C* [see: monoctanoin]

glycerol 1-octanoate *monoctanoin component A* [see: monoctanoin]

glycerol phosphate, manganese salt [see: manganese glycerophosphate]

glyceryl behenate NF *tablet and capsule lubricant*

glyceryl borate [see: boroglycerin]

glyceryl guaiacolate [now: guaifenesin]

glyceryl monostearate NF *emulsifying agent*

glyceryl triacetate [now: triacetin]

glyceryl trierucate *investigational (orphan) agent for adrenoleukodystrophy* [also: glyceryl trioleate]

glyceryl trinitrate BAN *coronary vasodilator* [also: nitroglycerin]

glyceryl trioleate *investigational (orphan) agent for adrenoleukodystrophy* [also: glyceryl trierucate]

glycerylaminophenaquine [see: glafenine]

Glyceryl-T capsules, oral liquid (discontinued 2007) ℞ *antiasthmatic; bronchodilator; expectorant* [theophylline; guaifenesin] 150•90 mg; 150•90 mg/15 mL

glycinato dihydroxyaluminum hydrate [see: dihydroxyaluminum aminoacetate]

glycine USP, INN *nonessential amino acid; urologic irrigant; symbols: Gly, G* [also: aminoacetic acid] 1.5% ⧆ Cleocin; Galzin; Quelicin

glycine aluminum-zirconium complex [see: aluminum zirconium tetrachlorohydrex gly; aluminum zirconium trichlorohydrex gly]

Glycine max medicinal herb [see: soy]

glycine2-human glucagon-like peptide-2, recombinant *investigational (orphan) for short bowel syndrome*

glycitein *one of several soy isoflavones that provide cell-protective effects* ⧆ colistin

glycitin *isoform precursor to glycitein* [q.v.]

glyclopyramide INN

glycobiarsol USP, INN [also: bismuth glycollylarsanilate]

glycocholate sodium [see: sodium glycocholate]

glycocoll [see: glycine]

glycol distearate USAN *thickening agent*

GlycoLax powder for oral solution ℞ *laxative* [polyethylene glycol–electrolyte solution (PEG 3350)] 17 g/dose ⧆ glucalox

glycolic acid *mild exfoliant and keratolytic*

glycolipodipsipeptides *a class of broad-spectrum antibiotics that are bactericidal against gram-positive aerobic and anaerobic bacteria*

***p*-glycolophenetidide** [see: fenacetinol]

glycopeptides *a class of antibiotic antineoplastics*

glycophenylate [see: mepenzolate bromide]

glycoprotein (GP) IIb/IIIa receptor antagonists *a class of platelet aggregation inhibitors for acute coronary syndrome, unstable angina, myocardial infarction, and cardiac surgery*

glycopyrrolate USAN, USP *GI antispasmodic; antisecretory; peptic ulcer adjunct* [also: glycopyrronium bromide] 1, 2 mg oral; 0.2 mg/mL injection

glycopyrrone bromide [see: glycopyrrolate]

glycopyrronium bromide INN, BAN *GI antispasmodic; antisecretory; peptic ulcer adjunct* [also: glycopyrrolate]

glycosaminoglycans *a class of anticoagulants used for the prophylaxis of postoperative deep vein thrombosis (DVT)*

glycosides, cardiac *a class of cardiovascular drugs that increase the force of cardiac contractions* [also called: digitalis glycosides]

glycyclamide INN, BAN

glycylcyclines *a class of bacteriostatic, antimicrobial antibiotics; a derivative of tetracyclines that have greater efficacy against tetracycline-resistant infections*

glycyrrhetinic acid [see: enoxolone]

glycyrrhiza NF

Glycyrrhiza glabra; G. palidiflora; G. uralensis *medicinal herb* [see: licorice]

glydanile sodium [now: glicetanile sodium]

glyhexamide USAN, INN *antidiabetic*

glyhexylamide [see: metahexamide]

Glylorin *investigational (Phase III, orphan) for nonbullous congenital ichthyosiform erythroderma (a.k.a. congenital primary ichthyosis)* [monolaurin]

glymidine BAN *antidiabetic* [also: glymidine sodium]

glymidine sodium USAN, INN *antidiabetic* [also: glymidine]

glymol [see: mineral oil]

Glynase PresTabs (micronized tablets) ℞ *sulfonylurea antidiabetic that stimulates insulin secretion in the pancreas* [glyburide] 1.5, 3, 6 mg

glyoctamide USAN, INN *antidiabetic*

Gly-Oxide *oral solution* OTC *antiseptic* [carbamide peroxide] 10% ⊘ gallic acid

glyparamide USAN *antidiabetic*

glyphylline [see: dyphylline]

glypinamide INN

Glypressin *investigational (orphan) for bleeding esophageal varices and hepatorenal syndrome* [terlipressin]

glyprothiazol INN ⊘ cloprothiazole

glyprothizol [see: glyprothiazol]

Glyquin *cream* ℞ *hyperpigmentation bleaching agent* [hydroquinone (in a sunscreen base)] 4% ⊘ Glaucon; Qualaquin

Glyquin-XM *cream* ℞ *hyperpigmentation bleaching agent* [hydroquinone (in a sunscreen base with vitamin E)] 4%

Glyset *tablets* ℞ *antidiabetic agent for type 2 diabetes; alpha-glucosidase inhibitor that delays the digestion of dietary carbohydrates* [miglitol] 25, 50, 100 mg ⊘ Calcet; Gelhist

glysobuzole INN [also: isobuzole]

GM-CSF (granulocyte-macrophage colony-stimulating factor) [see: regramostim; sargramostim; molgramostim]

Gnaphalium polycephalum; G. uliginosum *medicinal herb* [see: everlasting]

GNP Cold Head Congestion Daytime *caplets* OTC *antitussive; decongestant; analgesic; antipyretic* [dextromethorphan hydrobromide; phenylephrine HCl; acetaminophen] 10•5•325 mg

Gn-RH, GnRH (gonadotropin-releasing hormone) *an endogenous hormone, produced in the hypothalamus, which stimulates the release of luteinizing hormone (LH) and follicle-stimulating hormone (FSH) from the pituitary* [also known as: luteinizing hormone–releasing hormone (LH-RH)]

goatweed *medicinal herb* [see: St. John wort]

gold *element (Au)*

gold Au 198 USAN, USP *antineoplastic; liver imaging aid; radioactive agent*

Gold Bond Medicated Triple Action Relief lotion OTC *moisturizer; emollient; mild anesthetic; antipruritic; counterirritant* [dimethicone; menthol] 5%•0.15%

gold sodium thiomalate USP *antirheumatic (50% gold)* [also: sodium aurothiomalate] 50 mg/mL injection

gold sodium thiosulfate NF [also: sodium aurotiosulfate]

gold thioglucose [see: aurothioglucose]

gold thread (Coptis trifolia) root *medicinal herb used as an antiphlogistic, bitter tonic, and sedative*

golden senecio *medicinal herb* [see: life root]

goldenrod (Solidago nemoralis; S. odora; S. virgaurea) leaves and flowering tops *medicinal herb used as an astringent, carminative, diaphoretic, diuretic, and stimulant*

goldenseal (Hydrastis canadensis) rhizome and root *medicinal herb used as an antibiotic and antiseptic and for internal bleeding, colon inflammation, eye infections, liver disorders, menorrhagia, mouth sores, muscular pain, sciatic pain, and vaginitis*

golimumab *investigational (NDA filed, orphan) anti-TNF-alpha monoclonal antibody for chronic sarcoidosis, rheumatoid arthritis, psoriatic arthritis, and ankylosing spondylitis*

GoLYTELY powder for oral solution ℞ *pre-procedure bowel evacuant* [polyethylene glycol–electrolyte solution (PEG 3350)] 60 g/L

gonacrine [see: acriflavine]

gonadorelin INN, BAN *gonad-stimulating principle* [also: gonadorelin acetate]

gonadorelin acetate USAN *gonadotropin-releasing hormone for the induction of ovulation in women with hypothalamic amenorrhea (orphan); diagnostic aid for fertility* [also: gonadorelin]

gonadorelin HCl USAN *gonad-stimulating principle; synthetic luteinizing hormone–releasing hormone (LH-RH);* *in vivo diagnostic aid for anterior pituitary function*

gonadotrophin, chorionic INN, BAN *a hormone produced by human placenta (chorion) and extracted from the urine of pregnant women; used for prepubertal cryptorchidism or hypogonadism and to induce ovulation in anovulatory women; also used for rapid weight loss* [also: gonadotropin, chorionic]

gonadotrophin, serum INN

gonadotropin, chorionic USP *a hormone produced by human placenta (chorion) and extracted from the urine of pregnant women; used for prepubertal cryptorchidism or hypogonadism and to induce ovulation in anovulatory women; also used for rapid weight loss* [also: gonadotrophin, chorionic] 500, 1000, 2000 IU/mL injection

gonadotropin, serum [see: gonadotrophin, serum]

gonadotropin-releasing hormone (Gn-RH) *an endogenous hormone, produced in the hypothalamus, which stimulates the release of luteinizing hormone (LH) and follicle-stimulating hormone (FSH) from the pituitary* [also known as: luteinizing hormone–releasing hormone (LH-RH)]

gonadotropin-releasing hormone analogs *a class of hormonal antineoplastics*

gonadotropins *a class of hormones that stimulate the ovaries, including follicle-stimulating hormone and luteinizing hormone*

Gonak ophthalmic solution OTC *gonioscopic examination aid* [hydroxypropyl methylcellulose] 2.5% ⑨ Kank-a

Gonal-f subcu injection ℞ *recombinant follicle-stimulating hormone (FSH) for induction of ovulation or spermatogenesis (orphan); adjunct to assisted reproductive technologies (ART)* [follitropin alfa] 75, 450, 1050 IU

Gonal-f RFF Pen (prefilled syringes) ℞ *recombinant follicle-stimulating hormone (FSH) for induction of ovulation;*

adjunct to assisted reproductive technologies (ART) [follitropin alfa] 300, 450, 900 IU

Gonic powder for IM injection ℞ *a human-derived hormone used for pre-pubertal cryptorchidism or hypogonadism and to induce ovulation in anovulatory women* [chorionic gonadotropin] 1000 U/mL ⃞ Kank-a

***Goniopora* spp.** *natural material* [see: coral]

Gonioscopic Prism Solution Drop-Tainers (eye drops) OTC *agent for bonding gonioscopic prisms to the eye* [hydroxyethyl cellulose]

Goniosol ophthalmic solution OTC *gonioscopic examination aid* [hydroxypropyl methylcellulose] 2.5% ⃞ Gynazole-1; Konsyl

Gonozyme Diagnostic reagent kit for professional use ℞ *in vitro diagnostic aid for Neisseria gonorrhoeae*

Good Sense Pain Relief Allergy Sinus gelcaps (discontinued 2007) OTC *decongestant; antihistamine; analgesic; antipyretic* [pseudoephedrine HCl; chlorpheniramine maleate; acetaminophen] 30•2•500 mg

Good Sense Sinus caplets (discontinued 2007) OTC *decongestant; antihistamine; analgesic; antipyretic* [pseudoephedrine HCl; chlorpheniramine maleate; acetaminophen] 30•2•500 mg

Good Start; Good Start Essentials; Good Start Supreme oral liquid, powder for oral liquid OTC *total or supplementary infant feeding*

Goody's Body Pain oral powder OTC *analgesic; antipyretic; anti-inflammatory* [acetaminophen; aspirin] 325•500 mg/dose

Goody's Extra Strength oral powder OTC *analgesic; antipyretic; anti-inflammatory* [acetaminophen; aspirin; caffeine] 325•500•65 mg/dose

Goody's PM oral powder OTC *antihistamine; sleep aid; analgesic; antipyretic* [diphenhydramine citrate; acetaminophen] 38•500 mg/packet

goose grass *medicinal herb* [see: bedstraw; cinquefoil]

goose hair; gosling weed *medicinal herb* [see: bedstraw]

Gordobalm OTC *analgesic; mild anesthetic; antipruritic; counterirritant; antiseptic* [methyl salicylate; menthol; camphor; alcohol 16%]

Gordochom topical solution OTC *antifungal; antiseptic* [undecylenic acid; chloroxylenol] 25%•3%

Gordofilm topical liquid ℞ *keratolytic* [salicylic acid in flexible collodion] 16.7%

Gordogesic Creme OTC *analgesic; counterirritant* [methyl salicylate] 10%

Gordon's Urea 40% cream ℞ *for removal of dystrophic nails* [urea] 40% ⃞ Cardene SR

Gormel Creme OTC *moisturizer; emollient; keratolytic* [urea] 20%

goserelin USAN, INN, BAN *hormonal antineoplastic for prostate and breast cancer; luteinizing hormone-releasing hormone (LHRH) agonist* [also: goserelin acetate]

goserelin acetate JAN *hormonal antineoplastic for prostatic carcinoma, breast cancer, and endometriosis; luteinizing hormone-releasing hormone (LHRH) agonist* [also: goserelin]

gosling weed; goose grass; goose hair *medicinal herb* [see: bedstraw]

gossypol (*Gossypium* spp.) seed oil *medicinal herb for male and female contraception; not generally regarded as safe and effective as male sterility may be irreversible; investigational (orphan) for cancer of the adrenal cortex*

gotu kola (*Centella asiatica; Hydrocotyle asiatica*) entire plant *medicinal herb for abscesses, hypertension, contraception, leprosy, nervous breakdown, physical and mental fatigue, promoting wound healing, and rheumatism*

goutberry *medicinal herb* [see: blackberry]

govafilcon A USAN *hydrophilic contact lens material*

GP-500 tablets (discontinued 2007) ℞ *decongestant; expectorant* [pseudoephedrine HCl; guaifenesin] 120•500 mg

G/P 1200/60 sustained-release tablets (discontinued 2007) ℞ *expectorant; decongestant* [guaifenesin; pseudoephedrine HCl] 1200•60 mg

GP IIb/IIIa inhibitors [see: glycoprotein (GP) IIb/IIIa receptor antagonists]

gp100 adenoviral gene therapy *investigational (Phase III, orphan) theraccine for metastatic melanoma*

gp120 (glycoprotein 120) antigens *investigational (Phase I–III) vaccine for HIV* [also: AIDS vaccine]

gp160 (glycoprotein 160) antigens *investigational (orphan) antiviral (therapeutic, Phase II) and vaccine (preventative, Phase I) for HIV and AIDS*

gp96 heat shock protein-peptide complex *investigational (Phase III, orphan) antineoplastic for renal cell carcinoma and metastatic melanoma*

grace, herb of *medicinal herb* [see: rue]

Gradumet (trademarked dosage form) *controlled-release tablet*

graftskin *a living, bilayered skin construct for diabetic foot ulcers and pressure sores (the epidermal layer is living human keratinocytes; the dermal layer is living human fibroblasts)*

gramicidin USP, INN *antibacterial antibiotic*

gramicidin & neomycin sulfate & polymyxin B sulfate *topical antibiotic* 0.025 mg•1.75 mg•10 000 U per mL eye drops

gramicidin S INN

Graminis rhizoma *medicinal herb* [see: couch grass]

granisetron USAN, INN, BAN *serotonin 5-HT₃ receptor antagonist; antiemetic to prevent nausea and vomiting following chemotherapy, radiation, or surgery*

granisetron HCl USAN *serotonin 5-HT₃ receptor antagonist; antiemetic to prevent nausea and vomiting following chemotherapy, radiation, or surgery*

(base=89%) 1 mg oral; 2 mg/10 mL oral; 0.1, 1 mg/mL injection

Granisol oral solution ℞ *antiemetic to prevent nausea and vomiting following chemotherapy* [granisetron (as HCl)] 1 mg/5 mL ⬚ Chronosule

Granul-Derm aerosol spray ℞ *proteolytic enzyme for debridement of necrotic tissue; vulnerary* [trypsin; Peruvian balsam] 0.1•72.5 mg/0.82 mL

Granulex aerosol spray ℞ *proteolytic enzyme for debridement of necrotic tissue; vulnerary* [trypsin; Peruvian balsam] 0.1•72.5 mg/0.82 mL

granulocyte colony-stimulating factor (G-CSF), recombinant [see: filgrastim]

granulocyte-macrophage colony-stimulating factor (GM-CSF) [see: regramostim; sargramostim; molgramostim]

GranuMed aerosol spray ℞ *proteolytic enzyme for debridement of necrotic tissue; vulnerary* [trypsin; Peruvian balsam] 0.1•72.5 mg/0.82 mL

grape, bear's *medicinal herb* [see: uva ursi]

grape, Rocky Mountain; wild Oregon grape *medicinal herb* [see: Oregon grape]

grape seed (*Vitis coigetiae; V. vinifera*) oil *medicinal herb for dental caries; also used as a dietary source of essential fatty acids and tocopherols*

grape seed extract *natural free radical scavenger for inflammatory collagen disease and peripheral vascular disease; contains 92%–95% procyanidolic oligomers (PCOs)*

grapefruit (*Citrus paradisi*) *medicinal herb for potassium replacement; the pectin is used to help reduce cholesterol and promote regression of atherosclerosis*

grass burdock *medicinal herb* [see: burdock]

grass myrtle *medicinal herb* [see: calamus]

Gratiola officinalis *medicinal herb* [see: hedge hyssop]

gravelroot *medicinal herb* [see: queen of the meadow]

graybeard tree *medicinal herb* [see: fringe tree]

great wild valerian *medicinal herb* [see: valerian]

greater celandine *medicinal herb* [see: celandine]

green broom; greenweed *medicinal herb* [see: dyer's broom]

green hellebore *(Veratrum viride)* *medicinal herb* [see: hellebore]

green soap [see: soap, green]

green tea *(Camellia sinensis)* leaves *medicinal herb used as an antihyperlipidemic, antimicrobial, antineoplastic, and antioxidant; also used to promote longevity by attenuating severe fatal diseases* ☒ currant

Green Throat Spray; Red Throat Spray OTC *mild mucous membrane anaesthetic; antipruritic; counterirritant* [phenol] 1.4%

greenweed; green broom *medicinal herb* [see: dyer's broom]

grepafloxacin INN *broad-spectrum fluoroquinolone antibiotic*

grepafloxacin HCl USAN *broad-spectrum fluoroquinolone antibiotic*

Grifola frondosa *medicinal herb* [see: maitake mushrooms]

Grifols [see: Human Albumin Grifols]

Grindelia squarrosa *medicinal herb* [see: gum weed]

Gripe Water [see: Baby's Bliss Gripe Water; Colic-Ease Gripe Water; Wellements Organic Gripe Water]

Grisactin 250 capsules (discontinued 2004) ℞ *systemic antifungal* [griseofulvin (microsize)] 250 mg

Grisactin 500 tablets (discontinued 2004) ℞ *systemic antifungal* [griseofulvin (microsize)] 500 mg

Grisactin Ultra tablets (discontinued 2004) ℞ *systemic antifungal* [griseofulvin (ultramicrosize)] 250 mg

griseofulvin USP, INN, BAN *systemic antifungal* 125 mg/5 mL oral

Gris-PEG film-coated tablets ℞ *systemic antifungal* [griseofulvin (ultramicrosize)] 125, 250 mg

ground apple *medicinal herb* [see: chamomile]

ground berry *medicinal herb* [see: wintergreen]

ground holly *medicinal herb* [see: pipsissewa]

ground lemon *medicinal herb* [see: mandrake]

ground lily *medicinal herb* [see: birthroot]

ground raspberry *medicinal herb* [see: goldenseal]

ground squirrel pea *medicinal herb* [see: twin leaf]

ground thistle *medicinal herb* [see: carline thistle]

group B streptococcus immune globulin [see: streptococcus immune globulin, group B]

growth hormone, human (hGH) [see: somatropin]

growth hormone-releasing factor (GHRF; GH-RF) *investigational (orphan) for inadequate endogenous growth hormone in children*

G-strophanthin [see: ouabain]

GTI-2040 [see: antisense 20-mer phosphorothiolate oligonucleotide]

guabenxan INN

guacetisal INN

guafecainol INN

GUAI 800/DM 30 sustained-release tablets ℞ *expectorant; antitussive* [guaifenesin; dextromethorphan hydrobromide] 800•30 mg

guaiac

guaiacol NF ☒ guggul

p-**guaiacol** [see: mequinol]

guaiacol carbonate NF

guaiacol glyceryl ether [see: guaifenesin]

guaiactamine INN

guaiapate USAN, INN *antitussive*

guaiazulene soluble [see: sodium guaifenate]

guaietolin INN

Guaifed sustained-release capsules ℞ *decongestant; expectorant* [phenylephrine HCl; guaifenesin] 15•400 mg ⊠ CVAD; CVD

Guaifed syrup (discontinued 2007) OTC *decongestant; expectorant* [pseudoephedrine HCl; guaifenesin] 60•400 mg/10 mL ⊠ CVAD; CVD

Guaifed-PD sustained-release capsules ℞ *decongestant; expectorant* [phenylephrine HCl; guaifenesin] 7.5•200 mg

Guaifen DM extended-release tablets ℞ *antitussive; decongestant; expectorant* [dextromethorphan hydrobromide; phenylephrine HCl; guaifenesin] 20•40•1200 mg ⊠ C-Phen DM; G Phen DM; GFN 1000/DM 50

Guaifen PE extended-release tablets ℞ *decongestant; expectorant* [phenylephrine HCl; guaifenesin] 25•800 mg

guaifenesin USAN, USP, INN *expectorant* [also: guaiphenesin] 200, 400 mg oral; 100 mg/5 mL oral

guaifenesin & codeine phosphate *expectorant; narcotic antitussive; narcotic analgesic* 300•10 mg oral

guaifenesin & dextromethorphan hydrobromide *expectorant; antitussive* 500•30 mg oral

Guaifenesin DM extended-release caplets (discontinued 2007) ℞ *antitussive; expectorant* [dextromethorphan hydrobromide; guaifenesin] 30•600 mg

Guaifenesin DM syrup OTC *antitussive; expectorant* [dextromethorphan hydrobromide; guaifenesin] 10•100 mg/5 mL

Guaifenesin DM NR oral liquid ℞ *antitussive; expectorant* [dextromethorphan hydrobromide; guaifenesin] 10•100 mg/5 mL

guaifenesin & dyphylline *expectorant; antiasthmatic; bronchodilator* 200•200 mg oral

guaifenesin & hydrocodone bitartrate *expectorant; narcotic antitussive* 100•5 mg/5 mL oral

Guaifenesin NR oral liquid ℞ *expectorant* [guaifenesin] 100 mg/5 mL

guaifenesin & phenylephrine HCl *expectorant; decongestant* 600•15, 600•40, 900•25, 900•30, 1200•30 mg oral

guaifenesin & pseudoephedrine HCl *expectorant; decongestant* 500•60, 595•48, 795•85, 800•90, 1200•50 mg oral

guaifenesin & pseudoephedrine HCl & dextromethorphan hydrobromide *expectorant; decongestant; antitussive* 800•90•60 mg oral

Guaifenesn DM 1000/60 extended-release caplets ℞ *expectorant; antitussive* [guaifenesin; dextromethorphan hydrobromide] 1000•60 mg

Guaifenex DM extended-release caplets ℞ *antitussive; expectorant* [dextromethorphan hydrobromide; guaifenesin] 30•600 mg

Guaifenex G; Guaifenex LA extended-release caplets (discontinued 2004) ℞ *expectorant* [guaifenesin] 1200 mg; 600 mg

Guaifenex GP extended-release film-coated tablets ℞ *decongestant; expectorant* [pseudoephedrine HCl; guaifenesin] 120•1200 mg

Guaifenex PSE 60; Guaifenex PSE 85; Guaifenex PSE 120 extended-release caplets ℞ *decongestant; expectorant* [pseudoephedrine HCl; guaifenesin] 60•600 mg; 85•795 mg; 120•600 mg

Guaifenex-Rx extended-release tablets (AM and PM) (discontinued 2004) ℞ *decongestant; expectorant added* AM [guaifenesin; pseudoephedrine HCl (AM)] 600 mg AM; 600•60 mg PM

Guaifenex-Rx DM extended-release tablets (AM and PM) (discontinued 2004) ℞ *expectorant; decongestant added* AM; *antitussive added* PM [guifenesin; pseudoephedrine HCl (AM); dextromethorphan hydrobromide (PM)] 600•60 mg AM; 600•30 mg PM

guaifylline INN *bronchodilator; expectorant* [also: guaithylline]

GuaiMAX-D extended-release caplets ℞ *decongestant; expectorant* [pseudo-

ephedrine HCl; guaifenesin] 120•
600 mg

guaimesal INN ⍰ Kemsol

Guaimist DM syrup (discontinued 2007) ℞ *antitussive; decongestant; expectorant* [dextromethorphan hydrobromide; pseudoephrine HCl; guaifenesin] 15•40•100 mg/5 mL

Guaipax PSE sustained-release tablets ℞ *decongestant; expectorant* [pseudoephedrine HCl; guaifenesin] 120•
600 mg

guaiphenesin BAN *expectorant* [also: guaifenesin]

guaisteine INN

Guaitex PSE tablets ℞ *decongestant; expectorant* [pseudoephedrine HCl; guaifenesin] 120•500 mg

guaithylline USAN *bronchodilator; expectorant* [also: guaifylline]

Guai-Vent/PSE sustained-release tablets (discontinued 2006) ℞ *decongestant; expectorant* [pseudoephedrine HCl; guaifenesin] 120•600 mg

guamecycline INN, BAN

guanabenz USAN, INN *centrally acting antiadrenergic antihypertensive*

guanabenz acetate USAN, USP, JAN *centrally acting antiadrenergic antihypertensive* 4, 8 mg oral

guanacline INN, BAN *antihypertensive* [also: guanacline sulfate]

guanacline sulfate USAN *antihypertensive* [also: guanacline]

guanadrel INN *antihypertensive* [also: guanadrel sulfate]

guanadrel sulfate USAN, USP *antihypertensive* [also: guanadrel]

guanatol HCl [see: chloroguanide HCl]

guanazodine INN

guancidine INN *antihypertensive* [also: guancydine]

guancydine USAN *antihypertensive* [also: guancidine]

guanethidine INN, BAN *antihypertensive* [also: guanethidine monosulfate]

guanethidine monosulfate USAN, USP *antihypertensive; investigational (orphan) for reflex sympathetic dystrophy and causalgia* [also: guanethidine]

guanethidine sulfate USAN, USP, JAN *antihypertensive*

guanfacine INN, BAN *antihypertensive; antiadrenergic* [also: guanfacine HCl]

guanfacine HCl USAN *antihypertensive; antiadrenergic; selective α_{2A} receptor agonist; investigational (NDA filed) nonstimulant treatment for attention-deficit/hyperactivity disorder (ADHD); investigational (orphan) for fragile X syndrome* [also: guanfacine] 1, 2 mg oral

guanidine HCl *cholinergic muscle stimulant* 125 mg oral

guanisoquin sulfate USAN *antihypertensive* [also: guanisoquine]

guanisoquine INN *antihypertensive* [also: guanisoquin sulfate] ⍰ quinisocaine

guanoclor INN, BAN *antihypertensive* [also: guanoclor sulfate]

guanoclor sulfate USAN *antihypertensive* [also: guanoclor]

guanoctine INN *antihypertensive* [also: guanoctine HCl]

guanoctine HCl USAN *antihypertensive* [also: guanoctine]

guanoxabenz USAN, INN *antihypertensive*

guanoxan INN, BAN *antihypertensive* [also: guanoxan sulfate]

guanoxan sulfate USAN *antihypertensive* [also: guanoxan]

guanoxyfen INN *antihypertensive; antidepressant* [also: guanoxyfen sulfate]

guanoxyfen sulfate USAN *antihypertensive; antidepressant* [also: guanoxyfen]

Guaphenyl II capsules ℞ *decongestant; expectorant* [phenylephrine HCl; guaifenesin] 20•375 mg

Guaphenyl LA dual-release capsules ℞ *decongestant; expectorant* [phenylephrine HCl (extended release); guaifenesin (immediate release)] 30•400 mg

guar gum NF *dietary fiber supplement; tablet binder and disintegrant* ⍰ karaya gum

guarana (*Paullinia cupana; P. sorbilis*) seed paste *medicinal herb for dysentery, malaria, and weight reduction* ⍰ Choron-10; Creon 5

guaranine [see: caffeine]

guggul *(Commiphora mukul)* plant *medicinal herb for hypercholesterolemia and for arthritis and weight reduction in Ayurvedic medicine* ☑ guaiacol

Guiadrine DM sustained-release caplets (discontinued 2007) ℞ *antitussive; expectorant* [dextromethorphan hydrobromide; guaifenesin] 30•600 mg

Guiatuss syrup OTC *expectorant* [guaifenesin] 100 mg/5 mL

Guiatuss AC syrup ℞ *narcotic antitussive; expectorant* [codeine phosphate; guaifenesin; alcohol 3.5%] 10•100 mg/5 mL ☑ cat's claw

Guiatuss DAC syrup ℞ *narcotic antitussive; decongestant; expectorant* [codeine phosphate; pseudoephedrine HCl; guaifenesin; alcohol 1.9%] 10•30•100 mg/5 mL

Guiatuss DM syrup OTC *antitussive; expectorant* [dextromethorphan hydrobromide; guaifenesin] 10•100 mg/5 mL

Guiatuss PE oral liquid (discontinued 2005) OTC *decongestant; expectorant* [pseudoephedrine HCl; guaifenesin] 60•200 mg/10 mL

gum Arabic *medicinal herb* [see: acacia]

gum arabic [see: acacia]

gum ivy *medicinal herb* [see: English ivy]

gum myrrh tree *medicinal herb* [see: myrrh]

gum plant *medicinal herb* [see: comfrey; yerba santa]

gum senegal [see: acacia]

gum tree, hemlock *medicinal herb* [see: hemlock]

gum weed *(Grindelia squarrosa)* flowering top and leaves *medicinal herb for asthma, bronchitis, bladder infection, poison ivy and oak, and psoriasis and other skin disorders*

guncotton, soluble [see: pyroxylin]

gusperimus INN *immunosuppressant; investigational (orphan) for acute renal graft rejection* [also: gusperimus trihydrochloride; gusperimus HCl]

gusperimus HCl JAN *immunosuppressant* [also: gusperimus trihydrochloride; gusperimus]

gusperimus trihydrochloride USAN *immunosuppressant* [also: gusperimus; gusperimus HCl]

gutta percha USP *dental restoration agent*

GyMiso *investigational (orphan) for complete expulsion of the products of conception after intrauterine fetal death* [misoprostol]

gymnema *(Gymnema melicida; G. sylvestre)* leaves and roots *medicinal herb for diabetes, hyperactivity, and hypoglycemia*

Gynazole-1 vaginal cream in prefilled applicator ℞ *antifungal* [butoconazole nitrate] 2% ☑ Genasal; Goniosol; Konsyl

Gynecort Female Creme cream *corticosteroidal anti-inflammatory* [hydrocortisone acetate] 1%

Gyne-Lotrimin 3 vaginal inserts, vaginal cream, combination pack (inserts + cream) OTC *antifungal* [clotrimazole] 200 mg; 2%; 200 mg + 1%

Gyne-Lotrimin 7 vaginal cream OTC *antifungal* [clotrimazole] 1%

gynergon [see: estradiol]

Gynodiol tablets ℞ *estrogen replacement therapy for the treatment of postmenopausal symptoms and prevention of postmenopausal osteoporosis; palliative therapy for prostate and metastatic breast cancers* [estradiol] 0.5, 1, 1.5, 2 mg

gynoestryl [see: estradiol]

Gynol II Contraceptive vaginal gel, vaginal jelly OTC *spermicidal contraceptive (for use with a diaphragm)* [nonoxynol 9] 2%; 3%

Gynostemma pentaphyllum *medicinal herb* [see: jiaogulan]

Gynovite Plus tablets OTC *vitamin/mineral/calcium/iron supplement* [multiple vitamins & minerals; calcium; iron; folic acid; biotin] ±•83•3•0.067•≟ mg

Gy-Pak (trademarked packaging form) *unit-of-issue package* ☑ COPAC; CPB WC; CPC; K-Pek

gypsy weed *medicinal herb* [see: speed-well]

Gyrocap (trademarked dosage form) *timed-release capsule*

H 9600 SR sustained-release caplets (discontinued 2007) ℞ *decongestant; expectorant* [pseudoephedrine HCl; guaifenesin] 90•600 mg

H₁ blockers *a class of antihistamines* [also called: histamine H₁ antagonists]

H₂ blockers *a class of gastrointestinal antisecretory agents* [also called: histamine H₂ antagonists]

²H (deuterium) [see: deuterium oxide]

H₂¹⁵O [see: water O 15]

³H (tritium) [see: tritiated water]

HAART (highly active antiretroviral therapy) *multi-drug therapy given to HIV-positive patients to prevent progression to AIDS; a generic term applied to several different anti-HIV protocols*

hachimycin INN, BAN

HAD (hexamethylmelamine, Adriamycin, DDP) *chemotherapy protocol*

Haemophilus **b conjugate vaccine** (*Haemophilus influenzae* type b capsular polysaccharide, covalently bound to tetanus toxoid)

hafnium *element (Hf)*

Hair Booster Vitamin tablets OTC *vitamin/mineral/iron supplement* [multiple B vitamins & minerals; iron; folic acid] ≐•18•0.4 mg

halarsol [see: dichlorophenarsine HCl]

halazepam USAN, USP, INN, BAN *benzodiazepine anxiolytic; sedative*

halazone USP, INN *disinfectant; water purifier*

halcinonide USAN, USP, INN, BAN *topical corticosteroidal anti-inflammatory*

Halcion tablets ℞ *benzodiazepine sedative and hypnotic* [triazolam] 0.125, 0.25 mg

Haldol IM injection (discontinued 2006) ℞ *conventional (typical) butyrophenone antipsychotic; antispas-*

modic/antidyskinetic for Tourette syndrome; treatment for severe pediatric behavioral disorders such as aggression, combativeness, hyperexcitability, and poor impulse control [haloperidol lactate] 5 mg/mL

Haldol Decanoate 50; Haldol Decanoate 100 long-acting IM injection ℞ *conventional (typical) butyrophenone antipsychotic; antispasmodic/antidyskinetic for Tourette syndrome; treatment for severe pediatric behavioral disorders such as aggression, combativeness, hyperexcitability, and poor impulse control* [haloperidol decanoate] 50 mg/mL; 100 mg/mL

Halenol, Children's oral liquid (discontinued 2008) OTC *analgesic; antipyretic* [acetaminophen] 160 mg/5 mL

haletazole INN [also: halethazole]

halethazole BAN [also: haletazole]

Haley's M-O oral liquid OTC *saline/emollient laxative* [magnesium hydroxide; mineral oil] 900 mg•3.75 mL per 15 mL

HalfLytely Bowel Prep Kit enteric-coated delayed-release tablets + powder for oral solution ℞ *pre-procedure bowel evacuant* [bisacodyl + polyethylene glycol–electrolyte solution (PEG 3350)] 5 mg + 2 L

Halfprin; Halfprin 81 enteric-coated tablets OTC *analgesic; antipyretic; anti-inflammatory; antirheumatic* [aspirin] 165 mg; 81 mg

Hall's Plus lozenges OTC *mild anesthetic; antipruritic; counterirritant* [menthol] 10 mg

Hall's Sugar Free Mentho-Lyptus lozenges OTC *mild anesthetic; antipruritic; counterirritant; antiseptic* [menthol; eucalyptus oil] 5•2.8, 6•2.8 mg

Halls Zinc Defense lozenges OTC *antiseptic to relieve sore throat* [zinc acetate] 5 mg

hallucinogens *a class of agents that induce hallucinations*

halobetasol propionate USAN *topical corticosteroidal anti-inflammatory* [also: ulobetasol] 0.05% topical

halocarban INN *disinfectant* [also: cloflucarban]

halocortolone INN

halocrinic acid [see: brocrinat]

halofantrine INN, BAN *antimalarial* [also: halofantrine HCl]

halofantrine HCl USAN *antimalarial (orphan)* [also: halofantrine]

Halofed tablets OTC *nasal decongestant* [pseudoephedrine HCl] 30, 60 mg

halofenate USAN, INN, BAN *antihyperlipoproteinemic; uricosuric*

halofuginone INN, BAN *antiprotozoal* [also: halofuginone hydrobromide]

halofuginone hydrobromide USAN *antiprotozoal; investigational (orphan) for scleroderma* [also: halofuginone]

Halog ointment, cream, solution ℞ *corticosteroidal anti-inflammatory* [halcinonide] 0.1%

Halog-E cream ℞ *corticosteroidal anti-inflammatory* [halcinonide] 0.1%

halometasone INN

halonamine INN

halopemide USAN, INN *antipsychotic*

halopenium chloride INN, BAN

haloperidol USAN, USP, INN, BAN *conventional (typical) butyrophenone antipsychotic; antispasmodic/antidyskinetic for Tourette syndrome; treatment for severe pediatric behavioral disorders such as aggression, combativeness, hyperexcitability, and poor impulse control* 0.5, 1, 2, 5, 10, 20 mg oral

haloperidol decanoate USAN, BAN *conventional (typical) butyrophenone antipsychotic; antispasmodic/antidyskinetic for Tourette syndrome; treatment for severe pediatric behavioral disorders such as aggression, combativeness, hyperexcitability, and poor impulse control* 50, 100 mg/mL injection

haloperidol lactate *conventional (typical) butyrophenone antipsychotic; antispasmodic/antidyskinetic for Tourette syndrome; treatment for severe pediatric behavioral disorders such as aggression, combativeness, hyperexcitability, and poor impulse control* 2 mg/mL oral; 5 mg/mL injection

halopone chloride [see: halopenium chloride]

halopredone INN *topical anti-inflammatory* [also: halopredone acetate]

halopredone acetate USAN *topical anti-inflammatory* [also: halopredone]

haloprogesterone USAN, INN *progestin*

haloprogin USAN, USP, INN, JAN *antibacterial; antifungal*

halopyramine BAN [also: chloropyramine]

Halotex cream, solution (discontinued 2004) ℞ *antifungal for tinea pedis, tinea cruris, tinea corporis, tinea manuum, and tinea versicolor* [haloprogin] 1%

halothane USP, INN, BAN *inhalation general anesthetic* ② Hylutin

Halotussin syrup OTC *expectorant* [guaifenesin; alcohol 3.5%] 100 mg/5 mL

Halotussin AC oral liquid (discontinued 2005) ℞ *narcotic antitussive; expectorant* [codeine phosphate; guaifenesin] 20•200 mg/10 mL

haloxazolam INN

haloxon INN, BAN

halquinol BAN *topical anti-infective* [also: halquinols]

halquinols USAN *topical anti-infective* [also: halquinol]

Haltran tablets (discontinued 2005) OTC *analgesic; antiarthritic; antipyretic; nonsteroidal anti-inflammatory drug (NSAID) for mild to moderate pain, migraine headaches, and primary dysmenorrhea* [ibuprofen] 200 mg

HAM (hexamethylmelamine, Adriamycin, melphalan) *chemotherapy protocol*

HAM (hexamethylmelamine, Adriamycin, methotrexate) *chemotherapy protocol*

Hamamelis virginiana medicinal herb [see: witch hazel]

hamamelis water medicinal herb [see: witch hazel]

hamycin USAN, INN antifungal

HandiHaler (trademarked delivery device) inhalation powder dispenser

hard fat [see: fat, hard]

hardock medicinal herb [see: burdock]

hareburr medicinal herb [see: burdock]

Harpagophytum procumbens medicinal herb [see: devil's claw]

hashish *(Cannabis sativa)* euphoric/hallucinogenic street drug made from the resin of the flowering tops of the cannabis plant

Havrix adult IM injection, pediatric IM injection ℞ immunization against hepatitis A virus (HAV) [hepatitis A vaccine, inactivated] 1440 ELISA units (EL.U.)/mL; 720 EL.U./0.5 mL

haw medicinal herb [see: hawthorn]

Hawaiian Tropic Cool Aloe with I.C.E. gel OTC anesthetic; antipruritic; counterirritant [lidocaine; menthol]

hawthorn *(Crataegus laevigata; C. monogyna; C. oxyacantha)* flowers, leaves, and berries medicinal herb for angina pectoris, arrhythmias, arteriosclerosis, enlarged heart, high or low blood pressure, hypoglycemia, palpitations, and tachycardia; also used as an antiseptic ⏍ Hytrin

Hayfebrol oral liquid (discontinued 2007) OTC decongestant; antihistamine [pseudoephedrine HCl; chlorpheniramine maleate] 60•4 mg/10 mL

hazel, snapping; hazelnut medicinal herb [see: witch hazel]

H-BIG IV injection investigational (orphan) prophylaxis against hepatitis B reinfection in liver transplant patients [hepatitis B immune globulin]

HBIG (hepatitis B immune globulin) [q.v.]

hBNP (human B-type natriuretic peptide) [see: nesiritide; nesiritide citrate]

1% HC ointment ℞ corticosteroidal anti-inflammatory [hydrocortisone] 1%

HC (hydrocortisone) [q.v.]

4-HC (4-hydroperoxycyclophosphamide) [q.v.]

HC Derma-Pax topical liquid OTC corticosteroidal anti-inflammatory; antihistamine; antiseptic [hydrocortisone; pyrilamine maleate; chlorpheniramine maleate; chlorobutanol] 0.5%•0.44%•0.06%•25%

HCA (hydrocortisone acetate) [q.v.]

H-CAP (hexamethylmelamine, cyclophosphamide, Adriamycin, Platinol) chemotherapy protocol

hCG (human chorionic gonadotropin) [see: gonadotropin, chorionic]

HCT (hydrochlorothiazide) [q.v.]

HCTZ (hydrochlorothiazide) [q.v.]

HD 85 oral/rectal suspension ℞ radiopaque contrast medium for gastrointestinal imaging [barium sulfate] 85%

HD 200 Plus powder for oral suspension ℞ radiopaque contrast medium for gastrointestinal imaging [barium sulfate] 98%

HDCV (human diploid cell vaccine) [see: rabies vaccine]

HDMTX (high-dose methotrexate [with leucovorin rescue]) chemotherapy protocol for bone sarcoma

HDMTX-CF (high-dose methotrexate, citrovorum factor) chemotherapy protocol

HDMTX/LV (high-dose methotrexate, leucovorin [rescue]) chemotherapy protocol

HDPEB (high-dose PEB protocol) chemotherapy protocol [see: PEB]

HD-VAC (high-dose [methotrexate], vinblastine, Adriamycin, cisplatin) chemotherapy protocol

HE-2000 investigational (Phase II) cellular energy regulator for HIV and AIDS

Head & Shoulders; Head & Shoulders Dry Scalp shampoo OTC antiseborrheic; antibacterial; antifungal [pyrithione zinc] 1%

Head & Shoulders Intensive Treatment lotion/shampoo OTC antiseborrheic; dandruff treatment [selenium sulfide] 1%

heal-all *medicinal herb* [see: figwort; stone root; woundwort]

healing herb *medicinal herb* [see: comfrey]

Healon; Healon GV intraocular injection ℞ *viscoelastic agent for ophthalmic surgery* [hyaluronate sodium] 10 mg/mL; 14 mg/mL

Healon Yellow intraocular injection ℞ *viscoelastic agent for ophthalmic surgery; diagnostic agent* [hyaluronate sodium; fluorescein sodium] 10• 0.005 mg/mL

heart, mother's; shepherd's heart *medicinal herb* [see: shepherd's purse]

Heartline enteric-coated tablets OTC *analgesic; antipyretic; anti-inflammatory; antirheumatic* [aspirin] 81 mg

heather (Calluna vulgaris) flowering shoots *medicinal herb used as an antiseptic, cholagogue, diaphoretic, diuretic, expectorant, and vasoconstrictor*

heavy liquid petrolatum [see: mineral oil]

heavy water (D₂O) [see: deuterium oxide]

Hectorol capsules, bolus injection during dialysis ℞ *synthetic vitamin D analogue; serum calcium regulator for hyperparathyroidism due to chronic kidney disease* [doxercalciferol] 0.5, 2.5 mcg; 2 mcg/mL

hedaquinium chloride INN, BAN

Hedeoma pulegeoides *medicinal herb* [see: pennyroyal]

Hedera helix *medicinal herb* [see: English ivy]

hedge bindweed (Convolvulus sepium) flowering plant and roots *medicinal herb used as a cholagogue, febrifuge, and purgative*

hedge garlic (Sisymbrium alliaria) *medicinal herb* [see: garlic]

hedge hyssop (Gratiola officinalis) plant *medicinal herb used as a cardiac, diuretic, purgative, and vermifuge*

hedge-burs *medicinal herb* [see: bedstraw]

"hedgehog" proteins *a class of novel human proteins that induce the formation of regenerative tissue*

Heet Liniment OTC *analgesic; counterirritant; antiseptic* [methyl salicylate; camphor; capsaicin; alcohol 70%] 15%•3.6%•0.025%

hefilcon A USAN *hydrophilic contact lens material*

hefilcon B USAN *hydrophilic contact lens material*

hefilcon C USAN *hydrophilic contact lens material*

helenien [see: xantofyl palmitate]

Helianthemum canadense *medicinal herb* [see: rock rose]

helicon [see: aspirin]

Helicosol powder for oral solution ℞ *diagnostic aid for detection of* H. pylori *in the stomach* [carbon C 13 urea]

Helidac 14-day dose-pack ℞ *combination treatment for active duodenal ulcer with* H. pylori *infection* [bismuth subsalicylate (chewable tablets); metronidazole (tablets); tetracycline HCl (capsules)] 8 × 262.4 mg; 4 × 250 mg; 4 × 500 mg (per day)

heliomycin INN

heliox *helium-oxygen mixture used for respiratory distress* (usually an 80%• 20% mix)

Helistat sponge ℞ *hemostat for surgery* [absorbable collagen sponge]

helium USP *diluent for gases; element* (He)

Helixate FS powder for IV injection ℞ *systemic hemostatic; antihemophilic for the prevention and control of bleeding in classical hemophilia (hemophilia A) and von Willebrand disease (orphan)* [antihemophilic factor concentrate, recombinant] 250, 500, 1000 IU/vial

Helizide capsule *investigational (NDA filed) combination therapy for* H. pylori *infection* [biskalcitrate potassium; metronidazole; tetracycline HCl] 140•125•125 mg

hellebore (Helleborus spp.; Veratrum spp.) rhizome *medicinal herb used as an antihypertensive; not generally* *regarded as safe and effective for internal consumption due to toxicity*

Helleborus spp. *medicinal herb* [see: hellebore]

helmet flower *medicinal herb* [see: aconite; sandalwood; skullcap]

helmet pod *medicinal herb* [see: twin leaf]

HEMA (2-hydroxyethyl methacrylate) *contact lens material*

Hemabate IM injection ℞ *prostaglandin-type abortifacient; for postpartum uterine bleeding* [carboprost tromethamine] 250 mcg/mL

Hema-Check slide tests for home use OTC *in vitro diagnostic aid for fecal occult blood*

Hema-Combistix reagent strips *in vitro diagnostic aid for multiple urine products*

Hemaspan timed-release tablets (discontinued 2005) OTC *hematinic; vitamin/iron supplement; stool softener* [ferrous fumarate (source of iron); ascorbic acid; docusate sodium] 330 (110)•200•20 mg

Hemastix reagent strips for professional use ℞ *in vitro diagnostic aid for urine occult blood*

Hematest reagent tablets for professional use ℞ *in vitro diagnostic aid for fecal occult blood*

Hematide *investigational (Phase III) synthetic peptide–based erythropoiesis-stimulating agent (ESA) to increase RBC production for anemia of chronic renal failure*

hematin [now: hemin]

Hematinic tablets ℞ *hematinic* [ferrous fumarate; folic acid] 106 mg Fe•1 mg

Hematinic Plus tablets ℞ *hematinic; vitamin/mineral supplement* [multiple vitamins & minerals; ferrous fumarate; folic acid] ≛•106 mg Fe•1 mg

hematinics *a class of iron-containing agents for the prevention and treatment of iron-deficiency anemia*

hematopoietics *a class of antianemic agents that promote the formation of red blood cells*

Hematrol *synthetic progestin; investigational (orphan) for immune thrombocytopenic purpura (ITP)* [medroxyprogesterone acetate]

heme arginate *investigational (orphan) for acute symptomatic porphyria and myelodysplastic syndrome*

HemeSelect Collection kit for home use OTC *in vitro diagnostic aid for fecal occult blood* [for use with **HemeSelect Reagent kit**]

HemeSelect Reagent kit for professional use ℞ *in vitro diagnostic aid for fecal occult blood* [for use with **HemeSelect Collection kit**]

Hemex *investigational (orphan) for acute porphyric syndromes* [hemin; zinc mesoporphyrin]

hemiacidrin [see: citric acid, glucono-delta-lactone & magnesium carbonate]

hemin *enzyme inhibitor for acute intermittent porphyria (AIP), porphyria variegata, and hereditary coproporphyria (orphan)*

hemin & zinc mesoporphyrin *investigational (orphan) for acute porphyric syndromes*

hemlock (Tsuga canadensis) bark *medicinal herb used as an astringent, diaphoretic, and diuretic* 🔊 Humalog

Hemoccult slide tests for professional use, test tape for professional use ℞ *in vitro diagnostic aid for fecal occult blood*

Hemoccult II slide tests for professional use ℞ *in vitro diagnostic aid for fecal occult blood*

Hemoccult II Dispenserpak; Hemoccult II Dispenserpak Plus slide tests for home use OTC *in vitro diagnostic aid for fecal occult blood*

Hemoccult SENSA; Hemoccult II SENSA slide tests for professional use ℞ *in vitro diagnostic aid for fecal occult blood*

Hemocitrate *investigational (orphan) adjunct to leukapheresis procedures* [sodium citrate]

Hemocyte tablets OTC *hematinic; iron supplement* [ferrous fumarate (source of iron)] 324 mg (106 mg)

Hemocyte Plus elixir ℞ *hematinic* [polysaccharide-iron complex; multiple B vitamins & minerals; folic acid] 12•±•0.33 mg

Hemocyte Plus tablets ℞ *hematinic* [ferrous fumarate; multiple B vitamins & minerals; sodium ascorbate; folic acid] 106•±•200•1 mg

Hemocyte-F elixir ℞ *hematinic* [polysaccharide-iron complex; cyanocobalamin; folic acid] 100 mg Fe•25 mcg•1 mg per 5 mL

Hemocyte-F tablets ℞ *hematinic* [ferrous fumarate; folic acid] 106•1 mg

Hemofil M IV injection ℞ *systemic hemostatic; antihemophilic for the prevention and control of bleeding in classical hemophilia (hemophilia A) and von Willebrand disease (orphan)* [antihemophilic factor concentrate, human] (the actual number of AHF units is indicated on the vial)

hemoglobin crosfumaril USAN, INN *blood substitute*

Hemopad fiber ℞ *topical hemostat for surgery* [microfibrillar collagen hemostat] ⑨ Humibid

Hemophilus b conjugate vaccine *active bacterin for* Haemophilus influenzae *type b*

Hemorid for Women cream OTC *anesthetic and vasoconstrictor for hemorrhoids* [pramoxine HCl; phenylephrine HCl] 1%•0.25%

Hemorid for Women lotion OTC *emollient and protectant for hemorrhoids* [mineral oil; petrolatum; glycerin]

Hemorid for Women rectal suppositories OTC *vasoconstrictor and astringent for hemorrhoids* [zinc oxide; phenylephrine HCl] 11%•0.25%

Hemorrhoidal HC rectal suppositories ℞ *corticosteroidal anti-inflammatory for hemorrhoids* [hydrocortisone acetate] 25 mg

hemostatics *a class of therapeutic blood modifiers that arrest the flow of blood* [see also: astringents; styptics]

Hemotene fiber (discontinued 2008) ℞ *topical hemostat for surgery* [microfibrillar collagen hemostat] 1 g ⑨ Humatin

Hemovit film-coated tablets ℞ *hematinic* [multiple B vitamins; vitamin C; folic acid; biotin] ±•60•1•0.3 mg

Hemoxin *investigational (orphan) for sickle cell disease* [niprisan]

hemp *medicinal herb* [see: marijuana]

hemp agrimony (Eupatorium cannabinum) plant *medicinal herb used as a cholagogue, diaphoretic, diuretic, emetic, expectorant, and purgative*

hemp nettle (Galeopsis tetrahit) plant *medicinal herb used as an astringent, diuretic, and expectorant*

Hem-Prep anorectal ointment, rectal suppositories OTC *temporary relief of hemorrhoidal symptoms; vasoconstrictor; astringent; emollient* [phenylephrine HCl; zinc oxide] 0.025%•11%; 0.25%•11%

Hemril Uniserts (rectal suppositories) OTC *temporary relief of hemorrhoidal symptoms* [bismuth subgallate; bismuth resorcin compound; benzyl benzoate; Peruvian balsam; zinc oxide] 2.25%•1.75%•1.2%•1.8%•11%

Hemril-HC Uniserts (suppositories) ℞ *corticosteroidal anti-inflammatory for hemorrhoids* [hydrocortisone acetate] 25 mg

henbane (Hyoscyamus niger) plant *medicinal herb used as an anodyne, antispasmodic, calmative, and narcotic; primarily used externally because of its high toxicity*

heneicosafluorotripropylamine [see: perfluamine]

henna (Alkanna tinctoria) root *medicinal herb used as an astringent, antibiotic, and cosmetic dye; not generally regarded as safe and effective*

henna (Lawsonia inermis) leaves *medicinal herb used as an astringent*

HEOD (hexachloro-epoxy-octahy-dro-dimethanonaththalene) [see: dieldrin]

Hepacid *investigational (orphan) treatment for hepatocellular carcinoma* [pegylated arginine deiminase]

HepaGam B IM injection ℞ *treatment for acute exposure to blood containing hepatitis B surface antigen (HBsAg); prophylaxis against hepatitis B infection after maternal, social, or sexual exposure to hepatitis B* [hepatitis B immune globulin, solvent/detergent treated] 5% (50 mg/mL)

Hepandrin *investigational (orphan) anabolic steroid for alcoholic hepatitis* [oxandrolone]

heparin BAN *anticoagulant; antithrombotic* [also: heparin calcium]

heparin, 2-0-desulfated *investigational (orphan) for cystic fibrosis*

heparin, unfractionated *investigational (orphan) oral treatment for sickle cell disease*

heparin calcium USP *anticoagulant; antithrombotic* [also: heparin]

Heparin I.V. Flush prefilled syringe ℞ *IV flush for catheter patency (not therapeutic)* [heparin sodium] 1 U/mL

Heparin Lock Flush solution ℞ *IV flush for catheter patency (not therapeutic)* [heparin sodium] 10, 100 U/mL

heparin sodium USP, INN, BAN *anticoagulant; antithrombotic* 1000, 2000, 2500, 5000, 7500, 10 000, 20 000, 40 000 U/mL injection

Heparin Sodium in 5% Dextrose IV injection ℞ *anticoagulant* [heparin sodium] 40, 50 U/mL

heparin sodium & sodium chloride 0.45% *anticoagulant; antithrombotic* 12 500 U•250 mL, 25 000 U•250 mL, 25 000 U•500 mL

heparin sodium & sodium chloride 0.9% *anticoagulant; antithrombotic* 1000 U•500 mL, 2000 U•1000 mL

heparin sulfate [see: danaparoid sodium]

heparin whole blood [see: blood, whole]

HepatAmine IV infusion ℞ *nutritional therapy for hepatic failure and hepatic encephalopathy* [multiple branched-chain essential and nonessential amino acids; electrolytes]

HepatAssist *investigational (orphan) for severe liver failure* [xenogeneic hepatocytes]

hepatica (Hepatica acutiloba; H. triloba) leaves and flowers *medicinal herb used as a diuretic and pectoral*

Hepatic-Aid II Instant Drink powder OTC *enteral nutritional treatment for chronic liver disease* [multiple branched chain amino acids]

hepatics *a class of agents that affect the liver (a term used in folk medicine)*

hepatitis A vaccine, inactivated *active immunizing agent for the hepatitis A virus (HAV)*

hepatitis B immune globulin (HBIG) USP *passive immunizing agent; treatment for acute exposure to blood containing hepatitis B surface antigen (HBsAg); prophylaxis against hepatitis B infection after transplant (orphan), maternal, social, or sexual exposure to hepatitis B*

hepatitis B surface antigen (HBsAg) [see: hepatitis B virus vaccine, inactivated]

hepatitis B virus vaccine, inactivated USP *active immunizing agent for hepatitis B and D*

hepatitis C virus immune globulin, human *investigational (orphan) prophylaxis against hepatitis C infection in liver transplant patients*

HepeX-B *investigational (orphan) prophylaxis against hepatitis B reinfection in liver transplant patients*

Hepflush-10 solution ℞ *IV flush for catheter patency (not therapeutic)* [heparin sodium] 10 U/mL

Hep-Forte capsules OTC *geriatric dietary supplement* [multiple vitamins & food products; folic acid; biotin] ≛• 60• ≛ mcg

Heplisav *investigational (Phase III) active immunizing agent for hepatitis B* [hepatitis B surface antigen]

Hep-Lock; Hep-Lock U/P solution ℞ *IV flush for catheter patency (not therapeutic)* [heparin sodium] 10, 100 U/mL

HEPP (H-chain ε [IgE] pentapeptide) [see: pentigetide]

hepronicate INN

Hepsera tablets ℞ *antiviral for chronic hepatitis B virus (HBV) infection* [adefovir dipivoxil] 10 mg

heptabarb INN [also: heptabarbitone]

heptabarbital [see: heptabarb; heptabarbitone]

heptabarbitone BAN [also: heptabarb]

heptaminol INN, BAN

heptaminol HCl [see: heptaminol]

2-heptanamine [see: tuaminoheptane]

2-heptanamine sulfate [see: tuaminoheptane sulfate]

heptaverine INN

heptolamide INN

hepzidine INN

HER (human epidermal growth factor receptor) inhibitors [q.v.]

HER1 (human epidermal growth factor receptor 1) inhibitors *a class of antineoplastics that suppress the growth of lung and pancreatic cancers*

HER2 (human epidermal growth factor receptor 2) inhibitors *a class of antineoplastics, predominantly monoclonal antibodies, that suppress the growth of breast cancer*

Heracleum lanatum *medicinal herb* [see: masterwort]

herb of grace *medicinal herb* [see: rue]

HercepTest test kit *diagnostic aid for the HER2 protein, used to screen patients who may benefit from treatment with* **Herceptin**

Herceptin powder for IV infusion ℞ *monoclonal antibody antineoplastic for metastatic HER2-overexpressing breast cancer; investigational (orphan) for pancreatic cancer* [trastuzumab] 440 mg

Hercules woundwort *medicinal herb* [see: woundwort]

heroin *potent narcotic analgesic street drug which is highly addictive; banned in the U.S.* [medically known as diamorphine and diacetylmorphine HCl]

heroin HCl *(banned in the U.S.)* [see: diacetylmorphine HCl]

Herpecin L lip balm OTC *vulnerary; sunblock* [dimethicone; meradimate; octinoxate; octisalate; oxybenzone] 1%•5%•7.5%•5%•6%

herpes simplex virus, genetically modified (G207) *investigational (orphan) agent for malignant glioma*

herpes simplex virus gene *investigational (orphan) for primary and metastatic brain tumors*

Herrick Lacrimal Plug ℞ *blocks the puncta and canaliculus to eliminate tear loss in keratitis sicca* [silicone plug]

HES (hydroxyethyl starch) [see: hetastarch]

Hespan IV infusion ℞ *plasma volume expander for shock due to hemorrhage, burns, surgery* [hetastarch] 6 g/100 mL

hesperidin *a bioflavonoid (q.v.)*

hesperidin methyl chalcone [see: bioflavonoids]

hetacillin USAN, USP, INN, BAN *antibacterial*

hetacillin potassium USAN, USP *antibacterial*

hetaflur USAN, INN, BAN *dental caries prophylactic*

hetastarch USAN, BAN *plasma volume extender* [also: hydroxyethylstarch] 6% in normal saline

heteronium bromide USAN, INN, BAN *anticholinergic*

Hetrazan tablets (available for compassionate use only) ℞ *anthelmintic for Bancroft filariasis, onchocerciasis, tropical eosinophilia, and loiasis* [diethylcarbamazine citrate] 50 mg

hexaammonium molybdate tetrahydrate [see: ammonium molybdate]

Hexabrix injection ℞ *radiopaque contrast medium* [ioxaglate meglumine; ioxaglate sodium (54.3% total iodine)] 393•196 mg/mL (320 mg/mL)

HexaCAF; Hexa-CAF (hexamethylmelamine, cyclophosphamide, amethopterin, fluorouracil) *chemotherapy protocol for ovarian cancer*

hexacarbacholine bromide INN [also: carbolonium bromide]

hexachlorane [see: lindane]

hexachlorocyclohexane [see: lindane]

hexachlorophane BAN *topical anti-infective; detergent* [also: hexachlorophene]

hexachlorophene USP, INN *topical anti-infective; detergent* [also: hexachlorophane]

hexacyclonate sodium INN

hexacyprone INN

hexadecanoic acid [see: palmitic acid]

hexadecanoic acid, methylethyl ester [see: isopropyl palmitate]

hexadecanol [see: cetyl alcohol]

hexadecylamine hydrofluoride [see: hetaflur]

hexadecylpyridinium chloride [see: cetylpyridinium chloride]

hexadecyltrimethylammonium bromide [see: cetrimonium bromide]

hexadecyltrimethylammonium chloride [see: cetrimonium chloride]

2,4-hexadienoic acid, potassium salt [see: potassium sorbate]

hexadiline INN

hexadimethrine bromide INN, BAN

hexadiphane [see: prozapine]

Hexadrol tablets, elixir (discontinued 2004) ℞ *corticosteroidal anti-inflammatory* [dexamethasone] 1.5, 4 mg; 0.5 mg/5 mL

Hexadrol Phosphate intra-articular, intralesional, soft tissue, or IM injection ℞ *corticosteroidal anti-inflammatory* [dexamethasone sodium phosphate] 4, 10, 20 mg/mL

hexadylamine [see: hexadiline]

Hexafed sustained-release film-coated tablets (discontinued 2007) ℞ *decongestant; antihistamine* [pseudoephedrine HCl; dexchlorpheniramine maleate] 60•4 mg

hexafluorenium bromide USAN, USP *skeletal muscle relaxant; succinylcholine synergist* [also: hexafluronium bromide]

hexafluorodiethyl ether [see: flurothyl]

hexaflurone bromide [see: hexafluorenium bromide]

hexafluronium bromide INN *skeletal muscle relaxant; succinylcholine synergist* [also: hexafluorenium bromide]

Hexalen capsules ℞ *antineoplastic for advanced ovarian adenocarcinoma (orphan)* [altretamine] 50 mg

hexamarium bromide [see: distigmine bromide]

hexametazime BAN

hexamethone bromide [see: hexamethonium bromide]

hexamethonium bromide INN, BAN

hexamethylenamine [now: methenamine]

hexamethylenamine mandelate [see: methenamine mandelate]

hexamethylenetetramine [see: methenamine]

hexamethylmelamine (HMM; HXM) [see: altretamine]

hexamidine INN

hexamine hippurate BAN *urinary antibacterial* [also: methenamine hippurate]

hexamine mandelate [see: methenamine mandelate]

hexapradol INN

hexaprofen INN, BAN

hexapropymate INN, BAN

hexasonium iodide INN

hexavitamin USP

Hexavitamin tablets OTC *vitamin supplement* [multiple vitamins]

hexcarbacholine bromide INN [also: carbolonium bromide]

hexedine USAN, INN *antibacterial*

hexemal [see: cyclobarbital]

hexestrol NF, INN

hexetidine BAN

hexicide [see: lindane]

hexinol [see: cyclomenol]

hexobarbital USP, INN

hexobarbital sodium NF

hexobendine USAN, INN, BAN *vasodilator*

hexocyclium methylsulphate BAN [also: hexocyclium methylsulfate; hexocyclium metilsulfate]

hexocyclium metilsulfate INN [also: hexocyclium methylsulfate; hexocyclium methylsulphate]

hexoprenaline INN, BAN *tocolytic; bronchodilator* [also: hexoprenaline sulfate]

hexoprenaline sulfate USAN, JAN *tocolytic; bronchodilator* [also: hexoprenaline]

hexopyrimidine [see: hexetidine]

hexopyrrolate [see: hexopyrronium bromide]

hexopyrronium bromide INN

hexydaline [see: methenamine mandelate]

hexylcaine INN *local anesthetic* [also: hexylcaine HCl]

hexylcaine HCl USP *local anesthetic* [also: hexylcaine]

hexylene glycol NF *humectant; solvent*

hexylresorcinol USP *anthelmintic; topical antiseptic*

1-hexyltheobromine [see: pentifylline]

H-F Gel *investigational (orphan) emergency treatment for hydrofluoric acid burns* [calcium gluconate]

HFA-134a (hydrofluoroalkane) *propellant used in CFC-free aerosol delivery systems*

hFSH (human follicle-stimulating hormone) [now: menotropins]

HFZ (homofenazine) [q.v.]

^{197}**Hg** [see: chlormerodrin Hg 197]

^{197}**Hg** [see: merisoprol acetate Hg 197]

^{197}**Hg** [see: merisoprol Hg 197]

^{203}**Hg** [see: chlormerodrin Hg 203]

^{203}**Hg** [see: merisoprol acetate Hg 203]

hGH (human growth hormone) [see: somatropin]

hibenzate INN *combining name for radicals or groups* [also: hybenzate]

Hibiclens sponge/brush OTC *broad-spectrum antimicrobial; germicidal* [chlorhexidine gluconate; alcohol 4%] 4%

Hibiclens Antiseptic/AntiMicrobial Skin Cleanser topical liquid OTC *broad-spectrum antimicrobial; germicidal* [chlorhexidine gluconate; alcohol 4%] 4%

hibiscus (*Hibiscus sabdariffa* **and other species)** flowers and leaves *medicinal herb for cancer, edema, heart problems and nervous disorders; also used topically as an emollient; not generally regarded as safe and effective*

Hibistat Germicidal Hand Rinse topical liquid OTC *broad-spectrum antimicrobial; germicidal* [chlorhexidine gluconate; alcohol 70%] 0.5%

Hibistat Towelette OTC *broad-spectrum antimicrobial; germicidal* [chlorhexidine gluconate; alcohol 70%] 0.5%

HibTITER IM injection ℞ *vaccine for H. influenzae type b (HIB) infections in children 2–71 months* [Hemophilus b conjugate vaccine (with a diphtheria CRM$_{197}$ carrier)] 10•(25) mcg/0.5 mL

Hi-C DAZE (high-dose cytarabine, daunorubicin, azacitidine, etoposide) *chemotherapy protocol for acute myelogenous leukemia (AML)*

Hi-Cal VM nutrition bar OTC *enteral nutritional therapy for HIV and AIDS*

Hicon oral solution ℞ *radioactive antineoplastic for thyroid carcinoma; thyroid inhibitor for hyperthyroidism* [sodium iodide I 131] 1000 mCi/mL (250, 500, 1000 mCi/dose)

Hi-Cor 1.0; Hi-Cor 2.5 cream ℞ *corticosteroidal anti-inflammatory* [hydrocortisone] 1%; 2.5%

HIDA (hepatoiminodiacetic acid) [see: lidofenin]

HiDAC (high-dose ara-C) *chemotherapy protocol*

Hieracium pilosella medicinal herb [see: mouse ear]

high angelica *medicinal herb* [see: angelica]

high molecular weight dextran [see: dextran 70]

high osmolar contrast media (HOCM) *a class of older radiopaque* agents that have a high osmolar concentration of iodine (the contrast agent), which corresponds to a higher incidence of adverse reactions [also called: ionic contrast media]

High Potency N-Vites tablets OTC *vitamin supplement* [multiple B vitamins; vitamin C] ± • 500 mg

hilafilcon A USAN *hydrophilic contact lens material*

hilafilcon B USAN *hydrophilic contact lens material*

hillberry *medicinal herb* [see: wintergreen]

Hiltonol *investigational (orphan) agent for orthopoxvirus infections* [polyinosinic-polycytidilic acid]

Himalayan ginseng (Panax pseudoginseng) *medicinal herb* [see: ginseng]

hindheel *medicinal herb* [see: tansy]

hini *medicinal herb* [see: Culver root]

hioxifilcon A USAN *hydrophilic contact lens material*

Hipotest tablets OTC *dietary supplement* [multiple vitamins & minerals; multiple food products; calcium; iron; biotin] ± • 53.5 • 50 • 0.001 mg

Hi-Po-Vites tablets OTC *dietary supplement* [multiple vitamins & minerals; multiple food products; iron; folic acid; biotin] ± • 6 • 0.4 • 1 mg

Hiprex tablets R *urinary antibiotic* [methenamine hippurate] 1 g

Hirudo medicinalis *natural treatment* [see: leeches]

Histacol DM Pediatric oral drops (discontinued 2007) OTC *antitussive; antihistamine; decongestant; for children 1–18 months* [dextromethorphan hydrobromide; brompheniramine maleate; pseudoephedrine HCl] 4 • 1 • 15 mg/mL

Histacol DM Pediatric syrup R *antitussive; decongestant; antihistamine; expectorant* [dextromethorphan hydrobromide; pseudoephedrine HCl; brompheniramine maleate; guaifenesin] 5 • 30 • 2 • 50/5 mL

Histade sustained-release capsules (discontinued 2007) R *decongestant;*

antihistamine [pseudoephedrine HCl; chlorpheniramine maleate] 120 • 12 mg

Histamax D oral drops R *decongestant; antihistamine; for children 1–24 months* [phenylephrine HCl; carbinoxamine maleate] 1.5 • 1.5 mg/mL

histamine dihydrochloride USAN *histamine H_2 receptor agonist; investigational (NDA filed, orphan) adjuvant to interleukin-2 for stage IV malignant melanoma and acute myeloid leukemia (AML); investigational (Phase II) for hepatitis C and renal cell carcinoma*

histamine H_1 antagonists *a class of antihistamines* [also called: H_1 blockers]

histamine H_2 antagonists *a class of gastrointestinal antisecretory agents* [also called: H_2 blockers]

histamine phosphate USP *gastric secretory stimulant; diagnostic aid for pheochromocytoma*

histantin [see: chlorcyclizine HCl]

histapyrrodine INN

Histatab D tablets R *antihistamine; decongestant; anticholinergic to dry mucosal secretions* [dexchlorpheniramine maleate; pseudoephedrine HCl; methscopolamine nitrate] 3.5 • 45 • 1 mg

Histatab Plus tablets (discontinued 2007) OTC *decongestant; antihistamine* [phenylephrine HCl; chlorpheniramine maleate] 5 • 2 mg

Hista-Vent DA sustained-release caplets R *decongestant; antihistamine; anticholinergic to dry mucosal secretions* [phenylephrine HCl; chlorpheniramine maleate; methscopolamine nitrate] 20 • 8 • 2.5 mg

Histenol-Forte tablets (discontinued 2007) OTC *antitussive; decongestant; analgesic; antipyretic* [dextromethorphan hydrobromide; pseudoephedrine HCl; acetaminophen] 10 • 30 • 325 mg

Histex oral liquid R *decongestant; antihistamine* [pseudoephedrine HCl; chlorpheniramine maleate] 30 • 2 mg/5 mL

Histex I/E extended-release capsules ℞ *antihistamine for allergic rhinitis* [carbinoxamine maleate] 10 mg

Histex CT film-coated timed-release tablets ℞ *antihistamine for allergic rhinitis* [carbinoxamine maleate] 8 mg

Histex HC oral liquid ℞ *narcotic antitussive; antihistamine; decongestant* [hydrocodone bitartrate; carbinoxamine maleate; pseudoephedrine HCl] 5•2•30 mg/5 mL

Histex Pd oral liquid ℞ *antihistamine for allergic rhinitis* [carbinoxamine maleate] 4 mg/5 mL

Histex SR extended-release caplets, extended-release capsules ℞ *decongestant; antihistamine* [pseudoephedrine HCl; brompheniramine maleate] 120•10 mg

Histex SR film-coated, sustained-release tablets (discontinued 2007) ℞ *decongestant; antihistamine; analgesic; antipyretic* [phenylephrine HCl; chlorpheniramine maleate; acetaminophen] 40•8•500 mg

histidine (ʟ-histidine) USAN, USP, INN *amino acid (essential in infants and in renal failure, nonessential otherwise); symbols: His, H*

histidine monohydrochloride NF

495-ʟ-histidineglucosylceramidase [see: imiglucerase]

Histinex HC syrup ℞ *narcotic antitussive; antihistamine; decongestant* [hydrocodone bitartrate; chlorpheniramine maleate; phenylephrine HCl] 2.5•2•5 mg/5 mL

Histinex PV syrup ℞ *narcotic antitussive; antihistamine; decongestant* [hydrocodone bitartrate; chlorpheniramine maleate; pseudoephedrine HCl] 2.5•2•30 mg/5 mL

Histolyn-CYL intradermal injection ℞ *diagnostic aid for histoplasmosis* [histoplasmin (mycelial derivative)] 1:100

histoplasmin USP *dermal histoplasmosis test; Histoplasma capsulatum cultures in mycelial or yeast lysate form* 1:100 injection (yeast lysate form)

histrelin USAN, INN *LHRH agonist; investigational (orphan) for acute intermittent porphyria, hereditary coproporphyria, and variegate porphyria*

histrelin acetate *LHRH agonist for palliative treatment of advanced prostate cancer and central precocious puberty (orphan)*

Histussin D oral liquid (discontinued 2006) ℞ *narcotic antitussive; decongestant* [hydrocodone bitartrate; pseudoephedrine HCl] 5•60 mg/5 mL

Histussin HC oral liquid (discontinued 2007) ℞ *narcotic antitussive; antihistamine; decongestant* [hydrocodone bitartrate; dexbrompheniramine maleate; phenylephrine HCl] 2.5•1•5 mg/5 mL

HIV immune globulin (HIVIG) *investigational (Phase III, orphan) immunomodulator for AIDS and maternal/fetal HIV transfer*

HIV immunotherapeutic (HIV-IT); HIV therapeutic *investigational (Phase II) gene therapy for HIV; investigational (Phase I–III) antiviral for symptomatic HIV*

HIV protease inhibitors *a class of antivirals that block HIV replication*

HIV vaccine [see: AIDS vaccine]

HIV-1 LA test [see: Recombigen HIV-1 LA]

HIV-1 peptide vaccine *investigational (Phase I) vaccine for HIV*

HIVAB HIV-1 EIA; HIVAB HIV-1/ HIV-2 EIA; HIVAB HIV-2 EIA reagent kit for professional use ℞ *in vitro diagnostic aid for HIV antibodies* [enzyme immunoassay (EIA)]

HIVAG-1 reagent kit for professional use ℞ *in vitro diagnostic aid for HIV antibodies* [enzyme immunoassay (EIA)]

hive vine *medicinal herb* [see: squaw vine]

Hivid film-coated tablets (discontinued 2006) ℞ *antiviral for advanced HIV infection (orphan)* [zalcitabine] 0.375, 0.75 mg ⃞ Hyphed

HIV-IG *investigational (Phase III, orphan) immunomodulator for AIDS and maternal/fetal HIV transfer* [HIV immune globulin]

HIV-neutralizing antibodies *investigational (orphan) treatment for AIDS*

HLA-B7/beta2M DNA lipid complex *investigational (Phase II/III, orphan) for invasive and metastatic melanoma*

HMB (β-hydroxy-β-methylbutyrate) [q.v.]

HMB (homatropine methylbromide) [q.v.]

HMDP (hydroxymethylene diphosphonate) [see: oxidronic acid]

hMG (human menopausal gonadotropin) [see: menotropins]

HMG-CoA (3-hydroxy-3-methylglutaryl-coenzyme A) reductase inhibitors *a class of antihyperlipidemics that markedly reduce serum LDL and total cholesterol and, to a lesser extent, VLDL and triglycerides* [also called: "statins"]

HMM (hexamethylmelamine) [see: altretamine]

HMS *eye drop suspension (discontinued 2006)* ℞ *steroidal anti-inflammatory* [medrysone] 1%

HN₂ (nitrogen mustard) [see: mechlorethamine HCl]

HOAP-BLEO (hydroxydaunomycin, Oncovin, ara-C, prednisone, bleomycin) *chemotherapy protocol*

hoarhound *medicinal herb* [see: horehound]

hock heal *medicinal herb* [see: woundwort]

hog apple *medicinal herb* [see: mandrake; noni]

hogweed *medicinal herb* [see: broom; masterwort]

Hold DM *lozenges* OTC *antitussive* [dextromethorphan hydrobromide] 5 mg

holly *(Ilex aquifolium; I. opaca; I. vomitoria) leaves and berries medicinal herb used as a CNS stimulant and emetic; not generally regarded as safe and effective*

holly, ground *medicinal herb* [see: pipsissewa]

holly bay *medicinal herb* [see: magnolia]

holly-leaved barberry; holly mahonia *medicinal herb* [see: Oregon grape]

holmium *element* (Ho)

holy thistle; blessed cardus *medicinal herb* [see: blessed thistle]

homarylamine INN

homatropine BAN *ophthalmic anticholinergic* [also: homatropine hydrobromide] ⅀ HumatroPen

homatropine hydrobromide USP *ophthalmic anticholinergic; cycloplegic; mydriatic* [also: homatropine] 5% *eye drops*

homatropine methylbromide USP, INN, BAN *anticholinergic*

homatropine methylbromide & hydrocodone bitartrate *anticholinergic; narcotic antitussive* 1.5•5 mg/5 mL *oral*

Home Access; Home Access Express *test kit for home use* OTC *in vitro diagnostic aid for HIV in the blood*

Home Access Hepatitis C Check *test kit for home use* OTC *in vitro diagnostic aid for hepatitis C in the blood*

homidium bromide INN, BAN

Hominex-1 *powder* OTC *formula for infants with homocystinuria or hypermethioninemia*

Hominex-2 *powder* OTC *enteral nutritional therapy for homocystinuria or hypermethioninemia*

homochlorcyclizine INN, BAN

homofenazine (HFZ) INN

homoharringtonine *investigational (orphan) agent for chronic myelogenous leukemia*

homomenthyl salicylate [see: homosalate]

homopipramol INN

homosalate USAN, INN *ultraviolet sunscreen*

4-homosulfanilamide [see: mafenide]

homprenorphine INN, BAN

honey *natural remedy used as an antibacterial and wound healing agent and as a gargle to promote expectoration;*

not generally regarded as safe and effective for infants because of possible Clostridium botulinum contamination

honeybee venom natural remedy [see: bee venom]

honeybloom medicinal herb [see: dogbane]

hoodwart medicinal herb [see: skullcap]

HOP (hydroxydaunomycin, Oncovin, prednisone) chemotherapy protocol

hopantenic acid INN

hops (Humulus lupulus) flower medicinal herb for aiding digestion, appetite stimulation, bronchitis, cystitis, delirium, edema, headache, hyperactivity, insomnia, intestinal cramps, menstrual disorders, nervousness, pain, excessive sexual desire, and tuberculosis

hoquizil INN bronchodilator [also: hoquizil HCl]

hoquizil HCl USAN bronchodilator [also: hoquizil]

Hordeum vulgare medicinal herb [see: barley]

horehound (Marrubium vulgare) plant medicinal herb for asthma, colds and cough, croup, inducing diaphoresis and diuresis, intestinal parasites, lung disorders, promoting expectoration, and respiratory disorders

horse chestnut (Aesculus californica; A. glabra; A. hippocastanum) nuts and leaves medicinal herb for arthritis, colds and congestion, hemorrhoids, rheumatism, and varicose veins; not generally regarded as safe and effective for internal use as it is highly toxic

horse-elder; horseheal medicinal herb [see: elecampane]

horsefoot; horsehoof medicinal herb [see: coltsfoot]

horsemint (Monarda punctata) leaves and flowering tops medicinal herb used as a cardiac, carminative, diaphoretic, diuretic, emmenagogue, stimulant, and sudorific

horseradish (Armoracia lapathifolia; A. rusticana) root medicinal herb for appetite stimulation, colic, cough, edema, expelling afterbirth, hay fever, poor circulation, sciatic pain, sinus disorders, and skin and internal tumors; also used as a vermifuge

horsetail (Equisetum arvens) plant medicinal herb for bladder disorders, brittle nails, glandular disorders, internal bleeding, nosebleeds, poor circulation, tuberculosis, and urinary disorders

horseweed; fleabane (Erigeron canadensis) plant medicinal herb used as an astringent, diuretic, and hemostatic

ho-shou-wu; fo-ti (Polygonum multiflorum) root medicinal herb for atherosclerosis, blood cleansing, constipation, improving liver and kidney function, insomnia, malaria, muscle aches, tuberculosis, and weak bones; also used to increase fertility, prevent aging, and promote longevity

H.P. Acthar Gel IM or subcu injectable gel ℞ corticosteroid; anti-inflammatory; diagnostic aid for testing adrenocortical function; investigational (orphan) for infantile spasms [corticotropin, repository] 80 U/mL

HPA-23 investigational (orphan) treatment for AIDS

HPMCP (hydroxypropyl methylcellulose phthalate) [q.v.]

HPMPC (3-hydroxy-2-phosphonomethoxypropyl cytosine [dihydrate]) [see: cidofovir]

H-R Lubricating vaginal jelly OTC moisturizer/lubricant [hydroxypropyl methylcellulose]

HspE7 investigational (orphan) agent for recurrent respiratory papillomatosis

5-HT (5-hydroxytryptamine) [see: serotonin]

HT (human thrombin) [see: thrombin]

HT; 3-HT (3-hydroxytyramine) [see: dopamine]

5-HTP (5-hydroxytryptophan) [see: L-5 hydroxytryptophan]

huckleberry medicinal herb [see: bilberry]

Humalog vials, prefilled syringe cartridges, and disposable pen injectors for subcu injection ℞ *rapid-acting insulin analogue for diabetes* [insulin lispro, human (rDNA)] 100 U/mL; 150 U/1.5 mL, 300 U/3 mL; 300 U/3 mL ② hemlock

Humalog KwikPen disposable pen injectors for subcu injection ℞ *rapid-acting insulin analogue for diabetes* [insulin lispro, human (rDNA)] 100 U/mL

Humalog Mix 50/50 KwikPen disposable pen injectors for subcu injection ℞ *dual-acting insulin analogue for diabetes* [insulin lispro protamine; insulin lispro, human (rDNA)] 50%•50% (100 U/mL total)

Humalog Mix 75/25 vials and disposable pen injectors for subcu injection ℞ *dual-acting insulin analogue for diabetes* [insulin lispro protamine; insulin lispro, human (rDNA)] 75%•25% (100 U/mL total)

Humalog Mix 75/25 KwikPen disposable pen injectors for subcu injection ℞ *dual-acting insulin analogue for diabetes* [insulin lispro protamine; insulin lispro, human (rDNA)] 75%•25% (100 U/mL total)

human acid alpha-glucosidase [see: alglucosidase alfa]

Human Albumin Grifols IV infusion ℞ *blood volume expander for shock, burns, and hypoproteinemia* [human albumin] 25%

human amniotic fluid-derived surfactant [see: surfactant, human amniotic fluid derived]

human anti–transforming growth factor [see: anti–transforming growth factor; monoclonal antibody to transforming growth factor]

human B-type natriuretic peptide (hBNP) [see: nesiritide; nesiritide citrate]

human chorionic gonadotropin (hCG) [see: gonadotropin, chorionic]

human complement receptor [see: complement receptor type I, soluble recombinant human]

human diploid cell vaccine (HDCV) [see: rabies vaccine]

human epidermal growth factor receptor (HER) inhibitors *a class of antineoplastics, predominantly monoclonal antibodies, that suppress the growth of breast, colorectal, head, and neck cancers; includes HER1 (q.v.), HER2 (q.v.), HER3, and HER4* [also known as: epidermal growth factor receptor (EGFR) inhibitors]

human follicle-stimulating hormone (hFSH) [now: menotropins]

human growth hormone (hGH) JAN *growth hormone* [also: somatropin]

human growth hormone, recombinant (rhGH) [see: somatropin]

human growth hormone releasing factor (hGH-RF) [see: growth hormone-releasing factor (GH-RF)]

human immunodeficiency virus (HIV) immune globulin (HIVIG) [see: HIV immune globulin]

human insulin [see: insulin, human; insulin aspart; insulin aspart protamine]

human menopausal gonadotropin (hMG) [see: menotropins]

human monoclonal antibodies *antibodies cloned from a single human cell* [see: monoclonal antibodies]

human papillomavirus (HPV), recombinant *vaccine for genital warts (condylomata acuminata), cervical cancer, and precancerous or dysplastic vaginal, vulvar, or cervical intraepithelial neoplasia caused by HPV infections*

human papillomavirus (HPV) recombinant vaccine, bivalent *investigational (NDA filed) vaccine for cervical cancer and precancerous lesions caused by HPV types 16 and 18*

human papillomavirus (HPV) recombinant vaccine, quadrivalent *vaccine for genital warts (condylomata acuminata), cervical cancer, and precancerous or dysplastic vaginal, vulvar, or cervical intraepithelial neoplasia caused by HPV types 6, 11, 16, and*

18; *currently approved for women 9–26 years*

human retinal pigmented epithelial (RPE) cells on spherical cell-coated microcarriers (CCM) *investigational (Phase II, orphan) dopamine-producing brain implants for stage 3 and 4 Parkinson disease*

human serum albumin diethylene-triaminepentaacetic acid (DTPA) technetium (⁹⁹ᵐTc) JAN *radioactive agent* [also: technetium Tc 99m pentetate]

human superoxide dismutase (SOD) [see: superoxide dismutase, human]

Human Surf *investigational (orphan) agent for the prevention and treatment of respiratory distress syndrome (RDS) in premature infants* [surfactant, human amniotic fluid derived]

human T-cell inhibitor [see: muromonab-CD3]

human T-cell lymphotrophic virus type III (HTLV-III) [now: human immunodeficiency virus (HIV)]

Human T-Lymphotropic Virus Type I EIA *reagent kit for professional use* ℞ *in vitro diagnostic aid for HTLV I antibody in serum or plasma* [enzyme immunoassay (EIA)]

human transferrin [see: transferrin, human]

humanized monoclonal antibodies *antibodies cloned from a single murine (mouse/rat) cell, then genetically altered to prevent rejection by the human immune system* [see: monoclonal antibodies]

HumaPen Memoir (trademarked delivery device) ℞ *digital insulin self-injector with 16-dose memory, for use with* **Humalog** (insulin lispro)

Humate-P powder for IV injection ℞ *antihemophilic for von Willebrand disease (orphan)* [antihemophilic factor (AHF); von Willebrand factor (VWF)] 250•600, 500•1200, 1000•2400 U/vial

Humatin capsules ℞ *aminoglycoside antibiotic; amebicide for acute and chronic intestinal amebiasis* [paromomycin sulfate] 250 mg ② Hemotene

Humatrope powder for subcu or IM injection; prefilled cartridges for **HumatroPen** (self-injection device) ℞ *growth hormone for adults or children with congenital or endogenous growth hormone deficiency, children with Turner syndrome or renal-induced growth failure, or AIDS-wasting syndrome (orphan)* [somatropin] 5 mg (15 IU) per vial; 6, 12, 24 mg (18, 36, 72 IU) per cartridge

HumatroPen (trademarked delivery device) *subcu self-injector for* **Humatrope** ② homatropine

HuMax-CD4 *investigational (orphan) for mycosis fungoides* [monoclonal antibody to CD4, human]

Humibid extended-release tablets OTC *expectorant* [guaifenesin] 1200 mg ② Hemopad

Humibid CS tablets (discontinued 2007) OTC *antitussive; expectorant* [dextromethorphan hydrobromide; guaifenesin] 20•400 mg

Humibid DM extended-release capsules (discontinued 2007) ℞ *antitussive; decongestant; expectorant* [dextromethorphan hydrobromide; guaifenesin; potassium guaiacolsulfonate] 50•400•200 mg

Humibid DM sustained-release caplets (discontinued 2004) ℞ *antitussive; expectorant* [dextromethorphan hydrobromide; guaifenesin] 30•600 mg

Humibid E tablets OTC *expectorant* [guaifenesin] 400 mg ② Hemopad

Humibid L.A. sustained-release caplets (discontinued 2004) ℞ *expectorant* [guaifenesin; potassium guaiacolsulfonate] 600•300 mg

Humibid Pediatric sustained-release capsules (discontinued 2004) ℞ *expectorant* [guaifenesin] 300 mg

Humira subcu injection in prefilled syringes ℞ DMARD *for moderate to severe rheumatoid arthritis (RA), juvenile rheumatoid arthritis (JRA; orphan), psoriatic arthritis, and ankylosing spon-*

dylitis; immunostimulant for Crohn disease [adalimumab] 20, 40 mg

HuMist Moisturizing nasal mist OTC *nasal moisturizer* [sodium chloride (saline solution)] 0.65%

Humorsol Ocumeter (eye drops) (discontinued 2004) ℞ *antiglaucoma agent; reversible cholinesterase inhibitor miotic* [demecarium bromide] 0.125%, 0.25%

Humulin 50/50 subcu injection OTC *antidiabetic* [isophane human insulin (rDNA); human insulin (rDNA)] 100 U/mL

Humulin 70/30 prefilled cartridges for subcu injection (discontinued 2004) OTC *antidiabetic* [isophane human insulin (rDNA); human insulin (rDNA)] 150 U/1.5 mL

Humulin 70/30 vials and disposable pen injectors for subcu injection OTC *antidiabetic* [isophane human insulin (rDNA); human insulin (rDNA)] 100 U/mL; 300 U/3 mL

Humulin L subcu injection (discontinued 2005) OTC *antidiabetic* [insulin zinc, human (rDNA)] 100 U/mL

Humulin N prefilled cartridges for subcu injection (discontinued 2004) OTC *antidiabetic* [isophane human insulin (rDNA)] 100 U/1.5 mL

Humulin N vials and disposable pen injectors for subcu injection OTC *antidiabetic* [isophane human insulin (rDNA)] 100 U/mL; 300 U/3 mL

Humulin R vials and disposable pen injectors for subcu injection OTC *antidiabetic* [human insulin (rDNA)] 100 U/mL

Humulin R Regular U-500 (concentrated) subcu injection ℞ *antidiabetic* [insulin, human (rDNA)] 500 U/mL

Humulin U subcu injection (discontinued 2005) OTC *antidiabetic* [insulin zinc, extended human (rDNA)] 100 U/mL

Humulus lupulus medicinal herb [see: hops]

huperzine A *natural extract from Chinese club moss that enhances memory,* *focus, and concentration; prevents the breakdown of the neurotransmitter acetylcholine*

hurr-burr *medicinal herb* [see: burdock]

Hurricaine spray liquid, oral gel OTC *mucous membrane anesthetic* [benzocaine] 20%

Hurricaine topical liquid (discontinued 2007) OTC *mucous membrane anesthetic* [benzocaine] 20%

HXM (hexamethylmelamine) [see: altretamine]

Hyalgan intra-articular injection in vials and prefilled syringes ℞ *viscoelastic lubricant and "shock absorber" for osteoarthritis and temporomandibular joint syndrome* [hyaluronate sodium] 20 mg/2 mL

hyalosidase INN, BAN

hyaluronan *viscoelastic lubricant and "shock absorber" for osteoarthritis of the knee*

hyaluronate sodium USAN, JAN *ophthalmic surgical aid; treatment for osteoarthritis and TMJ syndrome; topical treatment for dermal ulcers, wounds, and burns; veterinary synovitis agent* [also: hyaluronic acid] 0.1% topical

hyaluronic acid BAN *ophthalmic surgical aid; treatment for osteoarthritis and TMJ syndrome; dermal filler for deep wrinkles and facial folds; veterinary synovitis agent; investigational (orphan) for emphysema due to alpha₁-antitrypsin (AaT) deficiency* [also: hyaluronate sodium]

hyaluronidase USP, INN, BAN *adjuvant to increase the absorption and dispersion of injected drugs, hypodermoclysis, and subcutaneous urography; investigational (NDA filed) agent to clear vitreous hemorrhage; also used for diabetic retinopathy*

hyaluronoglucosaminidase [see: hyalosidase]

hyamate [see: buramate]

Hyate:C (Porcine) powder for IV injection ℞ *systemic hemostatic; antihemophilic for the prevention and control of bleeding in classical hemophilia*

(hemophilia A) and von Willebrand disease (orphan) in patients with antibodies to human factor VIII [antihemophilic factor concentrate, porcine] (actual number of AHF units is indicated on the vial)

hybenzate USAN combining name for radicals or groups [also: hibenzate]

Hybri-CEAker radiodiagnostic monoclonal antibody to carcinoembryonic antigen (CEA); investigational (orphan) for the detection of colorectal carcinoma [indium In 111 altumomab pentetate]

Hybrid Capture II Chlamydia Test reagent kit for professional use R in vitro diagnostic aid for Chlamydia trachomatis

Hycamtin capsules R antineoplastic for small cell lung cancer (SCLC) [topotecan HCl] 0.25, 1 mg

Hycamtin powder for IV injection R antineoplastic for ovarian, cervical, and small cell lung cancers; also used for non–small cell lung cancer; investigational (Phase II) for AIDS-related progressive multifocal leukoencephalopathy (PML) [topotecan HCl] 4 mg/dose

hycanthone USAN, INN antischistosomal

hycanthone mesylate antischistosomal

Hycet oral liquid R narcotic analgesic; antipyretic [hydrocodone bitartrate; acetaminophen; alcohol 7%] 2.5•108 mg/5 mL

hyclate INN combining name for radicals or groups

Hycodan tablets, syrup R narcotic antitussive; anticholinergic [hydrocodone bitartrate; homatropine methylbromide] 5•1.5 mg; 5•1.5 mg/5 mL

Hycort cream, ointment R corticosteroidal anti-inflammatory [hydrocortisone] 1%

Hycosin Expectorant syrup (discontinued 2007) R narcotic antitussive; expectorant [hydrocodone bitartrate; guaifenesin; alcohol 10%] 5•100 mg/5 mL

Hycotuss Expectorant syrup R narcotic antitussive; expectorant [hydro-

codone bitartrate; guaifenesin; alcohol 10%] 5•100 mg/5 mL

hydantoins a class of anticonvulsants

Hydase solution for injection R adjuvant to increase the absorption and dispersion of injected drugs, hypodermoclysis, and subcutaneous urography [hyaluronidase (bovine)] 150 U/mL

Hydeltrasol IV, IM injection (discontinued 2008) R corticosteroid; anti-inflammatory [prednisolone sodium phosphate] 20 mg/mL

Hydergine sublingual tablets, tablets, oral liquid R cognition adjuvant for age-related mental capacity decline [ergoloid mesylates] 0.5, 1 mg; 1 mg; 1 mg/mL

Hydergine LC liquid-filled capsules (discontinued 2004) R cognition adjuvant for age-related mental capacity decline [ergoloid mesylates] 1 mg

Hydex PD oral liquid R narcotic antitussive; antihistamine; decongestant [hydrocodone bitartrate; dexchlorpheniramine maleate; phenylephrine HCl] 4•2•5 mg/5 mL

hydracarbazine INN

hydragogues a class of purgatives that produce abundant watery discharge from the bowels

hydralazine INN, BAN antihypertensive; peripheral vasodilator [also: hydralazine HCl]

hydralazine HCl USP, JAN antihypertensive; peripheral vasodilator; investigational (orphan) for severe intrapartum hypertension due to eclampsia or preeclampsia of pregnancy [also: hydralazine] 10, 25, 50, 100 mg oral; 20 mg/mL injection

hydralazine HCl & hydrochlorothiazide antihypertensive; peripheral vasodilator; diuretic 25•25, 50•50 mg oral

hydralazine polistirex USAN antihypertensive

Hydramine syrup, elixir (discontinued 2007) R antihistamine; sleep aid; antitussive [diphenhydramine HCl] 12.5 mg/5 mL

hydrangea (Hydrangea arborescens) leaves and root *medicinal herb for arthritis, bladder infections, gallstones, gonorrhea, gout, kidney stones, rheumatism, and urinary disorders*

Hydrap-ES tablets (discontinued 2007) ℞ *antihypertensive; vasodilator; diuretic* [hydrochlorothiazide; reserpine; hydralazine HCl] 15•0.1•25 mg

hydrargaphen INN, BAN

hydrastine USP

hydrastine HCl USP

hydrastinine HCl NF

Hydrastis canadensis medicinal herb [see: goldenseal]

Hydrate IV or IM injection (discontinued 2006) ℞ *antinauseant; antiemetic; antivertigo; motion sickness preventative* [dimenhydrinate] 50 mg/mL

hydrazinecarboximidamide monohydrochloride [see: pimagedine HCl]

hydrazinoxane [see: domoxin]

Hydrea capsules ℞ *antineoplastic for melanoma, squamous cell carcinoma, myelocytic leukemia, and ovarian cancer; sickle cell anemia treatment (orphan); also adjunctive therapy for HIV infections* [hydroxyurea] 500 mg

Hydrisalic gel ℞ *keratolytic* [salicylic acid] 6%

Hydrisea lotion OTC *moisturizer; emollient* [Dead Sea salts]

Hydrisinol cream, lotion OTC *moisturizer; emollient*

Hydro 40 aerosol foam ℞ *moisturizer; emollient; keratolytic* [urea] 40%

Hydro Cobex IM injection (discontinued 2008) ℞ *hematinic; vitamin B₁₂ supplement* [hydroxocobalamin] 1000 mcg/mL

Hydro GP oral liquid ℞ *narcotic antitussive; decongestant; expectorant* [hydrocodone bitartrate; phenylephrine HCl; guaifenesin] 2.5•7.5•50 mg/5 mL

hydrobentizide INN

hydrobutamine [see: butidrine]

Hydrocare Cleaning and Disinfecting solution OTC *chemical disinfecting solution for soft contact lenses* [thimerosal] 0.002%

Hydrocare Preserved Saline solution OTC *rinsing/storage solution for soft contact lenses* [sodium chloride (preserved saline solution)]

Hydrocerin cream base, lotion base OTC *nontherapeutic base for compounding various dermatological preparations*

Hydrocet capsules ℞ *narcotic analgesic; antipyretic* [hydrocodone bitartrate; acetaminophen] 5•500 mg

hydrochloric acid NF *acidifying agent*

hydrochloric acid, diluted NF *acidifying agent*

hydrochlorothiazide (HCT; HCTZ) USP, INN, BAN *antihypertensive; diuretic* 12.5, 25, 50, 100 mg oral

hydrochlorothiazide & benazepril HCl *antihypertensive; diuretic; angiotensin-converting enzyme (ACE) inhibitor* 6.25•5, 12.5•10, 12.5•20, 25•20 mg oral

hydrochlorothiazide & bisoprolol fumarate *antihypertensive; diuretic; β-blocker* 6.5•2.5, 6.5•5, 6.5•10 mg oral

hydrochlorothiazide & captopril *antihypertensive; diuretic; angiotensin-converting enzyme (ACE) inhibitor* 15•25, 25•25, 15•50, 25•50 mg oral

hydrochlorothiazide & enalapril maleate *antihypertensive; diuretic; angiotensin-converting enzyme (ACE) inhibitor* 12.5•5, 25•10 mg oral

hydrochlorothiazide & fosinopril sodium *antihypertensive; diuretic; angiotensin-converting enzyme (ACE) inhibitor* 12.5•10, 12.5•20 mg

hydrochlorothiazide & hydralazine HCl *antihypertensive; diuretic; peripheral vasodilator* 25•25, 50•50 mg oral

hydrochlorothiazide & lisinopril *antihypertensive; diuretic; angiotensin-converting enzyme (ACE) inhibitor* 12.5•10, 12.5•20, 25•20 mg oral

hydrochlorothiazide & methyldopa *antihypertensive; diuretic; central antiadrenergic* 15•250, 25•250, 30•500, 50•500 mg oral

hydrochlorothiazide & metoprolol tartrate *antihypertensive; diuretic; β-blocker* 25•50, 25•100, 50•100 mg oral

hydrochlorothiazide & moexipril HCl *antihypertensive; diuretic; angiotensin-converting enzyme (ACE) inhibitor* 12.5•7.5, 12.5•15, 25•15 mg oral

hydrochlorothiazide & propranolol HCl *antihypertensive; diuretic; antiadrenergic (β-blocker)* 25•40, 25•80 mg oral

hydrochlorothiazide & quinapril HCl *antihypertensive; diuretic; angiotensin-converting enzyme (ACE) inhibitor* 12.5•10, 12.5•20, 25•10, 25•20 mg oral

hydrochlorothiazide & triamterene *antihypertensive; potassium-sparing diuretic* 25•37.5 mg oral

hydrocholeretics *a class of gastrointestinal drugs that exert laxative effects and increase volume and water content of bile actions*

Hydrocil Instant powder OTC *bulk laxative* [psyllium hydrophilic mucilloid] 3.5 g/scoop

hydrocodone INN, BAN *antitussive* [also: hydrocodone bitartrate]

hydrocodone bitartrate USAN, USP *narcotic antitussive* [also: hydrocodone]

hydrocodone bitartrate & acetaminophen *narcotic antitussive; analgesic* 2.5•500, 5•325, 5•500, 7.5•650, 7.5•750, 10•325, 10•500, 10•650, 10•750 mg oral; 7.5•500, 10•325 mg/15 mL oral

hydrocodone bitartrate & guaifenesin *narcotic antitussive; expectorant* 5•100 mg/5 mL oral

hydrocodone bitartrate & homatropine methylbromide *narcotic antitussive; anticholinergic* 5•1.5 mg/5 mL oral

hydrocodone bitartrate & ibuprofen *narcotic antitussive; analgesic* 7.5•200 mg oral

hydrocodone bitartrate & pseudoephedrine HCl & brompheniramine maleate *narcotic antitussive; decongestant; antihistamine* 2.5•30•3 mg/5 mL oral

hydrocodone bitartrate & pseudoephedrine HCl & carbinoxamine maleate *narcotic antitussive; decongestant; antihistamine* 5•30•2 mg/5 mL oral

Hydrocodone CP syrup (discontinued 2007) ℞ *narcotic antitussive; antihistamine; decongestant* [hydrocodone bitartrate; chlorpheniramine maleate; phenylephrine HCl] 2.5•2•5 mg/5 mL

Hydrocodone GF syrup (discontinued 2007) ℞ *narcotic antitussive; expectorant* [hydrocodone bitartrate; guaifenesin] 5•100 mg/5 mL

Hydrocodone HD oral liquid (discontinued 2007) ℞ *narcotic antitussive; antihistamine; decongestant* [hydrocodone bitartrate; chlorpheniramine maleate; phenylephrine HCl] 3.33•4•10 mg/10 mL

hydrocodone polistirex USAN *narcotic antitussive*

hydrocodone tannate *narcotic antitussive*

Hydrocof-HC oral liquid (discontinued 2007) ℞ *narcotic antitussive; antihistamine; decongestant* [hydrocodone bitartrate; chlorpheniramine maleate; pseudoephedrine HCl] 3•2•15 mg/5 mL

Hydrocol adhesive dressings *occlusive wound dressing* [hydrocolloid gel]

hydrocolloid gel *dressings for wet wounds*

Hydrocort cream ℞ *corticosteroidal anti-inflammatory* [hydrocortisone] 2.5%

hydrocortamate INN

hydrocortamate HCl [see: hydrocortamate]

hydrocortisone (HC) USP, INN, BAN *corticosteroid; anti-inflammatory* 5, 10, 20 mg oral; 0.5%, 1%, 2.5% topical

hydrocortisone aceponate INN *corticosteroid; anti-inflammatory*

hydrocortisone acetate (HCA) USP, BAN *corticosteroid; anti-inflammatory*

1% topical; 25 mg suppositories; 25, 50 mg/mL injection

hydrocortisone acetate & lidocaine HCl *corticosteroidal anti-inflammatory; local anesthetic* 3%•0.5%, 2.5%•3% topical

hydrocortisone & acetic acid *corticosteroid; anti-inflammatory; acidifying agent* 1%•2% otic solution

hydrocortisone buteprate USAN [now: hydrocortisone probutate]

hydrocortisone butyrate BAN *topical corticosteroidal anti-inflammatory* [also: hydrocortisone probutate] 0.1% topical

hydrocortisone cyclopentylpropionate *corticosteroid; anti-inflammatory* [see: hydrocortisone cypionate]

hydrocortisone cypionate USP *corticosteroid; anti-inflammatory*

hydrocortisone hemisuccinate USP *corticosteroid; anti-inflammatory*

hydrocortisone & iodoquinol *corticosteroidal anti-inflammatory; amebicide; antimicrobial* 1%•1% topical

hydrocortisone & neomycin sulfate & polymyxin B sulfate *topical ophthalmic/otic corticosteroidal anti-inflammatory and antibiotic* 1%•0.35%•10 000 U/mL eye drops; 1%•10 000 U/mL•5 mg/mL ear drops

hydrocortisone probutate USAN, USP *topical corticosteroidal anti-inflammatory* [previously known as: hydrocortisone buteprate]

hydrocortisone sodium phosphate USP, BAN *corticosteroid; anti-inflammatory*

hydrocortisone sodium succinate USP, BAN *corticosteroid; anti-inflammatory*

hydrocortisone valerate USAN, USP *topical corticosteroidal anti-inflammatory* 0.2% topical

Hydrocortisone with Aloe ointment OTC *corticosteroidal anti-inflammatory; emollient* [hydrocortisone; aloe] 1%• $\frac{?}{}$

Hydrocortone tablets ℞ *corticosteroid; anti-inflammatory* [hydrocortisone] 10, 20 mg

Hydrocortone Acetate intralesional, intra-articular, or soft tissue injection ℞ *corticosteroid; anti-inflammatory* [hydrocortisone acetate] 25, 50 mg/mL

Hydrocortone Phosphate IV, subcu, or IM injection ℞ *corticosteroid; anti-inflammatory* [hydrocortisone sodium phosphate] 50 mg/mL

Hydrocotyle asiatica medicinal herb [see: gotu kola]

Hydrocream Base OTC *cream base*

Hydro-Crysti 12 IM injection (discontinued 2008) ℞ *hematinic; vitamin* B_{12} *supplement* [hydroxocobalamin] 1000 mcg/mL

HydroDIURIL tablets ℞ *antihypertensive; diuretic* [hydrochlorothiazide] 25 mg

Hydro-DP syrup (discontinued 2007) ℞ *narcotic antitussive; antihistamine; sleep aid; decongestant* [hydrocodone bitartrate; diphenhydramine HCl; phenylephrine HCl] 2•12.5•7.5 mg/5 mL

HydroFed syrup ℞ *narcotic antitussive; decongestant; expectorant* [hydrocodone bitartrate; phenylephrine HCl; guaifenesin] 2.5•6•150 mg/5 mL

hydrofilcon A USAN *hydrophilic contact lens material*

hydroflumethiazide USP, INN, BAN *antihypertensive; diuretic*

hydrofluoric acid dental *caries prophylactic*

hydrofluoroalkane (HFA) *propellant used in CFC-free aerosol delivery systems* [usually HFA-134a]

hydrogen *element (H)*

hydrogen peroxide USP *topical anti-infective*

hydrogen tetrabromoaurate [see: bromauric acid]

hydrogenated ergot alkaloids [now: ergoloid mesylates]

hydrogenated vegetable oil [see: vegetable oil, hydrogenated]

Hydrogesic capsules ℞ *narcotic analgesic; antipyretic* [hydrocodone bitartrate; acetaminophen] 5•500 mg

hydromadinone INN

Hydromet syrup (discontinued 2007) ℞ *narcotic antitussive; anticholinergic* [hydrocodone bitartrate; homatropine methylbromide] 5•1.5 mg/5 mL

Hydromide syrup (discontinued 2007) ℞ *narcotic antitussive; anticholinergic* [hydrocodone bitartrate; homatropine methylbromide] 5•1.5 mg/5 mL

hydromorphinol INN, BAN

hydromorphone INN, BAN *narcotic analgesic; widely abused as a street drug* [also: hydromorphone HCl]

hydromorphone HCl USP *narcotic analgesic; widely abused as a street drug* [also: hydromorphone] 2, 4, 8 mg oral; 1 mg/mL oral; 3 mg rectal; 1, 2, 4, 10 mg/mL injection

hydromorphone sulfate

Hydron CP oral liquid ℞ *narcotic antitussive; antihistamine; decongestant* [hydrocodone bitartrate; chlorpheniramine maleate; phenylephrine HCl] 5•2•10 mg/5 mL

Hydron EX; Hydron KGS oral liquid ℞ *narcotic antitussive; expectorant* [hydrocodone bitartrate; potassium guaiacolsulfonate] 2.5•120 mg/5 mL; 5•300 mg/5 mL

Hydron PSC oral liquid ℞ *narcotic antitussive; antihistamine; decongestant* [hydrocodone bitartrate; chlorpheniramine maleate; pseudoephedrine HCl] 5•2•30 mg/5 mL

Hydropane syrup (discontinued 2007) ℞ *narcotic antitussive; anticholinergic* [hydrocodone bitartrate; homatropine methylbromide] 5•1.5 mg/5 mL

Hydro-Par tablets ℞ *antihypertensive; diuretic* [hydrochlorothiazide] 25, 50 mg

Hydro-PC oral liquid (discontinued 2007) ℞ *narcotic antitussive; antihistamine; decongestant* [hydrocodone bitartrate; chlorpheniramine maleate; phenylephrine HCl] 2•2•5 mg/5 mL

Hydro-PC II oral liquid ℞ *narcotic antitussive; antihistamine; decongestant* [hydrocodone bitartrate; chlorphen-

iramine maleate; phenylephrine HCl] 2•2•7.5 mg/5 mL

Hydropel ointment OTC *skin protectant* [silicone; hydrophobic starch derivative] 30%•10%

Hydrophed tablets (discontinued 2007) ℞ *antiasthmatic; bronchodilator; decongestant; antihistamine* [theophylline; ephedrine sulfate; hydroxyzine HCl] 130•25•10 mg

Hydrophilic OTC *ointment base*

hydrophilic ointment [see: ointment, hydrophilic]

hydrophilic petrolatum [see: petrolatum, hydrophilic]

Hydropres-50 tablets (discontinued 2007) ℞ *antihypertensive; diuretic* [hydrochlorothiazide; reserpine] 50• 0.125 mg

hydroquinone USP *hyperpigmentation bleaching agent* 3%, 4% topical

hydroquinone methyl ether [see: mequinol]

Hydro-Serp tablets (discontinued 2007) ℞ *antihypertensive; diuretic* [hydrochlorothiazide; reserpine] 50• 0.125 mg

Hydroserpine #1; Hydroserpine #2 tablets (discontinued 2007) ℞ *antihypertensive; diuretic* [hydrochlorothiazide; reserpine] 25•0.125 mg; 50• 0.125 mg

HydroSkin cream, lotion OTC *corticosteroidal anti-inflammatory* [hydrocortisone] 1%

HydroSkin ointment (discontinued 2007) OTC *corticosteroidal anti-inflammatory* [hydrocortisone] 1%

hydrotalcite INN, BAN

Hydro-Tussin CBX syrup ℞ *decongestant; antihistamine* [pseudoephedrine HCl; carbinoxamine maleate] 25•2 mg/5 mL

Hydro-Tussin DM oral liquid ℞ *antitussive; expectorant* [dextromethorphan hydrobromide; guaifenesin] 20•200 mg/5 mL

Hydro-Tussin HC syrup ℞ *narcotic antitussive; antihistamine; decongestant* [hydrocodone bitartrate; chlorpheniramine maleate; pseudoephedrine HCl] 3•2•15 mg/5 mL

Hydro-Tussin HD oral liquid ℞ *narcotic antitussive; decongestant; expectorant* [hydrocodone bitartrate; pseudoephedrine HCl; guaifenesin] 2.5•30•100 mg/5 mL

Hydro-Tussin HG syrup ℞ *narcotic antitussive; expectorant* [hydrocodone bitartrate; guaifenesin] 3.5•100 mg/5 mL

Hydro-Tussin XP syrup ℞ *narcotic antitussive; decongestant; expectorant* [hydrocodone bitartrate; pseudoephedrine HCl; guaifenesin] 3•15•100 mg/5 mL

hydroxamethocaine BAN [also: hydroxytetracaine]

hydroxidione sodium succinate [see: hydroxydione sodium succinate]

hydroxindasate INN

hydroxindasol INN

hydroxizine chloride [see: hydroxyzine HCl]

hydroxocobalamin USAN, USP, INN, BAN, JAN *vitamin B₁₂; hematopoietic; antidote to acute cyanide poisoning (orphan)* [also: hydroxocobalamin acetate] 1 mg/mL injection

hydroxocobalamin acetate JAN *vitamin B₁₂; hematopoietic* [also: hydroxocobalamin]

hydroxocobalamin & sodium thiosulfate *investigational (orphan) for severe acute cyanide poisoning*

hydroxocobemine [see: hydroxocobalamin]

3-hydroxy-2-phosphonomethoxypropyl cytosine (HPMPC) dihydrate [see: cidofovir]

N-hydroxyacetamide [see: acetohydroxamic acid]

4′-hydroxyacetanilide [see: acetaminophen]

4′-hydroxyacetanilide salicylate [see: acetaminosalol]

hydroxyamfetamine INN *ophthalmic adrenergic; mydriatic* [also: hydroxyamphetamine hydrobromide; hydroxyamphetamine]

hydroxyamphetamine BAN *ophthalmic adrenergic; mydriatic* [also: hydroxyamphetamine hydrobromide; hydroxyamfetamine]

hydroxyamphetamine hydrobromide USP *ophthalmic adrenergic/vasoconstrictor; mydriatic* [also: hydroxyamfetamine; hydroxyamphetamine]

4-hydroxyanisole (4HA); p-hydroxyanisole [see: mequinol]

hydroxyapatite BAN *prosthetic aid* [also: durapatite; calcium phosphate, tribasic]

2-hydroxybenzamide [see: salicylamide]

2-hydroxybenzoic acid [see: salicylic acid]

o-hydroxybenzyl alcohol [see: salicyl alcohol]

hydroxybutanedioic acid [see: malic acid]

4-hydroxybutanoic acid [see: gamma hydroxybutyrate (GHB)]

4-hydroxybutanoic acid, sodium salt [see: sodium oxybate]

hydroxybutyrate sodium, gamma [see: sodium oxybate]

hydroxycarbamide INN *antineoplastic* [also: hydroxyurea]

hydroxychloroquine INN, BAN *antimalarial; lupus erythematosus suppressant* [also: hydroxychloroquine sulfate]

hydroxychloroquine sulfate USP *antimalarial; antirheumatic; lupus erythematosus suppressant* (base=77.5%) [also: hydroxychloroquine] 200 mg oral

25-hydroxycholecalciferol [see: calcifediol]

hydroxycincophene [see: oxycinchophen]

hydroxydaunomycin [see: doxorubicin]

14-hydroxydihydromorphine [see: hydromorphinol]

hydroxydione sodium succinate INN, BAN

1α-hydroxyergocalciferol [see: doxercalciferol]

hydroxyethyl cellulose NF *suspending and viscosity-increasing agent; ophthalmic aid*

2-hydroxyethyl methacrylate (HEMA) *contact lens material*

hydroxyethyl starch (HES) [see: hetastarch]

hydroxyethylstarch JAN *plasma volume extender* [also: hetastarch]

hydroxyhexamide

3-hydroxyisovalerate; β-hydroxyisovalerate [see: β-hydroxy-β-methylbutyrate (HMB)]

hydroxylapatite [see: durapatite; calcium phosphate, tribasic]

hydroxymagnesium aluminate [see: magaldrate]

hydroxymesterone [see: medrysone]

6-hydroxymethylacylfulvene *investigational (orphan) for advanced or metastatic pancreatic cancer*

β-hydroxy-β-methylbutyrate (HMB) *an endogenous metabolite of the amino acid L-leucine; a natural supplement taken to prevent exercise-induced muscle breakdown (proteolysis), resulting in larger muscle gains from resistance training; may have immunomodulatory effects*

hydroxymethylene diphosphonate (HMDP) [see: oxidronic acid]

hydroxymethylgramicidin [see: methocidin]

N-hydroxynaphthalimide diethyl phosphate [see: naftalofos]

hydroxypethidine INN, BAN

hydroxyphenamate USAN *minor tranquilizer* [also: oxyfenamate]

N-4-hydroxyphenylretinamide [see: fenretinide]

hydroxyprocaine INN, BAN

hydroxyprogesterone INN, BAN *synthetic progestin for amenorrhea, metrorrhagia, and dysfunctional uterine bleeding* [also: hydroxyprogesterone caproate]

hydroxyprogesterone caproate USP, INN, JAN *synthetic progestin for amenorrhea, metrorrhagia, and dysfunctional uterine bleeding* [also: hydroxyprogesterone] 125, 250 mg/mL IM injection (in oil)

2-hydroxypropanoic acid, calcium salt, hydrate [see: calcium lactate]

hydroxypropyl cellulose NF *topical protectant; emulsifying and coating agent* [also: hydroxypropylcellulose]

hydroxypropyl methylcellulose USP *suspending and viscosity-increasing agent; ophthalmic moisturizer and surgical aid; vaginal moisturizer/lubricant* [also: hypromellose; hydroxypropylmethylcellulose]

hydroxypropyl methylcellulose 1828 USP

hydroxypropyl methylcellulose phthalate (HPMCP) NF *tablet-coating agent* [also: hydroxypropylmethylcellulose phthalate]

hydroxypropyl methylcellulose phthalate 200731 NF *tablet-coating agent*

hydroxypropyl methylcellulose phthalate 220824 NF *tablet-coating agent*

hydroxypropylcellulose JAN *topical protectant; emulsifying and coating agent* [also: hydroxypropyl cellulose]

hydroxypropylmethylcellulose JAN *suspending and viscosity-increasing agent; ophthalmic surgical aid* [also: hydroxypropyl methylcellulose; hypromellose]

hydroxypropylmethylcellulose phthalate JAN *tablet-coating agent* [also: hydroxypropyl methylcellulose phthalate]

hydroxypyridine tartrate INN

hydroxyquinoline *topical antiseptic and protectant*

4′-hydroxysalicylanilide [see: osalmid]

hydroxystearin sulfate NF

hydroxystenozole INN

hydroxystilbamidine INN, BAN *antileishmanial* [also: hydroxystilbamidine isethionate]

hydroxystilbamidine isethionate USP *antileishmanial* [also: hydroxystilbamidine]

hydroxysuccinic acid [see: malic acid]

hydroxytetracaine INN [also: hydroxamethocaine]

hydroxytoluic acid INN, BAN

5-hydroxytryptamine₁ (5-HT₁) [see: serotonin]

5-hydroxytryptamine₃ (5-HT₃) receptor antagonists *a class of antinauseant and antiemetic agents used primarily after emetogenic cancer chemotherapy*

5-hydroxytryptophan (5-HTP) [see: L-5 hydroxytryptophan]

3-hydroxytyramine (HT; 3-HT) [see: dopamine]

hydroxyurea USAN, USP, BAN *antimetabolite antineoplastic for melanoma, squamous cell carcinoma, myelocytic leukemia, and ovarian cancer; sickle cell anemia treatment (orphan); also adjunctive therapy for HIV infections* [also: hydroxycarbamide] 250, 500 mg oral

1α-hydroxyvitamin D₂ [see: doxercalciferol]

hydroxyzine INN, BAN *anxiolytic; minor tranquilizer; antiemetic; piperazine antihistamine; antipruritic* [also: hydroxyzine HCl]

hydroxyzine HCl USP *anxiolytic; minor tranquilizer; antiemetic; piperazine antihistamine; antipruritic* [also: hydroxyzine] 10, 25, 50 mg oral; 10 mg/5 mL oral; 25, 50 mg/mL injection

hydroxyzine pamoate USP *anxiolytic; minor tranquilizer; antiemetic; piperazine antihistamine; antipruritic* 25, 50, 100 mg oral

Hyflex-650 tablets ℞ *analgesic; antipyretic; antihistamine; sleep aid* [acetaminophen; phenyltoloxamine citrate] 650•60 mg

Hygenic Cleansing anorectal pads OTC *moisturizer and cleanser for external rectal/vaginal areas; astringent* [witch hazel] 50%

Hygroton tablets ℞ *antihypertensive; diuretic* [chlorthalidone] 100 mg

Hy-KXP oral liquid ℞ *narcotic antitussive; expectorant* [hydrocodone bitartrate; potassium guaiacolsulfonate] 4.5•300 mg/5 mL

Hylaform gel for subcu injection in prefilled syringes ℞ *dermal filler for wrinkles and facial folds* [hylan B] 5.5 mg/mL

hylan B *hyaluronic acid gel–based dermal filler*

hylan G-F 20 *hyaluronic acid gel-fluid polymer mixture for osteoarthritis and TMJ syndrome*

Hylenex solution for injection ℞ *adjuvant to increase the absorption and dispersion of injected drugs, hypodermoclysis, and subcutaneous urography* [hyaluronidase (recombinant human)] 150 U/mL

Hylira gel ℞ *wound healing agent for skin irritations, dermal ulcers, wounds, and burns* [hyaluronate sodium] 0.2%

Hylorel tablets (discontinued 2008) ℞ *antihypertensive* [guanadrel sulfate] 10, 25 mg

Hylutin IM injection (discontinued 2004) ℞ *synthetic progestin for amenorrhea, metrorrhagia, and dysfunctional uterine bleeding* [hydroxyprogesterone caproate in oil] 125, 250 mg/mL

hymecromone USAN, INN *choleretic*

HyoMax-FT chewable tablets ℞ *GI/GU antispasmodic; anticholinergic* [hyoscyamine sulfate] 0.125 mg

hyoscine hydrobromide BAN *GI antispasmodic; prevent motion sickness; cycloplegic; mydriatic* [also: scopolamine hydrobromide]

hyoscine methobromide BAN *anticholinergic* [also: methscopolamine bromide]

hyoscyamine (L-hyoscyamine) USP, BAN *anticholinergic; urinary antispasmodic*

hyoscyamine hydrobromide USP *GI antispasmodic; anticholinergic*

hyoscyamine sulfate USP *GI/GU antispasmodic; antiparkinsonian; anticholinergic "drying agent" for allergic rhinitis and hyperhidrosis* [also: hyoscyamine sulphate] 0.125, 0.25, 0.375 mg oral; 0.125 mg/mL oral

hyoscyamine sulphate BAN *GI/GU antispasmodic; antiparkinsonian; anti-*

cholinergic "drying agent" for allergic rhinitis and hyperhidrosis [also: hyoscyamine sulfate]

Hyoscyamus niger medicinal herb [see: henbane]

Hyosophen tablets, elixir (discontinued 2008) ℞ *GI/GU anticholinergic/antispasmodic; sedative* [atropine sulfate; scopolamine hydrobromide; hyoscyamine hydrobromide; phenobarbital] 0.0194•0.0065•0.1037•16.2 mg; 0.0194•0.0065•0.1037•16.2 mg/5 mL

Hypaque-76 injection ℞ *radiopaque contrast medium* [diatrizoate meglumine; diatrizoate sodium (48.7% total iodine)] 660•100 mg/mL (370 mg/mL)

Hypaque-Cysto intracavitary instillation ℞ *radiopaque contrast medium for urological imaging* [diatrizoate meglumine (46.67% iodine)] 300 mg/mL (141 mg/mL)

Hypaque Meglumine 60% injection ℞ *radiopaque contrast medium* [diatrizoate meglumine (46.67% iodine)] 600 mg/mL (282 mg/mL)

Hypaque Sodium powder for oral/rectal solution ℞ *radiopaque contrast medium for gastrointestinal imaging* [diatrizoate sodium (59.87% iodine)] 1002 mg/g (600 mg/g)

Hypaque Sodium 50% injection ℞ *radiopaque contrast medium* [diatrizoate sodium (46.67% iodine)] 500 mg/mL (300 mg/mL)

HyperHEP B S/D IM injection ℞ *hepatitis B immunizing agent* [hepatitis B immune globulin, solvent/detergent treated] 0.5, 1, 5 mL

hypericin investigational (Phase III, orphan) antineoplastic for glioblastoma multiforme and cutaneous T-cell lymphoma

Hypericum perforatum medicinal herb [see: St. John's wort]

Hyperlyte CR IV admixture ℞ *intravenous electrolyte therapy* [combined electrolyte solution]

Hypermune RSV investigational (orphan) treatment for respiratory syncytial virus (RSV) infections [respiratory syncytial virus immune globulin (RSV-IG)]

hyperosmotic laxatives a subclass of laxatives that use the osmotic effect to retain water in the intestines, lowering colonic pH and increasing peristalsis [see also: laxatives]

HyperRab S/D IM injection ℞ *passive immunizing agent for use after rabies exposure* [rabies immune globulin, solvent/detergent treated] 150 IU/mL (300, 1500 IU/dose)

HyperRHO S/D Mini-Dose IM injection ℞ *obstetric Rh factor immunity suppressant* [Rh$_O$(D) immune globulin, solvent/detergent treated] 50 mcg

Hyperstat IV injection ℞ *vasodilator for hypertensive emergency* [diazoxide] 15 mg/mL

Hyphed syrup ℞ *narcotic antitussive; antihistamine; decongestant* [hydrocodone bitartrate; chlorpheniramine maleate; pseudoephedrine HCl; alcohol 5%] 2.5•2•30 mg/5 mL ② Hivid

Hy-Phen tablets ℞ *narcotic analgesic; antipyretic* [hydrocodone bitartrate; acetaminophen] 5•500 mg

hyphylline [see: dyphylline]

hypnogene [see: barbital]

hypnotics a class of agents that induce sleep

hypochlorous acid, sodium salt [see: sodium hypochlorite]

β-hypophamine [see: vasopressin]

α-hypophamine [see: oxytocin]

hypophosphorous acid NF *antioxidant*

Hyporet (trademarked delivery form) prefilled disposable syringe

HypoTears ophthalmic ointment OTC *moisturizer/lubricant* [white petrolatum; mineral oil]

HypoTears; HypoTears PF eye drops OTC *moisturizer/lubricant* [polyvinyl alcohol] 1%

hyprolose [see: hydroxypropyl cellulose]

hypromellose INN, BAN *suspending and viscosity-increasing agent* [also:

hydroxypropyl methylcellulose;
hydroxypropylmethylcellulose]

Hyskon uterine infusion ℞ *hysteroscopy aid* [dextran 70; dextrose] 32%•10%

Hysone cream OTC *corticosteroidal anti-inflammatory; antifungal; antibacterial* [hydrocortisone; clioquinol] 10•30 mg/g

hyssop (*Hyssopus officinalis*) leaves *medicinal herb for chronic hay fever, congestion, cough, lung ailments, promoting expectoration, and sore throat*

hyssop, hedge *medicinal herb* [see: hedge hyssop]

hyssop, Indian; wild hyssop *medicinal herb* [see: blue vervain]

hyssop, prairie *medicinal herb* [see: wild hyssop]

Hytakerol capsules (discontinued 2005) ℞ *vitamin D therapy for tetany and hypoparathyroidism* [dihydrotachysterol] 0.125 mg

HyTan oral suspension ℞ *narcotic antitussive; antihistamine* [hydrocodone tannate; chlorpheniramine tannate] 5•4 mg/5 mL

Hytinic capsules (discontinued 2006) OTC *hematinic; iron supplement* [polysaccharide-iron complex] 150 mg Fe

Hytinic IM injection (discontinued 2005) ℞ *hematinic* [ferrous gluconate; multiple B vitamins; procaine HCl] 3 mg/mL• ≝ •2%

Hytone cream, lotion, ointment ℞ *corticosteroidal anti-inflammatory* [hydrocortisone] 1%, 2.5%; 1%, 2.5%; 2.5%

Hytone 1% ointment, spray ℞ *corticosteroidal anti-inflammatory* [hydrocortisone] 1%

Hytrin soft capsules ℞ α_1-*adrenergic blocker for hypertension and benign prostatic hyperplasia (BPH)* [terazosin HCl] 1, 2, 5, 10 mg

Hytuss tablets (discontinued 2006) OTC *expectorant* [guaifenesin] 100 mg

Hytuss 2X capsules (discontinued 2006) OTC *expectorant* [guaifenesin] 200 mg

Hyzaar 50-12.5; Hyzaar 100-12.5; Hyzaar 100-25 film-coated tablets ℞ *antihypertensive; angiotensin II receptor antagonist; diuretic* [losartan potassium; hydrochlorothiazide] 50•12.5 mg; 100•12.5 mg; 100•25 mg

I

[123]I [see: iodohippurate sodium I 123]
[123]I [see: sodium iodide I 123]
[125]I [see: albumin, iodinated I 125 serum]
[125]I [see: diatrizoate sodium I 125]
[125]I [see: diohippuric acid I 125]
[125]I [see: diotyrosine I 125]
[125]I [see: fibrinogen I 125]
[125]I [see: insulin I 125]
[125]I [see: iodohippurate sodium I 125]
[125]I [see: iodopyracet I 125]
[125]I [see: iomethin I 125]
[125]I [see: iothalamate sodium I 125]
[125]I [see: liothyronine I 125]
[125]I [see: oleic acid I 125]

[125]I [see: povidone I 125]
[125]I [see: rose bengal sodium I 125]
[125]I [see: sodium iodide I 125]
[125]I [see: thyroxine I 125]
[125]I [see: triolein I 125]
[131]I [see: albumin, aggregated iodinated I 131 serum]
[131]I [see: albumin, iodinated I 131 serum]
[131]I [see: diatrizoate sodium I 131]
[131]I [see: diohippuric acid I 131]
[131]I [see: diotyrosine I 131]
[131]I [see: ethiodized oil I 131]
[131]I [see: insulin I 131]
[131]I [see: iodipamide sodium I 131]

^{131}I [see: iodoantipyrine I 131]
^{131}I [see: iodocholesterol I 131]
^{131}I [see: iodohippurate sodium I 131]
^{131}I [see: iodopyracet I 131]
^{131}I [see: iomethin I 131]
^{131}I [see: iothalamate sodium I 131]
^{131}I [see: iotyrosine I 131]
^{131}I [see: liothyronine I 131]
^{131}I [see: macrosalb (^{131}I)]
^{131}I [see: oleic acid I 131]
^{131}I [see: povidone I 131]
^{131}I [see: rose bengal sodium I 131]
^{131}I [see: sodium iodide I 131]
^{131}I [see: thyroxine I 131]
^{131}I [see: tolpovidone I 131]
^{131}I [see: triolein I 131]

ibacitabine INN

ibafloxacin USAN, INN, BAN *antibacterial*

ibandronate sodium USAN *bisphosphonate bone resorption inhibitor for the prevention and treatment of postmenopausal osteoporosis in women; also used for metastatic bone disease in breast cancer*

ibazocine INN

IBC (isobutyl cyanoacrylate) [see: bucrylate]

Iberet; Iberet-500 controlled-release Filmtabs (film-coated tablets) OTC *hematinic* [multiple B vitamins; ferrous sulfate; sodium ascorbate] ≛•105•150 mg; ≛•105•500 mg ☒ eyebright

Iberet-Folic-500 controlled-release Filmtabs (film-coated tablets) (discontinued 2008) ℞ *hematinic* [ferrous sulfate; multiple B vitamins; sodium ascorbate; folic acid] 105• ≛ •500•0.8 mg

iboga *(Tabernanthe iboga)* euphoric/ hallucinogenic street drug, the root of which is chewed or chopped into a fine powder and mixed with other drugs; doses high enough to induce hallucinations are also likely to cause death

ibopamine USAN, INN, BAN *peripheral dopaminergic agent; vasodilator*

ibritumomab tiuxetan USAN *radioimmunotherapy carrier; monoclonal antibody radiolabeled with indium In 111*

and yttrium Y 90 to treat non-Hodgkin B-cell lymphoma (orphan)

ibrotal [see: ibrotamide]

ibrotamide INN

IB-Stat oral spray ℞ *pediatric anticholinergic "drying agent" for allergic rhinitis and hyperhidrosis* [hyoscyamine sulfate] 0.125 mg/mL

ibudilast INN

Ibudone film-coated tablets ℞ *narcotic analgesic; antipyretic* [hydrocodone bitartrate; ibuprofen] 5•200, 10•200 mg ☒ Iopidine

ibufenac USAN, INN *analgesic; anti-inflammatory*

ibuprofen USAN, USP, INN, BAN *analgesic; antipyretic; antiarthritic; nonsteroidal anti-inflammatory drug (NSAID) for mild to moderate pain, migraine headaches, and primary dysmenorrhea* 200, 400, 600, 800 mg oral; 100 mg/ 5 mL oral; 40 mg/mL oral

ibuprofen aluminum USAN *analgesic; antipyretic; antiarthritic; nonsteroidal anti-inflammatory drug (NSAID) for mild to moderate pain, migraine headaches, and primary dysmenorrhea*

Ibuprofen Children's Cold oral suspension OTC *decongestant; analgesic; antipyretic* [pseudoephedrine HCl; ibuprofen] 15•100 mg/5 mL

ibuprofen & hydrocodone bitartrate *analgesic; narcotic antitussive* 200•7.5 mg oral

ibuprofen lysine *nonsteroidal antiinflammatory drug (NSAID) used to close a significant patent ductus arteriosus (PDA) in premature infants* (orphan) (base=58.5%)

ibuprofen & oxycodone HCl *narcotic analgesic* 400•5 mg oral

ibuprofen piconol USAN *topical anti-inflammatory*

ibuproxam INN

Ibutab tablets OTC *analgesic; antipyretic; antiarthritic; nonsteroidal anti-inflammatory drug (NSAID) for mild to moderate pain, migraine headaches, and primary dysmenorrhea* [ibuprofen] 200 mg

ibutamoren mesylate USAN *growth hormone for congenital growth hormone deficiency, musculoskeletal impairment, and hip fractures*

ibuterol INN

ibutilide INN *antiarrhythmic* [also: ibutilide fumarate]

ibutilide fumarate USAN *antiarrhythmic for atrial fibrillation/flutter* [also: ibutilide]

ibuverine INN ⊡ Epifrin

ibylcaine chloride [see: butethamine HCl]

ICA 17043 *investigational (Phase III) agent for sickle cell disease*

ICaps timed-release tablets OTC *vitamin/mineral supplement* [multiple vitamins & minerals] ⊡ Aquabase; Equipoise

ICaps Plus tablets OTC *vitamin/mineral supplement* [multiple vitamins & minerals]

Icar chewable tablets, oral suspension OTC *hematinic; iron supplement* [carbonyl iron] 15 mg; 15 mg/1.25 mL ⊡ agar

icatibant acetate USAN *investigational (NDA filed, orphan) competitive bradykinin receptor-2 antagonist for hereditary angioedema and burn-induced edema*

ICE (idarubicin, cytarabine, etoposide) *chemotherapy protocol for acute myelogenous leukemia (AML)*

ICE (ifosfamide [with mesna rescue], carboplatin, etoposide) *chemotherapy protocol for osteosarcoma and lung cancer* [also: MICE]

Iceland moss (Cetraria islandica) plant *medicinal herb for anemia, bronchitis, hay fever, congestion, cough, digestive disorders, and lung disorders*

ICE-T (ifosfamide [with mesna rescue], carboplatin, etoposide, Taxol) *chemotherapy protocol for sarcoma, breast cancer, and non–small cell lung cancer (NSCLC)* ⊡ Aceta

IC-Green powder for IV injection Ŗ *in vivo diagnostic aid for cardiac output, hepatic function, and ophthalmic*

angiography [indocyanine green] 25 mg ⊡ Wigraine

ichthammol USP, BAN *topical anti-infective* 10%, 20%

iclazepam INN

icodextrin INN, BAN *peritoneal dialysis solution for end-stage renal disease* (orphan)

icopezil maleate USAN *acetylcholinesterase inhibitor; cognition adjuvant for Alzheimer disease*

icosapent INN *omega-3 marine triglyceride* [also: eicosapentaenoic acid (EPA)]

icospiramide INN ⊡ oxiperomide

icotidine USAN *antagonist to histamine H_1 and H_2 receptors*

ictasol USAN *disinfectant*

Ictotest reagent tablets for professional use Ŗ *in vitro diagnostic aid for bilirubin in the urine*

Icy Hot balm, cream OTC *analgesic; mild anesthetic; antipruritic; counterirritant* [methyl salicylate; menthol] 29%•7.6%; 30%•10%

Icy Hot Back Pain Relief; Icy Hot Pop & Peel; Icy Hot Pro-Therapy transdermal patch OTC *mild anesthetic; antipruritic; counterirritant* [menthol] 5%

Icy Hot Chill Stick OTC *analgesic; mild anesthetic; antipruritic; counterirritant* [methyl salicylate; menthol] 30%•10%

IDA-based BF 12 (idarubicin, cytarabine, etoposide) *chemotherapy protocol for acute myelogenous leukemia (AML)*

Idamycin powder for IV injection (discontinued 2004) Ŗ *anthracycline antibiotic antineoplastic for acute myeloid leukemia (AML) (orphan); investigational (orphan) for myelodysplastic syndromes, acute and chronic myelogenous leukemia, and acute lymphoblastic leukemia in pediatric patients* [idarubicin HCl] 5, 10, 20 mg

Idamycin PFS powder for IV infusion Ŗ *anthracycline antibiotic antineoplastic for acute myeloid leukemia (AML)*

(orphan); investigational (orphan) for myelodysplastic syndromes, acute and chronic myelogenous leukemia, and acute lymphoblastic leukemia in pediatric patients [idarubicin HCl] 5, 10, 20 mg/vial

idarubicin (IDR) INN, BAN *anthracycline antibiotic antineoplastic* [also: idarubicin HCl]

idarubicin HCl USAN, INN *anthracycline antibiotic antineoplastic for acute myeloid leukemia (AML) (orphan); investigational (orphan) for myelodysplastic syndromes, acute and chronic myelogenous leukemia, and acute lymphoblastic leukemia in pediatric patients* [also: idarubicin] 5, 10, 20 mg/vial injection

idaverine INN

idazoxan INN, BAN

idebenone INN, JAN *investigational (orphan) for cardiomyopathy associated with Friedreich ataxia*

idenast INN

Identi-Dose (trademarked packaging form) *unit dose package*

idoxifene USAN *antihormone antineoplastic; osteoporosis treatment; estrogen receptor antagonist for hormone replacement therapy*

idoxuridine (IDU) USAN, USP, INN, BAN, JAN *ophthalmic antiviral; investigational (orphan) for nonparenchymatous sarcomas*

IDR (idarubicin) [q.v.]

idralfidine INN

idremcinal USAN, INN *motilin agonist to stimulate gastrointestinal motility*

idrobutamine [see: butidrine]

idrocilamide INN

idropranolol INN

IDU (idoxuridine) [q.v.]

iduronidase [now: laronidase]

idursulfase *iduronate-2-sulfatase enzyme to improve walking capacity in patients with Hunter syndrome (mucopolysaccharidosis II; MPS II; orphan)*

IE (ifosfamide [with mesna rescue], etoposide) *chemotherapy protocol for soft tissue sarcoma*

ifenprodil INN

ifetroban USAN *antithrombotic; anti-ischemic; antivasospastic*

ifetroban sodium USAN *antithrombotic; anti-ischemic; antivasospastic*

Ifex powder for IV injection ℞ *nitrogen mustard-type alkylating antineoplastic for testicular cancer (orphan); investigational (orphan) for bone and soft tissue sarcomas* [ifosfamide] 1, 3 g

IFN (interferon) [q.v.]

IFN-alpha 2 (interferon alfa-2) [see: interferon alfa-2b, recombinant]

ifosfamide USAN, USP, INN, BAN *nitrogen mustard-type alkylating antineoplastic for testicular cancer (orphan); investigational (orphan) for bone and soft tissue sarcomas* 1, 3 g injection

IfoVP (ifosfamide [with mesna rescue], VePesid) *chemotherapy protocol for osteosarcoma*

ifoxetine INN

IG (immune globulin) [see: globulin, immune]

IgE pentapeptide [see: pentigetide]

Igel 56 *hydrophilic contact lens material* [hefilcon C] ② OCL

IGF-1 (insulin-like growth factor-1) [now: mecasermin]

IGF-1/IGFBP-3 complex [see: mecasermin rinfabate]

IgG (immunoglobulin G) [see: globulin, immune]

IgG1 [see: immunoglobulin G1]

IGIM (immune globulin intramuscular) [see: globulin, immune; Rh$_O$D immune globulin]

IGIV (immune globulin intravenous) [see: globulin, immune; Rh$_O$D immune globulin]

igmesine HCl USAN *sigma receptor ligand antidepressant*

IGSC, SCIG (immune globulin subcutaneous) [see: globulin, immune]

IL-1, IL-2, etc. [see: interleukin-1, interleukin-2, etc.]

IL-2 (interleukin-2) [see: aldesleukin; teceleukin; celmoleukin]

IL-13-PE38QQR protein *investigational (orphan) for malignant glioma*

IL-4 pseudomonas toxin fusion protein *investigational (orphan) for astrocytic glioma*

ilepcimide USAN, INN *anticonvulsant; investigational (orphan) for drug-resistant generalized tonic-clonic epilepsy*

Iletin (U.S. products) [see: Lente Iletin II]

Ilex aquifolium; I. opaca; I. vomitoria medicinal herb [see: holly]

Ilex paraguariensis medicinal herb [see: yerba maté]

Ilex verticillata medicinal herb [see: winterberry]

Illicium anisatum; I. verum medicinal herb [see: star anise]

ilmofosine USAN, INN *antineoplastic*

ilodecakin USAN, INN *interleukin 10, human clone; immunomodulator for Crohn disease, ulcerative colitis, rheumatoid arthritis (RA), and psoriasis*

ilomastat USAN *matrix metalloproteinase (MMP) inhibitor for corneal ulcers, inflammation, and cancers*

ilonidap USAN, INN *anti-inflammatory*

Ilopan IM injection, IV infusion ℞ *postoperative ileus prophylactic* [dexpanthenol] 250 mg/mL

iloperidone USAN, INN *investigational (Phase III) selective serotonin and dopamine antagonist for schizophrenia*

iloprost INN, BAN *prostacyclin analogue for pulmonary arterial hypertension (orphan); investigational (orphan) intravenous treatment for thrombocytopenia and Raynaud phenomenon associated with systemic sclerosis*

Ilosone tablets, Pulvules (capsules), oral suspension (discontinued 2005) ℞ *macrolide antibiotic* [erythromycin estolate] 500 mg; 250 mg; 125, 250 mg/5 mL

Ilotycin ophthalmic ointment ℞ *antibiotic* [erythromycin] 0.5% ⊉ Altazine

Ilotycin Gluceptate IV injection ℞ *macrolide antibiotic* [erythromycin gluceptate] 1 g/vial

I-L-X elixir OTC *hematinic* [ferrous gluconate; liver concentrate 1:20; multiple B vitamins] 70•98• ± mg/15 mL ⊉ Aloxi; Olux

I-L-X B₁₂ caplets OTC *hematinic* [carbonyl iron; desiccated liver; multiple B vitamins; ascorbic acid] 37.5• 130• ± •120 mg

I-L-X B₁₂ elixir OTC *hematinic* [ferric ammonium citrate; liver fraction 1; multiple B vitamins] 102•98• ± mg/15 mL

imafen INN *antidepressant* [also: imafen HCl] ⊉ Imovane

imafen HCl USAN *antidepressant* [also: imafen]

Imager ac rectal suspension ℞ *radiopaque contrast medium for gastrointestinal imaging* [barium sulfate] 100%

imanixil INN

imatinib mesylate USAN *antineoplastic for chronic myeloid leukemia (orphan), acute lymphoblastic leukemia, chronic eosinophilic leukemia, myelodysplastic diseases, gastrointestinal stromal tumors (orphan), systemic mastitis, and dermatofibrosarcoma protuberans*

imazodan INN *cardiotonic* [also: imazodan HCl]

imazodan HCl USAN *cardiotonic* [also: imazodan]

imcarbofos USAN, INN *veterinary anthelmintic*

imciromab INN *monoclonal antibody Fab to myosin, murine* [also: imciromab pentetate]

imciromab pentetate USAN, BAN *monoclonal antibody Fab to myosin, murine* [also: imciromab; indium In 111 imciromab pentetate]

Imdur extended-release tablets ℞ *coronary vasodilator; antianginal* [isosorbide mononitrate] 30, 60, 120 mg ⊉ imidurea

imexon INN *investigational (orphan) for multiple myeloma, metastatic malignant melanoma, and pancreatic adenocarcinoma*

IMF (ifosfamide [with mesna rescue], methotrexate, fluorouracil) *chemotherapy protocol*

imiclopazine INN

imidapril INN, BAN

imidazole carboxamide [see: dacarbazine]

imidazole salicylate INN

imidecyl iodine USAN *topical anti-infective*

imidocarb INN, BAN *antiprotozoal (Babesia)* [also: imidocarb HCl]

imidocarb HCl USAN *antiprotozoal (Babesia)* [also: imidocarb]

imidoline INN *antipsychotic* [also: imidoline HCl] ☑ amedalin; omidoline

imidoline HCl USAN *antipsychotic* [also: imidoline]

imidurea NF *antimicrobial* ☑ Imdur

imiglucerase USAN, INN *glucocerebrosidase enzyme replacement for type 1 Gaucher disease (orphan); investigational (orphan) for types 2 and 3 Gaucher disease*

Imigran (foreign name for U.S. product **Imitrex**)

imiloxan INN *antidepressant* [also: imiloxan HCl] ☑ amalgucin

imiloxan HCl USAN *antidepressant* [also: imiloxan]

iminophenimide INN

iminostilbene anticonvulsants *a class of anticonvulsants with a chemical structure similar to tricyclic antidepressants*

imipemide [now: imipenem]

imipenem USAN, USP, INN, BAN, JAN *broad-spectrum carbapenem antibiotic*

imipramine INN, BAN *tricyclic antidepressant* [also: imipramine HCl] ☑ ampyrimine; embramine

imipramine HCl USP *tricyclic antidepressant; treatment for childhood enuresis* [also: imipramine] 10, 25, 50 mg oral

imipramine pamoate *tricyclic antidepressant* 75, 100, 125, 150 mg oral

imipraminoxide INN

imiquimod USAN, INN *topical immunomodulator for external genital and perianal warts (condylomata acuminata), actinic keratoses, and superficial basal cell carcinoma (sBCC)*

imirestat INN

Imitrex film-coated tablets ℞ *vascular serotonin 5-HT₁ receptor agonist for the acute treatment of migraine headaches* [sumatriptan succinate] 25, 50, 100 mg

Imitrex nasal spray ℞ *vascular serotonin 5-HT₁ receptor agonist for the acute treatment of migraine headaches* [sumatriptan] 5, 20 mg/dose

Imitrex subcu injection in vials, prefilled syringes, or STaTdose self-injector kits (two prefilled syringes) ℞ *vascular serotonin 5-HT₁ receptor agonist for the acute treatment of migraine and cluster headaches* [sumatriptan succinate] 4, 6 mg/0.5 mL dose

ImmTher *investigational (orphan) immunostimulant for pulmonary and hepatic metastases of colorectal adenocarcinoma, Ewing sarcoma, and osteosarcoma* [disaccharide tripeptide glycerol dipalmitoyl]

ImmuDyn *investigational (orphan) agent to increase platelet count in immune thrombocytopenic purpura* [Pseudomonas aeruginosa purified extract]

Immun-Aid powder OTC *enteral nutritional therapy for immunocompromised patients* ☑ Emend

immune globulin (IG) [see: globulin, immune]

immune globulin intramuscular (IGIM) [see: globulin, immune]

immune globulin intravenous (IGIV) [see: globulin, immune]

immune globulin intravenous pentetate USAN *radiodiagnostic imaging agent for inflammation and infection* [also: indium In 111 IGIV pentetate]

immune globulin subcutaneous [see: globulin, immune]

immune serum globulin (ISG) [see: globulin, immune]

Immunex CRP test kit for professional use ℞ *in vitro diagnostic aid for C-reactive protein (CRP) in blood to diagnose inflammatory conditions* [latex agglutination test]

Immuno-C *investigational (Phase II, orphan) treatment of cryptosporidiosis-*

induced diarrhea in immunocompromised patients [*Cryptosporidium parvum* bovine colostrum IgG concentrate]

Immunocal powder for oral solution OTC *enteral nutritional therapy* [milk-based formula] 10 g/pkt.

ImmunoCAP Specific IgE blood test kit for professional use ℞ *in vitro diagnostic aid for IgE detection* [316 different allergens]

immunoglobulin G1 (mouse monoclonal 7E11-C5.3 antihuman prostatic carcinoma cell) disulfide [see: capromab pendetide]

immunoglobulin G1 (mouse monoclonal ZCE025 antihuman antigen CEA) disulfide [see: indium In 111 altumomab pentetate; altumomab]

immunoglobulin G2 (human-mouse monoclonal HuM291 anti-CD3 antigen) disulfide [now: visilizumab]

immunosuppressants *a class of drugs used to suppress the immune response, used primarily after organ transplantation surgery*

Immupath *investigational (orphan) treatment for AIDS* [HIV-neutralizing antibodies]

ImmuRAID-AFP *investigational (orphan) for diagnostic aid for AFP-producing tumors, hepatoblastoma, and hepatocellular carcinoma* [monoclonal antibody to human alpha-fetoprotein (AFP), murine, radiolabeled with technetium Tc 99m]

ImmuRAIT-LL2 *investigational (orphan) treatment for B-cell leukemia and lymphoma* [monoclonal antibody IgG$_{2a}$ to B cell, murine, radiolabeled with iodine I 131]

Imodium capsules ℞ *antidiarrheal* [loperamide HCl] 2 mg

Imodium A-D caplets, oral liquid OTC *antidiarrheal* [loperamide HCl] 1 mg; 1 mg/5 mL, 1 mg/7.5 mL

Imodium Advanced chewable tablets OTC *antidiarrheal; antiflatulent* [loperamide HCl; simethicone] 2•125 mg

Imogam Rabies-HT IM injection ℞ *passive immunizing agent for use after rabies exposure* [rabies immune globulin, heat treated] 150 IU/mL (300, 1500 IU/vial)

imolamine INN, BAN

Imovax Rabies Vaccine IM injection ℞ *rabies vaccine for pre-exposure vaccination or post-exposure prophylaxis* [rabies vaccine, human diploid cell (HDCV)] ≥ 2.5 IU/mL

imoxiterol INN

impacarzine INN

Impact ready-to-use oral liquid OTC *enteral nutritional therapy* [lactose-free formula]

Impact Rubella slide test for professional use ℞ *in vitro diagnostic aid for detection of rubella virus antibodies in serum* [latex agglutination test]

Impatiens balsamina; I. biflora; I. capensis medicinal herb [see: jewelweed]

IMPE [see: etipirium iodide]

Implanon subdermal polymer implant ℞ *progestin; long-term (3 years) contraceptive* [etonogestrel] 68 mg

implitapide *investigational (orphan) for homozygous familial hypercholesterolemia and types I and V hyperlipoproteinemia*

impromidine INN, BAN *gastric secretion indicator* [also: impromidine HCl]

impromidine HCl USAN *gastric secretion indicator* [also: impromidine]

improsulfan INN

Improved Analgesic ointment (discontinued 2007) OTC *analgesic; mild anesthetic; antipruritic; counterirritant* [methyl salicylate; menthol] 18.3%•16%

imuracetam INN

Imuran IV injection ℞ *immunosuppressant for organ transplantation (orphan) and rheumatoid arthritis; investigational (orphan) for graft-versus-host (GVH) disease of the oral mucosa* [azathioprine sodium] 100 mg

Imuran tablets ℞ *immunosuppressant for organ transplantation (orphan) and rheumatoid arthritis; investigational*

(orphan) for graft-versus-host (GVH) disease of the oral mucosa [azathioprine] 50 mg

Imuthiol investigational (Phase II/III, orphan) immunomodulator for HIV and AIDS [diethyldithiocarbamate]

Imuvert investigational (orphan) for primary brain malignancies [Serratia marcescens extract (polyribosomes)]

^{111}**In** [see: indium In 111 altumomab pentetate]

^{111}**In** [see: indium In 111 imciromab pentetate]

^{111}**In** [see: indium In 111 murine anti-CEA monoclonal antibody]

^{111}**In** [see: indium In 111 murine monoclonal antibody]

^{111}**In** [see: indium In 111 oxyquinoline]

^{111}**In** [see: indium In 111 pentetate]

^{111}**In** [see: indium In 111 pentetreotide]

^{111}**In** [see: indium In 111 satumomab pendetide]

^{111}**In** [see: pentetate indium disodium In 111]

^{113m}**In** [see: indium chlorides In 113m]

inactivated mumps vaccine [see: mumps virus vaccine, inactivated]

inactivated poliomyelitis vaccine (IPV) [see: poliovirus vaccine, inactivated]

inactivated poliovirus vaccine (IPV) [see: poliovirus vaccine, inactivated]

inamrinone USAN cardiotonic [also: amrinone]

inamrinone lactate vasodilator for congestive heart failure

inaperisone INN

Inapsine IV or IM injection R general anesthetic; antiemetic [droperidol] 2.5 mg/mL ☑ InhibiZone

Increlex subcu injection R recombinant human insulin-like growth factor-1 (rhIGF-1) for children with primary IGF deficiency without concomitant growth hormone (GH) deficiency [mecasermin] 10 mg/mL

incretin mimetic agents a class of antidiabetic drugs that improve the body's normal glucose-sensing mechanisms by activating the glucagon-like peptide-1 (GLP-1) receptors

indacaterol investigational beta agonist to improve pulmonary airflow

indacrinic acid [see: indacrinone]

indacrinone USAN, INN antihypertensive; diuretic

indalpine INN, BAN

Indamix DM oral suspension R antitussive; antihistamine; decongestant [dextromethorphan tannate; dexchlorpheniramine tannate; pseudoephedrine tannate] 27.5•3•50 mg/5 mL

indanazoline INN

indanediones a class of anticoagulants that interfere with vitamin K–dependent clotting factors

indanidine INN

indanorex INN

indapamide USAN, INN, BAN antihypertensive; diuretic 1.25, 2.5 mg oral

indatraline INN

indecainide INN antiarrhythmic [also: indecainide HCl]

indecainide HCl USAN antiarrhythmic [also: indecainide]

indeloxazine INN antidepressant [also: indeloxazine HCl]

indeloxazine HCl USAN antidepressant [also: indeloxazine]

indenolol INN, BAN

Inderal IV injection R antianginal; antiarrhythmic; antihypertensive; antiadrenergic (β-blocker); migraine preventative [propranolol HCl] 1 mg/mL ☑ Anadrol-50

Inderal tablets (discontinued 2008) R antianginal; antiarrhythmic; antihypertensive; antiadrenergic (β-blocker); migraine preventative [propranolol HCl] 10, 20, 40, 60, 80 mg ☑ Anadrol-50

Inderal LA long-acting capsules R antianginal; antihypertensive; antiadrenergic (β-blocker); migraine preventative [propranolol HCl] 60, 80, 120, 160 mg ☑ Anadrol-50

Inderide 40/25 tablets (discontinued 2008) R antihypertensive; β-blocker;

diuretic [propranolol HCl; hydrochlorothiazide] 40•25 mg ℞ Android

Inderide 80/25 tablets (discontinued 2007) ℞ *antihypertensive; β-blocker; diuretic* [propranolol HCl; hydrochlorothiazide] 80•25 mg ℞ Android

Inderide LA 80/50; Inderide LA 120/50; Inderide LA 160/50 long-acting capsules (discontinued 2004) ℞ *antihypertensive; β-blocker; diuretic* [propranolol HCl; hydrochlorothiazide] 80•50 mg; 120•50 mg; 160•50 mg

Indian apple *medicinal herb* [see: mandrake]

Indian arrow; Indian arrow wood *medicinal herb* [see: wahoo]

Indian bark *medicinal herb* [see: magnolia]

Indian bay *medicinal herb* [see: laurel]

Indian corn (*Zea mays*) styles (silk) *medicinal herb used as an analgesic, diuretic, demulcent, and litholytic*

Indian cress (*Tropaeolum majus*) flowers, leaves, and seeds *medicinal herb used as an antiseptic and expectorant*

Indian elm *medicinal herb* [see: slippery elm]

Indian frankincense *medicinal herb* [see: frankincense]

Indian hemp *medicinal herb* [see: marijuana]

Indian hyssop *medicinal herb* [see: blue vervain]

Indian paint, red *medicinal herb* [see: bloodroot]

Indian paint, yellow *medicinal herb* [see: goldenseal]

Indian pipe *medicinal herb* [see: fit root]

Indian plant *medicinal herb* [see: bloodroot; goldenseal]

Indian poke (*Veratrum viride*) *medicinal herb* [see: hellebore]

Indian root *medicinal herb* [see: spikenard; wahoo]

Indian shamrock *medicinal herb* [see: birthroot]

Indian tobacco *medicinal herb* [see: lobelia]

Indiana protocol *chemotherapy protocol for ovarian cancer* [see: PAC-I]

indigo (*Indigofera* spp.) plant *medicinal herb for fever, hemorrhoids, inducing emesis, inflammation, liver cleansing, ovarian and stomach cancer, pain, scorpion bites, and worms; not generally regarded as safe and effective*

indigo, wild *medicinal herb* [see: wild indigo]

indigo carmine BAN *cystoscopy aid* [also: indigotindisulfonate sodium]

indigotindisulfonate sodium USP *cystoscopy aid* [also: indigo carmine]

indinavir USAN *antiviral protease inhibitor for HIV infection*

indinavir sulfate USAN *antiretroviral protease inhibitor for HIV infection* (base=80%)

indiplon *investigational (NDA filed) oral GABA-A receptor agonist for insomnia*

indium *element (In)*

indium (¹¹¹In) diethylenetriamine pentaacetate JAN *radionuclide cisternography aid; radioactive agent* [also: indium In 111 pentetate]

indium chlorides In 113m USAN, USP *radioactive agent*

Indium DTPA In 111 intrathecal injection ℞ *radiodiagnostic imaging agent for radionuclide cisternograpy* [pentetate indium disodium In 111] 37 MBq (1 mCi)/mL

indium In 111 altumomab pentetate USAN *radiodiagnostic monoclonal antibody to carcinoembryonic antigen (CEA); investigational (orphan) for the detection of colorectal carcinoma* [also: altumomab]

indium In 111 antimelanoma antibody XMMME-0001-DTPA [see: antimelanoma antibody]

indium In 111 capromab *radiolabeled monoclonal antibody; imaging agent for new or recurrent prostate cancer and its metastases* [compare: capromab pendetide]

indium In 111 CYT-103 [now: indium In 111 satumomab pendetide]

**indium In 111 ibritumomab tiuxe-
tan** *radioimmunotherapy for non-
Hodgkin B-cell lymphoma (orphan)*

indium In 111 IGIV pentetate *radiodiagnostic imaging agent for inflammation and infection* [also: immune globulin intravenous pentetate]

indium In 111 imciromab pentetate
*diagnostic monoclonal antibody Fab to
myosin, murine; investigational (orphan)
imaging agent for cardiac necrosis and
myocarditis*

indium In 111 oxyquinoline USAN,
USP *radioactive agent; diagnostic aid*

indium In 111 pentetate USP *radionuclide cisternography aid; radioactive
agent* [also: indium (^{111}In) diethylenetriamine pentaacetate]

indium In 111 pentetreotide USAN
*radioactive imaging agent for SPECT
scans of neuroendocrine tumors; investigational (orphan) radiotherapeutic
agent for somatostatin receptor–positive
neuroendocrine tumors*

**indium In 111 satumomab pende-
tide** USAN *radiodiagnostic imaging aid
for ovarian (orphan) and colorectal
carcinoma* [also: satumomab]

indobufen INN

indocate INN

Indocin capsules, suppositories (discontinued 2006) ℞ *nonsteroidal anti-
inflammatory drug (NSAID) for moderate to severe osteoarthritis, rheumatoid
arthritis, and ankylosing spondylitis, and
acute bursitis/tendinitis* [indomethacin]
25, 50 mg; 50 mg

Indocin oral suspension ℞ *nonsteroidal
anti-inflammatory drug (NSAID) for
moderate to severe osteoarthritis, rheumatoid arthritis, and ankylosing spondylitis, and acute bursitis/tendinitis* [indo-
methacin] 25 mg/5 mL

Indocin I.V. powder for IV injection
℞ *prostaglandin synthesis inhibitor for
neonatal closure of patent ductus arteriosus* [indomethacin sodium trihy-
drate] 1 mg

Indocin SR sustained-release capsules
℞ *nonsteroidal anti-inflammatory drug*

*(NSAID) for moderate to severe osteo-
arthritis, rheumatoid arthritis, and
ankylosing spondylitis, and acute bursi-
tis/tendinitis* [indomethacin] 75 mg

indocyanine green USP, JAN *in vivo
diagnostic aid for cardiac output,
hepatic function, and ophthalmic angiography* 25 mg injection

indolapril INN *antihypertensive* [also:
indolapril HCl]

indolapril HCl USAN *antihypertensive*
[also: indolapril]

indole 3-carbinol *natural phytochemi-
cal found in cruciferous vegetables;
antioxidant and estrogen blocker shown
effective against hormone-related cancers of the prostate, the uterus, and
especially the breast; restores the p21
tumor suppressor gene*

indolidan USAN, INN, BAN *cardiotonic*

indolones *a class of dopamine receptor
antagonists with conventional (typical)
antipsychotic activity* [also called:
dihydroindolones]

indometacin INN, JAN *antiarthritic;
nonsteroidal anti-inflammatory drug
(NSAID)* [also: indomethacin]

indometacin farnecil JAN *antiarthritic; nonsteroidal anti-inflammatory
drug (NSAID)* [also: indomethacin]

indomethacin USAN, USP, BAN *nonsteroidal anti-inflammatory drug (NSAID)
for moderate to severe osteoarthritis,
rheumatoid arthritis, ankylosing spondylitis, and acute bursitis/tendinitis*
[also: indometacin; indomethacin
farnecil] 25, 50, 75 mg oral; 50 mg
rectal suppositories

indomethacin sodium USAN *anti-
inflammatory* 1 mg injection

indomethacin sodium trihydrate *neonatal closure of patent ductus arteriosus*

indopanolol INN

indopine INN

indoprofen USAN, INN, BAN *analgesic;
anti-inflammatory*

indoramin USAN, INN, BAN *antihypertensive*

indoramin HCl USAN, BAN *antihypertensive*

indorenate INN *antihypertensive* [also: indorenate HCl]

indorenate HCl USAN *antihypertensive* [also: indorenate]

indoxole USAN, INN *antipyretic; anti-inflammatory*

indriline INN *CNS stimulant* [also: indriline HCl]

indriline HCl USAN *CNS stimulant* [also: indriline]

inductin [see: diphoxazide]

I-neb AAD (adaptive aerosol delivery) (trademarked delivery device) *oral inhalation solution dispenser*

Infalyte oral solution OTC *electrolyte replacement* [sodium, potassium, and chloride electrolytes] ⊃ Enfalyte

Infanrix IM injection ℞ *active immunizing agent for diphtheria, tetanus, and pertussis; Dtap (diphtheria predominant) vaccine used in the initial immunization series of infants and children 6 weeks to 6 years old* [diphtheria toxoid; tetanus toxoid; inactivated pertussis toxin] 25 Lf•10 Lf•25 mcg per 0.5 mL dose

Infantaire oral drops (discontinued 2008) OTC *analgesic; antipyretic* [acetaminophen] 100 mg/mL

Infasurf intratracheal suspension ℞ *agent for prophylaxis and treatment of respiratory distress syndrome (RDS) in premature infants* (orphan) [calfactant] 6 mL

Infatab (trademarked dosage form) *pediatric chewable tablet*

INFeD IV or IM injection ℞ *hematinic* [iron dextran] 100 mg Fe/dose ⊃ Unifed

Infergen subcu injection ℞ *consensus interferon for the treatment of chronic hepatitis C virus (HCV) infections* [interferon alfacon-1] 9, 15 mcg/0.3 mL dose

Inflamase Mild; Inflamase Forte eye drops (discontinued 2006) ℞ *corticosteroidal anti-inflammatory* [prednisolone sodium phosphate] 0.125%; 1%

infliximab *monoclonal antibody to TNFα (tumor necrosis factor alpha); anti-inflammatory for Crohn disease* (orphan)*, ulcerative colitis, rheumatoid and psoriatic arthritis, ankylosing spondylitis, and plaque psoriasis; investigational* (orphan) *for uveitis*

influenza purified surface antigen [see: influenza split-virus vaccine]

influenza split-virus vaccine *subcategory of influenza virus vaccine*

influenza subvirion vaccine [see: influenza split-virus vaccine]

influenza virus vaccine (injectable) USP *active immunizing agent for influenza* [virus strains for the 2008–2009 season: A/Brisbane/59/2007 (H1N1), A/Brisbane/10/2007 (H3N2), and B/Florida/4/2006]

influenza virus vaccine (intranasal) *active immunizing agent for influenza* [virus strains for the 2008–2009 season: A/South Dakota/6/2007 (H1N1), A/Brisbane/59/2007 (H3N2), A/Uruguay/16/2007 (H3N2), A/Brisbane/10/2007 (H3N2), and B/Florida/4/2006]

influenza virus vaccine, H5N1 *active immunizing agent for H5N1 influenza A (avian flu; bird flu) in adults 18–64 years; this vaccine is not available commercially but is being stockpiled by the U.S. government for future outbreaks* [virus strain: A/Vietnam/1203/2004 (H5N1, clade 1)] 90 mcg/mL injection (with 98.2 mcg/dose thimerosal preservative=50mcg/dose mercury)

influenza whole-virus vaccine *subcategory of influenza virus vaccine*

infraRUB cream (discontinued 2004) OTC *analgesic; mild anesthetic; antipruritic; counterirritant* [methyl salicylate; menthol] 35%•10%

Infumorph 200; Infumorph 500 concentrate for continuous microinfusion ℞ *narcotic analgesic; intraspinal microinfusion for intractable chronic pain* (orphan) [morphine sulfate] 10 mg/mL (200 mg/vial); 25 mg/mL (500 mg/vial)

Infuvite Adult IV infusion ℞ *multivitamin adjunct for adults receiving paren-*

teral nutrition [multiple vitamins; folic acid; biotin] $\pm$•600•60 mcg

Infuvite Pediatric IV infusion ℞ *multivitamin adjunct for infants and children receiving parenteral nutrition* [multiple vitamins; folic acid; biotin] $\pm$•140•20 mcg

INGN-201 *investigational (Phase III) gene therapy for head and neck cancers* [also: adenoviral p53 gene; p53 adenoviral gene]

INH (isonicotinic acid hydrazide) [see: isoniazid]

INH-A00021 *investigational (orphan) agent to reduce or prevent staphylococci-induced nosocomial bacteremia in very low birthweight infants*

Inhal-Aid (trademarked delivery device) *portable inhalation device*

inhalants *a class of street drugs that include nitrous oxide, volatile nitrites, and petroleum distillates* [see: nitrous oxide; volatile nitrites; petroleum distillate inhalants]

InhibiZone surface treatment ℞ *prophylactic antibiotic treatment for penile prostheses before implantation* [minocycline; rifampin] 3–10•9–25 mg (depending on prosthesis size) ☒ Inapsine

inicarone INN

Inject-all (trademarked delivery form) *prefilled disposable syringe*

Inlay-Tabs (trademarked dosage form) *tablets with contrasting inlay*

Innohep deep subcu injection ℞ *anticoagulant/antithrombotic for the prevention and treatment of deep vein thrombosis (DVT)* [tinzaparin sodium] 20 000 IU/mL

InnoLet prefilled disposable syringe OTC *device for self-administration of insulin* (available prefilled with **Novolin 70/30** or **Novolin N**) [insulin] 1–40 U/injection ☒ Ionil T

InnoPran XL long-acting capsules ℞ *antihypertensive; antiadrenergic (β-blocker)* [propranolol HCl] 80, 100, 120 mg

inocoterone INN *anti-acne* [also: inocoterone acetate]

inocoterone acetate USAN *anti-acne* [also: inocoterone]

inolimomab *investigational (orphan) for graft-versus-host disease*

INOmax inhalation gas ℞ *inhalation gas for neonatal hypoxic respiratory failure due to persistent pulmonary hypertension (orphan); investigational (orphan) for acute adult respiratory distress syndrome and to diagnose sarcoidosis* [nitric oxide] 100, 800 ppm

inosine INN, JAN ☒ Anacin; Enzone; Unasyn

inosine pranobex BAN, JAN *investigational (orphan) immunomodulator for subacute sclerosing panencephalitis*

inosiplex [now: inosine pranobex]

Inositech capsules OTC *vitamin B supplement* [inositol] 324 mg

inositol NF *dietary lipotropic supplement* 250, 500, 650 mg oral ☒ anisatil

inositol niacinate USAN *peripheral vasodilator* [also: inositol nicotinate]

inositol nicotinate INN, BAN *peripheral vasodilator* [also: inositol niacinate]

inotropes *a class of drugs that affect the force or energy of muscle contractions*

inprochone [see: inproquone]

inproquone INN, BAN

INSH (isonicotinoyl-salicylidene-hydrazine) [see: salinazid]

InspirEase (trademarked delivery device) *portable inhalation device*

Inspra film-coated tablets ℞ *aldosterone receptor antagonist for hypertension and congestive heart failure (CHF); improves survival after a cardiovascular event* [eplerenone] 25, 50 mg

Insta-Glucose oral gel OTC *blood glucose elevating agent for hypoglycemia* [glucose] 40%

insulin USP, JAN *antidiabetic*

insulin, biphasic INN, BAN *antidiabetic*

insulin, biphasic isophane BAN *antidiabetic*

insulin, dalanated USAN, INN *antidiabetic*

insulin, globin zinc USP [also: globin zinc insulin]

insulin, human USAN, USP, INN, BAN, JAN *antidiabetic*

insulin, human, isophane USP *antidiabetic*

insulin, human zinc USP *antidiabetic*

insulin, human zinc, extended USP *antidiabetic*

insulin, isophane USP, BAN, INN, JAN *antidiabetic*

insulin, neutral USAN, JAN *antidiabetic* [also: neutral insulin]

insulin, NPH (neutral protamine Hagedorn) [see: insulin, isophane]

insulin, protamine zinc (PZI) USP *antidiabetic* [also: insulin zinc protamine; protamine zinc insulin]

insulin argine INN *antidiabetic*

insulin aspart USAN, INN *rapid-acting insulin analogue for diabetes*

insulin aspart protamine *intermediate-acting insulin analogue for diabetes*

insulin defalan INN *antidiabetic*

insulin detemir USAN *antidiabetic; long-acting insulin formulation intended to provide continuous basal insulin levels through once- or twice-daily subcu injections*

insulin glargine INN *long-acting, once-daily basal insulin analogue for diabetes*

insulin glulisine *rapid-onset, short-acting insulin analogue for diabetes*

insulin I 125 USAN *radioactive agent*

insulin I 131 USAN *radioactive agent*

insulin lispro USAN, INN, BAN *rapid-acting insulin analogue for diabetes*

insulin lispro protamine *intermediate-acting insulin analogue for diabetes*

Insulin Reaction gel OTC *glucose elevating agent* [glucose] 40%

Insulin Reaction oral gel OTC *blood glucose elevating agent for hypoglycemia* [glucose] 40%

insulin zinc USP, INN, BAN, JAN *antidiabetic*

insulin zinc, extended USP *antidiabetic* [also: insulin zinc suspension (crystalline)]

insulin zinc, prompt USP *antidiabetic* [also: insulin zinc suspension (amorphous)]

insulin zinc protamine JAN *antidiabetic* [also: insulin, protamine zinc; protamine zinc insulin]

insulin zinc suspension (amorphous) INN, BAN, JAN *antidiabetic* [also: insulin zinc, prompt]

insulin zinc suspension (crystalline) INN, BAN, JAN *antidiabetic* [also: insulin zinc, extended]

insulin-like growth factor-1, recombinant human (rhIGF-1) [now: mecasermin]

Intal aerosol spray ℞ *anti-inflammatory; mast cell stabilizer for prophylactic treatment of allergy, asthma, and bronchospasm* [cromolyn sodium] 800 mcg/dose

Intal solution for nebulization (discontinued 2008) ℞ *anti-inflammatory; mast cell stabilizer for prophylactic treatment of allergy, asthma, and bronchospasm* [cromolyn sodium] 20 mg/2 mL ampule

Integrilin IV injection ℞ *platelet aggregation inhibitor for acute coronary syndrome, unstable angina, myocardial infarction, and cardiac surgery* [eptifibatide] 0.75, 2 mg/mL

Intelence tablets ℞ *non-nucleoside reverse transcriptase inhibitor (NNRTI) for drug-resistant HIV-1 infections* [etravirine] 100 mg

Intensol (trademarked dosage form) *concentrated oral solution*

α-2-interferon [see: interferon alfa-2b, recombinant]

interferon, fibroblast [now: interferon beta]

interferon, leukocyte [now: interferon alfa-n3]

interferon α2b [see: interferon alfa-2b]

interferon αA [see: interferon alfa-2a]

interferon alfa JAN *immunostimulant; investigational (orphan) for oral human papillomavirus (HPV) warts in HIV-infected patients*

interferon alfa (BALL-1) JAN

interferon alfa, human lympho-blastoid *immunostimulant; investigational (orphan) for oral human papillomavirus (HPV) warts in HIV-infected patients, polycythemia vera, and Behçet disease*

interferon alfa-1b *investigational (orphan) antineoplastic for multiple myeloma*

interferon alfa-2 & interleukin-2 (aldesleukin) *chemotherapy protocol for renal cell carcinoma*

interferon alfa-2a (IFN-αA; rIFN-A) USAN, INN, BAN, JAN *immunostimulant for hairy cell leukemia, hepatitis C, Kaposi sarcoma (orphan), and chronic myelogenous leukemia (orphan); investigational (orphan) for malignant melanoma and esophageal, renal, colorectal, and other cancers*

interferon alfa-2b (IFN-α2) USAN, INN, BAN *antineoplastic for hairy-cell leukemia, malignant melanoma, AIDS-related Kaposi sarcoma (orphan), and various other cancers; antiviral for condylomata acuminata and chronic hepatitis B and C infection*

interferon alfacon-1 USAN *bioengineered consensus interferon for the treatment of chronic hepatitis C virus (HCV) infections*

interferon alfa-n1 USAN, INN, BAN *antineoplastic; biological response modifier for chronic hepatitis C; investigational (orphan) for AIDS-related Kaposi sarcoma and human papillomavirus in severe respiratory papillomatosis*

interferon alfa-n3 USAN *immunomodulator and antiviral for condylomata acuminata; investigational (Phase III) cytokine for HIV, AIDS, and ARC*

interferon beta (IFN-B) BAN, JAN *antineoplastic; antiviral; immunomodulator*

interferon beta-1a USAN *immunomodulator for relapsing multiple sclerosis (orphan); investigational (orphan) for non-A, non-B hepatitis, juvenile rheumatoid arthritis, Kaposi sarcoma, brain tumors, and various other cancers*

interferon beta-1b USAN *immunomodulator for relapsing-remitting multiple sclerosis (orphan); investigational (orphan) for AIDS*

interferon gamma-1a JAN

interferon gamma-1b USAN, INN, BAN *immunoregulator for chronic granulomatous disease (orphan) and severe malignant osteopetrosis (orphan); investigational (orphan) for renal cell carcinoma and pulmonary fibrosis*

interferon gamma-2a [see: interferon gamma-1b]

α-interferons [see: interferon alfa-n1 and -n3]

Intergel *irrigating solution* ℞ *adhesion barrier for open gynecological and lower GI surgical procedures* [ferric hyaluronate] 0.5% ☒ Antrocol

interleukin-1 alpha, recombinant human *investigational (orphan) hematopoietic potentiator for aplastic anemia and bone marrow transplants*

interleukin-1 receptor antagonist, recombinant human [now: anakinra]

interleukin-1 Trap *investigational (orphan) for cold-induced autoinflammatory syndrome 1 (CIAS1)–associated periodic syndromes, Still disease, and juvenile rheumatoid arthritis*

interleukin-2 (aldesleukin) & interferon alfa-2 *chemotherapy protocol for renal cell carcinoma*

interleukin-2, liposome-encapsulated recombinant *investigational (orphan) for brain, central nervous system, kidney, and pelvic cancers*

interleukin-2, recombinant (IL-2) [see: aldesleukin; teceleukin; celmoleukin]

interleukin-3, recombinant human *investigational (orphan) adjunct to bone marrow transplants and Diamond-Blackfan anemia*

interleukin-10 (IL-10) [see: ilodecakin]

interleukin-11, recombinant human (rhIL-11) [see: oprelvekin]

interleukin-12 (IL-12) [see: edodekin alfa]

intermedine INN

Intestinex capsules OTC *natural intestinal bacteria; probiotic; dietary supplement; fever blister treatment* [*Lactobacillus acidophilus*] 100 million CFU

intoplicine INN *antineoplastic; topoisomerase I and II inhibitor*

Intrachol *investigational (orphan) for choline deficiency of long-term parenteral nutrition* [choline chloride]

IntraDose injectable gel *investigational (NDA filed, orphan) alkylating antineoplastic for squamous cell carcinoma of the head and neck; investigational (orphan) for metastatic malignant melanoma* [cisplatin; epinephrine]

Intralipid 10% IV infusion (discontinued 2008) ℞ *nutritional therapy* [fat emulsion]

Intralipid 20%; Intralipid 30% IV infusion ℞ *nutritional therapy* [fat emulsion]

IntraSite gel OTC *wound dressing* [graft T starch copolymer] 2% ⧉ Anatrast

intravascular perfluorochemical emulsion *synthetic blood oxygen carrier for PTCA*

intravenous fat emulsion [see: fat emulsion, intravenous]

intrazole USAN, INN *anti-inflammatory*

Intrinsa transdermal patch *investigational (Phase III) hormone replacement therapy for female sexual dysfunction (FSD) and hypoactive sexual desire disorder (HSDD) in women* [testosterone]

intrinsic factor concentrate *antianemic to enhance the body's utilization of vitamin B_{12}*

intriptyline INN *antidepressant* [also: intriptyline HCl]

intriptyline HCl USAN *antidepressant* [also: intriptyline]

Introlan Half-Strength oral liquid OTC *enteral nutritional therapy* [lactose-free formula]

Introlite oral liquid OTC *enteral nutritional therapy* [lactose-free formula]

Intron A subcu or IM injection ℞ *antineoplastic for hairy cell leukemia, malignant melanoma, Kaposi sarcoma (orphan), and various other cancers; antiviral for condylomata acuminata and chronic hepatitis B and C infection* [interferon alfa-2b] 3, 5, 10, 18, 25, 50 million IU/vial ⧉ Anturane

Intropaste oral paste ℞ *radiopaque contrast medium for esophageal imaging* [barium sulfate] 70%

Intropin IV injection (discontinued 2004) ℞ *vasopressor for cardiac, pulmonary, traumatic, septic, or renal shock* [dopamine HCl] 40, 80, 160 mg/mL

Intuniv *investigational (NDA filed) selective α_{2A} receptor agonist; nonstimulant treatment for attention-deficit/hyperactivity disorder (ADHD)* [guanfacine HCl]

Inula helenium *medicinal herb* [see: elecampane]

inulin USP *diagnostic aid for renal function; dietary fiber supplement* 100 mg/mL injection ⧉ Enlon

Invanz powder for IV or IM injection ℞ *broad-spectrum carbapenem antibiotic* [ertapenem sodium] 1 g/vial

Invega IM injection *investigational (NDA filed) once-monthly injectable antischizophrenic* [paliperidone palmitate]

Invega OROS (extended-release caplets) ℞ *once-daily antischizophrenic; investigational (Phase III) for bipolar mania* [paliperidone] 3, 6, 9 mg

invenol [see: carbutamide]

Inversine tablets ℞ *antiadrenergic; ganglionic blocker for severe hypertension; investigational (orphan) for Tourette syndrome* [mecamylamine HCl] 2.5 mg

invert sugar [see: sugar, invert]

Invirase tablets, capsules ℞ *antiretroviral protease inhibitor for HIV* [saquinavir mesylate] 500 mg; 200 mg

iobenguane (^{131}I) INN *radioactive agent* [also: iobenguane I 131]

iobenguane I 123 USP *radioactive agent*

iobenguane sulfate I 131 USAN *diagnostic aid for pheochromocytoma (orphan)*

iobenzamic acid USAN, INN, BAN *radiopaque contrast medium for cholecystography*

Iobid DM sustained-release tablets ℞ *antitussive; expectorant* [dextromethorphan hydrobromide; guaifenesin] 30•600 mg

iobutoic acid INN

iocanlidic acid I 123 USAN *cardiac diagnostic aid*

Iocare Balanced Salt ophthalmic solution OTC *intraocular irrigating solution* [sodium chloride (balanced saline solution)]

iocarmate meglumine USAN *radiopaque contrast medium* [also: meglumine iocarmate]

iocarmic acid USAN, INN, BAN *radiopaque contrast medium*

iocetamic acid USAN, USP, INN, BAN *oral radiopaque contrast medium for cholecystography (62% iodine)*

iodamide USAN, INN, BAN *radiopaque contrast medium*

iodamide meglumine USAN *radiopaque contrast medium*

iodecimol INN

iodecol [see: iodecimol]

iodetryl INN

Iodex; Iodex-P ointment OTC *broad-spectrum antimicrobial* [povidone-iodine] 4.7%; 10% ⊠ ADEKs; Adoxa; Edex

Iodex with Methyl Salicylate ointment OTC *analgesic; counterirritant; anti-infective* [methyl salicylate; iodine] 4.8%•4.7%

iodinated (^{125}I) human serum albumin INN *radioactive agent; blood volume test* [also: albumin, iodinated I 125 serum]

iodinated (^{131}I) human serum albumin INN, JAN *radioactive agent; intrathecal imaging agent; blood volume test* [also: albumin, iodinated I 131 serum]

iodinated glycerol [see: glycerol, iodinated]

iodinated I 125 albumin [see: albumin, iodinated I 125]

iodinated I 131 aggregated albumin [see: albumin, iodinated I 131 aggregated]

iodinated I 131 albumin [see: albumin, iodinated I 131]

iodine USP *broad-spectrum topical anti-infective; element (I)* 2% topical

iodine I 131 6B-iodomethyl-19-norcholesterol *investigational (orphan) for adrenal cortical imaging*

iodine I 131 metaiodobenzylguanidine sulfate [now: iobenguane sulfate I 131]

iodine I 131 tositumomab *monoclonal antibody to non-Hodgkin lymphoma (NHL), radiolabeled with iodine I 131, for the detection of NHL and targeted delivery of radiation (orphan)* [see also: tositumomab]

iodipamide USP, BAN *parenteral radiopaque contrast medium* [also: adipiodone]

iodipamide meglumine USP, BAN *parenteral radiopaque contrast medium (49.42% iodine)* [also: adipiodone meglumine]

iodipamide methylglucamine [see: iodipamide meglumine]

iodipamide sodium USP *parenteral radiopaque contrast medium*

iodipamide sodium I 131 USAN *radioactive agent*

iodisan [see: prolonium iodide]

iodixanol USAN, INN, BAN *parenteral radiopaque contrast medium (49.1% iodine)*

iodized oil NF

iodoalphionic acid NF [also: pheniodol sodium]

iodoantipyrine I 131 USAN *radioactive agent*

iodobehenate calcium NF

m-iodobenzylguanidine sulfate I 123 [see: iobenguane sulfate I 123]

iodocetylic acid (^{123}I) INN *diagnostic aid* [also: iodocetylic acid I 123]

iodocetylic acid I 123 USAN *diagnostic aid* [also: iodocetylic acid (^{123}I)]

iodochlorhydroxyquin [now: clioquinol]

iodocholesterol (^{131}I) INN *radioactive agent* [also: iodocholesterol I 131]

iodocholesterol I 131 USAN *radioactive agent* [also: iodocholesterol (^{131}I)]

iodoform NF

iodohippurate sodium I 123 USAN, USP *renal function test; radioactive agent*

iodohippurate sodium I 125 USAN *radioactive agent*

iodohippurate sodium I 131 USAN, USP *renal function test; radioactive agent* [also: sodium iodohippurate (^{131}I)]

iodohydroxyquin [see: clioquinol]

iodol USP

iodomethamate sodium NF

iodopanoic acid [see: iopanoic acid]

Iodopen IV injection ℞ *iodine supplement* [sodium iodide (85% elemental iodine)] 118 mcg/mL (100 mcg I/mL) 🔊 woodbine

iodophthalein, soluble [now: iodophthalein sodium]

iodophthalein sodium NF, INN

iodopyracet NF [also: diodone]

iodopyracet I 125 USAN *radioactive agent*

iodopyracet I 131 USAN *radioactive agent*

iodoquinol USAN, USP *antimicrobial; amebicide for intestinal amebiasis* [also: diiodohydroxyquinoline]

iodoquinol & hydrocortisone *amebicide; antimicrobial; corticosteroidal anti-inflammatory* 1%•1% topical

iodothiouracil INN, BAN

iodothymol [see: thymol iodide]

Iodotope capsules, oral solution ℞ *radioactive antineoplastic for thyroid carcinoma; thyroid inhibitor for hyperthyroidism* [sodium iodide I 131] 8, 15, 30, 50, 100 mCi; 7.05 mCi/mL (7, 14, 28, 70, 106 mCi/vial)

iodoxamate meglumine USAN, BAN *radiopaque contrast medium*

iodoxamic acid USAN, INN, BAN *radiopaque contrast medium*

iodoxyl [see: iodomethamate sodium]

iofendylate INN *radiopaque contrast medium* [also: iophendylate]

iofetamine (^{123}I) INN *diagnostic aid; radioactive agent* [also: iofetamine HCl I 123] 🔊 E-Vitamin

iofetamine HCl I 123 USAN *diagnostic aid; radioactive agent* [also: iofetamine (^{123}I)]

Iofoam (trademarked dosage form) *topical foam* 🔊 AFM

ioglicic acid USAN, INN, BAN *radiopaque contrast medium*

ioglucol USAN, INN *radiopaque contrast medium*

ioglucomide USAN, INN *radiopaque contrast medium*

ioglunide INN

ioglycamic acid USAN, INN, BAN *radiopaque contrast medium for cholecystography*

iogulamide USAN *radiopaque contrast medium* 🔊 aklomide

iohexol USAN, INN, BAN *parenteral radiopaque contrast medium (46.36% iodine)*

iolidonic acid INN

iolixanic acid INN

iomeglamic acid INN

iomeprol USAN, INN, BAN *radiopaque contrast medium*

iomethin I 125 USAN *neoplasm test; radioactive agent* [also: iometin (^{125}I)] 🔊 Amitone; emetine

iomethin I 131 USAN *neoplasm test; radioactive agent* [also: iometin (^{131}I)] 🔊 Amitone; emetine

iometin (^{125}I) INN *neoplasm test; radioactive agent* [also: iomethin I 125] 🔊 Amitone; emetine

iometin (^{131}I) INN *neoplasm test; radioactive agent* [also: iomethin I 131] 🔊 Amitone; emetine

iometopane I 123 USAN *diagnostic imaging aid for dopamine and serotonin transporter sites*

iomorinic acid INN

Ionamin capsules ℞ *anorexiant; CNS stimulant* [phentermine HCl resin complex] 15, 30 mg

Ionax foam OTC *medicated cleanser for acne* [benzalkonium chloride]

Ionax Astringent Skin Cleanser topical liquid OTC *keratolytic cleanser for acne* [salicylic acid; isopropyl alcohol]

Ionax Scrub OTC *abrasive medicated cleanser for acne* [benzalkonium chloride]

ionic contrast media *a class of older radiopaque agents that, in general, have a high osmolar concentration of iodine (the contrast agent), which corresponds to a higher incidence of adverse reactions* [also called: high osmolar contrast media (HOCM)]

Ionil shampoo OTC *antiseborrheic; keratolytic; antiseptic* [salicylic acid; benzalkonium chloride]

Ionil Plus shampoo OTC *antiseborrheic; keratolytic* [salicylic acid] 2%

Ionil T shampoo OTC *antiseborrheic; antipsoriatic* [coal tar] 1% ⊘ InnoLet

Ionil-T Plus shampoo OTC *antiseborrheic; antipsoriatic; antipruritic; antibacterial* [coal tar] 2%

Ionosol B and 5% Dextrose IV infusion ℞ *intravenous nutritional/electrolyte therapy* [combined electrolyte solution; dextrose] 500, 1000 mg/dose

Ionosol T and 5% Dextrose IV infusion ℞ *intravenous nutritional/electrolyte therapy* [combined electrolyte solution; dextrose]

ionphylline [see: aminophylline]

Ionsys transdermal patch with a patient-controlled dose release button ℞ *transdermal narcotic analgesic for short-term management of postoperative pain* [fentanyl HCl] 40 mcg/actuation (maximum 3.2 mg/24 hr.)

iopamidol USAN, USP, INN, BAN *parenteral radiopaque contrast medium (49% iodine)*

iopanoic acid USP, INN, BAN *oral radiopaque contrast medium for cholecystography (66.68% iodine)*

iopentol USAN, INN, BAN *radiopaque contrast medium*

Iophen tablets, elixir, drops ℞ *expectorant* [iodinated glycerol] 30 mg; 60 mg/5 mL; 50 mg/mL ⊘ Aveeno; Aviane

iophendylate USP, BAN *radiopaque contrast medium* [also: iofendylate]

iophenoic acid INN [also: iophenoxic acid]

iophenoxic acid USP [also: iophenoic acid]

Iophylline elixir (discontinued 2007) ℞ *antiasthmatic; bronchodilator; expectorant* [theophylline; iodinated glycerol] 120•30 mg/15 mL ⊘ Avolean

Iopidine Drop-Tainers (eye drops) ℞ *sympathomimetic antiglaucoma agent* [apraclonidine HCl] 0.5%, 1% ⊘ Ibudone

ioprocemic acid USAN, INN *radiopaque contrast medium*

iopromide USAN, INN, BAN *parenteral radiopaque contrast medium (39% iodine)*

iopronic acid USAN, INN, BAN *radiopaque contrast medium for cholecystography*

iopydol USAN, INN, BAN *radiopaque contrast medium for bronchography*

iopydone USAN, INN, BAN *radiopaque contrast medium for bronchography* ⊘ Ibudone

Iosal II sustained-release tablets ℞ *decongestant; expectorant* [pseudoephedrine HCl; guaifenesin] 60•600 mg ⊘ Wyseal

iosarcol INN

iosefamic acid USAN, INN *radiopaque contrast medium*

ioseric acid USAN, INN *radiopaque contrast medium*

iosimide INN

iosulamide INN *radiopaque contrast medium* [also: iosulamide meglumine] ⊘ osalmid

iosulamide meglumine USAN *radiopaque contrast medium* [also: iosulamide]

iosulfan blue *parenteral radiopaque contrast medium for lymphography*

iosumetic acid USAN, INN *radiopaque contrast medium*

iotalamic acid INN *radiopaque contrast medium* [also: iothalamic acid]

iotasul USAN, INN *radiopaque contrast medium*

iotetric acid USAN, INN *radiopaque contrast medium*

iothalamate meglumine USP *parenteral radiopaque contrast medium (47% iodine)* [also: meglumine iothalamate]

iothalamate sodium USP *parenteral radiopaque contrast medium (59.9% iodine)* [also: sodium iothalamate]

iothalamate sodium I 125 USAN *radioactive agent* [also: sodium iotalamate (^{125}I)]

iothalamate sodium I 131 USAN *radioactive agent* [also: sodium iotalamate (^{131}I)]

iothalamic acid USP, BAN *radiopaque contrast medium* [also: iotalamic acid]

iothiouracil sodium

iotranic acid INN

iotriside INN

iotrizoic acid INN

iotrol [now: iotrolan]

iotrolan USAN, INN, BAN *parenteral radiopaque contrast medium* ☒ Atralin

iotroxic acid USAN, INN, BAN *radiopaque contrast medium*

iotyrosine I 131 USAN *radioactive agent*

ioversol USAN, INN, BAN *parenteral radiopaque contrast medium (47.3% iodine)*

ioxabrolic acid INN

ioxaglate meglumine USAN *parenteral radiopaque contrast medium* [also: meglumine ioxaglate]

ioxaglate sodium USAN *parenteral radiopaque contrast medium* [also: sodium ioxaglate]

ioxaglic acid USAN, INN, BAN *radiopaque contrast medium*

ioxilan USAN, INN *diagnostic aid* ☒ Exelon

ioxitalamic acid INN

ioxotrizoic acid USAN, INN *radiopaque contrast medium*

iozomic acid INN

IPA (ifosfamide, Platinol, Adriamycin) *chemotherapy protocol for pediatric hepatoblastoma*

ipazilide fumarate USAN *antiarrhythmic*

ipecac USP *emetic*

ipecac, milk *medicinal herb* [see: birthroot; dogbane]

ipecac, powdered USP

ipexidine INN *dental caries prophylactic* [also: ipexidine mesylate]

ipexidine mesylate USAN, INN *dental caries prophylactic* [also: ipexidine]

Iplex subcu injection ℞ *recombinant human insulin-like growth factor-1 (rhIGF-1) for children with primary IGF deficiency without concomitant growth hormone (GH) deficiency* [mecasermin rinfabate]

ipodate calcium USP *oral radiopaque contrast medium for cholecystography (61.7% iodine)*

ipodate sodium USAN, USP *oral radiopaque contrast medium for cholecystography (61.4% iodine)* [also: sodium ipodate; sodium iopodate]

IPOL subcu injection ℞ *vaccine for poliovirus types 1, 2, and 3* [poliovirus vaccine, inactivated] 0.5 mL ☒ A.P.L.; apple; E-Pilo-1; OPAL

Ipomoea pandurata *medicinal herb* [see: wild jalap]

Ipomoea violacea **(morning glory)** *seeds contain lysergic acid amide, chemically similar to LSD, which produces hallucinations when ingested as a street drug* [see also: LSD]

ipragratine INN

ipramidil INN

ipratropium bromide USAN, INN, BAN *anticholinergic bronchodilator for bronchospasm, emphysema, and chronic obstructive pulmonary disease (COPD); antisecretory for rhinorrhea 0.02% inhalation; 0.03%, 0.06% nasal spray*

ipratropium bromide & albuterol sulfate *bronchodilator combination for bronchospasm, emphysema, and chronic obstructive pulmonary disease (COPD)* 0.017%•0.083% (0.5•3 mg/dose) inhaler

iprazochrome INN

iprazone [see: isoprazone]

ipriflavone INN

iprindole USAN, INN, BAN *antidepressant*

Iprivasc powder for subcu injection ℞ *anticoagulant; thrombin inhibitor for the prevention of deep vein thrombosis (DVT) in elective hip replacement surgery* [desirudin] 15 mg/dose

iprocinodine HCl USAN, BAN *veterinary antibacterial*

iproclozide INN, BAN

iprocrolol INN

iprofenin USAN *hepatic function test*

iproheptine INN

iproniazid INN, BAN

ipronidazole USAN, INN, BAN *antiprotozoal (Histomonas)*

ipropethidine [see: properidine]

iproplatin USAN, INN, BAN *antineoplastic*

iprotiazem INN

iproxamine INN *vasodilator* [also: iproxamine HCl]

iproxamine HCl USAN *vasodilator* [also: iproxamine]

iprozilamine INN

ipsalazide INN, BAN

ipsapirone INN, BAN *anxiolytic* [also: ipsapirone HCl]

ipsapirone HCl USAN *anxiolytic* [also: ipsapirone]

Ipstyl (name changed to **Somatuline Depot** upon marketing release in 2007)

IPTD (isopropyl-thiadiazol) [see: glyprothiazol]

IPV (inactivated poliomyelitis vaccine) [see: poliovirus vaccine, inactivated]

IPV (inactivated poliovaccine) [see: poliovirus vaccine, inactivated]

iquindamine INN

Iquix eye drops ℞ *fluoroquinolone antibiotic for corneal ulcers* [levofloxacin] 1.5%

¹⁹²Ir [see: iridium Ir 192]

irbesartan USAN *angiotensin II receptor antagonist for hypertension; treatment to delay the progression of diabetic nephropathy*

Ircon tablets OTC *hematinic; iron supplement* [carbonyl iron] 66 mg ☒ AeroCaine; argon

Ircon-FA tablets OTC *hematinic* [carbonyl iron; folic acid] 82 mg Fe•0.8 mg

Iressa film-coated tablets ℞ *antineoplastic for advanced or metastatic non–small cell lung cancer (NSCLC); investigational (Phase III) for head and neck cancers* [gefitinib] 250 mg

irgasan [see: triclosan]

iridium *element (Ir)*

iridium Ir 192 USAN *radioactive agent*

irindalone INN

irinotecan INN *topoisomerase I inhibitor; antineoplastic for metastatic colon and rectal cancers* [also: irinotecan HCl]

irinotecan HCl USAN, JAN *topoisomerase I inhibitor; antineoplastic for metastatic colorectal cancer* [also: irinotecan] 20 mg/mL injection

Iris florentina medicinal herb [see: orris root]

Iris versicolor medicinal herb [see: blue flag]

Irish broom *medicinal herb* [see: broom]

Irish moss (Chondrus crispus) plant *medicinal herb used as a demulcent*

irloxacin INN

irofulven USAN, INN *DNA synthesis inhibitor; apoptosis inducer; investigational (orphan) antineoplastic for renal cell carcinoma and ovarian cancer*

irolapride INN

Iromin-G tablets OTC *vitamin/iron supplement* [multiple vitamins; ferrous gluconate; folic acid] ≛•30•0.8 mg

iron *element (Fe)* ☒ Errin

iron carbohydrate complex [see: polyferose]

Iron Chews chewable tablets OTC *hematinic; iron supplement* [carbonyl iron] 15 mg

iron dextran USP *hematinic*

iron heptonate [see: gleptoferron]

iron hexacyanoferrate [see: ferric hexacyanoferrate]

iron hydroxide sucrose complex [see: iron sucrose; saccharated ferric oxide]

iron oxide, saccharated [see: iron sucrose; saccharated ferric oxide]

iron perchloride [see: ferric chloride]

iron polymalether [see: ferropolimaler]

Iron Protein Plus capsules OTC *hematinic; iron supplement* [iron protein succinylate] 300 mg (15 mg Fe)

iron protein succinylate *hematinic (5% elemental iron)*

iron saccharate [see: iron sucrose; saccharated ferric oxide]

iron sorbitex USAN, USP *hematinic*

iron sucrose USAN *hematinic for iron deficiency in patients with non-dialysis-dependent chronic kidney disease (NDD-CKD), hemodialysis-dependent chronic kidney disease (HDD-CKD), and peritoneal dialysis-dependent chronic kidney disease (PDD-CKD)* [also: saccharated ferric oxide]

iron sugar [see: iron sucrose; saccharated ferric oxide]

Iron-Folic 500 timed-release tablets OTC *hematinic* [ferrous sulfate; multiple B vitamins; sodium ascorbate; folic acid] 105•±•500•0.8 mg

Irrigate eye wash OTC *extraocular irrigating solution* [sterile isotonic solution] ⊡ ergot

irritant laxatives *a subclass of laxatives that work by direct action on the intestinal mucosa and nerve plexus to increase peristaltic action* [more commonly called stimulant laxatives]

irsogladine INN

irtemazole USAN, INN, BAN *uricosuric*

IS 5-MN (isosorbide 5-mononitrate) [see: isorbide mononitrate]

isaglidole INN

isamfazone INN

isamoltan INN

isamoxole USAN, INN, BAN *antiasthmatic*

isatoribine USAN *immunomodulator; cell growth regulator*

isaxonine INN

isbogrel INN

iseganan *antimicrobial* [also: iseganan HCl]

iseganan HCl USAN, INN *antimicrobial* [also: iseganan]

Isentress film-coated tablets ℞ *integrase inhibitor for drug-resistant HIV-1 infection* [raltegravir (as potassium)] 400 mg

isepamicin USAN, INN, BAN *aminoglycoside antibiotic*

isethionate USAN, BAN *combining name for radicals or groups* [also: isetionate]

isetionate INN *combining name for radicals or groups* [also: isethionate]

ISG (immune serum globulin) [see: globulin, immune]

ISIS 2503 *investigational (Phase II) Ha-ras selective antisense inhibitor for breast cancer*

Ismelin tablets (discontinued 2006) ℞ *antihypertensive; investigational (orphan) for reflex sympathetic dystrophy and causalgia* [guanethidine monosulfate] 25 mg

Ismo film-coated tablets ℞ *coronary vasodilator; antianginal* [isosorbide mononitrate] 20 mg

Ismotic solution ℞ *osmotic diuretic* [isosorbide] 45%

iso-alcoholic elixir NF

isoaminile INN, BAN

isoamyl *p*-methoxycinnamate [see: amiloxate]

isoamyl nitrate [see: amyl nitrite]

Iso-B capsules OTC *vitamin supplement* [multiple B vitamins; folic acid; biotin] ±•200•100 mcg

isobromindione INN

isobucaine HCl USP

isobutamben USAN, INN *topical anesthetic*

isobutane NF *aerosol propellant* ⊡ Aseptone 1; azapetine

isobutyl *p*-aminobenzoate [see: isobutamben]

isobutyl α-phenylcyclohexaneglycolate [see: ibuverine]

isobutyl 2-cyanoacrylate (IBC) [see: bucrylate]

isobutyl nitrite; butyl nitrite *amyl nitrite substitutes, sold as euphoric street drugs, which produce a quick but short-lived "rush"* [see also: amyl nitrite; volatile nitrites]

p-isobutylhydratropohydroxamic acid [see: ibuproxam]

isobutylhydrochlorothiazide [see: buthiazide]

isobutyramide *investigational (orphan) for sickle cell disease, beta-thalassemia syndrome, and beta-hemoglobinopathies*

isobuzole BAN [also: glysobuzole]

Isocal oral liquid OTC *enteral nutritional therapy* [lactose-free formula] ⊡ Asacol; Os-Cal 500

Isocal HCN ready-to-use oral liquid OTC *enteral nutritional therapy* [lactose-free formula]

Isocal HN oral liquid OTC *enteral nutritional therapy* [lactose-free formula]

isocarboxazid USP, INN, BAN *monoamine oxidase (MAO) inhibitor for depression*

Isochron extended-release tablets Ṛ *coronary vasodilator; antianginal* [isosorbide dinitrate] 40 mg

isoconazole USAN, INN, BAN *antibacterial; antifungal* ⊡ azaconazole

isocromil INN

Isocult for Bacteriuria culture paddles for professional use Ṛ *in vitro diagnostic aid for nitrate, uropathogens, or bacteria in the urine*

Isocult for Candida culture paddles for professional use Ṛ *in vitro diagnostic aid for* Candida albicans *in the vagina*

Isocult for N. gonorrhoeae and Candida culture test for professional use Ṛ *in vitro diagnostic aid for gonorrhea and Candida in various specimens*

Isocult for Neisseria gonorrhoeae culture paddles for professional use Ṛ *in vitro diagnostic aid for gonorrhea*

Isocult for Staphylococcus aureus culture paddles for professional use Ṛ *in vitro diagnostic aid for* Staphylococcus aureus *in exudate*

Isocult for Streptococcal pharyngitis culture paddles for professional use Ṛ *in vitro diagnostic test for streptococcal pharyngitis in throat swabs*

Isocult for T. vaginalis and Candida culture test for professional use Ṛ *in vitro diagnostic aid for Trichomonas and Candida in vaginal or urethral cultures*

isodapamide [see: zidapamide]

d-isoephedrine HCl [see: pseudoephedrine HCl]

isoetarine INN *sympathomimetic bronchodilator* [also: isoetharine] ⊡ estrone; oestrone

isoethadione [see: paramethadione]

isoetharine USAN, BAN *sympathomimetic bronchodilator* [also: isoetarine] ⊡ estrone; oestrone

isoetharine HCl USP, BAN *sympathomimetic bronchodilator* 1% inhalation

isoetharine mesylate USP, BAN *sympathomimetic bronchodilator*

isofezolac INN

isoflupredone INN, BAN *anti-inflammatory* [also: isoflupredone acetate]

isoflupredone acetate USAN *anti-inflammatory* [also: isoflupredone]

isoflurane USAN, USP, INN, BAN *inhalation general anesthetic*

isoflurophate USP *antiglaucoma agent; irreversible cholinesterase inhibitor miotic* [also: dyflos]

Isoject (trademarked delivery form) *prefilled disposable syringe*

Isolan oral liquid OTC *enteral nutritional therapy* [lactose-free formula] ⊡ Wycillin

isoleucine (L-isoleucine) USAN, USP, INN, JAN *essential amino acid; symbols: Ile, I*

isoleucine & leucine & valine *investigational (orphan) for hyperphenylalaninemia*

Isolyte E; Isolyte S; Isolyte S pH 7.4 IV infusion Ṛ *intravenous electrolyte therapy* [combined electrolyte solution] ⊡ esilate; esylate

Isolyte G (H; M; P; R; S) with 5% Dextrose IV infusion Ṛ *intravenous nutritional/electrolyte therapy* [combined electrolyte solution; dextrose]

Isolyte S pH 7.4 IV infusion Ṛ *intravenous electrolyte therapy* [combined electrolyte solution]

isomazole INN *cardiotonic* [also: isomazole HCl]

isomazole HCl USAN *cardiotonic* [also: isomazole]

isomeprobamate [see: carisoprodol]

isomer [def.] *One of a group of chemical compounds having the same molecular formula, but differing in either the arrangement of atoms or the bonds between atoms in the compound.* [see also: enantiomer]

isomerol USAN *antiseptic*

isometamidium BAN [also: isometamidium chloride]

isometamidium chloride INN [also: isometamidium]

isomethadone INN, BAN

isomethepdrine chloride [see: isometheptene]

isometheptene INN, BAN

isometheptene HCl [see: isometheptene]

isometheptene mucate USP *cerebral vasoconstrictor; "possibly effective" for migraine headaches*

isometheptene mucate & dichloralphenazone & acetaminophen *cerebral vasoconstrictor and analgesic for vascular and tension headaches; "possibly effective" for migraine headaches* 65•100•325 mg oral

Isomil oral liquid, powder for oral liquid OTC *hypoallergenic infant food* [soy protein formula] ☑ Esimil

Isomil DF ready-to-use oral liquid OTC *hypoallergenic infant food for management of diarrhea* [soy protein formula]

Isomil SF oral liquid OTC *hypoallergenic infant food* [soy protein formula, sucrose free]

isomolpan INN *antipsychotic; dopamine autoreceptor antagonist* [also: isomolpan HCl]

isomolpan HCl USAN *antipsychotic; dopamine autoreceptor antagonist* [also: isomolpan]

isomylamine HCl USAN *smooth muscle relaxant*

IsonaRif capsules *tuberculostatic* [rifampin; isoniazid] 300•150 mg

isoniazid USP, INN, BAN *bactericidal; primary tuberculostatic* 50, 100, 300 mg oral; 50 mg/5 mL oral; 100 mg/mL injection

isonicophen [see: aconiazide]

isonicotinic acid hydrazide (INH) [see: isoniazid]

isonicotinic acid vanillylidenehydrazide [see: ftivazide]

1-isonicotinoyl-2-salicylidenehydrazine (INSH) [see: salinazid]

isonicotinylhydrazine [see: isoniazid]

isonixin INN

isooctadecanol [see: isostearyl alcohol]

isooctadecyl alcohol [see: isostearyl alcohol]

Isopan oral liquid OTC *antacid* [magaldrate] 540 mg/5 mL ☑ azabon

Isopan Plus oral liquid OTC *antacid; antiflatulent* [magaldrate; simethicone] 540•40 mg/5 mL

isopentyl p-methoxycinnamate [see: amiloxate]

isopentyl nitrite [see: amyl nitrite]

isophenethanol [see: nifenalol]

isoprazone INN, BAN ☑ azaprocin

isoprednidene INN, BAN

isopregnenone [see: dydrogesterone]

isoprenaline INN, BAN *sympathomimetic bronchodilator; vasopressor for shock* [also: isoproterenol HCl]

L-isoprenaline [see: levisoprenaline]

isoprenaline HCl [see: isoproterenol HCl]

Isoprinosine *investigational (orphan) immunomodulator for subacute sclerosing panencephalitis* [inosine pranobex]

isoprofen INN

isopropamide iodide USP, INN, BAN *peptic ulcer adjunct*

isopropanol [see: isopropyl alcohol]

isopropicillin INN

isoproponum iodide [see: isopropamide iodide]

7-isopropoxyisoflavone [see: ipriflavone]

isopropyl alcohol USP *topical anti-infective/antiseptic; solvent*

isopropyl alcohol, rubbing USP *rubefacient*

N-isopropyl meprobamate [see: carisoprodol]

isopropyl myristate NF *emollient*

isopropyl palmitate NF *oleaginous vehicle*

isopropyl sebacate

isopropyl unoprostone [see: unoprostone isopropyl]

isopropylantipyrine [see: propyphenazone]

isopropylarterenol HCl [see: isoproterenol HCl]

isopropylarterenol sulfate [see: isoproterenol sulfate]

isoproterenol HCl USP *sympathomimetic bronchodilator; vasopressor for cardiac, hypovolemic, or septic shock; adjunct therapy for congestive heart failure (CHF)* [also: isoprenaline] 1:5000 (0.2 mg/mL) injection

isoproterenol sulfate USP *sympathomimetic bronchodilator*

Isoptin SR film-coated sustained-release tablets R *antihypertensive; antianginal; antiarrhythmic; calcium channel blocker* [verapamil HCl] 120, 180, 240 mg

Isopto Atropine Drop-Tainers (eye drops) R *cycloplegic; mydriatic* [atropine sulfate] 0.5%, 1%

Isopto Carbachol Drop-Tainers (eye drops) R *antiglaucoma agent; direct-acting miotic* [carbachol] 0.75%, 1.5%, 3%

Isopto Carpine Drop-Tainers (eye drops) R *antiglaucoma agent; direct-acting miotic* [pilocarpine HCl] 0.25%, 0.5%, 1%, 2%, 3%, 4%, 5%, 6%, 8%, 10%

Isopto Cetamide Drop-Tainers (eye drops) R *antibiotic* [sulfacetamide sodium] 15%

Isopto Homatropine Drop-Tainers (eye drops) R *cycloplegic; mydriatic* [homatropine hydrobromide] 2%, 5%

Isopto Hyoscine Drop-Tainers (eye drops) R *cycloplegic; mydriatic* [scopolamine hydrobromide] 0.25%

Isopto Plain; Isopto Tears Drop-Tainers (eye drops) OTC *moisturizer/lubricant* [hydroxypropyl methylcellulose] 0.5%

Isordil sublingual tablets (discontinued 2005) R *coronary vasodilator; antianginal* [isosorbide dinitrate] 2.5, 5, 10 mg

Isordil Tembid (sustained-release capsules and tablets) (discontinued 2004) R *coronary vasodilator; antianginal* [isosorbide dinitrate] 40 mg

Isordil Titradose (tablets) R *coronary vasodilator; antianginal* [isosorbide dinitrate] 5, 10, 20, 30, 40 mg

isosorbide USAN, USP, INN, BAN *osmotic diuretic; investigational (orphan) agent for Fabry disease*

isosorbide dinitrate USAN, USP, INN, BAN *coronary vasodilator; antianginal* 2.5, 5, 10, 20, 30, 40 mg oral

isosorbide mononitrate USAN, INN, BAN *coronary vasodilator; antianginal* 10, 20, 30, 60, 120 mg oral

Isosource; Isosource HN oral liquid OTC *enteral nutritional therapy* [lactose-free formula]

isospaglumic acid INN

isospirilene [see: spirilene]

isostearyl alcohol USAN *emollient; solvent*

isosulfamerazine [see: sulfaperin]

isosulfan blue USAN *lymphangiography aid* [also: sulphan blue]

isosulpride INN

Isotein HN powder OTC *enteral nutritional therapy* [lactose-free formula]

3-isothiocyanato-1-propene [see: allyl isothiocyanate]

isothiocyanic acid, allyl ester [see: allyl isothiocyanate]

isothipendyl INN, BAN

isothipendyl HCl [see: isothipendyl]

isotiquimide USAN, INN, BAN *antiulcerative*

Isotrate ER extended-release tablets (discontinued 2005) R *antianginal; vasodilator* [isosorbide dinitrate] 60 mg

isotretinoin USAN, USP, INN, BAN *first generation retinoid; systemic keratolytic for severe recalcitrant cystic acne; investigational (Phase III) for neuroblastoma*

isotretinoin anisatil USAN *keratolytic for acne vulgaris*

Isovorin ℞ *chemotherapy "rescue" agent (orphan)* [L-leucovorin] 🔲 acifran

Isovue-200; Isovue-250; Isovue-300; Isovue-370 injection ℞ *radiopaque contrast medium* [iopamidol (49% iodine)] 408 mg/mL (200 mg/mL); 510 mg/mL (250 mg/mL); 612 mg/mL (300 mg/mL); 755 mg/mL (370 mg/mL) 🔲 EZFE 200

Isovue-M 200; Isovue-M 300 intrathecal injection ℞ *radiopaque contrast medium for myelography* [iopamidol (49% iodine)] 408 mg/mL (200 mg/mL); 612 mg/mL (300 mg/mL)

isoxaprolol INN

isoxepac USAN, INN, BAN *anti-inflammatory*

isoxicam USAN, INN, BAN *nonsteroidal anti-inflammatory drug (NSAID); antiarthritic; analgesic; antipyretic*

isoxsuprine INN, BAN *peripheral vasodilator* [also: isoxsuprine HCl]

isoxsuprine HCl USP, JAN *peripheral vasodilator* [also: isoxsuprine] 10, 20 mg oral

I-Soyalac oral liquid OTC *hypoallergenic infant food* [soybean protein formula]

isradipine USAN, INN, BAN *antihypertensive; dihydropyridine calcium channel blocker* 2.5, 5 mg oral

isrodipine [see: isradipine]

Istalol eye drops ℞ *antiglaucoma agent (β-blocker)* [timolol maleate] 0.5%

Istin (EUR) (European name for U.S. product **Norvasc**) 🔲 acetone

istradefylline *selective adenosine A_{2A} receptor antagonist; modified xanthine derivative; investigational (NDA filed) levodopa/carbidopa potentiator to reduce the severity of dyskinesia and improve motor function in Parkinson disease*

Isuprel IV injection or infusion ℞ *vasopressor for cardiac, hypovolemic, or septic shock; adjunct therapy for congestive heart failure (CHF)* [isoproterenol HCl] 1:5000, 1:50 000 (0.2, 0.02 mg/mL) 🔲 Aspirol

itanoxone INN

itasetron USAN *anxiolytic; antidepressant; antiemetic; serotonin 5-HT_3 receptor antagonist*

itazigrel USAN, INN *platelet antiaggregatory agent*

itazogrel [see: itazigrel]

Itch Relief Gel Spritz spray OTC *poison ivy treatment* [camphor] 0.5%

itchweed (Veratrum viride) *medicinal herb* [see: hellebore]

Itch-X topical spray, gel OTC *anesthetic* [pramoxine HCl] 1%

itobarbital [see: butalbital]

itraconazole USAN, INN, BAN *systemic triazole antifungal* 100 mg oral

itramin tosilate INN [also: itramin tosylate]

itramin tosylate BAN [also: itramin tosilate]

itrocainide INN

iturelix USAN, INN *gonadotropin releasing hormone antagonist; ovarian and testicular steroid suppressant*

I-Valex-1 powder OTC *formula for infants with leucine catabolism disorder* 🔲 Avelox; Euflex

I-Valex-2 powder OTC *enteral nutritional therapy for leucine catabolism disorder* 🔲 Avelox; Euflex

Ivarest cream OTC *poison ivy treatment* [calamine; diphenhydramine HCl] 14%•2%

ivarimod INN

Iveegam EN powder for IV infusion ℞ *passive immunizing agent for HIV and Kawasaki syndrome; investigational (orphan) for acute myocarditis and juvenile rheumatoid arthritis* [immune globulin (IGIV)] 5 g/dose

ivermectin USAN, INN, BAN *antiparasitic; anthelmintic for strongyloidiasis and onchocerciasis*

ivermectin component B_{1a}
ivermectin component B_{1b}

IVIG (intravenous immunoglobulin) [q.v.]

ivoqualine INN 🔲 Evoclin

ivy *medicinal herb* [see: American ivy; English ivy; poison ivy]

Ivy Block lotion OTC *preventative for poison ivy, oak, or sumac; use before the risk of exposure* [bentoquatam] 5%

Ivy Cleanse medicated wipes OTC *to remove toxic oils from poison ivy, oak, or sumac* [isopropanol; cetyl alcohol]

Ivy Soothe cream OTC *poison ivy treatment; corticosteroidal anti-inflammatory* [hydrocortisone] 1% ⑳ Eovist; Evista

Ivy Stat gel OTC *poison ivy treatment; corticosteroidal anti-inflammatory* [hydrocortisone] 1%

Ivy Super Dry topical liquid OTC *poison ivy treatment* [zinc acetate; isopropanol; benzyl alcohol] 2%•35%•10%

Ivy-Dry lotion OTC *poison ivy treatment* [zinc acetate; isopropanol] 2%• 12.5% ⑳ ephedra

ixabepilone *antibiotic antineoplastic; epothilone microtubule inhibitor for advanced or metastatic breast cancer*

Ixel *investigational (Phase III) serotonin and norepinephrine reuptake inhibitor for depression and fibromyalgia syndrome* [milnacipran]

Ixempra powder for IV infusion ℞ *antibiotic antineoplastic; epothilone microtubule inhibitor for advanced or metastatic breast cancer* [ixabepilone] 15, 45 mg/vial

izonsteride USAN *antineoplastic 5α-reductase inhibitor for prostate cancer*

jalap *(Ipomoea jalapa) medicinal herb* [see: wild jalap]

Jamaica mignonette *medicinal herb* [see: henna *(Lawsonia)*]

Jamaica pepper *medicinal herb* [see: allspice]

Jamaica sarsaparilla *medicinal herb* [see: sarsaparilla]

Jamaica sorrel *medicinal herb* [see: hibiscus]

Jantoven tablets ℞ *coumarin-derivative anticoagulant for myocardial infarction, thromboembolic episodes, venous thrombosis, and pulmonary embolism* [warfarin sodium] 1, 2, 2.5, 3, 4, 5, 6, 7.5, 10 mg

Janumet film-coated caplets ℞ *combination product for type 2 diabetes that increases insulin production, decreases glucose production, and increases cellular response to insulin* [sitagliptin phosphate; metformin HCl] 50•500, 50•1000 mg

Januvia film-coated tablets ℞ *antidiabetic that enhances the function of the body's incretin system to increase insulin production in the pancreas and reduce glucose production in the liver* [sitagliptin phosphate] 25, 50, 100 mg

Japanese encephalitis (JE) virus vaccine, live attenuated *active immunizing agent (orphan)*

jasmine *(Jasminum officinale) flowers medicinal herb used as a calmative* ⑳ Yasmin

jaundice berry *medicinal herb* [see: barberry]

jaundice root *medicinal herb* [see: goldenseal]

java pepper *medicinal herb* [see: cubeb]

Jay-Phyl syrup ℞ *antiasthmatic; bronchodilator; expectorant* [dyphylline; guaifenesin] 200•100 mg/10 mL ⑳ Avail

Jeffersonia diphylla medicinal herb [see: twin leaf]

Jersey tea *medicinal herb* [see: New Jersey tea]

Jerusalem cowslip; Jerusalem sage *medicinal herb* [see: lungwort]

jessamine, yellow *medicinal herb* [see: gelsemium]

Jesuit's bark *medicinal herb* [see: quinine]

Jets chewable tablets OTC *dietary supplement* [lysine; multiple vitamins] 300•± mg ② A/T/S; oats

JE-VAX powder for subcu injection ℞ *active immunizing agent (orphan)* [Japanese encephalitis (JE) virus vaccine, live attenuated] 0.5 mL (1–3 years), 1 mL (≥ 4 years)

Jevity; Jevity 1.5 Cal ready-to-use oral liquid OTC *enteral nutritional therapy* [lactose-free formula] 237 mL cans ② Avita

jewelweed (Impatiens balsamina; I. biflora; I. capensis) juice *medicinal herb for prophylaxis and treatment of poison ivy rash*

Jew's harp plant *medicinal herb* [see: birthroot]

jiaogulan (Gynostemma pentaphyllum) leaves *medicinal herb used to regulate blood pressure and strengthen the immune system, and for its adaptogenic, antihyperlipidemic, antineoplastic, antioxidant, and cardio- and cerebrovascular protective effects* ② equilin

jimsonweed (Datura stramonium) leaves and flowering tops *medicinal herb used as an analgesic, antiasthmatic, antispasmodic, hypnotic, and narcotic; also abused as a street drug*

J-Max extended-release tablets, syrup ℞ *decongestant; expectorant* [phenylephrine HCl; guaifenesin] 35•1200 mg; 5•200 mg/5 mL

jodphthalein sodium [see: iodophthalein sodium]

joe-pye weed *medicinal herb* [see: queen of the meadow]

jofendylate [see: iophendylate]

Johnswort *medicinal herb* [see: St. John's wort]

Jolessa film-coated tablets (in packs of 91) ℞ *extended-cycle (3 month) monophasic oral contraceptive* [levonorgestrel; ethinyl estradiol] 0.15 mg•30 mcg × 84 days; counters × 7 days ② Alesse

Jolivette tablets (in packs of 28) ℞ *oral contraceptive (progestin only)* [norethindrone] 0.35 mg

jopanoic acid [see: iopanoic acid]

josamycin USAN, INN *antibacterial*

jotrizoic acid [see: iotrizoic acid]

J-Tan oral suspension ℞ *antihistamine* [brompheniramine tannate] 4 mg/5 mL ② Attain; 8 in 1

J-Tan D oral suspension ℞ *decongestant; antihistamine* [phenylephrine tannate; brompheniramine tannate] 5•4 mg/5 mL

J-Tann D PD oral drops ℞ *decongestant; antihistamine; for children 1–24 months* [pseudoephedrine HCl; brompheniramine maleate] 7.5•1 mg/mL

Juglans cinerea *medicinal herb* [see: butternut]

Juglans nigra *medicinal herb* [see: black walnut]

Juglans regia *medicinal herb* [see: English walnut]

Junel 21 Day 1/20; Junel 21 Day 1.5/30 tablets (in packs of 21) ℞ *monophasic oral contraceptive* [norethindrone acetate; ethinyl estradiol] 1 mg•20 mcg; 1.5 mg•30 mcg ② Inhal-Aid

Junel Fe 1/20 tablets (in packs of 28) ℞ *monophasic oral contraceptive; iron supplement* [norethindrone acetate; ethinyl estradiol; ferrous fumarate] 1 mg•20 mcg•75 mg × 21 days; 0•0•75 mg × 7 days ② One-Alpha

Junel Fe 1.5/30 tablets (in packs of 28) ℞ *monophasic oral contraceptive; iron supplement* [norethindrone acetate; ethinyl estradiol; ferrous fumarate] 1.5 mg•30 mcg•75 mg × 21 days; 0•0•75 mg × 7 days ② One-Alpha

"Junior Strength" products [see under product name]

juniper (Juniperus communis) berries *medicinal herb for arthritis, bleeding, bronchitis, colds, edema, infections, kidney infections, pancreatic disorders, uric acid build-up, urinary disorders, and water retention*

juniper, prickly (Juniperus oxycedrus) *medicinal herb* [see: juniper]

juniper tar USP *antieczematic*

Junovan *investigational (NDA filed, orphan) for high-grade osteosarcoma following surgical resection* [mifamurtide]

Jurnista OROS (extended-release tablets) *investigational (Phase III) delivery form for a narcotic analgesic* [hydromorphone]

Just Tears eye drops OTC *moisturizer/lubricant* [polyvinyl alcohol] 1.4% ⑨ Estrace

Juvederm 18; Juvederm 24 subcu injection (discontinued 2007) ℞ *transparent dermal filler for wrinkles and facial folds; increasing numbers indicate increasing density, from fluid for superficial wrinkles to gel for deep folds* [hyaluronic acid] 24 mg/mL

Juvederm 24HV; Juvederm 30; Juvederm 30HV subcu injection ℞ *transparent dermal filler for wrinkles and facial folds; increasing numbers indicate increasing density, from fluid for superficial wrinkles to gel for deep folds; "HV" indicates high viscosity* [hyaluronic acid] 24 mg/mL

K+ 8; K+ 10 film-coated extended-release tablets ℞ *potassium supplement* [potassium chloride] 600 mg (8 mEq K); 750 mg (10 mEq K)

K+ Care powder for oral solution ℞ *potassium supplement* [potassium chloride] 15, 20, 25 mEq K/pkt.

K+ Care ET effervescent tablets ℞ *potassium supplement* [potassium bicarbonate] 20, 25 mEq K

⁴²K [see: potassium chloride K 42]

k82 ImmunoCap test kit for professional use ℞ *in vitro diagnostic aid for specific latex allergies*

KAb201 [see: anti-CEA sheep-human chimeric monoclonal antibodies (MAb) radiolabeled with iodine I 131]

Kadian polymer-coated sustained-release pellets in capsules ℞ *narcotic analgesic* [morphine sulfate] 10, 20, 30, 50, 60, 80, 100, 200 mg ⑨ codeine; Quad Tann

kainic acid INN

Kala tablets OTC *natural intestinal bacteria; probiotic; dietary supplement; fever blister treatment; not generally regarded as safe and effective as an antidiarrheal* [Lactobacillus acidophilus (soy-based)] 200 million CFU

kalafungin USAN, INN *antifungal*

Kaletra film-coated tablets, oral solution ℞ *antiretroviral protease inhibitor combination for HIV infection* [lopinavir; ritonavir] 100•25, 200•50 mg; 80•20 mg/mL ⑨ Caltro; coal tar

Kaletra gelcaps (discontinued 2005) ℞ *antiviral protease inhibitor for HIV infection* [lopinavir; ritonavir] 133.3•33.3 mg ⑨ Caltro; coal tar

kallidinogenase INN, BAN

Kalmia latifolia *medicinal herb* [see: mountain laurel]

kalmopyrin [see: calcium acetylsalicylate]

kalsetal [see: calcium acetylsalicylate]

Kaltostat; Kaltostat Fortex pads OTC *wound dressing* [calcium alginate fiber]

kalumb *medicinal herb* [see: colombo]

kanamycin INN, BAN *aminoglycoside antibiotic; tuberculosis retreatment* [also: kanamycin sulfate]

kanamycin B [see: bekanamycin]

kanamycin sulfate USP *aminoglycoside antibiotic; tuberculosis retreatment* [also: kanamycin] 75, 500, 1000 mg/vial injection

Kank-a topical liquid/film OTC *mucous membrane anesthetic* [benzocaine] 20% ⑨ Gonak

kanna *(Sceletium tortuosum)* plant *medicinal herb used as a antidepressant, anxiolytic, relaxant, and euphoriant*

Kantrex capsules, IV or IM injection, pediatric injection ℞ *aminoglycoside antibiotic* [kanamycin sulfate] 500 mg; 500, 1000 mg; 75 mg

Kao Lectrolyte powder for pediatric oral solution OTC *electrolyte replenisher*

Kaodene Non-Narcotic oral liquid OTC *antidiarrheal; GI adsorbent; antacid* [kaolin; pectin; bismuth subsalicylate] 130•6.48•⅔ mg/mL

kaolin USP clay *natural material used topically as an emollient and drying agent and ingested for binding gastrointestinal toxins and controlling diarrhea* ⓓ Calan; Clenia; khellin

Kaon elixir ℞ *potassium supplement* [potassium gluconate] 20 mEq K/15 mL

Kaon-Cl; Kaon-Cl 10 extended-release tablets ℞ *potassium supplement* [potassium chloride] 500 mg (6.7 mEq K); 750 mg (10 mEq K)

Kaon-Cl 20% oral liquid ℞ *potassium supplement* [potassium chloride; alcohol 5%] 40 mEq K/15 mL

Kaopectate caplets, oral liquid OTC *antidiarrheal; antinauseant* [bismuth subsalicylate] 262 mg; 262, 575 mg/15 mL

Kaopectate, Children's oral liquid OTC *antidiarrheal; antinauseant* [bismuth subsalicylate] 261 mg/15 mL

Kaopectate II caplets (discontinued 2004) OTC *antidiarrheal* [loperamide HCl] 2 mg

Kaopectate Advanced Formula oral liquid (discontinued 2004) OTC *antidiarrheal; GI adsorbent* [attapulgite] 750 mg/15 mL

Kaopectate Maximum Strength caplets OTC *antidiarrheal; GI adsorbent* [attapulgite] 750 mg

Kao-Spen oral suspension OTC *GI adsorbent; antidiarrheal* [kaolin; pectin] 5.2 g•260 mg per 30 mL ⓓ Gas-Ban

Kao-Tin oral liquid OTC *antidiarrheal; antinauseant* [bismuth subsalicylate] 262 mg/15 mL ⓓ K-Tan

Kapectolin oral liquid, oral suspension OTC *GI adsorbent; antidiarrheal* [bismuth subsalicylate] 262 mg/15 mL

Kapseal (trademarked dosage form) *capsules sealed with a band*

karaya gum *(Sterculia tragacantha; S. urens; S. villosa)* *medicinal herb used as a topical astringent and bulk laxative* ⓓ guar gum

Karidium tablets, chewable tablets, drops ℞ *dental caries preventative* [sodium fluoride] 2.2 mg; 2.2 mg; 0.275 mg/drop ⓓ Geridium

Karigel; Karigel-N gel ℞ *dental caries preventative* [sodium fluoride] 1.1%

Kariva tablets (in packs of 28) ℞ *biphasic oral contraceptive* [desogestrel; ethinyl estradiol] ⓓ Geref
Phase 1 (21 days): 0.15 mg•20 mcg;
Phase 2 (5 days): 0•10 mcg;
Counters (2 days)

karyocyte growth factor [see: pegylated megakaryocyte growth and development factor, recombinant human]

kasal USAN *food additive* ⓓ Kay Ciel

kaugoed; kougoed *medicinal herb* [see: kanna]

kava kava *(Piper methysticum)* root *medicinal herb for insomnia and nervousness*

Kay Ciel oral liquid, powder for oral solution ℞ *potassium supplement* [potassium chloride] 20 mEq K/15 mL; 20 mEq K/pkt. ⓓ kasal

Kayexalate powder for oral or rectal suspension ℞ *potassium-removing agent for hyperkalemia* [sodium polystyrene sulfonate]

Kaylixir oral liquid ℞ *potassium supplement* [potassium gluconate; alcohol 5%] 20 mEq K/15 mL

K-C oral suspension OTC *antidiarrheal; GI adsorbent; antacid* [kaolin; pectin; bismuth subcarbonate] 5 g•260 mg•260 mg per 30 mL

KCl (potassium chloride) [q.v.]

K-Dur 10; K-Dur 20 controlled-release tablets ℞ *potassium supplement* [potassium chloride] 750 mg (10 mEq K); 1500 mg (20 mEq K)

kebuzone INN ② Capsin; Cubicin; quipazine

Keflex Pulvules (capsules), oral suspension ℞ *first-generation cephalosporin antibiotic* [cephalexin] 250, 333, 500, 750 mg; 125, 250 mg/5 mL

Keftab tablets (discontinued 2005) ℞ *first-generation cephalosporin antibiotic* [cephalexin HCl] 500 mg

kellofylline [see: visnafylline]

Kelnor 1/35 tablets (in packs of 28) ℞ *monophasic oral contraceptive* [ethynodiol diacetate; ethinyl estradiol] 1 mg•35 mcg × 21 days; counters × 7 days

kelp *(Fucus versiculosus)* plant *medicinal herb for brittle fingernails, cleaning arteries, colitis, eczema, goiter, obesity, and toning adrenal, pituitary, and thyroid glands* ② KLB6

kelp *(Laminaria digitata; L. japonica)* plant *medicinal herb for cervical dilation and cervical ripening* ② KLB6

Kemadrin tablets ℞ *anticholinergic; antiparkinsonian* [procyclidine HCl] 5 mg

Kemstro orally disintegrating tablets ℞ *skeletal muscle relaxant* [baclofen] 10, 20 mg

Kenaject-40 IM, intra-articular, intrabursal, intradermal injection (discontinued 2008) ℞ *corticosteroid; anti-inflammatory* [triamcinolone acetonide] 40 mg/mL

Kenalog ointment, cream, lotion, aerosol spray ℞ *corticosteroidal anti-inflammatory* [triamcinolone acetonide] 0.025%, 0.1%, 0.5%; 0.025%, 0.1%, 0.5%; 0.025%, 0.1%; ⚕

Kenalog in Orabase oral paste ℞ *corticosteroidal anti-inflammatory* [triamcinolone acetonide] 0.1%

Kenalog-10; Kenalog-40 IM, intra-articular, intrabursal, intradermal injection ℞ *corticosteroid; anti-inflammatory* [triamcinolone acetonide] 10 mg/mL; 40 mg/mL

Kenalog-H cream ℞ *corticosteroidal anti-inflammatory* [triamcinolone acetonide] 0.1%

Kendall compound A [see: dehydrocorticosterone]

Kendall compound B [see: corticosterone]

Kendall compound E [see: cortisone acetate]

Kendall compound F [see: hydrocortisone]

Kendall desoxy compound B [see: desoxycorticosterone acetate]

Kenonel cream ℞ *corticosteroidal anti-inflammatory* [triamcinolone acetonide] 1%

Kenwood Therapeutic oral liquid OTC *vitamin/mineral supplement* [multiple vitamins & minerals]

keoxifene HCl [now: raloxifene HCl]

Kepivance powder for IV injection ℞ *keratinocyte growth factor (KGF) for radiation- and chemotherapy-induced oral mucositis* [palifermin] 6.25 mg/dose

Keppra film-coated tablets, oral solution, IV injection ℞ *anticonvulsant for myoclonic, partial-onset, and generalized tonic-clonic seizures; oral forms are also used to treat migraine headaches and bipolar disorder* [levetiracetam] 250, 500, 750, 1000 mg; 100 mg/mL; 100 mg/mL ② CAPPr; copper

Keppra XR film-coated extended-release tablets ℞ *once-daily anticonvulsant for partial-onset seizures* [levetiracetam] 500 mg

keracyanin INN

Kerafoam topical foam ℞ *moisturizer; emollient; keratolytic* [urea] 30% ② CarraFoam; Geravim

Keralac cream, ointment ℞ *moisturizer; emollient; keratolytic* [urea] 50% ② garlic

Keralac lotion ℞ *moisturizer; emollient; keratolytic* [urea; lactic acid; vitamin E] 35%•⚕•⚕ ② garlic

Keralac Nail Gel ℞ *moisturizer; emollient; keratolytic* [urea] 50%

Keralac Nailstick topical solution ℞ *moisturizer; emollient; keratolytic* [urea] 50%

Kerasal ointment OTC *keratolytic and moisturizer/emollient for dry, rough, or cracked feet* [salicylic acid; urea] 5%• 10% ⊡ cresol; Cryselle

Kerasal AL cream OTC *moisturizer/ emollient for dry, rough, or cracked feet* [ammonium lactate] ⊡ carazolol

keratinocyte growth factor, recombinant human (rhKGF) *investigational (orphan) to reduce the incidence and severity of radiation-induced xerostomia*

keratolytics *a class of agents that cause sloughing of the horny layer of the epidermis and softening of the skin*

Keri; Keri Light lotion (discontinued 2004) OTC *moisturizer; emollient*

Keri Age Defy & Protect lotion OTC *moisturizer; emollient; sunscreen (SPF 15)* [octinoxate; oxybenzone] 7.5%• 2%

Keri Creme (discontinued 2004) OTC *moisturizer; emollient*

Keri Long Lasting cream OTC *moisturizer; emollient*

Keri Original; Keri Advanced; Keri Nourishing Shea Butter; Keri Renewal Milk Body; Keri Renewal Skin Firming; Keri Sensitive Skin; Keri Shave lotion OTC *moisturizer; emollient*

KeriCort-10 cream OTC *corticosteroidal anti-inflammatory* [hydrocortisone] 1%

Kerlone film-coated tablets ℞ *β-blocker for hypertension* [betaxolol HCl] 10, 20 mg

kernelwort *medicinal herb* [see: figwort]

Kerodex #51 cream OTC *skin protectant for dry or oily work* ⊡ Cardec-S; Kredex

Kerodex #71 cream OTC *water repellant skin protectant for wet work* ⊡ Cardec-S; Kredex

Kerol topical suspension ℞ *moisturizer; emollient; keratolytic* [urea (in a vehicle containing lactic acid and salicylic acid)] 50% ⊡ caraway oil; coral

Ketalar IV or IM injection ℞ *rapid-acting general anesthetic; sometimes abused as a street drug due to its "dissociative state" effects* [ketamine HCl] 10, 50, 100 mg/mL

ketamine INN, BAN *a rapid-acting general anesthetic; sometimes abused as a street drug due to its "dissociative state" effects* [also: ketamine HCl]

ketamine HCl USAN, USP, JAN *a rapid-acting general anesthetic; sometimes abused as a street drug due to its "dissociative state" effects* [also: ketamine]

ketanserin USAN, INN, BAN *serotonin antagonist*

ketazocine USAN, INN *analgesic*

ketazolam USAN, INN, BAN *minor tranquilizer*

Ketek film-coated tablets, Ketek Pak (10 film-coated tablets) ℞ *broad-spectrum ketolide antibiotic for community-acquired pneumonia (CAP); approval to treat other types of respiratory tract infections was withdrawn by the FDA in 2007* [telithromycin] 300, 400 mg; 400 mg

kethoxal USAN *antiviral* [also: ketoxal]

ketimipramine INN *antidepressant* [also: ketipramine fumarate]

ketimipramine fumarate [see: ketipramine fumarate]

ketipramine fumarate USAN *antidepressant* [also: ketimipramine]

7-KETO DHEA *investigational dehydroepiandrosterone (DHEA) derivative for Alzheimer disease*

ketobemidone INN, BAN

ketocaine INN ⊡ quatacaine

ketocainol INN

KetoCare reagent strips for home use OTC *in vitro diagnostic aid for acetone (ketones) in the urine*

ketocholanic acid [see: dehydrocholic acid]

ketoconazole USAN, USP, INN, BAN *broad-spectrum imidazole antifungal; topical treatment for tinea corporis, tinea cruris, tinea pedis, tinea versicolor, cutaneous candidiasis, and seborrheic dermatitis* 200 mg oral; 2% topical

ketoconazole & cyclosporine A
investigational (orphan) to diminish nephrotoxicity from organ transplantation

Keto-Diastix reagent strips *in vitro diagnostic aid for multiple urine products*

ketohexazine [see: cetohexazine]

ketolides *a class of oral antibiotics*

Ketonex-1 powder OTC *formula for infants with maple syrup urine disease (MSUD)*

Ketonex-2 powder *enteral nutritional therapy for maple syrup urine disease (MSUD)*

ketoprofen USAN, INN, BAN, JAN *analgesic; antipyretic; nonsteroidal anti-inflammatory drug (NSAID) for osteoarthritis, rheumatoid arthritis, and primary dysmenorrhea* 50, 75, 100, 150, 200 mg oral

ketorfanol USAN, INN *analgesic*

ketorolac INN, BAN *analgesic; nonsteroidal anti-inflammatory drug (NSAID) for moderately severe acute pain; investigational (Phase III) intranasal formulation* [also: ketorolac tromethamine]

ketorolac tromethamine USAN *analgesic; nonsteroidal anti-inflammatory drug (NSAID) for moderately severe acute pain; ocular treatment for allergic conjunctivitis, cataract extraction, and corneal refractive surgery* [also: ketorolac] 10 mg oral; 15, 30 mg/mL injection

Ketostix reagent strips for home use OTC *in vitro diagnostic aid for acetone (ketones) in the urine*

ketotifen INN, BAN *antihistamine; mast cell stabilizer* [also: ketotifen fumarate]

ketotifen fumarate USAN, JAN *antihistamine; mast cell stabilizer* (base=71.4%) [also: ketotifen] 0.025% eye drops

Ketotransdel *investigational (Phase III) topical nonsteroidal anti-inflammatory drug (NSAID)*

ketotrexate INN

ketoxal INN *antiviral* [also: kethoxal]

Key-Plex injection (discontinued 2006) ℞ *parenteral vitamin therapy* [multiple B vitamins; vitamin C] ± •50 mg/mL

Key-Pred 25; Key-Pred 50 IM injection (discontinued 2008) ℞ *corticosteroid; anti-inflammatory* [prednisolone acetate] 25 mg/mL; 50 mg/mL ⍰ capuride

Key-Pred-SP IV or IM injection (discontinued 2008) ℞ *corticosteroid; anti-inflammatory* [prednisolone sodium phosphate] 20 mg/mL

K-G Elixir ℞ *potassium supplement* [potassium gluconate] 20 mEq K/15 mL

KGF (keratinocyte growth factor) [q.v.]

KGHB (potassium gamma hydroxybutyrate) [see: gamma hydroxybutyrate (GHB)]

khellin INN ⍰ Calan; Clenia; kaolin

khelloside INN ⍰ Colazide

Kiacta oral *investigational (NDA filed, orphan) amyloid fibrinogen inhibitor for AA (secondary) amyloidosis* [eprodisate]

Kid Kare Children's Cough/Cold oral liquid OTC *antitussive; antihistamine; decongestant; for children 6–11 years* [dextromethorphan hydrobromide; chlorpheniramine maleate; pseudoephedrine HCl] 10•2•30 mg/10 mL

Kid Kare Nasal Decongestant oral drops OTC *nasal decongestant* [pseudoephedrine HCl] 7.5 mg/0.8 mL

kidney root *medicinal herb* [see: queen of the meadow]

KIE syrup (discontinued 2007) ℞ *bronchodilator; decongestant; expectorant* [ephedrine HCl; potassium iodide] 16•300 mg/10 mL

Kindercal oral liquid OTC *enteral nutritional therapy* [lactose-free formula]

Kinerase cream, lotion OTC *moisturizer; emollient* [N^6-furfuryladenine] 0.1%

Kinerase Intensive Eye Cream OTC *moisturizer; emollient* [kinetin; safflower oil] 0.125%• ±

Kineret subcu injection in prefilled syringes ℞ *interleukin-1 receptor antagonist (IL-1ra); nonsteroidal anti-inflam-*

matory drug (NSAID) for rheumatoid arthritis (RA) [anakinra] 100 mg

Kinevac powder for IV injection ℞ *diagnostic aid for gallbladder function* [sincalide] 1 mcg/mL

king's clover *medicinal herb* [see: melilot]

king's cure *medicinal herb* [see: pipsissewa]

king's fern *medicinal herb* [see: buckhorn brake]

kininase II inhibitors [see: angiotensin-converting enzyme inhibitors]

kinnikinnik *medicinal herb* [see: uva ursi]

Kinrix suspension for IM injection ℞ *active immunizing agent for diphtheria, tetanus, pertussis, hepatitis B and D, and three types of poliovirus* [diphtheria & tetanus toxoids & acellular pertussis (DTaP) vaccine; hepatitis B virus vaccine; inactivated poliovirus vaccine (IPV) Types 1, 2, and 3] 0.5 mL/dose

Kionex powder for oral or rectal suspension ℞ *potassium-removing agent for hyperkalemia* [sodium polystyrene sulfonate] 15 g/60 mL ⊘ Cognex

kitasamycin USAN, INN, BAN, JAN *antibacterial* [also: acetylkitasamycin; kitasamycin tartrate]

kitasamycin tartrate JAN *antibacterial* [also: kitasamycin; acetylkitasamycin]

Klamath weed *medicinal herb* [see: St. John's wort]

Klaron 10% lotion ℞ *antibiotic for acne* [sulfacetamide sodium] 10% ⊘ chlorine

KLB6; Ultra KLB6 softgels OTC *dietary supplement* [vitamin B₆; multiple food supplements] 3.5•± mg; 16.7•± mg ⊘ kelp

K-Lease extended-release capsules (discontinued 2004) ℞ *potassium supplement* [potassium chloride] 750 mg (10 mEq K) ⊘ Cal-Cee; Colace

Kleen-Handz solution (discontinued 2008) OTC *antiseptic* [ethyl alcohol] 62%

Klonopin tablets, Wafers (orally disintegrating tablets) ℞ *anticonvulsant; anxiolytic for panic disorder; also used for parkinsonian dysarthria, neuralgias, multifocal tics, and manic episodes of a bipolar disorder; investigational (orphan) for hyperexplexia (startle disease)* [clonazepam] 0.5, 1, 2 mg; 0.125, 0.25, 0.5, 1, 2 mg

K-Lor powder for oral solution ℞ *potassium supplement* [potassium chloride] 15, 20 mEq K/pkt.

Klor-Con; Klor-Con/25 powder for oral solution ℞ *potassium supplement* [potassium chloride] 20 mEq K/pkt.; 25 mEq K/pkt. ⊘ chloroquine

Klor-Con M10; Klor-Con M15; Klor-Con M20 extended-release tablets ℞ *potassium supplement* [potassium chloride] 750 mg (10 mEq K); 1125 mg (15 mEq K); 1500 mg (20 mEq K)

Klor-Con/EF effervescent tablets ℞ *potassium supplement* [potassium bicarbonate; potassium citrate] 25 mEq K

Klorvess oral liquid, effervescent granules, effervescent tablets ℞ *potassium supplement* [potassium chloride] 20 mEq K/15 mL; 20 mEq K/pkt.; 20 mEq K ⊘ Claravis

Klotrix film-coated controlled-release tablets ℞ *potassium supplement* [potassium chloride] 750 mg (10 mEq K) ⊘ Glutarex-1

Klout topical liquid, shampoo OTC *pesticide-free lice removal agent* [acetic acid; isopropanol; sodium laureth sulfate] ⊘ CoLyte; K-Lyte

K-Lyte; K-Lyte DS effervescent tablets ℞ *potassium supplement* [potassium bicarbonate; potassium citrate] 25 mEq K; 50 mEq K ⊘ CoLyte; Klout

K-Lyte/Cl powder for oral solution ℞ *potassium supplement* [potassium chloride] 25 mEq K/dose

K-Lyte/Cl; K-Lyte/Cl 50 effervescent tablets ℞ *potassium supplement* [potassium chloride] 25 mEq K; 50 mEq K

knitback; knitbone *medicinal herb* [see: comfrey]

knob grass; knob root *medicinal herb* [see: stone root]

K-Norm controlled-release capsules (discontinued 2004) ℞ *potassium supplement* [potassium chloride] 750 mg (10 mEq K)

knotted marjoram *medicinal herb* [see: marjoram]

knotweed *(Polygonum aviculare; P. hydropiper; P. persicaria; P. punctatum)* plant *medicinal herb used as an antiseptic, astringent, diaphoretic, diuretic, emmenagogue, rubefacient, and stimulant*

Koate-DVI (double viral inactivation) powder for IV injection ℞ *systemic hemostatic; antihemophilic for the prevention and control of bleeding in classical hemophilia (hemophilia A) and von Willebrand disease (orphan)* [antihemophilic factor concentrate, human] 250, 500, 1000 IU

Kof-Eze lozenges OTC *mild anesthetic; antipruritic; counterirritant* [menthol] 6 mg ☒ Coughtuss

Kogenate powder for IV injection (discontinued 2004) ℞ *antihemophilic for treatment of hemophilia A and presurgical prophylaxis of hemophiliacs (orphan)* [antihemophilic factor, recombinant]

Kogenate FS powder for IV injection ℞ *systemic hemostatic; antihemophilic for the prevention and control of bleeding in classical hemophilia (hemophilia A) and von Willebrand disease (orphan)* [antihemophilic factor, recombinant] 250, 500, 1000 IU

KOH (potassium hydroxide) [q.v.]

kola nut *(Cola acuminata)* seed *medicinal herb used as a stimulant; natural source of caffeine* ☒ Cal-Nate

Kolephrin caplets (discontinued 2007) OTC *decongestant; antihistamine; analgesic; antipyretic* [pseudoephedrine HCl; chlorpheniramine maleate; acetaminophen] 30•2•325 mg ☒ Calphron; Claforan

Kolephrin GG/DM oral liquid OTC *antitussive; expectorant* [dextromethorphan hydrobromide; guaifenesin] 10•150 mg/5 mL

Kolephrin/DM caplets (discontinued 2007) OTC *antitussive; antihistamine; decongestant; analgesic; antipyretic* [dextromethorphan hydrobromide; chlorpheniramine maleate; pseudoephedrine HCl; acetaminophen] 10•2•30•325 mg

kolfocon A USAN *hydrophobic contact lens material*

kolfocon B USAN *hydrophobic contact lens material*

kolfocon C USAN *hydrophobic contact lens material*

kolfocon D USAN *hydrophobic contact lens material*

Kolyum oral liquid ℞ *potassium supplement* [potassium gluconate; potassium chloride] 20 mEq K/15 mL ☒ gallium

kombucha (yeast/bacteria/fungus symbiont) fermented tea *natural treatment for aging, cancer, intestinal disorders, and rheumatism* ☒ Compack

Kondremul Plain emulsion OTC *emollient laxative* [mineral oil]

Konsyl powder for oral solution OTC *bulk laxative* [psyllium] 6 g/tsp. or pkt. ☒ Goniosol; Gynazole-1

Konsyl Easy Mix Formula powder for oral solution OTC *bulk laxative with electrolytes* [psyllium; electrolytes] 6•≛ g/tsp. or pkt.

Konsyl Fiber tablets OTC *bulk laxative; antidiarrheal* [calcium polycarbophil] 625 mg

Konsyl Orange powder for oral solution OTC *bulk laxative* [psyllium] 3.4 g/tbsp. or pkt.

Konsyl-D powder OTC *bulk laxative* [psyllium] 3.4 g/tsp.

Korean ginseng *(Panax ginseng; P. shin-seng)* *medicinal herb* [see: ginseng]

kougoed; kaugoed *medicinal herb* [see: kanna]

Kovia 6.5 ointment ℞ *proteolytic enzyme for debridement of necrotic tissue; vulnerary* [papain; urea] 650 000 IU/g•10%

Kovitonic oral liquid OTC *hematinic* [ferric pyrophosphate; multiple B vitamins; lysine; folic acid] 42•±• 10•0.1 mg/15 mL

K-Pek oral suspension (discontinued 2007) OTC *antidiarrheal* [bismuth subsalicylate] 262 mg/15 mL ⊠ COPAC; CPB WC; CPC; Gy-Pak

K-Pek II caplets OTC *antidiarrheal* [loperamide HCl] 2 mg ⊠ COPAC; CPB WC; CPC; Gy-Pak

K-Phos M.F. tablets ℞ *urinary acidifier* [potassium acid phosphate; sodium acid phosphate] 155•350 mg (1.1 mEq K, 2.9 mEq Na)

K-Phos Neutral film-coated caplets ℞ *urinary acidifier; phosphorus supplement* [sodium phosphate, dibasic; potassium phosphate, monobasic; sodium phosphate, monobasic] 250 mg P

K-Phos No. 2 tablets ℞ *urinary acidifier* [potassium acid phosphate; sodium acid phosphate] 305•700 mg (2.3 mEq K, 5.8 mEq Na)

K-Phos Original tablets ℞ *urinary acidifier* [potassium acid phosphate] 500 mg (3.7 mEq K)

K.P.N. tablets OTC *vitamin/mineral/calcium/iron supplement* [multiple vitamins & minerals; calcium; iron; folic acid] ±•333•11•0.27 mg

81mKr [see: krypton Kr 81m]

85Kr [see: krypton clathrate Kr 85]

Kredex ⓔ (European name for U.S. product **Coreg**) ⊠ Cardec-S; Kerodex

Kristalose powder for oral solution ℞ *hyperosmotic laxative* [lactulose] 10, 20 g/pkt.

Kronocap (trademarked dosage form) *sustained-release capsule*

Kronofed-A sustained-release capsules (discontinued 2007) ℞ *decongestant; antihistamine* [pseudoephedrine HCl; chlorpheniramine maleate] 120•8 mg

Kronofed-A Jr. sustained-release capsules (discontinued 2007) ℞ *decongestant; antihistamine* [pseudoephedrine HCl; chlorpheniramine maleate] 60•4 mg

krypton *element (Kr)*

krypton clathrate Kr 85 USAN *radioactive agent*

krypton Kr 81m USAN, USP *radioactive agent*

K-Tab film-coated extended-release tablets ℞ *potassium supplement* [potassium chloride] 750 mg (10 mEq K) ⊠ CTAB; Q-Tapp

K-Tan caplets ℞ *decongestant antihistamine; sleep aid* [phenylephrine tannate; pyrilamine tannate] 25•60 mg ⊠ Kao-Tin

K-Tan 4 oral suspension ℞ *decongestant; antihistamine; sleep aid* [phenylephrine tannate; pyrilamine tannate] 5•30 mg/5 mL ⊠ Kao-Tin

Kudrox oral suspension (discontinued 2004) OTC *antacid; antiflatulent* [aluminum hydroxide; magnesium hydroxide; simethicone] 500•450•40 mg/5 mL

kudzu (Pueraria lobata; P. thunbergiana) root *medicinal herb for the management of alcoholism*

kunecatechins *a class of natural polyphenolic antioxidants; topical treatment for external genital and perianal warts (condyloma acuminatum) in immunocompromised adults* [also known as: sinecatechins; see also: catechins; epicatechins]

Kuric cream ℞ *broad-spectrum antifungal for tinea corporis, tinea cruris, tinea pedis, tinea versicolor, cutaneous candidiasis, and seborrheic dermatitis* [ketoconazole] 2% ⊠ Carac; Coreg

Kutapressin subcu or IM injection (discontinued 2004) ℞ *claimed to be an anti-inflammatory for multiple dermatoses* [liver derivative complex] 25.5 mg/mL

Kutrase capsules ℞ *porcine-derived digestive enzymes* [lipase; protease; amylase] 2400•30 000•30 000 USP units

Kuvan tablets ℞ *phenylalanine hydroxylase (PAH) enzyme for mild to moderate phenylketonuria (PKU)* [sapropterin dihydrochloride] 100 mg ⊠ caffeine; C-Phen

Ku-Zyme capsules ℞ *porcine-derived digestive enzymes* [lipase; protease; amylase] 1200•15 000•15 000 USP units

Ku-Zyme HP capsules ℞ *porcine-derived digestive enzymes* [lipase; protease; amylase] 8000•30 000•30 000 USP units

K-vescent effervescent powder ℞ *potassium supplement* [potassium chloride] 20 mEq K/pkt.

Kwelcof oral liquid ℞ *narcotic antitussive; expectorant* [hydrocodone bitartrate; guaifenesin] 5•100 mg/5 mL

KwikPen (trademarked delivery device) *prefilled self-injection syringe for various* **Humalog** *products*

K-Y vaginal jelly OTC *moisturizer/lubricant* [glycerin; hydroxyethyl cellulose]

K-Y Plus vaginal gel OTC *spermicidal contraceptive (for use with a diaphragm)* [nonoxynol 9] 2.2%

kyamepromazin [see: cyamemazine]

Kybernin P IV *investigational (orphan) agent for thromboembolic episodes due to congenital aT-III deficiency* [antithrombin III concentrate]

Kynapid *investigational (NDA filed) selective ion channel blocker for the acute conversion of atrial fibrillation* [vernakalant]

Kytril film-coated tablets, oral solution, IV infusion ℞ *antiemetic to prevent nausea and vomiting following chemotherapy, radiation, or surgery* [granisetron HCl] 1.12 mg (1 mg base); 1.12 mg/5 mL (1 mg/5 mL base); 0.11, 1.12 mg/mL (0.1, 1 mg/mL base)

Kytril oral solution (discontinued 2008) ℞ *antiemetic to prevent nausea and vomiting following chemotherapy, radiation, or surgery* [granisetron HCl] 1.12 mg/5 mL (1 mg/5 mL base)

L

L-5 hydroxytryptophan (L-5HTP) *natural precursor to serotonin; investigational (orphan) for tetrahydrobiopterin deficiency; also used as a natural remedy for depression*

LA-12 IM injection (discontinued 2006) ℞ *hematinic; vitamin B₁₂ supplement* [hydroxocobalamin] 1000 mcg/mL

LAAM (*l*-acetyl-α-methadol [or] *l*-alpha-acetyl-methadol) [see: levomethadyl acetate]

labetalol INN, BAN *antihypertensive; antiadrenergic (α- and β-blocker)* [also: labetalol HCl]

labetalol HCl USAN, USP *antihypertensive; antiadrenergic (α- and β-blocker)* [also: labetalol] 100, 200, 300 mg oral; 5 mg/mL injection

labetuzumab *monoclonal antibody to carcinoembryonic antigen (CEA)*

Labrador tea (*Ledum groenlandicum; L. latifolium; L. palustre*) leaves *medicinal herb for bronchial infections, cough, diarrhea, headache, kidney disorders, lung infections, malignancies, rheumatism, and sore throat*

Labstix reagent strips *in vitro diagnostic aid for multiple urine products*

Lac-Hydrin cream, lotion ℞ *moisturizer; emollient* [ammonium lactate] 12%

Lac-Hydrin Five lotion OTC *moisturizer; emollient* [lactic acid]

LACI (lipoprotein-associated coagulation inhibitor) [see: tifacogin]

lacidipine USAN, INN, BAN *antihypertensive; calcium channel blocker*

LAC-Lotion ℞ *moisturizer; emollient* [ammonium lactate] 12%

lacosamide *investigational (Phase III) adjunctive therapy for adults with* uncontrolled partial seizures; investigational (Phase II) for diabetic neuropathy

Lacril eye drops OTC *moisturizer/lubricant* [hydroxypropyl methylcellulose] 0.5%

Lacri-Lube NP; Lacri-Lube S.O.P. ophthalmic ointment OTC *moisturizer/lubricant* [white petrolatum; mineral oil; lanolin]

Lacrisert ophthalmic insert OTC *ophthalmic moisturizer/lubricant* [hydroxypropyl cellulose] 5 mg

lactagogues *a class of agents that promote or increase the flow of breast milk* [also called: galactagogues]

LactAid oral liquid, tablets OTC *digestive aid for lactose intolerance* [lactase enzyme] 250 U/drop; 3000 U

lactalfate INN

lactase enzyme *digestive enzyme for lactose intolerance*

lactated potassic saline [see: potassic saline, lactated]

lactated Ringer (LR) injection [see: Ringer injection, lactated]

lactated Ringer (LR) solution [see: Ringer injection, lactated]

lactic acid USP *pH adjusting agent; investigational (orphan) for severe aphthous stomatitis in terminally immunocompromised patients*

Lactic Acid 10% E cream ℞ *emollient; moisturizer* [lactic acid; vitamin E] 10%•116.67 IU/g

lactic acid bacteria (Lactobacillus, Bifidobacterium, and Streptococcus sp.) *investigational (orphan) for chronic pouchitis*

LactiCare lotion OTC *emollient; moisturizer* [lactic acid]

LactiCare-HC lotion ℞ *corticosteroidal anti-inflammatory* [hydrocortisone] 1%, 2.5%

Lactinex granules, chewable tablets OTC *natural intestinal bacteria; probiotic; dietary supplement; not generally regarded as safe and effective as an antidiarrheal* [Lactobacillus acidophilus; L. bulgaricus]

Lactinol lotion ℞ *emollient; moisturizer* [lactic acid] 10%

Lactinol-E cream ℞ *emollient; moisturizer* [lactic acid; vitamin E] 10%•116.67 IU/g

lactitol INN, BAN

Lactobacillus acidophilus *natural intestinal bacteria; probiotic; dietary supplement; fever blister treatment; not generally regarded as safe and effective as an antidiarrheal* [also: acidophilus]

Lactobacillus bifidus *natural intestinal bacteria; probiotic; dietary supplement*

Lactobacillus bulgaricus *natural intestinal bacteria; probiotic; dietary supplement; not generally regarded as safe and effective as an antidiarrheal*

Lactobacillus sp. [see also: lactic acid bacteria]

lactobin *investigational (orphan) for AIDS-related diarrhea*

lactobionic acid, calcium salt, dihydrate [see: calcium lactobionate]

Lactocal-F film-coated tablets ℞ *vitamin/mineral/calcium/iron supplement* [multiple vitamins & minerals; calcium; iron; folic acid] ±•200•65•1 mg

lactoferrin alpha *investigational (orphan) for the prevention and treatment of graft-versus-host disease*

lactoflavin [see: riboflavin]

LactoFree oral liquid, powder for oral liquid OTC *hypoallergenic infant formula* [milk-based formula, lactose free]

LactoFree LIPIL oral liquid, powder for oral liquid OTC *hypoallergenic infant formula fortified with omega-3 fatty acids* [milk-based formula, lactose free]

Lacto-Key-100; Lacto-Key-600 capsules OTC *natural intestinal bacteria; probiotic; dietary supplement; fever blister treatment* [Lactobacillus acidophilus] ≥ 1 billion CFU; ≥ 6 billion CFU

β-lactone [see: propiolactone]

γ-lactone D-glucofuranuronic acid [see: glucurolactone]

lactose NF *tablet and capsule diluent; dietary supplement*

Lactrase capsules OTC *digestive aid for lactose intolerance* [lactase enzyme] 250 mg

Lactrex 12% cream ℞ *emollient; moisturizer* [lactic acid] 12%

Lactuca sativa medicinal herb [see: lettuce]

Lactuca virosa medicinal herb [see: wild lettuce]

lactulose USAN, USP, INN, BAN *hyperosmotic laxative; synthetic disaccharide used to prevent and treat portal-systemic encephalopathy* 10 g/15 mL oral or rectal

ladakamycin [now: azacitidine]

Lady Esther cream OTC *moisturizer; emollient* [mineral oil]

lady's mantle *(Alchemilla xanthochlora; A. vulgaris)* plant *medicinal herb for diarrhea and other digestive disorders; also used as an astringent, anti-inflammatory agent, menstrual cycle regulator, and muscle relaxant*

lady's slipper *(Cypripedium pubescens)* root *medicinal herb for chorea, hysteria, insomnia, nervousness, and restlessness*

Lagesic extended-release caplets ℞ *analgesic; antipyretic; antihistamine; sleep aid* [acetaminophen; phenyltoloxamine citrate] 600•66 mg ⚠ Luxiq

laidlomycin INN *veterinary growth stimulant* [also: laidlomycin propionate potassium]

laidlomycin propionate potassium USAN *veterinary growth stimulant* [also: laidlomycin]

Laki-Lorand factor [see: factor XIII]

L-All 12 oral suspension (discontinued 2008) ℞ *antitussive; decongestant* [carbetapentane tannate; phenylephrine tannate] 30•30 mg/5 mL

lamb mint medicinal herb [see: peppermint; spearmint]

Lambda (name changed to **Fosrenol** upon marketing release in 2004)

lamb's quarter medicinal herb [see: birthroot]

Lamictal tablets, chewable/dispersible tablets ℞ *phenyltriazine anticonvul-*

sant; adjunctive treatment for partial seizures, Lennox-Gastaut syndrome (orphan), primary generalized tonic-clonic (PGTC) seizures, and bipolar disorder [lamotrigine] 25, 100, 150, 200 mg; 2, 5, 25 mg

Lamictal XR extended-release tablets *investigational (NDA filed) once-daily dosing* [lamotrigine]

lamifiban USAN, INN *glycoprotein (GP) IIb/IIIa receptor inhibitor; antiplatelet/antithrombotic agent for unstable angina*

lamifiban HCl USAN *glycoprotein (GP) IIb/IIIa receptor inhibitor; antiplatelet/antithrombotic agent for unstable angina*

Laminaria digitata; L. japonica medicinal herb [see: kelp]

Lamisil tablets, granules for oral suspension ℞ *systemic allylamine antifungal for onychomycosis* [terbinafine HCl] 250 mg; 125, 187.5 mg/pkt

Lamisil AF Defense topical powder OTC *antifungal* [tolnaftate] 1%

Lamisil aT cream, gel, spray, drops OTC *allylamine antifungal* [terbinafine HCl] 1%

Lamium album medicinal herb [see: blind nettle]

lamivudine USAN, INN, BAN *nucleoside reverse transcriptase inhibitor; antiviral for HIV and chronic hepatitis B infections*

lamivudine & stavudine *combination nucleoside reverse transcriptase inhibitor (NRTI) for HIV and AIDS* 150•30, 150•40 mg oral

lamivudine & stavudine & nevirapine *combination nucleoside reverse transcriptase inhibitor (NRTI) and non-nucleoside reverse transcriptase inhibitor (NNRTI) for HIV and AIDS* 30•6•50, 60•12•100, 150•30•200, 150•40•200 mg oral

lamivudine & zidovudine & abacavir sulfate *nucleoside reverse transcriptase inhibitor (NRTI) combination for HIV and AIDS* 150•300•300 mg oral

lamotrigine USAN, INN, BAN *phenyltriazine anticonvulsant; adjunctive treatment for partial seizures, Lennox-Gas-*

taut syndrome (orphan), *primary generalized tonic-clonic (PGTC) seizures,
and bipolar disorder* 5, 25 mg oral

Lampit (available only from the Centers for Disease Control) ℞ *anti-infective for Chagas disease* [nifurtimox]

Lamprene capsules ℞ *bactericidal;
tuberculostatic; leprostatic (orphan);
available only to physicians enrolled in
the National Hansen Disease Program
through the FDA* [clofazimine] 50 mg

lamtidine INN, BAN

Lanabiotic ointment OTC *antibiotic;
anesthetic* [polymyxin B sulfate; neomycin sulfate; bacitracin zinc; lido-
caine] 10 000 U•3.5 mg•500 U•40
mg per g

Lanacane spray, cream OTC *anesthetic;
antiseptic* [benzocaine; benzethonium
chloride] 20%•0.1%; 6%•0.1% ☒
lignocaine

Lanacaps (trademarked dosage form)
timed-release capsules

Lanacort 5 cream, ointment OTC *corticosteroidal anti-inflammatory* [hydro-
cortisone acetate] 0.5% ☒ lungwort

Lanacort 10 cream OTC *corticosteroidal
anti-inflammatory* [hydrocortisone
acetate] 1% ☒ lungwort

Lanaphilic cream OTC *moisturizer;
emollient; keratolytic* [urea] 20%

Lanaphilic OTC *ointment base*

Lanaphilic with Urea OTC *ointment
base* [urea] 10%

Lanatabs (trademarked dosage form)
sustained-release tablets

lanatoside NF, INN, BAN

Laniazid tablets ℞ *tuberculostatic* [iso-
niazid] 50 mg

Laniazid C.T. tablets ℞ *tuberculostatic*
[isoniazid] 300 mg

lanolin USP *ointment base; water-in-oil
emulsion; emollient/protectant*

lanolin, anhydrous USP *absorbent
ointment base*

lanolin alcohols *ointment base ingredient*

Lanolor cream OTC *moisturizer; emollient*

Lanophyllin elixir (discontinued
2008) ℞ *antiasthmatic; bronchodilator*
[theophylline] 80 mg/15 mL

lanoteplase USAN *thrombolytic; tissue
plasminogen activator (tPA)*

Lanoxicaps capsules (discontinued
2008) ℞ *cardiac glycoside to increase
cardiac output; antiarrhythmic*
[digoxin] 0.05, 0.1, 0.2 mg

Lanoxin tablets, pediatric elixir, IV or
IM injection ℞ *cardiac glycoside to
increase cardiac output; antiarrhythmic*
[digoxin] 0.125, 0.25 mg; 0.05
mg/mL; 0.1, 0.25 mg/mL ☒ Lincocin

lanreotide acetate USAN *somatostatin
analogue; antineoplastic; reduces endogenous growth hormone (GH) and insulin growth factor-1 (IGF-1) levels to
treat acromegaly (orphan)* (base=77%)

lansoprazole USAN, INN, BAN *proton
pump inhibitor for gastric and duodenal
ulcers, erosive esophagitis, GERD, and
other gastroesophageal disorders*

lanthanum *element (La)*

lanthanum carbonate *phosphate binder
for hyperphosphatemia in end-stage
renal disease (ESRD)*

Lantus vials, OptiClik cartridges, and
SoloStar prefilled syringes for subcu
injection ℞ *long-acting, once-daily
basal insulin analogue for diabetes* [insu-
lin glargine (rDNA)] 100 U/mL; 300
IU/3 mL; 300 U/3 mL

Lapacho colorado; L. morado medicinal
herb [see: pau d'arco]

lapatinib ditosylate *tyrosine kinase
inhibitor; antineoplastic for advanced or
metastatic breast cancer; investigational
for kidney, head, and neck cancers*

lapirium chloride INN *surfactant* [also:
lapyrium chloride]

**LAPOCA (L-asparaginase, Oncovin,
cytarabine, Adriamycin)** *chemotherapy protocol* ☒ Lobac

laprafylline INN

lapyrium chloride USAN *surfactant*
[also: lapirium chloride]

laramycin [see: zorbamycin]

larch (*Larix americana; L. europaea*)
bark, resin, young shoots, and needles
*medicinal herb used as an anthelmintic,
diuretic, laxative, and vulnerary; pow-*

dered bark is 98% arabinogalactans [see also: arabinogalactans]

Largon IV or IM injection (discontinued 2004) ℞ *sedative; analgesic adjunct* [propiomazine HCl] 20 mg/mL

Lariam tablets ℞ *antimalarial for acute chloroquine-resistant malaria (orphan)* [mefloquine HCl] 250 mg

Larix americana; L. europaea medicinal herb [see: larch]

Larodopa capsules ℞ *dopamine precursor for Parkinson disease* [levodopa] 100, 250 mg

Larodopa tablets ℞ *dopamine precursor for Parkinson disease* [levodopa] 100, 250, 500 mg

laronidase *enzyme replacement therapy for mucopolysaccharidosis I (MPS I) (orphan)*

laropiprant *investigational (NDA filed) prostaglandin D_2 (PGD_2) inhibitor to reduce flushing during niacin therapy*

laroxyl [see: amitriptyline]

Larrea divaricata; L. glutinosa; L. tridentata medicinal herb [see: chaparral]

lasalocid USAN, INN, BAN *coccidiostat for poultry*

Lasix tablets, oral solution, IM or IV injection ℞ *antihypertensive; loop diuretic* [furosemide] 20, 40, 80 mg; 10 mg/mL; 10 mg/mL

lasofoxifene tartrate USAN *second-generation selective estrogen receptor modulator (SERM); investigational (NDA filed) for osteoporosis and the reduction of LDL cholesterol; investigational (Phase III) for breast cancer*

Lassar paste [betanaphthol (q.v.) + zinc oxide (q.v.)]

latamoxef INN, BAN *anti-infective* [also: moxalactam disodium]

latamoxef disodium [see: moxalactam disodium]

latanoprost USAN, INN *topical prostaglandin agonist for glaucoma and ocular hypertension*

latex agglutination test *in vitro diagnostic aid*

Latrodectus **immune F(ab)2** *investigational (orphan) treatment for black widow spider bites*

laudexium methylsulfate [see: laudexium metilsulfate; laudexium methylsulphate]

laudexium methylsulphate BAN [also: laudexium metilsulfate]

laudexium metilsulfate INN [also: laudexium methylsulphate]

lauralkonium chloride INN

laurel *(Laurus nobilis)* leaves and fruit *medicinal herb used as an aromatic, astringent, carminative, and stomachic*

laurel, mountain; rose laurel; sheep laurel *medicinal herb* [see: mountain laurel]

laurel, red; swamp laurel *medicinal herb* [see: magnolia]

laurel, spurge; spurge olive *medicinal herb* [see: mezereon]

laureth 4 USAN *surfactant*

laureth 9 USAN *spermaticide; surfactant*

laureth 10S USAN *spermaticide*

lauril INN *combining name for radicals or groups*

laurilsulfate INN *combining name for radicals or groups* [also: sodium lauryl sulfate]

laurixamine INN

laurocapram USAN, INN *excipient*

lauroguadine INN

laurolinium acetate INN, BAN

lauromacrogol 400 INN

Laurus nobilis medicinal herb [see: laurel]

Laurus persea medicinal herb [see: avocado]

lauryl isoquinolinium bromide USAN *anti-infective*

lavender *(Lavandula* spp.) flowers, leaves, and oil *medicinal herb for acne, bile flow stimulation, diabetes, edema, flatulence, hyperactivity, insomnia, intestinal spasms, migraine headache, and stimulating menstrual flow*

lavender oil NF

lavoltidine INN *antiulcerative; histamine H_2-receptor blocker* [also: lavoltidine succinate; loxtidine]

lavoltidine succinate USAN *antiulcerative; histamine H_2-receptor blocker* [also: lavoltidine; loxtidine]

lawrencium *element (Lr)*

Lawsonia inermis *medicinal herb* [see: henna]

Laxative & Stool Softener softgels OTC *stimulant laxative; stool softener* [casanthranol; docusate sodium] 30• 100 mg

laxatives *a class of agents that promote evacuation of the bowels or have a mild purgative effect; subclasses: saline, stimulant, bulk-producing, emollient, stool-softening, and hyperosmotic* [see also: cathartics; purgatives; various subclasses]

Lax-Pills tablets OTC *stimulant laxative* [sennosides] 15, 25 mg

lazabemide USAN, INN *antiparkinsonian*

lazabemide HCl USAN *antiparkinsonian*

lazaroids *a class of potent antioxidants that can protect against oxygen radical–mediated lipid peroxidation and progressive neuronal degeneration following brain or spinal trauma, subarachnoid hemorrhage, or stroke* [also called: 21-aminosteroids]

Lazer Creme OTC *moisturizer; emollient* [vitamins A and E] 3333.3• 116.67 U/g

Lazer Formalyde solution ℞ *anhidrotic for hyperhidrosis and bromhidrosis* [formaldehyde] 10%

LazerSporin-C ear drops ℞ *corticosteroidal anti-inflammatory; antibiotic* [hydrocortisone; neomycin sulfate; polymyxin B sulfate] 1%•5 mg• 10 000 U per mL

LC-65 solution OTC *cleaning solution for hard, soft, or rigid gas permeable contact lenses*

L-Carnitine tablets, capsules OTC *dietary amino acid* [levocarnitine] 500 mg; 250 mg

LCD (liquor carbonis detergens) [see: coal tar]

LCR (leurocristine) [see: vincristine]

LCx *Neisseria gonorrhoeae* **Assay** reagent kit for professional use ℞ *in vitro diagnostic aid for Neisseria gonorrhoeae infection*

lead *element (Pb)*

lecimibide USAN *hypocholesterolemic; antihyperlipidemic*

lecithin NF *emulsifier; surfactant; natural phospholipid mixture of various phosphatidylcholines used as an antihypercholesterolemic and cognition enhancer for Alzheimer and other dementias* 420, 1200 mg oral

lecithol *natural remedy* [see: lecithin]

LED (liposome-encapsulated doxorubicin) [see: doxorubicin HCl, liposome-encapsulated]

Lederject (trademarked delivery form) *prefilled disposable syringe*

ledoxantrone trihydrochloride USAN *antineoplastic; topoisomerase II inhibitor*

Ledum groenlandicum; L. latifolium; L. palustre *medicinal herb* [see: Labrador tea]

leeches (Hirudo medicinalis) *natural adjunct to postsurgical wound management*

leek (Allium porrum) *bulb, lower stem, and leaves medicinal herb used as an appetite stimulant, decongestant, and diuretic*

Leena tablets (in packs of 28) ℞ *triphasic oral contraceptive* [norethindrone; ethinyl estradiol] Phase 1 (7 days): 0.5 mg•35 mcg; Phase 2 (9 days): 1 mg•35 mcg; Phase 3 (5 days): 0.5 mg•35 mcg

lefetamine INN

leflunomide USAN, INN *anti-inflammatory for rheumatoid arthritis and benign prostatic hypertrophy (BPH); investigational (orphan) for malignant glioma, ovarian cancer, and prevention of organ transplant rejection* 10, 20 mg oral

Legalon *investigational (orphan) antitoxin for Amanita phalloides (mushroom) intoxication* [disodium silibinin dihemisuccinate]

Legatrin PM caplets OTC *prevention and treatment of nocturnal leg cramps*

[diphenhydramine HCl; acetamino-phen] 50•500 mg

legs, red *medicinal herb* [see: bistort]

leiopyrrole INN

lemidosul INN

lemon *(Citrus limon)* fruit and peel *medicinal herb used as an astringent, refrigerant, and source of vitamin C*

lemon, ground; wild lemon *medicinal herb* [see: mandrake]

lemon balm *(Melissa officinalis)* plant *medicinal herb used as an antispasmodic and sedative; also used for Graves disease and cold sores*

lemon oil NF

lemon verbena *(Aloysiatriphylla spp.)* leaves and flowers *medicinal herb for fever, flatulence, gastrointestinal spasms and other disorders, and sedation*

lemon walnut *medicinal herb* [see: butternut]

lemongrass *(Andropogon citratus; Cymbopogon citratus)* leaves *medicinal herb for colds, cough, fever, gastrointestinal spasm and other disorders, nervousness, pain, and rheumatism; also used as an antiemetic*

Lemotussin-DM oral liquid (discontinued 2007) ℞ *antitussive; antihistamine; decongestant; expectorant* [dextromethorphan hydrobromide; chlorpheniramine maleate; pseudoephedrine HCl; guaifenesin; potassium guaiacolsulfonate] 7.5•2•10•50•50 mg

lenalidomide *immunomodulator for multiple myeloma and transfusion-dependent anemia in patients with myelodysplastic syndrome (orphan); thalidomide analogue*

lenampicillin INN

lenercept USAN *tumor necrosis factor (TNF) receptor antagonist for septic shock, multiple sclerosis, inflammatory bowel disease, and rheumatoid arthritis*

leniquinsin USAN, INN *antihypertensive*

lenitzol [see: amitriptyline]

lenograstim USAN, INN, BAN *immunomodulator; antineutropenic; hematopoietic stimulant*

lenperone USAN, INN *antipsychotic*

Lens Drops solution OTC *rewetting solution for hard or soft contact lenses*

Lens Lubricant solution OTC *rewetting solution for hard or soft contact lenses*

Lens Plus Daily Cleaner solution OTC *surfactant cleaning solution for soft contact lenses*

Lens Plus Oxysept products [see: Oxysept]

Lens Plus Rewetting Drops OTC *rewetting solution for soft contact lenses*

Lens Plus Sterile Saline aerosol solution OTC *rinsing/storage solution for soft contact lenses* [sodium chloride (saline solution)]

Lente Iletin II vials for subcu injection OTC *antidiabetic* [insulin zinc (pork)] 100 U/mL

lentin [see: carbachol]

lentinan JAN *immunomodulator*

Lentinula edodes *medicinal herb* [see: shiitake mushrooms]

Leontodon taraxacum *medicinal herb* [see: dandelion]

Leonurus cardiaca *medicinal herb* [see: motherwort]

leopard's bane *medicinal herb* [see: arnica]

Lepidium meyenii *medicinal herb* [see: maca]

lepirudin *anticoagulant for heparin-associated thrombocytopenia (orphan)*

leprostatics *a class of drugs effective against leprosy*

leptacline INN

leptandra; purple leptandra *medicinal herb* [see: Culver root]

lergotrile USAN, INN *prolactin enzyme inhibitor*

lergotrile mesylate USAN *prolactin enzyme inhibitor*

leridistim USAN *interleukin-3 and granulocyte colony-stimulating factor receptor agonist for chemotherapy-induced neutropenia and thrombocytopenia*

Lescol capsules ℞ *HMG-CoA reductase inhibitor for hypercholesterolemia, hypertriglyceridemia, mixed dyslipidemia, atherosclerosis, and coronary heart* *disease (CHD)* [fluvastatin sodium] 20, 40 mg

Lescol XL film-coated extended-release tablets ℞ *HMG-CoA reductase inhibitor for hypercholesterolemia, hypertriglyceridemia, mixed dyslipidemia, atherosclerosis, and coronary heart disease (CHD)* [fluvastatin (as sodium)] 80 mg

lesopitron INN *anxiolytic*

lesser centaury *medicinal herb* [see: centaury]

Lessina film-coated tablets (in packs of 21 or 28) ℞ *monophasic oral contraceptive; emergency postcoital contraceptive* [levonorgestrel; ethinyl estradiol] 0.1 mg•20 mcg ⊠ leucine; lysine

Letairis film-coated tablets ℞ *endothelin receptor antagonist (ERA) vasodilator for pulmonary arterial hypertension (PAH)* [ambrisentan] 5, 10 mg ⊠ LTRAs

leteprinim potassium USAN *nerve growth factor*

letimide INN *analgesic* [also: letimide HCl]

letimide HCl USAN *analgesic* [also: letimide]

letosteine INN

letrazuril INN *investigational (Phase II) treatment for AIDS-related cryptosporidial diarrhea*

letrozole USAN, INN *aromatase inhibitor; estrogen antagonist; antineoplastic for early, advanced, or metastatic breast cancer in postmenopausal women* 2.5 mg oral

lettuce (Lactuca sativa) juice and leaves *medicinal herb used as an anodyne, antispasmodic, expectorant, and sedative (for herbal medical use, common garden lettuce is harvested after it has gone to seed, and a milky juice is extracted)*

Leucanthemum parthenium *medicinal herb* [see: feverfew]

leucarsone [see: carbarsone]

leucine (L-leucine) USAN, USP, INN, JAN *essential amino acid; symbols: Leu, L* ⊠ Lessina; lysine

leucine & isoleucine & valine *investigational (orphan) for hyperphenylalaninemia*

L-leucine & L-tyrosine & L-serine *investigational (orphan) for hepatocellular carcinoma*

leucinocaine INN

leucocianidol INN

Leucomax ⓔⓤⓡ (available in 36 foreign countries) *investigational (orphan) antineutropenic and hematopoietic stimulant for bone marrow transplants, chronic lymphocytic leukemia (CLL), myelodysplastic syndrome, aplastic anemia, and AIDS-related neutropenia* [molgramostim]

leucomycin [see: kitasamycin; spiramycin]

L-leucovorin *chemotherapy "rescue" agent (orphan)*

leucovorin calcium USP *antianemic; folate replenisher; antidote to folic acid antagonist; chemotherapy "rescue" agent (orphan)* [also: calcium folinate] 5, 15, 25 mg oral; 3, 10 mg injection; 50, 100, 200, 350 mg/vial injection

leucovorin & fluorouracil *antineoplastic for metastatic colorectal cancer (orphan)*

leucovorin & methotrexate *antineoplastic for osteosarcoma (orphan)*

Leukeran film-coated tablets ℞ *nitrogen mustard-type alkylating antineoplastic for multiple leukemias, lymphomas, and neoplasms* [chlorambucil] 2 mg

Leukine powder for IV infusion ℞ *antineutropenic for bone marrow transplant and graft delay (orphan)* [sargramostim] 250, 500 mcg

leukocyte interferon [now: interferon alfa-n3]

leukocyte protease inhibitor [see: secretory leukocyte protease inhibitor]

leukocyte typing serum USP *in vitro blood test*

leukopoietin [see: sargramostim]

Leukotac *investigational (orphan) for graft-versus-host disease* [inolimomab]

leukotriene receptor antagonists (LTRAs); leukotriene receptor

inhibitors *a class of antiasthmatics that inhibit bronchoconstriction when used prophylactically (will not reverse bronchospasm)*

leupeptin *investigational (orphan) aid to microsurgical peripheral nerve repair*

leuprolide acetate USAN *gonadotropin suppressant; antihormonal antineoplastic for various cancers; LHRH agonist for central precocious puberty (orphan), endometriosis, and uterine fibroids* [also: leuprorelin] 5 mg/mL injection

leuprorelin INN, BAN *testosterone suppressant; antihormonal antineoplastic for various cancers* [also: leuprolide acetate]

leurocristine (LCR) [see: vincristine]

leurocristine sulfate [see: vincristine sulfate]

Leustatin IV infusion ℞ *antineoplastic for hairy-cell leukemia (orphan); investigational (orphan) for chronic lymphocytic leukemia, myeloid leukemia, multiple sclerosis, and non-Hodgkin lymphoma* [cladribine] 1 mg/mL

Leuvectin *investigational (Phase I/II, orphan) gene-based therapy for advanced metastatic renal cell carcinoma*

Levacet caplets OTC *analgesic; antipyretic; antihistamine* [aspirin; acetaminophen; salicylamide; phenyltoloxamine citrate; caffeine] 400•400•150•50•40 mg

levacetylmethadol INN *narcotic analgesic* [also: levomethadyl acetate]

levalbuterol *sympathomimetic bronchodilator; single isomer of albuterol*

levalbuterol HCl USAN *sympathomimetic bronchodilator; single isomer of albuterol* 0.021%, 0.042%, 0.0103% inhalation solution

levalbuterol sulfate USAN *sympathomimetic bronchodilator; single isomer of albuterol*

levalbuterol tartrate USAN *sympathomimetic bronchodilator; single isomer of albuterol*

Levall oral liquid ℞ *antitussive; decongestant; expectorant* [carbetapentane citrate; phenylephrine HCl; guaifenesin] 15•5•100 mg/5 mL

Levall 5.0 oral liquid ℞ *narcotic antitussive; decongestant; expectorant* [hydrocodone bitartrate; phenylephrine HCl; guaifenesin] 2.5•5•100 mg/5 mL

Levall 12 oral suspension ℞ *antitussive; decongestant* [carbetapentane tannate; phenylephrine tannate] 30•25 mg/5 mL

levallorphan INN, BAN [also: levallorphan tartrate]

levallorphan tartrate USP [also: levallorphan]

levamfetamine INN *anorectic* [also: levamfetamine succinate; levamphetamine]

levamfetamine succinate USAN *anorectic* [also: levamfetamine; levamphetamine]

levamisole INN, BAN *biological response modifier; antineoplastic; veterinary anthelmintic* [also: levamisole HCl] ⧉ lofemizole

levamisole HCl USAN, USP *biological response modifier; antineoplastic; veterinary anthelmintic* [also: levamisole] ⧉ lofemizole HCl

levamphetamine BAN *anorectic* [also: levamfetamine succinate; levamfetamine]

levant berry (Anamirta cocculus; A. paniculata) leaves and berries *medicinal herb for epilepsy, lice, malaria, morphine poisoning, and worms; not generally regarded as safe and effective for ingestion or topical application on abraded skin*

Levaquin film-coated tablets, oral solution, IV infusion ℞ *broad-spectrum fluoroquinolone antibiotic* [levofloxacin] 250, 500, 750 mg; 25 mg/mL; 250, 500, 750 mg

Levaquin Leva-pak (5 tablets) ℞ *broad-spectrum fluoroquinolone antibiotic for acute bacterial sinusitis* [levofloxacin] 750 mg

levarterenol [see: norepinephrine bitartrate]

levarterenol bitartrate [now: norepinephrine bitartrate]

Levatol caplets ℞ *β-blocker for hypertension* [penbutolol sulfate] 20 mg

Levbid extended-release tablets ℞ *GI/ GU antispasmodic; antiparkinsonian; anticholinergic "drying agent" for allergic rhinitis or hyperhidrosis* [hyoscyamine sulfate] 0.375 mg

levcromakalim USAN, INN, BAN *antiasthmatic; antihypertensive*

levcycloserine USAN, INN *enzyme inhibitor*

levdobutamine INN *cardiotonic* [also: levdobutamine lactobionate]

levdobutamine lactobionate USAN *cardiotonic* [also: levdobutamine]

levdropropizine INN

Levemir vials, prefilled syringes, and PenFill cartridges for subcu injection ℞ *antidiabetic; long-acting insulin formulation intended to provide continuous basal insulin levels through once- or twice-daily dosing* [insulin detemir (rDNA)] 100 U/mL; 300 U/3 mL; 300 U/3 mL

levemopamil INN *treatment for stroke*

levetiracetam USAN, INN *anticonvulsant for myoclonic, partial-onset, and generalized tonic-clonic seizures; oral forms are also used to treat migraine headaches and bipolar disorder*

levisoprenaline INN

Levisticum officinale medicinal herb [see: lovage]

Levitra film-coated tablets ℞ *phosphodiesterase type 5 (PDE5) inhibitor; selective vasodilator for erectile dysfunction (ED)* [vardenafil HCl] 2.5, 5, 10, 20 mg

Levlen tablets (in Slidecases of 28) (discontinued 2008) ℞ *monophasic oral contraceptive; emergency postcoital contraceptive* [levonorgestrel; ethinyl estradiol] 0.15 mg•30 mcg × 21 days; counters × 7 days ☑ Lufyllin

Levlite tablets (in Slidecases of 28) (discontinued 2008) ℞ *monophasic oral contraceptive* [levonorgestrel; eth-

inyl estradiol] 0.1 mg•20 mcg × 21 days; counters × 7 days ☑ Lypholyte

levlofexidine INN

levmetamfetamine USAN, USP *nasal decongestant*

levobetaxolol INN *topical antiglaucoma agent (β-blocker)* [also: levobetaxolol HCl]

levobetaxolol HCl USAN *topical antiglaucoma agent (β-blocker)* [also: levobetaxolol]

levobunolol INN, BAN *topical antiglaucoma agent (β-blocker)* [also: levobunolol HCl]

levobunolol HCl USAN, USP *topical antiglaucoma agent (β-blocker)* [also: levobunolol] 0.25%, 0.5% eye drops

levobupivacaine HCl USAN *long-acting local anesthetic*

levocabastine INN, BAN *antihistamine* [also: levocabastine HCl]

levocabastine HCl USAN *antihistamine; investigational (orphan) ophthalmic suspension for vernal keratoconjunctivitis* [also: levocabastine]

levocarbinoxamine tartrate [see: rotoxamine tartrate]

levocarnitine USAN, USP, INN *dietary amino acid for primary and secondary genetic carnitine deficiency (orphan) and end-stage renal disease (orphan); investigational (orphan) for pediatric cardiomyopathy* 100, 300 mg/mL oral; 200 mg/mL injection

levocetirizine dihydrochloride *second-generation piperazine antihistamine for allergic rhinitis and chronic idiopathic urticaria; isomer of cetirizine*

levodopa USAN, USP, INN, BAN, JAN *dopamine precursor for Parkinson disease*

levodopa & carbidopa *dopamine precursor plus potentiator for Parkinson disease (orphan)* 100•10, 100•25, 200•50, 250•25 mg oral

Levo-Dromoran tablets, IV, IM, or subcu injection ℞ *narcotic analgesic* [levorphanol tartrate] 2 mg; 2 mg/mL

levofacetoperane INN

levofenfluramine INN

levofloxacin USAN, INN, JAN *broad-spectrum fluoroquinolone antibiotic*

levofuraltadone USAN, INN *antibacterial; antiprotozoal*

levoglutamide INN [now: glutamine]

Levolet tablets ℞ *synthetic thyroid hormone (T_4 fraction only)* [levothyroxine sodium] ② Lypholyte

levoleucovorin calcium USAN *antidote to folic acid antagonists; chemotherapy "rescue agent" for osteosarcoma and colon cancer* (base=78%) 64 mg (50 mg base) injection

levomenol INN

levomepate [see: atromepine]

levomepromazine INN *analgesic* [also: methotrimeprazine]

levomethadone INN

levomethadyl acetate USAN *narcotic analgesic* [also: levacetylmethadol]

levomethadyl acetate HCl USAN *narcotic analgesic for management of opiate addiction* (orphan)

levomethorphan INN, BAN

levometiomeprazine INN

levomoprolol INN

levomoramide INN, BAN

levonantradol INN, BAN *analgesic* [also: levonantradol HCl]

levonantradol HCl USAN *analgesic* [also: levonantradol]

levonordefrin USP *adrenergic; vasoconstrictor* [also: corbadrine]

levonorgestrel USAN, USP, INN, BAN *progestin; oral contraceptive; contraceptive intrauterine device (IUD); emergency postcoital ("morning after") contraceptive*

Levophed IV infusion ℞ *vasopressor for acute hypotensive shock* [norepinephrine bitartrate] 1 mg/mL

levophenacylmorphan INN, BAN

levopropicillin INN *antibacterial* [also: levopropylcillin potassium]

levopropicillin potassium [see: levopropylcillin potassium]

levopropoxyphene INN, BAN *antitussive* [also: levopropoxyphene napsylate]

levopropoxyphene napsylate USAN *antitussive* [also: levopropoxyphene]

levopropylcillin potassium USAN *antibacterial* [also: levopropicillin]

levopropylhexedrine INN

levoprotiline INN

Levora tablets (in packs of 28) ℞ *monophasic oral contraceptive* [levonorgestrel; ethinyl estradiol] 0.15 mg• 30 mcg × 21 days; counters × 7 days

levorin INN

levorotatory alkaloids of belladonna *a subclass of belladonna alkaloids (q.v.)* [also known as: belladonna L-alkaloids]

levorphanol INN, BAN *narcotic analgesic* [also: levorphanol tartrate]

levorphanol tartrate USP *narcotic analgesic* [also: levorphanol] 2 mg oral

levosimendan USAN *investigational (Phase III) calcium sensitizer and vasodilator for decompensated heart failure*

Levo-T tablets ℞ *synthetic thyroid hormone (T_4 fraction only)* [levothyroxine sodium] 25, 50, 75, 88, 100, 112, 125, 137, 150, 175, 200, 300 mcg

Levothroid caplets, powder for injection ℞ *synthetic thyroid hormone (T_4 fraction only)* [levothyroxine sodium] 25, 50, 75, 88, 100, 112, 125, 150, 175, 200, 300 mcg; 200 mcg

levothyroxine sodium USP, INN *synthetic thyroid hormone (T_4 fraction only)* [also: thyroxine] 25, 50, 75, 88, 100, 112, 125, 137, 150, 175, 200, 300 mcg oral; 200, 500 mcg injection

levoxadrol INN *local anesthetic; smooth muscle relaxant* [also: levoxadrol HCl]

levoxadrol HCl USAN *local anesthetic; smooth muscle relaxant* [also: levoxadrol]

Levoxyl tablets ℞ *synthetic thyroid hormone (T_4 fraction only)* [levothyroxine sodium] 25, 50, 75, 88, 100, 112, 125, 137, 150, 175, 200, 300 mcg

LEV/PSE/GG extended-release capsules ℞ *decongestant; expectorant* [pseudoephedrine HCl; guaifenesin] 90•400 mg

Levsin IV, IM, or subcu injection ℞ *GI/GU antispasmodic to reduce motility during radiologic imaging; preopera-*

tive antimuscarinic to reduce salivary and gastric secretions [hyoscyamine sulfate] 0.5 mg/mL

Levsin tablets, drops, elixir ℞ *GI/GU antispasmodic; antiparkinsonian; anticholinergic "drying agent" for allergic rhinitis and hyperhidrosis* [hyoscyamine sulfate] 0.125 mg; 0.125 mg/mL; 0.125 mg/5 mL

Levsin PB drops (discontinued 2008) ℞ *GI/GU anticholinergic/antispasmodic; sedative* [hyoscyamine sulfate; phenobarbital; alcohol 5%] 0.125•15 mg/mL

Levsin with Phenobarbital tablets ℞ *GI/GU antispasmodic; anticholinergic; sedative* [hyoscyamine sulfate; phenobarbital] 0.125•15 mg

Levsinex Timecaps (timed-release capsules) ℞ *GI/GU antispasmodic; antiparkinsonian; anticholinergic "drying agent" for allergic rhinitis or hyperhidrosis* [hyoscyamine sulfate] 0.375 mg

Levsin/SL sublingual tablets (also may be chewed or swallowed) ℞ *GI/GU antispasmodic; anticholinergic* [hyoscyamine sulfate] 0.125 mg

Levulan Kerastick topical solution ℞ *photosensitizer for photodynamic therapy of precancerous actinic keratoses of the face and scalp (used with the* **BLU-U Blue Light Photodynamic Therapy Illuminator)** [aminolevulinic acid HCl] 20%

levulose BAN *nutrient; caloric replacement* [also: fructose]

Lexapro film-coated tablets, oral solution ℞ *selective serotonin reuptake inhibitor (SSRI) for major depression and generalized anxiety disorder; also used for panic disorder* [escitalopram oxalate] 5, 10, 20 mg; 5 mg/5 mL

lexipafant USAN *platelet activating factor (PAF) antagonist*

Lexiscan IV injection ℞ *coronary vasodilator to induce pharmacological stress for myocardial perfusion imaging* [regadenoson] 0.08 mg/mL

lexithromycin USAN, INN *antibacterial*

Lexiva film-coated caplets, oral suspension ℞ *antiretroviral; HIV-1 protease inhibitor* [fosamprenavir calcium (converts to amprenavir)] 700 mg (600 mg); 50 mg/mL (43 mg/mL)

lexofenac INN

Lexxel film-coated dual-release tablets (discontinued 2007) ℞ *antihypertensive; angiotensin-converting enzyme (ACE) inhibitor; calcium channel blocker* [enalapril maleate (immediate release); felodipine (extended release)] 5•2.5 mg

Lexxel film-coated dual-release tablets (discontinued 2008) ℞ *antihypertensive; angiotensin-converting enzyme (ACE) inhibitor; calcium channel blocker* [enalapril maleate (immediate release); felodipine (extended release)] 5•5 mg

LH (luteinizing hormone) [see: lutropin alfa]

LH-RF (luteinizing hormone–releasing factor) acetate hydrate [see: gonadorelin acetate]

LH-RF diacetate tetrahydrate [now: gonadorelin acetate]

LH-RF dihydrochloride [now: gonadorelin HCl]

LH-RF HCl [see: gonadorelin HCl]

LH-RH (luteinizing hormone–releasing hormone) *an endogenous hormone, produced in the hypothalamus, which stimulates the release of luteinizing hormone (LH) and follicle-stimulating hormone (FSH) from the pituitary* [also known as: gonadotropin-releasing hormone (Gn-RH)]

Lialda film-coated delayed-release tablets ℞ *once-daily anti-inflammatory for mild to moderate ulcerative colitis* [mesalamine (5-aminosalicylic acid)] 1.2 g

liarozole INN, BAN *antipsoriatic; aromatase inhibitor* [also: liarozole fumarate] ⑨ Lioresal

liarozole fumarate USAN *antipsoriatic; aromatase inhibitor; investigational (orphan) for congenital ichthyosis* [also: liarozole]

liarozole HCl USAN *antineoplastic for prostate cancer; aromatase inhibitor*

liatermin USAN *dopaminergic neuronal growth stimulator for Parkinson disease*

Liatris scariosa; L. spicata; L. squarrosa *medicinal herb* [see: blazing star]

libecillide INN

libenzapril USAN, INN *antihypertensive; angiotensin-converting enzyme (ACE) inhibitor*

LibiGel gel *androgen; investigational (Phase III) for female sexual dysfunction* [testosterone]

Librax capsules ℞ *GI/GU anticholinergic/antispasmodic; anxiolytic* [clidinium bromide; chlordiazepoxide HCl] 2.5•5 mg ⑨ Loprox

Librium capsules, powder for IM or IV injection ℞ *benzodiazepine anxiolytic; sedative; alcohol withdrawal aid; sometimes abused as a street drug* [chlordiazepoxide HCl] 5, 10, 25 mg; 100 mg ⑨ Lipram 4500

Lice Asphyxiator liquid emulsion *investigational (Phase III) nontoxic, insecticide-free treatment for head lice*

licofelone *investigational (Phase III) analgesic/antiarthritic/nonsteroidal anti-inflammatory drug (NSAID) with low gastric side effects*

licorice (*Glycyrrhiza glabra; G. pallidiflora; G. uralensis*) root *medicinal herb for Addison disease, blood cleansing, colds, cough, drug withdrawal, female disorders, hoarseness, hypoglycemia, lung disorders, sore throat, and stomach ulcers; also used as an expectorant and to increase energy*

licostinel USAN *NMDA receptor antagonist*

licryfilcon A USAN *hydrophilic contact lens material*

licryfilcon B USAN *hydrophilic contact lens material*

LidaMantle cream ℞ *anesthetic* [lidocaine HCl] 3%

LidaMantle HC cream ℞ *corticosteroidal anti-inflammatory; anesthetic* [hydrocortisone acetate; lidocaine] 0.5%•3%

lidamidine INN *antiperistaltic* [also: lidamidine HCl]

lidamidine HCl USAN *antiperistaltic* [also: lidamidine]

Lidex cream, ointment, topical solution ℞ *corticosteroidal anti-inflammatory* [fluocinonide] 0.05%

Lidex-E cream ℞ *corticosteroidal anti-inflammatory; emollient* [fluocinonide] 0.05%

lidimycin INN *antifungal* [also: lydimycin]

lidocaine USP, INN *topical/local anesthetic; transdermal delivery for postherpetic neuralgia (orphan)* [also: lignocaine]

lidocaine benzyl benzoate [see: denatonium benzoate]

lidocaine HCl USP *topical/local anesthetic; mucous membrane anesthetic; antiarrhythmic for acute ventricular arrhythmias* [also: lignocaine HCl] 2%, 3%, 4%, 5% topical; 1%, 2% IV injection; 4%, 10%, 20% IV admixture

Lidocaine HCl in Dextrose injection, IV infusion ℞ *local anesthetic for obstetric use; IV infusion for acute ventricular arrhythmias* [lidicaine HCl; dextrose] 1.5%•7.5%, 5%•7.5%; 0.2%, 0.4%, 0.8%

lidocaine HCl & epinephrine *injectable local anesthetic; vasoconstrictor* 0.5%•1:200 000, 1%•1:100 000, 1%•1:200 000, 1.5%•1:200 000, 2%•1:50 000, 2%•1:100 000, 2%•1:200 000 injection

lidocaine HCl & hydrocortisone acetate *local anesthetic; corticosteroidal anti-inflammatory* 0.5%•3%, 3%•2.5% topical

lidocaine & prilocaine *local anesthetic* 2.5%•2.5% topical

Lidocaine/Hydrocortisone Rectal cream in prefilled applicator ℞ *corticosteroidal anti-inflammatory; anesthetic* [hydrocortisone acetate; lidocaine HCl] 0.5%•3%

Lidoderm transdermal patch R *anesthetic for post-herpetic neuralgia (orphan)* [lidocaine] 5%

lidofenin USAN, INN *hepatic function test*

lidofilcon A USAN *hydrophilic contact lens material*

lidofilcon B USAN *hydrophilic contact lens material*

lidoflazine USAN, INN, BAN *coronary vasodilator*

LidoPen auto-injector (automatic IM injection device) R *emergency injection for cardiac arrhythmias* [lidocaine HCl] 300 mg/3 mL dose

Lidosense 4 cream OTC *anesthetic* [lidocaine] 4%

Lidosite Topical System transdermal patch R *local anesthetic* [lidocaine HCl; epinephrine] 10%•0.1%

lifarizine USAN, INN, BAN *platelet aggregation inhibitor*

life everlasting *medicinal herb* [see: everlasting]

Life Extension Booster; Life Extension Super Booster softgels OTC *vitamin/mineral supplement* [multiple vitamins & minerals]

Life Extension Herbal Mix powder for oral solution OTC *dietary supplement*

Life Extension Mix; Life Extension Mix with Niacin; Life Extension Mix without Copper caplets, capsules, powder for oral solution OTC *vitamin/mineral supplement* [multiple vitamins & minerals]

Life Extension Two-Per-Day tablets OTC *vitamin/mineral supplement* [multiple vitamins & minerals]

life root (*Senecio aureus*; *S. jacoboea*; *S. vulgaris*) *medicinal herb for childbirth pain, diaphoresis, edema, fever, and stimulation of labor and menses; not generally regarded as safe and effective for ingestion because of hepatotoxicity*

LifeCare bags (delivery form) *premixed IV infusion bags*

life-of-man *medicinal herb* [see: spikenard]

lifibrate USAN, INN *antihyperlipoproteinemic*

lifibrol USAN, INN *antihyperlipidemic*

LIG (lymphocyte immune globulin) [q.v.]

light mineral oil [see: mineral oil, light]

lignocaine BAN *topical/local anesthetic* [also: lidocaine] ☒ Lanacane

lignocaine HCl BAN *local anesthetic; antiarrhythmic* [also: lidocaine HCl]

lignosulfonic acid, sodium salt [see: polignate sodium]

lilopristone INN

lily, conval; May lily *medicinal herb* [see: lily of the valley]

lily, ground *medicinal herb* [see: birthroot]

lily, white pond; sweet water lily; sweet-scented pond lily; sweet-scented water lily; white water lily; toad lily *medicinal herb* [see: white pond lily]

lily of the valley (*Convallaria majalis*) flower, leaves, and rhizome *medicinal herb for arrhythmias, edema, epilepsy, and heart disorders*

limaprost INN

limarsol [see: acetarsone]

Limbitrol DS tablets R *antidepressant; anxiolytic* [chlordiazepoxide; amitriptyline HCl] 10•25 mg

Limbrel capsules R *natural COX-2 inhibitor; analgesic and anti-inflammatory for the dietary management of osteoarthritis* [flavocoxid] 250, 500 mg

lime USP *pharmaceutic necessity*

lime, sulfurated (calcium polysulfide, calcium thiosulfate) USP *wet dressing/soak for cystic acne and seborrhea*

lime tree *medicinal herb* [see: linden tree]

linarotene USAN, INN *antikeratinizing agent*

Lincocin capsules (discontinued 2008) R *lincosamide antibiotic* [lincomycin (as HCl)] 500 mg ☒ Lanoxin

Lincocin IV or IM injection R *lincosamide antibiotic* [lincomycin (as HCl)] 300 mg/mL ☒ Lanoxin

lincomycin USAN, INN, BAN *lincosamide antibiotic*

lincomycin HCl USP *lincosamide antibiotic*

Lincorex IV or IM injection (discontinued 2008) ℞ *lincosamide antibiotic* [lincomycin (as HCl)] 300 mg/mL

lincosamides *a class of antimicrobial antibiotics with potentially serious side effects, to which bacterial resistance has been shown*

lindane USAN, USP, INN, BAN *pediculicide for lice; scabicide* 1% topical

linden tree *(Tilia americana; T. cordata; T. europaea; T. platyphyllos) flowers medicinal herb for diaphoresis, diarrhea, headache, hypertension, indigestion, nasal congestion, nervousness, skin moisturizer, stomach disorders, and throat irritation*

linezolid USAN *oxazolidinone antibiotic for gram-positive bacterial infections*

Linguets (trademarked dosage form) *buccal tablets*

Linker protocol (daunorubicin, vincristine, prednisone, asparaginase, teniposide, cytarabine, methotrexate [with leucovorin rescue]) *chemotherapy protocol for acute lymphocytic leukemia (ALL)*

linogliride USAN, INN *antidiabetic*

linogliride fumarate USAN *antidiabetic*

linolexamide [see: clinolamide]

Linomide *investigational (orphan) bone marrow transplant adjunct for leukemia* [roquinimex]

linopiridine USAN, INN *cognition enhancer for Alzheimer disease*

linseed *medicinal herb* [see: flaxseed]

linsidomine INN

lint bells *medicinal herb* [see: flaxseed]

lintopride INN

lintuzumab *investigational (orphan) for acute myelogenous leukemia*

Linum usitatissimum *medicinal herb* [see: flaxseed]

lion's ear; lion's tail *medicinal herb* [see: motherwort]

lion's tooth *medicinal herb* [see: dandelion]

Lioresal caplets ℞ *skeletal muscle relaxant* [baclofen] 10, 20 mg ☒ liarozole

Lioresal intrathecal injection ℞ *skeletal muscle relaxant for intractable spasticity due to multiple sclerosis or spinal cord injury (orphan); investigational (orphan) for trigeminal neuralgia and cerebral palsy* [baclofen] 0.05 mg/0.5 mL (50 mcg/mL), 10 mg/20 mL (500 mcg/mL), 10 mg/5 mL (2000 mcg/mL)

liothyronine INN, BAN *radioactive agent* [also: liothyronine I 125]

liothyronine I 125 USAN *radioactive agent* [also: liothyronine]

liothyronine I 131 USAN *radioactive agent*

liothyronine sodium USP, BAN *synthetic thyroid hormone (T_3 fraction only); treatment of myxedema coma or precoma (orphan)* 10 mcg injection

liotrix USAN, USP *synthetic thyroid hormone (a 4:1 mixture of T_4 and T_3)*

Lip Medex oral ointment OTC *mild mucous membrane anesthetic; antipruritic; counterirritant* [camphor; phenol] 1%•0.54%

lipancreatin [see: pancrelipase]

lipase *digestive enzyme (digests fats)* [24 IU/mg in pancrelipase; 2 IU/mg in pancreatin]

lipase of pancreas [see: pancrelipase]

lipase triacylglycerol [see: pancrelipase]

lipid/DNA human cystic fibrosis gene *investigational (orphan) for cystic fibrosis*

Lipil [see: Enfamil LIPIL; LactoFree LIPIL; ProSobee LIPIL]

Lipisorb powder OTC *enteral nutritional therapy* [lactose-free formula]

Lipitor film-coated tablets ℞ *HMG-CoA reductase inhibitor for hypercholesterolemia, dysbetalipoproteinemia, hypertriglyceridemia, mixed dyslipidemia, and the prevention of cardiovascular disease and stroke in high-risk patients* [atorvastatin calcium] 10, 20, 40, 80 mg

Lipofen capsules ℞ *antihyperlipidemic for primary hypercholesterolemia, hypertriglyceridemia, and mixed dyslip-*

idemia; also used for hyperuricemia [fenofibrate] 50, 150 mg

Lipoflavonoid capsules OTC *dietary lipotropic with vitamin supplementation* [choline; inositol; multiple B vitamins; vitamin C; lemon bioflavonoids] 111.3•111.3• ± •100•100 mg

Lipogen capsules, caplets OTC *dietary lipotropic with vitamin supplementation* [choline; inositol; multiple vitamins] 111•111• ± mg

α-lipoic acid; lipoicin *natural antioxidant* [see: alpha lipoic acid]

Lipomul oral liquid OTC *dietary fat supplement* [corn oil] 10 g/15 mL

Lipo-Nicin/100 tablets ℞ *peripheral vasodilator; antihyperlipidemic* [niacin; niacinamide; multiple vitamins] 100•75• ± mg

Lipo-Nicin/300 timed-release capsules ℞ *peripheral vasodilator; antihyperlipidemic* [niacin; multiple vitamins] 300• ± mg

Liponol capsules OTC *dietary lipotropic with vitamin supplementation* [choline; inositol; methionine; multiple B vitamins] 115•83•110• ± mg

lipopeptides [see: cyclic lipopeptides]

Lipo-PGE1 *vasodilator; platelet aggregation inhibitor; investigational (orphan) for ischemic ulcerations due to peripheral arterial disease* [alprostadil lipid emulsion]

lipoprotein-associated coagulation inhibitor (LACI) [see: tifacogin]

liposomal amphotericin B [see: amphotericin B lipid complex (ABLC)]

liposomal cyclosporin A [see: cyclosporine, liposomal]

liposomal gentamicin [see: gentamicin liposome]

liposomal nystatin [see: nystatin, liposomal]

liposomal prostaglandin E1 [see: alprostadil lipid emulsion]

liposome-encapsulated doxorubicin HCl (LED) [see: doxorubicin HCl, liposome-encapsulated]

liposome-encapsulated recombinant interleukin-2 [see: interleukin-2, liposome-encapsulated recombinant]

liposome-encapsulated T4 endonuclease V (T4N5) [see: T4 endonuclease V, liposome encapsulated]

Liposyn II 10%; Liposyn II 20%; Liposyn III 10%; Liposyn III 20%; Liposyn III 30% IV infusion ℞ *nutritional therapy* [fat emulsion]

Lipotriad caplets OTC *dietary lipotropic with vitamin supplementation* [choline; inositol; multiple vitamins] 111• ± • ± mg

lipotropics *a class of oral nutritional supplements*

Lipram 4500 delayed-release capsules containing enteric-coated microspheres ℞ *porcine-derived digestive enzymes* [lipase; protease; amylase] 4500•25 000•20 000 USP units ⑨ Librium

Lipram-CR5; Lipram-CR10; Lipram-CR20 delayed-release capsules containing enteric-coated microspheres ℞ *porcine-derived digestive enzymes* [lipase; protease; amylase] 5000•18 750•16 600 USP units; 10 000•37 500•33 200 USP units; 20 000•75 000•66 400 USP units

Lipram-PN10; Lipram-PN16; Lipram-PN20 delayed-release capsules containing enteric-coated microspheres ℞ *porcine-derived digestive enzymes* [lipase; protease; amylase] 10 000•30 000•30 000 USP units; 16 000•48 000•48 000 USP units; 20 000•44 000•56 000 USP units

Lipram-UL12; Lipram-UL18; Lipram-UL20 delayed-release capsules containing enteric-coated microspheres ℞ *porcine-derived digestive enzymes* [lipase; protease; amylase] 12 000•39 000•39 000 USP units; 18 000•58 500•58 500 USP units; 20 000•65 000•65 000 USP units

Li-Q-Nol *natural enzyme cofactor; investigational (orphan) for Huntington disease, pediatric CHF, and mitochon-*

drial cytopathies [coenzyme Q10 (as ubiquinol)]

Liquadd oral solution ℞ *CNS stimulant for attention-deficit/hyperactivity disorder (ADHD)* [dextroamphetamine sulfate] 5 mg/5 mL ☑ Locoid

liquefied phenol [see: phenol, liquefied]

Liquibid sustained-release tablet ℞ *expectorant* [guaifenesin] 400 mg

Liquibid 1200 sustained-release tablet (discontinued 2004) ℞ *expectorant* [guaifenesin] 1200 mg

Liquibid-D dual-release caplets ℞ *decongestant; expectorant* [phenylephrine HCl (extended release); guaifenesin (38% immediate release; 62% extended release)] 40•650 mg

Liquibid-D 1200 dual-release caplets ℞ *decongestant; expectorant* [phenylephrine HCl (25% immediate release; 75% extended release); guaifenesin (33% immediate release; 67% extended release)] 40•1200 mg

Liquibid-PD dual-release tablets ℞ *decongestant; expectorant* [phenylephrine HCl; guaifenesin] 20•315 mg (5•120 mg immediate release; 15• 195 mg extended release)

LiquiCaps; Liqui-caps (dosage form) *soft liquid-filled gelcaps*

Liquicet oral liquid ℞ *narcotic analgesic; antipyretic* [hydrocodone bitartrate; acetaminophen] 10•500 mg/15 mL

Liqui-Char oral liquid OTC *adsorbent antidote for poisoning* [activated charcoal] 12.5 g/60 mL, 15 g/75 mL, 25 g/120 mL, 30 g/120 mL, 50 g/240 mL

Liqui-Coat HD concentrated oral suspension ℞ *radiopaque contrast medium for gastrointestinal imaging* [barium sulfate] 210%

Liquicough DM oral liquid OTC *antitussive; decongestant; expectorant* [dextromethorphan hydrobromide; pseudoephedrine HCl; guaifenesin] 15•32•175 mg/5 mL

Liquid Caps (dosage form) *soft liquid-filled gelcaps*

liquid glucose [see: glucose, liquid]

liquid petrolatum [see: mineral oil]

Liquid Pred syrup (discontinued 2008) ℞ *corticosteroid; anti-inflammatory* [prednisone; alcohol 5%] 5 mg/5 mL

Liquid Tabs (dosage form) *liquid-filled tablets*

Liquidambar orientalis; L. styraciflua medicinal herb [see: storax]

Liqui-Doss emulsion OTC *emollient laxative* [mineral oil]

Liquifilm Tears; Liquifilm Forte eye drops OTC *moisturizer/lubricant* [polyvinyl alcohol] 1.4%; 3%

Liquifilm Wetting solution OTC *wetting solution for hard contact lenses*

Liqui-Gels; Liqui-gels (trademarked dosage form) *soft liquid-filled gelcaps*

Liquimat lotion OTC *antiseptic and keratolytic for acne* [sulfur] 4%

Liquiprin Drops for Children (discontinued 2008) OTC *analgesic; antipyretic* [acetaminophen] 80 mg/1.66 mL

Liquitab (trademarked dosage form) *chewable tablet*

LiquiVent investigational (Phase III, orphan) *treatment for acute respiratory distress syndrome (ARDS) in adults* [perflubron]

liquor carbonis detergens (LCD) [see: coal tar]

liraglutide *glucagon-like peptide-1 (GLP-1); investigational (NDA filed) for type 2 diabetes; investigational (Phase II) for weight loss*

liroldine INN

lisadimate USAN, INN *sunscreen*

lisdexamfetamine dimesylate *CNS stimulant; oral treatment for attention-deficit/hyperactivity disorder (ADHD)*

lisinopril USAN, INN, BAN *antihypertensive; angiotensin-converting enzyme (ACE) inhibitor; adjunctive treatment for congestive heart failure (CHF)* 2.5, 5, 10, 20, 30, 40 mg oral

lisinopril & hydrochlorothiazide *antihypertensive; angiotensin-converting enzyme (ACE) inhibitor; diuretic* 10•12.5, 20•12.5, 20•25 mg oral

lisofylline (LSF) USAN *acetyltransferase inhibitor; investigational (Phase III,* *orphan) immunomodulator and cytokine inhibitor for acute myeloid leukemia*

Listerine; Cool-Mint Listerine; FreshBurst Listerine; Natural Citrus Listerine; Tartar Control Listerine mouthwash/gargle OTC *analgesic; mild anesthetic; antipruritic; counterirritant; antiseptic* [methyl salicylate; eucalyptol; thymol; menthol; alcohol 22%–26%] 0.06%•0.09%•0.06%•0.04% ② Loestrin 21 1/20

Listerine Tooth Defense oral rinse OTC *dental caries preventative* [sodium fluoride; alcohol 21.6%] 0.0221% (0.01% fluoride)

Listermint Arctic Mint mouthwash/gargle OTC *oral antiseptic*

lisuride INN [also: lysuride]

lithium *element (Li); antipsychotic for manic episodes* 8 mEq/5 mL oral

lithium benzoate NF

lithium carbonate USAN, USP *antimanic; immunity booster in chemotherapy and AIDS* (150 mg=4 mEq lithium) 150, 300, 450, 600 mg oral

lithium citrate USP *antimanic; immunity booster in chemotherapy and AIDS* 300 mg/5 mL oral

lithium hydroxide USP *antimanic*

lithium hydroxide monohydrate [see: lithium hydroxide]

Lithium QD *investigational (Phase III) once-daily antipsychotic for manic episodes of a bipolar disorder* [lithium carbonate]

lithium salicylate NF

Lithobid slow-release tablets ℞ *antipsychotic for manic episodes* [lithium carbonate] 300 mg

litholytics *a class of agents that dissolve stones or calculi* [see also: antilithics]

Lithonate capsules ℞ *antipsychotic for manic episodes* [lithium carbonate] 300 mg

Lithostat tablets ℞ *adjunctive therapy in chronic urea-splitting urinary tract infections* [acetohydroxamic acid] 250 mg

Lithotabs film-coated tablets ℞ *antipsychotic for manic episodes* [lithium carbonate] 300 mg

litracen INN ② Lotrisone

Little Colds Cough Formula oral drops OTC *antitussive for children 2–3 years* [dextromethorphan hydrobromide] 7.5 mg/mL

Little Colds for Infants and Children oral drops OTC *nasal decongestant* [phenylephrine HCl] 0.25%

Little Noses Gentle Formula, Infants and Children nose drops OTC *nasal decongestant* [phenylephrine HCl] 0.125%

Little Tummys Laxative oral drops OTC *stimulant laxative* [sennosides] 8.8 mg/mL

liver, desiccated; liver extracts *source of vitamin B$_{12}$*

Liver Combo No. 5 IM injection (discontinued 2004) ℞ *hematinic; vitamin B supplement* [liver extracts; vitamin B$_{12}$; folic acid] 10 mcg•100 mcg•0.4 mg per mL

liver derivative complex *claimed to be an anti-inflammatory for various dermatological conditions*

liver lily *medicinal herb* [see: blue flag]

liverleaf; liverwort *medicinal herb* [see: hepatica]

Livial ⓔⓤⓡ (available in Europe, Asia, and South America) *investigational (NDA filed) synthetic steroid for osteoporosis and other postmenopausal symptoms* [tibolone]

lividomycin INN

Livitrinsic-f capsules ℞ *hematinic* [ferrous fumarate; cyanocobalamin; ascorbic acid; intrinsic factor concentrate; folic acid] 110 mg•15 mcg•75 mg•240 mg•0.5 mg

Livostin eye drop suspension (discontinued 2005) ℞ *antihistamine for allergic conjunctivitis* [levocabastine HCl] 0.05%

lixazinone sulfate USAN *cardiotonic; phosphodiesterase inhibitor*

lixivaptan USAN *selective vasopressin V$_2$–receptor antagonist for nonhypovolemic hyponatremia*

LKV Infant Drops powder + liquid
OTC *vitamin supplement* [multiple
vitamins; biotin] ±•75 mcg/0.6 mL
LLD factor [see: cyanocobalamin]
10% LMD IV injection ℞ *plasma volume expander for shock due to hemorrhage, burns, or surgery* [dextran 40]
10%
**LMD (low molecular weight dex-
tran)** [see: dextran 40]
**LMF (Leukeran, methotrexate, flu-
orouracil)** *chemotherapy protocol*
**LMWD (low molecular weight dex-
tran)** [see: dextran 40]
L·M·X4 cream OTC *anesthetic* [lido-
caine, liposome-encapsulated] 4%
L·M·X5 anorectal cream OTC *anesthetic* [lidocaine, liposome-encapsu-
lated] 5%
Lobac capsules ℞ *skeletal muscle relaxant; antihistamine; sleep aid; analgesic;
antipyretic* [salicylamide; phenyltoloxamine; acetaminophen] 200•20•
300 mg ⚇ LAPOCA
Lobana Body lotion OTC *moisturizer;
emollient*
**Lobana Body Shampoo; Lobana
Liquid Lather** topical liquid OTC
soap-free therapeutic skin cleanser
[chloroxylenol]
Lobana Derm-Ade cream OTC *moisturizer; emollient* [vitamins A, D, and E]
Lobana Peri-Garde ointment OTC
moisturizer; emollient; antiseptic [vita-
mins A, D, and E; chloroxylenol]
lobelia (Lobelia inflata) plant (tincture) *medicinal herb for arthritis,
asthma, bronchitis, hay fever, colds,
cough, ear infections, epilepsy, fever,
food poisoning, lockjaw, nervousness,
pain, pneumonia, preventing miscarriage, whooping cough, and worms*
lobeline INN *nicotine withdrawal aid*
[also: lobeline HCl]
lobeline HCl JAN *nicotine withdrawal
aid* [also: lobeline]
lobendazole USAN, INN *veterinary anthelmintic*
lobenzarit INN *antirheumatic* [also:
lobenzarit sodium]

lobenzarit sodium USAN *antirheumatic*
[also: lobenzarit]
lobradimil USAN *receptor-mediated per-
meability reducer; investigational (Phase III)
blood-brain barrier permeability-enhancing agent for carrying carboplatin to
brain tumors*
lobucavir USAN, INN *antiviral*
lobuprofen INN
LoCholest; LoCholest Light powder
for oral suspension (discontinued
2005) ℞ *cholesterol-lowering antihyperlipidemic; also used for biliary obstruction* [cholestyramine resin] 4 g/dose
locicortolone dicibate INN
locicortone [see: locicortolone dicibate]
Locoid cream, ointment, solution,
lotion ℞ *corticosteroidal anti-inflammatory* [hydrocortisone butyrate]
0.1% ⚇ Liquadd
Locoid Lipocream ℞ *corticosteroidal
anti-inflammatory* [hydrocortisone
butyrate (in an oil-in-water emulsion)] 0.1% (70% oil•30% water)
locust plant *medicinal herb* [see: senna]
lodaxaprine INN
lodazecar INN
lodelaben USAN, INN *antiarthritic;
emphysema therapy adjunct*
lodenosine USAN *reverse transcriptase
antiviral*
Lodine film-coated tablets, capsules
(discontinued 2006) ℞ *analgesic;
nonsteroidal anti-inflammatory drug
(NSAID) for osteoarthritis, rheumatoid
arthritis, juvenile rheumatoid arthritis,
and other chronic pain* [etodolac] 400,
500 mg; 200 mg
Lodine XL film-coated extended-
release tablets (discontinued 2006)
℞ *analgesic; nonsteroidal anti-inflammatory drug (NSAID) for osteoarthritis, rheumatoid arthritis, juvenile rheumatoid arthritis, and other chronic pain*
[etodolac] 400, 500, 600 mg
lodinixil INN
lodiperone INN
Lodosyn tablets ℞ *decarboxylase inhibitor; levodopa potentiator for Parkinson*

disease (no effect when given alone) [carbidopa] 25 mg

lodoxamide INN, BAN *antiallergic; antiasthmatic* [also: lodoxamide ethyl]

lodoxamide ethyl USAN *antiallergic; antiasthmatic* [also: lodoxamide]

lodoxamide trometamol BAN *antiallergic; antiasthmatic* [also: lodoxamide tromethamine]

lodoxamide tromethamine USAN *antiasthmatic; antiallergic for vernal keratoconjunctivitis (orphan)* [also: lodoxamide trometamol]

Lodrane oral liquid ℞ *decongestant; antihistamine* [pseudoephedrine HCl; brompheniramine maleate] 60•4 mg/5 mL

Lodrane 12 D; Lodrane 24 D sustained-release tablets ℞ *decongestant; antihistamine* [pseudoephedrine HCl; brompheniramine maleate] 45•6 mg; 90•12 mg

Lodrane 12 Hour extended-release tablets ℞ *antihistamine* [brompheniramine maleate] 6 mg

Lodrane 24 extended-release capsules ℞ *antihistamine* [brompheniramine maleate] 12 mg

Lodrane D oral suspension ℞ *decongestant; antihistamine* [pseudoephedrine tannate; brompheniramine tannate] 90•8 mg/5 mL

Lodrane LD sustained-release capsules (discontinued 2007) ℞ *decongestant; antihistamine* [pseudoephedrine HCl; brompheniramine maleate] 60•6 mg

Lodrane XR oral suspension ℞ *antihistamine* [brompheniramine tannate] 8 mg/5 mL

Loestrin 21 1/20; Loestrin 21 1.5/30 tablets (in packs of 21) ℞ *monophasic oral contraceptive* [norethindrone acetate; ethinyl estradiol] 1 mg•20 mcg; 1.5 mg•30 mcg ② Listerine

Loestrin 24 Fe tablets (in packs of 28) ℞ *monophasic oral contraceptive; iron supplement* [norethindrone acetate; ethinyl estradiol; ferrous fumarate] 1•0.02•75 mg × 24 days; 0•0•75 mg × 4 days

Loestrin Fe 1/20 tablets (in packs of 28) ℞ *monophasic oral contraceptive; iron supplement* [norethindrone acetate; ethinyl estradiol; ferrous fumarate] 1 mg•20 mcg•75 mg × 21 days; 0•0•75 mg × 7 days

Loestrin Fe 1.5/30 tablets (in packs of 28) ℞ *monophasic oral contraceptive; iron supplement* [norethindrone acetate; ethinyl estradiol; ferrous fumarate] 1.5 mg•30 mcg•75 mg × 21 days; 0•0•75 mg × 7 days

lofemizole INN *anti-inflammatory; analgesic; antipyretic* [also: lofemizole HCl] ② levamisole

lofemizole HCl USAN *anti-inflammatory; analgesic; antipyretic* [also: lofemizole] ② levamisole HCl

lofendazam INN, BAN

lofentanil INN, BAN *narcotic analgesic* [also: lofentanil oxalate]

lofentanil oxalate USAN *narcotic analgesic* [also: lofentanil]

lofepramine INN, BAN *antidepressant* [also: lofepramine HCl]

lofepramine HCl USAN *antidepressant* [also: lofepramine]

lofexidine INN, BAN *antihypertensive* [also: lofexidine HCl]

lofexidine HCl USAN *centrally acting alpha-2-adrenergic agonist for hypertension; investigational (Phase III) treatment for opiate withdrawal syndrome* [also: lofexidine]

Lofibra capsules, tablets ℞ *antihyperlipidemic for primary hypercholesterolemia, hypertriglyceridemia, and mixed dyslipidemia; also used for hyperuricemia* [fenofibrate] 67, 134, 200 mg; 54, 160 mg

loflucarban INN

Logen tablets ℞ *antidiarrheal* [diphenoxylate HCl; atropine sulfate] 2.5•0.025 mg ② Leukine

LoHist 12 Hour extended-release tablets ℞ *antihistamine* [brompheniramine tannate] 6 mg

LoHist 12D extended-release tablets ℞ *decongestant; antihistamine* [pseudoephedrine HCl; brompheniramine maleate] 45•6 mg

LoHist-LQ oral liquid ℞ *decongestant; antihistamine* [pseudoephedrine HCl; brompheniramine maleate] 60•4 mg/5 mL

LoHist-PD Pediatric oral drops ℞ *decongestant; antihistamine; for children 1–24 months* [pseudoephedrine HCl; brompheniramine maleate] 12.5•1 mg/mL

LoKara lotion ℞ *corticosteroidal anti-inflammatory* [desonide] 0.05%

LOMAC (leucovorin, Oncovin, methotrexate, Adriamycin, cyclophosphamide) *chemotherapy protocol*

Lomanate oral liquid ℞ *antidiarrheal* [diphenoxylate HCl; atropine sulfate] 2.5•0.025 mg/5 mL

lombazole INN, BAN

lomefloxacin USAN, INN, BAN *broad-spectrum fluoroquinolone antibiotic*

lomefloxacin HCl USAN *broad-spectrum fluoroquinolone antibiotic*

lomefloxacin mesylate USAN *antibacterial*

lometraline INN *antipsychotic; antiparkinsonian* [also: lometraline HCl]

lometraline HCl USAN *antipsychotic; antiparkinsonian* [also: lometraline]

lometrexol INN *antineoplastic* [also: lometrexol sodium]

lometrexol sodium USAN *antineoplastic* [also: lometrexol]

lomevactone INN

lomifylline INN

lomofungin USAN *antifungal*

Lomotil tablets, oral liquid ℞ *antidiarrheal* [diphenoxylate HCl; atropine sulfate] 2.5•0.025 mg; 2.5•0.025 mg/5 mL

lomustine USAN, INN, BAN *nitrosourea-type alkylating antineoplastic for brain tumors and Hodgkin disease*

lonafarnib *investigational (Phase III) antineoplastic for lung cancer*

Lonalac powder OTC *enteral nutritional therapy* [milk-based formula]

lonapalene USAN *antipsoriatic*

lonaprofen INN

lonazolac INN

lonidamine INN, BAN *investigational (Phase II) indazole-3-carboxylic acid for benign prostatic hyperplasia (BPH)*

Loniten tablets ℞ *antihypertensive; vasodilator* [minoxidil] 2.5, 10 mg

Lonox tablets ℞ *antidiarrheal* [diphenoxylate HCl; atropine sulfate] 2.5•0.025 mg

loop diuretics *a class of diuretic agents that inhibit the reabsorption of sodium and chloride*

Lo/Ovral tablets (in Pilpaks of 21 or 28) ℞ *monophasic oral contraceptive; emergency postcoital contraceptive* [norgestrel; ethinyl estradiol] 0.3 mg•30 mcg

loperamide INN, BAN *antiperistaltic; antidiarrheal* [also: loperamide HCl]

loperamide HCl USAN, USP, JAN *antiperistaltic; antidiarrheal* [also: loperamide] 2 mg oral; 1 mg/5 mL oral

loperamide oxide INN, BAN *antiperistaltic; antidiarrheal*

Lophophora williamsii *a flowering Mexican cactus whose heads (mescal buttons) are used to produce mescaline, a hallucinogenic street drug*

Lopid film-coated tablets ℞ *triglyceride-lowering antihyperlipidemic for hypertriglyceridemia (types IV and V hyperlipidemia) and coronary heart disease* [gemfibrozil] 600 mg (300 mg capsules available in Canada)

lopinavir USAN *antiviral protease inhibitor for HIV infection*

lopirazepam INN

loprazolam INN, BAN

lopremone [now: protirelin]

Lopressor tablets, IV injection ℞ *antianginal; antihypertensive; β-blocker* [metoprolol tartrate] 50, 100 mg; 1 mg/mL

Lopressor HCT 50/25; Lopressor HCT 100/25; Lopressor HCT 100/50 tablets ℞ *antihypertensive; β-blocker; diuretic* [metoprolol tartrate; hydrochlorothiazide] 50•25 mg; 100•25 mg; 100•50 mg

loprodiol INN

Loprox cream, gel, topical suspension, shampoo ℞ *antifungal for tinea pedis, tinea cruris, tinea corporis, tinea versicolor, candidiasis, and seborrheic dermatitis* [ciclopirox] 0.77% ⚲ Librax

Lorabid Pulvules (capsules), powder for oral suspension (discontinued 2007) ℞ *second-generation cephalosporin antibiotic* [loracarbef] 200, 400 mg; 100, 200 mg/5 mL

loracarbef USAN, INN *second-generation cephalosporin antibiotic*

lorajmine INN *antiarrhythmic* [also: lorajmine HCl]

lorajmine HCl USAN *antiarrhythmic* [also: lorajmine]

Loramyc ⓔᵁᴿ buccal tablet (available in France) *investigational (Phase III) antifungal for oropharyngeal candidiasis* [miconazole]

lorapride INN

loratadine USAN, INN, BAN *second-generation peripherally selective piperidine antihistamine for allergic rhinitis; also used for chronic idiopathic urticaria* 10 mg oral; 5 mg/5 mL oral

lorazepam USAN, USP, INN, BAN *benzodiazepine anxiolytic; preanesthetic sedative; anticonvulsant* 0.5, 1, 2 mg oral; 2, 4 mg/mL injection

Lorazepam Intensol oral drops ℞ *benzodiazepine anxiolytic; sedative; anticonvulsant* [lorazepam] 2 mg/mL

lorbamate USAN, INN *muscle relaxant*

lorcainide INN, BAN *antiarrhythmic* [also: lorcainide HCl]

lorcainide HCl USAN *antiarrhythmic* [also: lorcainide]

lorcaserin HCl *investigational (Phase III) 5-HT$_{2c}$ serotonin receptor agonist for the treatment of obesity*

Lorcet Plus; Lorcet 10/650 tablets ℞ *narcotic analgesic; antipyretic* [hydrocodone bitartrate; acetaminophen] 7.5•650 mg; 10•650 mg

Lorcet-HD capsules ℞ *narcotic analgesic; antipyretic* [hydrocodone bitartrate; acetaminophen] 5•500 mg

lorcinadol USAN, INN, BAN *analgesic*

loreclezole USAN, INN, BAN *antiepileptic*

Lorenzo oil (erucic acid and oleic acid) *natural treatment for childhood adrenoleukodystrophy and adrenomyeloneuropathy in adults*

lorglumide INN

lormetazepam USAN, INN, BAN *sedative; hypnotic*

lornoxicam USAN, INN, BAN *analgesic; anti-inflammatory*

Lorothidol (available only from the Centers for Disease Control) ℞ *anti-infective for paragonimiasis and fascioliasis* [bithionol]

lorpiprazole INN

Lortab elixir ℞ *narcotic analgesic; antipyretic* [hydrocodone bitartrate; acetaminophen] 2.5•167 mg/5 mL

Lortab 2.5/500; Lortab 5/500; Lortab 7.5/500; Lortab 10/500 tablets ℞ *narcotic analgesic; antipyretic* [hydrocodone bitartrate; acetaminophen] 2.5•500 mg; 5•500 mg; 7.5•500 mg; 10•500 mg

Lortab ASA tablets ℞ *narcotic analgesic; antipyretic* [hydrocodone bitartrate; aspirin] 5•500 mg

lortalamine USAN, INN *antidepressant*

Lortuss DM oral liquid OTC *antitussive; antihistamine; decongestant* [dextromethorphan hydrobromide; brompheniramine maleate; phenylephrine HCl] 15•2•7.5 mg/5 mL

Lortuss HC oral liquid ℞ *narcotic antitussive; decongestant* [hydrocodone bitartrate; phenylephrine HCl] 3.75•7.5 mg/5 mL

lorzafone USAN, INN *minor tranquilizer*

losartan INN *antihypertensive; angiotensin II receptor antagonist; treatment to delay the progression of diabetic nephropathy* [also: losartan potassium]

losartan potassium USAN *angiotensin II receptor antagonist for hypertension; treatment to delay the progression of diabetic nephropathy* [also: losartan] 25, 50, 100 mg oral

losigamone INN

losindole INN

losmiprofen INN

losoxantrone INN *antineoplastic* [also: losoxantrone HCl]

losoxantrone HCl USAN *antineoplastic* [also: losoxantrone]

losulazine INN *antihypertensive* [also: losulazine HCl]

losulazine HCl USAN *antihypertensive* [also: losulazine]

Lotemax eye drop suspension ℞ *corticosteroidal anti-inflammatory* [loteprednol etabonate] 0.5%

Lotensin tablets ℞ *antihypertensive; angiotensin-converting enzyme (ACE) inhibitor; also used for nondiabetic neuropathy* [benazepril HCl] 5, 10, 20, 40 mg

Lotensin HCT 5/6.25; Lotensin HCT 10/12.5; Lotensin HCT 20/12.5; Lotensin HCT 20/25 tablets ℞ *antihypertensive; angiotensin-converting enzyme (ACE) inhibitor; diuretic* [benazepril HCl; hydrochlorothiazide] 5•6.25 mg; 10•12.5 mg; 20•12.5 mg; 20•25 mg

loteprednol INN *corticosteroidal anti-inflammatory* [also: loteprednol etabonate]

loteprednol etabonate USAN *topical ophthalmic corticosteroidal anti-inflammatory* [also: loteprednol]

lotifazole INN

lotrafiban HCl USAN *platelet aggregation inhibitor; GP IIb/IIIa receptor antagonist*

Lotrel capsules ℞ *antihypertensive; angiotensin-converting enzyme (ACE) inhibitor; calcium channel blocker* [amlodipine besylate; benazepril HCl] 2.5•10, 5•10, 5•20, 5•40, 10•20, 10•40 mg

lotrifen INN

Lotrimin AF cream, topical solution, lotion OTC *antifungal* [clotrimazole] 1%

Lotrimin AF powder, spray powder, spray liquid OTC *antifungal for tinea pedis, tinea cruris, and tinea corporis* [miconazole nitrate] 2%

Lotrimin Ultra cream OTC *benzylamine antifungal* [butenafine HCl] 1%

Lotrisone cream, lotion ℞ *corticosteroidal anti-inflammatory; antifungal* [betamethasone dipropionate; clotrimazole] 0.05%•1% ⑨ litracen

Lotronex film-coated tablets ℞ *serotonin 5-HT₃ receptor antagonist for diarrhea-predominant irritable bowel syndrome (IBS) in women* [alosetron HCl] 0.562, 1.124 mg (0.5, 1 mg base)

lotucaine INN

lousewort *medicinal herb* [see: betony; feverweed]

lovage (Angelica levisticum; Levisticum officinale) leaves and roots *medicinal herb for bad breath, boils, edema, flatulence, and sore throat; also used topically as a skin emollient*

Lovasa capsules OTC *dietary supplement* [eicosapentaenoic acid (EPA); docosahexaenoic acid (DHA)] 465•375 mg

lovastatin USAN, INN, BAN *HMG-CoA reductase inhibitor for hypercholesterolemia, hyperlipidemia, atherosclerosis, and the prevention and treatment of coronary heart disease (CHD)* 10, 20, 40 mg oral

Lovaza gelcaps ℞ *adjunct to diet restriction for hypertriglyceridemia; investigational (orphan) for immunoglobulin A nephropathy* [omega-3 acid ethyl esters (source of eicosapentaenoic acid and docosahexanoic acid); vitamin E] 1000•4 mg (465 mg EPA; 375 mg DHA)

Lovenox deep subcu injection, prefilled syringes ℞ *anticoagulant/antithrombotic for prevention of deep vein thrombosis (DVT) following knee, hip, or abdominal surgery, unstable angina, and myocardial infarction* [enoxaparin sodium] 100 mg/mL; 30, 40, 60, 80, 100, 120, 150 mg

loviride USAN, INN *non-nucleoside reverse transcriptase inhibitor (NNRTI) antiviral*

low molecular weight dextran (LMD; LMWD) [see: dextran 40]

low molecular weight heparins *a class of anticoagulants used for the prophylaxis or treatment of thromboembolic* *complications of surgery and ischemic complications of unstable angina or myocardial infarction*

low osmolar contrast media (LOCM) *a class of newer radiopaque agents that have a low osmolar concentration of iodine (the contrast agent), which corresponds to a lower incidence of adverse reactions* [also called: nonionic contrast media]

Lowila Cake bar OTC *soap-free therapeutic skin cleanser*

Low-Ogestrel tablets (in packs of 28) ℞ *monophasic oral contraceptive; emergency postcoital contraceptive* [norgestrel; ethinyl estradiol] 0.3 mg•30 mcg × 21 days; counters × 7 days

Lowsium Plus oral suspension OTC *antacid; antiflatulent* [magaldrate; simethicone] 540•40 mg/5 mL

loxanast INN

loxapine USAN, INN, BAN *minor tranquilizer; conventional (typical) dibenzoxazepine antipsychotic for schizophrenia*

loxapine HCl *minor tranquilizer; conventional (typical) dibenzoxazepine antipsychotic for schizophrenia*

loxapine succinate USAN *minor tranquilizer; conventional (typical) dibenzoxazepine antipsychotic for schizophrenia* (base=73.4%) 5, 10, 25, 50 mg oral (as base)

loxiglumide INN

Loxitane capsules ℞ *conventional (typical) dibenzoxazepine antipsychotic for schizophrenia* [loxapine succinate] 6.8, 13.6, 34, 68.1 mg (5, 10, 25, 50 mg base)

loxoprofen INN

loxoribine USAN, INN *immunostimulant; vaccine adjuvant; investigational (orphan) for common variable immunodeficiency*

loxotidine [now: lavoltidine succinate]

loxtidine BAN *antiulcerative; histamine H_2-receptor blocker* [also: lavoltidine succinate; lavoltidine]

lozilurea INN

Lozi-Tabs (trademarked dosage form) *lozenges*

Lozol film-coated tablets ℞ *antihypertensive; diuretic* [indapamide] 1.25, 2.5 mg

L-PAM (L-phenylalanine mustard) [see: melphalan]

LR (lactated Ringer) solution [see: Ringer injection, lactated]

LSD (lysergic acid diethylamide) *hallucinogenic street drug associated with disorders of sensory and temporal perception, depersonalization, and ataxia* [medically known as lysergide]

LSF (lisofylline) [q.v.]

LTA 360 Kit topical solution ℞ *anesthetic* [lidocaine HCl] 4%

LTRAs (leukotriene receptor antagonists) *a class of antiasthmatics* ⧉ Letairis

Lu texaphyrin [see: motexafin lutetium]

lubeluzole USAN, INN *neuroprotector*

lubiprostone *selective chloride channel activator to increase fluid secretion in the small intestine for the treatment of chronic idiopathic constipation in adults and irritable bowel syndrome (IBS) in women*

Lubricating Jelly OTC *vaginal moisturizer/lubricant* [glycerin; propylene glycol]

Lubricoat (trademarked ingredient) *surgical aid* [ferric hyaluronate]

Lubriderm cream, lotion (discontinued 2004) OTC *moisturizer; emollient*

Lubriderm Bath Oil (discontinued 2004) OTC *bath emollient*

Lubriderm Daily Moisture with SPF 15 lotion OTC *moisturizer; emollient; sunscreen* [octinoxate; octisalate; oxybenzone] 7.5%•4%•3%

Lubriderm Skin Nourishing with Sea Kelp Extract lotion OTC *moisturizer; emollient*

LubriFresh P.M. ophthalmic ointment OTC *ocular moisturizer/lubricant* [white petrolatum; mineral oil] 83%•15%

Lubrin vaginal inserts OTC *lubricant for sexual intercourse* [glycerin; caprylic triglyceride] ⧉ Lupron

Lubriskin lotion OTC *moisturizer; emollient*

LubriTears eye drops OTC *moisturizer/lubricant* [hydroxypropyl methylcellulose] 0.3%

LubriTears ophthalmic ointment OTC *ocular moisturizer/lubricant* [white petrolatum; mineral oil; lanolin]

lucanthone INN, BAN *antischistosomal* [also: lucanthone HCl]

lucanthone HCl USAN, USP *antischistosomal* [also: lucanthone]

lucartamide INN

Lucassin *investigational (NDA filed, orphan) hormone to improve renal function in patients with hepatorenal syndrome (HRS)* [terlipressin]

lucensomycin [see: lucimycin]

Lucentis ophthalmic intravitreal injection *vascular endothelial growth factor (VEGF-A) inhibitor for neovascular (wet) age-related macular degeneration (AMD)* [ranibizumab] 10 mg/mL (0.5 mg/dose)

Lucidex enteric-coated tablets OTC *CNS stimulant; analeptic* [caffeine] 100 mg

Lucilia caesar natural treatment [see: maggots]

lucimycin INN

lucinactant *investigational (Phase II/III, orphan) for respiratory distress syndrome in adults and premature infants and meconium aspiration in newborn infants* [also: KL4 surfactant]

Luer-lock (trademarked delivery form) *prefilled self-injection syringe*

lufironil USAN, INN *collagen inhibitor*

lufuradom INN

Lufyllin elixir, IM injection (discontinued 2005) Ṝ *antiasthmatic; bronchodilator* [dyphylline] 100 mg/15 mL; 250 mg/mL ⊕ Levlen

Lufyllin tablets Ṝ *antiasthmatic; bronchodilator* [dyphylline] 200 mg ⊕ Levlen

Lufyllin 400 tablets Ṝ *antiasthmatic; bronchodilator* [dyphylline] 400 mg ⊕ Levlen

Lufyllin-EPG tablets, elixir (discontinued 2007) Ṝ *antiasthmatic; bronchodilator; decongestant; expectorant; sedative* [dyphylline; ephedrine HCl; guaifenesin; phenobarbital] 100•16•200•16 mg; 150•24•300•24 mg/15 mL

Lufyllin-GG elixir Ṝ *antiasthmatic; bronchodilator; expectorant* [dyphylline; guaifenesin] 100•100 mg/15 mL

Lufyllin-GG tablets (discontinued 2007) Ṝ *antiasthmatic; bronchodilator; expectorant* [dyphylline; guaifenesin] 200•200 mg

Lugol solution Ṝ *thyroid-blocking therapy* [iodine; potassium iodide] 5%•10%

Lumenax (name changed to **Xifaxan** upon marketing release in 2004)

Lumigan eye drops Ṝ *synthetic prostamide analogue for glaucoma and ocular hypertension* [bimatoprost] 0.03%

Luminal Sodium IV or IM injection Ṝ *long-acting barbiturate sedative, hypnotic, and anticonvulsant; also abused as a street drug* [phenobarbital sodium; alcohol 10%] 60, 130 mg/mL

lumiracoxib *investigational (Phase III) antiarthritic for osteoarthritis; analgesic for acute pain; COX-2 inhibitor; nonsteroidal anti-inflammatory drug (NSAID)*

Lumirem ⓔ (European name for U.S. product **GastroMARK**)

Lunelle IM injection Ṝ *once-monthly injectable contraceptive* [estradiol cypionate; medroxyprogesterone acetate] 5•25 mg/0.5 mL

Lunesta film-coated tablets Ṝ *nonbarbiturate sedative and hypnotic for chronic insomnia* [eszopiclone] 1, 2, 3 mg

lung surfactant, synthetic [see: colfosceril palmitate]

lungwort (*Pulmonaria officinalis*) flowering plant *medicinal herb used as an astringent, demulcent, emollient, expectorant, and pectoral* ⊕ Lanacort

Lunivia ⓔ (European name for U.S. product **Lunesta**)

2,6-lupetidine [see: nanofin]

lupitidine INN *veterinary antagonist to histamine H₂ receptors* [also: lupitidine HCl]

lupitidine HCl USAN *veterinary antagonist to histamine H₂ receptors* [also: lupitidine]

Lupron; Lupron Pediatric subcu injection (daily) ℞ *hormonal antineoplastic for prostatic cancer and central precocious puberty (orphan)* [leuprolide acetate] 5 mg/mL ② Lubrin

Lupron Depot microspheres for IM injection (monthly) ℞ *hormonal antineoplastic for prostatic cancer, endometriosis, and uterine fibroids* [leuprolide acetate] 3.75, 7.5 mg

Lupron Depot–3 month; Lupron Depot–4 month microspheres for IM injection ℞ *hormonal antineoplastic for prostatic cancer, endometriosis, and uterine fibroids* [leuprolide acetate] 11.5, 22.5 mg; 30 mg

Lupron Depot-Ped microspheres for IM injection (monthly) ℞ *hormonal antineoplastic for central precocious puberty (orphan)* [leuprolide acetate] 7.5, 11.25, 15 mg

luprostiol INN, BAN

Luride Lozi-Tabs (chewable tablets), drops, gel ℞ *dental caries preventative* [sodium fluoride] 0.25, 1.1, 2.2 mg; 1.1 mg/mL; 1.2%

Luride SF Lozi-Tabs (lozenges) ℞ *dental caries preventative* [sodium fluoride] 2.2 mg

lurosetron mesylate USAN *antiemetic*

lurtotecan dihydrochloride USAN *antineoplastic; topoisomerase I inhibitor*

Lusonal oral liquid (discontinued 2007) ℞ *nasal decongestant* [pseudoephedrine HCl] 15 mg/10 mL

Lustra; Lustra-AF cream ℞ *hyperpigmentation bleaching agent* [hydroquinone] 4%

lutein *natural carotenoid used to prevent and treat age-related macular degeneration (AMD), retinitis pigmentosa (RP), and other retinal dysfunction*

luteinizing hormone, recombinant human (rhLH) [see: lutropin alfa]

luteinizing hormone–releasing factor acetate hydrate [see: gonadorelin acetate]

luteinizing hormone–releasing factor diacetate tetrahydrate [now: gonadorelin acetate]

luteinizing hormone–releasing factor dihydrochloride [now: gonadorelin HCl]

luteinizing hormone–releasing factor HCl [see: gonadorelin HCl]

luteinizing hormone–releasing hormone (LH-RH) *an endogenous hormone, produced in the hypothalamus, which stimulates the release of luteinizing hormone (LH) and follicle-stimulating hormone (FSH) from the pituitary* [also known as: gonadotropin-releasing hormone (Gn-RH)]

Lutera tablets (in packs of 28) ℞ *monophasic oral contraceptive* [levonorgestrel; ethinyl estradiol] 0.1 mg• 20 mcg × 21 days; counters × 7 days

lutetium *element (Lu)*

lutetium texaphyrin [now: motexafin lutetium]

lutrelin INN *luteinizing hormone-releasing hormone (LHRH) agonist* [also: lutrelin acetate]

lutrelin acetate USAN *luteinizing hormone-releasing hormone (LHRH) agonist* [also: lutrelin]

Lutrepulse powder for continuous ambulatory infusion (discontinued 2007) ℞ *gonadotropin-releasing hormone for the induction of ovulation in women with hypothalamic amenorrhea (orphan)* [gonadorelin acetate] 0.8, 3.2 mg

lutropin alfa USAN *gonadotropin; recombinant human luteinizing hormone (rhLH) for the induction of ovulation in hypogonadal women (orphan)*

Luveris powder for subcu injection ℞ *gonadotropin; recombinant human luteinizing hormone (rhLH) for the induction of ovulation in hypogonadal women (orphan)* [lutropin alfa] 75 IU/dose

Luvox film-coated tablets ℞ *selective serotonin reuptake inhibitor (SSRI) for obsessive-compulsive disorder (OCD)* [fluvoxamine maleate] 25, 50, 100 mg

Luvox CR extended-release capsules ℞ *selective serotonin reuptake inhibitor (SSRI) for obsessive-compulsive disorder (OCD) and social anxiety disorder (SAD)* [fluvoxamine maleate] 100, 150 mg

luxabendazole INN, BAN

Luxiq foam ℞ *corticosteroidal anti-inflammatory for scalp dermatoses* [betamethasone valerate] 0.12%

L-VAM (leuprolide acetate, vinblastine, Adriamycin, mitomycin) *chemotherapy protocol*

lyapolate sodium USAN *anticoagulant* [also: sodium apolate]

Lybrel film-coated tablets ℞ *non-cyclic (continuous-use) oral contraceptive that completely eliminates menstrual cycles; investigational (Phase III) for premenstrual dysphoric disorder (PMDD)* [levonorgestrel; ethinyl estradiol] 0.9 mg•20 mcg

lycetamine USAN *topical antimicrobial*

lycine HCl [see: betaine HCl]

lycopene *natural substance found in high concentration in ripe tomatoes; a member of the carotene family; used as an antineoplastic and antioxidant*

Lycopodium clavatum *medicinal herb* [see: club moss]

Lycopus virginicus *medicinal herb* [see: bugleweed]

lydimycin USAN *antifungal* [also: lidimycin]

lymecycline INN, BAN

Lymphazurin 1% subcu injection ℞ *radiopaque contrast medium for lymphography* [isosulfan blue] 10 mg/mL (1%)

lymphoblastoid interferon alfa [see: interferon alfa, human lymphoblastoid]

LymphoCide *investigational (Phase III, orphan) monoclonal antibody for AIDS-related non-Hodgkin lymphoma* [epratuzumab, radiolabeled with yttrium Y 90]

lymphocyte immune globulin (LIG) *passive immunizing agent to prevent allograft rejection of renal transplants; treatment for aplastic anemia; investigational (orphan) for organ and bone marrow transplants* [also: antithymocyte globulin (aTG)]

lymphogranuloma venereum antigen USP

LymphoScan *monoclonal antibody IgG_{2a} to B cell, murine; investigational (Phase III, orphan) diagnostic aid for non-Hodgkin B-cell lymphoma, AIDS-related lymphomas, and other acute and chronic B-cell leukemias* [technetium Tc 99m bectumomab]

LymphoStat-B *investigational (Phase III) human monoclonal antibody to B-lymphocyte for active systemic lupus erythematosus (SLE)* [belimumab]

lynestrenol USAN, INN *progestin* [also: lynoestrenol]

lynoestrenol BAN *progestin* [also: lynestrenol]

Lyo-Ject (trademarked delivery form) *prefilled dual-chambered syringe with lyophilized powder and diluent*

Lypholized Vitamin B Complex & Vitamin C with B_{12} injection ℞ *parenteral vitamin therapy* [multiple B vitamins; vitamin C] ≛•50 mg/mL

Lypholyte; Lypholyte II IV admixture ℞ *intravenous electrolyte therapy* [combined electrolyte solution] ⑨ Levlite

lypressin USAN, USP, INN, BAN *posterior pituitary hormone; antidiuretic; vasoconstrictor*

Lyrica capsules ℞ *anticonvulsant; agent for the management of neuropathic pain from diabetic peripheral neuropathy (DPN), postherpetic neuralgia (PHN), and fibromyalgia; investigational (NDA filed) for generalized anxiety disorder (GAD)* [pregabalin] 25, 50, 75, 100, 150, 200, 225, 300 mg

lysergic acid diethylamide (LSD) *street drug* [see: LSD; lysergide]

lysergide INN, BAN

lysine (L-lysine) USAN, INN *essential amino acid; symbols: Lys, K; natural remedy for the prophylaxis and treatment of recurrent oral and genital herpes simplex outbreaks; inhibits HSV replication* 312, 500, 1000 mg oral ⊡ Lessina; leucine
lysine acetate USP *amino acid*
DL-lysine acetylsalicylate [see: aspirin DL-lysine]
lysine HCl USAN, USP *amino acid*
L-lysine monoacetate [see: lysine acetate]

L-lysine monohydrochloride [see: lysine HCl]
8-L-lysine vasopressin [see: lypressin]
Lysodase *investigational (orphan) chronic enzyme replacement therapy for Gaucher disease* [PEG-glucocerebrosidase]
Lysodren tablets ℞ *antibiotic antineoplastic for inoperable adrenal cortical carcinoma and Cushing syndrome* [mitotane] 500 mg
lysostaphin USAN *antibacterial enzyme*
lysuride BAN [also: lisuride]

M-CSF (macrophage colony-stimulating factor) [now: cilmostim]
M-2 protocol (vincristine, carmustine, cyclophosphamide, prednisone, melphalan) *chemotherapy protocol for multiple myeloma*
MAA (macroaggregated albumin) [see: albumin, aggregated]
Maalox oral suspension OTC *antacid* [aluminum hydroxide; magnesium hydroxide] 225•200 mg/5 mL
Maalox; Maalox Multi-Symptom oral liquid OTC *antacid; antiflatulent* [aluminum hydroxide; magnesium hydroxide; simethicone] 200•200•20 mg; 400•400•40 mg
Maalox Antacid/Calcium Supplement chewable tablets OTC *antacid; calcium supplement* [calcium carbonate] 600 mg
Maalox Anti-Gas chewable tablets OTC *antiflatulent* [simethicone] 80 mg
Maalox Anti-Gas, Extra Strength oral suspension OTC *antacid; antiflatulent* [aluminum hydroxide; magnesium hydroxide; simethicone] 500•450•40 mg/5 mL
Maalox Children's chewable tablets OTC *antacid* [calcium carbonate] 400 mg

Maalox Max chewable tablets OTC *antacid; antiflatulent; calcium supplement* [calcium carbonate; simethicone; calcium] 1000•60•400 mg
Maalox Plus Antacid Junior chewable tablets OTC *antacid; antiflatulent* [calcium carbonate; simethicone] 400•24 mg
Maalox Quick Dissolve chewable tablets OTC *antacid; calcium supplement* [calcium carbonate] 600, 1000 mg
Maalox TC oral suspension OTC *antacid* [aluminum hydroxide; magnesium hydroxide] 600•300 mg/5 mL
Maalox Total Stomach Relief oral suspension OTC *antidiarrheal; antinauseant* [bismuth subsalicylate] 525 mg/15 mL
MAb; MAB (monoclonal antibodies) [q.v.]
MABOP (Mustargen, Adriamycin, bleomycin, Oncovin, prednisone) *chemotherapy protocol* ⊡ Māpap; MOBP; MOP-BAP
MabThera (EUR) (European name for the U.S. product **Rituxan**)
mabuterol INN
MAC (methotrexate, actinomycin D, chlorambucil) *chemotherapy protocol*

MAC; MAC III (methotrexate, acti-nomycin D, cyclophosphamide) *chemotherapy protocol for gestational trophoblastic neoplasm*

MAC (mitomycin, Adriamycin, cyclophosphamide) *chemotherapy protocol*

maca (Lepidium meyenii) *root medicinal herb used as an adaptogen, aphrodisiac in males, fertility aid in females, and to relieve stress*

MACC (methotrexate, Adriamycin, cyclophosphamide, CCNU) *chemotherapy protocol for non–small cell lung cancer (NSCLC)*

mace (Myristica fragrans) *dried nutmeg aril (the fleshy network surrounding the seed) medicinal herb* [see: nutmeg]

MACHO (methotrexate, asparaginase, cyclophosphamide, hydroxydaunomycin, Oncovin) *chemotherapy protocol*

MACOP-B (methotrexate, Adriamycin, cyclophosphamide, Oncovin, prednisone, bleomycin) *chemotherapy protocol for non-Hodgkin lymphoma* ☑ MCP; Mega-B

macroaggregated albumin (MAA) [see: albumin, aggregated]

macroaggregated iodinated (^{131}I) human albumin [see: macrosalb (^{131}I)]

Macrobid capsules ℞ *urinary antibiotic* [nitrofurantoin (macrocrystals); nitrofurantoin monohydrate] 25•75 mg

Macrodantin capsules ℞ *urinary antibiotic* [nitrofurantoin (macrocrystals)] 25, 50, 100 mg

Macrodex IV infusion ℞ *plasma volume expander for shock due to hemorrhage, burns, or surgery* [dextran 70] 6%

macrogol 4000 INN, BAN [also: polyethylene glycol 4000]

macrogol ester 2000 INN *surfactant* [also: polyoxyl 40 stearate]

macrogol ester 400 INN *surfactant* [also: polyoxyl 8 stearate]

macrolides *a class of antibiotics that are bacteriostatic or bactericidal, depending on drug concentration*

macrophage, incubated autologous *investigational (orphan) agent to improve motor and sensory outcome in spinal cord injury*

macrophage colony-stimulating factor (M-CSF) [now: cilmostim]

macrophage-targeted β-glucocerebrosidase [now: alglucerase]

macrosalb (^{131}I) INN, BAN

macrosalb (^{99m}Tc) INN, BAN [also: technetium (^{99m}Tc) labeled macro-aggregated human ...]

Macrotys actaeoides *medicinal herb* [see: black cohosh]

Macugen intravitreous injection in prefilled syringes ℞ *pegylated VEGF (vascular endothelial growth factor) antagonist for neovascular (wet) age-related macular degeneration (AMD); also used for diabetic macular edema* [pegaptanib sodium] 0.3 mg/dose ☑ Mycogen II

MAD (MeCCNU, Adriamycin) *chemotherapy protocol*

mad-dog weed; mad weed *medicinal herb* [see: skullcap]

MADDOC (mechlorethamine, Adriamycin, dacarbazine, DDP, Oncovin, cyclophosphamide) *chemotherapy protocol* ☑ Myadec

madnep; madness *medicinal herb* [see: masterwort]

maduramicin USAN, INN *anticoccidal*

mafenide USAN, INN, BAN *bacteriostatic; adjunct to burn therapy*

mafenide acetate USP *broad-spectrum bacteriostatic to prevent meshed autograft loss on second- and third-degree burns (orphan)*

mafenide HCl

mafilcon A USAN *hydrophilic contact lens material* ☑ mefloquine

mafoprazine INN

mafosfamide INN *investigational (orphan) for neoplastic meningitis*

Mag-200 tablets OTC *magnesium supplement* [magnesium oxide] 200 mg Mg

magaldrate USAN, USP, INN *antacid* 540 mg/5 mL oral

Magaldrate Plus oral suspension OTC *antacid; antiflatulent* [magaldrate; simethicone] 540•40 mg/5 mL

Magalox Plus chewable tablets OTC *antacid; antiflatulent* [aluminum hydroxide; magnesium hydroxide; simethicone] 200•200•25 mg

Magan tablets ℞ *analgesic; antirheumatic* [magnesium salicylate] 545 mg

Mag-Cal tablets OTC *dietary supplement* [calcium carbonate; vitamin D; multiple minerals] 416.7 mg•66.7 IU• ±

Mag-Cal Mega tablets OTC *mineral supplement* [magnesium; calcium] 800•400 mg

Mag-Caps capsules OTC *magnesium supplement* [magnesium oxide] 140 mg (85 mg Mg)

Mag-G tablets OTC *magnesium supplement* [magnesium gluconate dihydrate] 500 mg (27 mg Mg)

maggots *(Lucilia caesar; Phaenicia sericata; Pharmia regina) natural treatment for debriding necrotic tissue in abscesses, burns, cellulitis, gangrene, osteomyelitis, and ulcers*

magic mouthwash *a slang term for the combination of a local anesthetic plus one or more of the following: an antihistamine, a corticosteroid, an antifungal, an antibiotic—with or without an antacid used as a carrier*

Maginex enteric-coated tablets (discontinued 2004) OTC *magnesium supplement* [magnesium-L-aspartate HCl] 615 mg (61 mg Mg)

Maginex DS powder for oral liquid (discontinued 2004) OTC *magnesium supplement* [magnesium-L-aspartate HCl] 1230 mg (122 mg Mg)/pkt.

Magnacal ready-to-use oral liquid OTC *enteral nutritional therapy* [lactose-free formula] ⑨ Monocal

Magnacet caplets ℞ *narcotic analgesic; antipyretic* [oxycodone HCl; acetaminophen] 2.5•400, 5•400, 7.5•400, 10•400 mg ⑨ Menest

Magnaprin; Magnaprin Arthritis Strength Captabs film-coated tablets (discontinued 2007) OTC *analgesic; antipyretic; anti-inflammatory; antirheumatic* [aspirin (buffered with aluminum hydroxide, magnesium hydroxide, and calcium carbonate)] 325 mg ⑨ minaprine

MagneBind 200; MagneBind 300 tablets OTC *calcium/magnesium supplement that binds dietary phosphate* [magnesium carbonate; calcium carbonate] 200•400 mg; 300•250 mg

MagneBind 400 Rx tablets ℞ *calcium/magnesium supplement that binds dietary phosphate* [magnesium carbonate; calcium carbonate; folic acid] 400•200•1 mg

magnesia, milk of USP *antacid; saline laxative* [also: magnesium hydroxide] 400 mg/5 mL oral

magnesia magma [now: magnesia, milk of]

magnesium *element (Mg)*

magnesium aluminosilicate hydrate [see: almasilate]

magnesium aluminum silicate NF *suspending agent*

magnesium amino acid chelate *dietary magnesium supplement*

magnesium aspartate [see: potassium aspartate & magnesium aspartate]

magnesium carbonate USP *antacid; dietary magnesium supplement*

magnesium carbonate hydrate [see: magnesium carbonate]

magnesium chloride USP *electrolyte replenisher* 1.97 mEq/mL (20%) injection

magnesium chloride hexahydrate [see: magnesium chloride]

magnesium citrate USP *dietary magnesium supplement; saline laxative* 100 mg Mg oral; 1.75 g/30 mL oral

magnesium clofibrate INN

magnesium D-gluconate dihydrate [see: magnesium gluconate]

magnesium D-gluconate hydrate [see: magnesium gluconate]

magnesium EDTA (ethylene diamine tetraacetic acid) [see: edetate magnesium disodium]

magnesium gluconate USP *dietary magnesium supplement* 12.7 mg Mg oral

magnesium glycinate USAN

magnesium hydroxide USP *antacid; saline laxative* [also: magnesia, milk of]

magnesium hydroxycarbonate *anti-urolithic*

magnesium oxide USP *antacid; sorbent; magnesium supplement* (base= 60.3%) 400 mg (241.3 mg Mg) oral

magnesium phosphate USP *antacid*

magnesium phosphate pentahydrate [see: magnesium phosphate]

magnesium salicylate USP *analgesic; antipyretic; anti-inflammatory; antirheumatic*

magnesium salicylate tetrahydrate [see: magnesium salicylate]

magnesium silicate NF *tablet excipient*

magnesium silicate hydrate [see: magnesium trisilicate]

magnesium stearate NF *tablet and capsule lubricant*

magnesium sulfate USP, JAN *anticonvulsant used for eclampsia or pre-eclampsia; controls hypertension and convulsions due to acute nephritis in children; saline laxative; electrolyte replenisher; magnesium supplement; also used as a tocolytic for preterm labor* 4%, 8%, 12.5%, 50% (0.325, 0.65, 1, 4 mEq/mL) injection

magnesium sulfate heptahydrate [see: magnesium sulfate]

magnesium trisilicate USP *antacid*

magnesium-L-aspartate HCl *dietary magnesium supplement*

Magnevist IV injection ℞ *radiopaque contrast medium for imaging of the head and neck, and to enhance MRIs of the brain, spine, and other CNS tissue* [gadopentetate dimeglumine] 469 mg/mL

magnolia (Magnolia glauca) bark *medicinal herb used as an antiperiodic,* *aromatic, astringent, diaphoretic, febrifuge, stimulant, and tonic*

Magnox oral suspension OTC *antacid* [aluminum hydroxide; magnesium hydroxide] 225•200 mg/5 mL ⑨ Minox

Magonate tablets, oral liquid OTC *magnesium supplement* [magnesium gluconate dihydrate] 500 mg (27 mg Mg); 1 g (54 mg Mg)/5 mL

Magonate Natal pediatric oral drops OTC *magnesium supplement* [magnesium gluconate] 3.52 mg Mg/mL

Mag-Ox 400 tablets OTC *antacid; magnesium supplement* [magnesium oxide] 400 mg (241 mg Mg)

Magsal tablets (discontinued 2006) ℞ *analgesic; antipyretic; anti-inflammatory; antihistamine; sleep aid* [magnesium salicylate; phenyltoloxamine citrate] 600•25 mg ⑨ Mucosil-10

Mag-Tab SR sustained-release caplets OTC *magnesium supplement* [magnesium lactate dihydrate] 84 mg Mg

Magtrate tablets OTC *magnesium supplement* [magnesium gluconate] 500 mg (29 mg Mg)

mahogany birch; mountain mahogany *medicinal herb* [see: birch]

Mahonia aquifolium *medicinal herb* [see: Oregon grape]

ma-huang *medicinal herb* [see: ephedra]

MAID (mesna [rescue], Adriamycin, ifosfamide, dacarbazine) *chemotherapy protocol for soft tissue and bone sarcomas*

maitake mushrooms (Grifola frondosa) cap and stem *medicinal herb for cancer, diabetes, hypercholesterolemia, hypertension, obesity, and stimulation of the immune system*

maitansine INN *antineoplastic* [also: maytansine]

Maitec injection *investigational (orphan) agent for disseminated* Mycobacterium avium-intracellulare *infection* [gentamicin sulfate, liposomal]

Majorana hortensis *medicinal herb* [see: marjoram]

Major-Con chewable tablets OTC *anti-flatulent* [simethicone] 80 mg

Major-gesic tablets (discontinued 2007) OTC *antihistamine; sleep aid; analgesic; antipyretic* [phenyltolox-amine citrate; acetaminophen] 30•325 mg

malaleuca *medicinal herb* [see: tea tree oil]

Malarone; Malarone Pediatric film-coated tablets ℞ *malaria prophylaxis and treatment* [atovaquone; proguanil HCl (chloroguanide HCl)] 250•100 mg; 62.5•25 mg ⊡ Myleran

malathion USP, BAN *pediculicide for lice* ⊡ Miltown

maletamer INN *antiperistaltic* [also: malethamer]

malethamer USAN *antiperistaltic* [also: maletamer]

maleylsulfathiazole INN

malic acid NF *acidifying agent*

malidone [see: aloxidone]

Mallamint chewable tablets OTC *antacid* [calcium carbonate] 420 mg

Mallazine eye drops (discontinued 2006) OTC *decongestant; vasoconstric-tor* [tetrahydrozoline HCl] 0.05%

mallow (Malva rotundifolia; M. syl-vestris) plant *medicinal herb used as an astringent, demulcent, emollient, and expectorant*

mallow, marsh (Althaea officinalis) *medicinal herb* [see: marsh mallow]

malonal [see: barbital]

malotilate USAN, INN *liver disorder treatment* ⊡ Multilyte-20

Malpighia glabra; M. punicifolia *medicinal herb* [see: acerola]

Maltsupex coated tablets, powder, oral liquid OTC *bulk laxative* [barley malt soup extract] 750 mg; 8 g/scoop; 16 g/tbsp.

Malva rotundifolia; M. sylvestris *medicinal herb* [see: mallow]

Mammol ointment OTC *emollient for nipples of nursing mothers* [bismuth subnitrate] 40%

m-AMSA (acridinylamine methane-sulphon anisidide) [see: amsacrine]

Mandameth enteric-coated tablets ℞ *urinary antibiotic* [methenamine man-delate] 0.5, 1 g

Mandelamine film-coated tablets ℞ *urinary antibiotic* [methenamine man-delate] 0.5, 1 g

mandelic acid NF

mandrake (Mandragora officinarium; Podophyllum peltatum) root and resin *medicinal herb for cancer, condy-lomata, constipation, fever, indigestion, liver disorders, lower bowel disorders, warts, and worms; not generally regarded as safe and effective for chil-dren or pregnant women*

mangafodipir trisodium USAN *paren-teral radiopaque contrast agent to enhance MRIs of the liver*

manganese *element* (Mn)

manganese chloride USP *dietary man-ganese supplement* 0.1 mg/mL injection

manganese chloride tetrahydrate [see: manganese chloride]

manganese citrate *dietary manganese supplement (30% elemental manganese)*

manganese gluconate (manganese D-gluconate) USP *dietary manganese supplement*

manganese glycerophosphate NF

manganese hypophosphite NF

manganese phosphinate [see: man-ganese hypophosphite]

manganese sulfate USP *dietary man-ganese supplement* 0.1 mg/mL injection

manganese sulfate monohydrate [see: manganese sulfate]

mangofodipir trisodium *MRI contrast medium for liver imaging*

manidipine 6300 INN

manna sugar [see: mannitol]

mannite [see: mannitol]

mannitol (D-mannitol) USP *renal function test aid; antihypertensive; osmotic diuretic; urologic irrigant; investigational (orphan) mucolytic for bronchiectasis and cystic fibrosis* 10%, 15%, 20%, 25% injection

mannitol hexanitrate INN

mannityl nitrate [see: mannitol hexa-nitrate]

D-mannoheptulose *the active principle in avocado that suppresses excess insulin production by the pancreas; investigational treatment for obesity and type 2 diabetes* [also: avocado sugar extract]

mannomustine INN, BAN

mannopentaose phosphate sulfate *investigational (orphan) for high-risk, advanced melanoma*

mannosulfan INN

manozodil INN

Mantoux test [see: tuberculin]

MAO inhibitors (monoamine oxidase inhibitors) [q.v.]

Maolate tablets (discontinued 2007) ℞ *skeletal muscle relaxant* [chlorphenesin carbamate] 400 mg ⧆ Multi 75

Maox 420 tablets OTC *antacid* [magnesium oxide] 420 mg ⧆ Megace; M-oxy

MAP (mitomycin, Adriamycin, Platinol) *chemotherapy protocol*

Māpap tablets, caplets, capsules, rapid-release gelcaps OTC *analgesic; antipyretic* [acetaminophen] 325 mg; 500 mg; 500 mg; 500 mg ⧆ MABOP; MOBP; MOP-BAP

Māpap, Children's chewable tablets, elixir OTC *analgesic; antipyretic* [acetaminophen] 80 mg; 160 mg/5 mL

Māpap, Junior chewable tablets OTC *analgesic; antipyretic* [acetaminophen] 160 mg

Māpap Arthritis Pain extended-release tablets OTC *analgesic; antipyretic* [acetaminophen] 650 mg

Māpap Cold Formula Multi-Symptom tablets OTC *antitussive; decongestant; analgesic; antipyretic* [dextromethorphan hydrobromide; phenylephrine HCl; acetaminophen] 10•5•325 mg

Māpap Infant Drops OTC *analgesic; antipyretic* [acetaminophen] 100 mg/mL

Māpap Sinus geltabs OTC *decongestant; analgesic; antipyretic* [pseudoephedrine HCl; acetaminophen] 30•500 mg

Māpap Sinus Congestion and Pain caplets OTC *decongestant; analgesic; antipyretic* [phenylephrine HCl; acetaminophen] 5•325 mg

maple lungwort *medicinal herb* [see: lungwort]

maprotiline USAN, INN *tetracyclic antidepressant*

maprotiline HCl USP *tetracyclic antidepressant* 25, 50, 75 mg oral

Maranox tablets (discontinued 2008) OTC *analgesic; antipyretic* [acetaminophen] 325 mg

maraviroc *cellular chemokine receptor 5 (CCR5) inhibitor; twice-daily oral antiretroviral for early-stage HIV infections*

Marax tablets (discontinued 2007) ℞ *antiasthmatic; bronchodilator; decongestant* [theophylline; ephedrine sulfate] 130•25 mg

Marax-DF pediatric syrup (discontinued 2007) ℞ *antiasthmatic; bronchodilator; decongestant; antihistamine* [theophylline; ephedrine sulfate; hydroxyzine HCl] 97.5•18.75•7.5 mg/15 mL

Marblen tablets, oral liquid OTC *antacid* [calcium carbonate; magnesium carbonate] 520•400 mg; 540•400 mg/5 mL

Marcaine injection ℞ *local anesthetic* [bupivacaine HCl] 0.25%, 0.5%, 0.75%

Marcaine with Epinephrine injection ℞ *local anesthetic* [bupivacaine HCl; epinephrine] 0.25%•1:200 000, 0.5%•1:200 000, 0.75%•1:200 000

Marcof Expectorant syrup ℞ *narcotic antitussive; expectorant* [hydrocodone bitartrate; potassium guaiacolsulfonate] 5•350 mg/5 mL

mare's tail *medicinal herb* [see: fleabane; horseweed]

Marezine tablets OTC *antiemetic; anticholinergic; antihistamine; motion sickness preventative* [cyclizine HCl] 50 mg ⧆ morazone

Margesic capsules ℞ *barbiturate sedative; analgesic; antipyretic* [butalbital; acetaminophen; caffeine] 50•325•40 mg

Margesic H capsules ℞ *narcotic analgesic; antipyretic* [hydrocodone bitartrate; acetaminophen] 5•500 mg

maribavir USAN *investigational (Phase III) benzimidazole riboside antiviral for cytomegalovirus disease in stem cell transplants*

maridomycin INN

marigold (Calendula officinalis) florets *medicinal herb for bruises, cuts, dysmenorrhea, eye infections, fever, and skin diseases; not generally regarded as safe and effective*

marijuana; marihuana (Cannabis sativa) *euphoric/hallucinogenic street drug made from the dried leaves and flowering tops of the cannabis plant; medicinal herb for asthma, analgesia, leprosy, and loss of appetite; investigational (orphan) for HIV-wasting syndrome*

marimastat USAN *antineoplastic; matrix metalloproteinase (MMP) inhibitor*

Marine Lipid Concentrate softgels OTC *dietary supplement* [omega-3 fatty acids] 1200 mg

Marinol oil-filled gelcaps ℞ *antiemetic for chemotherapy; appetite stimulant for AIDS patients (orphan)* [dronabinol] 2.5, 5, 10 mg ◻ Moranyl

mariptiline INN

marjoram (Majorana hortensis; Origanum vulgare) plant *medicinal herb for abdominal cramps, colic, headache, indigestion, respiratory problems, and violent cough*

Marlin Salt System tablets OTC *rinsing/storage solution for soft contact lenses* [sodium chloride (normal saline solution)] 250 mg

Marlin Salt System II tablets OTC *rinsing/storage solution for soft contact lenses* [sodium chloride (normal saline solution)] 250 mg

Marmine IV or IM injection ℞ *antinauseant; antiemetic; antivertigo; motion sickness preventative* [dimenhydrinate] 50 mg/mL

Marmine tablets OTC *antinauseant; antiemetic; antivertigo; motion sickness preventative* [dimenhydrinate] 50 mg

Marnatal-F film-coated tablets ℞ *vitamin/mineral/calcium/iron supplement* [multiple vitamins & minerals; calcium; iron; folic acid] ≝•250•60•1 mg

Marogen *investigational (orphan) hematinic for anemia of end-stage renal disease* [epoetin beta]

maroxepin INN

Marplan tablets ℞ *monoamine oxidase (MAO) inhibitor for depression* [isocarboxazid] 10 mg

Marpres tablets (discontinued 2007) ℞ *antihypertensive; vasodilator; diuretic* [hydrochlorothiazide; reserpine; hydralazine HCl] 15•0.1•25 mg

Marrubium vulgare *medicinal herb* [see: horehound]

marsh clover; marsh trefoil *medicinal herb* [see: buckbean]

marsh mallow (Althaea officinalis) root *medicinal herb for asthma, boils, bronchial infections, cough, emphysema, infected wounds, kidney disorders, lung congestion, sore throat, and urinary bleeding*

Mar-Spas orally disintegrating caplets ℞ *GI antispasmodic; anticholinergic "drying agent" for allergic rhinitis* [L-hyoscyamine sulfate] 0.25 mg

MARstem *investigational (orphan) agent for myelodysplastic syndrome and neutropenia due to bone marrow transplantation* [angiotensin 1-7]

MART-1 adenoviral gene therapy *investigational (orphan) for metastatic malignant melanoma*

Marten-Tab caplets ℞ *barbiturate sedative; analgesic; antipyretic* [butalbital; acetaminophen] 50•325 mg

Marthritic tablets ℞ *analgesic; antipyretic; anti-inflammatory; antirheumatic* [salsalate] 750 mg

Masophen tablets, capsules OTC *analgesic; antipyretic* [acetaminophen] 325, 500 mg; 500 mg

masoprocol USAN, INN *antineoplastic for actinic keratoses (AK)*

Massé Breast cream OTC *moisturizer and emollient for nipples of nursing women*

Massengill Baking Soda Freshness vaginal solution OTC *cleanser and deodorizer; acidity modifier* [sodium bicarbonate]

Massengill Disposable Douche vaginal solution OTC *antiseptic/germicidal cleanser and deodorizer; acidity modifier* [cetylpyridinium chloride; lactic acid; sodium lactate]

Massengill Disposable Douche; Massengill Vinegar & Water Extra Mild vaginal solution OTC *acidity modifier; cleanser and deodorizer* [vinegar (acetic acid)]

Massengill Douche solution concentrate OTC *vaginal cleanser and deodorizer; acidity modifier* [lactic acid; sodium lactate; sodium bicarbonate]

Massengill Douche vaginal powder OTC *cleanser and deodorizer; analgesic; mild anesthetic; antipruritic; counterirritant* [methyl salicymate; ammonium alum; phenol; menthol; thymol]

Massengill Feminine Cleansing Wash topical liquid OTC *for external perivaginal cleansing*

Massengill Medicated towelettes OTC *corticosteroidal anti-inflammatory* [hydrocortisone] 0.5%

Massengill Medicated Douche with Cepticin; Massengill Medicated Disposable Douche with Cepticin vaginal solution OTC *antiseptic/germicidal cleanser and deodorizer* [povidone-iodine] 12%; 10%

Massengill Vinegar & Water Extra Cleansing with Puraclean vaginal solution OTC *antiseptic/germicidal cleanser and deodorizer; acidity modifier* [cetylpyridinium chloride; vinegar (acetic acid)]

mast cell stabilizers *a class of topical agents that inhibit the antigen-induced release of inflammatory mediators (e.g., various histamines and leukotrienes) from human mast cells; used on* nasal, ophthalmological, and gastrointestinal mucosa [also known as: mediator release inhibitors]

masterwort (*Heracleum lanatum*) root and seed *medicinal herb used as an antispasmodic, carminative, and stimulant*

Mastisol topical liquid OTC *adhesive for securing dressings, IV lines, etc. on the skin*

maté *medicinal herb* [see: yerba maté]

Matricaria chamomilla *medicinal herb* [see: chamomile]

matrix metalloproteinase (MMP) inhibitors *a class of investigational (orphan) agents to treat corneal ulcers*

Matulane capsules ℞ *antineoplastic for Hodgkin disease; investigational (orphan) for malignant glioma; also used for other lymphomas, melanoma, brain tumors, and lung cancer* [procarbazine HCl] 50 mg

Mavik tablets ℞ *antihypertensive; angiotensin-converting enzyme (ACE) inhibitor; treatment for congestive heart failure* [trandolapril] 1, 2, 4 mg 🔲 MVAC

maxacalcitol USAN *vitamin D_3 analogue*

MaxAdFVIII *investigational (orphan) for hemophilia A* [antihemophilic factor (FVIII)]

Maxair Autohaler (breath-activated metered-dose inhaler) ℞ *sympathomimetic bronchodilator for asthma and bronchospasm* [pirbuterol acetate] 0.2 mg/dose

Maxalt caplets ℞ *vascular serotonin 5-$HT_{1B/1D}$ receptor agonist for the acute treatment of migraine* [rizatriptan benzoate] 5, 10 mg

Maxalt-MLT orally disintegrating tablets ℞ *vascular serotonin 5-$HT_{1B/1D}$ receptor agonist for the acute treatment of migraine* [rizatriptan benzoate] 5, 10 mg

Maxamine *investigational (NDA filed, orphan) adjuvant to interleukin-2 for stage IV malignant melanoma and acute myeloid leukemia (AML); investigational (Phase II) for hepatitis C and renal cell carcinoma* [histamine dihydrochloride]

Maxaquin film-coated tablets ℞ *broad-spectrum fluoroquinolone antibiotic* [lomefloxacin HCl] 400 mg

MaxEPA soft capsules OTC *dietary supplement* [omega-3 fatty acids; multiple vitamins & minerals] 1000• ± mg

Maxibolin *an anabolic steroid abused as a street drug* [see: ethylestrenol]

Maxidex Drop-Tainers (eye drop/ear drop suspension) ℞ *corticosteroidal anti-inflammatory for corneal injury, ophthalmic inflammation, and otic inflammation* [dexamethasone sodium phosphate] 0.1%

Maxidone caplets ℞ *narcotic analgesic; antipyretic* [hydrocodone bitartrate; acetaminophen] 10•750 mg ☒ mixidine

Maxifed caplets ℞ *decongestant; expectorant* [pseudoephedrine HCl; guaifenesin] 60•400 mg

Maxifed DM; Maxifed DMX sustained-release caplets OTC *antitussive; decongestant; expectorant* [dextromethorphan hydrobromide; pseudoephedrine HCl; guaifenesin] 20•40•400 mg; 20•60•400 mg

Maxifed-G sustained-release caplets OTC *decongestant; expectorant* [pseudoephedrine HCl; guaifenesin] 60•580 mg

Maxiflor cream, ointment ℞ *corticosteroidal anti-inflammatory* [diflorasone diacetate] 0.05%

Maxiflu G tablets ℞ *antitussive; decongestant; expectorant; analgesic; antipyretic* [dextromethorphan hydrobromide; pseudoephedrine HCl; guaifenesin; acetaminophen] 30•60•600•500 mg

Maxilube vaginal jelly OTC *moisturizer/lubricant*

Maximum Blue Label; Maximum Green Label tablets OTC *vitamin/mineral supplement* [multiple vitamins & minerals; folic acid; biotin] ± • 130•50 mcg

Maximum D3 capsules OTC *vitamin supplement* [cholecalciferol (vitamin D₃)] 10 000 IU

Maximum Red Label tablets OTC *vitamin/mineral/iron supplement* [multiple vitamins & minerals; iron; folic acid; biotin] ± •3.3 mg•0.13 mg•50 mcg

"Maximum Strength" products [see under product name]

Maxiphen DM; Maxiphen-G DM extended-release caplets ℞ *antitussive; decongestant; expectorant* [dextromethorphan hydrobromide; phenylephrine HCl; guaifenesin] 20•10•400 mg; 30•20•1000 mg

Maxiphen-G extended-release caplets ℞ *decongestant; expectorant* [phenylephrine HCl; guaifenesin] 20•1000 mg

Maxipime powder for IV or IM injection ℞ *fourth-generation cephalosporin antibiotic* [cefepime HCl] 0.5, 1, 2 g

Maxitrol eye drop suspension, ophthalmic ointment ℞ *corticosteroidal anti-inflammatory; antibiotic* [dexamethasone; neomycin sulfate; polymyxin B sulfate] 0.1%•0.35%•10 000 U/mL; 0.1%•0.35%•10 000 U/g

Maxi-Tuss DM oral liquid (discontinued 2007) ℞ *antitussive; expectorant* [dextromethorphan hydrobromide; guaifenesin] 20•200 mg/5 mL

Maxi-Tuss HC oral liquid (discontinued 2007) ℞ *narcotic antitussive; antihistamine; decongestant* [hydrocodone bitartrate; chlorpheniramine maleate; phenylephrine HCl] 2.5•4•10 mg/5 mL

Maxi-Tuss HCG oral liquid ℞ *narcotic antitussive; expectorant* [hydrocodone bitartrate; guaifenesin] 6•200 mg/5 mL

Maxi-Tuss HCX oral liquid ℞ *narcotic antitussive; antihistamine; decongestant* [hydrocodone bitartrate; chlorpheniramine maleate; phenylephrine HCl] 6•2•12 mg/5 mL

Maxivate lotion (discontinued 2004) ℞ *corticosteroidal anti-inflammatory* [betamethasone dipropionate] 0.05%

Maxivate ointment, cream ℞ *cortico-steroidal anti-inflammatory* [betamethasone dipropionate] 0.05%

Maxi-Vite tablets OTC *vitamin/mineral/calcium/iron supplement* [multiple vitamins & minerals; calcium; iron; folic acid; biotin] ±•53.5•1.5•0.4•0.001 mg

Maxolon tablets ℞ *antiemetic for chemotherapy and postoperative nausea and vomiting; GI stimulant for diabetic gastroparesis and symptomatic gastroesophageal reflux; also used as a radiosensitizer and to stimulate lactation* [metoclopramide HCl] 10 mg

Maxovite sustained-release tablets OTC *vitamin/mineral supplement* [multiple vitamins & minerals; folic acid; biotin] ±•330•11.7 mcg

Maxzide tablets ℞ *antihypertensive; diuretic* [triamterene; hydrochlorothiazide] 37.5•25, 75•50 mg

May apple *medicinal herb* [see: mandrake]

May bells; May lily *medicinal herb* [see: lily of the valley]

May bush; May tree *medicinal herb* [see: hawthorn]

May lily *medicinal herb* [see: lily of the valley]

maytansine USAN *antineoplastic* [also: maitansine]

mazapertine succinate USAN *antipsychotic; dopamine receptor antagonist*

mazaticol INN

MAZE (*m*-AMSA, azacitidine, etoposide) *chemotherapy protocol*

mazindol USAN, USP, INN, BAN *anorexiant; CNS stimulant; investigational (orphan) treatment for Duchenne muscular dystrophy*

mazipredone INN

MB (methylene blue) [q.v.]

m-BACOD; M-BACOD (methotrexate, bleomycin, Adriamycin, cyclophosphamide, Oncovin, dexamethasone) *chemotherapy protocol for non-Hodgkin lymphoma* ("m" is 200 mg/m^2; "M" is 3 g/m^2)

m-BACOD reduced dose (methotrexate, bleomycin, Adriamycin, cyclophosphamide, Oncovin, dexamethasone) *chemotherapy protocol for HIV-associated non-Hodgkin lymphoma*

M-BACOS (methotrexate, bleomycin, Adriamycin, cyclophosphamide, Oncovin, Solu-Medrol) *chemotherapy protocol*

MBC (methotrexate, bleomycin, cisplatin) *chemotherapy protocol for head and neck cancer*

MBD (methotrexate, bleomycin, DDP) *chemotherapy protocol*

MBR (methylene blue, reduced) [see: methylene blue]

MC (mitoxantrone, cytarabine) *chemotherapy protocol for acute myelocytic leukemia (AML)*

M-Caps capsules ℞ *urinary acidifier to control ammonia production* [racemethionine] 200 mg

MCBP (melphalan, cyclophosphamide, BCNU, prednisone) *chemotherapy protocol*

MCC (mycobacterial cell wall complex) [see: urocidin]

MCH (microfibrillar collagen hemostat) [q.v.]

M-Clear Jr syrup (discontinued 2007) ℞ *narcotic antitussive; expectorant* [hydrocodone bitartrate; potassium guaiacolsulfonate] 2.5•175 mg/5 mL

M-Clear WC oral liquid ℞ *narcotic antitussive; expectorant* [codeine phosphate; guaifenesin] 6.3•100 mg/5 mL

MCP (melphalan, cyclophosphamide, prednisone) *chemotherapy protocol*

M-CSF (macrophage colony-stimulating factor) [now: cilmostim]

MCT oil OTC *dietary fat supplement* [medium chain triglycerides from coconut oil]

MCT (medium chain triglycerides) [q.v.]

MCV (methotrexate, cisplatin, vinblastine) *chemotherapy protocol*

MD-76 R injection ℞ *radiopaque contrast medium* [diatrizoate meglumine; diatrizoate sodium (48.7% total iodine)] 660•100 mg/mL (370 mg/mL)

MDA (methylenedioxyamphetamine) [see: MDMA, MDEA]

MDEA (3,4-methylenedioxyethamphetamine) *a hallucinogenic amphetamine derivative closely related to MDMA, abused as a street drug, which causes dependence* [see also: amphetamines; MDMA]

MD-Gastroview oral solution (discontinued 2005) ℞ *radiopaque contrast medium for gastrointestinal imaging* [diatrizoate meglumine; diatrizoate sodium (48.29% total iodine)] 660•100 mg/mL (367 mg/mL)

MDI (delivery device) *metered-dose inhaler*

MDMA (3,4-methylenedioxymethamphetamine) *widely abused hallucinogenic street drug that is chemically related to amphetamines and mescaline and causes dependence; investigational euphoric to counteract suicidal ideations and feelings of hopelessness in terminal cancer patients* [see also: amphetamines; mescaline; MDEA]

MDP (methylene diphosphonate) [now: medronate disodium]

MDX-240 *investigational (Phase II) virus-specific antibody for AIDS*

MEA (mercaptoethylamine) [see: mercaptamine]

meadow cabbage *medicinal herb* [see: skunk cabbage]

meadow sorrel *medicinal herb* [see: sorrel]

meadowsweet (Filipendula ulmaria) plant *medicinal herb used for ulcers and upper respiratory problems; also used as an astringent, diaphoretic, and diuretic*

mealberry *medicinal herb* [see: uva ursi]

mealy starwort *medicinal herb* [see: star grass]

measles immune globulin USP

measles virus vaccine, live USP *active immunizing agent for measles (rubeola)*

measles & rubella virus vaccine, live USP *active immunizing agent for measles (rubeola) and rubella*

measles, mumps, & rubella virus vaccine, live USP *active immunizing agent for measles (rubeola), mumps, and rubella*

measles, mumps, rubella, & varicella virus vaccine, live attenuated *active immunizing agent for measles (rubeola), mumps, rubella, and varicella*

Mebadin (available only from the Centers for Disease Control) ℞ *investigational anti-infective for amebiasis and amebic dysentery* [dehydroemetine]

meballymal [see: secobarbital]

mebamoxine [see: benmoxin]

mebanazine INN, BAN

Mebaral tablets ℞ *long-acting barbiturate sedative, hypnotic, and anticonvulsant* [mephobarbital] 32, 50, 100 mg

mebendazole USAN, USP, INN *anthelmintic for trichuriasis, enterobiasis, ascariasis, and uncinariasis* 100 mg oral

mebenoside INN

mebeverine INN *smooth muscle relaxant* [also: mebeverine HCl]

mebeverine HCl USAN *smooth muscle relaxant* [also: mebeverine]

mebezonium iodide INN, BAN

mebhydrolin INN, BAN

mebiquine INN

mebolazine INN

mebrofenin USAN, INN *hepatobiliary function test*

mebrophenhydramine HCl [see: embramine HCl]

mebubarbital [see: pentobarbital]

mebumal [see: pentobarbital]

mebutamate USAN, INN *antihypertensive*

mebutizide INN

mecamylamine INN *antiadrenergic; ganglionic blocker for severe hypertension* [also: mecamylamine HCl]

mecamylamine HCl USP *antiadrenergic; ganglionic blocker for severe hypertension; investigational (orphan) for Tourette syndrome* [also: mecamylamine]

mecamylamine HCl & nicotine
*investigational (Phase III) transdermal
patch for smoking cessation*

mecarbinate INN

mecarbine [see: mecarbinate]

mecasermin USAN, INN, BAN *recombinant human insulin-like growth factor-1
(rhIGF-1) for children with primary
IGF deficiency without concomitant
growth hormone (GH) deficiency;
investigational (NDA filed, orphan) for
amyotrophic lateral sclerosis; investigational (orphan) for postpoliomyelitis
syndrome*

**mecasermin & insulin-like growth
factor binding protein-3** *recombinant human insulin-like growth factor-1
(rhIGF-1) plus a binding protein; investigational (orphan) for severe burns*

mecasermin rinfabate *recombinant
human insulin-like growth factor-1
(rhIGF-1) for children with primary
IGF deficiency without concomitant
growth hormone (GH) deficiency;
investigational (orphan) for GH-insen-
sitivity syndrome and extreme insulin-
resistance syndromes*

**MeCCNU (methyl chloroethyl-
cyclohexyl-nitrosourea)** [see:
semustine]

mecetronium ethylsulfate USAN *antiseptic* [also: mecetronium etilsulfate]

mecetronium etilsulfate INN *antiseptic* [also: mecetronium ethylsulfate]

mechlorethamine HCl USP *nitrogen
mustard-type alkylating antineoplastic;
investigational (orphan) for mycosis
fungoides* [also: chlormethine; mustine; nitrogen mustard N-oxide HCl]

meciadanol INN

mecillinam INN, BAN *antibacterial*
[also: amdinocillin]

mecinarone INN

meclizine HCl USP *antiemetic; antihistamine; anticholinergic; motion sickness
relief* [also: meclozine] 12.5, 25, 50
mg oral

meclocycline USAN, INN, BAN *topical
antibiotic* ☒ meglucycline

meclocycline sulfosalicylate USAN,
USP *topical antibiotic*

meclofenamate sodium USAN, USP
*analgesic; antiarthritic; nonsteroidal
anti-inflammatory drug (NSAID) for
osteoarthritis, rheumatoid arthritis, primary dysmenorrhea, and other mild to
moderate pain* 50, 100 mg oral

meclofenamic acid USAN, INN *nonsteroidal anti-inflammatory drug (NSAID)*

meclofenoxate INN, BAN

meclonazepam INN

mecloqualone USAN, INN *sedative;
hypnotic*

mecloralurea INN

meclorisone INN, BAN *topical anti-
inflammatory* [also: meclorisone dibu-
tyrate]

meclorisone dibutyrate USAN *topical
anti-inflammatory* [also: meclorisone]

mecloxamine INN

meclozine INN, BAN *antiemetic; antihistamine; anticholinergic; motion sickness relief* [also: meclizine HCl] ☒
Miacalcin

mecobalamin USAN, INN *vitamin;
hematopoietic*

mecrilate INN *tissue adhesive* [also:
mecrylate]

mecrylate USAN *tissue adhesive* [also:
mecrilate]

**MECY (methotrexate, cyclophos-
phamide)** *chemotherapy protocol*

mecysteine INN

Meda Cap capsules (discontinued
2006) OTC *analgesic; antipyretic* [acet-
aminophen] 500 mg

Meda Tab tablets (discontinued 2006)
OTC *analgesic; antipyretic* [acetamino-
phen] 325 mg

Medacote lotion OTC *antihistamine;
astringent* [pyrilamine maleate; zinc
oxide] 1%• ² ☒ Modecate

Medalone 40; Medalone 80 [see:
depMedalone 40; depMedalone 80]

medazepam INN *minor tranquilizer*
[also: medazepam HCl]

medazepam HCl USAN *minor tranquilizer* [also: medazepam]

medazomide INN

medazonamide [see: medazomide]

Medebar Plus rectal suspension ℞ *radiopaque contrast medium for gastrointestinal imaging* [barium sulfate] 100%

Medent-DM sustained-release tablets ℞ *antitussive; decongestant; expectorant* [dextromethorphan hydrobromide; pseudoephedrine HCl; guaifenesin] 30•60•800 mg

Medent-PE extended-release tablets ℞ *decongestant; expectorant* [phenylephrine HCl; guaifenesin] 12.5•600 mg

Mederma gel OTC *moisturizer and emollient for scars* [PEG-4; onion extract; xanthan gum; allantoin]

Medescan oral suspension ℞ *radiopaque contrast medium for gastrointestinal imaging* [barium sulfate] 2.3%

medetomidine INN, BAN *veterinary analgesic; veterinary sedative* [also: medetomidine HCl]

medetomidine HCl USAN *veterinary analgesic; veterinary sedative* [also: medetomidine]

mediator release inhibitors *a class of topical agents that inhibit the antigen-induced release of inflammatory mediators (e.g., various histamines and leukotrienes) from human mast cells; used on nasal, ophthalmological, and gastrointestinal mucosa* [also known as: mast cell stabilizers]

medibazine INN

Medicago sativa *medicinal herb* [see: alfalfa]

medical air [see: air, medical]

Medicated Acne Cleanser OTC *antiseptic, antifungal, and keratolytic for acne* [colloidal sulfur; resorcinol] 4%•2%

Medicidin-D tablets OTC *decongestant; antihistamine; analgesic; antipyretic* [phenylephrine HCl; chlorpheniramine maleate; acetaminophen] 5•2•325 mg

medicinal zinc peroxide [see: zinc peroxide, medicinal]

Medicone anorectal ointment OTC *anesthetic* [benzocaine] 20% ⃰ Modicon

Medicone rectal suppositories (discontinued 2004) OTC *vasoconstrictor for hemorrhoids* [phenylephrine HCl] 0.25% ⃰ Modicon

Medi-First Sinus Decongestant tablets OTC *nasal decongestant* [pseudoephedrine HCl] 30 mg

medifoxamine INN

Medigesic capsules ℞ *barbiturate sedative; analgesic; antipyretic* [butalbital; acetaminophen; caffeine] 50•325•40 mg

medinal [see: barbital sodium]

Mediotic-HC ear drops ℞ *corticosteroidal anti-inflammatory; local anesthetic; antiseptic* [hydrocortisone; pramoxine HCl; chloroxylenol; benzalkonium chloride] 1%•1%•0.1%•0.01%

Mediplast plaster OTC *keratolytic* [salicylic acid] 40%

Mediplex Tabules (tablets) OTC *vitamin/mineral supplement* [multiple vitamins & minerals]

Mediplex Plus tablets OTC *vitamin/mineral supplement* [multiple vitamins & minerals; folic acid] ≐ •0.4 mg

Medi-Quik topical spray, topical aerosol spray OTC *anesthetic; antiseptic* [lidocaine; benzalkonium chloride] 2%•0.13%

medium chain triglycerides (MCT) *dietary lipid supplement*

medorinone USAN, INN *cardiotonic*

medorubicin INN

Medotar ointment OTC *antipsoriatic; antiseborrheic; astringent; antiseptic* [coal tar; zinc oxide] 1%• ≐

medrogestone USAN, INN, BAN *progestin*

Medrol tablets, Dosepak (unit of use package) ℞ *corticosteroid; anti-inflammatory; immunosuppressant* [methylprednisolone] 2, 4, 8, 16, 24, 32 mg

medronate disodium USAN *pharmaceutic aid*

medronic acid USAN, INN, BAN *pharmaceutic aid*

medroxalol USAN, INN, BAN *antihypertensive*

medroxalol HCl USAN *antihypertensive*

medroxiprogesterone acetate [see: medroxyprogesterone acetate]

medroxyprogesterone INN, BAN *synthetic progestin for secondary amenorrhea or abnormal uterine bleeding; hormonal antineoplastic* [also: medroxyprogesterone acetate]

medroxyprogesterone acetate USP *synthetic progestin for secondary amenorrhea, abnormal uterine bleeding, and endometrial hyperplasia; hormonal antineoplastic; investigational (orphan) for immune thrombocytopenic purpura (ITP)* [also: medroxyprogesterone] 2.5, 5, 10 mg oral; 150 mg/mL depot injection

MED-Rx DM controlled-release tablets (14-day, 56-tablet regimen) (discontinued 2005) ℞ *expectorant; decongestant added* AM; *antitussive added* PM [guifenesin; pseudoephedrine HCl (AM); dextromethorphan hydrobromide (PM)] 600•60 mg AM; 600•30 mg PM

medrylamine INN

medrysone USAN, USP, INN *ophthalmic corticosteroidal anti-inflammatory*

mefeclorazine INN

mefenamic acid USAN, USP, INN, BAN *analgesic; nonsteroidal anti-inflammatory drug (NSAID) for mild to moderate pain and primary dysmenorrhea* 250 mg oral

mefenidil USAN, INN *cerebral vasodilator*

mefenidil fumarate USAN *cerebral vasodilator*

mefenidramium metilsulfate INN

mefenorex INN *anorectic* [also: mefenorex HCl]

mefenorex HCl USAN *anorectic* [also: mefenorex]

mefeserpine INN

mefexamide USAN, INN *CNS stimulant*

mefloquine USAN, INN, BAN *antimalarial* ⊠ mafilcon A

mefloquine HCl USAN *antimalarial for acute chloroquine-resistant malaria (orphan)* 250 mg oral

Mefoxin powder or frozen premix for IV or IM injection ℞ *cephamycin antibiotic* [cefoxitin sodium] 1, 2, 10 g

mefruside USAN, INN *diuretic*

Mega VM-80 tablets OTC *geriatric vitamin/mineral supplement* [multiple vitamins & minerals; folic acid; biotin] ±•400•80 mcg

Mega-B tablets OTC *vitamin supplement* [multiple B vitamins; folic acid; biotin] ±•100•100 mcg ⊠ MACOP-B; MCP

Megace tablets ℞ *synthetic progestin; hormonal antineoplastic for advanced carcinoma of the breast or endometrium* [megestrol acetate] 40 mg ⊠ Maox 420; M-oxy

Megace; Megace ES oral suspension ℞ *synthetic progestin; treatment for AIDS-related anorexia and cachexia (orphan)* [megestrol acetate] 40 mg/mL; 125 mg/mL ⊠ Maox; M-oxy

Megagen *investigational (orphan) adjunct to hematopoietic stem cell transplantation* [megakaryocyte growth and development factor, pegylated, recombinant human]

megakaryocyte growth and development factor, pegylated, recombinant human *investigational (orphan) adjunct to hematopoietic stem cell transplantation*

megallate INN *combining name for radicals or groups*

megalomicin INN *antibacterial* [also: megalomicin potassium phosphate]

megalomicin potassium phosphate USAN *antibacterial* [also: megalomicin]

Megaton elixir (discontinued 2006) ℞ *vitamin/mineral supplement* [multiple B vitamins & minerals; folic acid] ±•0.1 mg ⊠ Micatin

megestrol INN, BAN *synthetic progestin; hormonal antineoplastic for breast or endometrial cancer; investigational (Phase III) for liver cancer* [also: megestrol acetate]

megestrol acetate USAN, USP *synthetic progestin; hormonal antineoplastic for breast or endometrial cancer; therapy* for AIDS-related anorexia and cachexia (orphan) [also: megestrol] 20, 40 mg oral; 40 mg/mL oral

meglitinide INN

meglitinides a class of antidiabetic agents that stimulate insulin production in the pancreas

meglucycline INN ⑨ meclocycline

meglumine USP, INN radiopaque contrast medium

meglumine diatrizoate BAN oral/ parenteral radiopaque contrast medium (46.67% iodine) [also: diatrizoate meglumine]

meglumine iocarmate BAN radiopaque contrast medium [also: iocarmate meglumine]

meglumine iothalamate BAN parenteral radiopaque contrast medium (47% iodine) [also: iothalamate meglumine]

meglumine ioxaglate BAN radiopaque contrast medium [also: ioxaglate meglumine]

meglutol USAN, INN antihyperlipoproteinemic ⑨ miglitol

mel B [see: melarsoprol]

mel W [see: melarsonyl potassium]

Melacine investigational (NDA filed, orphan) theraccine (therapeutic vaccine) for invasive stage IIB–IV melanoma [melanoma vaccine]

meladrazine INN, BAN

melafocon A USAN hydrophobic contact lens material

melagatran parenteral anticoagulant and direct thrombin inhibitor

Melaleuca alternifolia medicinal herb [see: tea tree oil]

Melanocid investigational (orphan) treatment for invasive malignant melanoma [pegylated arginine deiminase]

melanoma vaccine investigational (NDA filed, orphan) theraccine (therapeutic vaccine) for invasive stage IIB–IV melanoma

melarsonyl potassium INN, BAN

melarsoprol INN, BAN investigational anti-infective for trypanosomiasis

Melatonex time-release tablets OTC natural supplement to aid the sleep cycle

[melatonin; vitamin B₆; calcium; iron] 3•10•31•1 mg

melatonin natural sleep aid; investigational (orphan) for circadian rhythm sleep disorders in blind people with no light perception

melengestrol INN antineoplastic; progestin [also: melengestrol acetate]

melengestrol acetate USAN antineoplastic; progestin [also: melengestrol]

meletimide INN

melfalan [see: melphalan]

Melfiat-105 Unicelles (sustained-release capsules) ℞ anorexiant; CNS stimulant [phendimetrazine tartrate] 105 mg

Melia azedarach medicinal herb [see: pride of China]

melilot (Melilotus alba; M. officinalis) flowering plant medicinal herb used as an antispasmodic, diuretic, emollient, expectorant, and vulnerary

Melimmune investigational (orphan) for invasive cutaneous melanoma [monoclonal antibody to anti-idiotype melanoma-associated antigen, murine]

melinamide INN

Melissa officinalis medicinal herb [see: lemon balm]

melitracen INN antidepressant [also: melitracen HCl]

melitracen HCl USAN antidepressant [also: melitracen]

melizame USAN, INN sweetener

Mellaril tablets, concentrate for oral solution (discontinued 2004) ℞ conventional (typical) phenothiazine antipsychotic for schizophrenia; sedative; also used for agitation or psychosis due to Alzheimer or other dementias [thioridazine HCl] 15, 100, 200 mg; 30 mg/mL

meloxicam USAN, INN, BAN COX-2 inhibitor; analgesic; antipyretic; nonsteroidal anti-inflammatory drug (NSAID) for osteoarthritis, rheumatoid arthritis, and juvenile rheumatoid arthritis; also used for ankylosing spondylitis and acute bursitis/tendinitis 7.5, 15 mg oral; 7.5 mg/5 mL oral

Melpaque HP cream ℞ *hyperpigmentation bleaching agent* [hydroquinone (in a sunscreen base)] 4%

melperone INN, BAN

melphalan (MPL) USAN, USP, INN, BAN, JAN *nitrogen mustard-type alkylating antineoplastic for multiple myeloma (orphan) and ovarian cancer; investigational (orphan) for metastatic melanoma; also used for breast and testicular cancers and bone marrow transplantation*

Melquin HP cream ℞ *hyperpigmentation bleaching agent* [hydroquinone] 4%

memantine INN *NMDA (N-methyl-D-aspartate) antagonist; neuroprotective agent* [also: memantine HCl]

memantine HCl *NMDA (N-methyl-D-aspartate) antagonist for Alzheimer disease; investigational (Phase III) neuroprotective agent for AIDS dementia* [also: memantine]

Memoir (trademarked delivery device) *a battery-powered self-injector for insulin with a memory chip that tracks the last 16 doses*

Memorette (trademarked packaging form) *patient compliance package*

memotine INN *antiviral* [also: memotine HCl]

memotine HCl USAN *antiviral* [also: memotine]

menabitan INN *analgesic* [also: menabitan HCl]

menabitan HCl USAN *analgesic* [also: menabitan]

Menactra IM injection ℞ *meningitis vaccine for children, adolescents, and adults 2–55 years* [meningococcal polysaccharide vaccine, groups A, C, Y, and W-135, conjugated to diphtheria toxoid] 4•4•4•4•48 mcg per 0.5 mL dose

menadiol BAN *vitamin K_4; prothrombogenic* [also: menadiol sodium diphosphate]

menadiol sodium diphosphate USP *vitamin K_4; prothrombogenic* [also: menadiol]

menadiol sodium sulfate INN

menadione USP *vitamin K_3; prothrombogenic* ② Minidyne

menadione sodium bisulfite USP, INN

Menadol captabs OTC *analgesic; antipyretic; antiarthritic; nonsteroidal anti-inflammatory drug (NSAID) for mild to moderate pain, migraine headaches, and primary dysmenorrhea* [ibuprofen] 200 mg

menaphthene [see: menadione]

menaphthone [see: menadione]

menaphthone sodium bisulfite [see: menadione sodium bisulfite]

menaquinone *vitamin K_2; prothrombogenic*

menatetrenone INN

menbutone INN, BAN

M-End oral liquid ℞ *narcotic antitussive; antihistamine; decongestant* [hydrocodone bitartrate; brompheniramine maleate; pseudoephedrine HCl] 2.5•2•15 mg/5 mL

M-End Max oral liquid ℞ *narcotic antitussive; antihistamine; decongestant* [hydrocodone bitartrate; brompheniramine maleate; phenylephrine HCl] 5•2•7.5 mg/5 mL

M-End WC oral liquid ℞ *narcotic antitussive; antihistamine; decongestant* [codeine phosphate; brompheniramine maleate; pseudoephedrine HCl] 6.3•1.3•10 mg/5 mL

mendelevium *element (Md)*

Menest film-coated tablets ℞ *a mixture of equine estrogens for the treatment of postmenopausal symptoms; palliative therapy for prostate and breast cancers* [esterified estrogens] 0.3, 0.625, 1.25, 2.5 mg ② Magnacet

menfegol INN

menglytate INN

menichlopholan [see: niclofolan]

Meni-D capsules ℞ *anticholinergic; antivertigo agent; motion sickness preventative* [meclizine HCl] 25 mg

meningococcal polysaccharide vaccine, group A USP *active bacterin for meningitis (Neisseria meningitidis)*

meningococcal polysaccharide vaccine, group C USP *active bacterin for meningitis* (Neisseria meningitidis)

meningococcal polysaccharide vaccine, group W-135 *active bacterin for meningitis* (Neisseria meningitidis)

meningococcal polysaccharide vaccine, group Y *active bacterin for meningitis* (Neisseria meningitidis)

Menispermum cocculus; M. lacunosum medicinal herb [see: levant berry]

menitrazepam INN

menoctone USAN, INN *antimalarial*

menogaril USAN, INN *antibiotic antineoplastic*

Menomune-A/C/Y/W-135 powder for subcu injection ℞ *meningitis vaccine* [meningococcal polysaccharide vaccine, groups A, C, Y, and W-135] 50 mcg of each group per 0.5 mL dose

Menopur powder or pellet for IM injection ℞ *gonadotropin; follicle-stimulating hormone (FSH) and luteinizing hormone (LH) for the induction of ovulation in women and spermatogenesis in men; adjunct to assisted reproductive technologies (ART)* [menotropins] 75 FSH units + 75 LH units

Menostar transdermal patch ℞ *estrogen replacement therapy for postmenopausal symptoms* [estradiol-17β] 14 mcg/day

menotropins USAN, USP *gonadotropin; follicle-stimulating hormone (FSH) and luteinizing hormone (LH) for the induction of ovulation in women and spermatogenesis in men; adjunct to assisted reproductive technologies (ART)* [also: follitropin beta]

Men-Phor lotion OTC *mild anesthetic; antipruritic; counterirritant* [menthol; camphor] 0.5%•0.5%

Mentax cream ℞ *benzylamine antifungal* [butenafine HCl] 1% ⓓ Mintox

Mentha piperita medicinal herb [see: peppermint]

Mentha pulegium medicinal herb [see: pennyroyal]

Mentha spicata medicinal herb [see: spearmint]

menthol USP *mild topical anesthetic; antipruritic; counterirritant* ⓓ Mynatal

Menthol Cough Drops lozenges OTC *mild anesthetic; antipruritic; counterirritant* [menthol] 6.5 mg

Mentholatum vaporizing ointment OTC *mild anesthetic; antipruritic; counterirritant* [menthol; camphor] 9%•1.3%

Mentholatum Cherry Chest Rub for Kids vaporizing ointment OTC *mild anesthetic; antipruritic; counterirritant; antiseptic* [menthol; camphor; eucalyptus oil] 4.7%•2.6%•1.2%

menthyl anthranilate [see: meradimate]

Menyanthes trifoliata medicinal herb [see: buckbean]

meobentine INN *antiarrhythmic* [also: meobentine sulfate]

meobentine sulfate USAN *antiarrhythmic* [also: meobentine]

mepacrine INN *anthelmintic; antimalarial* [also: quinacrine HCl]

mepacrine HCl [see: quinacrine HCl]

meparfynol [see: methylpentynol]

mepartricin USAN, INN *antifungal; antiprotozoal*

mepazine acetate [see: pecazine]

mepenzolate bromide USP, INN *GI antispasmodic; anticholinergic; peptic ulcer adjunct*

mepenzolate methylbromide [see: mepenzolate bromide]

mepenzolone bromide [see: mepenzolate bromide]

Mepergan injection (discontinued 2004) ℞ *narcotic analgesic; sedative* [meperidine HCl; promethazine HCl] 25•25 mg/mL

Mepergan Fortis capsules (discontinued 2004) ℞ *narcotic analgesic; sedative* [meperidine HCl; promethazine HCl] 50•25 mg

meperidine HCl USP *narcotic analgesic; also abused as a street drug* [also: pethidine] 50, 100 mg oral; 50 mg/5 mL oral; 10, 25, 50, 75, 100 mg/mL injection

meperidine HCl & promethazine HCl *narcotic analgesic; sedative* 50•25 mg oral

Mephaquin ℞ *antimalarial for acute chloroquine-resistant malaria (orphan)* [mefloquine HCl]

mephenesin NF, INN

mephenhydramine [see: moxastine]

mephenoxalone INN

mephentermine INN *adrenergic; vasoconstrictor; vasopressor for hypotensive shock* [also: mephentermine sulfate]

mephentermine sulfate USP *adrenergic; vasoconstrictor; vasopressor for hypotensive shock* [also: mephentermine]

mephenytoin USAN, USP, INN *hydantoin anticonvulsant* [also: methoin]

mephobarbital USP, JAN *anticonvulsant; sedative* [also: methylphenobarbital; methylphenobarbitone]

Mephyton tablets ℞ *coagulant to correct anticoagulant-induced prothrombin deficiency; vitamin K supplement* [phytonadione] 5 mg

mepicycline [see: pipacycline]

MEPIG (mucoid exopolysaccharide *Pseudomonas* [hyper]immune globulin) [q.v.]

mepindolol INN, BAN

mepiperphenidol bromide

mepiprazole INN, BAN

mepirizole [see: epirizole]

mepiroxol INN

mepitiostane INN

mepivacaine INN *local anesthetic* [also: mepivacaine HCl]

mepivacaine HCl USP *local anesthetic* [also: mepivacaine] 3% injection

mepivacaine HCl & levonordefrin *injectable local anesthetic; vasoconstrictor* 2%•1:20 000 injection

mepixanox INN

mepolizumab USAN, INN *immunomodulator; investigational (orphan) for hypereosinophilic syndrome*

mepramidil INN

meprednisone USAN, USP, INN

meprobamate USP, INN, BAN, JAN *anxiolytic; sedative; hypnotic; minor tranquilizer; also abused as a street drug* 200, 400 mg oral

Mepron oral suspension ℞ *antiprotozoal for AIDS-related* Pneumocystis pneumonia (PCP) *(orphan); investigational (orphan) for AIDS-related* Toxoplasma gondii *encephalitis* [atovaquone] 750 mg/5 mL

meproscillarin INN, BAN

meprothixol BAN [also: meprotixol]

meprotixol INN [also: meprothixol]

meprylcaine INN *local anesthetic* [also: meprylcaine HCl]

meprylcaine HCl USP *local anesthetic* [also: meprylcaine]

meptazinol INN, BAN *analgesic* [also: meptazinol HCl]

meptazinol HCl USAN *analgesic* [also: meptazinol]

mepyramine INN, BAN *antihistamine* [also: pyrilamine maleate]

mepyramine maleate [see: pyrilamine maleate]

mepyrium [see: amprolium]

mepyrrotazine [see: dimelazine]

mequidox USAN, INN *antibacterial*

mequinol USAN, INN *hyperpigmentation bleaching agent* ② Micanol; Myconel

mequitamium iodide INN

mequitazine INN, BAN

mequitazium iodide [see: mequitamium iodide]

meradimate USAN *ultraviolet A sunscreen*

meragidone sodium

meralein sodium USAN, INN *topical anti-infective*

meralluride NF, INN

merbaphen USP

merbromin NF, INN *general antiseptic*

mercaptamine INN *antiurolithic* [also: cysteamine]

mercaptoarsenical [see: arsthinol]

mercaptoarsenol [see: arsthinol]

mercaptoethylamine (MEA) [see: mercaptamine]

mercaptomerin (MT6) INN [also: mercaptomerin sodium]

mercaptomerin sodium USP [also: mercaptomerin]

mercaptopurine (6-MP) USP, INN *antimetabolite antineoplastic for acute lymphocytic, lymphoblastic, myelogenous, and myelomonocytic leukemias* 50 mg oral

mercuderamide INN

mercufenol chloride USAN *topical anti-infective*

mercumatilin sodium INN

mercuric oxide, yellow NF *ophthalmic antiseptic (FDA ruled it "not safe and effective" in 1992)*

mercuric salicylate NF

mercuric succinimide NF

mercurobutol INN

mercurophylline NF, INN

mercurous chloride [see: calomel]

mercury *element (Hg)*

mercury, ammoniated USP *topical antiseptic; antipsoriatic*

mercury amide chloride [see: mercury, ammoniated]

mercury oleate NF

merethoxylline procaine

mergocriptine INN

Meridia capsules ℞ *anorexiant for the treatment of obesity* [sibutramine HCl] 5, 10, 15 mg

merisoprol acetate Hg 197 USAN *radioactive agent*

merisoprol acetate Hg 203 USAN *radioactive agent*

merisoprol Hg 197 USAN *renal function test; radioactive agent*

Meritene powder OTC *enteral nutritional therapy* [milk-based formula]

meropenem USAN, INN, BAN *broad-spectrum carbapenem antibiotic for bacterial meningitis in children, intra-abdominal infections, and complicated skin and skin structure infections (SSSIs); investigational (orphan) for acute pulmonary episodes in cystic fibrosis*

Merrem I.V. powder for IV infusion ℞ *broad-spectrum carbapenem antibiotic for bacterial meningitis in children, intra-abdominal infections, and complicated skin and skin structure infections (SSSIs); investigational (orphan) for*

acute pulmonary episodes in cystic fibrosis [meropenem] 500, 1000 mg

mersalyl INN

mersalyl sodium [see: mersalyl]

Mersol solution, tincture OTC *antiseptic; antibacterial; antifungal* [thimerosal] 1:1000 ⊡ Murocel

mertiatide INN

Meruvax II powder for subcu injection ℞ *rubella vaccine* [rubella virus vaccine, live] 0.5 mL ⊡ M-R-Vax II

mesabolone INN

Mesafem *investigational (Phase III) selective serotonin reuptake inhibitor (SSRI) for postmenopausal hot flashes and other vasomotor symptoms* [paroxetine mesylate]

mesalamine USAN *anti-inflammatory for ulcerative colitis and proctitis* [also: mesalazine] 4 g/60 mL enema ⊡ mezilamine; muzolimine

mesalazine INN, BAN *anti-inflammatory; treatment of ulcerative colitis and proctitis* [also: mesalamine]

mescaline *hallucinogenic street drug derived from the flowering heads (mescal buttons) of a Mexican cactus*

Mescolor sustained-release film-coated tablets (discontinued 2005) ℞ *decongestant; antihistamine; anticholinergic to dry mucosal secretions* [pseudoephedrine HCl; chlorpheniramine maleate; methscopolamine nitrate] 120•8•2.5 mg

meseclazone USAN, INN *anti-inflammatory*

mesembryanthemum *medicinal herb* [see: kanna]

mesifilcon A USAN *hydrophilic contact lens material*

mesilate INN *combining name for radicals or groups* [also: mesylate]

mesna USAN, INN, BAN *prophylaxis for ifosfamide-induced hemorrhagic cystitis (orphan); investigational (orphan) treatment for cyclophosphamide-induced hemorrhagic cystitis* 100 mg/mL injection, 400 mg oral

Mesnex film-coated caplets, IV injection ℞ *prophylaxis for ifosfamide-*

*induced hemorrhagic cystitis (orphan);
investigational (orphan) treatment for
cyclophosphamide-induced hemorrhagic
cystitis* [mesna] 400 mg; 100 mg/mL

mesocarb INN

meso-inositol [see: inositol]

**meso-NDGA (nordihydroguaiaretic
acid)** [see: masoprocol]

**meso-nordihydroguaiaretic acid
(NDGA)** [see: masoprocol]

mesoridazine USAN, INN *phenothiazine
antipsychotic*

mesoridazine besylate USP *conventional (typical) phenothiazine antipsychotic for schizophrenia*

mespiperone C 11 USAN *radiopharmaceutical imaging aid for PET scans of the
brain (produced at bedside for immediate administration)*

mespirenone INN

mestanolone INN, BAN

mestenediol [see: methandriol]

mesterolone USAN, INN, BAN *androgen; also abused as a street drug*

Mestinon tablets, Timespan (extended-release tablets), syrup, IM or IV injection ℞ *cholinergic/anticholinesterase
muscle stimulant; muscle relaxant
reversal; treatment for myasthenia
gravis* [pyridostigmine bromide] 60
mg; 180 mg; 60 mg/5 mL; 5 mg/mL

mestranol USAN, USP, INN *estrogen*

mesudipine INN

mesulergine INN

mesulfamide INN

mesulfen INN [also: mesulphen]

mesulphen BAN [also: mesulfen]

mesuprine INN *vasodilator; smooth
muscle relaxant* [also: mesuprine HCl]

mesuprine HCl USAN *vasodilator;
smooth muscle relaxant* [also: mesuprine]

mesuximide INN *succinimide anticonvulsant for petit mal (absence) seizures*
[also: methsuximide]

mesylate USAN, USP, BAN *combining
name for radicals or groups* [also:
mesilate]

metabromsalan USAN, INN *disinfectant*

metabutethamine HCl NF

metabutoxycaine HCl NF

metacetamol INN, BAN

metaclazepam INN

metacycline INN *antibacterial* [also:
methacycline]

Metadate CD dual-release capsules
(30% immediate release, 70%
extended release) ℞ *CNS stimulant;
once-daily treatment for attention-deficit/hyperactivity disorder (ADHD)*
[methylphenidate HCl] 10, 20, 30,
40, 50, 60 mg

Metadate ER extended-release tablets
℞ *CNS stimulant for attention-deficit/
hyperactivity disorder (ADHD) and
narcolepsy* [methylphenidate HCl]
10, 20 mg

Metafolin (trademarked ingredient)
bioactive form of folic acid [L-methylfolate]

Metaglip film-coated tablets ℞ *antidiabetic combination for type 2 diabetes
that stimulates insulin secretion in the
pancreas, decreases hepatic glucose production, and increases cellular response
to insulin* [glipizide; metformin HCl]
2.5•250, 2.5•500, 5•500 mg

metaglycodol INN

metahexamide INN

metahexanamide [see: metahexamide]

Metahydrin tablets (discontinued
2006) ℞ *diuretic; antihypertensive*
[trichlormethiazide] 4 mg

metalkonium chloride INN

metallibure INN *anterior pituitary activator for swine* [also: methallibure]

metalol HCl USAN *antiadrenergic (β-receptor)*

metamelfalan INN

metamfazone INN [also: methamphazone]

metamfepramone INN [also: dimepropion]

metamfetamine INN *CNS stimulant;
widely abused as a street drug* [also:
methamphetamine HCl]

metamizole sodium INN *analgesic;
antipyretic* [also: dipyrone]

metampicillin INN

Metamucil capsules OTC *bulk laxative* [psyllium husk] 520 mg

Metamucil effervescent powder OTC *bulk laxative; antacid* [psyllium hydrophilic mucilloid; sodium bicarbonate; potassium bicarbonate] 3.4• 2•2 g/pkt.

Metamucil wafers OTC *bulk laxative* [psyllium husk] 3.4 g

Metamucil Original Texture; Metamucil Smooth Texture; Berry Burst! Metamucil powder OTC *bulk laxative* [psyllium husk] 3.4 g/dose

metandienone INN [also: methandrostenolone; methandienone]

metanixin INN

Metanx tablets ℞ *vitamin B supplement* [vitamins B_6 and B_{12}; folic acid] 25• 2•2.8 mg

metaoxedrine chloride [see: phenylephrine HCl]

metaphosphoric acid, potassium salt [see: potassium metaphosphate]

metaphosphoric acid, trisodium salt [see: sodium trimetaphosphate]

metaphyllin [see: aminophylline]

metapramine INN

metaproterenol polistirex USAN *sympathomimetic bronchodilator* [also: orciprenaline]

metaproterenol sulfate USAN, USP *sympathomimetic bronchodilator* 10, 20 mg oral; 10 mg/5 mL oral; 0.4%, 0.6%, 5% inhalation solution

metaradrine bitartrate [see: metaraminol bitartrate]

metaraminol INN *adrenergic; vasopressor for acute hypotensive shock, anaphylaxis, or traumatic shock* [also: metaraminol bitartrate]

metaraminol bitartrate USP *adrenergic; vasopressor for acute hypotensive shock, anaphylaxis, or traumatic shock* [also: metaraminol]

Metaret injection *investigational (NDA filed, orphan) growth factor antagonist for prostate cancer* [suramin hexasodium] 600 mg

Metastron IV injection ℞ *analgesic for metastatic bone pain* [strontium chloride Sr 89] 10.9–22.6 mg/mL (4 mCi)

Metatensin #2; Metatensin #4 tablets (discontinued 2007) ℞ *antihypertensive* [trichlormethiazide; reserpine] 2•0.1 mg; 4•0.1 mg

metaterol INN

metaxalone USAN, INN, BAN *skeletal muscle relaxant*

metazamide INN

metazepium iodide [see: buzepide metiodide]

metazide INN

metazocine INN, BAN

metbufen INN

metcaraphen HCl

metembonate INN *combining name for radicals or groups*

meteneprost USAN, INN *oxytocic; prostaglandin*

metenolone INN *anabolic steroid; also abused as a street drug* [also: methenolone acetate; methenolone; metenolone acetate]

metenolone acetate JAN *anabolic steroid; also abused as a street drug* [also: methenolone acetate; metenolone; methenolone]

metenolone enanthate JAN *anabolic steroid; also abused as a street drug* [also: methenolone enanthate]

metergoline INN, BAN

metergotamine INN

metescufylline INN

metesculetol INN

metesind glucuronate USAN *specific thymidylate synthase (TS) inhibitor antineoplastic*

metethoheptazine INN

metetoin INN *anticonvulsant* [also: methetoin] ② mitotane

metformin USAN, INN, BAN *biguanide antidiabetic for type 2 diabetes that decreases hepatic glucose production and increases cellular response to insulin* [also: metformin HCl]

Metformin ER extended-release caplets (discontinued 2007) ℞ *biguanide antidiabetic that decreases hepatic glu-*

cose production and increases cellular response to insulin [metformin HCl] 500 mg

metformin HCl USAN, JAN *biguanide antidiabetic for type 2 diabetes that decreases hepatic glucose production and increases cellular response to insulin* [also: metformin] 500, 750, 850, 1000 mg oral

metformin HCl & glipizide *antidiabetic combination for type 2 diabetes that stimulates insulin secretion in the pancreas, decreases hepatic glucose production, and increases cellular response to insulin* 250•2.5, 500•2.5, 500•5 mg

metformin HCl & glyburide *antidiabetic combination for type 2 diabetes that decreases hepatic glucose production, increases cellular response to insulin, and stimulates insulin secretion in the pancreas* 250•1.25, 500•2.5, 500•5 mg oral

methacholine bromide NF

methacholine chloride USP, INN *cholinergic; bronchoconstrictor for in vivo pulmonary challenge tests*

methacrylic acid copolymer NF *tablet-coating agent*

methacycline USAN *antibacterial* [also: metacycline]

methacycline HCl USP *gram-negative and gram-positive bacteriostatic; antirickettsial*

methadol [see: dimepheptanol]

methadone INN *narcotic analgesic; narcotic addiction detoxicant; often abused as a street drug* [also: methadone HCl]

methadone HCl USP *narcotic analgesic; narcotic addiction detoxicant; often abused as a street drug* [also: methadone] 5, 10, 40 mg oral; 5, 10 mg/5 mL oral; 10 mg/mL oral; 10 mg/mL injection

methadonium chloride [see: methadone HCl]

Methadose tablets, dispersible tablets, oral concentrate ℞ *narcotic analgesic; narcotic addiction detoxicant; often abused as a street drug* [methadone HCl] 5, 10 mg; 40 mg; 10 mg/mL

methadyl acetate USAN *narcotic analgesic* [also: acetylmethadol]

methafilcon B USAN *hydrophilic contact lens material*

Methagual OTC *analgesic; counterirritant* [methyl salicylate; guaiacol] 8%•2%

Methalgen cream OTC *analgesic; mild anesthetic; antipruritic; counterirritant* [methyl salicylate; menthol; camphor; mustard oil]

methallenestril INN

methallenestrol [see: methallenestril]

methallibure USAN *anterior pituitary activator for swine* [also: metallibure]

methalthiazide USAN *diuretic; antihypertensive*

methamoctol

methamphazone BAN [also: metamfazone]

methamphetamine HCl USP *CNS stimulant; widely abused as a street drug* [also: metamfetamine] 5 mg oral

methampyrone [now: dipyrone]

methanabol [see: methandriol]

methandienone BAN [also: methandrostenolone; metandienone]

methandriol

methandrostenolone USP *steroid; discontinued for human use, but the veterinary product is still available and sometimes abused as a street drug* [also: metandienone; methandienone]

methaniazide INN

methanol [see: methyl alcohol]

methantheline bromide USP *peptic ulcer adjunct* [also: methanthelinium bromide]

methanthelinium bromide INN, BAN *anticholinergic* [also: methantheline bromide]

methaphenilene INN, BAN [also: methaphenilene HCl]

methaphenilene HCl NF [also: methaphenilene]

methapyrilene INN [also: methapyrilene fumarate]

methapyrilene fumarate USP [also: methapyrilene]

methapyrilene HCl USP

methaqualone USAN, USP, INN, BAN *hypnotic; sedative; widely abused as a street drug, which leads to dependence*

methaqualone HCl USP

metharbital USP, INN, JAN *anticonvulsant* [also: metharbitone]

metharbitone BAN *anticonvulsant* [also: metharbital]

methastyridone INN

Methatropic capsules OTC *dietary lipotropic with vitamin supplementation* [choline; inositol; methionine; multiple B vitamins] 115•83•110• ± mg

methazolamide USP, INN *carbonic anhydrase inhibitor for glaucoma* 25, 50 mg oral 🔳 mitozolomide

Methblue 65 tablets ℞ *urinary anti-infective and antiseptic; antidote to cyanide poisoning* [methylene blue] 65 mg

methcathinone *a highly addictive manufactured street drug similar to cathinone, with amphetamine-like effects* [see also: cathinone; *Catha edulis*]

methdilazine USP, INN *phenothiazine antihistamine; antipruritic*

methdilazine HCl USP *phenothiazine antihistamine; antipruritic*

methenamine USP, INN *urinary antibiotic*

methenamine hippurate USAN, USP *urinary antibiotic* [also: hexamine hippurate]

methenamine mandelate USP *urinary antibiotic* 0.5, 1 g oral; 0.5 g/5 mL oral

methenamine sulfosalicylate *topical antipsoriatic*

methenolone BAN *anabolic steroid; also abused as a street drug* [also: methenolone acetate; metenolone; metenolone acetate]

methenolone acetate USAN *anabolic steroid; also abused as a street drug* [also: metenolone; methenolone; metenolone acetate]

methenolone enanthate USAN *anabolic steroid; also abused as a street drug* [also: metenolone enanthate]

metheptazine INN

Methergine coated tablets, IV or IM injection ℞ *oxytocic for induction of labor, control of postpartum uterine atony, and postpartum hemorrhage* [methylergonovine maleate] 0.2 mg; 0.2 mg/mL

methestrol INN

methetharimide [see: bemegride]

methetoin USAN *anticonvulsant* [also: metetoin] 🔳 mitotane

methicillin sodium USAN, USP *penicillinase-resistant penicillin antibiotic* [also: meticillin]

methimazole USP *thyroid inhibitor* [also: thiamazole] 5, 10 mg oral

methindizate BAN [also: metindizate]

methiodal sodium USP, INN

methiomeprazine INN

methiomeprazine HCl [see: methiomeprazine]

methionine (DL-methionine) NF, JAN *urinary acidifier* [also: racemethionine] 500 mg oral

methionine (L-methionine) USAN, USP, INN, JAN *essential amino acid; symbols: Met, M; investigational (orphan) for AIDS myelopathy*

methionyl neurotropic factor, brain-derived, recombinant *investigational (orphan) for amyotrophic lateral sclerosis (ALS)*

methionyl stem cell factor, recombinant human *investigational (orphan) for primary bone marrow failure*

N-methionylleptin (human) [see: metreleptin]

methiothepin [see: metitepine]

methisazone USAN *antiviral* [also: metisazone]

methisoprinol [now: inosine pranobex]

Methitest tablets ℞ *synthetic androgen for hypogonadism or testosterone deficiency in men, delayed puberty in boys, and metastatic breast cancer in women; hormone replacement therapy (HRT) for postandropausal symptoms; also abused as a street drug* [methyltestosterone] 10, 25 mg

methitural INN

methixene HCl USAN *smooth muscle relaxant* [also: metixene]

methocamphone methylsulfate
[see: trimethidinium methosulfate]

methocarbamol USP, INN, BAN, JAN
skeletal muscle relaxant 500, 750 mg
oral

methocidin INN

methohexital USP, INN *barbiturate general anesthetic* [also: methohexitone]

methohexital sodium USP *barbiturate general anesthetic*

methohexitone BAN *barbiturate general anesthetic* [also: methohexital]

methoin BAN *anticonvulsant* [also: mephenytoin]

methonaphthone [see: menbutone]

methophedrine [see: methoxyphedrine]

methophenazine [see: metofenazate]

methopholine USAN *analgesic* [also: metofoline]

methoprene INN

methopromazine INN

methopromazine maleate [see: methopromazine]

methopyrimazole [see: epirizole]

d-**methorphan** [see: dextromethorphan]

d-**methorphan hydrobromide** [see: dextromethorphan hydrobromide]

methoserpidine INN, BAN

methotrexate (MTX) USAN, USP, INN, BAN, JAN *antimetabolite antineoplastic for leukemia, lymphoma, and various solid tumors; systemic antipsoriatic; antirheumatic for adult and juvenile rheumatoid arthritis (orphan)* 2.5 mg oral

methotrexate & laurocapram *investigational (orphan) for topical treatment of mycosis fungoides*

methotrexate & leucovorin *antineoplastic for osteosarcoma (orphan)*

Methotrexate LPF Sodium preservative-free injection ℞ *antimetabolite antineoplastic for leukemia, lymphoma, various solid tumors, and osteogenic sarcoma (orphan); systemic antipsoriatic; antirheumatic* [methotrexate sodium] 2.5 mg/mL

methotrexate sodium USP *antirheumatic; systemic antipsoriatic; antime-*

tabolite antineoplastic for leukemia, lymphoma, various solid tumors, and osteogenic sarcoma (orphan) 20, 1000 mg/vial injection; 2.5 mg/mL injection

methotrimeprazine USAN, USP *central analgesic; CNS depressant* [also: levomepromazine]

methotrimeprazine maleate *CNS depressant; neuroleptic*

methoxamine INN *adrenergic; vasoconstrictor; vasopressor for hypotensive shock during surgery* [also: methoxamine HCl]

methoxamine HCl USP *adrenergic; vasoconstrictor; vasopressor for hypotensive shock during surgery* [also: methoxamine]

methoxiflurane [see: methoxyflurane]

methoxsalen (8-methoxsalen) USP *repigmentation agent for vitiligo; antipsoriatic; palliative treatment for cutaneous T-cell lymphoma (CTCL); investigational (orphan) for diffuse systemic sclerosis and cardiac allografts*

methoxy polyethylene glycol [see: polyethylene glycol monomethyl ether]

8-methoxycarbonyloctyl oligosaccharides *investigational (Phase III, orphan)* E. coli *neutralizer for traveler's diarrhea and hemolytic uremic syndrome (HUS)*

2-methoxyestradiol *investigational (orphan) for multiple myeloma and ovarian cancer*

methoxyfenoserpin [see: mefeserpine]

methoxyflurane USAN, USP, INN, BAN *inhalation general anesthetic*

methoxyphedrine INN

p-**methoxyphenacyl** [see: anisatil]

methoxyphenamine INN [also: methoxyphenamine HCl]

methoxyphenamine HCl USP [also: methoxyphenamine]

4-methoxyphenol [see: mequinol]

o-**methoxyphenyl salicylate acetate** [see: guacetisal]

methoxypromazine maleate [see: methopromazine]

8-methoxypsoralen (8-MOP) [see: methoxsalen]

5-methoxyresorcinol [see: flamenol]

methphenoxydiol [see: guaifenesin]

methscopolamine bromide USP *GI antispasmodic; peptic ulcer adjunct* [also: hyoscine methobromide] 2.5, 5 mg oral

methscopolamine nitrate *anticholinergic; respiratory antisecretory*

methsuximide USP, BAN *succinimide anticonvulsant for petit mal (absence) seizures* [also: mesuximide]

methyclothiazide USAN, USP, INN *antihypertensive; diuretic* 2.5, 5 mg oral

methydromorphine [see: methyldihydromorphine]

methyl alcohol NF *solvent*

methyl aminolevulinate HCl *photosensitizer for photodynamic therapy of precancerous actinic keratoses of the face and scalp; for use with* CureLight BroadBand Model 01 *(red-light illumination)*

methyl benzoquate BAN *coccidiostat for poultry* [also: nequinate]

methyl cresol [see: cresol]

methyl cysteine [see: mecysteine]

methyl p-hydroxybenzoate [see: methylparaben]

methyl isobutyl ketone NF *alcohol denaturant*

methyl nicotinate USAN

methyl palmoxirate USAN *antidiabetic*

methyl phthalate [see: dimethyl phthalate]

methyl salicylate NF *topical analgesic; mild topical anesthetic; counterirritant; flavoring agent*

methyl sulfoxide [see: dimethyl sulfoxide]

methyl violet [see: gentian violet]

l-methylaminoethanolcatechol [see: epinephrine]

methylaminopterin [see: methotrexate]

methylandrostenediol [see: methandriol]

methylatropine nitrate USAN *anticholinergic* [also: atropine methonitrate]

methylbenactyzium bromide INN

methylbenzethonium chloride USP, INN *topical anti-infective/antiseptic*

α-methylbenzylhydrazine [see: mebanazine]

methylbicyclone *investigational (orphan) for cystic fibrosis*

methylcarbamate of salicylanilide [see: anilamate]

methyl-CCNU (chloroethyl-cyclohexyl-nitrosourea) [see: semustine]

methylcellulose USP, INN *ophthalmic moisturizer; suspending and viscosity-increasing agent; bulk laxative*

methylcellulose, propylene glycol ether of [see: hydroxypropyl methylcellulose]

methylchromone INN, BAN

N-methyl-D-aspartate (NMDA) *an endogenous neurotransmitter similar to glutamate; an NMDA inhibitor blocks the action of glutamate, which can overstimulate the receptors and become neurotoxic in excessive amounts, causing various dementias and CNS disorders*

methyldesorphine INN, BAN

methyldigoxin [see: metildigoxin]

methyldihydromorphine INN

methyldihydromorphinone HCl [see: metopon]

methyldinitrobenzamide [see: dinitolmide]

methyldioxatrine [see: meletimide]

N-methyldiphenethylamine [see: demelverine]

α-methyl-DL-thyroxine ethyl ester [see: etiroxate]

methyldopa USAN, USP, INN, BAN, JAN *centrally acting antiadrenergic antihypertensive* 250, 500 mg oral

α-methyldopa [now: methyldopa]

methyldopa & hydrochlorothiazide *antihypertensive; central antiadrenergic; diuretic* 250•15, 250•25, 500•30, 500•50 mg oral

methyldopate BAN *centrally acting antiadrenergic antihypertensive* [also: methyldopate HCl]

methyldopate HCl USAN, USP *centrally acting antiadrenergic antihyper-*

tensive [also: methyldopate] 50 mg/mL injection

methylene blue (MB) USP *antimethemoglobinemic; GU antiseptic; antidote to cyanide poisoning; diagnostic aid for gastric secretions* [also: methylthioninium chloride] 65 mg oral; 10 mg/mL injection

methylene chloride NF *solvent*

methylene diphosphonate (MDP) [now: medronate disodium]

methylenedioxyamphetamine (MDA) [see: MDMA, MDEA]

3,4-methylenedioxyethamphetamine (MDEA) [q.v.]

3,4-methylenedioxymethamphetamine (MDMA) [q.v.]

6-methyleneoxytetracycline (MOTC) [see: methacycline]

methylenprednisolone [see: prednylidene]

methylergometrine INN *oxytocic* [also: methylergonovine maleate]

methylergometrine maleate [see: methylergonovine maleate]

methylergonovine maleate USP *oxytocic for induction of labor, control of postpartum uterine atony, and postpartum hemorrhage* [also: methylergometrine]

methylergonovinium bimaleate [see: methylergonovine maleate]

methylergotamine [see: metergotamine]

methylestrenolone [see: normethandrone]

L-methylfolate *bioactive form of folic acid* [see: folic acid]

methyl-GAG (methylglyoxal-*bis*-guanylhydrazone) [see: mitoguazone]

methylglyoxal-*bis*-guanylhydrazone (methyl-GAG; MGBG) [see: mitoguazone]

1-methylhexylamine [see: tuaminoheptane]

1-methylhexylamine sulfate [see: tuaminoheptane sulfate]

N-methylhydrazine [see: procarbazine]

Methylin tablets, chewable tablets, oral liquid R̥ *CNS stimulant for attention-deficit/hyperactivity disorder (ADHD) and narcolepsy* [methylphenidate HCl] 5, 10, 20 mg; 2.5, 5, 10 mg; 5, 10 mg/5 mL

Methylin ER extended-release tablets R̥ *CNS stimulant for attention-deficit/hyperactivity disorder (ADHD) and narcolepsy* [methylphenidate HCl] 10, 20 mg

methylmorphine [see: codeine]

methylnaltrexone bromide *opioid receptor antagonist for opioid-induced constipation (orphan); investigational (NDA filed) for postoperative ileus*

methyl-nitro-imidazole [see: carnidazole]

methylnortestosterone [see: normethandrone]

methylparaben USAN, NF *antifungal agent; preservative*

methylparaben sodium USAN, NF *antimicrobial preservative*

methylparafynol [see: meparfynol]

methylpentynol INN, BAN

methylperidol [see: moperone]

(+)-methylphenethylamine [see: dextroamphetamine]

(–)-methylphenethylamine [see: levamphetamine]

methylphenethylamine HCl [see: amphetamine HCl]

methylphenethylamine phosphate [see: amphetamine phosphate]

(–)-methylphenethylamine succinate [see: levamfetamine succinate]

methylphenethylamine sulfate [see: amphetamine sulfate]

(+)-methylphenethylamine sulfate [see: dextroamphetamine sulfate]

methylphenidate INN, BAN *CNS stimulant for attention-deficit/hyperactivity disorder (ADHD) and narcolepsy; also abused as a street drug* [also: methylphenidate HCl]

methylphenidate HCl (MPH) USP, JAN *CNS stimulant for attention-deficit/hyperactivity disorder (ADHD) and narcolepsy; also abused as a street drug* [also: methylphenidate] 5, 10, 20 mg oral

methylphenobarbital INN *anticonvul-sant; sedative* [also: mephobarbital; methylphenobarbitone]

methylphenobarbitone BAN *anticon-vulsant; sedative* [also: mephobarbi-tal; methylphenobarbital]

d-**methylphenylamine sulfate** [see: dextroamphetamine sulfate]

methylphytyl napthoquinone [see: phytonadione]

methylprednisolone USP, INN, BAN, JAN *corticosteroid; anti-inflammatory; immunosuppressant* 4, 8, 16, 32 mg oral

methylprednisolone aceponate INN

methylprednisolone acetate USP, JAN *corticosteroid; anti-inflammatory; immunosuppressant* 20, 40, 80 mg/mL injection

methylprednisolone hemisuccinate USP *corticosteroid; anti-inflammatory*

methylprednisolone sodium phos-phate USAN *corticosteroid; anti-inflammatory* 40, 125, 500, 1000 mg/ vial injection

methylprednisolone sodium succi-nate USP, JAN *corticosteroid; anti-inflammatory; immunosuppressant* 40, 125, 500, 1000 mg injection

methylprednisolone suleptanate USAN, INN *corticosteroid; anti-inflam-matory*

methylpromazine

4-methylpyrazole (4-MP) [see: fome-pizole]

methylrosaniline chloride [now: gentian violet]

methylrosanilinium chloride INN *top-ical anti-infective* [also: gentian violet]

methylscopolamine bromide [see: methscopolamine bromide]

methylsulfate USP *combining name for radicals or groups* [also: metilsulfate]

methylsulfonylmethane (MSM) *natural source of sulfur; promotes an increase in collagen and the endogenous antioxidant glutathione*

methyltestosterone USP, INN, BAN *synthetic androgen for hypogonadism or testosterone deficiency in men, delayed puberty in boys, and metastatic breast cancer in women; hormone replacement therapy (HRT) for postandropausal symptoms; also abused as a street drug* 10, 25 mg oral

methyltestosterone & esterified estrogens *combination synthetic androgen and equine estrogen; hor-mone replacement therapy for post-menopausal symptoms* 1.25•0.625, 2.5•1.25 mg oral

methyltheobromine [see: caffeine]

methylthionine chloride [see: meth-ylene blue]

methylthionine HCl [see: methylene blue]

methylthioninium chloride INN *anti-methemoglobinemic; antidote to cya-nide poisoning* [also: methylene blue]

methylthiouracil USP, INN

methyltrienolone [see: metribolone]

methynodiol diacetate USAN *proges-tin* [also: metynodiol]

methyprylon USP, INN *sedative; hyp-notic* [also: methprylone]

methyprylone BAN *sedative* [also: methyprylon]

methyridene BAN [also: metyridine]

methysergide USAN, INN, BAN *migraine-specific vasoconstrictor and peripheral serotonin antagonist for the prophylaxis of vascular headaches*

methysergide maleate USP *migraine-specific vasoconstrictor and peripheral serotonin antagonist for the prophylaxis of vascular headaches*

metiamide USAN, INN *antagonist to his-tamine H_2 receptors*

metiapine USAN, INN *antipsychotic*

metiazinic acid INN

metibride INN

meticillin INN *penicillinase-resistant penicillin antibiotic* [also: methicillin sodium]

meticillin sodium *penicillinase-resis-tant penicillin antibiotic* [see: methi-cillin sodium]

Meticorten tablets (discontinued 2008) ℞ *corticosteroid; anti-inflammatory; immunosuppressant* [prednisone] 1 mg

meticrane INN

metildigoxin INN

metilsulfate INN *combining name for radicals or groups* [also: methylsulfate]

Metimyd eye drop suspension, ophthalmic ointment ℞ *corticosteroidal anti-inflammatory; antibiotic* [prednisolone acetate; sulfacetamide sodium] 0.5%•10%

metindizate INN [also: methindizate]

metioprim USAN, INN, BAN *antibacterial*

metioxate INN

metipirox INN

metipranolol USAN, INN, BAN *topical antiglaucoma agent (β-blocker)*

metipranolol HCl *topical antiglaucoma agent (β-blocker)* 0.3% eye drops

metiprenaline INN

metirosine INN *antihypertensive* [also: metyrosine]

metisazone INN *antiviral* [also: methisazone]

metitepine INN

metixene INN *smooth muscle relaxant* [also: methixene HCl]

metixene HCl [see: methixene HCl]

metizoline INN *adrenergic; vasoconstrictor* [also: metizoline HC]

metizoline HCl USAN *adrenergic; vasoconstrictor* [also: metizoline]

metkefamide INN *analgesic* [also: metkephamid acetate]

metkefamide acetate [see: metkephamid acetate]

metkephamid acetate USAN *analgesic* [also: metkefamide]

metochalcone INN

metocinium iodide INN

metoclopramide INN, BAN, JAN *antiemetic for chemotherapy; GI stimulant; antidopaminergic; radiosensitizer* [also: metoclopramide HCl]

metoclopramide HCl USAN, USP, JAN *antidopaminergic; antiemetic for chemotherapy and postoperative nausea and vomiting; GI stimulant for diabetic gastroparesis and symptomatic gastroesophageal reflux; also used as a radiosensitizer and to stimulate lactation* [also: metoclopramide] 5, 10 mg oral; 5 mg/5 mL oral; 5 mg/mL injection

metoclopramide monohydrochloride monohydrate [see: metoclopramide HCl]

metocurine iodide USAN, USP *neuromuscular blocker; muscle relaxant* 2 mg/mL injection

metofenazate INN

metofoline INN *analgesic* [also: methopholine]

metogest USAN, INN *hormone*

metolazone USAN, INN *antihypertensive; diuretic* 2.5, 5, 10 mg oral

metomidate INN, BAN

metopimazine USAN, INN *antiemetic*

Metopirone softgels ℞ *diagnostic aid for testing hypothalamic-pituitary adrenocorticotropic hormone (ACTH) function* [metyrapone] 250 mg

metopon INN

metopon HCl [see: metopon]

metoprine USAN *antineoplastic*

metoprolol USAN, INN, BAN *antianginal; antihypertensive; antiadrenergic (β-receptor)*

metoprolol fumarate USAN *antianginal; antihypertensive; antiadrenergic (β-receptor)*

metoprolol succinate USAN *antianginal; antihypertensive; antiadrenergic (β-receptor)* 25, 50, 100, 200 mg oral

metoprolol tartrate USAN, USP *antianginal; antihypertensive; antiadrenergic (β-receptor)* 25, 50, 100 mg oral; 1 mg/mL injection

metoprolol tartrate & hydrochlorothiazide *antihypertensive; β-blocker; diuretic* 50•25, 100•25, 100•50 mg oral

metoquizine USAN, INN *anticholinergic*

metoserpate INN *veterinary sedative* [also: metoserpate HCl]

metoserpate HCl USAN *veterinary sedative* [also: metoserpate]

metostilenol INN

metoxepin INN

metoxiestrol [see: moxestrol]

metrafazoline INN

metralindole INN

metrazifone INN

metreleptin USAN, INN *metabolic regulator for obesity; investigational (orphan) for metabolic disorders due to generalized or familial lipodystrophy*

metrenperone USAN, INN, BAN *veterinary myopathic*

metribolone INN

metrifonate USAN, INN *veterinary anthelmintic* [also: trichlorfon; metriphonate]

metrifudil INN

metriphonate BAN *veterinary anthelmintic* [also: trichlorfon; metrifonate]

metrizamide USAN, INN *parenteral radiopaque contrast medium (48.25% iodine)*

metrizoate sodium USAN *radiopaque contrast medium* [also: sodium metrizoate]

Metro I.V. ready-to-use injection ℞ *antibiotic; antiprotozoal; amebicide* [metronidazole] 500 mg/100 mL

MetroCream cream ℞ *antibacterial for rosacea* [metronidazole] 0.75%

MetroCream; MetroGel; MetroLotion ℞ *antibiotic for rosacea (orphan); investigational (orphan) for decubitus ulcers and perioral dermatitis* [metronidazole] 0.75%

MetroGel gel ℞ *antibacterial for rosacea; investigational (orphan) for perioral dermatitis* [metronidazole] 1%

MetroGel 1% Kit gel + skin cleanser ℞ *antibacterial for rosacea* [metronidazole; **Cetaphil** cleansing solution (q.v.)] 1%•4 oz.

MetroGel Vaginal gel ℞ *antibacterial for bacterial vaginosis* [metronidazole] 0.75%

MetroLotion lotion ℞ *antibacterial for rosacea* [metronidazole] 0.75%

metronidazole USAN, USP, INN, BAN *antibiotic; antiprotozoal/amebicide; acne rosacea treatment (orphan); investigational (orphan) for perioral dermatitis and advanced decubitus ulcers* 250, 375, 500, 750 mg oral; 500 mg/100 mL injection; 0.75% topical/vaginal

metronidazole benzoate *antiprotozoal (Trichomonas)*

metronidazole HCl USAN *antibiotic; antiprotozoal; amebicide*

metronidazole phosphate USAN *antibacterial; antiprotozoal*

MET-Rx food bar, powder for drink OTC *enteral nutritional therapy* 100 g; 72 g 🔊 Mytrex

Metubine Iodide IV injection (discontinued 2004) ℞ *neuromuscular blocker; anesthesia adjunct* [metocurine iodide] 2 mg/mL

metuclazepam [see: metaclazepam]

meturedepa USAN, INN *antineoplastic*

Metvixia cream ℞ *photosensitizer for photodynamic therapy of precancerous actinic keratoses of the face and scalp; for use with* **CureLight BroadBand Model 01** *(red-light illumination)* [methyl aminolevulinate HCl] 16.8%

metynodiol INN *progestin* [also: methynodiol diacetate]

metynodiol diacetate [see: methynodiol diacetate]

metyrapone USAN, USP, INN *diagnostic aid for testing hypothalamic-pituitary adrenocorticotropic hormone (ACTH) function*

metyrapone tartrate USAN *pituitary function test*

metyridine INN [also: methyridene]

metyrosine USAN, USP *antihypertensive; pheochromocytomic agent*

Mevacor tablets ℞ *HMG-CoA reductase inhibitor for hypercholesterolemia, atherosclerosis, and the prevention and treatment of coronary heart disease (CHD)* [lovastatin] 20, 40 mg

mevastatin INN

mevinolin [now: lovastatin]

mexafylline INN

mexazolam INN

mexenone INN, BAN

mexiletine INN, BAN *antiarrhythmic* [also: mexiletine HCl]

mexiletine HCl USAN, USP *antiarrhythmic* [also: mexiletine] 150, 200, 150 mg

mexiprostil INN

Mexitil capsules ℞ *antiarrhythmic* [mexiletine HCl] 150, 200, 250 mg

mexoprofen INN

mexrenoate potassium USAN, INN *aldosterone antagonist*

Mexsana Medicated powder OTC *diaper rash treatment* [kaolin; zinc oxide; eucalyptus oil; camphor; cornstarch]

mezacopride INN

mezepine INN

mezereon (*Daphne mezereum*) bark *medicinal herb used as a cathartic, diuretic, emetic, and rubefacient; eating the berries can be fatal, and people have been poisoned by eating birds that ate the berries*

mezilamine INN 🔄 mesalamine; muzolimine

Mezlin powder for IV or IM injection (discontinued 2004) ℞ *extended-spectrum penicillin antibiotic* [mezlocillin sodium] 1, 2, 3, 4, 20 g/vial 🔄 Mysoline

mezlocillin USAN, INN *extended-spectrum penicillin antibiotic*

mezlocillin sodium USP *extended-spectrum penicillin antibiotic*

MF (methotrexate [with leucovorin rescue], fluorouracil) *chemotherapy protocol for breast cancer*

MF (mitomycin, fluorouracil) *chemotherapy protocol*

MFP (melphalan, fluorouracil, medroxyprogesterone acetate) *chemotherapy protocol*

MG Cold Sore Formula topical solution OTC *mucous membrane anesthetic; antipruritic; counterirritant* [lidocaine; menthol] 2•1%

MG217 Medicated ointment OTC *antipsoriatic; antiseborrheic; antifungal; keratolytic; antiseptic* [coal tar solution; colloidal sulfur; salicylic acid] 2%•1.1%•1.5%

MG217 Medicated Tar lotion, ointment OTC *antipsoriatic; antiseborrheic* [coal tar solution] 1%; 2%

MG217 Medicated Tar shampoo OTC *antiseborrheic; antipsoriatic; antipruritic; antibacterial* [coal tar] 3%

MG217 Medicated Tar-Free shampoo OTC *antiseborrheic; keratolytic; antiseptic* [sulfur; salicylic acid] 5%•3%

MG217 Sal-Acid ointment OTC *antipsoriatic; keratolytic* [salicylic acid] 3%

MG400 shampoo OTC *antiseborrheic; keratolytic; antiseptic* [salicylic acid; sulfur] 3%•5%

MGA (melengestrol acetate) [q.v.]

MGBG (methylglyoxal-*bis*-guanylhydrazone) [see: mitoguazone]

MGW (magnesium sulfate + glycerin + water) enema [q.v.]

MHP-A tablets ℞ *urinary antibiotic; antiseptic; analgesic; antispasmodic* [methenamine; phenyl salicylate; methylene blue; benzoic acid; atropine sulfate; hyoscyamine sulfate] 40.8•18.1•5.4•4.5•0.03•0.03 mg

Miacalcin metered-dose nasal spray ℞ *calcium regulator for postmenopausal osteoporosis; investigational (orphan) for Paget disease* [calcitonin (salmon)] 200 IU/0.09 mL dose

Miacalcin subcu or IM injection ℞ *calcium regulator for Paget disease (orphan), hypercalcemia, and postmenopausal osteoporosis* [calcitonin (salmon)] 200 IU/mL 🔄 meclozine

Mi-Acid gelcaps OTC *antacid* [calcium carbonate; magnesium carbonate] 311•232 mg

Mi-Acid; Mi-Acid II oral liquid OTC *antacid; antiflatulent* [aluminum hydroxide; magnesium hydroxide; simethicone] 200•200•20 mg/5 mL; 400•400•40 mg/5 mL

mianserin INN, BAN *serotonin inhibitor; antihistamine* [also: mianserin HCl]

mianserin HCl USAN, JAN *serotonin inhibitor; antihistamine* [also: mianserin]

mibefradil INN *vasodilator and calcium channel blocker for hypertension and chronic stable angina* [also: mibefradil dihydrochloride]

mibefradil dihydrochloride USAN *vasodilator and calcium channel blocker for hypertension and chronic stable angina* [also: mibefradil]

M¹³¹IBG [now: iobenguane sulfate I 131]

MIBG-I-123 [see: iobenguane sulfate I 123]

mibolerone USAN, INN *anabolic; androgen*

micafungin sodium *systemic echinocandin antifungal for prophylaxis and treatment of esophageal candidiasis and prophylaxis of candidiasis in patients undergoing hemopoietic stem cell transplantation (HSCT)*

Micardis tablets ℞ *antihypertensive; angiotensin II receptor antagonist* [telmisartan] 20, 40, 80 mg

Micardis HCT tablets ℞ *long-acting antihypertensive; angiotensin II receptor antagonist; diuretic* [telmisartan; hydrochlorothiazide] 40•12.5, 80•12.5, 80•25 mg

Micatin cream, powder, spray powder, spray liquid OTC *antifungal for tinea pedis, tinea cruris, and tinea corporis* [miconazole nitrate] 2% ☒ Megaton

MICE (mesna [rescue], ifosfamide, carboplatin, etoposide) *chemotherapy protocol for osteosarcoma and lung cancer* [also: ICE]

micinicate INN

Miconal cream ℞ *antipsoriatic* [anthralin] 1% ☒ mequinol; Myconel

miconazole USP, INN, BAN, JAN *fungicidal*

Miconazole 7 vaginal suppositories (discontinued 2007) OTC *antifungal* [miconazole nitrate] 100 mg

miconazole nitrate USAN, USP, JAN *antifungal; topical treatment for tinea pedis, tinea cruris, and tinea corporis* 2% topical

Micrainin tablets ℞ *analgesic; antipyretic; anti-inflammatory; anxiolytic; sedative* [aspirin; meprobamate] 325•200 mg

MICRhoGAM IM injection, prefilled syringes ℞ *obstetric Rh factor immunity suppressant* [Rh₀(D) immune globulin (gamma globulin)] 50 mcg (5%)

microbubble contrast agent *investigational (orphan) neurosonographic diagnostic aid for intracranial tumors*

Microcaps (trademarked dosage form) *fast-melting tablets*

microcrystalline cellulose [see: cellulose, microcrystalline]

microcrystalline wax [see: wax, microcrystalline]

microfibrillar collagen hemostat (MCH) *topical hemostat*

Microgestin Fe 1/20 tablets (in packs of 28) ℞ *monophasic oral contraceptive; iron supplement* [norethindrone acetate; ethinyl estradiol; ferrous fumarate] 1 mg•20 mcg•75 mg × 21 days; 0•0•75 mg × 7 days

Microgestin Fe 1.5/30 tablets (in packs of 28) ℞ *monophasic oral contraceptive; iron supplement* [norethindrone acetate; ethinyl estradiol; ferrous fumarate] 1.5 mg•30 mcg•75 mg × 21 days; 0•0•75 mg × 7 days

Micro-K; Micro-K 10 Extencaps (controlled-release capsules) ℞ *potassium supplement* [potassium chloride] 600 mg (8 mEq K); 750 mg (10 mEq K)

Micro-K LS extended-release powder for oral solution ℞ *potassium supplement* [potassium chloride] 20 mEq K/pkt.

MicroKlenz topical liquid OTC *antiseptic wound cleanser* [acemannan]

Microlipid emulsion OTC *dietary fat supplement* [safflower oil] 50%

Micronase tablets ℞ *sulfonylurea antidiabetic that stimulates insulin secretion in the pancreas* [glyburide] 1.25, 2.5, 5 mg

microNefrin solution for inhalation OTC *sympathomimetic bronchodilator for bronchial asthma and COPD; vasopressor for shock* [racepinephrine HCl] 2.25%

micronized aluminum *astringent*

Micronized Glyburide tablets ℞ *sulfonylurea antidiabetic that stimulates insulin secretion in the pancreas* [glyburide] 1.5, 3 mg

micronomicin INN

Micronor [see: Ortho Micronor]
microplasmin, recombinant human *investigational (orphan) adjunct to vitrectomy in pediatric patients*
Microstix-3 reagent strips for professional use ℞ *in vitro diagnostic aid for nitrate, uropathogens, or bacteria in the urine*
MicroTrak *Chlamydia trachomatis* slide test for professional use ℞ *in vitro diagnostic aid for* Chlamydia trachomatis
MicroTrak HSV 1/HSV 2 Culture Identification/Typing Test culture test for professional use ℞ *in vitro diagnostic aid for herpes simplex virus in tissue cultures*
MicroTrak HSV 1/HSV 2 Direct Specimen Identification/Typing Test slide test for professional use ℞ *in vitro diagnostic aid for herpes simplex virus in external lesions*
MicroTrak *Neisseria gonorrhoeae* **Culture Confirmation Test** reagent kit for professional use ℞ *in vitro diagnostic aid for* Neisseria gonorrhoeae
Microzide capsules ℞ *antihypertensive; diuretic* [hydrochlorothiazide] 12.5 mg
mictine [see: aminometradine]
midaflur USAN, INN *sedative*
midaglizole INN
midalcipran [see: milnacipran]
midamaline INN
Midamor tablets ℞ *antihypertensive; potassium-sparing diuretic* [amiloride HCl] 5 mg
midazogrel INN
midazolam INN, BAN, JAN *short-acting benzodiazepine general anesthetic* [also: midazolam HCl]
midazolam HCl USAN *short-acting benzodiazepine general anesthetic* [also: midazolam] 2 mg/mL oral; 1, 5 mg/mL injection
midazolam maleate USAN *intravenous anesthetic*
midecamycin INN
midodrine INN, BAN *antihypotensive; vasoconstrictor; vasopressor for ortho-*

static hypotension (OH) [also: midodrine HCl]
midodrine HCl USAN, JAN *antihypotensive; vasoconstrictor; vasopressor for orthostatic hypotension (orphan); also used for urinary incontinence* [also: midodrine] 2.5, 5 mg oral
Midol Cramp Formula tablets OTC *analgesic; antipyretic; nonsteroidal anti-inflammatory drug (NSAID) for mild to moderate pain of primary dysmenorrhea* [ibuprofen] 200 mg
Midol Extended Relief caplets OTC *analgesic; nonsteroidal anti-inflammatory drug (NSAID) for osteoarthritis, rheumatoid arthritis, juvenile arthritis, ankylosing spondylitis, primary dysmenorrhea, bursitis/tendinitis, and other mild to moderate pain* [naproxen sodium] 220 mg (200 mg base)
Midol Maximum Strength Menstrual caplets, gelcaps OTC *analgesic; antipyretic; antihistamine; sleep aid* [acetaminophen; caffeine; pyrilamine maleate] 500•60•15 mg
Midol PM caplets OTC *analgesic; antipyretic; antihistamine; sleep aid* [acetaminophen; diphenhydramine] 500•25 mg
Midol PMS caplets, gelcaps OTC *analgesic; antipyretic; diuretic; antihistamine; sleep aid* [acetaminophen; pamabrom; pyrilamine maleate] 500•25•15 mg
Midol Teen caplets OTC *analgesic; antipyretic; diuretic* [acetaminophen; pamabrom] 500•25 mg
Midrin capsules ℞ *cerebral vasoconstrictor and analgesic for vascular and tension headaches; "possibly effective" for migraine headaches* [isometheptene mucate; dichloralphenazone; acetaminophen] 65•100•325 mg ② Mudrane
Midstream Pregnancy Test kit for home use OTC *in vitro diagnostic aid; urine pregnancy test*
MIFA (mitomycin, fluorouracil, Adriamycin) chemotherapy protocol
Mifadren; Mifedren *progesterone antagonist; investigational (orphan) for Cushing syndrome* [mifepristone]

mifamurtide *liposomal muramyl tripeptide phosphatidylethanolamine (MTP-PE); investigational (NDA filed, orphan) for high-grade osteosarcoma following surgical resection*

mifarmonab [see: imciromab pentetate]

Mifegyne ⓔ (European name for U.S. product **Mifeprex**) ⊞ Mephaquin

mifentidine INN

Mifeprex tablets ℞ (not available in pharmacies; administered only by a physician in an office, clinic, or hospital setting) *abortifacient for intrauterine pregnancy; postcoital contraceptive; progesterone antagonist; also used for uterine leiomyomata* [mifepristone] 200 mg

mifepristone USAN, INN, BAN *progesterone antagonist; abortifacient for the termination f intrauterine pregnancy; postcoital contraceptive; investigational (Phase III) GR-II antagonist to reduce abnormal cortisol release in psychotic major depression; investigational (orphan) for Cushing syndrome*

mifobate USAN, INN *antiatherosclerotic*

Migergot suppositories ℞ *migraine treatment; vasoconstrictor* [ergotamine tartrate; caffeine] 2•100 mg

miglitol USAN, INN, BAN *antidiabetic agent for type 2 diabetes; alpha-glucosidase inhibitor that delays the digestion of dietary carbohydrates* ⊞ meglutol

miglustat *glucosylceramide synthase inhibitor; substrate reduction therapy (SRT) to reduce the glycosphingolipid (GSL) production in type I Gaucher disease (orphan)*

mignonette, Jamaica *medicinal herb* [see: henna (Lawsonia)]

Migranal nasal spray ℞ *ergot alkaloid for the rapid control of migraine and other vascular headaches* [dihydroergotamine mesylate] 0.5 mg/spray

MigraTen capsules ℞ *cerebral vasoconstrictor and analgesic for migraine and tension headaches* [isometheptene mucate; acetaminophen; caffeine] 65•325•100 mg

Migratine capsules (discontinued 2008) ℞ *cerebral vasoconstrictor and analgesic for vascular and tension headaches; "possibly effective" for migraine headaches* [isometheptene mucate; dichloralphenazone; acetaminophen] 65•100•325 mg

mikamycin INN, BAN

MiKasome *investigational (Phase II) antibiotic liposomal formulation for complicated urinary tract infections and AIDS-related mycobacterial infections* [amikacin]

milacemide INN *anticonvulsant; antidepressant* [also: milacemide HCl]

milacemide HCl USAN *anticonvulsant; antidepressant* [also: milacemide]

milameline HCl USAN *partial muscarinic agonist for Alzheimer disease*

mild silver protein [see: silver protein, mild]

milenperone USAN, INN, BAN *antipsychotic*

Miles Nervine caplets OTC *antihistamine; sleep aid* [diphenhydramine HCl] 25 mg

milfoil *medicinal herb* [see: yarrow]

milipertine USAN, INN *antipsychotic*

milk ipecac *medicinal herb* [see: birthroot; dogbane]

milk of bismuth [see: bismuth, milk of]

milk of magnesia (MOM) [see: magnesia, milk of]

Milk of Magnesia-Cascara, Concentrated oral suspension OTC *antacid; saline/stimulant laxative* [milk of magnesia; aromatic cascara fluidextract; alcohol 7%] 30•5 mL/15 mL

milk thistle (Silybum marianum) seeds *medicinal herb for Amanita mushroom poisoning, bronchitis, gallbladder disorders, hemorrhage, liver damage, peritonitis, spleen disorders, stomach disorders, and varicose veins*

milkweed (Asclepias syriaca) roots *medicinal herb used as a diuretic, emetic, purgative, and tonic*

Millipred oral solution ℞ *corticosteroid; anti-inflammatory* [prednisolone] 15 mg/5 mL

milnacipran INN *investigational (Phase III) serotonin and norepinephrine reuptake inhibitor for depression and fibromyalgia syndrome*

milodistim USAN *antineutropenic; hematopoietic stimulant; granulocyte macrophage colony-stimulating factor (GM-CSF) + interleukin 3*

miloxacin INN

milrinone USAN, INN, BAN *cardiotonic*

milrinone lactate *vasodilator for congestive heart failure* 1 mg/mL injection

miltefosine INN *anthelmintic for leishmaniasis; investigational for HIV infections*

Miltown tablets ℞ *anxiolytic; also abused as a street drug* [meprobamate] 200, 400 mg

milverine INN

mimbane INN *analgesic* [also: mimbane HCl]

mimbane HCl USAN *analgesic* [also: mimbane]

Mimyx cream ℞ *emollient for various dermatoses* [betaine; olive oil; glycerin]

minalrestat USAN *aldose reductase inhibitor for diabetic neuropathy and other long-term diabetic complications*

minaprine USAN, INN, BAN *psychotropic* ⟳ Magnaprin

minaprine HCl USAN *antidepressant*

minaxolone USAN, INN *anesthetic*

mindodilol INN

mindolic acid [see: clometacin]

mindoperone INN

MINE (mesna [rescue], ifosfamide, Novantrone, etoposide) *chemotherapy protocol for non-Hodgkin lymphoma*

MINE-ESHAP (alternating cycles of MINE and ESHAP) *chemotherapy protocol for non-Hodgkin lymphoma*

minepentate INN, BAN

Mineral Ice [see: Therapeutic Mineral Ice]

mineral oil USP *emollient/protectant; moisturizer/lubricant; laxative; solvent*

mineral oil, light NF *tablet and capsule lubricant; vehicle*

mineralocorticoids *a class of adrenal cortical steroids that are used for partial replacement therapy in adrenocortical insufficiency*

Mini Two-Way Action tablets OTC *bronchodilator; decongestant; expectorant* [ephedrine HCl; guaifenesin] 12.5●200, 25●200 mg

MiniAdFVIII *investigational (orphan) agent for hemophilia A* [adenovirus-based vector Factor VIII complementary DNA to somatic cells]

mini-BEAM (BCNU, etoposide, ara-C, melphalan) *chemotherapy protocol for Hodgkin lymphoma*

mini-COAP (cyclophosphamide, Oncovin, ara-C, prednisone) *chemotherapy protocol*

Minidyne solution OTC *broad-spectrum antimicrobial* [povidone-iodine] 10% ⟳ menadione

Min-I-Mix (delivery form) *dual-chambered prefilled syringe*

Minipress capsules ℞ *antihypertensive; α_1-adrenergic blocker* [prazosin HCl] 1, 2, 5 mg

Minirin nasal spray ℞ *posterior pituitary hormone for hemophilia A (orphan), von Willebrand disease (orphan), central diabetes insipidus, and nocturnal enuresis* [desmopressin acetate; chlorobutanol] 10●500 mcg/dose

Minitran transdermal patch ℞ *coronary vasodilator; antianginal; also used for acute myocardial infarction, erectile dysfunction, and Raynaud disease* [nitroglycerin] 0.1, 0.2, 0.4, 0.6 mg/hr. (9, 18, 36, 54 mg total)

Minit-Rub OTC *analgesic; mild anesthetic; antipruritic; counterirritant* [methyl salicylate; menthol; camphor] 15%●3.5%●2.3%

Minizide 1; Minizide 2; Minizide 5 capsules (discontinued 2007) ℞ *antihypertensive; α-blocker; diuretic* [prazosin HCl; polythiazide] 1●0.5 mg; 2●0.5 mg; 5●0.5 mg ⟳ Monocid

Minocin pellet-filled capsules, oral suspension ℞ *tetracycline antibiotic for gram-negative and gram-positive bacteria; antirickettsial; investigational (orphan) for chronic malignant pleural*

effusion [minocycline HCl] 50, 100 mg; 50 mg/5 mL

Minocin powder for IV injection ℞ *tetracycline antibiotic for gram-negative and gram-positive bacteria; antirickettsial; investigational (orphan) for chronic malignant pleural effusion* [minocycline] 100 mg/vial

Minocin PAC (Professional Acne Care) 60 capsules plus 3 skin care products ℞ *tetracycline antibiotic for acne* [minocycline HCl] 50, 100 mg

minocromil USAN, INN, BAN *prophylactic antiallergic*

minocycline USAN, INN, BAN *tetracycline antibiotic for gram-negative and gram-positive bacteria; antirickettsial; adjunct to scaling and root planing for periodontitis*

minocycline HCl USP *tetracycline antibiotic for gram-negative and gram-positive bacteria; antirickettsial; investigational (orphan) for chronic malignant pleural effusion* 50, 75, 100 mg oral

minoxidil USAN, USP, INN, BAN *antihypertensive; peripheral vasodilator; topical hair growth stimulant* 2.5, 10 mg oral

Minoxidil for Men topical solution OTC *hair growth stimulant* [minoxidil; alcohol 30%] 5%

Minreal Freez gel OTC *mild anesthetic; antipruritic; counterirritant* [menthol] 2%

mint; lamb mint; mackerel mint; Our Lady's mint *medicinal herb* [see: spearmint]

mint, brandy; lamb mint *medicinal herb* [see: peppermint]

mint, mountain *medicinal herb* [see: marjoram; Oswego tea]

mint, squaw *medicinal herb* [see: pennyroyal]

Mintezol chewable tablets, oral suspension ℞ *anthelmintic for strongyloidiasis (threadworm), larva migrans, and trichinosis* [thiabendazole] 500 mg; 500 mg/5 mL

Mintox chewable tablets OTC *antacid* [aluminum hydroxide; magnesium hydroxide] 200•200 mg ▣ Mentax

Mintox oral suspension OTC *antacid; antiflatulent* [aluminum hydroxide; magnesium hydroxide; simethicone] 200•200•20 mg/5 mL ▣ Mentax

Mintox Plus oral liquid OTC *antacid; antiflatulent* [aluminum hydroxide; magnesium hydroxide; simethicone] 500•450•40 mg/5 mL

Mintuss MR syrup (discontinued 2007) ℞ *narcotic antitussive; antihistamine; sleep aid; decongestant* [hydrocodone bitartrate; pyrilamine maleate; phenylephrine HCl] 10•10•10 mg/10 mL

Minute-Gel ℞ *dental caries preventative* [acidulated phosphate fluoride] 1.23%

Miochol-E solution ℞ *direct-acting miotic for ophthalmic surgery* [acetylcholine chloride] 1:100

mioflazine INN, BAN *coronary vasodilator* [also: mioflazine HCl]

mioflazine HCl USAN *coronary vasodilator* [also: mioflazine]

Miostat solution ℞ *direct-acting miotic for ophthalmic surgery* [carbachol] 0.01%

miotics *a class of drugs that cause the pupil of the eye to contract*

mipafilcon A USAN *hydrophilic contact lens material*

mipimazole INN

mipomersen *investigational (Phase III) treatment for familial hypercholesterolemia*

MiraFlow solution OTC *cleaning solution for hard or soft contact lenses*

MiraForte [see: Super MiraForte with Chrysin]

MiraLAX powder for oral solution OTC (previously ℞) *hyperosmotic laxative; pre-procedure bowel evacuant* [polyethylene glycol 3350] 17 g/dose

Mirapex tablets ℞ *dopamine agonist for idiopathic Parkinson disease; treatment for primary restless legs syndrome (RLS)* [pramipexole dihydrochloride] 0.125, 0.25, 0.5, 0.75, 1, 1.5 mg

Miraphen PSE extended-release tablets (discontinued 2007) ℞ *deconges-*

tant; expectorant [pseudoephedrine HCl; guaifenesin] 120•600 mg

MiraSept Step 2 solution OTC *rinsing/ storage solution for soft contact lenses* [sodium chloride (preserved saline solution)]

MiraSept System solutions OTC *two-step chemical disinfecting system for soft contact lenses* [hydrogen peroxide–based]

Miraxion *investigational (Phase III) for Huntington disease* [semi-synthetic derivative of eicosapentaenoic acid (EPA)]

Mircera IV injection in single-use vials and prefilled syringes ℞ *erythropoiesis-stimulating agent (ESA) for the treatment of anemia due to chronic renal failure (orphan)* [epoetin beta (in methoxy PEG)] 50, 75, 100, 150, 200, 250, 300, 400, 600, 800, 1000 mcg

Mircette tablets (in packs of 28) ℞ *biphasic oral contraceptive* [desogestrel; ethinyl estradiol]
Phase 1 (21 days): 0.15 mg•20 mcg;
Phase 2 (5 days): 0•10 mcg;
Counters (2 days)

Mirena intrauterine device (IUD) ℞ *long-term (5 year) contraceptive insert* [levonorgestrel] 20 mcg/day ⊡ Murine

mirfentanil INN *analgesic* [also: mirfentanil HCl]

mirfentanil HCl USAN *analgesic* [also: mirfentanil]

mirincamycin INN *antibacterial; antimalarial* [also: mirincamycin HCl]

mirincamycin HCl USAN *antibacterial; antimalarial* [also: mirincamycin]

mirisetron maleate USAN *anxiolytic*

miristalkonium chloride INN

miroprofen INN

mirosamicin INN

mirostipen USAN *myeloprotectant*

mirtazapine USAN, INN *tetracyclic antidepressant; serotonin 5-HT$_{1A}$ agonist* 7.5, 15, 30, 45 mg oral

misonidazole USAN, INN *antiprotozoal (Trichomonas)*

misoprostol USAN, INN, BAN *prevents NSAID-induced gastric ulcers; has been*

used for cervical ripening and induction of labor; use by pregnant women can cause abortion, premature birth, or birth defects; investigational (orphan) for complete expulsion of the products of conception 100, 200 mcg oral

Mission Prenatal; Mission Prenatal F.A.; Mission Prenatal H.P. tablets OTC *vitamin/iron supplement* [multiple vitamins; ferrous gluconate; folic acid] ≗•30•0.4 mg; ≗•30•0.8 mg; ≗•30•0.8 mg

Mission Prenatal Rx tablets ℞ *vitamin/calcium/iron supplement* [multiple vitamins; calcium; iron; folic acid] ≗•175•29.5•1 mg

Mission Surgical Supplement tablets OTC *vitamin/iron supplement* [multiple vitamins; ferrous gluconate] ≗•27 mg

mistletoe (*Phoradendron flavescens; P. serotinum; P. tomentosum; Viscum album*) plant *medicinal herb for cancer, chorea, epilepsy, hypertension, internal hemorrhages, menstrual disorders, nervousness, poor circulation, and spleen disorders; not generally regarded as safe and effective for ingestion as it is highly toxic*

Mistometer (trademarked delivery form) *metered-dose inhalation aerosol*

Mitchella repens *medicinal herb* [see: squaw vine]

mithramycin [now: plicamycin]

mitindomide USAN, INN *antineoplastic*

mitobronitol INN, BAN

mitocarcin USAN, INN *antineoplastic*

mitoclomine INN, BAN

mitocromin USAN *antineoplastic*

mitoflaxone INN

mitogillin USAN, INN *antineoplastic*

mitoguazone INN *investigational (orphan) antineoplastic for non-Hodgkin lymphoma*

mitolactol INN *investigational (orphan) antineoplastic for brain tumors and recurrent or metastatic cervical squamous cell carcinoma*

mitomalcin USAN, INN *antineoplastic*

mitomycin USAN, USP, INN, BAN *antibiotic antineoplastic for disseminated* adenocarcinoma of the stomach or pancreas; investigational (orphan) for refractory glaucoma and glaucoma surgery 5, 20, 40 mg injection

mitomycin C (MTC) [see: mitomycin]

mitonafide INN

mitopodozide INN, BAN

mitoquidone INN, BAN

mitosper USAN, INN antineoplastic

mitotane USAN, USP, INN antibiotic antineoplastic for inoperable adrenal cortical carcinoma and Cushing syndrome ☒ metetoin

mitotenamine INN, BAN

mitotic inhibitors a class of antineoplastics that inhibit cell division (mitosis)

mitoxantrone INN antibiotic antineoplastic [also: mitoxantrone HCl; mitozantrone]

mitoxantrone HCl USAN antibiotic antineoplastic for prostate cancer (orphan) and acute nonlymphocytic leukemia (ANLL) (orphan); immunomodulator for progressive and relapsing-remitting multiple sclerosis (orphan) [also: mitoxantrone; mitozantrone] 2 mg/mL injection

mitozantrone BAN antineoplastic [also: mitoxantrone HCl; mitoxantrone]

mitozolomide INN, BAN

Mitrolan chewable tablets (discontinued 2004) OTC bulk laxative; antidiarrheal [calcium polycarbophil] 625 mg

mitronal [see: cinnarizine]

mitumomab USAN antineoplastic monoclonal antibody for G_{D3} ganglioside–expressing tumors; investigational (Phase III) for small cell lung cancer

Mivacron IV infusion (discontinued 2006) ℞ muscle relaxant; adjunct to anesthesia [mivacurium chloride] 0.5, 2 mg/mL

mivacurium chloride USAN, INN, BAN neuromuscular blocking agent

mivobulin isethionate USAN antineoplastic; mitotic inhibitor; tubulin binder

Mixed E 400; Mixed E 1000 softgels OTC vitamin supplement [vitamin E] 400 IU; 1000 IU

mixed tocopherols [see: vitamin E]

mixidine USAN, INN coronary vasodilator ☒ Maxidone

Mix-O-Vial (trademarked delivery form) two-compartment vial

mizoribine INN

MK-518 investigational (Phase III) antiretroviral HIV-1 integrase inhibitor to prevent HIV replication

MKC-442 investigational (Phase III) non-nucleoside reverse transcriptase inhibitor (NNRTI) for HIV and AIDS

MM (mercaptopurine, methotrexate) chemotherapy protocol

MMOPP (methotrexate, mechlorethamine, Oncovin, procarbazine, prednisone) chemotherapy protocol

MMP (matrix metalloproteinase) inhibitors [q.v.]

MMR (measles, mumps & rubella vaccines) [q.v.]

M-M-R II powder for subcu injection ℞ measles, mumps, and rubella vaccine [measles, mumps, and rubella virus vaccine, live; neomycin] 1000 U•20 000 U•1000 U•25 mcg/0.5 mL dose

MOB (mechlorethamine, Oncovin, bleomycin) chemotherapy protocol

MOB-III (mitomycin, Oncovin, bleomycin, cisplatin) chemotherapy protocol

Moban tablets ℞ conventional (typical) dihydroindolone antipsychotic for schizophrenia [molindone HCl] 5, 10, 25, 50 mg

mobecarb INN

mobenzoxamine INN

Mobic tablets, oral suspension ℞ once-daily analgesic; antipyretic; nonsteroidal anti-inflammatory drug (NSAID) for osteoarthritis, rheumatoid arthritis, and juvenile rheumatoid arthritis; also used for ankylosing spondylitis and acute bursitis/tendinitis [meloxicam] 7.5, 15 mg; 7.5 mg/5 mL ☒ MBC

Mobidin tablets ℞ analgesic; antipyretic; anti-inflammatory; antirheumatic [magnesium salicylate] 600 mg

Mobigesic tablets OTC analgesic; antipyretic; anti-inflammatory; antihistamine;

sleep aid [magnesium salicylate; phenyltoloxamine citrate] 325•30 mg

Mobisyl Creme OTC *analgesic* [trolamine salicylate] 10%

MOBP (mitomycin, Oncovin, bleomycin, Platinol) *chemotherapy protocol for cervical cancer* ② MABOP; Māpap; MOP-BAP

moccasin snake antivenin [see: antivenin (Crotalidae) polyvalent]

mocimycin INN

mociprazine INN

mock pennyroyal *medicinal herb* [see: pennyroyal]

moclobemide USAN, INN, BAN *antidepressant; MAO inhibitor*

moctamide INN

Moctanin biliary infusion (discontinued 2005) ℞ *anticholelithogenic for dissolution of cholesterol gallstones (orphan)* [monoctanoin]

modafinil USAN, INN *analeptic for excessive daytime sleepiness due to narcolepsy (orphan), obstructive sleep apnea, or shift work sleep disorder (SWSD); also used for fatigue associated with multiple sclerosis*

modaline INN *antidepressant* [also: modaline sulfate]

modaline sulfate USAN *antidepressant* [also: modaline]

Modane enteric-coated tablets OTC *stimulant laxative* [bisacodyl] 5 mg

modecainide USAN, INN *antiarrhythmic*

Modicon tablets (in Dialpaks and Veridates of 28) ℞ *monophasic oral contraceptive* [norethindrone; ethinyl estradiol] 0.5 mg•35 mcg × 21 days; counters × 7 days ② Medicone

modified Bagshawe protocol *chemotherapy protocol* [see: CHAMOCA]

modified bovine lung surfactant extract [see: beractant]

modified Burow solution [see: aluminum acetate solution]

modified cellulose gum [now: croscarmellose sodium]

modified Shohl solution (sodium citrate & citric acid) *urinary alkalinizer; compounding agent*

Modiodal (foreign name for U.S. product **Provigil**)

Modical powder OTC *carbohydrate caloric supplement* [glucose polymers]

Moduretic tablets ℞ *antihypertensive; diuretic* [amiloride HCl; hydrochlorothiazide] 5•50 mg

moexipril INN, BAN *antihypertensive; angiotensin-converting enzyme (ACE) inhibitor*

moexipril HCl USAN *antihypertensive; angiotensin-converting enzyme (ACE) inhibitor* 7.5, 15 mg oral

moexipril HCl & hydrochlorothiazide *antihypertensive; angiotensin-converting enzyme (ACE) inhibitor; diuretic* 7.5•12.5, 15•12.5, 15•25 mg oral

moexiprilat INN

MOF (MeCCNU, Oncovin, fluorouracil) *chemotherapy protocol*

mofebutazone INN

mofedione [see: oxazidione]

mofegiline INN *antiparkinsonian* [also: mofegiline HCl]

mofegiline HCl USAN *antiparkinsonian* [also: mofegiline]

mofetil USAN, INN *combining name for radicals or groups*

mofloverine INN

mofoxime INN

MOF-STREP; MOF-Strep (MeCCNU, Oncovin, fluorouracil, streptozocin) *chemotherapy protocol*

moguisteine INN

Moist Again vaginal gel OTC *moisturizer/lubricant* [glycerin; aloe vera]

Moi-Stir throat spray, Swabsticks OTC *saliva substitute*

Moisture Drops eye drops OTC *moisturizer/lubricant* [hydroxypropyl methylcellulose] 0.5%

Moisture Eyes eye drops OTC *moisturizer/lubricant* [propylene glycol] 0.95%

mold allergenic extracts *diagnosis and treatment of allergies*

molfarnate INN

molgramostim USAN, INN, BAN *antineutropenic and hematopoietic stimulant; investigational (orphan) for bone marrow transplants, chronic lympho-*

cytic leukemia (CLL), myelodysplastic syndrome, aplastic anemia, and AIDS-related neutropenia

molinazone USAN, INN *analgesic*

molindone INN *conventional (typical) dihydroindolone antipsychotic for schizophrenia* [also: molindone HCl]

molindone HCl USAN *conventional (typical) dihydroindolone antipsychotic for schizophrenia* [also: molindone]

Mollifene Ear Wax Removing Formula ear drops OTC *cerumenolytic to emulsify and disperse ear wax* [carbamide peroxide] 6.5%

molracetam INN

molsidomine USAN, INN *antianginal; coronary vasodilator*

molybdenum *element (Mo)*

Molypen IV injection ℞ *intravenous nutritional therapy* [ammonium molybdate tetrahydrate] 25 mcg/mL

MOM (milk of magnesia) [see: magnesia, milk of]

Momentum caplets OTC *analgesic; antipyretic; anti-inflammatory; antihistamine; sleep aid* [aspirin; phenyltoloxamine citrate] 500•15 mg

Momentum Muscular Backache Formula caplets OTC *analgesic; antipyretic; anti-inflammatory* [magnesium salicylate] 580 mg

mometasone INN, BAN *topical corticosteroidal anti-inflammatory* [also: mometasone furoate]

mometasone furoate USAN *topical corticosteroidal anti-inflammatory; oral inhalation aerosol for chronic asthma; nasal aerosol for allergic rhinitis and nasal polyps* [also: mometasone] 0.1% topical

Momordica charantia medicinal herb [see: bitter melon]

MOMP (mechlorethamine, Oncovin, methotrexate, prednisone) *chemotherapy protocol*

monalazone disodium INN

monalium hydrate [see: magaldrate]

Monarc-M powder for IV injection ℞ *systemic hemostatic; antihemophilic for the prevention and control of bleeding* in classical hemophilia (hemophilia A) and von Willebrand disease (orphan) [antihemophilic factor concentrate] 2–15 IU/mg

Monarda didyma medicinal herb [see: Oswego tea]

Monarda fistulosa medicinal herb [see: wild bergamot]

Monarda punctata medicinal herb [see: horsemint]

monarsen *investigational (orphan) for myasthenia gravis*

monascus yeast (Monascus purpureus) *natural remedy for gastric disorders, indigestion, lowering cholesterol, and poor circulation*

monatepil INN *antianginal; antihypertensive* [also: monatepil maleate]

monatepil maleate USAN *antianginal; antihypertensive* [also: monatepil]

monensin USAN, INN *antiprotozoal; antibacterial; antifungal*

Monistat cream OTC *antifungal* [miconazole nitrate] 2%

Monistat 1 vaginal ointment in prefilled applicator OTC *antifungal* [tioconazole] 6.5%

Monistat 1 Combination Pack vaginal inserts + cream OTC *antifungal* [miconazole nitrate] 200 mg + 2%

Monistat 1-Day vaginal ointment in prefilled applicator OTC *antifungal* [tioconazole] 6.5%

Monistat 3 vaginal cream, combination pack (vaginal inserts + cream), cream combination pak (vaginal cream in prefilled applicators + external cream) OTC *antifungal* [miconazole nitrate] 2%; 200 mg + 2%; 4% + 2%

Monistat 7 vaginal inserts, vaginal cream, combination pack (inserts + cream) OTC *antifungal* [miconazole nitrate] 100 mg; 2%; 100 mg + 2%

Monistat-Derm cream (discontinued 2008) ℞ *antifungal for tinea pedis, tinea cruris, and tinea corporis* [miconazole nitrate] 2%

mono- & di-acetylated monoglycerides NF *plasticizer*

mono- & di-glycerides NF *emulsifying agent*

monoamine oxidase (MAO) inhibitors (MAOIs) *a class of antidepressants that increase CNS monoamine neurotransmitters (epinephrine, norepinephrine, and serotonin)*

monobactams *a class of bactericidal antibiotics effective against gram-negative aerobic pathogens*

monobasic potassium phosphate [see: potassium phosphate, monobasic]

monobasic sodium phosphate [see: sodium phosphate, monobasic]

monobenzone USP, INN *depigmenting agent for vitiligo*

monobenzyl ether of hydroquinone [see: monobenzone]

monobromated camphor [see: camphor, monobromated]

Monocal tablets OTC *calcium/fluoride supplement* [calcium; fluoride] 250•3 mg ⑦ Magnacal

monocalcium phosphate [see: calcium phosphate, dibasic]

Monocaps tablets OTC *vitamin/mineral/iron supplement* [multiple vitamins & minerals; ferrous fumarate; folic acid; biotin] ±•14 mg•0.1 mg•15 mcg

Mono-Chlor topical liquid R̆ *cauterant; keratolytic* [monochloroacetic acid] 80%

monochloroacetic acid *strong keratolytic/cauterant*

monochlorothymol [see: chlorothymol]

monochlorphenamide [see: clofenamide]

Monocid powder for IV or IM injection (discontinued 2004) R̆ *second-generation cephalosporin antibiotic* [cefonicid sodium] 1, 10 g ⑦ Minizide

Monoclate P powder for IV injection R̆ *systemic hemostatic; antihemophilic for the prevention and control of bleeding in classical hemophilia (hemophilia A) and von Willebrand disease* (orphan) [antihemophilic factor concentrate,

human] (actual number of AHF units is indicated on the vial)

monoclonal antibodies (MAb; MAB) *a class of biological agents that have been cloned (exact copies produced asexually in vitro or in vivo) from a single cell harvested from a human, mouse, or rat; cloning multiplies the number of antibodies attacking the target* [compare: chimeric, human, humanized, and murine variants]

monoclonal antibody 1D10, humanized *investigational (orphan) agent for non-Hodgkin B-cell lymphoma*

monoclonal antibody 5A8 to CD4 *investigational (orphan) for post-exposure prophylaxis to occupational HIV exposure*

monoclonal antibody 5c8, recombinant humanized [now: ruplizumab]

monoclonal antibody 5G1.1, humanized *investigational (orphan) C5 complement inhibitor for dermatomyositis*

monoclonal antibody 7E3 [see: abciximab]

monoclonal antibody 7E3 [see: abciximab]

monoclonal antibody to alpha-fetoprotein (AFP), murine, radiolabeled with iodine I 123 *investigational (orphan) diagnostic aid for AFP-producing tumors, hepatocellular carcinoma, and hepatoblastoma*

monoclonal antibody to alpha-fetoprotein (AFP), murine, radiolabeled with iodine I 131 *investigational (orphan) for AFP-producing tumors, hepatocellular carcinoma, and hepatoblastoma*

monoclonal antibody to alpha-fetoprotein (AFP), murine, radiolabeled with technetium Tc 99m *investigational (orphan) diagnostic aid for AFP-producing tumors, hepatoblastoma, and hepatocellular carcinoma*

monoclonal antibody to anti-idiotype melanoma-associated antigen, murine *investigational (orphan) for invasive cutaneous melanoma*

monoclonal antibody to B4, ricin (blocked) conjugated murine *investigational (orphan) for B-cell lymphoma, leukemia, and treatment of bone marrow in non-T-cell acute lymphocytic leukemia*

monoclonal antibody B43.13 *investigational (orphan) for epithelial ovarian cancer*

monoclonal antibody to B-cell lymphoma, murine or human *investigational (orphan) for B-cell lymphoma*

monoclonal antibody to cA2, chimeric [see: infliximab]

monoclonal antibody to carcinoembryonic antigen (CEA), chimeric (sheep-human) [now: labetuzumab]

monoclonal antibody to carcinoembryonic antigen (CEA), chimeric (sheep-human), radiolabeled with yttrium Y 90 [now: yttrium Y 90 labetuzumab]

monoclonal antibody to carcinoembryonic antigen (CEA), humanized [now: altumomab; altumomab pentetate]

monoclonal antibody to carcinoembryonic antigen (CEA), humanized, radiolabeled with indium In 111 [now: indium In 111 altumomab pentetate]

monoclonal antibody to CD2, humanized *investigational (orphan) for graft-versus-host disease and prevention of renal transplant rejection*

monoclonal antibody to CD3 [see: muromonab-CD3; teplizumab; visilizumab]

monoclonal antibody to CD4, human *investigational (orphan) for mycosis fungoides*

monoclonal antibody to CD6, ricin (blocked) conjugated murine *investigational (orphan) for T-cell leukemias, lymphomas, and other mature T-cell malignancies*

monoclonal antibody to CD16, humanized *investigational (Phase III) for adult immune thrombocytopenic purpura (ITP)*

monoclonal antibody to CD22 antigen on B-cells [now: epratuzumab]

monoclonal antibody to CD23 immunoglobulin G1 (IgG1) kappa *investigational (orphan) for chronic lymphocytic leukemia*

monoclonal antibody to CD30, human *investigational (orphan) for Hodgkin disease and T-cell lymphomas*

monoclonal antibody to CD40 *investigational (orphan) for multiple myeloma*

monoclonal antibody to CD45 *investigational (orphan) to prevent acute graft rejection of human organ transplants*

monoclonal antibody to CD55 *investigational (orphan) for gastric tumors*

monoclonal antibody to cytomegalovirus (CMV), human *investigational (orphan) to prevent or treat CMV retinitis and other CMV infections due to bone marrow transplants, organ transplants, or AIDS*

monoclonal antibody to endotoxin E5 [now: edobacomab]

monoclonal antibody to epidermal growth factor receptor (EGFR) protein [see: cetuximab; gefitinib; panitumumab]

monoclonal antibody Fab to myosin, murine [now: imciromab pentetate]

monoclonal antibody Fab to myosin, murine, radiolabeled with indium In 111 [now: indium In 111 imciromab pentetate]

monoclonal antibody to fibrin [now: biciromab]

monoclonal antibody G250 to IgG, chimeric (human-murine) *investigational (orphan) agent for renal cell carcinoma*

monoclonal antibody to gpIIb/IIIa [now: abciximab]

monoclonal antibody to hepatitis B virus, human [now: tuvirumab]

monoclonal antibody to hsp90, recombinant human [now: efungumab]

monoclonal antibody HuM291, chimeric (human-mouse) [now: visilizumab]

monoclonal antibody to human chorionic gonadotropin (hCG), murine, radiolabeled with iodine I 123 *investigational (orphan) diagnostic aid for hCG-producing tumors*

monoclonal antibody to human chorionic gonadotropin (hCG), murine, radiolabeled with iodine I 131 *investigational (orphan) for hCG-producing tumors*

monoclonal antibody to human chorionic gonadotropin (hCG), murine, radiolabeled with technetium Tc 99m *investigational (orphan) diagnostic aid for hCG-producing tumors such as germ cell and trophoblastic cell tumors*

monoclonal antibody to human epidermal growth factor receptor 2 (HER2) protein [see: trastuzumab]

monoclonal antibody IDEC-131 to CD40L, humanized *investigational (Phase II, orphan) for systemic lupus erythematosus (SLE)*

monoclonal antibody IgG$_{1k}$ to CTLA-4, human *investigational (orphan) for high-risk stages II, III, and IV melanoma*

monoclonal antibody IgG$_{2a}$ to B cell, murine [now: bectumomab]

monoclonal antibody IgG$_{2a}$ to B cell, murine, radiolabeled with iodine I 131 *investigational (orphan) for B-cell leukemia and lymphoma*

monoclonal antibody IgG$_{2a}$ to B cell, murine, radiolabeled with technetium Tc 99m [now: technetium Tc 99m bectumomab]

monoclonal antibody IgM (C-58) to cytomegalovirus (CMV) *investigational (orphan) treatment and prophylaxis of CMV infections in allogenic bone marrow transplants*

monoclonal antibody to integrin receptor avb3/avb5, human *investigational (orphan) for high-risk stages II, III, and IV malignant melanoma*

monoclonal antibody to interleukin-6 receptors, humanized [see: tocilizumab]

monoclonal antibody to leukocyte function–associated antigen-1 (LFA-1), recombinant humanized [now: efalizumab]

monoclonal antibody LL2, humanized [now: epratuzumab]

monoclonal antibody to lupus nephritis *investigational (orphan) for immunization against lupus nephritis*

monoclonal antibody to Lym-1, radiolabeled with iodine I 131 *investigational (Phase III, orphan) treatment for non-Hodgkin B-cell lymphoma*

monoclonal antibody to melanoma, murine, radiolabeled with technetium Tc 99m *investigational (orphan) for diagnostic imaging agent for metastases of malignant melanoma*

monoclonal antibody M-T412 IgG to CD4, chimeric (human-murine) [now: priliximab]

monoclonal antibody to MY9, ricin (blocked) conjugated murine *investigational (orphan) for myeloid leukemia (including acute myelogenous leukemia [AML]), ex vivo treatment of autologous bone marrow in AML, and blast crisis in chronic myeloid leukemia (CML)*

monoclonal antibody to N901, ricin (blocked) conjugated murine *investigational (orphan) for small cell lung cancer*

monoclonal antibody to non-Hodgkin lymphoma (NHL) [now: tositumomab]

monoclonal antibody to non-Hodgkin lymphoma (NHL), radiolabeled with iodine I 131 [now: iodine I 131 tositumomab]

monoclonal antibody to pan T lymphocyte [now: zolimomab aritox]

monoclonal antibody to platelet-derived growth factor D, human *investigational (orphan) to slow the progression of IgA nephropathy and delay kidney failure*

monoclonal antibody to polymor-phic epithelial mucin, murine *investigational (Phase III, orphan) adjunctive treatment for ovarian cancer*

monoclonal antibody SC-1 [see: monoclonal antibody to CD55]

monoclonal antibody to Shiga-like toxin II, humanized *investigational (orphan) for the treatment of hemolytic uremic syndrome due to Shiga-like toxin–producing E. coli*

monoclonal antibody to Staphylococ-cus, chimeric, humanized *investigational (orphan) prophylaxis of S. epidermidis sepsis in low birthweight infants*

monoclonal antibody to TNF (tumor necrosis factor) [now: nerelimomab]

monoclonal antibody to TNF, chimeric A2 (human-murine) IgG [now: infliximab]

monoclonal antibody to TNFα (tumor necrosis factor alpha) [now: infliximab]

monoclonal antibody to transform-ing growth factor beta 1, human *investigational (orphan) for systemic sclerosis* [compare: anti–transforming growth factor B1,2,3]

monoclonal antibody tumor necro-sis treatment (TNT-1B), chimeric, radiolabeled with iodine I 131 *investigational (orphan) treatment for malignant glioblastoma multiforme and anaplastic astrocytoma*

monoclonal antibody to vascular endothelial growth factor, recom-binant human (rhuMAb-VEGF) [now: bevacizumab]

monoclonal antibody vehicles [see: targeted monoclonal antibody vehi-cles (T-MAVs)]

monoclonal antibody XMMEn-0e5 to endotoxin [now: edobacomab]

monoclonal factor IX [see: factor IX complex]

monoctanoin USAN, BAN *anticholelithogenic for dissolution of cholesterol gallstones (orphan)*

monoctanoin component A

monoctanoin component B

monoctanoin component C

monoctanoin component D

Mono-Diff reagent kit for professional use ℞ *in vitro diagnostic aid for mononucleosis*

Monodox capsules ℞ *tetracycline antibiotic* [doxycycline monohydrate] 50, 100 mg

Mono-Drop (trademarked delivery form) *prefilled eye drop dispenser*

monoethanolamine NF *surfactant*

monoethanolamine oleate INN *sclerosing agent* [also: ethanolamine oleate]

Mono-Gesic film-coated tablets (discontinued 2004) ℞ *analgesic; antipyretic; anti-inflammatory; antirheumatic* [salsalate] 750 mg

Monoket tablets ℞ *coronary vasodilator; antianginal* [isosorbide mononitrate] 10, 20 mg

Mono-Latex reagent kit for professional use ℞ *in vitro diagnostic aid for mononucleosis*

monolaurin *investigational (Phase III, orphan) for nonbullous congenital ichthyosiform erythroderma (a.k.a. congenital primary ichthyosis)*

monometacrine INN

Mononessa tablets (in packs of 28) ℞ *monophasic oral contraceptive* [norgestimate; ethinyl estradiol] 0.25 mg• 35 mcg × 21 days; counters × 7 days

Mononine powder for IV infusion ℞ *systemic hemostatic; antihemophilic for factor IX deficiency (hemophilia B; Christmas disease) (orphan)* [factor IX concentrate] 250, 500, 1000 U

monooctanoin [see: monoctanoin]

monophenylbutazone [see: mofebutazone]

monophosphothiamine INN

Mono-Plus reagent kit for professional use ℞ *in vitro diagnostic aid for mononucleosis*

monopotassium 4-aminosalicylate [see: aminosalicylate potassium]

monopotassium carbonate [see: potassium bicarbonate]

monopotassium D-gluconate [see: potassium gluconate]

monopotassium monosodium tartrate tetrahydrate [see: potassium sodium tartrate]

monopotassium phosphate [see: potassium phosphate, monobasic]

Monopril tablets ℞ *antihypertensive; angiotensin-converting enzyme (ACE) inhibitor; adjunctive treatment for congestive heart failure (CHF)* [fosinopril sodium] 10, 20, 40 mg

Monopril·HCT tablets ℞ *antihypertensive; angiotensin-converting enzyme (ACE) inhibitor; diuretic* [fosinopril sodium; hydrochlorothiazide] 10•12.5, 20•12.5 mg

monosodium p-aminohippurate [see: aminohippurate sodium]

monosodium 4-aminosalicylate dihydrate [see: aminosalicylate sodium]

monosodium carbonate [see: sodium bicarbonate]

monosodium D-gluconate [see: sodium gluconate]

monosodium D-thyroxine hydrate [see: dextrothyroxine sodium]

monosodium glutamate NF *flavoring agent; perfume*

monosodium L-ascorbate [see: sodium ascorbate]

monosodium L-thyroxine hydrate [see: levothyroxine sodium]

monosodium phosphate dihydrate [see: sodium phosphate, monobasic]

monosodium phosphate monohydrate [see: sodium phosphate, monobasic]

monosodium salicylate [see: sodium salicylate]

monosodium sulfite [see: sodium bisulfite]

Monospot slide test for professional use ℞ *in vitro diagnostic aid for mononucleosis*

monostearin [see: glyceryl monostearate]

Monosticon Dri-Dot slide test for professional use ℞ *in vitro diagnostic aid for mononucleosis*

monosulfiram BAN [also: sulfiram]

Mono-Sure slide test for professional use ℞ *in vitro diagnostic aid for mononucleosis*

Mono-Test slide test for professional use ℞ *in vitro diagnostic aid for mononucleosis*

monothioglycerol NF *preservative*

Monotropa uniflora medicinal herb [see: fit root]

Monovial (trademarked packaging form) *single-use vial with transfer needle set*

monoxerutin INN

monoxychlorosene *germicidal mouthwash*

Monsel solution [see: ferric subsulfate]

montelukast sodium USAN *leukotriene receptor inhibitor for allergic rhinitis, exercise-induced bronchoconstriction (EIB), and the prophylaxis and chronic treatment of asthma; also used for chronic urticaria and atopic dermatitis*

monteplase INN ⏷ Mynate 90 Plus

montirelin INN

montmorillonite (redmond clay) *natural remedy for bug bites and stings and other skin problems*

Montreal BCG vaccine [see: BCG vaccine]

Monuril ⓔᵁᴿ (foreign name for U.S. product **Monurol**)

Monurol granules for oral solution ℞ *broad-spectrum bactericidal antibiotic for urinary tract infections* [fosfomycin tromethamine] 3 g/pkt.

moose elm *medicinal herb* [see: slippery elm]

8-MOP capsules ℞ *systemic psoralens for psoriasis, repigmentation of idiopathic vitiligo, and cutaneous T-cell lymphoma (CTCL); used to increase tolerance to sunlight and enhance pigmentation* [methoxsalen] 10 mg

MOP (mechlorethamine, Oncovin, prednisone) *chemotherapy protocol*

MOP (mechlorethamine, Oncovin, procarbazine) *chemotherapy protocol for pediatric brain tumors*

8-MOP (8-methoxypsoralen) [see: methoxsalen]

MOP-BAP (mechlorethamine, Oncovin, procarbazine, bleomycin, Adriamycin, prednisone) *chemotherapy protocol* ☒ MABOP; Māpap; MOBP

moperone INN

mopidamol INN

mopidralazine INN

MOPP (mechlorethamine, Oncovin, procarbazine, prednisone) *chemotherapy protocol for Hodgkin lymphoma and brain cancer (medulloblastoma)*

MOPP (mustine HCl, Oncovin, procarbazine, prednisone) *chemotherapy protocol*

MOPP/ABV (mechlorethamine, Oncovin, procarbazine, prednisone, Adriamycin, bleomycin, vinblastine) *chemotherapy protocol for Hodgkin lymphoma*

MOPP/ABVD (alternating cycles of MOPP and ABVD) *chemotherapy protocol for Hodgkin lymphoma*

MOPP-BLEO; MOPP-Bleo (mechlorethamine, Oncovin, procarbazine, prednisone, bleomycin) *chemotherapy protocol*

MOPPHDB (mechlorethamine, Oncovin, procarbazine, prednisone, high-dose bleomycin) *chemotherapy protocol*

MOPPLDB (mechlorethamine, Oncovin, procarbazine, prednisone, low-dose bleomycin) *chemotherapy protocol*

MOPr (mechlorethamine, Oncovin, procarbazine) *chemotherapy protocol*

moprolol INN

moquizone INN

MORAb-009 *investigational (orphan) monoclonal antibody to mesothelin for the treatment of pancreatic cancer*

moracizine INN, BAN *antiarrhythmic* [also: moricizine]

morantel INN *anthelmintic* [also: morantel tartrate]

morantel tartrate USAN *anthelmintic* [also: morantel]

Moranyl (available only from the Centers for Disease Control) ℞ *antiparasitic for African trypanosomiasis and onchocerciasis* [suramin sodium] ☒ Marinol

morazone INN, BAN ☒ Marezine

morclofone INN

More-Dophilus powder OTC *natural intestinal bacteria; probiotic; dietary supplement; fever blister treatment; not generally regarded as safe and effective as an antidiarrheal* [*Lactobacillus acidophilus*] 4 billion CFU/g

morforex INN

moricizine USAN *antiarrhythmic* [also: moracizine]

moricizine HCl *antiarrhythmic for severe ventricular arrhythmias*

morinamide INN

Morinda citrifolia *medicinal herb* [see: noni]

Mormon tea *medicinal herb* [see: ephedra]

morniflumate USAN, INN *anti-inflammatory*

morning glory (Ipomoea violacea) seeds *contain lysergic acid amide, chemically similar to LSD, which produce hallucinations when ingested as a street drug* [see also: LSD]

morocromen INN

moroxydine INN, BAN

morphazinamide [see: morinamide]

morpheridine INN, BAN

morphine BAN *narcotic analgesic; widely abused as a street drug, which leads to dependence* [also: morphine sulfate] ☒ myrophine

morphine dinicotinate ester [see: nicomorphine]

Morphine ER extended-release tablets ℞ *narcotic analgesic* [morphine sulfate] 100, 200 mg

morphine HCl USP *narcotic analgesic preferred in Germany and England;*

widely abused as a street drug, which leads to dependence

morphine sulfate (MS) USP *narcotic analgesic preferred in the U.S.; intraspinal microinfusion for intractable chronic pain (orphan); widely abused as a street drug, which leads to dependence* [also: morphine] 15, 30, 60, 100, 200 mg oral; 2, 4, 20 mg/mL oral; 0.5, 1, 2, 4, 5, 8, 10, 15, 25, 50 mg/mL injection; 5, 10, 20, 30 mg rectal

Morphine Sulfate in 5% Dextrose IV, IM, or subcu injection ℞ *narcotic analgesic* [morphine sulfate] 1 mg/mL

4-morpholinecarboximidoylguanidine [see: moroxydine]

2-morpholinoethylrutin [see: ethoxazorutoside]

3-morpholinosydnoneimine [see: linsidomine]

morpholinyl succinimide [see: morsuximide]

morpholinylethyl morphine [see: pholcodine]

morrhuate sodium USP *sclerosing agent for varicose veins* [also: sodium morrhuate] 50 mg/mL injection

morsuximide INN

morsydomine [see: molsidomine]

mortification root *medicinal herb* [see: marsh mallow]

Morton Salt Substitute; Morton Seasoned Salt Substitute OTC *salt substitute* [potassium chloride] 64 mEq K/5 g; 56 mEq K/5 g

Morus nigra; M. rubra medicinal herb [see: mulberry]

Moschus moschiferus natural remedy [see: deer musk]

Mosco topical liquid OTC *keratolytic* [salicylic acid in flexible collodion] 17.6%

mosquito plant *medicinal herb* [see: pennyroyal]

motapizone INN

MOTC (methyleneoxytetracycline) [see: methacycline]

motexafin gadolinium USAN *investigational (NDA filed, orphan) radiosensitizer for non-small cell lung cancer patients with brain metastases*

motexafin lutetium USAN *radiosensitizer*

mother of thyme *medicinal herb* [see: thyme]

motherwort (Leonurus cardiaca) flowering tops and leaves *medicinal herb used as an antispasmodic, astringent, calmative, cardiac, emmenagogue, hepatic, laxative, nervine, and stomachic*

Motofen tablets ℞ *antidiarrheal* [difenoxin HCl; atropine sulfate] 1•0.025 mg

motrazepam INN

motretinide USAN, INN *keratolytic*

Motrin tablets (discontinued 2008) ℞ *analgesic; antiarthritic; antipyretic; nonsteroidal anti-inflammatory drug (NSAID) for moderate pain, migraine headaches, and primary dysmenorrhea* [ibuprofen] 400, 600, 800 mg

Motrin, Children's chewable tablets, oral suspension OTC *analgesic; antipyretic; nonsteroidal anti-inflammatory drug (NSAID) for minor aches and pains* [ibuprofen] 50 mg; 100 mg/5 mL

Motrin, Infants' oral drops OTC *analgesic; antipyretic; nonsteroidal anti-inflammatory drug (NSAID) for minor aches and pains* [ibuprofen] 40 mg/mL

Motrin, Junior Strength tablets, chewable tablets OTC *analgesic; antipyretic; nonsteroidal anti-inflammatory drug (NSAID) for minor aches and pains* [ibuprofen] 100 mg

Motrin Children's Cold oral suspension OTC *decongestant; analgesic; antipyretic* [pseudoephedrine HCl; ibuprofen] 15•100 mg/5 mL

Motrin IB tablets, gelcaps OTC *analgesic; antipyretic; antiarthritic; nonsteroidal anti-inflammatory drug (NSAID) for mild to moderate pain, migraine headaches, and primary dysmenorrhea* [ibuprofen] 200 mg

Motrin Migraine Pain caplets OTC *analgesic; antipyretic; nonsteroidal anti-inflammatory drug (NSAID) for mild to moderate pain of migraine headaches* [ibuprofen] 200 mg

Motrin Sinus Headache caplets (discontinued 2007) OTC *decongestant; analgesic; antipyretic* [pseudoephedrine HCl; ibuprofen] 30•200 mg

mountain ash *(Sorbus americana; S. aucuparia)* fruit *medicinal herb used as an aperient, astringent, and diuretic*

mountain balm *medicinal herb* [see: yerba santa]

mountain box; mountain cranberry *medicinal herb* [see: uva ursi]

mountain laurel *(Kalmia latifolia)* leaves *medicinal herb used as an astringent and sedative*

mountain mahogany *medicinal herb* [see: birch]

mountain mint *medicinal herb* [see: marjoram; Oswego tea]

mountain snuff; mountain tobacco *medicinal herb* [see: arnica]

mountain sorrel *medicinal herb* [see: wood sorrel]

mountain strawberry *medicinal herb* [see: strawberry]

mountain sumach *medicinal herb* [see: sumach]

mountain sweet *medicinal herb* [see: New Jersey tea]

mountain tea *medicinal herb* [see: wintergreen]

mouse ear *(Hieracium pilosella)* plant *medicinal herb used as an astringent, cholagogue, and diuretic* ⑨ MSIR

MouthKote throat spray OTC *saliva substitute*

MouthKote O/R mouthwash OTC *mild anesthetic; antipruritic; counterirritant; antiseptic* [menthol; benzyl alcohol]

MouthKote O/R oral solution OTC *topical antihistamine* [diphenhydramine] 1.25%

MouthKote P/R oral solution, ointment (discontinued 2004) OTC *topical antihistamine* [diphenhydramine HCl] 1.25%; 25%

mouthroot *medicinal herb* [see: gold thread]

moveltipril INN

MoviPrep oral liquid ℞ *pre-procedure bowel evacuant for colonoscopy* [PEG 3350; sodium sulfate; sodium chloride; potassium chloride; ascorbic acid; sodium ascorbate] 100•7.5•2.691•1.015•4.7•5.9 g/2 L dose

moxadolen INN

moxalactam disodium USAN, USP *cephalosporin antibiotic* [also: latamoxef]

moxantrazole [now: teloxantrone HCl]

moxaprindine INN

moxastine INN

Moxatag extended-release film-coated tablets ℞ *aminopenicillin antibiotic* [amoxicillin] 775 mg

moxaverine INN, BAN

moxazocine USAN, INN *analgesic; antitussive*

moxestrol INN

moxicoumone INN

moxidectin USAN, INN *veterinary antiparasitic*

moxifloxacin HCl USAN *broad-spectrum fluoroquinolone antibiotic*

moxilubant maleate USAN *leukotriene B₄ receptor antagonist for rheumatoid arthritis and psoriasis*

moxipraquine INN, BAN

moxiraprine INN

moxisylyte INN [also: thymoxamine]

moxnidazole USAN, INN *antiprotozoal (Trichomonas)*

moxonidine USAN, INN *centrally acting sympatholytic for hypertension, congestive heart failure, and type 2 diabetes*

M-oxy tablets ℞ *narcotic analgesic* [oxycodone HCl] 5 mg ⑨ Maox; Megace

MP (melphalan, prednisone) *chemotherapy protocol for multiple myeloma*

MP (mitoxantrone, prednisone) *chemotherapy protocol for prostate cancer*

4-MP (4-methylpyrazole) [see: fomepizole]

6-MP (6-mercaptopurine) [see: mercaptopurine]

MPA (medroxyprogesterone acetate) [q.v.]

MPA (mycophenolic acid) [q.v.]

MPF [see: Mucoprotective Factor]

m-PFL (methotrexate, Platinol, flu-orouracil, leucovorin [rescue]) *chemotherapy protocol*

MPH (methylphenidate HCl) [q.v.]

MPIF-1 (myeloid progenitor inhibi-tory factor 1) [see: mirostipen]

MPL (melphalan) [q.v.]

MPL + PRED (melphalan, predni-sone) *chemotherapy protocol*

M-Prednisol-40; M-Prednisol-80 intralesional, soft tissue, and IM injection (discontinued 2004) ℞ *corticosteroid; anti-inflammatory; immunosuppressant* [methylpredniso-lone acetate] 40 mg/mL; 80 mg/mL

MRV (mixed respiratory vaccine) [q.v.]

M-R-Vax II powder for subcu injec-tion (discontinued 2004) ℞ *measles and rubella vaccine* [measles & rubella virus vaccine, live; neomycin] 1000 U•1000 U•25 mcg/0.5 mL dose ⊘ Meruvax II

MS (magnesium salicylate) [q.v.]

MS (morphine sulfate) [q.v.]

MS Contin controlled-release tablets ℞ *narcotic analgesic; preoperative sed-ative and anxiolytic* [morphine sulfate] 15, 30, 60, 100, 200 mg

MSIR tablets (discontinued 2005) ℞ *narcotic analgesic; preoperative sedative and anxiolytic* [morphine sulfate] 15, 30 mg ⊘ mouse ear

MSIR oral solution, oral concentrate ℞ *narcotic analgesic; preoperative sedative and anxiolytic* [morphine sulfate] 10, 20 mg/5 mL; 20 mg/mL ⊘ mouse ear

MSM (methylsulfonylmethane) *natural source of sulfur; promotes an increase in collagen and the endogenous antioxidant glutathione*

MSTA (Mumps Skin Test Antigen) intradermal injection ℞ *diagnostic aid to assess immune system compe-tency (not effective in testing immunity to mumps virus)* [mumps skin test antigen] 0.1 mL (4 U/0.1 mL)

MT6 (mercaptomerin) [q.v.]

M-Tabs (trademarked dosage form) *orally disintegrating tablets*

MTC (mitomycin C) [see: mitomycin]

MTC-DOX (magnetically targeted carrier with doxorubicin) *investi-gational (orphan) delivery system for hepatocellular carcinoma*

M.T.E.-4; M.T.E.-4 Concentrated; M.T.E.-5; M.T.E.-5 Concentrated; M.T.E.-6; M.T.E.-6 Concentrated; M.T.E.-7 IV injection ℞ *intravenous nutritional therapy* [multiple trace ele-ments (metals)]

mTHPC [see: temoporfin]

MTP-PE (muramyl tripeptide phos-phatidylethanolamine) [see: mifa-murtide]

MTX (methotrexate) [q.v.]

MTX + MP + CTX (methotrexate, mercaptopurine, cyclophospha-mide) *chemotherapy protocol*

MTX/6-MP (methotrexate, mercap-topurine) *chemotherapy protocol for acute lymphocytic leukemia (ALL); the ongoing continuation protocol* [also: 1DMTX/6-MP (the first-day initia-tion protocol)]

MTX/6-MP/VP (methotrexate, mercaptopurine, vincristine, prednisone) *chemotherapy protocol for acute lymphocytic leukemia (ALL)*

MTX-CDDPAdr (methotrexate [with leucovorin rescue], CDDP, Adriamycin) *chemotherapy protocol for pediatric osteosarcoma*

Mucinex extended-release tablets, dual-release tablets OTC *expectorant* [guaifenesin] 600, 1200 mg; 600 mg (100 mg immediate release, 500 mg extended release)

Mucinex Children's oral liquid OTC *expectorant* [guaifenesin] 100 mg/5 mL

Mucinex D extended-release tablets OTC *decongestant; expectorant* [pseu-doephedrine HCl; guaifenesin] 60• 600, 120•1200 mg

Mucinex DM extended-release tab-lets OTC *antitussive; expectorant* [dex-tromethorphan hydrobromide; guai-fenesin] 30•600 mg

Mucinex Mini-Melts Children's; Mucinex Mini-Melts Junior oral granules OTC *expectorant* [guaifenesin] 50 mg/packet; 100 mg/packet

Mucinex with Codeine extended-release tablets *investigational (NDA filed) narcotic antitussive; expectorant* [codeine phosphate; guaifenesin] 30•600, 60•1200 mg

Muco-Fen; Muco-Fen 800; Muco-Fen 1200 timed-release tablets (discontinued 2004) ℞ *expectorant* [guaifenesin] 1000 mg; 800 mg; 1200 mg

Muco-Fen DM sustained-release tablets (discontinued 2007) ℞ *antitussive; expectorant* [dextromethorphan hydrobromide; guaifenesin] 60•1000 mg

mucoid exopolysaccharide *Pseudomonas* hyperimmune globulin (MEPIG) *investigational (orphan) for the prevention and treatment of pulmonary infections of cystic fibrosis*

mucolytics *a class of respiratory inhalant drugs that destroy or inhibit mucin*

Mucomyst solution for nebulization or intratracheal instillation ℞ *mucolytic* [acetylcysteine sodium] 10%, 20%

Mucomyst 10 IV *investigational (orphan) for severe acetaminophen overdose* [acetylcysteine]

Mucoprotective Factor (MPF) (trademarked ingredient) *aromatic flavored syrup* [eriodictyon]

Mucosil-10; Mucosil-20 solution for nebulization or intratracheal instillation (discontinued 2004) ℞ *mucolytic* [acetylcysteine sodium] 10%; 20% ▣ Magsal

MucusRelief Sinus tablets OTC *decongestant; expectorant* [phenylephrine HCl; guaifenesin] 10•400 mg

Mudrane tablets (discontinued 2007) ℞ *antiasthmatic; bronchodilator; decongestant; expectorant; sedative* [aminophylline; ephedrine HCl; potassium iodide; phenobarbital] 111•16•195•8 mg ▣ Midrin

Mudrane GG tablets (discontinued 2007) ℞ *antiasthmatic; decongestant; expectorant; sedative* [theophylline; ephedrine HCl; guaifenesin; phenobarbital] 111•16•100•8 mg

Mudrane GG-2 tablets (discontinued 2007) ℞ *antiasthmatic; bronchodilator; expectorant* [theophylline; guaifenesin] 111•100 mg

mugwort (*Artemisia vulgaris*) root and plant *medicinal herb used as a diaphoretic, emmenagogue, and laxative*

muira puama (*Ptychopetalum olacoides*) stem *medicinal herb used as an aphrodisiac and treatment for impotence in South America; clinical trials in France confirm these effects*

mulberry (*Morus nigra*; *M. rubra*) bark *medicinal herb used as an anthelmintic and cathartic*

mullein (*Verbascum nigrum*; *V. phlomoides*; *V. thapsiforme*; *V. thapsus*) plant *medicinal herb for asthma, bleeding in bowel and lungs, bronchitis, pain, bruises, cough, croup, diarrhea, hemorrhoids, earache, gout, insomnia, lymphatic system, nervousness, pleurisy, sinus congestion, and tuberculosis* ▣ Myolin

Multaq film-coated tablets *investigational (Phase III) antiarrhythmic for atrial fibrillation* [dronedarone] 400 mg

MulTE-Pak-4; MulTE-Pak-5 IV injection ℞ *intravenous nutritional therapy* [multiple trace elements (metals)]

Multi 75 timed-release tablets OTC *vitamin/mineral supplement* [multiple vitamins & minerals; folic acid; biotin] ±•0.4•2 mg ▣ Maolate

Multi Vit with Iron drops OTC *vitamin/iron supplement* [multiple vitamins; iron] ±•10 mg/mL

Multi Vitamin Concentrate injection ℞ *parenteral vitamin supplement* [multiple vitamins]

Multi-Day tablets OTC *vitamin supplement* [multiple vitamins; folic acid] ±•0.4 mg

Multi-Day Plus Iron tablets OTC *vitamin/iron supplement* [multiple vitamins; iron; folic acid] ±•18•0.4 mg

Multi-Day Plus Minerals tablets OTC *vitamin/mineral/iron supplement* [multiple vitamins & minerals; iron; folic acid; biotin] ± • 18 mg•0.4 mg•30 mcg

Multi-Day with Calcium and Extra Iron tablets OTC *vitamin/calcium/iron supplement* [multiple vitamins; calcium; iron; folic acid] ± • ± • 27•0.4 mg

Multifol caplets ℞ *vitamin/calcium/iron supplement* [multiple vitamins; calcium; iron (as ferrous fumarate); folic acid] ± • 125•65•1 mg

MultiHance IV injection ℞ *parenteral radiopaque contrast medium to enhance MRIs of the brain, spine, and other CNS tissue* [gadobenate dimeglumine] 529 mg/mL

MultiKine injection *investigational (Phase III) antineoplastic for prostate cancer; investigational (Phase I) immunotherapeutic agent for HIV and HPV infections* [multiple leukocytes and interleukins]

Multilex; Multilex-T & M tablets OTC *vitamin/mineral/iron supplement* [multiple vitamins & minerals; iron] ± • 15 mg

Multilyte-20; Multilyte-40 IV admixture ℞ *intravenous electrolyte therapy* [combined electrolyte solution] ⑨ malotilate

Multi-Mineral tablets OTC *mineral supplement* [multiple minerals]

Multiple Trace Element Neonatal; Multiple Trace Element with Selenium; Multiple Trace Element with Selenium Concentrated IV injection ℞ *intravenous nutritional therapy* [multiple trace elements (metals)]

Multistix; Multistix 2; Multistix 7; Multistix 8 SG; Multistix 9; Multistix 9 SG; Multistix 10 SG; Multistix SG reagent strips OTC *in vitro diagnostic aid for multiple urine products*

Multistix PRO reagent strips for professional use ℞ *in vitro diagnostic aid for urine protein/creatinine ratio*

Multitest CMI single-use intradermal skin test device (discontinued 2004) ℞ *skin test for multiple allergen sensitivity* [skin test antigens (seven different); glycerin (one for test control)]

Multitrace-5 Concentrate IV injection ℞ *intravenous nutritional therapy* [multiple trace elements (metals)]

multivitamin infusion, neonatal formula *investigational (orphan) total parenteral nutrition for very low birthweight infants*

Multi-Vitamin Mineral with Beta-Carotene tablets OTC *vitamin/mineral/iron supplement* [multiple vitamins & minerals; ferrous fumarate; folic acid; biotin] ± • 27•0.4•0.45 mg

Multivitamin with Fluoride pediatric oral drops ℞ *vitamin supplement; dental caries preventative* [multiple vitamins; fluoride] ± • 0.25, ± • 0.5 mg/mL

Multivitamins capsules OTC *vitamin supplement* [multiple vitamins]

Mulvidren-F Softabs (pediatric chewable tablets) ℞ *vitamin supplement; dental caries preventative* [multiple vitamins; fluoride] ± • 1 mg

mumps skin test antigen (MSTA) USP *diagnostic aid to assess immune system competency*

mumps vaccine [see: mumps virus vaccine, inactivated]

mumps virus vaccine, inactivated NF

mumps virus vaccine, live USP *active immunizing agent for mumps*

Mumpsvax powder for subcu injection ℞ *mumps vaccine* [mumps virus vaccine, live] 0.5 mL

mupirocin USAN, INN, BAN *topical antibiotic* 2% topical

mupirocin calcium USAN *topical antibiotic* (base=93%)

muplestim USAN *progenitor cell stimulator for neutropenia and thrombocytopenia*

murabutide INN

muraglitazar *peroxisome proliferator–activated receptor (PPAR)–alpha and –gamma agonist; antidiabetic to control blood glucose levels, lower triglycerides, and raise HDL*

muramyl tripeptide phosphatidyl-ethanolamine (MTP-PE) [see: mifamurtide]

Murine eye drops OTC *moisturizer/lubricant* [polyvinyl alcohol] 0.5% ☒ Mirena

Murine Ear ear drops OTC *cerumenolytic to emulsify and disperse ear wax; antiseptic* [carbamide peroxide; alcohol] 6.5%•6.3%

Murine Earigate spray OTC *ear wash* [purified water]

murine monoclonal antibodies *antibodies cloned from a single mouse or rat cell* [see: monoclonal antibodies]

Murine Tears Plus eye drops OTC *decongestant; vasoconstrictor; moisturizer/lubricant* [tetrahydrozoline HCl; polyvinyl alcohol; povidone] 0.05%•0.5%•0.6%

Muro 128 eye drops, ophthalmic ointment OTC *corneal edema-reducing agent* [sodium chloride (hypertonic saline solution)] 2%, 5%; 5%

murocainide INN

Murocel eye drops OTC *moisturizer/lubricant* [methylcellulose] 1% ☒ Mersol

Murocoll-2 eye drops ℞ *cycloplegic; mydriatic* [scopolamine hydrobromide; phenylephrine HCl] 0.3%•10%

murodermin INN

muromonab-CD3 USAN, INN *monoclonal antibody to CD3; immunosuppressant for renal, hepatic, and cardiac transplants*

Muroptic-5 eye drops OTC *corneal edema-reducing agent* [sodium chloride (hypertonic saline solution)] 5%

muscarinic agonists *a class of investigational analgesics*

Muse single-use intraurethral suppository ℞ *vasodilator for erectile dysfunction* [alprostadil] 125, 150, 500, 1000 mcg

musk *natural remedy* [see: deer musk]

mustaral oil [see: allyl isothiocyanate]

mustard (Brassica alba; Sinapis alba) seeds and oil *medicinal herb for indigestion and liver and lung disorders; also used as an appetizer, diuretic, emetic, and soak for aching feet, arthritis, and rheumatism*

mustard oil [see: allyl isothiocyanate]

Mustargen powder for IV or intracavitary injection ℞ *nitrogen mustard-type alkylating antineoplastic for multiple carcinomas, lymphomas and leukemias, mycosis fungoides, and polycythemia vera* [mechlorethamine HCl] 10 mg

Musterole Deep Strength Rub OTC *analgesic; mild anesthetic; antipruritic; counterirritant* [methyl salicylate; methyl nicotinate; menthol] 30%•0.5%•3%

Musterole Extra Strength OTC *mild topical anesthetic; antipruritic; counterirritant* [camphor; menthol] 5%•3%

mustine BAN *nitrogen mustard-type alkylating antineoplastic* [also: mechlorethamine HCl; chlormethine; nitrogen mustard N-oxide HCl]

mustine HCl [see: mechlorethamine HCl]

Mutamycin powder for IV injection (discontinued 2008) ℞ *antibiotic antineoplastic for disseminated adenocarcinoma of the stomach or pancreas* [mitomycin] 5, 20, 40 mg

muzolimine USAN, INN *diuretic; antihypertensive* ☒ mesalamine; mezilamine

MV (mitomycin, vinblastine) *chemotherapy protocol for breast cancer*

MV (mitoxantrone, VePesid) *chemotherapy protocol for acute myelocytic leukemia (ALL)*

MVAC; M-VAC (methotrexate, vinblastine, Adriamycin, cisplatin) *chemotherapy protocol for bladder cancer* ☒ Mavik

M-Vax *investigational (Phase III, orphan) theraccine for postsurgical stage III malignant melanoma* [DNP-conjugated tumor vaccine]

MVF (mitoxantrone, vincristine, fluorouracil) *chemotherapy protocol*

M.V.I. Neonatal IV infusion *investigational (orphan) total parenteral nutrition for very low birthweight infants* [multiple vitamins]

M.V.I. Pediatric injection ℞ *parenteral vitamin supplement* [multiple vitamins; folic acid; biotin] ±•140• 20 mcg/5 mL

M.V.I.-12 injection ℞ *parenteral vitamin supplement* [multiple vitamins; folic acid; biotin] ±•400•60 mcg/5 mL

M.V.M. capsules OTC *vitamin/mineral/iron supplement* [multiple vitamins & minerals; iron; folic acid; biotin] ±• 3.6 mg•0.08 mg•160 mcg

MVP (mitomycin, vinblastine, Platinol) *chemotherapy protocol for non–small cell lung cancer (NSCLC)*

MVPP (mechlorethamine, vinblastine, procarbazine, prednisone) *chemotherapy protocol for Hodgkin lymphoma* ▣ MFP; MVVPP

MVT (mitoxantrone, VePesid, thiotepa) *chemotherapy protocol*

MVVPP (mechlorethamine, vincristine, vinblastine, procarbazine, prednisone) *chemotherapy protocol* ▣ MFP; MVP

Myadec tablets OTC *vitamin/mineral/iron supplement* [multiple vitamins & minerals; iron; folic acid; biotin] ±•18 mg•0.4 mg•30 mcg ▣ MADDOC

Myambutol film-coated tablets ℞ *tuberculostatic* [ethambutol HCl] 100, 400 mg

Mycamine powder for IV infusion ℞ *systemic echinocandin antifungal for prophylaxis and treatment of esophageal candidiasis and prophylaxis of candidiasis in patients undergoing hemopoietic stem cell transplantation (HSCT)* [micafungin sodium] 50, 100 mg/dose

Mycelex troches ℞ *antifungal; oral candidiasis prophylaxis or treatment* [clotrimazole] 10 mg

Mycelex-3 vaginal cream in prefilled applicator OTC *antifungal* [butoconazole nitrate] 2%

Mycelex-7 vaginal cream, combination pack (vaginal inserts + cream)

OTC *antifungal* [clotrimazole] 1%; 100 mg + 1%

Mycifradin Sulfate oral solution ℞ *aminoglycoside antibiotic* [neomycin sulfate] 125 mg/5 mL

Mycinaire Saline Mist nasal spray OTC *nasal moisturizer* [sodium chloride (saline solution)] 0.65%

Mycinette throat spray OTC *mild mucous membrane anesthetic; antiseptic; astringent* [phenol; alum] 1.4%•0.3%

Mycinettes lozenges OTC *mucous membrane anesthetic* [benzocaine] 15 mg

"mycins" *brief term for a class of antibiotics derived from various strains of the fungus-like bacteria* Streptomyces, *or their synthetic analogues, whose generic names end in "mycin," such as lincomycin* [properly called: aminoglycosides]

Myci-Spray nasal spray OTC *decongestant; antihistamine* [phenylephrine HCl; pyrilamine maleate] 0.25%• 0.15%

mycobacterial cell wall complex (MCC) [see: urocidin]

Mycobacterium avium **sensitin RS-10** *investigational (orphan) diagnostic aid for* Mycobacterium avium *infection in immunocompromised patients*

Myco-Biotic II cream ℞ *corticosteroidal anti-inflammatory; antibiotic; antifungal* [triamcinolone acetonide; neomycin sulfate; nystatin] 0.1%• 0.5%•100 000 U per g

Mycobutin capsules ℞ *antiviral/antibacterial for prevention of* Mycobacterium avium *complex (MAC) in advanced HIV patients (orphan)* [rifabutin] 150 mg

Mycocide NS topical solution OTC *antiseptic* [benzalkonium chloride]

Mycogen II cream, ointment ℞ *corticosteroidal anti-inflammatory; antifungal* [triamcinolone acetonide; nystatin] 0.1%•100 000 U per g ▣ Macugen

Mycograb *investigational (Phase III, orphan) for invasive candidiasis and other severe fungal infections* [efungumab]

Mycolog-II cream, ointment R *corticosteroidal anti-inflammatory; antifungal* [triamcinolone acetonide; nystatin] 0.1%•100 000 U per g

Myconel cream R *corticosteroidal anti-inflammatory; antifungal* [triamcinolone acetonide; nystatin] 0.1%• 100 000 U per g ② mequinol; Micanol

mycophenolate mofetil USAN *purine biosynthesis inhibitor; immunosuppressant for allogenic renal, hepatic, or cardiac transplants (orphan); investigational (Phase III, orphan) treatment for myasthenia gravis* 250, 500 mg oral

mycophenolate mofetil HCl USAN *purine biosynthesis inhibitor; immunosuppressant for allogenic renal, hepatic, or cardiac transplants*

mycophenolate sodium [see: mycophenolic acid]

mycophenolic acid (MPA) USAN, INN *immunosuppressant for allogenic renal transplants*

Mycostatin cream, ointment, powder R *antifungal* [nystatin] 100 000 U/g; 100 000 U/g; 100 000 U/g

Mycostatin film-coated tablets R *systemic antifungal* [nystatin] 500 000 U

Mycostatin oral suspension (discontinued 2004) R *antifungal; oral candidiasis treatment* [nystatin] 100 000 U/mL

Mycostatin Pastilles (troches) R *antifungal; oral candidiasis treatment* [nystatin] 200 000 U

Myco-Triacet II cream, ointment R *corticosteroidal anti-inflammatory; antifungal* [triamcinolone acetonide; nystatin] 0.1%•100 000 U per g

mydeton [see: tolperisone]

MyDex extended-release caplets R *decongestant; expectorant* [phenylephrine HCl; guaifenesin] 30•900 mg

Mydfrin 2.5% eye drops R *decongestant; vasoconstrictor; mydriatic* [phenylephrine HCl] 2.5%

Mydriacyl Drop-Tainers (eye drops) R *cycloplegic; mydriatic* [tropicamide] 0.5%, 1%

mydriatics *a class of drugs that cause the pupil of the eye to dilate*

myelin *investigational (orphan) for multiple sclerosis*

myeloid progenitor inhibitory factor 1 (MPIF-1) [see: mirostipen]

myelosan [see: busulfan]

myfadol INN

Myfortic film-coated delayed-release tablets R *immunosuppressant for allogenic renal transplants* [mycophenolic acid] 180, 360 mg

Mygel; Mygel II oral suspension OTC *antacid; antiflatulent* [aluminum hydroxide; magnesium hydroxide; simethicone] 200•200•20 mg/5 mL; 400•400•40 mg/5 mL

MyHist-DM oral liquid R *antitussive; antihistamine; sleep aid; decongestant* [dextromethorphan hydrobromide; pyrilamine maleate; phenylephrine HCl] 15•12.5•7.5 mg/5 mL

MyHist-PD oral liquid R *decongestant; antihistamine; sleep aid* [phenylephrine HCl; chlorpheniramine maleate; pyrilamine maleate] 7.5•2• 12.5 mg/5 mL

Mykrox tablets (discontinued 2008) R *antihypertensive; diuretic* [metolazone] 0.5 mg

Mylagen gelcaps OTC *antacid* [calcium carbonate; magnesium carbonate] 311•232 mg

Mylagen; Mylagen II oral liquid OTC *antacid; antiflatulent* [aluminum hydroxide; magnesium hydroxide; simethicone] 200•200•20 mg/5 mL; 400•400•40 mg/5 mL

Mylanta chewable tablets, oral liquid OTC *antacid; antiflatulent* [aluminum hydroxide; magnesium hydroxide; simethicone] 200•200•20, 400• 400•40 mg; 200•200•20, 400•400• 40 mg/5 mL

Mylanta lozenges OTC *antacid* [calcium carbonate] 600 mg

Mylanta, Children's oral liquid, chewable tablets OTC *antacid* [calcium carbonate] 400 mg/5 mL; 400 mg

Mylanta Antacid gelcaps OTC *antacid* [calcium carbonate; magnesium hydroxide] 550•125 mg

Mylanta Gas chewable tablets, capsules OTC *antiflatulent* [simethicone] 40, 80, 125 mg; 125 mg

Mylanta Supreme oral liquid OTC *antacid* [calcium carbonate; magnesium hydroxide] 400•135 mg/5 mL

Mylanta Ultra chewable tablets OTC *antacid* [calcium carbonate; magnesium hydroxide] 700•300 mg

Myleran film-coated tablets ℞ *alkylating antineoplastic for chronic myelogenous leukemia (CML)* [busulfan] 2 mg ⓓ Malarone

Mylicon drops OTC *antiflatulent* [simethicone] 40 mg/0.6 mL

Mylinax *investigational (orphan) agent for chronic progressive multiple sclerosis* [cladribine]

Mylocel film-coated caplets ℞ *antineoplastic for melanoma, squamous cell carcinoma, myelocytic leukemia, and ovarian cancer; also adjunctive therapy for HIV infections* [hydroxyurea] 1000 mg

Mylotarg powder for IV infusion ℞ *monoclonal antibody–targeted chemotherapy agent for acute myeloid leukemia (orphan)* [gemtuzumab ozogamicin] 5 mg

Mylovenge *investigational (orphan) agent for multiple myeloma* [antigen-presenting cells pulsed with tumor immunoglobulin idiotype]

Mynatal capsules ℞ *vitamin/mineral/calcium/iron supplement* [multiple vitamins & minerals; calcium; iron; folic acid; biotin] ≚•300•65•1•0.03 mg

Mynatal FC caplets ℞ *vitamin/mineral/calcium/iron supplement* [multiple vitamins & minerals; calcium; iron; folic acid; biotin] ≚•250•60•1•0.03 mg

Mynatal P.N. captabs ℞ *vitamin/calcium/iron supplement* [multiple vitamins; calcium; iron; folic acid] ≚• 125•60•1 mg

Mynatal P.N. Forte caplets ℞ *vitamin/mineral/calcium/iron supplement* [mul-

tiple vitamins & minerals; calcium; iron; folic acid] ≚•250•60•1 mg

Mynatal Rx caplets ℞ *vitamin/mineral/calcium/iron supplement* [multiple vitamins & minerals; calcium; iron; folic acid; biotin] ≚•200•60•1•0.03 mg

Mynate 90 Plus delayed-release caplets ℞ *vitamin/calcium/iron supplement* [multiple vitamins; calcium; iron; folic acid] ≚•250•90•1 mg ⓓ monteplase

Myobloc injection ℞ *neurotoxin complex for symptomatic treatment of cervical dystonia (orphan)* [botulinum toxin, type B] 5000 U/mL

Myochrysine IM injection ℞ *antirheumatic* [gold sodium thiomalate] 50 mg/mL

Myocide NS topical solution OTC *antiseptic* [benzalkonium chloride]

Myoflex Creme OTC *analgesic* [trolamine salicylate] 10%

Myolin IV or IM injection ℞ *skeletal muscle relaxant* [orphenadrine citrate] 30 mg/mL ⓓ mullein

Myoscint ⒠ (approved in Europe) *monoclonal antibody Fab to myosin, murine; investigational (orphan) imaging agent for cardiac necrosis and myocarditis* [indium In 111 imciromab pentetate]

Myotrophin injection *investigational (NDA filed, orphan) for amyotrophic lateral sclerosis* [mecasermin]

Myoview ℞ *cardiovascular imaging aid* [technetium Tc 99m tetrofosmin]

Myozyme IV infusion ℞ *exogenous source of the acid alpha-glucosidase enzyme; enzyme replacement therapy for patients with Pompe disease (glycogenosis type 2; glycogen storage disease type II; GSDII) (orphan)* [alglucosidase alfa] 50 mg ⓓ MSM; MZM

Myphetane DX Cough syrup ℞ *antitussive; antihistamine; decongestant* [dextromethorphan hydrobromide; brompheniramine maleate; pseudoephedrine HCl; alcohol 1%] 10•2• 30 mg/5 mL

Myrac film-coated tablets ℞ *tetracycline antibiotic for gram-negative and*

gram-positive bacteria; antirickettsial [minocycline HCl] 50, 75, 100 mg

myralact INN, BAN

Myrica cerifera medicinal herb [see: bayberry]

myricodine [see: myrophine]

Myristica fragrans medicinal herb [see: nutmeg; mace]

myristica oil [see: nutmeg oil]

myristyl alcohol NF *stiffening agent*

myristyltrimethylammonium bromide *antiseborrheic*

myrophine INN, BAN ⑫ morphine

Myroxylon balsamum; M. pereirae medicinal herb [see: Peruvian balsam]

myrrh (Commiphora abssynica; C. molmol; C. myrrha) *seeds medicinal herb for bad breath, bronchitis, cancer, constipation, hay fever, hemorrhoids, leprosy, lung diseases, mouth and skin sores, sore throat, syphilis, and stimulating menses; also used as an antiseptic and astringent*

myrtecaine INN

Myrtilli fructus medicinal herb [see: bilberry]

myrtle *medicinal herb* [see: periwinkle]

myrtle, bog *medicinal herb* [see: buckbean]

myrtle, wax *medicinal herb* [see: bayberry]

myrtle flag; grass myrtle; sweet myrtle *medicinal herb* [see: calamus]

Mysoline oral suspension (discontinued 2004) ℞ *anticonvulsant for grand mal, psychomotor, or focal epileptic seizures* [primidone] 250 mg/5 mL ⑫ Mezlin

Mysoline tablets ℞ *anticonvulsant for grand mal, psychomotor, and focal epileptic seizures; also used for essential tremor and benign familial tremor* [primidone] 50, 250 mg ⑫ Mezlin

myspamol [see: proquamezine]

Mytelase caplets ℞ *anticholinesterase muscle stimulant; myasthenia gravis treatment* [ambenonium chloride] 10 mg

Mytrex cream, ointment (discontinued 2004) ℞ *corticosteroidal anti-inflammatory; antifungal* [triamcinolone acetonide; nystatin] 0.1%• 100 000 U/g ⑫ MET-Rx

Mytussin AC Cough syrup (discontinued 2007) ℞ *narcotic antitussive; expectorant* [codeine phosphate; guaifenesin; alcohol 3.5%] 10•100 mg/5 mL

Mytussin DAC oral liquid ℞ *narcotic antitussive; decongestant; expectorant* [codeine phosphate; pseudoephedrine HCl; guaifenesin; alcohol 1.7%] 10•30•100 mg/5 mL

Mytussin DM syrup (discontinued 2007) OTC *antitussive; expectorant* [dextromethorphan hydrobromide; guaifenesin] 10•100 mg/5 mL

myuizone [see: thioacetazone; thiacetazone]

My-Vitalife capsules OTC *vitamin/mineral/calcium/iron supplement* [multiple vitamins & minerals; calcium; iron; folic acid; biotin] ≟•130•27•0.4• 0.03 mg

MZM tablets ℞ *carbonic anhydrase inhibitor for glaucoma* [methazolamide] 25, 50 mg

MZM (methazolamide) [q.v.]

M-Zole 3 Combination Pack vaginal suppositories + cream OTC *antifungal* [miconazole nitrate] 200 mg; 2%

M-Zole 7 Dual Pack vaginal suppositories + cream OTC *antifungal* [miconazole nitrate] 100 mg; 2%

N₂ (nitrogen) [q.v.]

N-3 polyunsaturated fatty acids
[see: doconexent; icosapent; omega-3 marine triglycerides]

Na PCA; sodium PCA (sodium pyrrolidone carboxylic acid) [q.v.]

²²Na [see: sodium chloride Na 22]

nabazenil USAN, INN *anticonvulsant*

Nabi-HB IM injection ℞ *immunizing agent following exposure to hepatitis B surface antigen; investigational (orphan) prophylaxis against hepatitis B reinfection in liver transplant patients* [hepatitis B immune globulin] 1, 5 mL

nabilone USAN, INN, BAN *synthetic cannabinoid; antiemetic for nausea and vomiting associated with cancer chemotherapy; restricted use due to the high possibility of disturbing psychomimetic reactions and psychological dependence*

nabitan INN *analgesic* [also: nabitan HCl]

nabitan HCl USAN *analgesic* [also: nabitan]

naboctate INN *antiglaucoma agent; antinauseant* [also: naboctate HCl]

naboctate HCl USAN *antiglaucoma agent; antinauseant* [also: naboctate]

nabumetone USAN, INN, BAN *analgesic; nonsteroidal anti-inflammatory drug (NSAID) for osteoarthritis and rheumatoid arthritis* 500, 750 mg oral

nabutan HCl [now: nabitan HCl]

NAC (N-acetyl cysteine) *natural source of cysteine; promotes an increase in the endogenous antioxidant glutathione* [see also: acetylcysteine]

NAC (nitrogen mustard, Adriamycin, CCNU) *chemotherapy protocol*

nacartocin INN

N¹-acetylsulfanilamide [see: sulfacetamide]

NaCl (sodium chloride) [q.v.]

Nacystelyn dry powder for inhalation *investigational (orphan) for cystic fibrosis* [N-acetylcysteinate lysine]

NAD (nicotinamide-adenine dinucleotide) [see: nadide]

nadide USAN, INN *antagonist to alcohol and narcotics*

nadisan [see: carbutamide]

nadolol USAN, USP, INN, BAN *antianginal; antihypertensive; antiadrenergic (β-blocker)* 20, 40, 80, 120, 160 mg oral

nadolol & bendroflumethiazide *antihypertensive; β-blocker; diuretic* 40•5, 80•5 mg oral

nadoxolol INN

nadroparin calcium INN, BAN *low molecular weight heparin; anticoagulant/antithrombotic for prevention of deep vein thrombosis (DVT) after surgery, clotting during hemodialysis, unstable angina, and myocardial infarction*

naepaine HCl NF

nafamostat INN *anticoagulant; antifibrinolytic* [also: nafamostat mesylate; nafamostat mesilate]

nafamostat mesilate JAN *anticoagulant; antifibrinolytic* [also: nafamostat mesylate; nafamostat]

nafamostat mesylate USAN *anticoagulant; antifibrinolytic* [also: nafamostat; nafamostat mesilate]

nafarelin INN, BAN *luteinizing hormone-releasing hormone (LHRH) agonist* [also: nafarelin acetate]

nafarelin acetate USAN *luteinizing hormone-releasing hormone (LHRH) agonist for central precocious puberty (orphan) and endometriosis* [also: nafarelin]

Nafazair eye drops (discontinued 2006) ℞ *decongestant; vasoconstrictor* [naphazoline HCl] 0.1%

nafazatrom INN, BAN

nafcaproic acid INN

nafcillin INN *penicillinase-resistant penicillin antibiotic* [also: nafcillin sodium] ② naphazoline

nafcillin sodium USAN, USP *penicillinase-resistant penicillin antibiotic* [also: nafcillin] 1, 2 g IV infusion

nafenodone INN

nafenopin USAN, INN *antihyperlipoproteinemic*

nafetolol INN

nafimidone INN *anticonvulsant* [also: nafimidone HCl]

nafimidone HCl USAN *anticonvulsant* [also: nafimidone]

nafiverine INN

naflocort USAN, INN *topical adrenocortical steroid*

nafomine INN *muscle relaxant* [also: nafomine malate] ⑨ Novamine

nafomine malate USAN *muscle relaxant* [also: nafomine]

nafoxadol INN

nafoxidine HCl USAN, INN *antiestrogen*

nafronyl oxalate USAN *vasodilator* [also: naftidrofuryl]

naftalofos USAN, INN *veterinary anthelmintic*

naftazone INN, BAN

naftidrofuryl INN *vasodilator* [also: nafronyl oxalate]

naftifine INN, BAN *broad-spectrum antifungal* [also: naftifine HCl]

naftifine HCl USAN *broad-spectrum antifungal; topical treatment for tinea pedis, tinea cruris, and tinea corporis* [also: naftifine]

Naftin cream, gel ℞ *broad-spectrum antifungal for tinea pedis, tinea cruris, and tinea corporis* [naftifine HCl] 1%

naftopidil INN

naftoxate INN

naftypramide INN *antibacterial*

naganol [see: suramin sodium]

NaGHB (sodium gamma hydroxybutyrate) [see: gamma hydroxybutyrate (GHB); sodium oxybate]

Naglazyme IV infusion ℞ *recombinant human enzyme for the treatment of mucopolysaccharidosis VI (MPS VI; Maroteaux-Lamy syndrome)(orphan)* [galsulfase] 1 mg/mL

nagrestipen USAN *stem cell inhibitory protein*

nalazosulfamide [see: salazosulfamide]

nalbuphine INN, BAN *narcotic agonist-antagonist analgesic for moderate to severe pain; adjunct to obstetric and surgical analgesia* [also: nalbuphine HCl]

nalbuphine HCl USAN *narcotic agonist-antagonist analgesic for moderate to severe pain; adjunct to obstetric and surgical analgesia* [also: nalbuphine] 10, 20 mg/mL injection

Naldecon Senior EX oral liquid OTC *expectorant* [guaifenesin] 200 mg/5 mL

NalDex caplets ℞ *decongestant; antihistamine* [phenylephrine HCl; dexchlorpheniramine maleate] 18.5•3.5 mg

Nalex AC syrup ℞ *narcotic antitussive; antihistamine* [codeine phosphate; brompheniramine maleate] 10•2 mg/5 mL

Nalex Expectorant oral liquid ℞ *narcotic antitussive; decongestant; expectorant* [hydrocodone bitartrate; pseudoephedrine HCl; guaifenesin; alcohol 12.5%] 5•60•200 mg/5 mL

Nalex-A caplets, oral liquid ℞ *decongestant; antihistamine; sleep aid* [phenylephrine HCl; chlorpheniramine maleate; phenyltoloxamine citrate] 20•4•40 mg; 5•2.5•7.5 mg/5 mL

Nalex-A 12 oral suspension ℞ *decongestant; antihistamine; sleep aid* [phenylephrine tannate; chlorpheniramine tannate; pyrilamine tannate] 5•2•12.5 mg/5 mL

Nalex-DH oral liquid ℞ *narcotic antitussive; decongestant* [hydrocodone bitartrate; phenylephrine HCl] 5•10 mg/10 mL

Nalfon Pulvules (capsules) ℞ *analgesic; nonsteroidal anti-inflammatory drug (NSAID) for osteoarthritis, rheumatoid arthritis, and other mild to moderate pain; also used for juvenile rheumatoid arthritis, migraine headaches, and sunburn pain* [fenoprofen calcium] 200, 300 mg

nalidixane [see: nalidixic acid]

nalidixate sodium USAN *antibacterial*

nalidixic acid USAN, USP, INN *quinolone antibiotic for urinary tract infections (UTIs)*

nalmefene USAN, INN, BAN *narcotic antagonist; antidote to opioid overdose; postanesthesia "stir-up"*

nalmefene HCl *narcotic antagonist; antidote to opioid overdose; postanesthesia "stir-up"*

nalmetrene [now: nalmefene]

nalmexone INN *analgesic; narcotic antagonist* [also: nalmexone HCl]

nalmexone HCl USAN *analgesic; narcotic antagonist* [also: nalmexone]

nalorphine INN [also: nalorphine HCl]

nalorphine HCl USP [also: nalorphine]

naloxiphane tartrate [see: levallorphan tartrate]

naloxone INN, BAN *narcotic antagonist* [also: naloxone HCl]

naloxone HCl USAN, USP, JAN *narcotic antagonist* [also: naloxone] 0.4 mg/mL injection

naloxone HCl & pentazocine *narcotic agonist-antagonist analgesic* 0.5 • 50 mg oral

naltrexone USAN, INN, BAN *narcotic antagonist*

naltrexone HCl *narcotic antagonist for opiate blockage and maintenance in formerly opiate-dependent individuals (orphan); treatment for alcoholism; investigational (Phase III) for irritable bowel syndrome (IBS); also used for eating disorders and postconcussional syndrome* 50 mg oral

Namenda *film-coated caplets, oral solution NMDA (N-methyl-D-aspartate) antagonist for Alzheimer disease; investigational (Phase III) neuroprotective agent for AIDS dementia* [memantine HCl] 5, 10 mg; 2 mg/mL

naminterol INN

[¹³N] ammonia [see: ammonia N 13]

namoxyrate USAN, INN *analgesic*

namuron [see: cyclobarbitone]

nanafrocin INN

nandrolone BAN *anabolic* [also: nandrolone cyclotate]

nandrolone cyclotate USAN *anabolic* [also: nandrolone]

nandrolone decanoate USAN, USP *androgen/anabolic steroid for anemia of renal insufficiency; also used for AIDS-wasting syndrome; sometimes abused as a street drug*

nandrolone phenpropionate USP *androgen/anabolic steroid for metastatic breast cancer in women; sometimes abused as a street drug*

naniopine [see: nanofin]

NanobacTEST-S *for professional use* ℞ *blood serum test for the presence of nanobacterial antigens and antibodies*

NanobacTEST-U/A *for professional use* ℞ *rapid screening urine test for the presence of live, uncalcified nanobacteria by visual color comparison* [ELISA test]

nanofin INN

nanterinone INN, BAN

nantradol INN *analgesic* [also: nantradol HCl]

nantradol HCl USAN *analgesic* [also: nantradol]

NAPA (N-acetyl-p-aminophenol) [see: acetaminophen]

NAPA (N-acetyl-procainamide) [see: acecainide HCl]

napactadine INN *antidepressant* [also: napactadine HCl]

napactadine HCl USAN *antidepressant* [also: napactadine]

napadisilate INN *combining name for radicals or groups* [also: napadisylate]

napadisylate BAN *combining name for radicals or groups* [also: napadisilate]

napamezole INN *antidepressant* [also: napamezole HCl]

napamezole HCl USAN *antidepressant* [also: napamezole]

Na-PCA *topical spray* OTC *natural skin moisturizing factor; humectant* [sodium pyrrolidone carboxylic acid; aloe vera]

naphazoline INN, BAN *topical ophthalmic decongestant and vasoconstrictor; nasal decongestant* [also: naphazoline HCl; naphazoline nitrate] ⚕ nafcillin

naphazoline HCl USP *topical ophthalmic decongestant and vasoconstrictor; nasal decongestant* [also: naphazoline; naphazoline nitrate] 0.1% eye drops

naphazoline HCl & antazoline phosphate *topical ophthalmic decongestant and antihistamine* 0.05% • 0.5%

naphazoline HCl & pheniramine maleate *topical ophthalmic deconges-*

tant and antihistamine 0.025%•0.3% eye drops

naphazoline nitrate JAN *topical ophthalmic vasoconstrictor; nasal decongestant* [also: naphazoline HCl; naphazoline]

Naphazoline Plus eye drops OTC *decongestant; antihistamine* [naphazoline HCl; pheniramine maleate] 0.025%•0.3%

Naphcon eye drops OTC *decongestant; vasoconstrictor* [naphazoline HCl] 0.012% ☒ nefocon A; Novocain

Naphcon Forte Drop-Tainers (eye drops) (discontinued 2006) ℞ *decongestant; vasoconstrictor* [naphazoline HCl] 0.1%

Naphcon-A Drop-Tainers (eye drops) OTC *decongestant; antihistamine* [naphazoline HCl; pheniramine maleate] 0.025%•0.3% ☒ nefocon; Novocain

Naphoptic-A eye drops ℞ *decongestant; antihistamine* [naphazoline HCl; pheniramine maleate] 0.025%•0.3%

2-naphthol [see: betanaphthol]

naphthonone INN

naphthypramide [see: naftypramide]

Naphuride (available only from the Centers for Disease Control) ℞ *antiparasitic for African trypanosomiasis and onchocerciasis* [suramin sodium]

napirimus INN

napitane mesylate USAN *antidepressant; α-adrenergic blocker; norepinephrine uptake antagonist*

Naprelan controlled-release caplets ℞ *once-daily analgesic; nonsteroidal anti-inflammatory drug (NSAID) for osteoarthritis, rheumatoid arthritis, juvenile arthritis, and ankylosing spondylitis* [naproxen sodium] 412.5, 550 mg (375, 500 mg base)

naprodoxime INN

Naprosyn tablets, oral suspension ℞ *analgesic; nonsteroidal anti-inflammatory drug (NSAID) for osteoarthritis, rheumatoid arthritis, juvenile arthritis, ankylosing spondylitis, primary dysmenorrhea, bursitis/tendinitis, and other mild to moderate pain*

[naproxen] 250, 375, 500 mg; 125 mg/5 mL ☒ niaprazine

Naprosyn EC [see: EC-Naprosyn]

naproxen USAN, USP, INN, BAN, JAN *analgesic; nonsteroidal anti-inflammatory drug (NSAID) for osteoarthritis, rheumatoid arthritis, juvenile arthritis, ankylosing spondylitis, primary dysmenorrhea, bursitis/tendinitis, and other mild to moderate pain* 250, 375, 500 mg oral; 125 mg/5 mL oral ☒ nibroxane

naproxen sodium USAN, USP *analgesic; nonsteroidal anti-inflammatory drug (NSAID) for osteoarthritis, rheumatoid arthritis, juvenile arthritis, ankylosing spondylitis, primary dysmenorrhea, bursitis/tendinitis, and other mild to moderate pain* (base=91%) 220, 275, 550 mg oral

naproxol USAN, INN *anti-inflammatory; analgesic; antipyretic*

napsagatran USAN, INN *antithrombotic*

napsilate INN *combining name for radicals or groups* [also: napsylate]

napsylate USAN, BAN *combining name for radicals or groups* [also: napsilate]

Naqua tablets (discontinued 2006) ℞ *diuretic; antihypertensive* [trichlormethiazide] 2, 4 mg

naranol INN *antipsychotic* [also: naranol HCl] ☒ Norinyl 1 + 35

naranol HCl USAN *antipsychotic* [also: naranol]

narasin USAN, INN, BAN *coccidiostat; veterinary growth stimulant* ☒ Norzine

naratriptan INN, BAN *vascular serotonin 5-HT$_{1D}$ receptor agonist for the acute treatment of migraine* [also: naratriptan HCl]

naratriptan HCl USAN *vascular serotonin 5-HT$_{1D}$ receptor agonist for the acute treatment of migraine* [also: naratriptan]

Narcan IV, IM, or subcu injection ℞ *narcotic antagonist for opiate dependence or overdose; hypotension treatment* [naloxone HCl] 0.4 mg/mL

narcotic agonist-antagonists *a class of opioid or morphine-like analgesics* *with lower abuse potential than pure narcotic agonist analgesics*

narcotic agonists; narcotics *a class of opioid or morphine-like analgesics that relieve pain and induce sleep*

narcotine [see: noscapine]

narcotine HCl [see: noscapine HCl]

nard *medicinal herb* [see: spikenard]

Nardil film-coated tablets ℞ *MAO inhibitor for atypical, nonendogenous, or neurotic depression; also used for bulimia, post-traumatic stress disorders (PTSD), chronic migraine, and social anxiety disorder (SAD)* [phenelzine sulfate] 15 mg

Nariz oral liquid ℞ *decongestant; expectorant* [phenylephrine HCl; guaifenesin] 15•400 mg/10 mL

Naropin injection ℞ *long-acting local or regional anesthetic for surgery; epidural block for cesarean section* [ropivacaine HCl] 0.2%, 0.5%, 0.75%, 1%

narrow dock *medicinal herb* [see: yellow dock]

Nasabid SR long-acting tablets ℞ *decongestant; expectorant* [pseudoephedrine HCl; guaifenesin] 90•600 mg

Nasacort AQ nasal spray in a metered-dose pump ℞ *corticosteroidal anti-inflammatory for seasonal or perennial allergic rhinitis* [triamcinolone acetonide] 55 mcg/dose

Nasacort HFA pressurized metered-dose inhaler (pMDI) with a CFC-free propellant (discontinued 2008) ℞ *corticosteroidal anti-inflammatory for seasonal or perennial allergic rhinitis* [triamcinolone acetonide] 55 mcg/dose

NāSal nasal spray, nose drops OTC *nasal moisturizer* [sodium chloride (saline solution)] 0.65% ⊠ Neosol

Nasal Decongestant pediatric oral drops OTC *nasal decongestant* [pseudoephedrine HCl] 7.5 mg/0.8 mL

Nasal Decongestant spray OTC *nasal decongestant* [oxymetazoline HCl] 0.05%

Nasal Decongestant, Children's Non-Drowsy oral liquid OTC *nasal decongestant* [pseudoephedrine HCl] 15 mg/5 mL

Nasal Decongestant Sinus Non-Drowsy tablets (discontinued 2007) OTC *decongestant; analgesic; antipyretic* [pseudoephedrine HCl; acetaminophen] 30•500 mg

Nasal Moist nasal spray OTC *nasal moisturizer* [sodium chloride (saline solution)] 0.65%

Nasal Relief nasal spray OTC *nasal decongestant* [oxymetazoline HCl] 0.05%

Nasal Spray OTC *nasal moisturizer* [sodium chloride (saline solution)]

NasalCrom nasal spray OTC *anti-inflammatory/mast cell stabilizer for the prophylaxis of allergic rhinitis* [cromolyn sodium] 4% (5.2 mg/dose)

NasalCrom A nasal spray + tablets OTC *anti-inflammatory/mast cell stabilizer for the prophylaxis of allergic rhinitis; antihistamine* [cromolyn sodium; chlorpheniramine maleate] 4% (5.2 mg/dose); 4 mg

NasalCrom CA nasal spray + tablets OTC *anti-inflammatory/mast cell stabilizer for the prophylaxis of allergic rhinitis; decongestant; analgesic; antipyretic* [cromolyn sodium; pseudoephedrine HCl; acetaminophen] 4% (5.2 mg/dose); 30 mg•500 mg

Nasal-Ease with Zinc nasal gel OTC *nasal moisturizer and anti-infective* [zinc acetate]

Nasal-Ease with Zinc Gluconate nasal spray OTC *nasal moisturizer and anti-infective* [zinc gluconate]

Nasalide nasal spray (discontinued 2004) ℞ *corticosteroidal anti-inflammatory for seasonal or perennial rhinitis* [flunisolide] 0.025% (25 mcg/dose)

Nasarel metered dose nasal spray ℞ *corticosteroidal anti-inflammatory for seasonal or perennial rhinitis* [flunisolide] 0.025% (29 mcg/dose) ⊠ Nizoral

Nasatab LA long-acting caplets ℞ *decongestant; expectorant* [pseudoephedrine HCl; guaifenesin] 120•500 mg

Nascobal nasal gel in metered-dose applicator (discontinued 2007) ℞ *maintenance administration following intramuscular vitamin B₁₂ therapy* [cyanocobalamin] 500 mcg/0.1 mL dose

Nascobal nasal spray ℞ *once-weekly maintenance administration following intramuscular vitamin B₁₂ therapy* [cyanocobalamin] 500 mcg/0.1 mL dose

Nasex; Nasex-G extended-release caplets (discontinued 2008) ℞ *decongestant; expectorant* [phenylephrine HCl; guaifenesin] 25•650 mg; 25•835 mg

NASHA (non-animal stabilized hyaluronic acid) [see: hyaluronic acid]

Nashville Rabbit Antithymocyte Serum *investigational (orphan) passive immunizing agent to prevent allograft rejection of solid organ and bone marrow transplants* [antithymocyte globulin, rabbit]

Nasofed oral suspension ℞ *decongestant* [pseudoephedrine tannate] 50 mg/5 mL

Nasohist oral drops ℞ *decongestant; antihistamine* [phenylephrine HCl; chlorpheniramine maleate] 2•1 mg/mL

Nasohist DM oral drops ℞ *antitussive; antihistamine; decongestant* [dextromethorphan hydrobromide; chlorpheniramine maleate; phenylephrine HCl] 3•1•2 mg/mL

Nasonex nasal spray in a metered-dose pump ℞ *corticosteroidal anti-inflammatory for allergic rhinitis and nasal polyps* [mometasone furoate] 50 mcg/dose

Nasop orally disintegrating tablets ℞ *nasal decongestant* [phenylephrine HCl] 10 mg

Nasturtium officinale medicinal herb [see: watercress]

NaT (novel acting thrombolytic) [q.v.]

NataChew chewable tablets ℞ *prenatal vitamin/mineral supplement* [multiple vitamins & minerals; ferrous fumarate; folic acid] ≛•29•1 mg

Natacyn eye drop suspension ℞ *antifungal* [natamycin] 5%

NataFort film-coated tablets ℞ *prenatal vitamin/iron supplement* [multiple vitamins; ferrous sulfate; folic acid] ≛•60•1 mg

NatalCare Plus; NatalCare Three film-coated tablets ℞ *vitamin/mineral/calcium/iron supplement* [multiple vitamins & minerals; calcium; iron; folic acid] ≛•200•27•1 mg

natalizumab *humanized monoclonal antibody (huMAb) anti-inflammatory for treatment of multiple sclerosis and Crohn disease; investigational (Phase III) for rheumatoid arthritis; (withdrawn from the market in 2005 due to safety concerns, reintroduced in 2006)*

natamycin USAN, USP, INN, BAN *ophthalmic fungicidal antibiotic* [also: pimaricin]

Natarex Prenatal tablets ℞ *vitamin/calcium/iron supplement* [multiple vitamins; calcium; iron; folic acid; biotin] ≛•200•60•1•0.03 mg

NataTab CFe film-coated tablets (discontinued 2008) ℞ *prenatal vitamin/mineral supplement* [multiple vitamins & minerals]

NataTab FA; NataTab Rx film-coated tablets ℞ *prenatal vitamin/mineral supplement* [multiple vitamins & minerals]

nateglinide USAN *amino acid–derivative; meglitinide antidiabetic for type 2 diabetes that stimulates the release of insulin from the pancreas*

Natelle-EZ caplets ℞ *vitamin/mineral/calcium/iron supplement* [multiple vitamins & minerals; calcium; iron; folic acid biotin] ≛•100•25•1•0.3 mg

Natrecor powder for IV injection ℞ *human B-type natriuretic peptide (hBNP); vasodilator for acute congestive heart failure* [nesiritide citrate] 1.58 mg/vial

Natru-Vent nasal spray OTC *nasal decongestant* [xylometazoline HCl] 0.05%, 0.1%

Natural Fiber Laxative powder OTC *bulk laxative* [psyllium hydrophilic mucilloid] 3.4 g/dose

natural killer cell stimulatory factor [see: edodekin alfa]

Natural Psyllium Fiber powder OTC *bulk laxative* [psyllium hydrophilic mucilloid] 3.4 g/tsp.

Naturalyte oral solution OTC *electrolyte replacement* [sodium, potassium, and chloride electrolytes] 240 mL, 1 L ☑ Nutrilyte

Nature Throid tablets ℞ *natural thyroid replacement for hypothyroidism or thyroid cancer* [thyroid, desiccated (porcine)] 16.25, 32.4, 64.8, 129.6, 194.4 mg

Nature's Remedy tablets OTC *stimulant laxative* [cascara sagrada; aloe] 150•100 mg

Nature's Tears eye drops OTC *moisturizer/lubricant* [hydroxypropyl methylcellulose] 0.4%

Naturetin tablets (discontinued 2008) ℞ *antihypertensive; diuretic* [bendroflumethiazide] 5 mg

Naturvus *hydrophilic contact lens material* [hefilcon B] ☑ Neutra-Phos

Nausea Relief oral solution OTC *antiemetic for nausea associated with influenza, morning sickness, motion sickness, inhalation anesthesia, or food and drink indiscretions* [phosphorated carbohydrate solution (dextrose, fructose, and phosphoric acid)] 1.87 g•1.87 g•21.5 mg per dose

Nausetrol oral solution OTC *antiemetic for nausea associated with influenza, morning sickness, motion sickness, inhalation anesthesia, or food and drink indiscretions* [phosphorated carbohydrate solution (fructose, dextrose, and orthophosphoric acid)] 118 mL (1870•1870•21.5 mg)

Navane capsules ℞ *conventional (typical) thioxanthene antipsychotic for*

schizophrenia [thiothixene] 1, 2, 5, 10, 20 mg

Navane oral concentrate ℞ *conventional (typical) thioxanthene antipsychotic for schizophrenia* [thiothixene HCl] 5 mg/mL

Navelbine IV injection ℞ *antineoplastic for Hodgkin disease and lung, breast and ovarian cancer* [vinorelbine tartrate] 10 mg/mL

naxagolide INN *antiparkinsonian; dopamine agonist* [also: naxagolide HCl]

naxagolide HCl USAN *antiparkinsonian; dopamine agonist* [also: naxagolide]

naxaprostene INN

naxifylline USAN *treatment of edema due to congestive heart failure*

Nazarin oral liquid (discontinued 2008) ℞ *decongestant; expectorant* [phenylephrine HCl; guaifenesin] 15•400 mg/10 mL

Nazarin HC oral liquid ℞ *narcotic antitussive; decongestant; expectorant* [hydrocodone bitartrate; phenylephrine HCl; guaifenesin] 2.5•7.5•150 mg/5 mL

9-NC (9-nitrocamptothecin) [see: rubitecan]

ND Clear sustained-release capsules (discontinued 2007) ℞ *decongestant; antihistamine* [pseudoephedrine HCl; chlorpheniramine maleate] 120•8 mg

nealbarbital INN [also: nealbarbitone]

nealbarbitone BAN [also: nealbarbital]

nebacumab USAN, INN, BAN *antiendotoxin monoclonal antibody; investigational (orphan) for gram-negative bacteremia in endotoxin shock*

Nebcin IV or IM injection, pediatric injection, powder for injection ℞ *aminoglycoside antibiotic* [tobramycin sulfate] 10, 40 mg/mL; 10 mg/mL; 1.2 g

Nebido injection *investigational (NDA filed) long-acting hormone replacement for male hypogonadism* [testosterone]

nebidrazine INN

nebivolol HCl USAN, INN *cardioselective β_1-blocker for hypertension*

nebracetam INN

nebramycin USAN, INN *antibacterial*

nebramycin factor 6 [see: tobramycin]

NebuPent inhalation aerosol ℞ *antiprotozoal; treatment and prophylaxis of* Pneumocystis *pneumonia (PCP) (orphan)* [pentamidine isethionate] 300 mg

Necon 0.5/35; Necon 1/35 tablets (in packs of 21 or 28) ℞ *monophasic oral contraceptive* [norethindrone; ethinyl estradiol] 0.5 mg•35 mcg; 1 mg•35 mcg

Necon 1/50 tablets (in packs of 21 or 28) ℞ *monophasic oral contraceptive* [norethindrone; mestranol] 1 mg• 50 mcg

Necon 10/11 tablets (in packs of 21 or 28) ℞ *biphasic oral contraceptive* [norethindrone; ethinyl estradiol] Phase 1 (10 days): 500•35 mcg; Phase 2 (11 days): 1000•35 mcg

Necon 7/7/7 tablets (in packs of 28) ℞ *triphasic oral contraceptive* [norethindrone; ethinyl estradiol] Phase 1 (7 days): 0.5 mg•35 mcg; Phase 2 (7 days): 0.75 mg•35 mcg; Phase 3 (7 days): 1 mg•35 mcg

nedocromil USAN, INN, BAN *antiinflammatory; prophylactic antiallergic; mast cell stabilizer*

nedocromil calcium USAN *antiinflammatory; prophylactic antiallergic; mast cell stabilizer*

nedocromil sodium USAN *anti-inflammatory; mast cell stabilizer; antiasthmatic; prophylactic antiallergic*

neem tree (*Azadirachta indica*) fruit, leaves, root, and oil *medicinal herb for contraception, diabetes, heart disease, malaria, skin diseases, ulcers, and worms; also used as a pesticide and insect repellent; not generally regarded as safe and effective for infants as it may cause death*

nefazodone INN *antidepressant; selective serotonin and norepinephrine reuptake inhibitor (SSNRI)* [also: nefazodone HCl]

nefazodone HCl USAN *antidepressant; selective serotonin and norepinephrine reuptake inhibitor (SSNRI); FDA* approval for use in children and adolescents was withdrawn in 2004 due to safety concerns [also: nefazodone] 50, 100, 150, 200, 250 mg oral

neflumozide INN *antipsychotic* [also: neflumozide HCl]

neflumozide HCl USAN *antipsychotic* [also: neflumozide]

nefocon A USAN *hydrophobic contact lens material* ⊡ Naphcon; Novocain

nefopam INN *analgesic* [also: nefopam HCl]

nefopam HCl USAN *analgesic* [also: nefopam]

nefrolan [see: clorexolone]

Negaban *investigational (orphan) antibiotic for pulmonary* Burkholderia cepacia *infections* [temocillin sodium]

NegGram caplets ℞ *quinolone antibiotic for urinary tract infections (UTIs)* [nalidixic acid] 500 mg

NegGram oral suspension (discontinued 2005) ℞ *quinolone antibiotic for urinary tract infections (UTIs)* [nalidixic acid] 250 mg/5 mL

nelarabine USAN *DNA synthesis inhibitor; antineoplastic for T-cell acute lymphoblastic leukemia (T-ALL; orphan) and T-cell lymphoblastic lymphoma (T-LBL; orphan); nucleoside analogue; prodrug of ara-G*

neldazosin INN

nelezaprine INN *muscle relaxant* [also: nelezaprine maleate]

nelezaprine maleate USAN *muscle relaxant* [also: nelezaprine]

nelfilcon A USAN *hydrophilic contact lens material*

nelfinavir mesylate USAN *antiretroviral; protease inhibitor for HIV-1 infection*

nemadectin USAN, INN *veterinary antiparasitic*

nemazoline INN *nasal decongestant* [also: nemazoline HCl]

nemazoline HCl USAN *nasal decongestant* [also: nemazoline]

Nembutal elixir (discontinued 2006) ℞ *sedative; hypnotic; also abused as a street drug* [pentobarbital] 20 mg/5 mL

Nembutal Sodium capsules, IV or IM injection, suppositories ℞ *sedative; hypnotic; also abused as a street drug* [pentobarbital sodium] 50, 100 mg; 50 mg/mL; 30, 60, 120, 200 mg

Neo DM oral drops ℞ *antitussive; antihistamine; decongestant; for children 3–24 months* [dextromethorphan hydrobromide; chlorpheniramine maleate; phenylephrine HCl] 2.75•0.75•1.75 mg/mL

Neo DM oral suspension ℞ *antitussive; antihistamine; decongestant* [dextromethorphan tannate; bromphen-iramine tannate; phenylephrine tannate] 30•10•25 mg/5 mL

Neo DM syrup ℞ *antitussive; antihistamine; decongestant* [dextromethorphan hydrobromide; bromphen-amine maleate; pseudoephedrine HCl] 30•3•50 mg/5 mL

Neo HC syrup ℞ *narcotic antitussive; decongestant; antihistamine* [hydrocodone bitartrate; phenylephrine HCl; chlorpheniramine maleate] 5•7.5•3 mg/5 mL

neoarsphenamine NF, INN

Neoasma caplets ℞ *antiasthmatic; bronchodilator; expectorant* [theophylline; guaifenesin] 125•100 mg

NeoBenz Micro; NeoBenz Micro SD cream ℞ *keratolytic for acne* [benzoyl peroxide] 3.5%, 5.5%, 8.5%

neocarzinostatin [now: zinostatin]

Neocate One + ready-to-use pediatric oral liquid OTC *enteral nutritional therapy* [lactose-free formula] 237 mL ☒ nicotine

Neocera (trademarked ingredient) *suppository base* [polyethylent glycol 400, 1450, and 8000; polysorbate 60]

neocid [see: chlorphenothane]

neocinchophen NF, INN

NeoDecadron Ocumeter (eye drops), ophthalmic ointment ℞ *corticosteroidal anti-inflammatory; antibiotic* [dexamethasone sodium phosphate; neomycin sulfate] 0.1%•0.35%; 0.05%•0.35%

Neo-Dexair eye drops ℞ *corticosteroidal anti-inflammatory; antibiotic* [dexamethasone sodium phosphate; neomycin sulfate] 0.1%•0.35%

Neo-Dexameth eye drops ℞ *corticosteroidal anti-inflammatory; antibiotic* [dexamethasone sodium phosphate; neomycin sulfate] 0.1%•0.35%

Neo-Diaral capsules OTC *antidiarrheal* [loperamide] 2 mg

neodymium *element (Nd)*

Neo-fradin oral solution ℞ *aminoglycoside antibiotic* [neomycin sulfate] 125 mg/5 mL ☒ nifuradene

Neofrin eye drops ℞ *decongestant; vasoconstrictor; mydriatic* [phenylephrine HCl] 2.5%, 10% ☒ Nephron

Neoloid oral emulsion OTC *stimulant laxative* [castor oil] 36.4%

Neomark *investigational (NDA filed, orphan) radiosensitizer for primary brain tumors* [broxuridine]

neo-mercazole [see: carbimazole]

neomycin INN, BAN *antibacterial* [also: neomycin palmitate] ☒ nimazone; Numoisyn

neomycin B [see: framycetin]

neomycin palmitate USAN *antibacterial* [also: neomycin]

neomycin sulfate USP *aminoglycoside antibiotic* 500 mg oral

neomycin sulfate & polymyxin B sulfate & bacitracin zinc *topical antibiotic* 5 mg•10 000 U•400 U per g ophthalmic

neomycin sulfate & polymyxin B sulfate & dexamethasone *topical ophthalmic antibiotic and corticosteroidal anti-inflammatory* 0.35%•10 000 U/mL•0.1% eye drops

neomycin sulfate & polymyxin B sulfate & gramicidin *topical antibiotic* 1.75 mg•10 000 U•0.025 mg per mL eye drops

neomycin sulfate & polymyxin B sulfate & hydrocortisone *topical ophthalmic/otic antibiotic and corticosteroidal anti-inflammatory* 0.35%•10 000 U/mL•1% eye drops; 5 mg/mL•10 000 U/mL•1% ear drops

neomycin undecenoate [see: neomycin undecylenate]

neomycin undecylenate USAN *antibacterial; antifungal*

neon *element (Ne)*

Neopap suppositories (discontinued 2008) OTC *analgesic; antipyretic* [acetaminophen] 125 mg

neopenyl [see: clemizole penicillin]

NeoProfen IV injection ℞ *nonsteroidal anti-inflammatory drug (NSAID) for neonatal closure of patent ductus arteriosus (orphan)* [ibuprofen lysine] 17.1 mg/mL (10 mg/mL base)

neoquate [see: nequinate]

Neoral gelcaps, oral solution ℞ *immunosuppressant for allogenic kidney, liver, and heart transplants (orphan), rheumatoid arthritis, and psoriasis* [cyclosporine; alcohol 11.9%] 25, 100 mg; 100 mg/mL ☐ Norel LA

Neosar powder for IV injection ℞ *nitrogen mustard-type alkylating antineoplastic for multiple leukemias, lymphomas, blastomas, sarcomas, and organ cancers* [cyclophosphamide] 100 mg

Neosol orally disintegrating tablets ℞ *GI/GU antispasmodic; antiparkinsonian; anticholinergic "drying agent" for allergic rhinitis and hyperhidrosis* [hyoscyamine sulfate] 0.125 mg ☐ NāSal

Neosporin Drop Dose (eye drops) ℞ *antibiotic* [polymyxin B sulfate; neomycin sulfate; gramicidin] 10 000 U•1.75 mg•0.025 mg per mL

Neosporin ophthalmic ointment ℞ *antibiotic* [polymyxin B sulfate; neomycin sulfate; bacitracin zinc] 10 000 U•5 mg•400 U per g

Neosporin AF cream, spray liquid OTC *antifungal for tinea pedis, tinea cruris, and tinea corporis* [miconazole nitrate] 2%

Neosporin G.U. Irrigant solution ℞ *antibiotic* [neomycin sulfate; polymyxin B sulfate] 40 mg•200 000 U per mL

Neosporin Original ointment OTC *antibiotic* [polymyxin B sulfate; neomycin sulfate; bacitracin zinc] 5000 U•3.5 mg•400 U per g

Neosporin Plus Pain Relief cream OTC *antibiotic; local anesthetic* [polymyxin B sulfate; neomycin sulfate; pramoxine HCl] 10 000 U•3.5 mg•10 mg per g

Neosporin Plus Pain Relief ointment OTC *antibiotic; local anesthetic* [polymyxin B sulfate; neomycon sulfate; bacitracin zinc; pramoxine HCl] 10 000 U•3.5 mg•500 U•10 mg per g

neostigmine BAN *cholinergic/anticholinesterase muscle stimulant* [also: neostigmine bromide]

neostigmine bromide USP, INN, BAN *cholinergic/anticholinesterase muscle stimulant* [also: neostigmine] 15 mg oral

neostigmine methylsulfate USP *cholinergic/anticholinesterase muscle stimulant; urinary stimulant for postsurgical urinary retention; treatment for myasthenia gravis; antidote to neuromuscular blockers* 1:1000 (1 mg/mL), 1:2000 (0.5 mg/mL) injection

Neostrata Skin Lightening gel OTC *hyperpigmentation bleaching agent* [hydroquinone] 2%

Neo-Synephrine eye drops, viscous solution (discontinued 2006) ℞ *decongestant; vasoconstrictor; mydriatic* [phenylephrine HCl] 2.5%, 10%; 10%

Neo-Synephrine IV, IM, or subcu injection ℞ *vasopressor for hypotensive or cardiac shock* [phenylephrine HCl] 1% (10 mg/mL)

Neo-Synephrine 4-Hour Mild Formula nasal spray (name changed to **Neo-Synephrine Mild Strength** in 2008)

Neo-Synephrine 12-Hour; Neo-Synephrine 12-Hour Extra Moisturizing nasal spray OTC *nasal decongestant* [oxymetazoline HCl] 0.05%

Neo-Synephrine Mild Strength; Neo-Synephrine Regular Strength; Neo-Synephrine Extra Strength

nasal spray, nose drops OTC *nasal decongestant* [phenylephrine HCl] 0.25%; 0.5%; 1%

Neo-Tabs tablets ℞ *aminoglycoside antibiotic* [neomycin sulfate] 500 mg

Neotrace-4 IV injection ℞ *intravenous nutritional therapy* [multiple trace elements (metals)] ⊡ Nu-Tears

Neotricin HC ophthalmic ointment ℞ *corticosteroidal anti-inflammatory; antibiotic* [hydrocortisone acetate; neomycin sulfate; bacitracin zinc; polymyxin B sulfate] 1%•3.5%•400 U/g•10 000 U/g

Neovastat *investigational (Phase III) shark cartilage–based angiogenesis inhibitor for osteoarthritis, rheumatoid arthritis, and various cancers; investigational (orphan) for renal cell carcinoma* [AE-941 (code name—generic name not yet assigned)]

nepafenac USAN *nonsteroidal anti-inflammatory drug (NSAID) for pain and inflammation following cataract extraction surgery*

Nepeta cataria *medicinal herb* [see: catnip]

Nephplex Rx tablets ℞ *vitamin/zinc supplement* [multiple B vitamins; ascorbic acid; folic acid; biotin; zinc] ±•60•1•0.3•12.5 mg

NephrAmine 5.4% IV infusion ℞ *nutritional therapy for renal failure* [multiple essential amino acids; electrolytes]

nephritics *a class of agents that affect the kidney (a term used in folk medicine)*

Nephro-Calci tablets OTC *calcium supplement* [calcium carbonate] 1500 mg (600 mg Ca)

Nephrocaps capsules ℞ *vitamin supplement* [multiple B vitamins; vitamin C; folic acid; biotin] ±•100 mg•1 mg•150 mcg

Nephro-Fer tablets OTC *hematinic; iron supplement* [ferrous fumarate (source of iron)] 350 mg (115 mg)

Nephro-Fer Rx film-coated tablets (discontinued 2004) ℞ *hematinic* [ferrous fumarate; folic acid] 106.9•1 mg

Nephron solution for inhalation OTC *sympathomimetic bronchodilator; vasopressor for shock* [racepinephrine HCl] 2.25% ⊡ Neofrin

Nephron FA tablets ℞ *hematinic* [ferrous fumarate; multiple B vitamins; ascorbic acid; folic acid; biotin; docusate sodium] 66.6•±•40•1•0.3•75 mg

Nephro-Vite Rx film-coated tablets ℞ *vitamin supplement* [multiple B vitamins; vitamin C; folic acid; biotin] ±•60 mg•1 mg•300 mcg

Nephro-Vite Rx + Fe film-coated tablets (discontinued 2004) ℞ *hematinic* [ferrous fumarate; multiple B vitamins; ascorbic acid; folic acid; biotin] 100•±•60•1•0.3 mg

Nephro-Vite Vitamin B Complex and C Supplement tablets OTC *vitamin supplement* [multiple B vitamins; vitamin C; folic acid; biotin] ±•60•0.8•0.3 mg

Nephrox oral suspension OTC *antacid; laxative* [aluminum hydroxide; mineral oil 10%] 320 mg/5 mL ⊡ Niferex

nepicastat HCl USAN *dopamine β-hydroxylase inhibitor for congestive heart failure*

Nepro oral liquid OTC *enteral nutritional therapy for acute or chronic renal failure* [lactose-free formula] 240 mL

neptamustine INN *antineoplastic* [also: pentamustine]

Neptazane tablets (discontinued 2004) ℞ *carbonic anhydrase inhibitor for glaucoma* [methazolamide] 25, 50 mg

neptunium *element (Np)*

nequinate USAN, INN *coccidiostat for poultry* [also: methyl benzoquate] ⊡ Nu-knit

neramexane *investigational (Phase III) NMDA (N-methyl-D-aspartate)-receptor antagonist for Alzheimer disease*

neraminol INN

nerbacadol INN

nerelimomab USAN *monoclonal antibody to tumor necrosis factor (TNF); cytokine modulator*

neridronic acid INN

Nerium indicum; N. oleander medicinal herb [see: oleander]

nerve growth factor, recombinant human (rhNGF) *investigational (orphan) for HIV-associated sensory neuropathy*

nervines *a class of agents that have a calming or soothing effect on the nerves (a term used in folk medicine)*

Nesacaine; Nesacaine MPF injection ℞ *local anesthetic; central or peripheral nerve block, including lumbar and epidural block* [chloroprocaine HCl] 1%, 2%; 2%, 3% ⊠ New-Skin

nesapidil INN

nesiritide USAN *human B-type natriuretic peptide (hBNP); vasodilator for acute congestive heart failure*

nesiritide citrate *human B-type natriuretic peptide (hBNP); vasodilator for acute congestive heart failure*

nesosteine INN

Nestabs tablets (name changed to **Vitelle Nestabs** OTC upon status change to OTC in 2000)

Nestabs CBF; Nestabs FA tablets ℞ *vitamin/calcium/iron supplement for pregnancy and lactation* [multiple vitamins; calcium; iron; folic acid] ≗•200•50•1 mg; ≗•200•29•1 mg

Nestlé Good Start [see: Good Start]

Nestlé VHC 2.25 oral liquid OTC *enteral nutritional therapy* [lactose-free formula]

nethalide [see: pronetalol]

netilmicin INN, BAN *aminoglycoside antibiotic* [also: netilmicin sulfate]

netilmicin sulfate USAN, USP *aminoglycoside antibiotic* [also: netilmicin]

netobimin USAN, INN, BAN *veterinary anthelmintic*

netrafilcon A USAN *hydrophilic contact lens material*

nettle (*Urtica dioica; U. urens*) leaves and root *medicinal herb for blood cleansing, bronchitis, diarrhea, edema, hypertension, bleeding, and rheumatism;* ⊠ Nytol

nettle, hemp; bee nettle; dog nettle; hemp dead nettle *medicinal herb* [see: hemp nettle]

nettle flowers; dead nettle; stingless nettle; white nettle *medicinal herb* [see: blind nettle]

Neulasta subcu injection in prefilled syringe ℞ *hematopoietic stimulant for severe chronic neutropenia following cancer chemotherapy* [pegfilgrastim] 6 mg/0.6 mL

Neumega powder for subcu injection ℞ *platelet growth factor for prevention of thrombocytopenia following chemotherapy or radiation (orphan)* [oprelvekin] 5 mg

Neupogen IV or subcu injection, prefilled syringes ℞ *hematopoietic stimulant for severe chronic neutropenia (orphan); investigational (Phase III, orphan) cytokine for AIDS-related cytomegalovirus retinitis; investigational (orphan) for myelodysplastic syndrome* [filgrastim] 300 mcg/mL; 300, 480 mcg

Neuprex injection *investigational (Phase III, orphan) agent for gram-negative sepsis, hemorrhagic shock, and meningococcemia* [bactericidal and permeability-increasing protein, recombinant (rBPI-21)]

Neupro transdermal patch ℞ *once-daily treatment for early-stage Parkinson disease; investigational (NDA filed) for restless legs syndrome (RLS)* [rotigotine] 2, 4, 6 mg/24 h.

neural dopaminergic cells (or precursors), porcine fetal *investigational (orphan) intracerebral implant for stage 4 and 5 Parkinson disease*

neural gabaergic cells (or precursors), porcine fetal *investigational (orphan) intracerebral implant for Huntington disease*

NeuRecover-DA; NeuRecover-SA capsules OTC *dietary supplement* [multiple vitamins & minerals; multiple amino acids; folic acid] ≗•0.067 mg; ≗•0.067 mg

Neurelan *investigational (orphan) agent for multiple sclerosis and spinal cord injury* [fampridine]

NeuroCell-HD *investigational (orphan) intracerebral implant for Huntington disease* [neural gabaergic cells, porcine fetal]

NeuroCell-PD *investigational (Phase II/III, orphan) intracerebral implant for advanced Parkinson disease* [neural dopaminergic cells, porcine fetal]

Neurodep injection ℞ *parenteral vitamin therapy* [multiple B vitamins; vitamin C] ± •50 mg/mL

Neurodep-Caps capsules OTC *vitamin supplement* [vitamins B_1, B_6, and B_{12}] 125•125•1 mg

Neurolite injection ℞ *imaging aid for SPECT brain scans* [technetium Tc 99m bicisate]

Neurontin capsules, film-coated caplets, oral solution ℞ *anticonvulsant for partial-onset seizures; treatment for postherpetic neuralgia; investigational (orphan) for amyotrophic lateral sclerosis* [gabapentin] 100, 300, 400 mg; 600, 800 mg; 250 mg/5 mL

neurosin [see: calcium glycerophosphate]

NeuroSlim capsules OTC *dietary supplement* [multiple vitamins & minerals; multiple amino acids; folic acid; biotin] ± •0.066•0.05 mg

neurotrophic growth factor [see: methionyl neurotrophic factor]

neurotrophin-1 *investigational (orphan) for motor neuron disease and amyotrophic lateral sclerosis*

neustab [see: thioacetazone; thiacetazone]

Neut IV or subcu injection ℞ *pH buffer for metabolic acidosis; urinary alkalinizer* [sodium bicarbonate] 4% (0.48 mEq Na/mL)

Neutra-Caine liquid ℞ *mixed with injectable local anesthetics to reduce stinging pain at the injection site* [sodium bicarbonate] 7.5% ⊉ Nutricon

NeutraGard Advanced dental gel ℞ *caries preventative* [sodium fluoride] 1.1%

neutral acriflavine [see: acriflavine]

neutral insulin INN, BAN, JAN *antidiabetic* [also: insulin, neutral]

neutramycin USAN, INN *antibacterial*

Neutra-Phos powder for oral solution OTC *phosphorus supplement* [monobasic sodium phosphate; monobasic potassium phosphate; dibasic sodium phosphate; dibasic potassium phosphate] 250 mg P/pkt. ⊉ Naturvus

Neutra-Phos-K powder for oral solution OTC *phosphorus supplement* [monobasic potassium phosphate; dibasic potassium phosphate] 250 mg P/pkt.

NeuTrexin powder for IV injection (discontinued 2008) ℞ *antiprotozoal for AIDS-related* Pneumocystis *pneumonia (PCP) (orphan); investigational (orphan) antineoplastic for multiple cancers* [trimetrexate glucuronate] 25 mg

neutroflavine [see: acriflavine]

Neutrogena Antiseptic Cleanser for Acne-Prone Skin topical liquid OTC *cleanser for acne* [benzethonium chloride]

Neutrogena Body lotion, oil OTC *moisturizer; emollient*

Neutrogena Clear Pore topical liquid OTC *keratolytic cleansing mask for acne* [benzoyl peroxide] 3.5%

Neutrogena Drying gel OTC *astringent and antiseptic for acne* [hamamelis water (witch hazel); isopropyl alcohol]

Neutrogena Moisture lotion OTC *moisturizer; emollient* ⊉ nitrogen mustard

Neutrogena Non-Drying Cleansing lotion OTC *soap-free therapeutic skin cleanser*

Neutrogena Norwegian Formula Hand cream OTC *moisturizer; emollient*

Neutrogena Oil-Free Acne Wash topical liquid OTC *keratolytic cleanser for acne* [salicylic acid] 2%

Neutrogena Soap; Neutrogena Cleansing for Acne-Prone Skin; Neutrogena Baby Cleansing For-

mula Soap; **Neutrogena Dry Skin Soap; Neutrogena Oily Skin Soap** bar OTC *therapeutic skin cleanser*

Neutrogena T/Gel Original shampoo OTC *antiseborrheic; antipsoriatic; antipruritic; antibacterial* [coal tar extract] 2%

Neutrogena T/Sal shampoo OTC *antiseborrheic; antipsoriatic; antipruritic; antibacterial* [salicylic acid; coal tar] 2%•2%

neutrophil inhibitor, recombinant human (rhNI) *investigational (orphan) for cystic fibrosis*

Nevanac eye drop suspension ℞ *nonsteroidal anti-inflammatory drug (NSAID) for pain and inflammation following cataract extraction surgery* [nepafenac] 0.1%

nevirapine USAN, INN *antiviral nonnucleoside reverse transcriptase inhibitor (NNRTI) for HIV-1*

nevirapine & lamivudine & stavudine *combination nucleoside reverse transcriptase inhibitor (NRTI) and non-nucleoside reverse transcriptase inhibitor (NNRTI) for HIV and AIDS* 50•30•6, 100•60•12, 200•150•30, 200•150•40 mg oral

Nevis tablets *investigational (NDA filed) synthetic progestin/estrogen; hormone replacement therapy for postmenopausal symptoms* [norethindrone acetate; ethinyl estradiol] 1 mg•5 mcg

New Jersey tea (*Ceanothus americanus*) root bark *medicinal herb used as an astringent, expectorant, and sedative*

New Zealand green-lipped mussel (*Perna canaliculus*) freeze-dried body or gonads *natural treatment for osteoarthritis and rheumatoid arthritis*

new-estranol 1 [see: diethylstilbestrol]

new-oestranol 1 [see: diethylstilbestrol]

new-oestranol 11 [see: diethylstilbestrol dipropionate]

NewPaks (trademarked delivery form) *ready-to-use closed system containers*

NewPhase Complete caplets OTC *natural/herbal supplement for the relief or postmenopausal symptoms* [multiple vitamins and minerals; isoflavones; phytoestrogens]

New-Skin topical liquid, spray OTC *skin protectant; antiseptic* [hydroxyquinoline] ② Nesacaine

NexACT (trademarked delivery device) *topical delivery system*

Nexavar film-coated tablets ℞ *multikinase inhibitor; antineoplastic for advanced renal cell carcinoma (orphan) and hepatocellular carcinoma* [sorafenib tosylate] 274 mg (200 mg base)

nexeridine INN *analgesic* [also: nexeridine HCl]

nexeridine HCl USAN *analgesic* [also: nexeridine]

Nexium delayed-release entericcoated pellets in capsules ℞ *proton pump inhibitor for gastric and duodenal ulcers, erosive esophagitis, GERD, and other gastroesophageal disorders* [esomeprazole magnesium] 20, 40 mg

Nexium delayed-release oral suspension ℞ *proton pump inhibitor for gastric and duodenal ulcers, erosive esophagitis, GERD, and other gastroesophageal disorders* [esomeprazole magnesium] 10, 20, 40 mg

Nexium I.V. powder for infusion ℞ *proton pump inhibitor for the shortterm treatment of GERD in patients who cannot take the drug orally* [esomeprazole sodium] 20, 40 mg/dose

Nexrutine capsules OTC *dietary supplement; selective COX-2 inhibitor; antiinflammatory; antipyretic* [Phellodendron amurense extract] 250 mg

NFL (Novantrone, fluorouracil, leucovorin [rescue]) *chemotherapy protocol for breast cancer*

NG-29 *investigational (orphan) diagnostic aid for pituitary release of growth hormone*

NGF (nerve growth factor) [q.v.]

N-Graft *investigational (orphan) intracerebral implant for advanced Parkinson disease (for co-implantation with fetal neural cells)* [Sertoli cells, porcine]

N.G.T. cream ℞ *corticosteroidal antiinflammatory; antifungal* [triamcino-

lone acetonide; nystatin] 0.1%•
100 000 U per g

NI (neutrophil inhibitor) [q.v.]

niacin (vitamin B₃) USP *water-soluble
vitamin; peripheral vasodilator; antihyperlipidemic for hypertriglyceridemia
(types IV and V hyperlipidemia) and
hypercholesterolemia* [also: nicotinic
acid] 50, 100, 125, 250, 400, 500 mg
oral

niacinamide (vitamin B₃) USP *water-
soluble vitamin; enzyme cofactor; treatment for vitamin B₃ deficiency; also
used for several dermatologic conditions, including psoriasis* [also: nicoti-
namide] 100, 500 mg oral

niacinamide hydroiodide *expectorant*

Niacor immediate-release tablets ℞
*vitamin B₃ therapy; peripheral vasodila-
tor; antihyperlipidemic for hypertriglyceridemia (types IV and V hyperlipidemia) and hypercholesterolemia* [niacin]
500 mg

nialamide NF, INN

niaprazine INN ⊡ Naprosyn

Niaspan enteric-coated, extended-
release caplets ℞ *vitamin B₃ therapy;
peripheral vasodilator; antihyperlipidemic for hypertriglyceridemia (types IV
and V hyperlipidemia) and hypercholesterolemia* [niacin] 500, 750, 1000 mg

Niaspan CF extended-release caplets
*investigational (NDA filed) reduced-
flushing formulation* [niacin] 1000 mg

nibroxane USAN, INN *topical antimicrobial* ⊡ naproxen

Nicabate ⓔ (European name for U.S.
product **Nicoderm**)

nicafenine INN

nicainoprol INN

nicametate INN, BAN

nicaraven INN

nicarbazin BAN

nicardipine INN, BAN *vasodilator for
chronic stable angina; calcium channel
blocker for hypertension* [also: nicardipine HCl]

nicardipine HCl USAN *vasodilator for
chronic stable angina; calcium channel
blocker for hypertension* [also: nicardi-

pine] 20, 30 mg oral; 2.5 mg/mL
injection

NicCheck I reagent strips *in vitro
diagnostic aid for urine nicotine, used
to determine the smoking status of the
subject*

N'Ice throat spray OTC *mild anesthetic;
antipruritic; counterirritant* [menthol]
0.12%

N'Ice; N'Ice 'n Clear lozenges OTC
*mild anesthetic; antipruritic; counterir-
ritant* [menthol] 5 mg

N'Ice Vitamin C Drops (lozenges)
OTC *vitamin C supplement* [ascorbic
acid] 60 mg

nicergoline USAN, INN *vasodilator*

niceritrol INN, BAN

nicethamide BAN [also: nikethamide]

niceverine INN

nickel *element* (Ni)

niclofolan INN, BAN

niclosamide USAN, INN *anthelmintic
for cestodiasis (tapeworm)*

nicoboxil INN

nicoclonate INN

nicocodine INN, BAN

nicocortonide INN

**Nicoderm CQ Step 1; Nicoderm
CQ Step 2; Nicoderm CQ Step 3**
transdermal patch OTC *smoking cessation aid for the relief of nicotine withdrawal symptoms* [nicotine] 21 mg/
day; 14 mg/day; 7 mg/day

nicodicodine INN, BAN

**nicoduozide (isoniazid + nicothia-
zone)**

nicofibrate INN

nicofuranose INN

nicofurate INN

nicogrelate INN

Nicomide tablets ℞ *vitamin/mineral
supplement* [nicotinamide; zinc
oxide; cupric oxide; folic acid] 750•
25•1.5•0.5 mg

nicomol INN

nicomorphine INN, BAN

nicopholine INN

nicorandil USAN, INN *coronary vasodilator*

Nicorette chewing gum OTC *smoking cessation aid for the relief of nicotine withdrawal symptoms* [nicotine polacrilex] 2, 4 mg

Nicosyn lotion ℞ *antibiotic and keratolytic for acne* [sulfacetamide sodium; sulfur] 10%•5%

nicothiazone INN

nicotinaldehyde thiosemicarbazone [see: nicothiazone]

nicotinamide (vitamin B₃) INN, BAN, JAN *water-soluble vitamin; enzyme cofactor; treatment for vitamin B₃ deficiency; also used for several dermatologic conditions, including psoriasis* [also: niacinamide] 100, 500 mg oral

nicotinamide-adenine dinucleotide (NAD) [now: nadide]

nicotine *a poisonous alkaloid used as an insecticide and external parasiticide; the active principle in tobacco; smoking cessation aid for the relief of nicotine withdrawal symptoms* [see also: tobacco] 7, 14, 21 mg/day transdermal ▣ Neocate One +

nicotine bitartrate USAN *smoking cessation aid for the relief of nicotine withdrawal symptoms*

nicotine & mecamylamine HCl *investigational (Phase III) transdermal patch for smoking cessation*

nicotine polacrilex USAN *smoking cessation aid for the relief of nicotine withdrawal symptoms* 2, 4 mg oral

nicotine resin complex [see: nicotine polacrilex]

Nicotinex elixir (discontinued 2004) OTC *vitamin B₃ supplement; antihyperlipidemic* [niacin] 50 mg/5 mL

nicotinic acid (vitamin B₃) INN, BAN, JAN *water-soluble vitamin; peripheral vasodilator; antihyperlipidemic for hypertriglyceridemia (types IV and V hyperlipidemia) and hypercholesterolemia* [also: niacin] 50, 100, 125, 250, 400, 500 mg oral

nicotinic acid amide [see: niacinamide; nicotinamide]

nicotinic acid 1-oxide [see: oxiniacic acid]

nicotinohydroxamic acid [see: nicoxamat]

6-nicotinoyl dihydrocodeine [see: nicodicodine]

6-nicotinoylcodeine [see: nicocodine]

4-nicotinoylmorpholine [see: nicopholine]

nicotinyl alcohol USAN, BAN *peripheral vasodilator*

nicotinyl tartrate

Nicotrol oral inhaler ℞ *smoking cessation aid for the relief of nicotine withdrawal symptoms* [nicotine] 10 mg (4 mg delivered) per cartridge

Nicotrol NS nasal spray ℞ *smoking cessation aid for the relief of nicotine withdrawal symptoms* [nicotine] 0.5 mg/spray

Nicotrol Step 1; Nicotrol Step 2; Nicotrol Step 3 transdermal patch OTC *smoking cessation aid for the relief of nicotine withdrawal symptoms* [nicotine] 15 mg/day; 10 mg/day; 5 mg/day

nicotylamide [see: niacinamide]

nicoumalone BAN [also: acenocoumarol]

nicoxamat INN

nictiazem INN

nictindole INN

Nidran ℞ *alkylating antineoplastic* [nimustin HCl]

nidroxyzone INN

Nifediac CC film-coated extended-release tablets ℞ *calcium channel blocker for hypertension; also used for anal fissures* [nifedipine] 30, 60, 90 mg

Nifedical XL film-coated sustained-release tablets ℞ *coronary vasodilator for angina with or without vasospasm; calcium channel blocker for hypertension; also used for anal fissures* [nifedipine] 30, 60 mg

nifedipine USAN, USP, INN, BAN *coronary vasodilator for angina with or without vasospasm; calcium channel blocker for hypertension; also used for anal fissures; investigational (orphan) for interstitial cystitis* 10, 20, 30, 60, 90 mg oral

nifenalol INN

nifenazone INN, BAN

Niferex tablets, elixir OTC *hematinic; iron supplement* [polysaccharide-iron complex] 50 mg Fe; 100 mg Fe/5 mL ⧉ Nephrox

Niferex-150 capsules OTC *hematinic; vitamin/iron supplement* [iron; vitamin C; succinic acid] 150•50•50 mg ⧉ Nephrox

Niferex-150 Forte capsules ℞ *hematinic* [iron; vitamin C; cyanocobalamin; folic acid] 150 mg•60.8 mg•25 mcg•1 mg

Niferex-PN film-coated tablets ℞ *prenatal vitamin/iron supplement* [polysaccharide-iron complex; multiple vitamins & minerals; folic acid] 60•± •1 mg

Niferex-PN Forte film-coated tablets ℞ *prenatal vitamin/mineral/calcium/iron supplement* [multiple vitamins & minerals; calcium; polysaccharide-iron complex; folic acid] ± •250•60•1 mg

niflumic acid INN

nifluridide USAN *ectoparasiticide*

nifungin USAN, INN

nifuradene USAN, INN *antibacterial* ⧉ Neo-fradin

nifuralazine [see: furalazine]

nifuraldezone USAN, INN *antibacterial*

nifuralide INN

nifuramizone [see: nifurethazone]

nifuratel USAN, INN *antibacterial; antifungal; antiprotozoal (Trichomonas)*

nifuratrone USAN, INN *antibacterial*

nifurazolidone [see: furazolidone]

nifurdazil USAN, INN *antibacterial*

nifurethazone INN

nifurfoline INN

nifurhydrazone [see: nihydrazone]

nifurimide USAN, INN *antibacterial*

nifurizone INN

nifurmazole INN

nifurmerone USAN, INN *antifungal*

nifuroquine INN

nifuroxazide INN

nifuroxime NF, INN

nifurpipone (NP) INN

nifurpirinol USAN, INN *antibacterial*

nifurprazine INN

nifurquinazol USAN, INN *antibacterial*

nifursemizone USAN, INN *antiprotozoal for poultry (Histomonas)*

nifursol USAN, INN *antiprotozoal for poultry (Histomonas)*

nifurthiazole USAN, INN *antibacterial*

nifurthiline [see: thiofuradene]

nifurtimox INN, BAN *anti-infective for Chagas disease* (available only from the Centers for Disease Control and Prevention)

nifurtoinol INN

nifurvidine INN

nifurzide INN

Night Time Multi-Symptom Cold/ Flu Relief liquid-filled gelcaps OTC *antitussive; antihistamine; sleep aid; decongestant; analgesic; antipyretic* [dextromethorphan hydrobromide; doxylamine succinate; pseudoephedrine HCl; acetaminophen] 15•6.25•30•325 mg

nightshade; nightshade vine *medicinal herb* [see: bittersweet nightshade]

nightshade, American *medicinal herb* [see: pokeweed]

nightshade, deadly *medicinal herb* [see: belladonna]

nightshade, fetid; stinking nightshade *medicinal herb* [see: henbane]

nightshade, three-leaved *medicinal herb* [see: birthroot]

Nighttime Cold softgels (discontinued 2007) OTC *antitussive; antihistamine; sleep aid; decongestant; analgesic; antipyretic* [dextromethorphan hydrobromide; doxylamine succinate; pseudoephedrine HCl; acetaminophen] 10•6.25•30•250 mg

niguldipine INN

nihydrazone INN

nikethamide NF, INN [also: nicethamide]

Nilandron tablets ℞ *antiandrogen antineoplastic for metastatic prostate cancer* [nilutamide] 50, 150 mg

nileprost INN

nilestriol INN *estrogen* [also: nylestriol]

nilotinib HCl *kinase inhibitor antineo-plastic for Philadelphia chromosome–positive chronic myeloid leukemia (CML)*

nilprazole INN

Nilstat cream, ointment ℞ *antifungal* [nystatin] 100 000 U/g

Nilstat oral suspension, powder for oral suspension ℞ *antifungal; oral candidiasis treatment* [nystatin] 100 000 U/mL; 150 million, 500 million, 1 billion, 2 billion U

niludipine INN

nilutamide USAN, INN, BAN *antiandrogen antineoplastic adjunct to surgical or chemical castration for metastatic prostate cancer*

nilvadipine USAN, INN, JAN *calcium channel antagonist*

nimazone USAN, INN *anti-inflammatory* ② neomycin; Numoisyn

Nimbex IV infusion ℞ *nondepolarizing neuromuscular blocking agent for anesthesia* [cisatracurium besylate] 2, 10 mg/mL

Nimbus; Nimbus Quick Strip test kit for home use OTC *in vitro diagnostic aid; urine pregnancy test* [monoclonal antibody-based enzyme immunoassay]

Nimbus Plus test kit for professional use ℞ *in vitro diagnostic aid; urine pregnancy test*

nimesulide INN, BAN

nimetazepam INN

nimidane USAN, INN *veterinary acaricide*

nimodipine USAN, INN, BAN *vasodilator; calcium channel blocker for subarachnoid hemorrhage (SAH)* 30 mg oral

nimorazole INN, BAN

Nimotop soft liquid-filled capsules ℞ *calcium channel blocker for subarachnoid hemorrhage (SAH)* [nimodipine] 30 mg

nimotuzumab *investigational (orphan) monoclonal antibody for malignant glioma*

nimustine INN *alkylating neoplastic*

nimustine HCl *alkylating neoplastic*

niobium *element (Nb)*

niometacin INN ② Pneumotussin

Nion B Plus C caplets OTC *vitamin supplement* [multiple B vitamins; vitamin C] ± • 300 mg

Nipent powder for IV injection ℞ *antibiotic antineoplastic for hairy cell leukemia (orphan); investigational (orphan) for chronic lymphocytic leukemia and cutaneous and peripheral T-cell lymphomas; investigational (Phase III) for AIDS-related non-Hodgkin lymphoma* [pentostatin] 10 mg

niperotidine INN

nipradilol INN

Nipride (brand discontinued 1992) [see: sodium nitroprusside]

niprisan *investigational (orphan) for sickle cell disease*

niprofazone INN

Niravam orally disintegrating tablets ℞ *benzodiazepine anxiolytic; sedative; treatment for panic disorders and agoraphobia* [alprazolam] 0.25, 0.5, 1, 2 mg

niridazole USAN, INN *antischistosomal*

nisbuterol INN *bronchodilator* [also: nisbuterol mesylate]

nisbuterol mesylate USAN *bronchodilator* [also: nisbuterol]

nisobamate USAN, INN *minor tranquilizer*

nisoldipine USAN, INN, BAN, JAN *coronary vasodilator; calcium channel blocker for hypertension* 20, 30, 40 mg oral

nisoxetine USAN, INN *antidepressant*

nisterime INN *androgen* [also: nisterime acetate]

nisterime acetate USAN *androgen* [also: nisterime]

nitarsone USAN, INN *antiprotozoal (Histomonas)*

nitazoxanide (NTZ) INN *antiprotozoal for pediatric diarrhea due to Cryptosporidium parvum and Giardia lamblia infections (orphan); investigational (orphan) for intestinal amebiasis*

Nite Time Children's Liquid (discontinued 2007) OTC *antitussive; antihistamine; decongestant* [dextromethorphan hydrobromide; chlorpheniramine maleate; pseudoephedrine HCl] 15•2•30 mg/15 mL

Nite Time Cold Formula for Adults oral liquid (discontinued 2007) oTc *antitussive; antihistamine; sleep aid; decongestant; analgesic; antipyretic* [dextromethorphan hydrobromide; doxylamine succinate; pseudoephedrine HCl; acetaminophen; alcohol 10%] 30•12.5•60•1000 mg/30 mL

nithiamide USAN *veterinary antibacterial* [also: aminitrozole; acinitrazole]

nitisinone *adjunctive treatment for hereditary tyrosinemia type 1 (HT-1), a pediatric liver disease (orphan); investigational (orphan) for alkaptonuria*

nitracrine INN

nitrafudam INN *antidepressant* [also: nitrafudam HCl]

nitrafudam HCl USAN *antidepressant* [also: nitrafudam]

nitralamine HCl USAN *antifungal*

nitramisole INN *anthelmintic* [also: nitramisole HCl]

nitramisole HCl USAN *anthelmintic* [also: nitramisole]

nitraquazone INN

nitrates *a class of antianginal agents that cause the relaxation of vascular smooth muscles*

nitratophenylmercury [see: phenylmercuric nitrate]

nitrazepam USAN, INN, BAN, JAN *benzodiazepine sedative; anxiolytic; anticonvulsant; hypnotic*

nitre, sweet spirit of [see: ethyl nitrite]

nitrefazole INN, BAN

Nitrek transdermal patch ℞ *coronary vasodilator; antianginal; also used for acute myocardial infarction, erectile dysfunction, and Raynaud disease* [nitroglycerin] 0.2, 0.4, 0.6 mg/hr. (22.4, 44.8, 67.2 mg total)

nitrendipine USAN, INN, BAN, JAN *antihypertensive; calcium channel blocker*

nitric acid NF *acidifying agent*

nitric oxide *inhalation gas for neonatal hypoxic respiratory failure due to persistent pulmonary hypertension (orphan); investigational (orphan) for acute adult respiratory distress syndrome and to diagnose sarcoidosis*

nitricholine perchlorate INN

"nitro paste"; "nitropaste" *a brief term for "nitroglycerin paste"* [properly called: nitroglycerin ointment]

p-**nitrobenzenearsonic acid** [see: nitarsone]

Nitro-Bid ointment ℞ *coronary vasodilator; antianginal; also used for acute myocardial infarction, chronic anal fissure pain, erectile dysfunction, and Raynaud disease* [nitroglycerin] 2% (15 mg/inch)

Nitro-Bid IV infusion (discontinued 2005) ℞ *coronary vasodilator; antianginal; perioperative antihypertensive; treatment for congestive heart failure with myocardial infarction* [nitroglycerin] 5 mg/mL

9-nitrocamptothecin (9-NC); 9-nitro-20-(S)-camptothecin [now: rubitecan]

nitroclofene INN

nitrocycline USAN, INN *antibacterial*

nitrodan USAN, INN *anthelmintic*

Nitrodisc transdermal patch (discontinued 2005) ℞ *coronary vasodilator; antianginal* [nitroglycerin] 0.2, 0.3, 0.4 mg/hr. (16, 24, 32 mg total)

Nitro-Dur transdermal patch ℞ *coronary vasodilator; antianginal; also used for acute myocardial infarction, erectile dysfunction, and Raynaud disease* [nitroglycerin] 0.1, 0.2, 0.3, 0.4, 0.6, 0.8 mg/hr. (20, 40, 60, 80, 120, 160 mg total)

nitroethanolamine [see: aminoethyl nitrate]

nitrofuradoxadone [see: furmethoxadone]

nitrofural INN *broad-spectrum bactericidal; adjunct to burn treatment* [also: nitrofurazone]

nitrofurantoin USP, INN *urinary antibiotic* 50, 100 mg oral

nitrofurantoin sodium *urinary antibiotic*

nitrofurazone USP, BAN *broad-spectrum bactericidal; adjunct to burn treatment and skin grafting* [also: nitrofural] 0.2% topical

nitrofurmethone [see: furaltadone]

nitrofuroxizone [see: nidroxyzone]

Nitrogard transmucosal extended-release tablets (discontinued 2005) ℞ *coronary vasodilator; antianginal* [nitroglycerin] 2, 3 mg

nitrogen (N₂) NF *air displacement agent; element (N)* ☒ Neutra-Caine; Nutri-con

nitrogen monoxide [see: nitrous oxide]

nitrogen mustard N-oxide HCl JAN *alkylating antineoplastic* [also: mechlorethamine HCl; chlormethine; mustine] ☒ Neutrogena Moisture

nitrogen mustards *a class of alkylating antineoplastics* ☒ Neutrogena Moisture

nitrogen oxide (N₂O) [see: nitrous oxide]

nitroglycerin USP *coronary vasodilator; antianginal; antihypertensive; investigational (NDA filed) topical treatment for anal fissures* [also: glyceryl trinitrate] 0.3, 0.4, 0.6 mg sublingual; 2.5, 6.5, 9 mg oral; 5 mg/mL injection; 0.1, 0.2, 0.4, 0.6 mg/hr. transdermal; 2% topical

Nitroglycerin in Dextrose injection ℞ *coronary vasodilator; antianginal; antihypertensive* [nitroglycerin] 100 mcg/mL•5%, 200 mcg/mL•5%, 400 mcg/mL•5%

Nitroglyn extended-release capsules (discontinued 2004) ℞ *coronary vasodilator; antianginal; antihypertensive* [nitroglycerin] 2.5, 6.5, 9, 13 mg

nitrohydroxyquinoline [see: nitroxoline]

Nitrolan oral liquid OTC *enteral nutritional therapy* [lactose-free formula] ☒ Nutrilan

Nitrolingual Pumpspray CFC-free translingual aerosol ℞ *coronary vasodilator; emergency antianginal* [nitroglycerin; alcohol 20%] 0.4 mg/metered dose

nitromannitol [see: mannitol hexanitrate]

nitromersol USP *topical anti-infective*

nitromide USAN *coccidiostat for poultry; antibacterial*

nitromifene INN

nitromifene citrate USAN *antiestrogen*

NitroMist translingual aerosol ℞ *coronary vasodilator; emergency antianginal* [nitroglycerin] 400 mcg/spray

Nitrong sustained-release tablets (discontinued 2004) ℞ *coronary vasodilator; antianginal; antihypertensive* [nitroglycerin] 2.6, 6.5, 9 mg

"nitropaste"; "nitro paste" *a brief term for "nitroglycerin paste"* [properly called: nitroglycerin ointment]

Nitropress powder for IV injection, flip-top vials ℞ *vasodilator for hypertensive emergency* [sodium nitroprusside] 50 mg/dose

nitroprusside sodium [see: sodium nitroprusside]

NitroQuick sublingual tablets ℞ *coronary vasodilator; emergency antianginal* [nitroglycerin] 0.3, 0.4, 0.6 mg (1/200, 1/150, 1/100 gr.)

nitroscanate USAN, INN *veterinary anthelmintic*

nitrosoureas *a class of alkylating antineoplastics*

Nitrostat sublingual tablets ℞ *coronary vasodilator; emergency antianginal* [nitroglycerin] 0.3, 0.4, 0.6 mg (1/200, 1/150, 1/100 gr.)

nitrosulfathiazole INN [also: para-nitrosulfathiazole]

NitroTab sublingual tablets ℞ *coronary vasodilator; emergency antianginal* [nitroglycerin] 0.3, 0.4, 0.6 mg (1/200, 1/150, 1/100 gr.)

Nitro-Time extended-release capsules ℞ *coronary vasodilator; antianginal; antihypertensive* [nitroglycerin] 2.5, 6.5, 9 mg

nitrous acid, sodium salt [see: sodium nitrite]

nitrous oxide (N₂O) USP *a weak inhalation general anesthetic; sometimes* *abused as a street drug to create a dreamy or floating sensation*

nitroxinil INN

nitroxoline INN, BAN

nivacortol INN *corticosteroid; anti-inflammatory* [also: nivazol]

nivadipine [see: nilvadipine]

nivaquine [see: chloroquine phosphate]

nivazol USAN *corticosteroid; anti-inflammatory* [also: nivacortol] ② Novasal

Nivea After Tan; Nivea Moisturizing; Nivea Moisturizing Extra Enriched lotion OTC *moisturizer; emollient*

Nivea Moisturizing; Nivea Skin oil OTC *moisturizer; emollient*

Nivea Moisturizing Creme Soap bar OTC *therapeutic skin cleanser*

Nivea Ultra Moisturizing Creme OTC *moisturizer; emollient*

nivimedone sodium USAN *antiallergic*

Nix creme rinse OTC *pediculicide for lice; scabicide* [permethrin; alcohol 20%] 1%

nixylic acid INN

nizatidine USAN, USP, INN, BAN, JAN *histamine H_2 antagonist for gastric and duodenal ulcers and gastroesophageal reflux disease (GERD); also used to prevent NSAID-induced gastric ulcers* 150, 300 mg oral

nizofenone INN

Nizoral cream R̸ *antifungal for tinea corporis, tinea cruris, tinea pedis, tinea versicolor, cutaneous candidiasis, and seborrheic dermatitis* [ketoconazole] 2% ② Nasarel

Nizoral shampoo R̸ (available OTC in Canada) *antifungal for dandruff* [ketoconazole] 2% ② Nasarel

Nizoral tablets R̸ *systemic imidazole antifungal* [ketoconazole] 200 mg ② Nasarel

Nizoral A-D shampoo OTC *antifungal for dandruff* [ketoconazole] 1%

NMDA (N-methyl-D-aspartate) [q.v.]

N-Multistix; N-Multistix SG reagent strips *in vitro diagnostic aid for multiple urine products*

NNRTIs (non-nucleoside reverse transcriptase inhibitors) [see: reverse transcriptase inhibitors]

No Pain-HP roll-on OTC *analgesic; counterirritant* [capsaicin] 0.075%

nobelium *element (No)*

noberastine USAN, INN, BAN *antihistamine*

noble yarrow *medicinal herb* [see: yarrow]

nocebo effect [L. I will harm] *a perceived adverse effect from an inert substance* [compare to: placebo effect]

nocloprost INN

nocodazole USAN, INN *antineoplastic*

nodding wakerobin *medicinal herb* [see: birthroot]

NōDōz coated caplets OTC *CNS stimulant; analeptic* [caffeine] 200 mg

nofecainide INN

nofetumomab merpentan *monoclonal antibody imaging agent for small cell lung cancer*

nogalamycin USAN, INN *antineoplastic*

NoHist extended-release caplets R̸ *decongestant; antihistamine* [phenylephrine HCl; chlorpheniramine maleate] 20•8 mg ② Nuhist

NoHist A oral liquid R̸ *decongestant; antihistamine; sleep aid* [phenylephrine HCl; chlorpheniramine maleate; phenyltoloxamine citrate] 5•2.5•7.5 mg/5 mL ② Nuhist

NoHist DMX extended-release caplets R̸ *antitussive; antihistamine; decongestant* [dextromethorphan hydrobromide; chlorpheniramine maleate; phenylephrine HCl] 30•8•20 mg

NoHist EXT extended-release tablets R̸ *antihistamine; anticholinergic to dry mucosal secretions* [chlorpheniramine maleate; methscopolamine nitrate] 8•2.5 mg

NoHist Plus chewable caplets R̸ *decongestant; antihistamine; anticholinergic to dry mucosal secretions* [phenylephrine HCl; chlorpheniramine maleate; methscopolamine nitrate] 10•2•1.25 mg

Nolahist tablets OTC *nonselective piperidine antihistamine for allergic rhinitis* [phenindamine tartrate] 25 mg

nolatrexed dihydrochloride *thymidylate synthase inhibitor that disrupts DNA replication; investigational (Phase III, orphan) for inoperable primary liver cancer*

nolinium bromide USAN, INN *antisecretory; antiulcerative*

Nolvadex tablets (discontinued 2006) ℞ *antiestrogen antineoplastic for the treatment of breast cancer and the reduction of breast cancer incidence in high-risk women* [tamoxifen citrate] 10, 20 mg

nomegestrol INN

nomelidine INN

nomifensine INN *antidepressant* [also: nomifensine maleate]

nomifensine maleate USAN *antidepressant* [also: nomifensine]

Nomuc-PE extended-release capsules ℞ *decongestant; expectorant* [pseudoephedrine HCl; guaifenesin] 60•200 mg

nonabine INN, BAN

nonabsorbable surgical suture [see: suture, nonabsorbable surgical]

nonachlazine [now: azaclorzine HCl]

nonacog alfa USAN, INN *synthetic human blood coagulation factor IX; antihemophilic for hemophilia B and Christmas disease (orphan)* [also: factor IX complex]

nonanedioic acid [see: azelaic acid]

nonaperone INN

nonapyrimine INN

Non-Aspirin caplets OTC *analgesic; antipyretic* [acetaminophen] 500 mg

nonathymulin INN

nondestearinated cod liver oil [see: cod liver oil, nondestearinated]

Non-drowsy Allergy Relief orally disintegrating tablets OTC *nonsedating antihistamine for allergic rhinitis* [loratadine] 10 mg

Non-Drowsy Allergy Relief for Kids syrup OTC *nonsedating antihistamine for allergic rhinitis* [loratadine] 5 mg/5 mL

Non-Habit Forming Stool Softener capsules OTC *laxative; stool softener* [docusate sodium] 100 mg

noni *(Morinda citrifolia)* berries *medicinal herb for arthritis, bacterial infections, diabetes, drug addiction, headache, hypertension, liver and skin disorders, pain, and slowing aging; also used as an antioxidant*

nonionic contrast media *a class of newer radiopaque agents that, in general, have a low osmolar concentration of iodine (the contrast agent), which corresponds to a lower incidence of adverse reactions* [also called: low osmolar contrast media (LOCM)]

nonivamide INN

non-nucleoside reverse transcriptase inhibitors (NNRTIs) [see: reverse transcriptase inhibitors]

nonoxinol 4 INN *surfactant* [also: nonoxynol 4]

nonoxinol 9 INN *wetting and solubilizing agent; spermicide* [also: nonoxynol 9]

nonoxinol 15 INN *surfactant* [also: nonoxynol 15]

nonoxinol 30 INN *surfactant* [also: nonoxynol 30]

nonoxynol 4 USAN *surfactant* [also: nonoxinol 4]

nonoxynol 9 USAN, USP *wetting and solubilizing agent; spermicide* [also: nonoxinol 9]

nonoxynol 10 NF *surfactant*

nonoxynol 15 USAN *surfactant* [also: nonoxinol 15]

nonoxynol 30 USAN *surfactant* [also: nonoxinol 30]

nonsteroidal anti-inflammatory drugs (NSAIDs) *a class of anti-inflammatory drugs that have analgesic and antipyretic effects*

nonylphenoxypolyethoxyethanol [see: nonoxynol 4, 9, 15, & 30]

Nootropil ℞ *cognition adjuvant; investigational (orphan) for myoclonus* [piracetam]

nopal plant *medicinal herb for cleansing the lymphatic system, diabetes, diges-*

tion, obesity, neutralizing toxins, and preventing arteriosclerosis

Nora-BE tablets (in packs of 28) ℞ *oral contraceptive (progestin only)* [norethindrone] 0.35 mg

noracymethadol INN *analgesic* [also: noracymethadol HCl]

noracymethadol HCl USAN *analgesic* [also: noracymethadol]

noradrenaline bitartrate [see: norepinephrine bitartrate]

noramidopyrine methanesulfonate sodium [see: dipyrone]

norandrostenolone phenylpropionate [see: nandrolone phenpropionate]

norbolethone USAN *anabolic* [also: norboletone]

norboletone INN *anabolic* [also: norbolethone]

norbudrine INN [also: norbutrine]

norbutrine BAN [also: norbudrine]

norclostebol INN

Norco tablets ℞ *narcotic analgesic; antipyretic* [hydrocodone bitartrate; acetaminophen] 5•325, 7.5•325, 10•325 mg

norcodeine INN, BAN

Norcuron powder for IV injection ℞ *nondepolarizing neuromuscular blocker; adjunct to anesthesia* [vecuronium bromide] 10, 20 mg/vial

norcycline [see: sancycline]

nordazepam INN

nordefrin HCl NF

Nordette-28 tablets (in Pilpaks of 28) ℞ *monophasic oral contraceptive; emergency postcoital contraceptive* [levonorgestrel; ethinyl estradiol] 0.15 mg•30 mcg

nordinone INN

NordiPen (trademarked delivery device) *subcu self-injector for* **Norditropin**

Norditropin powder for subcu injection (discontinued 2008) ℞ *growth hormone for children and adults with congenital or endogenous growth hormone deficiency (GHD), short bowel syndrome, or AIDS-wasting syndrome;*

for children with Turner syndrome, Prader-Willi syndrome, or renal-induced growth failure [somatropin] 4, 8 mg (12, 24 IU) per vial

Norditropin prefilled cartridges for **NordiPen** (self-injection device) ℞ *growth hormone for children and adults with congenital or endogenous growth hormone deficiency (GHD), short bowel syndrome, or AIDS-wasting syndrome; for children with Turner syndrome, Prader-Willi syndrome, or renal-induced growth failure* [somatropin] 5, 10, 15 mg (15, 30, 45 IU) per 1.5 mL cartridge

Norditropin NordiFlex pen (self-injection device) ℞ *growth hormone for children and adults with congenital or endogenous growth hormone deficiency (GHD), short bowel syndrome, or AIDS-wasting syndrome; for children with Turner syndrome, Prader-Willi syndrome, or renal-induced growth failure* [somatropin] 5, 10, 15 mg (15, 30, 45 IU)

Norel DM oral liquid ℞ *antitussive; antihistamine; decongestant* [dextromethorphan hydrobromide; chlorpheniramine maleate; phenylephrine HCl] 15•4•10 mg/5 mL

Norel EX dual-release caplets ℞ *decongestant; expectorant* [phenylephrine HCl (extended release); guaifenesin (50% immediate release; 50% extended release)] 40•800 mg

Norel LA extended-release tablets (discontinued 2007) ℞ *decongestant; antihistamine* [phenylephrine HCl; carbinoxamine maleate] 40•8 mg ②
Neoral

Norel SR extended-release tablets ℞ *decongestant; antihistamine; sleep aid; analgesic* [phenylephrine HCl; chlorpheniramine maleate; phenyltoloxamine citrate; acetaminophen] 40•8•50•325 mg

norelgestromin USAN *progestin-type contraceptive*

norephedrine HCl [see: phenylpropanolamine HCl]

norepinephrine INN *adrenergic; vaso-constrictor; vasopressor for shock* [also: norepinephrine bitartrate]

norepinephrine bitartrate USAN, USP *adrenergic; vasoconstrictor; vasopressor for acute hypotensive shock* [also: norepinephrine] 1 mg/mL injection

norethandrolone NF, INN

norethindrone USP *synthetic progestin for amenorrhea, abnormal uterine bleeding, and endometriosis* [also: norethisterone]

norethindrone acetate USP *synthetic progestin for amenorrhea, abnormal uterine bleeding, and endometriosis* 5 mg oral

norethindrone acetate & estradiol *a mixture of synthetic and natural hormones; hormone replacement therapy for postmenopausal symptoms* 0.5•1 mg oral

norethisterone INN, BAN, JAN *progestin* [also: norethindrone]

norethynodrel USAN, USP *progestin* [also: noretynodrel]

noretynodrel INN *progestin* [also: norethynodrel]

noreximide INN

norfenefrine INN

Norflex IV or IM injection ℞ *skeletal muscle relaxant; analgesic; anticholinergic* [orphenadrine citrate] 30 mg/mL

Norflex sustained-release tablets (discontinued 2006) ℞ *skeletal muscle relaxant; analgesic; anticholinergic; also used at bedtime for quinine-resistant leg cramps* [orphenadrine citrate] 100 mg

norfloxacin USAN, USP, INN, BAN, JAN *broad-spectrum fluoroquinolone antibiotic*

norfloxacin succinil INN

norflurane USAN, INN *inhalation anesthetic*

Norforms vaginal suppositories OTC *moisturizer/lubricant* [polyethylene glycol]

Norgesic; Norgesic Forte tablets ℞ *skeletal muscle relaxant; analgesic; antipyretic* [orphenadrine citrate;

aspirin; caffeine] 25•385•30 mg; 50•770•60 mg

norgesterone INN

norgestimate USAN, INN, BAN *progestin*

norgestomet USAN, INN *progestin*

norgestrel USAN, USP, INN *progestin*

d-norgestrel (*incorrect enantiomer designation*) [now: levonorgestrel]

D-norgestrel [see: levonorgestrel]

norgestrienone INN

Norinyl 1 + 35 tablets (in Wallettes of 28) ℞ *monophasic oral contraceptive* [norethindrone; ethinyl estradiol] 1 mg•35 mcg × 21 days; counters × 7 days ② naranol

Norinyl 1 + 50 tablets (in Wallettes of 28) ℞ *monophasic oral contraceptive* [norethindrone; mestranol] 1 mg•50 mcg × 21 days; counters × 7 days ② naranol

Noritate cream ℞ *antibiotic for rosacea* [metronidazole] 1%

norletimol INN

norleusactide INN [also: pentacosactride]

norlevorphanol INN, BAN

norlupinanes *a class of antibiotics* [also called: quinolizidines]

½ normal saline (½ NS; 0.45% sodium chloride) *electrolyte replacement*

normal saline (NS; 0.9% sodium chloride) *electrolyte replacement* [also: saline solution]

normal serum albumin [see: albumin, human]

Normaline tablets OTC *sodium chloride replacement; dehydration preventative* [sodium chloride] 250 mg

normethadone INN, BAN

normethandrolone [see: normethandrone]

normethandrone

normethisterone [see: normethandrone]

Normix *investigational (orphan) antibacterial for hepatic encephalopathy* [rifaximin]

Normodyne film-coated tablets (discontinued 2004) ℞ *antihypertensive;*

antiadrenergic (α- and β-blocker) [labetalol HCl] 100, 200, 300 mg

Normodyne IV infusion ℞ *antihypertensive; antiadrenergic (α- and β-blocker)* [labetalol HCl] 5 mg/mL

normorphine INN, BAN

Normosang *investigational (orphan) for acute symptomatic porphyria and myelodysplastic syndrome* [heme arginate]

Normosol-M IV infusion ℞ *intravenous electrolyte therapy* [combined electrolyte solution] 1000 mL

Normosol-M and 5% Dextrose; Normosol-R and 5% Dextrose IV infusion ℞ *intravenous nutritional/ electrolyte therapy* [combined electrolyte solution; dextrose]

Normosol-R; Normosol-R pH 7.4 IV infusion ℞ *intravenous electrolyte therapy* [combined electrolyte solution]

Noroxin film-coated tablets ℞ *broad-spectrum fluoroquinolone antibiotic* [norfloxacin] 400 mg

Norpace capsules ℞ *antiarrhythmic* [disopyramide phosphate] 100, 150 mg

Norpace CR controlled-release capsules ℞ *antiarrhythmic* [disopyramide phosphate] 100, 150 mg

norpipanone INN, BAN

Norpramin film-coated tablets ℞ *tricyclic antidepressant* [desipramine HCl] 10, 25, 50, 75, 100, 150 mg

norpseudoephedrine [see: cathine]

Nor-QD tablets (in packs of 28) ℞ *oral contraceptive (progestin only)* [norethindrone] 0.35 mg

Nortemp, Children's oral suspension OTC *analgesic; antipyretic* [acetaminophen] 160 mg/5 mL

nortestosterone phenylpropionate [see: nandrolone phenpropionate]

Nor-Tet capsules ℞ *broad-spectrum antibiotic* [tetracycline HCl] 250, 500 mg

nortetrazepam INN

Northyx tablets ℞ *thyroid inhibitor* [methimazole] 5, 10, 15, 20 mg

Nortrel 0.5/35; Nortrel 1/35 tablets (in packs of 21 or 28) ℞ *monophasic oral contraceptive* [norethindrone; ethinyl estradiol] 0.5 mg•35 mcg; 1 mg•35 mcg

nortriptyline HCl USAN, USP, INN *tricyclic antidepressant* [10, 25, 50, 75 mg oral; 10 mg/5 mL oral]

Norvasc tablets ℞ *antianginal; antihypertensive; calcium channel blocker* [amlodipine besylate] 2.5, 5, 10 mg

norvinisterone INN

norvinodrel [see: norgesterone]

Norvir softgels, oral solution ℞ *antiretroviral protease inhibitor for HIV infection* [ritonavir] 100 mg; 80 mg/mL

Norway pine; Norway spruce *medicinal herb* [see: spruce]

Norwich coated tablets OTC *analgesic; antipyretic; anti-inflammatory; antirheumatic* [aspirin] 325, 500 mg

Norzine IM injection, suppositories, tablets ℞ *antiemetic* [thiethylperazine maleate] 5 mg/mL; 10 mg; 10 mg ☒ narasin

nosantine INN, BAN

noscapine USP, INN *antitussive*

noscapine HCl NF

Nose Better gel OTC *emollient; moisturizer; protectant; mild anesthetic; antipruritic; counterirritant* [allantoin; camphor; menthol] 0.5%•0.75%•0.5%

nosebleed *medicinal herb* [see: yarrow]

nosiheptide USAN, INN *veterinary growth stimulant*

Nōstrilla 12-Hour nasal spray OTC *nasal decongestant* [oxymetazoline HCl] 0.05%

notensil maleate [see: acepromazine]

Notuss-AC oral liquid ℞ *narcotic antitussive; antihistamine* [codeine phosphate; chlorpheniramine maleate] 10•2 mg/5 mL

Notuss-DC oral liquid ℞ *narcotic antitussive; decongestant* [codeine phosphate; pseudoephedrine HCl] 10•30 mg/5 mL

Notuss-Forte syrup ℞ *narcotic antitussive; decongestant; antihistamine* [hydrocodone bitartrate; pseudoephedrine HCl; chlorpheniramine maleate] 5•40•4 mg/5 mL

Notuss-PD oral liquid (discontinued 2007) ℞ *narcotic antitussive; decongestant; antihistamine* [hydrocodone bitartrate; phenylephrine HCl; dexchlorpheniramine maleate] 4•5•2 mg/5 mL

Nouriva Repair cream OTC *emollient/ protectant* [petrolatum; paraffin; mineral oil]

NovaCare film-coated tablets ℞ *prenatal vitamin/mineral/calcium/iron supplement* [multiple vitamins & minerals; calcium; iron; folic acid] ≛• 250•40•1 mg

Novacet lotion ℞ *antibiotic and keratolytic for acne* [sulfacetamide sodium; sulfur] 10%•5%

Novacort gel ℞ *corticosteroidal anti-inflammatory; local anesthetic* [hydrocortisone acetate; pramoxine] 2%• 1%

Nova-Dec tablets OTC *vitamin/mineral/ iron supplement* [multiple vitamins & minerals; iron; folic acid; biotin] ≛• 30 mg•0.4 mg•30 mcg

Novagest Expectorant with Codeine oral liquid (discontinued 2007) ℞ *narcotic antitussive; decongestant; expectorant* [codeine phosphate; pseudoephedrine HCl; guaifenesin; alcohol 1.4%] 10•30•100 mg/5 mL

Novahistine DH oral liquid ℞ *narcotic antitussive; antihistamine; decongestant* [dihydrocodeine bitartrate; chlorpheniramine maleate; phenylephrine HCl] 7.25•5•2 mg/5 mL

Novahistine DMX oral liquid (discontinued 2007) OTC *antitussive; decongestant; expectorant* [dextromethorphan hydrobromide; pseudoephedrine HCl; guaifenesin; alcohol 5%] 10•30•100 mg/5 mL

novamidon [see: aminopyrine]

Novamine; Novamine 15% IV infusion ℞ *total parenteral nutrition; peripheral parenteral nutrition* [multiple essential and nonessential amino acids] ⑨ nafomine

Novantrone IV infusion ℞ *antibiotic antineoplastic for prostate cancer*

(orphan) and acute nonlymphocytic leukemia (ANLL) (orphan); immunomodulator for progressive and relapsing-remitting multiple sclerosis (orphan) [mitoxantrone HCl] 2 mg/mL

Novarel powder for IM injection ℞ *a human-derived hormone used for prepubertal cryptorchidism or hypogonadism and to induce ovulation in anovulatory women* [chorionic gonadotropin] 1000 U/mL

Novasal film-coated tablets ℞ *analgesic; antipyretic; anti-inflammatory* [magnesium salicylate tetrahydrate] 600 mg ⑨ nivazol

NovaSource Renal oral liquid OTC *nutritional therapy for renal failure* [multiple vitamins & minerals] 237 mL/pkt.

novel (atypical) antipsychotics *a class of agents with a high affinity to the serotonin receptors and varying degrees of affinity to other neurotransmitter receptors; "atypical" due to the low incidence of extrapyramidal side effects (EPS)* [compare to: conventional (typical) antipsychotics]

novel acting thrombolytic (NaT) *investigational (orphan) for peripheral arterial occlusion*

novobiocin INN, BAN *bacteriostatic antibiotic* [also: novobiocin calcium]

novobiocin calcium USP *bacteriostatic antibiotic* [also: novobiocin]

novobiocin sodium USP *bacteriostatic antibiotic*

Novocain injection ℞ *local anesthetic for central or peripheral nerve block* [procaine HCl] 1%, 10% ⑨ Naphcon; nefocon A

Novolin 70/30 vials for subcu injection OTC *antidiabetic* [isophane human insulin (rDNA); human insulin (rDNA)] 100 U/mL

Novolin 70/30 PenFill NovoPen cartridge OTC *antidiabetic* [isophane human insulin (rDNA); human insulin (rDNA)] 150 U/1.5 mL, 300 U/3 mL

Novolin 70/30 Prefilled syringes OTC *antidiabetic* [isophane human insulin (rDNA); human insulin (rDNA)] 150 U/1.5 mL

Novolin N vials for subcu injection OTC *antidiabetic* [isophane human insulin (rDNA)] 100 U/mL

Novolin N PenFill NovoPen cartridge OTC *antidiabetic* [isophane human insulin (rDNA)] 150 U/1.5 mL, 300 U/3 mL

Novolin N Prefilled syringes OTC *antidiabetic* [isophane human insulin (rDNA)] 150 U/1.5 mL

Novolin R vials for subcu injection OTC *antidiabetic* [human insulin (rDNA)] 100 U/mL

Novolin R PenFill NovoPen cartridges OTC *antidiabetic* [human insulin (rDNA)] 150 U/1.5 mL, 300 U/3 mL

Novolin R Prefilled syringes OTC *antidiabetic* [human insulin (rDNA)] 150 U/1.5 mL

NovoLog vials for subcu injection R̥ *rapid-acting insulin analogue for diabetes* [insulin aspart, human (rDNA)] 100 U/mL

NovoLog FlexPen self-injector for subcu injection R̥ *rapid-acting insulin analogue for diabetes* [insulin aspart, human (rDNA)] 300 U/3 mL

NovoLog Mix 50/50 subcu injection R̥ *dual-acting insulin analogue for diabetes* [insulin aspart protamine; insulin aspart, human (rDNA)] 50%•50% (100 U/mL total)

NovoLog Mix 70/30 FlexPen self-injector for subcu injection R̥ *dual-acting insulin analogue for diabetes* [insulin aspart protamine; insulin aspart, human (rDNA)] 70%•30% (100 U/mL total)

NovoLog Mix 70/30 PenFill Novo-Pen cartridges for subcu injection R̥ *dual-acting insulin analogue for diabetes* [insulin aspart protamine; insulin aspart, human (rDNA)] 70%•30% (100 U/mL total)

NovoLog PenFill NovoPen cartridges for subcu injection R̥ *rapid-acting insulin analogue for diabetes* [insulin aspart, human (rDNA)] 300 U/3 mL

NovoNorm ⓔ (European name for U.S. product **Prandin**)

NovoPen 1.5; NovoPen Junior pre-filled reusable syringe *uses* **Novolin PenFill** *cartridges and* **NovoFine** *30-gauge disposable needles* [insulin (several types available)] 1–40 U/injection

NovoSeven powder for IV injection R̥ *coagulant for hemophilia A and B (orphan); investigational (orphan) for Glanzmann thrombasthenia* [factor VIIa, recombinant] 1.2, 2.4, 4.8 mg/vial

NOVP (Novantrone, Oncovin, vinblastine, prednisone) *chemotherapy protocol for Hodgkin lymphoma*

Noxafil oral suspension R̥ *broad-spectrum triazole antifungal for treatment of oropharyngeal candidiasis and prophylaxis of serious invasive fungal infections in immunocompromised patients* [posaconazole] 200 mg/5 mL

noxiptiline INN [also: noxiptyline]

noxiptyline BAN [also: noxiptiline]

noxythiolin BAN [also: noxytiolin]

noxytiolin INN [also: noxythiolin]

NP (nifurpipone) [q.v.]

NPH (neutral protamine Hagedorn) insulin [see: insulin, isophane]

NPH Iletin II vials for subcu injection (discontinued 2005) OTC *antidiabetic* [isophane insulin (pork)] 100 U/mL

NPI 32101 *investigational (Phase III) nanocrystalline silver for use as a topical antimicrobial barrier*

Nplate subcu injection R̥ *thrombopoietin (TPO) receptor agonist to increase platelet production in immune thrombocytopenic purpura (ITP)* [romiplostim] 250, 500 mcg

NRTIs (nucleoside reverse transcriptase inhibitors) [see: reverse transcriptase inhibitors]

NS (normal saline) [q.v.]

NSAIDs (nonsteroidal anti-inflammatory drugs) [q.v.]

NTZ (nitazoxanide) [q.v.]

Nubain IV, IM, or subcu injection ℞ *narcotic agonist-antagonist analgesic for moderate to severe pain; adjunct to obstetric and surgical analgesia* [nalbuphine HCl] 10, 20 mg/mL

nucleoside reverse transcriptase inhibitors (NRTI) *a class of antiretroviral drugs that inhibits the activity of reverse transcriptase (polymerase) in viral cells, causing a termination of DNA chain elongation, which prevents replication of the cells* [see: reverse transcriptase inhibitors]

nuclomedone INN

nuclotixene INN

Nucofed capsules ℞ *narcotic antitussive; decongestant* [codeine phosphate; pseudoephedrine HCl] 20•60 mg

Nucofed syrup (discontinued 2007) ℞ *narcotic antitussive; decongestant* [codeine phosphate; pseudoephedrine HCl] 20•60 mg/5 mL

Nucofed Expectorant syrup (discontinued 2007) ℞ *narcotic antitussive; decongestant; expectorant* [codeine phosphate; pseudoephedrine HCl; guaifenesin; alcohol 12.5%] 20•60•200 mg/5 mL

Nucofed Pediatric Expectorant syrup (discontinued 2007) ℞ *narcotic antitussive; decongestant; expectorant; for children 2–11 years* [codeine phosphate; pseudoephedrine HCl; guaifenesin; alcohol 6%] 10•30•100 mg/5 mL

Nucotuss Expectorant syrup (discontinued 2007) ℞ *narcotic antitussive; decongestant; expectorant* [codeine phosphate; pseudoephedrine HCl; guaifenesin; alcohol 12.5%] 20•60•200 mg/5 mL

Nucotuss Pediatric Expectorant syrup (discontinued 2007) ℞ *narcotic antitussive; decongestant; expectorant; for children 2–11 years* [codeine phosphate; pseudoephedrine HCl; guaifenesin; alcohol 6%] 10•30•100 mg/5 mL

nufenoxole USAN, INN *antiperistaltic*

Nuhist oral suspension (discontinued 2007) ℞ *decongestant; antihistamine* [phenylephrine tannate; chlorpheniramine tannate] 5•4.5 mg/5 mL ⊘ NoHist

Nu-Iron elixir (discontinued 2005) OTC *hematinic; iron supplement* [polysaccharide-iron complex] 100 mg Fe/5 mL

Nu-Iron 150 capsules OTC *hematinic; iron supplement* [polysaccharide-iron complex] 150 mg Fe

Nu-Iron Plus elixir ℞ *hematinic* [polysaccharide-iron complex; cyanocobalamin; folic acid] 300 mg•75 mcg•3 mg per 15 mL

Nu-Iron V film-coated tablets ℞ *vitamin/iron supplement* [polysaccharide-iron complex; multiple vitamins; folic acid] 60• ± •1 mg

Nu-knit (trademarked dosage form) *oxidized cellulose hemostatic pad* ⊘ nequinate

NuLev orally disintegrating tablets ℞ *GI/GU antispasmodic; antiparkinsonian; anticholinergic "drying agent" for allergic rhinitis* [hyoscyamine sulfate] 0.125 mg

NuLytely powder for oral solution ℞ *pre-procedure bowel evacuant* [polyethylene glycol–electrolyte solution (PEG 3350)] 60, 105 g/L

Numby Stuff topical liquid ℞ *anesthetic* [lidocaine HCl; epinephrine] 2%•1:100 000

Numoisyn lozenges ℞ *saliva substitute* ⊘ neomycin; nimazone

Numorphan IV, IM, or subcu injection (name changed to **Opana** in 2007)

Numorphan suppositories (discontinued 2006) ℞ *narcotic analgesic for moderate to severe pain and for preoperative support of anesthesia* [oxymorphone HCl] 5 mg

Numzident oral gel OTC *mucous membrane anesthetic* [benzocaine] 10%

Numzit Teething lotion OTC *mucous membrane anesthetic; antiseptic* [benzocaine; alcohol 12.1%] 0.2%

Numzit Teething oral gel OTC *mucous membrane anesthetic* [benzocaine] 7.5%

Nu-Natal Advanced film-coated tablets ℞ *vitamin/mineral/calcium/iron supplement; stool softener* [multiple vitamins & minerals; calcium; iron; folic acid; docusate sodium] ≟•200•90•1•50 mg

Nupercainal cream (discontinued 2005) OTC *anesthetic* [dibucaine] 0.5%

Nupercainal ointment OTC *anesthetic* [dibucaine] 1%

Nupercainal rectal suppositories OTC *emollient; astringent* [cocoa butter; zinc oxide] 2.1•0.25 g

Nuprin tablets, caplets OTC *analgesic; antiarthritic; antipyretic; nonsteroidal anti-inflammatory drug (NSAID) for mild to moderate pain, migraine headaches, and primary dysmenorrhea* [ibuprofen] 200 mg

Nuprin Backache caplets OTC *analgesic; antipyretic; anti-inflammatory* [magnesium salicylate] 580 mg

Nuquin HP cream ℞ *hyperpigmentation bleaching agent* [hydroquinone (in a sunscreen base)] 4%

Nuromax IV injection (discontinued 2004) ℞ *nondepolarizing neuromuscular blocker; adjunct to anesthesia* [doxacurium chloride] 1 mg/mL

Nursette (trademarked delivery form) *prefilled disposable bottle*

Nu-Salt OTC *salt substitute* [potassium chloride] 68 mEq K/5 g

nut, oil *medicinal herb* [see: butternut]

Nu-Tears eye drops OTC *moisturizer/lubricant* [polyvinyl alcohol] 1.4% ▨ Neotrace-4

Nu-Tears II eye drops OTC *moisturizer/lubricant* [polyvinyl alcohol; polyethylene glycol 400] 1%•1% ▨ Neotrace-4

nutmeg (*Myristica fragrans*) seed and aril *medicinal herb for diarrhea, flatulence, inducing expectoration, insomnia, mouth sores, rheumatism, salivary stimulation, and stimulating menstruation*

nutmeg oil NF

Nutracort cream ℞ *corticosteroidal anti-inflammatory* [hydrocortisone] 1%

Nutraderm cream, lotion OTC *moisturizer; emollient*

Nutraderm OTC *lotion base*

Nutraderm Bath Oil OTC *bath emollient*

Nutraloric powder OTC *enteral nutritional therapy* [milk-based formula]

Nutrament oral liquid OTC *enteral nutritional therapy* 12 oz. cans

Nutramigen oral liquid, powder for oral liquid OTC *hypoallergenic infant food* [enzymatically hydrolyzed protein formula]

Nutraplus cream, lotion OTC *moisturizer; emollient; keratolytic* [urea] 10%

Nutra-Soothe bath oil OTC *bath emollient* [colloidal oatmeal; light mineral oil]

Nutren 1.0 oral liquid OTC *enteral nutritional therapy* [lactose-free formula]

Nutren 1.5 oral liquid OTC *enteral nutritional therapy* [lactose-free formula]

Nutren 2.0 ready-to-use oral liquid OTC *enteral nutritional therapy* [lactose-free formula]

Nutr-E-Sol oral liquid OTC *vitamin supplement* [vitamin E] 798 IU/30 mL

NutreStore *investigational (orphan) agent used with human growth hormone (hGH) to treat short bowel syndrome* [glutamine]

Nutricon tablets OTC *vitamin/mineral/calcium/iron supplement* [multiple vitamins & minerals; calcium; iron; folic acid; biotin] ≟•200•20•0.4•0.15 mg ▨ Neutra-Caine

Nutrifac ZX caplets ℞ *vitamin/mineral supplement* [multiple vitamins & minerals; folic acid; biotin] ≟•1•0.2 mg

NutriFocus ready-to-use oral liquid OTC *enteral nutritional therapy* [milk-based formula] 237 mL cans

NutriHeal ready-to-use oral liquid OTC *enteral nutritional therapy* [milk-based formula] 250 mL cans

Nutrilan ready-to-use oral liquid OTC *enteral nutritional therapy* [lactose-free formula] ▨ Nitrolan

Nutrilyte; Nutrilyte II IV admixture ℞ *intravenous electrolyte therapy*

[combined electrolyte solution] ⑤ Naturalyte

Nutrineal *investigational (orphan) nutritional supplement for continuous ambulatory peritoneal dialysis patients* [peritoneal dialysis solution with 1.1% amino acids]

Nutropin powder for subcu injection (discontinued 2008) Ŗ *growth hormone for children and adults with congenital or endogenous growth hormone deficiency (GHD), short bowel syndrome, or AIDS-wasting syndrome; for children with Turner syndrome, Prader-Willi syndrome, or renal-induced growth failure* [somatropin] 5, 10 mg (15, 30 IU) per vial

Nutropin AQ subcu injection, prefilled pen self-injector Ŗ *growth hormone for children and adults with congenital or endogenous growth hormone deficiency (GHD), short bowel syndrome, or AIDS-wasting syndrome; for children with Turner syndrome, Prader-Willi syndrome, or renal-induced growth failure* [somatropin] 10 mg (30 IU) per vial; 10 mg (30 IU) per 2 mL cartridge

Nutropin Depot sustained-release injectable suspension (discontinued 2006) Ŗ *once- or twice-monthly dose-form of growth hormone (orphan)* [somatropin] 13.5, 18, 22.5 mg

Nutrox capsules OTC *dietary supplement* [multiple vitamins & minerals; multiple amino acids]

NuvaRing vaginal ring Ŗ *self-administered one-month contraceptive insert* [ethinyl estradiol; etonogestrel] 15• 120 mcg/day

nuvenzepine INN

Nuvigil tablets Ŗ *analeptic for excessive daytime sleepiness due to narcolepsy (orphan), obstructive sleep apnea, or shift work sleep disorder (SWSD)* [armodafinil] 50, 150, 250 mg

NXY-059 *investigational (Phase III) neuroprotectant for acute ischemic stroke*

nyctal [see: carbromal]

nydrane [see: benzchlorpropamid]

Nydrazid IM injection Ŗ *tuberculostatic* [isoniazid] 100 mg/mL

nylestriol USAN *estrogen* [also: nilestriol]

nylidrin HCl USP *peripheral vasodilator* [also: buphenine]

Nymphaea odorata *medicinal herb* [see: white pond lilly]

Nyotran *investigational (NDA filed, orphan) systemic antifungal for Aspergillus fumigatus and other invasive fungal infections* [nystatin, liposomal]

NyQuil Cold & Cough Relief, Children's oral liquid (discontinued 2007) OTC *antitussive; antihistamine; for adults and children ≥ 6 years* [dextromethorphan hydrobromide; chlorpheniramine maleate] 15•2 mg/15 mL

NyQuil Cough syrup OTC *antitussive; antihistamine; sleep aid* [dextromethorphan hydrobromide; doxylamine succinate] 30•12.5 mg/30 mL

NyQuil Multi-Symptom Cold & Flu Relief LiquiCaps (liquid-filled gelcaps) OTC *antitussive; antihistamine; sleep aid; analgesic; antipyretic* [dextromethorphan hydrobromide; doxylamine succinate; acetaminophen] 15•6.25•325 mg

NyQuil Multi-Symptom Cold/Flu Relief oral liquid OTC *antitussive; antihistamine; sleep aid; analgesic; antipyretic* [dextromethorphan hydrobromide; doxylamine succinate; acetaminophen] 30•12.5•1000 mg/30 mL

NyQuil Sinus LiquiCaps (liquid-filled gelcaps) OTC *antitussive; antihistamine; sleep aid; decongestant; analgesic; antipyretic* [doxylamine succinate; phenylephrine HCl; acetaminophen] 6.25•5•325 mg

nystatin USP, INN, BAN, JAN *polyene antifungal* 500 000 U/mL oral; 100 000 mg vaginal; 100 000 U/g topical

nystatin, liposomal *investigational (NDA filed, orphan) systemic antifungal for Aspergillus fumigatus and other invasive fungal infections*

Nystop powder Ŗ *antifungal* [nystatin] 100 000 U/g

Nytol tablets OTC *antihistamine; sleep aid* [diphenhydramine HCl] 25, 50 mg ⊡ nettle

NZGLM (New Zealand green-lipped mussel) [q.v.]

O₂ (oxygen) [q.v.]

oak *medicinal herb* [see: white oak]

OAP (Oncovin, ara-C, prednisone) *chemotherapy protocol*

Oasis mouthwash, throat spray OTC *saliva substitute*

oatmeal, colloidal *demulcent*

oats (Avena sativa) *grain and straw medicinal herb for dry itchy skin, hyperlipidemia, indigestion, insomnia, nervousness, opium addiction, reducing the desire to smoke, and strengthening the heart* ⊡ A/T/S

OB Complete caplets ℞ *vitamin/mineral/iron supplement* [multiple vitamins & minerals; folic acid; iron] ± •1.25•50 mg

OB Complete with DHA softgels ℞ *vitamin/mineral/iron supplement; omega-3 supplement* [multiple vitamins & minerals; folic acid; iron; docosahexaenoic acid (DHA)] ± • 1.25•28•200 mg

obecalp *placebo (spelled backward)* [q.v.]

obidoxime chloride USAN, INN *cholinesterase reactivator*

oblimersen sodium *antisense antineoplastic; investigational (NDA filed, orphan) for malignant melanoma; investigational (Phase III, orphan) for multiple myeloma and chronic lymphocytic leukemia (CLL)*

Obstetrix-100 tablets ℞ *prenatal vitamin/mineral/calcium/iron supplement; stool softener* [multiple vitamins; calcium; iron; folic acid; zinc; docusate sodium] ±•250•100•1•25•50 mg

Obtrex tablets ℞ *prenatal vitamin/mineral supplement; stool softener* [multiple vitamins and minerals; docusate sodium] ±•50 mg

O-Cal f.a. tablets ℞ *vitamin/mineral/calcium/iron supplement and dental caries preventative* [multiple vitamins & minerals; calcium; iron; folic acid; sodium fluoride] ±•200•66•1•1.1 mg

O-Cal Prenatal tablets ℞ *vitamin/mineral/calcium/iron supplement* [multiple vitamins & minerals; calcium; iron; folic acid] ±•200•15•1 mg

ocaperidone USAN, INN, BAN *antipsychotic*

Occlusal-HP topical liquid OTC *keratolytic* [salicylic acid in polyacrylic vehicle] 17%

Occucoat ophthalmic solution ℞ *ophthalmic surgical aid* [hydroxypropyl methylcellulose] 2% ⊡ OcuCoat

Ocean; Ocean for Kids nasal spray OTC *nasal moisturizer* [sodium chloride (saline solution)] 0.65% ⊡ Aceon; Aczone

ocfentanil INN *narcotic analgesic* [also: ocfentanil HCl]

ocfentanil HCl USAN *narcotic analgesic* [also: ocfentanil]

ociltide INN

Ocimum basilicum *medicinal herb* [see: basil]

ocinaplon USAN *anxiolytic*

OCL oral solution ℞ *pre-procedure bowel evacuant* [polyethylene glycol–electrolyte solution (PEG 3350)] 60 g/L

ocrase INN

ocrilate INN *tissue adhesive* [also: ocrylate]

ocrylate USAN *tissue adhesive* [also: ocrilate]

OCT (22-oxacalcitriol) [see: maxacalcitol]

octabenzone USAN, INN *ultraviolet screen*

octacaine INN

octacosactrin BAN [also: tosactide]

octacosanol *natural extract of wheat germ used to treat hypercholesterolemia; effective for lowering LDL-cholesterol, raising HDL-cholesterol, stopping the formation of arterial lesions and plaque deposits, and inhibiting clot formation*

octadecafluorodecehydronaphtha-lene [see: perflunafene]

octadecanoic acid, calcium salt [see: calcium stearate]

octadecanoic acid, sodium salt [see: sodium stearate]

octadecanoic acid, zinc salt [see: zinc stearate]

1-octadecanol [see: stearyl alcohol]

9-octadecenylamine hydrofluoride [see: dectaflur]

octafonium chloride INN

Octagam IV infusion ℞ *passive immunizing agent for primary immune deficient diseases and severe combined immunodeficiencies* [immune globulin (IGIV)] 5% (1, 2.5, 5, 10 g/dose)

Octamide PFS IV or IM injection ℞ *antiemetic for chemotherapy and post-operative nausea and vomiting; GI stimulant for diabetic gastroparesis and symptomatic gastroesophageal reflux; also used as a radiosensitizer and to stimulate lactation* [metoclopramide HCl] 5 mg/mL

octamoxin INN

octamylamine INN

octanoic acid USAN, INN *antifungal*

octapinol INN

Octastatin *antineoplastic; synthetic octapeptide analogue of somatostatin; investigational (orphan) for GI and pancreatic fistulas* [vapreotide acetate]

octastine INN

octatropine methylbromide INN, BAN *anticholinergic; peptic ulcer adjunct* [also: anisotropine methylbromide]

octatropone bromide [see: anisotropine methylbromide]

octaverine INN, BAN

octazamide USAN, INN *analgesic* ⑨ actisomide

octenidine INN, BAN *topical anti-infective* [also: octenidine HCl]

octenidine HCl USAN *topical anti-infective* [also: octenidine]

octenidine saccharin USAN *dental plaque inhibitor*

Octicare ear drops, ear drop suspension ℞ *corticosteroidal anti-inflammatory; antibiotic* [hydrocortisone; neomycin sulfate; polymyxin B sulfate] 1%•5 mg•10 000 U per mL

octicizer USAN *plasticizer*

octil INN *combining name for radicals or groups*

octimibate INN

octinoxate USAN *ultraviolet B sunscreen*

octisalate USAN *ultraviolet sunscreen*

octisamyl [see: octamylamine]

Octocaine HCl injection ℞ *local anesthetic* [lidocaine HCl; epinephrine] 2%•1:50 000, 2%•1:100 000

octoclothepine [see: clorotepine]

octocrilene INN *ultraviolet screen* [also: octocrylene]

octocrylene USAN *ultraviolet screen* [also: octocrilene]

octodecactide [see: codactide]

octodrine USAN, INN *adrenergic; vasoconstrictor; local anesthetic*

octopamine INN

octotiamine INN

octoxinol INN *surfactant/wetting agent* [also: octoxynol 9]

octoxynol 9 USAN, NF *surfactant/wetting agent; spermicide* [also: octoxinol]

OctreoScan injection ℞ *radioactive imaging agent for SPECT scans of neuroendocrine tumors* [indium In 111 pentetreotide] 10 mcg/vial

octreotide USAN, INN, BAN *somatostatin analogue; gastric antisecretory for acromegaly and severe diarrhea due to VIPomas and other tumors (orphan)*

octreotide acetate USAN *somatostatin analogue; gastric antisecretory for acromegaly and severe diarrhea due to VIPomas and other tumors (orphan)* (base=89.3%) 0.05, 0.1, 0.2, 0.5, 1 mg/mL injection

octreotide pamoate USAN *antineoplastic*

octriptyline INN *antidepressant* [also: octriptyline phosphate]

octriptyline phosphate USAN *antidepressant* [also: octriptyline]

octrizole USAN, INN *ultraviolet screen*

octyl methoxycinnamate [see: octinoxate]

octyl salicylate [see: octisalate]

S-octyl thiobenzoate [see: tioctilate]

octyl-2-cyanoacrylate [see: ocrylate]

octyldodecanol NF *oleaginous vehicle*

OcuCaps caplets OTC *vitamin/mineral supplement* [vitamins A, C, and E; multiple minerals] 5000 IU•400 mg•182 mg•±

OcuClear eye drops (discontinued 2006) OTC *decongestant; vasoconstrictor* [oxymetazoline HCl] 0.025%

OcuCoat prefilled syringe OTC *ophthalmic surgical aid* [hydroxypropyl methylcellulose] 2% ⊡ Occucoat

OcuCoat; OcuCoat PF eye drops OTC *moisturizer/lubricant* [hydroxypropyl methylcellulose] 0.8% ⊡ Occucoat

Ocudose (trademarked delivery form) *single-use eye drop dispenser*

Ocufen eye drops Ŗ *nonsteroidal antiinflammatory drug (NSAID); intraoperative miosis inhibitor* [flurbiprofen sodium] 0.03%

ocufilcon A USAN *hydrophilic contact lens material*

ocufilcon B USAN *hydrophilic contact lens material*

ocufilcon C USAN *hydrophilic contact lens material*

ocufilcon D USAN *hydrophilic contact lens material*

ocufilcon F USAN *hydrophilic contact lens material*

Ocuflox eye drops Ŗ *fluoroquinolone antibiotic for bacterial conjunctivitis and corneal ulcers (orphan)* [ofloxacin] 0.3%

Ocumeter (trademarked delivery form) *prefilled eye drop dispenser*

Ocupress eye drops Ŗ *antiglaucoma agent (β-blocker)* [carteolol HCl] 1%

Ocusert Pilo-20; Ocusert Pilo-40 continuous-release ocular wafer Ŗ *antiglaucoma agent; direct-acting miotic* [pilocarpine] 20 mcg/hr.; 40 mcg/hr.

OCuSOFT solution OTC *eyelid cleanser for blepharitis or contact lenses*

OcuSoft VMS film-coated tablets OTC *vitamin/mineral supplement* [vitamins A, C, and E; multiple minerals] 5000 IU•60 mg•30 mg•±

Ocusulf-10 eye drops Ŗ *antibiotic* [sulfacetamide sodium] 10% ⊡ AK-Sulf

Ocutricin ophthalmic ointment Ŗ *antibiotic* [polymyxin B sulfate; neomycin sulfate; bacitracin zinc] 10 000 U•3.5 mg•400 U per g ⊡ AK-Tracin

Ocuvite; Ocuvite PreserVision film-coated tablets OTC *vitamin/mineral supplement* [vitamins A, C, and E; multiple minerals] 5000 IU•60 mg•30 IU•±; 7160 IU•113 mg•100 IU•± ⊡ Aquavit-E

Ocuvite Extra tablets OTC *vitamin/mineral supplement* [vitamins A, C, and E; multiple B vitamins; multiple minerals; lutein] 1000 IU•300 mg•100 IU•±•±•2 mg

Ocuvite Lutein capsules OTC *vitamin/mineral supplement* [vitamins C and E; multiple minerals; lutein] 60 mg•30 IU•±•6 mg

Odor Free ArthriCare [see: ArthriCare, Odor Free]

Oenothera biennis *medicinal herb* [see: evening primrose]

OEP (oil of evening primrose) [see: evening primrose]

oestradiol BAN *estrogen replacement therapy for the treatment of postmenopausal disorders and prevention of postmenopausal osteoporosis; palliative therapy for prostatic and breast cancers* [also: estradiol]

oestradiol benzoate BAN [also: estradiol benzoate]

oestradiol valerate BAN *estrogen* [also: estradiol valerate]

Oestring (EUR) (Swedish name for U.S. product **Estring**)

oestriol succinate BAN *estrogen* [also: estriol; estriol succinate]

oestrogenine [see: diethylstilbestrol]

oestromenin [see: diethylstilbestrol]

oestrone BAN *estrogen replacement therapy for postmenopausal disorders; palliative therapy for prostatic and breast cancers* [also: estrone] ② isoetarine

Off-Ezy Corn & Callus Remover kit (topical liquid + cushion pads) OTC *keratolytic* [salicylic acid in a collodion-like vehicle] 17%

Off-Ezy Wart Remover topical liquid OTC *keratolytic* [salicylic acid in a collodion-like vehicle] 17%

ofloxacin USAN, INN, BAN, JAN *broad-spectrum fluoroquinolone antibiotic; topical corneal ulcer treatment* (orphan) 200, 300, 400 mg oral; 0.3% eye drops; 0.3% ear drops

ofornine USAN, INN *antihypertensive*

oftasceine INN

Ogen tablets ℞ *bioidentical human estrogen replacement therapy for the treatment of postmenopausal symptoms and prevention of postmenopausal osteoporosis* [estrone (from estropipate)] 0.625, 1.25, 2.5 (0.75, 1.5, 3) mg ② A.C.N.; Yocon

Ogen Vaginal cream (discontinued 2006) ℞ *natural estrogen replacement for postmenopausal atrophic vaginitis* [estropipate] 1.5 mg/g

Ogestrel 0.5/50 tablets (in packs of 28) ℞ *monophasic oral contraceptive; emergency postcoital contraceptive* [norgestrel; ethinyl estradiol] 0.5 mg• 50 mcg × 21 days; counters × 7 days ② Oxytrol

oglufanide disodium USAN *immunomodulator; investigational* (orphan) *angiogenesis inhibitor antineoplastic for ovarian cancer*

oil nut *medicinal herb* [see: butternut]

oil of evening primrose (OEP) [see: evening primrose]

oil of mustard [see: allyl isothiocyanate]

Oil of Olay Foaming Face Wash topical liquid OTC *cleanser for acne*

oil ricini [see: castor oil]

Oilatum Soap bar OTC *therapeutic skin cleanser*

ointment, hydrophilic USP *ointment base; oil-in-water emulsion*

ointment, white USP *oleaginous ointment base*

ointment, yellow USP *ointment base*

olaflur USAN, INN, BAN *dental caries prophylactic*

olamine USAN, INN *combining name for radicals or groups*

olanexidine HCl USAN *topical antibiotic for nosocomial or wound infections*

olanzapine USAN, INN *novel (atypical) thienobenzodiazepine antipsychotic for schizophrenia and manic episodes of a bipolar disorder* (available as a generic drug in Canada) ② elanzepine

olaquindox INN, BAN

old man's beard *medicinal herb* [see: fringe tree; woodbine]

old tuberculin (OT) [see: tuberculin]

Olea europaea *medicinal herb* [see: olive]

oleander (Nerium indicum; N. oleander) plant *medicinal herb for asthma, cancer, corns, epilepsy, and heart disease; not generally regarded as safe and effective in any form as it is very toxic*

oleandomycin INN [also: oleandomycin phosphate]

oleandomycin, triacetate ester [see: troleandomycin]

oleandomycin phosphate NF [also: oleandomycin]

oleic acid NF *emulsion adjunct*

oleic acid I 125 USAN *radioactive agent*

oleic acid I 131 USAN *radioactive agent*

oleovitamin A [now: vitamin A]

oleovitamin A & D USP *source of vitamins A and D*

oleovitamin D, synthetic [now: ergocalciferol]

olethytan 20 [see: polysorbate 80]

oletimol INN

oleum caryophylii [see: clove oil]

oleum gossypii seminis [see: cottonseed oil]

oleum maydis [see: corn oil]

oleum ricini [see: castor oil]

oleyl alcohol NF *emulsifying agent; emollient*

oligomycin D [see: rutamycin]

olive (*Olea europaea*) leaves, bark, and fruit *medicinal herb used as an antiseptic, astringent, cholagogue, demulcent, emollient, febrifuge, hypoglycemic, laxative, and tranquilizer* ☑ Aleve; Aluvia; ELF

olive, spurge; spurge laurel *medicinal herb* [see: mezereon]

olive oil NF *pharmaceutic aid* ☑ Elavil

olivomycin INN

olmesartan USAN *antihypertensive; angiotensin II receptor antagonist*

olmesartan medoxomil USAN, INN *antihypertensive; angiotensin II receptor antagonist*

olmidine INN

olopatadine INN *antiallergic; antiasthmatic*

olopatadine HCl USAN *antihistamine and mast cell stabilizer for allergic conjunctivitis and seasonal allergic rhinitis*

olpimedone INN

olsalazine INN, BAN *GI anti-inflammatory* [also: olsalazine sodium]

olsalazine sodium USAN *anti-inflammatory for ulcerative colitis* [also: olsalazine]

oltipraz INN

Olux; Olux-E topical foam ℞ *corticosteroidal anti-inflammatory for scalp dermatoses and plaque psoriasis* [clobetasol propionate; alcohol 60%] 0.05% ☑ Aloxi; I-L-X

olvanil USAN, INN *analgesic*

OM 401 *investigational (orphan) for sickle cell disease*

omaciclovir USAN *antiviral DNA polymerase inhibitor for herpes zoster*

Omacor gelcaps (U.S. name changed to **Lovaza** in 2008) ☑ Amicar

OMAD (Oncovin, methotrexate/citrovorum factor, Adriamycin, dactinomycin) *chemotherapy protocol*

omalizumab *recombinant humanized monoclonal antibody (rhuMAb) to*

immunoglobulin E (anti-IgE) for treatment of moderate to severe asthma

omega-3 acid ethyl esters *ethyl esters of docosahexaenoic acid (q.v.) and eicosapentaenoic acid (q.v.); adjunct to diet restriction for hypertriglyceridemia; investigational (orphan) for immunoglobulin A nephropathy*

omega-3 fatty acids [see: docosahexaenoic acid; doconexent; eicosapentaenoic acid; icosapent]

omega-3 fatty acids with all double bonds in the *cis* configuration *investigational (orphan) preventative for organ graft rejection*

omega-3 marine triglycerides BAN [12% docosahexaenoic acid (q.v.) + 18% eicosapentaenoic acid (q.v.)]

omeprazole USAN, INN, BAN, JAN *proton pump inhibitor for gastric and duodenal ulcers, erosive esophagitis, gastroesophageal reflux disease (GERD), upper GI bleeding, and other gastroesophageal disorders* 10, 20, 40 mg oral

omeprazole magnesium USAN *proton pump inhibitor for gastric and duodenal ulcers, erosive esophagitis, GERD, and other gastroesophageal disorders* (base= 97%)

omeprazole sodium USAN *gastric antisecretory*

omidoline INN ☑ amedalin; imidoline

Omnaris nasal spray ℞ *corticosteroidal anti-inflammatory for seasonal or perennial allergic rhinitis* [ciclesonide] 50, 200 mcg/spray

Omnicef capsules, oral suspension ℞ *third-generation cephalosporin antibiotic* [cefdinir] 300 mg; 125, 250 mg/5 mL

Omnigest EZ caplets OTC *herbal supplement to aid digestion* [multiple plant-derived digestive enzymes]

OmniHIB powder for IM injection, prefilled syringes ℞ Haemophilus influenzae *type b (HIB) vaccine* [Hemophilus b conjugate vaccine; tetanus toxoid] 10•24 mcg/0.5 mL

OMNIhist L.A. II long-acting tablets ℞ *decongestant; antihistamine; anticholinergic to dry mucosal secretions*

[phenylephrine HCl; chlorpheniramine maleate; methscopolamine nitrate] 25•8•2.5 mg

Omnipaque 140; Omnipaque 240; Omnipaque 300; Omnipaque 350 injection ℞ *radiopaque contrast medium* [iohexol (46.36% iodine)] 302 mg/mL (140 mg/mL); 518 mg/mL (240 mg/mL); 647 mg/mL (300 mg/mL); 755 mg/mL (350 mg/mL)

Omnipaque 180 injection (discontinued 2008) ℞ *radiopaque contrast medium* [iohexol (46.36% iodine)] 388 mg/mL (180 mg/mL)

Omniscan IV injection ℞ *radiopaque contrast medium for thoracic, abdominal, pelvic, and retroperitoneal imaging and to enhance MRIs of the brain, spine, and other CNS tissue* [gadodiamide] 287 mg/mL

Omnitrope powder for subcu injection, prefilled cartridges ℞ *growth hormone for children and adults with congenital or endogenous growth hormone deficiency (GHD), short bowel syndrome, or AIDS-wasting syndrome; for children with Turner syndrome, Prader-Willi syndrome, or renal-induced growth failure* [somatropin] 1.5, 5.8 mg (4.5, 17.4 IU) per vial; 5 mg (15 IU)

omoconazole INN *antifungal*

omoconazole nitrate USAN *antifungal*

omonasteine INN

Omr-IgG-am 5% [WNV] *investigational (orphan) passive immunizing agent for the West Nile virus* [immune globulin with high titers of West Nile virus antibodies]

onapristone INN *antineoplastic for hormone-dependent cancers*

Oncaspar IV or IM injection ℞ *antineoplastic for acute lymphocytic leukemia (orphan) and acute lymphoblastic leukemia* [pegaspargase] 750 IU/mL

Oncolym *investigational (Phase III, orphan) treatment for non-Hodgkin B-cell lymphoma* [monoclonal antibody to Lym-1, radiolabeled with iodine I 131]

Oncomun *investigational (orphan) for malignant glioma* [phosphorothiolate antisense oligodeoxynucleotide, TGF(β)2-specific]

Onconase *investigational (Phase III) antineoplastic for unresectable malignant mesothelioma (UMM) and small cell lung cancer (SCLC)* [ranpirnase]

Oncophage *investigational (Phase III, orphan) antineoplastic for renal cell carcinoma and metastatic melanoma* [gp96 heat shock protein-peptide complex]

OncoRad OV103 *investigational (orphan) antineoplastic for ovarian cancer*

OncoScint CR/OV (discontinued 2006) ℞ *radiodiagnostic imaging aid for ovarian (orphan) and colorectal cancer* [indium In 111 satumomab pendetide]

Onco-TCS *investigational (Phase III) antineoplastic for advanced non-Hodgkin lymphoma* [vincristine liposomal]

OncoTrac imaging kit *investigational (orphan) for diagnostic imaging agent for metastasis of malignant melanoma* [monoclonal antibodies to melanoma, murine, radiolabeled with technetium Tc 99m]

Oncovin IV injection, Hyporets (prefilled syringes) ℞ *antineoplastic for lung and breast cancers, various leukemias, lymphomas, and sarcomas* [vincristine sulfate] 1 mg/mL

Oncovite tablets OTC *vitamin supplement* [multiple vitamins]

ondansetron INN, BAN *serotonin 5-HT₃ receptor antagonist; antiemetic to prevent nausea and vomiting following chemotherapy, radiation, or surgery* [also: ondansetron HCl]

ondansetron HCl USAN *serotonin 5-HT₃ receptor antagonist; antiemetic to prevent nausea and vomiting following chemotherapy, radiation, or surgery* [also: ondansetron] 4, 8, 16, 24 mg oral; 4 mg/5 mL oral; 0.64, 2 mg/mL injection

Ondrox sustained-release tablets OTC *vitamin/mineral/calcium supplement* [multiple vitamins & minerals; multiple amino acids; calcium; folic acid; biotin] ± • ± • 50 • 0.2 • 0.015 mg ⧉ Androxy

1+1-F Creme ℞ *corticosteroidal anti-inflammatory; antifungal; antibacterial; anesthetic* [hydrocortisone; clioquinol; pramoxine] 1% • 3% • 1%

1% HC ointment ℞ *corticosteroidal anti-inflammatory* [hydrocortisone] 1%

One Touch reagent strips for home use OTC *in vitro diagnostic aid for blood glucose* ⧉ Ontak

109.881 *investigational (Phase III) taxoid for breast cancer*

166Ho-DOTMP *investigational (orphan) for multiple myeloma*

One-A-Day 55 Plus tablets OTC *geriatric vitamin/mineral supplement* [multiple vitamins & minerals; folic acid; biotin] ± • 400 • 30 mcg

One-A-Day Essential tablets OTC *vitamin supplement* [multiple vitamins; folic acid] ± • 400 mcg

One-A-Day Extras Antioxidant softgel capsules OTC *vitamin/mineral supplement* [vitamins A, C, and E; multiple minerals] 5000 IU • 250 mg • 200 IU • ±

One-A-Day Kids chewable tablets OTC *vitamin/mineral/iron supplement* [multiple vitamins & minerals; iron; folic acid; biotin] ± • 18 • 0.4 • 0.03 mg

One-A-Day Kids Scooby-Doo! Fizzy Vites chewable tablets OTC *vitamin/mineral/calcium/iron supplement* [multiple vitamins & minerals; calcium; iron (as ferrous fumarate); folic acid; biotin] ± • 50 • 9 • 0.2 • 0.02 mg

One-A-Day Maximum Formula tablets OTC *vitamin/mineral/iron supplement* [multiple vitamins & minerals; iron; folic acid; biotin] ± • 18 • 0.4 • 0.03 mg

One-A-Day Men's Vitamins tablets OTC *vitamin supplement* [multiple vitamins; folic acid] ± • 400 mcg

One-A-Day WeightSmart tablets OTC *vitamin/mineral/calcium/iron supplement* [multiple vitamins & minerals; calcium; iron (as ferrous fumarate); folic acid] ± • 300 • 18 • 0.4 mg

One-A-Day Women's Formula tablets OTC *vitamin/calcium/iron supplement* [multiple vitamins; calcium; iron; folic acid] ± • 450 • 27 • 0.4 mg

one.click (trademarked delivery device) *subcutaneous auto-injector*

1DMTX/6-MP (methotrexate [with leucovorin rescue], mercaptopurine) *chemotherapy protocol for acute lymphocytic leukemia (ALL); the first-day initiation protocol* [also: MTX/6-MP (the ongoing continuation protocol)]

One-Tablet-Daily OTC *vitamin supplement* [multiple vitamins; folic acid] ± • 400 mcg

One-Tablet-Daily with Iron OTC *vitamin/iron supplement* [multiple vitamins; iron; folic acid] ± • 18 • 0.4 mg

One-Tablet-Daily with Minerals OTC *vitamin/mineral/iron supplement* [multiple vitamins & minerals; iron; folic acid; biotin] ± • 18 • 0.4 • 0.03 mg

Onglyza *investigational (Phase III) antidiabetic that enhances the function of the body's incretin system to increase insulin production in the pancreas and reduce glucose production in the liver* [saxagliptin]

onion (Allium cepa) bulb *medicinal herb used as an anthelmintic, antiseptic, antispasmodic, carminative, diuretic, expectorant, and stomachic*

Onkolox *investigational (orphan) for renal cell carcinoma* [coumarin]

Onset Forte micro-coated tablets OTC *decongestant; antihistamine; analgesic; antipyretic* [phenylephrine HCl; chlorpheniramine maleate; acetaminophen] 5 • 2 • 162.5 mg

Ontak frozen solution for IV injection ℞ *antineoplastic for recurrent or persistent cutaneous T-cell lymphoma (orphan)* [denileukin diftitox] 150 mcg/mL ⧉ One Touch

ontazolast USAN *antiasthmatic; leukotriene biosynthesis inhibitor*

ontianil INN

Onxol IV infusion ℞ *antineoplastic for AIDS-related Kaposi sarcoma (orphan), breast and ovarian cancers, and non–small cell lung cancer (NSCLC)* [paclitaxel] 6 mg/mL

Ony-Clear topical solution OTC *antifungal* [benzalkonium chloride] 1%

OPA (Oncovin, prednisone, Adriamycin) *chemotherapy protocol for pediatric Hodgkin lymphoma*

OPAL (Oncovin, prednisone, L-asparaginase) *chemotherapy protocol* ⍨ A.P.L.; apple; E-Pilo-1; IPOL

Opana tablets, IV, IM, or subcu injection ℞ *narcotic analgesic for moderate to severe pain and for preoperative support of anesthesia; investigational (orphan) for intractable pain in narcotic-tolerant patients* [oxymorphone HCl] 5, 10 mg; 1 mg/mL

Opana ER extended-release film-coated tablets ℞ *narcotic analgesic for long-term treatment of moderate to severe pain* [oxymorphone HCl] 5, 7.5, 10, 15, 20, 30, 40 mg

Opaxio *investigational (Phase III) taxane antineoplastic for non–small cell lung cancer (NSCLC)* [polyglutamate paclitaxel]

Opcon-A eye drops OTC *decongestant; antihistamine; moisturizer/lubricant* [naphazoline HCl; pheniramine maleate; hydroxypropyl methylcellulose] 0.027%•0.315%•0.5% ⍨ Apokyn

OPEN (Oncovin, prednisone, etoposide, Novantrone) *chemotherapy protocol* ⍨ ouabain

Operand solution, prep pads, swab sticks, surgical scrub, perineal wash concentrate, aerosol, Iofoam skin cleanser, ointment OTC *broad-spectrum antimicrobial* [povidone-iodine] 1%; 1%; 1%; 7.5%; 1%; 0.5%; 1%; 1%

Operand Douche vaginal concentrate OTC *antiseptic/germicidal cleanser and deodorizer* [povidone-iodine]

Ophena *investigational (Phase III) selective estrogen receptor modulator (SERM) for the relief of postmenopausal symptoms* [ospemifene]

Ophthetic eye drops ℞ *topical anesthetic* [proparacaine HCl] 0.5%

Ophthifluor antecubital venous injection ℞ *ophthalmic diagnostic agent* [fluorescein sodium] 10%

opiniazide INN

opipramol INN *antidepressant; antipsychotic* [also: opipramol HCl]

opipramol HCl USAN *antidepressant; antipsychotic* [also: opipramol]

opium USP *narcotic analgesic; antiperistaltic; used in neonatal opioid withdrawal programs; widely abused as a street drug, which is highly addictive* 10 mg/mL oral

opium, powdered USP *narcotic analgesic*

Opium Tincture, Deodorized oral liquid ℞ *narcotic analgesic; antiperistaltic; used in neonatal opioid withdrawal programs; widely abused as a street drug, which is highly addictive* [opium; alcohol 19%] 10 mg/mL

Oplopanax horridus *medicinal herb* [see: devil's club]

OPP (Oncovin, procarbazine, prednisone) *chemotherapy protocol*

OPPA (Oncovin, prednisone, procarbazine, Adriamycin) *chemotherapy protocol for pediatric Hodgkin lymphoma*

oprelvekin USAN *platelet growth factor for prevention of thrombocytopenia following chemotherapy or radiation (orphan)* [also: interleukin 11, recombinant human]

Opteform moldable bone paste ℞ *human allograft material for orthopedic surgery* [demineralized bone powder; cortical bone chips]

Opticare PMS tablets OTC *vitamin/mineral supplement; digestive enzymes* [multiple vitamins & minerals; iron; folic acid; biotin; amylase; protease; lipase] ±•2.5 mg•0.033 mg•10.4 mcg•2500 U•2500 U•200 U

Opti-Clean solution OTC *cleaning solution for hard, soft, or rigid gas permeable contact lenses*

Opti-Clean II solution OTC *cleaning solution for hard or soft contact lenses*

Opti-Clean II Especially for Sensitive Eyes solution OTC *cleaning solution for rigid gas permeable contact lenses*

Opti-Clear eye drops OTC *decongestant; vasoconstrictor* [tetrahydrozoline HCl] 0.05%

OptiClik (trademarked insulin delivery device) *cartridge-type subcu injector for* **Lantus**

Opticrom 4% eye drops ℞ *mast cell stabilizer for vernal keratoconjunctivitis (orphan)* [cromolyn sodium]

Opticyl eye drops ℞ *cycloplegic; mydriatic* [tropicamide] 0.5%, 1%

Opti-Free solution OTC *chemical disinfecting solution for soft contact lenses* [note: one of four different products with the same name]

Opti-Free solution OTC *rewetting solution for soft contact lenses* [note: one of four different products with the same name]

Opti-Free solution OTC *surfactant cleaning solution for soft contact lenses* [note: one of four different products with the same name]

Opti-Free tablets OTC *enzymatic cleaner for soft contact lenses* [pork pancreatin] [note: one of four different products with the same name]

Opti-Free Express Multi-Purpose solution OTC *chemical disinfecting solution for soft contact lenses* [myristamidopropyl dimethylamine; polyquaternium-1] 0.0005%•0.001%

Optigene ophthalmic solution OTC *extraocular irrigating solution* [sterile isotonic solution] ⊡ aptocaine

Optigene 3 eye drops OTC *decongestant; vasoconstrictor* [tetrahydrozoline HCl] 0.05% ⊡ aptocaine

Optilets-500 Filmtabs (film-coated tablets) OTC *vitamin supplement* [multiple vitamins]

Optilets-M-500 Filmtabs (film-coated tablets) OTC *vitamin/mineral/iron supplement* [multiple vitamins & minerals; iron] ±•20 mg

OptiMARK IV injection ℞ *parenteral radiopaque contrast medium to enhance MRIs of the brain, head, and spine and liver structure and vascularity* [gadoversetamide] 330.9 mg

Optimental oral liquid OTC *enteral nutritional therapy* 237 mL

Optimmune *investigational (orphan) tear stimulant for severe keratoconjunctivitis sicca in Sjögren syndrome* [cyclosporine]

Optimox Prenatal tablets OTC *vitamin/mineral/calcium/iron supplement* [multiple vitamins & minerals; calcium; iron; folic acid] ±•100•5•0.133 mg

Optinate Omega-3 L-Vcaps tablets + capsules ℞ *calcium/iron supplement + omega-3 fatty acid supplement* [multiple vitamins & minerals; calcium citrate; carbonyl iron; folic acid; docusate sodium + docosahexaenoic acid (DHA)] ±•200•90•1•50 mg (tablets) + 250 mg (capsules)

Opti-One solution OTC *rewetting solution for soft contact lenses*

Opti-One Multi-Purpose solution OTC *chemical disinfecting solution for soft contact lenses* [EDTA; polyquaternium-1] 0.05%•0.001%

OptiPen One (trademarked insulin delivery device) *cartridge-type subcu injector*

OptiPranolol eye drops ℞ *antiglaucoma agent (β-blocker)* [metipranolol HCl] 0.3%

Optiray 160; Optiray 240; Optiray 300; Optiray 320; Optiray 350 injection ℞ *radiopaque contrast medium* [ioversol (47.3% iodine)] 339 mg/mL (160 mg/mL); 509 mg/mL (240 mg/mL); 636 mg/mL (300 mg/mL); 678 mg/mL (320 mg/mL); 741 mg/mL (350 mg/mL)

Opti-Soft Especially for Sensitive Eyes solution OTC *rinsing/storage*

solution for soft contact lenses [sodium chloride (preserved saline solution)]

Optison suspension for IV injection ℞ *radiopaque contrast medium to enhance echocardiography* [perflutren protein] 0.33–1 mg/3 mL vial

Opti-Tears solution OTC *rewetting solution for hard or soft contact lenses*

Optivar eye drops ℞ *antihistamine; mast cell stabilizer* [azelastine HCl] 0.05%

Optive eye drops OTC *moisturizer; emollient* [carboxymethylcellulose sodium; glycerin] 0.5%•0.9%

Optivite P.M.T. tablets OTC *geriatric vitamin/mineral supplement* [multiple vitamins & minerals; folic acid; biotin] ±•30•≟ mcg

OptiZen eye drops OTC *moisturizer/lubricant* [polysorbate 80] 0.5%

Opti-Zyme Enzymatic Cleaner Especially for Sensitive Eyes tablets OTC *enzymatic cleaner for soft or rigid gas permeable contact lenses* [pork pancreatin]

OPV (oral poliovirus vaccine) [see: poliovirus vaccine, live oral]

ORA5 topical liquid OTC *oral anti-infective* [copper sulfate; iodine; potassium iodide]

Orabase oral gel (discontinued 2007) OTC *mucous membrane anesthetic* [benzocaine] 15%

Orabase Baby oral gel OTC *mucous membrane anesthetic* [benzocaine] 7.5%

Orabase HCA oral paste ℞ *corticosteroidal anti-inflammatory* [hydrocortisone acetate] 0.5%

Orabase Lip Healer cream OTC *mucous membrane anesthetic; antipruritic; counterirritant; vulnerary* [benzocaine; menthol; allantoin] 5%• 0.5%•1.5%

Orabase Soothe-N-Seal topical liquid OTC *mucous membrane sealant and protectant for canker and mouth sores* [cyanoacrylate]

Orabase-B oral paste OTC *mucous membrane anesthetic* [benzocaine] 20%

Orabase-Plain oral paste OTC *relief from minor oral irritations* [plasticized hydrocarbon gel]

Oracea dual-release capsules (75% immediate release, 25% delayed release) ℞ *tetracycline antibiotic for the once-daily treatment for rosacea* [doxycycline] 40 mg ⑦ Aerius; EarEze; OROS; Urso 250

Oracit solution ℞ *urinary alkalinizing agent* [sodium citrate; citric acid] 490•640 mg/5 mL

Orajel topical liquid OTC *mucous membrane anesthetic* [benzocaine; alcohol 44.2%] 20% ⑦ Erygel

Orajel; Orajel Brace-aid; Orajel/d; Denture Orajel; Baby Orajel Nighttime Formula oral gel OTC *mucous membrane anesthetic* [benzocaine] 20%; 20%; 10%; 10%; 10% ⑦ Erygel

Orajel, Baby topical liquid, oral gel OTC *mucous membrane anesthetic* [benzocaine] 7.5%

Orajel Mouth-Aid topical liquid, oral gel OTC *mucous membrane anesthetic* [benzocaine] 20%

Orajel Perioseptic oral liquid OTC *antiseptic for braces* [carbamide peroxide] 15%

Orajel P.M. Nighttime Formula Toothache Pain Relief cream OTC *mucous membrane anesthetic* [benzocaine] 20%

Orajel Tooth & Gum Cleanser, Baby gel OTC *removes plaque-like film* [poloxamer 407; simethicone] 2%• 0.12%

Oral Wound Rinse mouthwash OTC *hydrogel wound treatment* [acemannan]

Oralet (trademarked dosage form) *oral lozenge/lollipop* ⑦ Aurolate

Oral-lyn (approved in India and Ecuador) *investigational (Phase III) oral insulin spray*

Oralone Dental paste ℞ *corticosteroidal anti-inflammatory* [triamcinolone acetonide] 0.1%

OraMagic oral rinse OTC *mucous membrane anesthetic* [benzocaine] 10%

Oramorph SR sustained-release tablets ℞ *narcotic analgesic* [morphine sulfate] 15, 30, 60, 100 mg

orange flower oil NF *flavoring agent; perfume*

orange flower water NF

orange oil NF

orange peel tincture, sweet NF

orange root *medicinal herb* [see: goldenseal]

orange spirit, compound NF

orange swallow wort *medicinal herb* [see: pleurisy root]

orange syrup NF

Orap tablets ℞ *antispasmodic/antidyskinetic for Tourette syndrome* [pimozide] 1, 2 mg (4 mg available in Canada)

Oraphen-PD elixir (discontinued 2008) OTC *analgesic; antipyretic* [acetaminophen] 120 mg/5 mL

Orapred oral solution ℞ *corticosteroidal anti-inflammatory for asthma* [prednisolone sodium phosphate; alcohol 2%] 20.2 mg/5 mL (15 mg/5 mL base)

Orapred ODT (orally disintegrating tablets) ℞ *corticosteroidal anti-inflammatory for asthma* [prednisolone sodium phosphate] 13.4, 20.2, 40.3 mg (10, 15, 30 mg base)

OraQuick Advance HIV-1/2 Antibody Test reagent kit for professional use ℞ *in vitro diagnostic aid for HIV-1 and HIV-2 antibodies in oral fluid, whole blood, or plasma*

OraQuick Rapid HIV-1 Antibody Test reagent kit for home use OTC *in vitro diagnostic aid for HIV-1 and HIV-2 antibodies in a fingerstick blood sample and HIV-1 antibodies in oral fluid*

orarsan [see: acetarsone]

Orasept throat spray OTC *mucous membrane anesthetic; antiseptic* [benzocaine; methylbenzethonium chloride] 0.996%•1.037% ☑ Aricept

Orasept topical liquid OTC *oral astringent; antiseptic* [tannic acid; methylbenzethonium chloride; alcohol 53.31%] 12.16%•1.53% ☑ Aricept

Orasol topical liquid OTC *mucous membrane anesthetic; antipruritic; counterirritant; antiseptic* [benzocaine; phenol; alcohol 70%] 6.3%•0.5% ☑ Eryzole; uracil

Orasone tablets (discontinued 2008) ℞ *corticosteroid; anti-inflammatory; immunosuppressant* [prednisone] 1, 5, 10, 20, 50 mg ☑ AeroZoin; Ureacin-10

OraSure reagent kit for home use OTC *in vitro diagnostic aid for HIV antibodies*

OraSure HIV-1 reagent kit for professional use ℞ *in vitro diagnostic aid for HIV antibodies using oral mucosal transudate* [single-sample, three-test kit: two ELISA assays + Western Blot assay]

Oraxyl capsules ℞ *antimicrobial adjunct to scaling and root planing to reduce pocket depth in periodontitis* [doxycycline hyclate] 20 mg

orazamide INN

Orazinc capsules, tablets OTC *zinc supplement* [zinc sulfate] 220 mg; 110 mg ☑ arsenic

orBec investigational (Phase III, orphan) *oral treatment for intestinal graft vs. host disease* [beclomethasone dipropionate]

orbofiban acetate USAN *platelet aggregation inhibitor; fibrinogen receptor antagonist*

orbutopril INN

orchanet *medicinal herb* [see: henna (Alkanna)]

orciprenaline INN, BAN *bronchodilator* [also: metaproterenol polistirex]

orciprenaline polistirex [see: metaproterenol polistirex]

orciprenaline sulfate [see: metaproterenol sulfate]

orconazole INN *antifungal* [also: orconazole nitrate]

orconazole nitrate USAN *antifungal* [also: orconazole]

oregano *medicinal herb* [see: marjoram]

Oregon grape (Mahonia aquifolium) rhizome and root *medicinal herb for acne, blood disorders, eczema, jaundice, liver disorders, promoting digestion, psoriasis, and staphylococcal infections*

Orencia powder for IV infusion ℞ *immunomodulator for rheumatoid arthritis (RA) and juvenile idiopathic arthritis* [abatacept] 250 mg ☒ errhines; Orinase

orestrate INN

orestrol [see: diethylstilbestrol dipropionate]

Oretic tablets (discontinued 2006) ℞ *antihypertensive; diuretic* [hydrochlorothiazide] 25, 50 mg ☒ Wartec

Orexin chewable tablets OTC *vitamin supplement* [vitamins B_1, B_6, and B_{12}] 8.1 mg•4.1 mg•25 mcg

Orfadin capsules ℞ *adjunctive treatment for hereditary tyrosinemia type 1 (HT-1), a pediatric liver disease (orphan)* [nitisinone] 2, 5, 10 mg

Organidin NR tablets, oral liquid ℞ *expectorant* [guaifenesin] 200 mg; 100 mg/5 mL

organoclay [see: bentoquatam]

Orgaran deep subcu injection (discontinued 2004) ℞ *anticoagulant/antithrombotic for prevention of deep vein thrombosis (DVT) following hip replacement surgery* [danaparoid sodium] 750 anti–factor Xa U/0.6 mL

orgotein USAN, INN, BAN *anti-inflammatory; antirheumatic; investigational (orphan) for amyotrophic lateral sclerosis and to prevent donor organ reperfusion injury* [previously known as superoxide dismutase (SOD)]

orienticine A; orienticine D [see: orientiparcin]

orientiparcin INN [a mixture of orienticine A and orienticine D]

Origanum vulgare medicinal herb [see: marjoram]

Orimune oral suspension (discontinued 2004) ℞ *vaccine for poliovirus types 1, 2, and 3* [poliovirus vaccine, live oral trivalent] 0.5 mL ☒ Aramine

Orinase tablets ℞ *sulfonylurea antidiabetic that stimulates insulin secretion in the pancreas* [tolbutamide] 500 mg ☒ errhines; Orencia

Orinase Diagnostic powder for IV injection ℞ *in vivo diagnostic aid for pancreatic islet cell adenoma* [tolbutamide sodium] 1 g

oritavancin diphosphate USAN *antibiotic; peptidoglycan synthesis inhibitor*

Orlaam IV injection (discontinued 2004) ℞ *narcotic analgesic for management of opiate addiction (orphan)* [levomethadyl acetate HCl] 10 mg/mL

orlipastat [see: orlistat]

orlistat USAN, INN *lipase inhibitor to suppress the absorption of dietary fats, leading to weight loss; preventative for type 2 diabetes*

ormaplatin USAN *antineoplastic*

ormetoprim USAN, INN *antibacterial*

Ornex No Drowsiness caplets OTC *decongestant; analgesic; antipyretic* [pseudoephedrine HCl; acetaminophen] 30•325, 30•500 mg

ornidazole USAN, INN *anti-infective*

Ornidyl IV injection concentrate ℞ *antiprotozoal for Trypanosoma brucei gambiense (sleeping sickness) infection (orphan); investigational (orphan) for AIDS-related Pneumocystis pneumonia (PCP)* [eflornithine HCl] 200 mg/mL

ornipressin INN

ornithine (L-ornithine) INN ☒ aranotin

ornithine vasopressin [see: ornipressin]

ornoprostil INN

OROS (trademarked dosage form) *extended- or patterned-release tablets* ☒ Aerius; Ear-Eze; Oracea; Urso 250

orotic acid INN

orotirelin INN

orpanoxin USAN, INN *anti-inflammatory*

orphenadine citrate [see: orphenadrine citrate]

orphenadrine INN, BAN *skeletal muscle relaxant; analgesic; anticholinergic* [also: orphenadrine citrate]

orphenadrine citrate USP *skeletal muscle relaxant; analgesic; anticholinergic; also used at bedtime for quinine-resistant leg cramps* [also: orphenadrine] 100 mg oral; 30 mg/mL injection

orphenadrine HCl *anticholinergic; antiparkinsonian*

Orphengesic; Orphengesic Forte
tablets ℞ *skeletal muscle relaxant;
analgesic; antipyretic* [orphenadrine
citrate; aspirin; caffeine] 25•385•30
mg; 50•770•60 mg

orpressin [see: ornipressin]

orris root (Iris florentina) *medicinal
herb used as a diuretic and stomachic*

ortetamine INN

orthesin [see: benzocaine]

Ortho Evra transdermal patch ℞
once-weekly contraceptive [norelges-
tromin; ethinyl estradiol] 150•20
mcg/day

Ortho Micronor tablets (in Dialpaks
of 28) ℞ *oral contraceptive (progestin
only)* [norethindrone] 0.35 mg

Ortho Tri-Cyclen tablets (in Dialpaks and Veridates of 28) ℞ *triphasic
oral contraceptive; treatment for acne
vulgaris in females* [norgestimate; ethinyl estradiol]
Phase 1 (7 days): 0.18 mg•35 mcg;
Phase 2 (7 days): 0.215 mg•35 mcg;
Phase 3 (7 days): 0.25•35 mcg

Ortho Tri-Cyclen Lo tablets (in
Dialpaks and Veridates of 28) ℞ *tri-
phasic oral contraceptive* [norgesti-
mate; ethinyl estradiol]
Phase 1 (7 days): 0.18 mg•25 mcg;
Phase 2 (7 days): 0.215 mg•25 mcg;
Phase 3 (7 days): 0.25 mg•25 mcg

Ortho-Cept tablets (in Dialpaks and
Veridates of 28) ℞ *monophasic oral
contraceptive* [desogestrel; ethinyl
estradiol] 0.15 mg•30 mcg × 21
days; counters × 7 days

Orthoclone OKT3 IV injection ℞
*immunosuppressant for renal, cardiac,
and hepatic transplants* [muromonab-
CD3] 5 mg/5 mL

orthocresol NF

Ortho-Cyclen tablets (in Dialpaks
and Veridates of 28) ℞ *monophasic
oral contraceptive* [norgestimate; ethinyl estradiol] 0.25 mg•35 mcg × 21
days; counters × 7 days

Ortho-Est tablets (discontinued 2008)
℞ *bioidentical human estrogen replacement therapy for the treatment of postmenopausal symptoms and prevention
of postmenopausal osteoporosis* [estrone
(from estropipate)] 0.625, 1.25
(0.75, 1.5) mg

Ortho-Gynol vaginal gel OTC *spermicidal contraceptive (for use with a diaphragm)* [octoxynol 9] 1%

Ortho-Novum 1/35 tablets (in Dialpaks and Veridates of 28) ℞ *monophasic oral contraceptive* [norethin-
drone; ethinyl estradiol] 1 mg•
35 mcg × 21 days; counters × 7 days

Ortho-Novum 1/50 tablets (in Dialpaks of 28) ℞ *monophasic oral contraceptive* [norethindrone; mestranol] 1
mg•50 mcg × 21 days; counters × 7
days

Ortho-Novum 7/7/7 tablets (in Dialpaks and Veridates of 28) ℞ *triphasic
oral contraceptive* [norethindrone;
ethinyl estradiol]
Phase 1 (7 days): 0.5 mg•35 mcg;
Phase 2 (7 days): 0.75 mg•35 mcg;
Phase 3 (7 days): 1 mg•35 mcg

Ortho-Novum 10/11 tablets (in
Dialpaks of 28) ℞ *biphasic oral con-
traceptive* [norethindrone; ethinyl
estradiol]
Phase 1 (10 days): 500•35 mcg;
Phase 2 (11 days): 1000•35 mcg

Ortho-Prefest [see: Prefest]

orthotolidine

Orthovisc intra-articular injection in
prefilled syringes ℞ *viscoelastic lubricant and "shock absorber" for osteoarthritis of the knee* [hyaluronan] 30 mg/
2 mL syringe

OrthoWash oral rinse ℞ *dental caries
preventative* [sodium fluoride (as acidulated phosphate solution)] 0.044%

Or-Tyl IM injection ℞ *gastrointestinal
anticholinergic/antispasmodic for irritable bowel syndrome (IBS)* [dicyclo-
mine HCl] 10 mg/mL

Orudis capsules (discontinued 2004)
℞ *analgesic; antipyretic; nonsteroidal
anti-inflammatory drug (NSAID) for
osteoarthritis, rheumatoid arthritis, and
primary dysmenorrhea* [ketoprofen]
25, 50, 75 mg

Orudis KT tablets (discontinued 2006) OTC *analgesic; antipyretic; nonsteroidal anti-inflammatory drug (NSAID) for osteoarthritis, rheumatoid arthritis, and primary dysmenorrhea* [ketoprofen] 12.5 mg

Oruvail sustained-release pellets in capsules (discontinued 2006) ℞ *once-daily analgesic; antipyretic; nonsteroidal anti-inflammatory drug (NSAID) for osteoarthritis, rheumatoid arthritis, and primary dysmenorrhea* [ketoprofen] 100, 150, 200 mg ⚕ Ureaphil

oryzanol A, B, and C *medicinal herb* [see: rice bran oil]

osalmid INN ⚕ iosulamide

osarsal [see: acetarsone]

Os-Cal 250+D; Os-Cal 500+D film-coated tablets OTC *dietary supplement* [calcium (as carbonate); vitamin D] 250 mg•125 IU; 500 mg•400 IU

Os-Cal 500 tablets, chewable tablets OTC *calcium supplement* [calcium carbonate] 1250 mg (500 mg Ca) ⚕ Asacol; Isocal

Os-Cal Fortified tablets OTC *vitamin/mineral/calcium/iron supplement* [multiple vitamins & minerals; calcium (as carbonate); iron (as ferrous fumarate)] ≝•250•5 mg

Os-Cal Ultra tablets OTC *vitamin/mineral/calcium supplement* [multiple vitamins & minerals; calcium (as carbonate)] ≝•600 mg

oseltamivir phosphate USAN *antiviral neuraminidase inhibitor for the prophylaxis and treatment of influenza A and B infections*

osmadizone INN

Osmitrol IV infusion ℞ *antihypertensive; osmotic diuretic* [mannitol] 5%, 10%, 15%, 20%

osmium *element (Os)*

Osmoglyn solution ℞ *osmotic diuretic* [glycerin] 50%

Osmolite; Osmolite HN oral liquid OTC *enteral nutritional therapy* [lactose-free formula]

OsmoPrep tablets ℞ *saline laxative; pre-procedure bowel evacuant* [sodium phosphate (monobasic and dibasic)] 1.5 g (1.102•0.398 g)

Osmorhiza longistylis *medicinal herb* [see: sweet cicely]

osmotic diuretics *a class of diuretics that increase excretion of sodium and chloride and decrease tubular absorption of water*

Osmunda cinnamomea; O. regalis *medicinal herb* [see: buckhorn brake]

ospemifene *investigational (Phase III) selective estrogen receptor modulator (SERM) for the relief of postmenopausal symptoms*

Ostavir *investigational (orphan) prophylaxis of hepatitis B reinfection following liver transplants* [tuvirumab]

Osteocalcin subcu or IM injection (discontinued 2006) ℞ *calcium regulator for Paget disease (orphan), hypercalcemia, and postmenopausal osteoporosis* [calcitonin (salmon)] 200 IU/mL

Osteo-D *investigational (orphan) calcium regulator for familial hypophosphatemic rickets* [secalciferol]

Osteofil injectable bone paste ℞ *human allograft material for orthopedic surgery* [demineralized bone powder]

OsteoMax effervescent powder for oral solution OTC *dietary supplement* [calcium citrate; vitamin D; magnesium] 500 mg•200 IU•200 mg

Osteo-Mins powder OTC *dietary supplement* [multiple minerals; vitamins C and D] ≝•500 mg•100 IU ⚕ Oesto-Mins

Ostiderm lotion OTC *for hyperhidrosis and bromhidrosis* [aluminum sulfate; zinc oxide] 14.5• ≝ mg/g

Ostiderm roll-on OTC *for hyperhidrosis and bromhidrosis* [aluminum chlorohydrate; camphor; alcohol] ≝ • ≝ • ≝

OstiGen Melts orally disintegrating tablets OTC *calcium supplement; vitamin and mineral supplement* [calcium; vitamin D; multiple vitamins & minerals] 350 mg•150 IU• ≝

ostreogrycin INN, BAN

osvarsan [see: acetarsone]

Oswego tea *(Monarda didyma)* leaves and flowers *medicinal herb used as a calmative, rubefacient, and stimulant*

OT (old tuberculin) [see: tuberculin]

Otic Domeboro ear drops ℞ *antibacterial; antifungal; antiseptic; astringent* [acetic acid; aluminum acetate] 2%•≗

Oticair ear drop suspension ℞ *corticosteroidal anti-inflammatory; antibiotic* [hydrocortisone; neomycin sulfate; polymyxin B sulfate] 1%•5 mg•10 000 U per mL ⍰ Outgro

Otic-Care ear drops, otic suspension (discontinued 2006) ℞ *corticosteroidal anti-inflammatory; antibiotic* [hydrocortisone; neomycin sulfate; polymyxin B sulfate] 1%•5 mg•10 000 U per mL ⍰ Outgro

otilonium bromide INN, BAN

Oti-Med ear drops (discontinued 2006) ℞ *corticosteroidal anti-inflammatory; antibacterial; antiseptic; anesthetic* [hydrocortisone; chloroxylenol; pramoxine HCl] 10•1•10 mg/mL

otimerate sodium INN

OtiTricin otic suspension (discontinued 2006) ℞ *corticosteroidal anti-inflammatory; antibiotic* [hydrocortisone; neomycin sulfate; polymyxin B sulfate] 1%•5 mg•10 000 U per mL

Otobiotic Otic ear drops (discontinued 2006) ℞ *corticosteroidal anti-inflammatory; antibiotic* [hydrocortisone; polymyxin B sulfate] 0.5%•10 000 U per mL

Otocain ear drops ℞ *anesthetic* [benzocaine] 20%

Otocalm ear drops (discontinued 2006) ℞ *anesthetic; analgesic* [benzocaine; antipyrine] 1.4%•5.4%

Otocort ear drops, otic suspension (discontinued 2006) ℞ *corticosteroidal anti-inflammatory; antibiotic* [hydrocortisone; neomycin sulfate; polymyxin B sulfate] 1%•5 mg•10 000 U per mL

Otomar-HC ear drops ℞ *corticosteroidal anti-inflammatory; local anesthetic; antiseptic* [hydrocortisone; pra-moxine HCl; chloroxylenol] 10•10•1 mg/mL

Otomycin-HPN Otic ear drops (discontinued 2006) ℞ *corticosteroidal anti-inflammatory; antibiotic* [hydrocortisone; neomycin sulfate; polymyxin B sulfate] 1%•5 mg•10 000 U per mL

Otosporin ear drops ℞ *corticosteroidal anti-inflammatory; antibiotic* [hydrocortisone; neomycin sulfate; polymyxin B sulfate] 1%•5 mg•10 000 U per mL

Otrivin nasal spray, nose drops, pediatric nose drops OTC *nasal decongestant* [xylometazoline HCl] 0.1%; 0.1%; 0.05% ⍰ etorphine; Etrafon

ouabain USP ⍰ OPEN

Our Lady's mint *medicinal herb* [see: spearmint]

Outgro solution OTC *pain relief for ingrown toenails* [tannic acid; chlorobutanol; isopropyl alcohol 83%] 25%•5% ⍰ Oticair

Ovace foam ℞ *antibiotic for acute and chronic seborrheic dermatitis and secondary bacterial infections of the scalp and skin* [sulfacetamide sodium] 10%

ovandrotone albumin INN, BAN

OvaRex *investigational (Phase II, orphan) therapeutic vaccine for epithelial ovarian cancer* [monoclonal antibody B43.13]

Ovastat *investigational (orphan) for ovarian cancer* [treosulfan]

O-Vax *investigational (Phase III, orphan) therapeutic vaccine for adjuvant treatment of ovarian cancer* [autologous cell (AC) vaccine]

Ovcon 35 caplets, chewable tablets (in packs of 21 or 28) ℞ *monophasic oral contraceptive* [norethindrone; ethinyl estradiol] 0.4 mg•35 mcg

Ovcon 35 Fe chewable tablets (name changed to **Femcon Fe** in 2007)

Ovcon 50 caplets (in packs of 28) ℞ *monophasic oral contraceptive* [norethindrone; ethinyl estradiol] 1 mg•50 mcg × 21 days; counters × 7 days

Ovide lotion ℞ *pediculicide for lice* [malathion; isopropyl alcohol 78%] 0.5% ② Ovoid

Ovidrel prefilled syringes for subcu injection ℞ *fertility stimulant for anovulatory women; adjuvant therapy for cryptorchidism* [choriogonadotropin alfa] 250 mcg/0.5 mL

ovine corticotropin-releasing hormone [see: corticorelin ovine triflutate]

Ovitrelle ⓔⓤⓡ (European name for U.S. product **Ovidrel**)

Ovoid (trademarked dosage form) *sugar-coated tablet* ② Ovide

Ovral tablets (in Pilpaks of 21 and 28) ℞ *monophasic oral contraceptive; emergency postcoital contraceptive* [norgestrel; ethinyl estradiol] 0.5 mg•50 mcg

Ovrette tablets (in Pilpaks of 28) (discontinued 2008) ℞ *oral contraceptive (progestin only)* [norgestrel] 0.075 mg

OvuGen test kit (discontinued 2004) *in vitro diagnostic aid to predict ovulation time* ② Ovcon 35

OvuKIT Self-Test kit for home use (discontinued 2004) OTC *in vitro diagnostic aid to predict ovulation time*

Ovulation Scope kit for home use OTC *in vitro diagnostic aid to predict ovulation time from a saliva sample*

OvuLite kit for home use OTC *in vitro diagnostic aid to predict ovulation time from a saliva sample*

OvuQuick Self-Test kit for home use (discontinued 2004) OTC *in vitro diagnostic aid to predict ovulation time*

[¹⁵O] water [see: water O 15]

ox bile extract [see: bile salts]

oxabolone cipionate INN

oxabrexine INN

22-oxacalcitriol (OCT) [see: maxacalcitol]

oxaceprol INN

oxacillin INN *penicillinase-resistant penicillin antibiotic* [also: oxacillin sodium]

oxacillin sodium USAN, USP *penicillinase-resistant penicillin antibiotic* [also:

oxacillin] 250 mg/5 mL oral; 0.5, 1, 2, 10 g injection

oxadimedine INN

oxadimedine HCl [see: oxadimedine]

oxadoddy *medicinal herb* [see: Culver root]

oxaflozane INN

oxaflumazine INN

oxafuradene [see: nifuradene]

oxagrelate USAN, INN *platelet antiaggregatory agent*

oxalinast INN

oxaliplatin USAN, INN *alkylating antineoplastic for advanced or metastatic colorectal cancers; also used for non-Hodgkin lymphoma and advanced ovarian cancer (orphan); investigational (Phase III) for pancreatic cancer*

Oxalis acetosella medicinal herb [see: wood sorrel]

oxamarin INN *hemostatic* [also: oxamarin HCl]

oxamarin HCl USAN *hemostatic* [also: oxamarin]

oxametacin INN

oxamisole INN *immunoregulator* [also: oxamisole HCl]

oxamisole HCl USAN *immunoregulator* [also: oxamisole]

oxamniquine USAN, USP, INN *antischistosomal; anthelmintic for schistosomiasis (flukes)*

oxamphetamine hydrobromide [see: hydroxyamphetamine hydrobromide]

oxamycin [see: cycloserine]

oxanamide INN

Oxandrin caplets ℞ *anabolic steroid for bone pain due to osteoporosis; investigational (Phase III, orphan) for AIDS-wasting syndrome; investigational (orphan) for muscular dystrophy and growth delay; also abused as a street drug* [oxandrolone] 2.5, 10 mg

oxandrolone USAN, USP, INN, BAN, JAN *anabolic steroid for bone pain due to osteoporosis; investigational (Phase III, orphan) for AIDS-wasting syndrome; investigational (orphan) for muscular dystrophy, alcoholic hepatitis, and growth delay; also abused as a* *street drug to increase muscle mass* 2.5, 10 mg oral

oxantel INN *anthelmintic* [also: oxantel pamoate]

oxantel pamoate USAN *anthelmintic* [also: oxantel]

oxantrazole HCl [see: piroxantrone HCl]

oxapadol INN

oxapium iodide INN

oxaprazine

oxapropanium iodide INN

oxaprotiline INN *antidepressant* [also: oxaprotiline HCl]

oxaprotiline HCl USAN *antidepressant* [also: oxaprotiline]

oxaprozin USAN, INN, BAN *analgesic; nonsteroidal anti-inflammatory drug (NSAID) for osteoarthritis and rheumatoid arthritis* 600 mg oral

oxaprozin potassium *analgesic; nonsteroidal anti-inflammatory drug (NSAID) for osteoarthritis and rheumatoid arthritis* (base=88.5%)

oxarbazole USAN, INN *antiasthmatic*

oxarutine [see: ethoxazorutoside]

oxatomide USAN, INN *antiallergic; antiasthmatic*

oxazafone INN

oxazepam USAN, USP, INN *benzodiazepine anxiolytic; sedative; alcohol withdrawal aid* 10, 15, 30 mg oral

oxazidione INN

oxazolam INN

oxazolidin [see: oxyphenbutazone]

oxazolidinediones *a class of anticonvulsants (no longer used)*

oxazorone INN ② oxisuran

oxcarbazepine INN *anticonvulsant for partial seizures in adults or children; also used for bipolar disorder and diabetic neuropathy* 150, 300, 600 mg oral

oxdralazine INN

oxeladin INN, BAN

oxendolone USAN, INN *antiandrogen for benign prostatic hypertrophy*

oxepinac INN

oxerutins BAN

oxetacaine INN *topical anesthetic* [also: oxethazaine]

oxetacillin INN

2-oxetanone [see: propiolactone]

oxethazaine USAN, BAN *topical anesthetic* [also: oxetacaine] ② oxytocin

oxetorone INN *migraine-specific analgesic* [also: oxetorone fumarate]

oxetorone fumarate USAN *migraine-specific analgesic* [also: oxetorone]

oxfenamide [see: oxiramide]

oxfendazole USAN, INN *anthelmintic*

oxfenicine USAN, INN, BAN *vasodilator*

oxibendazole USAN, INN *anthelmintic*

oxibetaine INN

oxibuprocaine chloride [see: benoxinate HCl]

oxichlorochine sulfate [see: hydroxychloroquine sulfate]

oxicinchophen [see: oxycinchophen]

oxiconazole INN, BAN *broad-spectrum topical antifungal* [also: oxiconazole nitrate]

oxiconazole nitrate USAN *broad-spectrum topical antifungal* [also: oxiconazole]

oxicone [see: oxycodone]

oxidized cellulose [see: cellulose, oxidized]

oxidized cholic acid [see: dehydrocholic acid]

oxidized regenerated cellulose [see: cellulose, oxidized regenerated]

oxidopamine USAN, INN *ophthalmic adrenergic*

oxidronate sodium *parenteral radiopaque contrast medium*

oxidronic acid USAN, INN, BAN *calcium regulator* ② Excedrin Extra Strength

oxifenamate [see: hydroxyphenamate]

oxifentorex INN

Oxi-Freeda tablets OTC *dietary supplement* [multiple vitamins & minerals; multiple amino acids]

oxifungin INN *antifungal* [also: oxifungin HCl]

oxifungin HCl USAN *antifungal* [also: oxifungin]

oxilorphan USAN, INN *narcotic antagonist*

oximetazoline HCl [see: oxymetazoline HCl]

oximetholone [see: oxymetholone]

oximonam USAN, INN *antibacterial*

oximonam sodium USAN *antibacterial*

oxindanac INN

oxiniacic acid INN

oxiperomide USAN, INN *antipsychotic* ② icospiramide

oxipertine [see: oxypertine]

oxipethidine [see: hydroxypethidine]

oxiphenbutazone [see: oxyphenbutazone]

oxiphencyclimine chloride [see: oxyphencyclimine HCl]

Oxipor VHC lotion OTC *antipsoriatic; antiseborrheic; keratolytic* [coal tar; alcohol 79%] 5%

Oxiprim *investigational (NDA filed, orphan) xanthine oxidase inhibitor for hyperuricemia* [oxypurinol sodium]

oxiprocaine [see: hydroxyprocaine]

oxiprogesterone caproate [see: hydroxyprogesterone caproate]

oxipurinol INN *xanthine oxidase inhibitor* [also: oxypurinol]

oxiracetam INN, BAN *treatment for Alzheimer disease*

oxiramide USAN, INN *antiarrhythmic*

oxisopred INN

Oxistat cream, lotion ℞ *broad-spectrum antifungal* [oxiconazole nitrate] 1%

oxistilbamidine isethionate [see: hydroxystilbamidine isethionate]

oxisuran USAN, INN *antineoplastic* ② oxazorone

oxitefonium bromide INN

oxitetracaine [see: hydroxytetracaine]

oxitetracycline [see: oxytetracycline]

oxitriptan INN

oxitriptyline INN

oxitropium bromide INN, BAN

oxmetidine INN, BAN *antagonist to histamine H_2 receptors* [also: oxmetidine HCl]

oxmetidine HCl USAN *antagonist to histamine H_2 receptors* [also: oxmetidine]

oxmetidine mesylate USAN *antagonist to histamine H_2 receptors*

oxodipine INN

oxogestone INN *progestin* [also: oxogestone phenpropionate]

oxogestone phenpropionate USAN *progestin* [also: oxogestone]

oxoglurate INN *combining name for radicals or groups*

oxolamine INN

oxolinic acid USAN, INN *antibacterial*

oxomemazine INN

oxonazine INN

4-oxopentanoic acid, calcium salt [see: calcium levulinate]

oxophenarsine INN [also: oxophenarsine HCl]

oxophenarsine HCl USP [also: oxophenarsine]

5-oxoproline [see: pidolic acid]

oxoprostol INN, BAN

oxothiazolidine carboxylate (L-2-oxothiazolidine-4-carboxylic acid) *investigational (orphan) immunomodulator for adult respiratory distress syndrome and amyotrophic lateral sclerosis*

oxozepam [see: oxazepam]

oxpentifylline BAN *peripheral vasodilator; hemorheologic agent* [also: pentoxifylline]

oxpheneridine INN

oxprenoate potassium INN

oxprenolol INN *coronary vasodilator* [also: oxprenolol HCl]

oxprenolol HCl USAN, USP *coronary vasodilator* [also: oxprenolol]

OxSODrol *anti-inflammatory; antirheumatic; investigational (orphan) to prevent donor organ reperfusion injury* [orgotein (previously known as superoxide dismutase, or SOD)]

Oxsoralen lotion ℞ *psoralens for repigmentation of idiopathic vitiligo* [methoxsalen] 1%

Oxsoralen-Ultra gelcaps ℞ *systemic psoralens for the treatment of severe recalcitrant psoriasis* [methoxsalen] 10 mg

oxtriphylline USP *bronchodilator* (theophylline=64%) [also: choline theophyllinate] 100, 200 mg oral; 50, 100 mg/5 mL oral

Oxy Medicated Cleanser & Pads
OTC *keratolytic cleanser for acne* [salicylic acid; alcohol] 0.5%•22%, 0.5%•40%, 2%•50%

Oxy Medicated Soap bar OTC *medicated cleanser for acne* [triclosan] 1%

Oxy Night Watch; Oxy Night Watch for Sensitive Skin lotion OTC *keratolytic for acne* [salicylic acid] 2%; 1%

Oxy Oil-Free Acne Wash topical liquid OTC *keratolytic for acne* [benzoyl peroxide] 10%

oxybenzone USAN, USP, INN *ultraviolet screen*

oxybuprocaine INN, BAN *topical anesthetic* [also: benoxinate HCl; oxybuprocaine HCl]

oxybuprocaine HCl JAN *topical anesthetic* [also: benoxinate HCl; oxybuprocaine]

oxybutynin USAN, INN, BAN *anticholinergic; smooth muscle relaxant; urinary antispasmodic* [also: oxybutynin chloride]

oxybutynin chloride USAN, USP *anticholinergic; smooth muscle relaxant; urinary antispasmodic for urge urinary incontinence and frequency* [also: oxybutynin] 5, 10, 15 mg oral; 5 mg/5 mL oral

oxybutynin HCl *investigational (Phase III) topical gel delivery form for overactive bladder*

Oxycel pads, pledgets, strips R *local hemostat for surgery* [cellulose, oxidized] ⊘ Exsel; Oxizole

oxychlorosene USAN *topical antiseptic*

oxychlorosene sodium USAN *topical antiseptic*

oxycinchophen INN, BAN

oxyclipine INN *anticholinergic* [also: propenzolate HCl]

oxyclipine HCl [see: propenzolate HCl]

oxyclozanide INN, BAN

oxycodone USAN, INN, BAN *narcotic analgesic; also abused as a street drug*

oxycodone HCl USAN, USP *narcotic analgesic; also abused as a street drug*

oxycodone HCl & acetaminophen *narcotic analgesic* 7.5•325, 7.5•500, 10•325, 10•650 mg oral

oxycodone HCl & ibuprofen *narcotic analgesic* 5•400 mg oral

oxycodone terephthalate USP *narcotic analgesic; also abused as a street drug*

OxyContin controlled-release tablets R *narcotic analgesic* [oxycodone HCl] 10, 15, 20, 30, 40, 60, 80, 160 mg

Oxydess II tablets R *CNS stimulant; amphetamine* [dextroamphetamine sulfate] 10 mg

oxydimethylquinazine [see: antipyrine]

oxydipentonium chloride INN

oxyethyltheophylline [see: etofylline]

OxyFast oral drops R *narcotic analgesic* [oxycodone HCl] 20 mg/mL

oxyfedrine INN, BAN

oxyfenamate INN *minor tranquilizer* [also: hydroxyphenamate]

oxyfilcon A USAN *hydrophilic contact lens material*

oxygen (O_2) USP *medicinal gas; element (O)*

oxygen, polymeric *investigational (orphan) for sickle cell anemia*

oxygen 93 percent USP *medicinal gas*

OxyIR immediate-release capsules R *narcotic analgesic* [oxycodone HCl] 5 mg

oxymesterone INN, BAN

oxymetazoline INN, BAN *topical ocular vasoconstrictor; nasal decongestant* [also: oxymetazoline HCl]

oxymetazoline HCl USAN, USP *topical ocular vasoconstrictor; nasal decongestant* [also: oxymetazoline] 0.05% nasal

oxymetholone USAN, USP, INN, BAN *androgen; anabolic steroid for anemia; also abused as a street drug*

oxymethylene urea [see: polynoxylin]

oxymorphone INN, BAN *narcotic analgesic* [also: oxymorphone HCl]

oxymorphone HCl USP *narcotic analgesic for moderate to severe pain and for preoperative support of anesthesia;*

investigational (orphan) for intractable pain in narcotic-tolerant patients [also: oxymorphone]

oxypendyl INN

oxypertine USAN, INN *antidepressant*

oxyphenbutazone USP, INN *anti-inflammatory; antirheumatic; antipyretic; analgesic*

oxyphencyclimine INN *anticholinergic* [also: oxyphencyclimine HCl]

oxyphencyclimine HCl USP *peptic ulcer adjunct* [also: oxyphencyclimine]

oxyphenhydrazine [see: carsalam]

oxyphenisatin BAN *laxative* [also: oxyphenisatin acetate; oxyphenisatine]

oxyphenisatin acetate USAN *laxative* [also: oxyphenisatine; oxyphenisatin]

oxyphenisatine INN *laxative* [also: oxyphenisatin acetate; oxyphenisatin]

oxyphenonium bromide

oxyphylline [see: etofylline]

oxypurinol USAN *xanthine oxidase inhibitor for hyperuricemia; metabolite of allopurinol* [also: oxipurinol]

oxypurinol sodium *investigational (NDA filed, orphan) xanthine oxidase inhibitor for hyperuricemia; metabolite of allopurinol*

oxypyrronium bromide INN

oxyquinoline USAN *disinfectant/antiseptic*

oxyquinoline benzoate [see: benzoxiquine]

oxyquinoline sulfate USAN, NF *complexing agent; antiseptic*

oxyridazine INN

Oxysept solution + tablets OTC *two-step chemical disinfecting system for soft contact lenses* [hydrogen peroxide–based]

Oxysept 2 solution OTC *rinsing/storage solution for soft contact lenses* [sodium chloride (saline solution)]

oxysonium iodide INN

oxytetracycline USP, INN *broad-spectrum tetracycline antibiotic; antirickettsial*

oxytetracycline calcium USP *tetracycline antibiotic; antirickettsial*

oxytetracycline HCl USP *tetracycline antibiotic; antirickettsial*

oxytocics *a class of posterior pituitary hormones that stimulate contraction of the myometrium (uterine muscle)*

oxytocin USP, INN *posterior pituitary hormone; oxytocic for induction of labor* 10 U/mL injection

Oxytrol transdermal patch ℞ *urinary antispasmodic for urge urinary incontinence and frequency* [oxybutynin chloride] 36 mg (3.9 mg/day)

Oxyzal Wet Dressing topical liquid OTC *antiseptic dressing for minor infections* [oxyquinoline sulfate; benzalkonium chloride]

Oysco 500 chewable tablets OTC *calcium supplement* [calcium carbonate] 1250 mg (500 mg Ca) ☒ Easy A1C

Oyst-Cal 500 film-coated tablets OTC *calcium supplement* [calcium carbonate] 1250 mg (500 mg Ca)

Oyst-Cal-D film-coated tablets OTC *dietary supplement* [calcium carbonate; vitamin D] 250 mg•125 IU

Oyster Calcium tablets OTC *dietary supplement* [calcium carbonate; vitamins A and D] 375 mg•800 IU•200 IU

Oyster Calcium 500 + D tablets OTC *dietary supplement* [calcium carbonate; vitamin D] 500 mg•125 IU

Oyster Calcium with Vitamin D tablets OTC *dietary supplement* [calcium carbonate; vitamin D] 250 mg•125 IU

Oyster Shell Calcium tablets OTC *calcium supplement* [calcium carbonate] 1250 mg (500 mg Ca)

Oyster Shell Calcium with Vitamin D tablets OTC *dietary supplement* [calcium carbonate; vitamin D] 250 mg•125 IU

Oystercal-D 250 tablets OTC *dietary supplement* [calcium carbonate; vitamin D] 250 mg•125 IU ☒ Astroglide

oz; gamma-oz *medicinal herb* [see: rice bran oil]

ozagrel INN *antiasthmatic* [also: ozagrel sodium] ☒ Ascor L 500

ozagrel sodium JAN *antiasthmatic* [also: ozagrel]

ozolinone USAN, INN *diuretic*

P

P Chlor GG oral drops ℞ *decongestant; antihistamine; expectorant; for children 2–24 months* [phenylephrine HCl; chlorpheniramine maleate; guaifenesin] 2•1•20 mg/mL

P & S shampoo OTC *antiseborrheic; keratolytic* [salicylic acid] 2%

P & S topical liquid OTC *antimicrobial hair dressing* [phenol]

³²P [see: chromic phosphate P 32]

³²P [see: polymetaphosphate P 32]

³²P [see: sodium phosphate P 32]

p53 adenoviral gene *investigational (Phase III) gene therapy for head and neck cancer* [also: adenoviral p53 gene]

P_1E_1; P_2E_1; P_4E_1; P_6E_1 Drop-Tainers (eye drops) (discontinued 2004) ℞ *antiglaucoma agent* [pilocarpine HCl; epinephrine bitartrate] 1%•1%; 2%•1%; 4%•1%; 6%•1%

PA MAb *investigational (orphan) treatment for anthrax exposure*

PAB (para-aminobenzoate) [see: aminobenzoic acid]

PABA (para-aminobenzoic acid) [now: aminobenzoic acid]

PABA sodium [see: aminobenzoate sodium]

PAB-Esc-C (Platinol, Adriamycin, bleomycin, escalating doses of cyclophosphamide) *chemotherapy protocol*

pabestrol D [see: diethylstilbestrol dipropionate]

PAC; PAC-I (Platinol, Adriamycin, cyclophosphamide) *chemotherapy protocol for ovarian and endometrial cancer; "I" stands for "Indiana protocol," used for ovarian cancer only*

P-A-C Analgesic tablets OTC *analgesic; antipyretic; anti-inflammatory* [aspirin; caffeine] 400•32 mg

PACE (Platinol, Adriamycin, cyclophosphamide, etoposide) *chemotherapy protocol*

Pacerone tablets ℞ *antiarrhythmic for acute ventricular tachycardia and fibrillation (orphan)* [amiodarone HCl] 100, 200 mg

PA-CI (Adriamycin, cisplatin) *chemotherapy protocol for pediatric hepatoblastoma*

Pacis powder for intravesical instillation (discontinued 2004) ℞ *antineoplastic for urinary bladder cancer* [BCG vaccine, Montreal strain] 120 mg (2.4–12 × 10⁸ CFU)

Packer's Pine Tar soap OTC *antiseborrheic; antipsoriatic; antipruritic; antibacterial* [pine tar]

paclitaxel USAN, INN, BAN *antineoplastic for AIDS-related Kaposi sarcoma (orphan), breast and ovarian cancers, and non–small cell lung cancer; investigational (orphan) for urothelial cancer* 6 mg/mL injection

paclitaxel & carboplatin & etoposide *chemotherapy protocol for primary adenocarcinoma and small cell lung cancer (SCLC)*

paclitaxel tocosol *investigational (Phase III) formulation of paclitaxel in a vitamin E–based emulsion for the treatment of metastatic breast cancer*

paclitaxel & trastuzumab *chemotherapy protocol for breast cancer*

paclitaxel & vinorelbine tartrate *chemotherapy protocol for breast cancer*

pacrinolol INN

pactimibe *acyl-CoA cholesterol acyltransferase (ACaT) inhibitor; investigational (Phase III) antiatherosclerotic; keeps cholesterol from sticking to artery walls*

padimate INN *ultraviolet screen* [also: padimate A]

padimate A USAN *ultraviolet screen* [also: padimate]

padimate O USAN *ultraviolet screen*

Paeonia officinalis *medicinal herb* [see: peony]

pafenolol INN ② befunolol

paflufocon A USAN *hydrophobic contact lens material*

paflufocon B USAN *hydrophobic contact lens material*

paflufocon C USAN *hydrophobic contact lens material*

paflufocon D USAN *hydrophobic contact lens material*

paflufocon E USAN *hydrophobic contact lens material*

pafuramidine maleate *investigational (Phase III) treatment for AIDS-related pneumocystis pneumonia (PCP)*

pagoclone USAN *nonsedating anxiolytic*

PAH (para-aminohippurate) [see: aminohippuric acid]

PAHA (para-aminohippuric acid) [see: aminohippuric acid]

Pain and Fever tablets, caplets OTC *analgesic; antipyretic* [acetaminophen] 325, 500 mg; 500 mg

Pain and Fever, Children's chewable tablets, oral liquid, oral drops OTC *analgesic; antipyretic* [acetaminophen] 80 mg; 160 mg/5 mL; 100 mg/mL

Pain Bust-R II cream OTC *analgesic; mild anesthetic; antipruritic; counterirritant* [methyl salicylate; menthol] 17%•12%

Pain Doctor cream OTC *analgesic; mild anesthetic; antipruritic; counterirritant* [methyl salicylate; menthol; capsaicin] 25%•10%•0.025%

Pain Gel Plus OTC *mild anesthetic; antipruritic; counterirritant* [menthol] 4%

Pain Relief caplets OTC *analgesic; antipyretic* [acetaminophen] 500 mg

Pain Reliever tablets OTC *analgesic; antipyretic* [acetaminophen] 325, 500 mg

Painaid tablets OTC *analgesic; antipyretic; anti-inflammatory* [acetaminophen; aspirin; salicylamide; caffeine] 110•162•152•32.4 mg

Painaid BRF (Back Relief Formula) tablets OTC *analgesic; antipyretic; anti-inflammatory* [magnesium salicylate tetrahydrate; acetaminophen] 250•250 mg

Painaid ESF (Extra Strength Formula) tablets OTC *analgesic; antipyretic;*

anti-inflammatory [acetaminophen; aspirin; caffeine] 250•250•65 mg

Painaid PMF (Premenstrual Formula) tablets OTC *analgesic; antipyretic; diuretic* [acetaminophen; pamabrom] 500•25 mg

Pain-gesic tablets OTC *analgesic; antipyretic; antihistamine; sleep aid* [acetaminophen; phenyltoloxamine citrate] 325•30 mg

paint, Indian *medicinal herb* [see: bloodroot]

paint, yellow Indian *medicinal herb* [see: goldenseal]

paint root, red *medicinal herb* [see: bloodroot]

Pain-X gel OTC *analgesic; mild anesthetic; antipruritic; counterirritant* [capsaicin; menthol; camphor] 0.05%•5%•4% ☑ Panokase; Pin-X

PALA disodium [see: sparfosate sodium]

Paladin ointment OTC *diaper rash treatment* [zinc oxide; petrolatum; lanolin; vitamins A & D] ☑ belladonna; Polydine

palatrigine INN, BAN

Palcaps 10; Palcaps 20 delayed-release capsules ℞ *porcine-derived digestive enzymes* [lipase; protease; amylase] 10 000•37 500•33 200 USP units; 20 000•75 000•66 400 USP units

paldimycin USAN, INN *antibacterial*

paldimycin A [see: paldimycin]

paldimycin B [see: paldimycin]

pale gentian *medicinal herb* [see: gentian]

palestrol [see: diethylstilbestrol]

Palgic tablets, oral liquid ℞ *antihistamine* [carbinoxamine maleate] 4 mg; 4 mg/5 mL

Palgic-D extended-release caplets (discontinued 2007) ℞ *decongestant; antihistamine* [pseudoephedrine HCl; carbinoxamine maleate] 80•8 mg

Palgic-DS syrup (discontinued 2007) ℞ *decongestant; antihistamine* [pseudoephedrine HCl; carbinoxamine maleate] 25•2 mg/5 mL

palifermin *keratinocyte growth factor (KGF) for radiation- and chemotherapy-induced oral mucositis*

palinavir USAN *antiviral; HIV-1 protease inhibitor*

palinum [see: cyclobarbitone]

paliperidone *oral benzisoxazole antischizophrenic; dopamine D_2 and serotonin 5-HT_{2A} receptor antagonist; investigational (Phase III) for bipolar mania; active metabolite of risperidone*

paliperidone palmitate *investigational (Phase III) long-acting injectable antischizophrenic; dopamine D_2 and serotonin $5HT_{2A}$ receptor antagonist; active metabolite of risperidone*

palivizumab *monoclonal antibody for prophylaxis of respiratory syncytial virus (RSV) in infants*

palladium *element (Pd)*

palladium Pd 103 *radioactive "seeds" for ultrasound-guided brachytherapy for adenocarcinoma of the prostate*

Palladone *extended-release pellets in capsules (withdrawn from the market in 2005 due to safety concerns)* ℞ *narcotic analgesic* [hydromorphone HCl] 12, 16, 24, 32 mg ℞ belladonna; Polydine

palm, dwarf; dwarf palmetto; pan palm *medicinal herb* [see: saw palmetto]

palmidrol INN

Palmitate-A 5000 *tablets* OTC *vitamin supplement* [vitamin A palmitate] 5000 IU

palmitic acid USAN *ultrasound contrast medium for echocardiography*

palmoxirate sodium USAN *antidiabetic* [also: palmoxiric acid]

palmoxiric acid INN *antidiabetic* [also: palmoxirate sodium]

Palomar "E" *ointment* OTC *emollient* [vitamin E]

palonosetron HCl USAN *selective serotonin 5-HT_3 antagonist; antiemetic to prevent chemotherapy-induced and postoperative nausea and vomiting*

PALS *coated tablets* OTC *systemic deodorant for ostomy, breath, and body*

odors [chlorophyllin copper complex] 100 mg ℞ Blue Ice; Boil-Ease

PAM; L-PAM (phenylalanine mustard) [see: melphalan]

2-PAM (2-pyridine aldoxime methylchloride) [see: pralidoxime chloride]

pamabrom USAN *nonprescription diuretic*

pamaqueside USAN *hypocholesterolemic; cholesterol absorption inhibitor; antiatherosclerotic*

pamaquine naphthoate NF

pamatolol INN *antiadrenergic (β-receptor)* [also: pamatolol sulfate] ℞ bometolol

pamatolol sulfate USAN *antiadrenergic (β-receptor)* [also: pamatolol]

Pamelor *capsules, oral solution* ℞ *tricyclic antidepressant* [nortriptyline HCl] 10, 25, 50, 75 mg; 10 mg/5 mL

pamidronate disodium USAN *bisphosphonate bone resorption inhibitor for Paget disease, hypercalcemia of malignancy (HCM), and bone metastases of breast cancer and multiple myeloma; also used for postmenopausal osteoporosis* 30, 60, 90 mg/vial injection

pamidronic acid INN, BAN

Pamine; Pamine Forte *tablets* ℞ *GI antispasmodic; anticholinergic; peptic ulcer treatment* [methscopolamine bromide] 2.5 mg; 5 mg ℞ BAMON

Pamine FQ Kit *tablets + capsules* ℞ *GI antispasmodic; anticholinergic; peptic ulcer treatment* [methscopolamine bromide (tablets); **Flora-Q** (capsules)] 5 mg; 8 million CFU

Pamisyl *investigational (orphan) for ulcerative colitis* [aminosalicylic acid]

pamoate USAN, USP *combining name for radicals or groups* [also: embonate]

Pamprin, Nighttime *powder* OTC *antihistamine; sleep aid; analgesic; antipyretic* [diphenhydramine HCl; acetaminophen] 50•650 mg

Pamprin Maximum Pain Relief *caplets* OTC *analgesic; antipyretic; diuretic* [acetaminophen; magnesium salicylate; pamabrom] 250•250•25 mg

Pamprin Multi-Symptom caplets, tablets OTC *analgesic; antipyretic; diuretic; antihistamine; sleep aid* [acetaminophen; pamabrom; pyrilamine maleate] 500•25•15 mg

Pan C Ascorbate tablets (discontinued 2007) OTC *vitamin C supplement with multiple bioflavonoids* [vitamin C; citrus bioflavonoids; hesperidin] 200•100•100 mg

Pan C-500 tablets OTC *vitamin C supplement with multiple bioflavonoids* [vitamin C; citrus bioflavonoids; hesperidin] 500•100•100 mg

PAN-2400 capsules OTC *digestive enzymes* [lipase; protease; amylase] 9816•60 214•75 900 U

Panacet 5/500 tablets ℞ *narcotic analgesic; antipyretic* [hydrocodone bitartrate; acetaminophen] 5•500 mg ⚕ boneset; poinsettia

panadiplon USAN, INN *anxiolytic*

Panadol tablets, caplets (discontinued 2008) OTC *analgesic; antipyretic* [acetaminophen] 500 mg ⚕ buniodyl

Panadol, Children's chewable tablets, oral liquid (discontinued 2008) OTC *analgesic; antipyretic* [acetaminophen] 80 mg; 160 mg/5 mL

Panadol, Infants' drops (discontinued 2008) OTC *analgesic; antipyretic* [acetaminophen] 100 mg/mL

Panadol, Junior caplets (discontinued 2008) OTC *analgesic; antipyretic* [acetaminophen] 160 mg

Panafil ointment, spray ℞ *proteolytic enzyme for debridement of necrotic tissue; vulnerary; wound deodorant* [papain; urea; chlorophyllin copper complex] 521 700 U/g•10%•0.5% ⚕ PenFill

Panafil SE spray ℞ *proteolytic enzyme for debridement of necrotic tissue; vulnerary; wound deodorant* [papain; urea; chlorophyllin copper complex] 405 900 U/g•10%•0.5%

Panafil White ointment ℞ *enzyme for wound debridement; vulnerary* [papain; urea] 10%•10%

Panalgesic cream OTC *analgesic; mild anesthetic; antipruritic; counterirritant* [methyl salicylate; menthol] 35%•4%

Panalgesic Gold liniment OTC *analgesic; mild anesthetic; antipruritic; counterirritant; antiseptic* [methyl salicylate; camphor; menthol; alcohol 22%] 55%•3.1%•1.25%

Panasal 5/500 tablets ℞ *narcotic analgesic; antipyretic* [hydrocodone bitartrate; aspirin] 5•500 mg

Panasol-S tablets (discontinued 2008) ℞ *corticosteroid; anti-inflammatory; immunosuppressant* [prednisone] 1 mg

Panatuss DX oral liquid (discontinued 2005) ℞ *decongestant; antihistamine; antitussive; expectorant* [phenylephrine HCl; dexchlorpheniramine maleate; dextromethorphan hydrobromide; guaifenesin] 5•1•15•100 mg/5 mL

Panax ginseng; P. shin-seng (Korean ginseng) *medicinal herb* [see: ginseng]

Panax horridum *medicinal herb* [see: devil's club]

Panax pseudoginseng (Chikusetsu ginseng; Himalayan ginseng; Sanchi ginseng; Zhuzishen) *medicinal herb* [see: ginseng]

Panax quinquefolia (American ginseng) *medicinal herb* [see: ginseng]

Panax spp. *medicinal herb* [see: ginseng]

Panax trifolius (dwarf ginseng) *medicinal herb* [see: ginseng]

Pancof syrup (discontinued 2007) ℞ *narcotic antitussive; antihistamine; decongestant* [dihydrocodeine bitartrate; chlorpheniramine maleate; pseudoephedrine HCl] 7.5•2•15 mg/5 mL

Pancof-EXP syrup (discontinued 2007) ℞ *narcotic antitussive; decongestant; expectorant* [dihydrocodeine bitartrate; pseudoephedrine HCl; guaifenesin] 7.5•15•100 mg/5 mL

Pancof-HC oral liquid (discontinued 2007) ℞ *narcotic antitussive; antihistamine; decongestant* [hydrocodone bitartrate; chlorpheniramine maleate; pseudoephedrine HCl] 3•2•15 mg/5 mL ⚕ Bancap HC

Pancof-HC syrup (discontinued 2007) ℞ *narcotic antitussive; decongestant* [hydrocodone bitartrate; pseudoephedrine HCl] 3•15 mg/5 mL ⊡ Bancap HC

Pancof-PD syrup ℞ *narcotic antitussive; antihistamine; decongestant* [dihydrocodeine bitartrate; chlorpheniramine maleate; phenylephrine HCl] 3•2•7.5 mg/5 mL

Pancof-XP oral liquid (discontinued 2007) ℞ *narcotic antitussive; decongestant; expectorant* [hydrocodone bitartrate; pseudoephedrine HCl; guaifenesin] 3•15•100 mg/5 mL

Pancof-XP syrup (discontinued 2007) ℞ *narcotic antitussive; expectorant* [hydrocodone bitartrate; guaifenesin] 3•90 mg/5 mL

pancopride USAN, INN *antiemetic; anxiolytic; peristaltic stimulant*

Pancrease; Pancrease MT 4; Pancrease MT 10; Pancrease MT 16; Pancrease MT 20 capsules containing enteric-coated microtablets (discontinued 2006) ℞ *porcine-derived digestive enzymes* [lipase; protease; amylase] 4.5•25•25; 4•12•12; 10•30•30; 16•48•48; 20•44•56 thousand USP units

pancreatin USP *porcine-derived digestive enzymes; a combination of lipase, protease, and amylase*

Pancrecarb MS-4; Pancrecarb MS-8; Pancrecarb MS-16 delayed-release capsules containing enteric-coated microspheres ℞ *porcine-derived digestive enzymes* [lipase; protease; amylase] 4000•25 000•25 000 USP units; 8000•45 000•40 000 USP units; 16 000•52 000•52 000 USP units

pancrelipase USAN, USP *porcine-derived digestive enzymes; a combination of lipase, protease, and amylase* 4.5•25•20, 8•30•30, 16•48•48, 16•60•60 thousand USP units

pancuronium bromide USAN, INN *nondepolarizing neuromuscular blocking agent; muscle relaxant; adjunct to tracheal intubation for general anesthesia or mechanical ventilation* 1, 2 mg/mL injection

Pandel cream ℞ *corticosteroidal antiinflammatory* [hydrocortisone probutate] 0.1% ⊡ buniodyl

Panfil G capsules, syrup ℞ *antiasthmatic; bronchodilator; expectorant* [dyphylline; guaifenesin] 200•100 mg; 100•50 mg/5 mL

pangamic acid [now: dimethylglycine HCl]

Pangestyme CN-10 delayed-release capsules ℞ *porcine-derived digestive enzymes* [lipase; protease; amylase] 10 000•37 500•33 200 USP units

Pangestyme CN-20 delayed-release capsules ℞ *porcine-derived digestive enzymes* [lipase; protease; amylase] 20 000•75 000•66 400 USP units

Pangestyme EC delayed-release capsules ℞ *porcine-derived digestive enzymes* [lipase; protease; amylase] 4500•25 000•20 000 USP units

Pangestyme MT16 delayed-release capsules ℞ *porcine-derived digestive enzymes* [lipase; protease; amylase] 16 000•48 000•48 000 USP units

Pangestyme UL12 delayed-release capsules ℞ *porcine-derived digestive enzymes* [lipase; protease; amylase] 12 000•39 000•39 000 USP units

Pangestyme UL18 delayed-release capsules ℞ *porcine-derived digestive enzymes* [lipase; protease; amylase] 18 000•58 500•58 500 USP units

Pangestyme UL20 delayed-release capsules ℞ *porcine-derived digestive enzymes* [lipase; protease; amylase] 20 000•65 000•65 000 USP units

Panglobulin NF powder for IV infusion (discontinued 2007) ℞ *passive immunizing agent for HIV and idiopathic thrombocytopenic purpura (ITP)* [immune globulin] 1, 3, 6, 12 g

Panhematin powder for IV injection ℞ *enzyme inhibitor for acute intermittent porphyria (AIP), porphyria variegata, and hereditary coproporphyria (orphan)* [hemin] 301 mg/vial

panidazole INN, BAN ☒ bendazol

Panitone-500 tablets (discontinued 2008) OTC *analgesic; antipyretic* [acetaminophen] 500 mg ☒ Ben-Tann

panitumumab *monoclonal antibody IgG2 to human epidermal growth factor receptor (EGFR) for metastatic colorectal cancer*

Panixine DisperDose tablets for oral suspension ℞ *first-generation cephalosporin antibiotic* [cephalexin] 125, 250 mg

Panlor DC capsules ℞ *narcotic antitussive; analgesic; antipyretic* [dihydrocodeine bitartrate; acetaminophen; caffeine] 16•356.4•30 mg

Panlor SS tablets ℞ *narcotic analgesic; antipyretic* [dihydrocodeine bitartrate; acetaminophen; caffeine] 32•712.8•60 mg

PanMist-DM extended-release caplets, syrup (discontinued 2007) ℞ *antitussive; decongestant; expectorant* [dextromethorphan hydrobromide; pseudoephedrine HCl; guaifenesin] 32•48•595 mg; 15•40•100 mg/5 mL

PanMist-JR extended-release caplets (discontinued 2007) ℞ *decongestant; expectorant* [pseudoephedrine HCl; guaifenesin] 48•595 mg

PanMist-LA extended-release caplets (discontinued 2007) ℞ *decongestant; expectorant* [pseudoephedrine HCl; guaifenesin] 85•795 mg

PanMist-S syrup (discontinued 2007) ℞ *decongestant; expectorant* [pseudoephedrine HCl; guaifenesin] 40•200 mg/5 mL

Pannaz sustained-release tablets (discontinued 2007) ℞ *decongestant; antihistamine; anticholinergic to dry mucosal secretions* [pseudoephedrine HCl; carbinoxamine maleate; methscopolamine bromide] 90•8•2.5 mg ☒ Benz 42

Pannaz S syrup (discontinued 2007) ℞ *decongestant; antihistamine; anticholinergic to dry mucosal secretions* [pseudoephedrine HCl; carbinoxa-

mine maleate; methscopolamine nitrate] 15•2•1.25 mg/5 mL

Panocaps; Panocaps MT 16; Panocaps MT 20 delayed-release capsules ℞ *porcine-derived digestive enzymes* [lipase; protease; amylase] 4500•25 000•20 000 USP units; 16 000•48 000•48 000 USP units; 20 000•44 000•56 000 USP units

Panokase tablets ℞ *porcine-derived digestive enzymes* [lipase; protease; amylase] 8000•30 000•30 000 USP units ☒ Pain-X; Pin-X

panomifene INN

Panorex *investigational (orphan) antineoplastic adjunct for pancreatic cancer* [edrecolomab]

Panoxyl cleansing bar OTC *keratolytic for acne* [benzoyl peroxide] 5%, 10%

Panoxyl 5; Panoxyl 10 gel ℞ *keratolytic and antiseptic for acne* [benzoyl peroxide; alcohol] 5%•12%; 10%•20%

Panoxyl AQ 2½; Panoxyl AQ 5; Panoxyl AQ 10 gel ℞ *keratolytic for acne* [benzoyl peroxide] 2.5%; 5%; 10%

Panretin capsules *investigational (Phase III, orphan) treatment for acute promyelocytic leukemia (APL); investigational (orphan) to prevent retinal detachment due to proliferative vitreoretinopathy* [alitretinoin]

Panretin gel ℞ *retinoid for cutaneous lesions of AIDS-related Kaposi sarcoma (orphan)* [alitretinoin] 0.1%

Panscol lotion, ointment OTC *keratolytic* [salicylic acid] 3%

pansy (Viola tricolor) plant *medicinal herb used as an anodyne, demulcent, diaphoretic, diuretic, expectorant, laxative, and vulnerary* ☒ Benz 42

pantenicate INN

panthenol USAN, USP, INN *B complex vitamin*

D-panthenol [see: dexpanthenol]

Panthoderm cream OTC *antipruritic; vulnerary; emollient* [dexpanthenol] 2%

pantoprazole USAN, INN, BAN *proton pump inhibitor for erosive esophagitis associated with gastroesophageal reflux disease (GERD)*

pantoprazole sodium USAN *proton pump inhibitor for erosive esophagitis associated with gastroesophageal reflux disease (GERD) and Zollinger-Ellison syndrome* (base=89%) 20, 40 mg oral

pantothenic acid (vitamin B₅) BAN *water-soluble vitamin; coenzyme A precursor* [also: calcium pantothenate] 92, 200, 500 mg oral

DL-pantothenic acid [see: calcium pantothenate, racemic]

pantothenol [see: dexpanthenol]

pantothenyl alcohol [see: panthenol]

D-pantothenyl alcohol [see: dexpanthenol]

panuramine INN, BAN

Panvac-VF *investigational (Phase III) antineoplastic vaccine for metastatic pancreatic cancer*

Panzem *investigational (orphan) for multiple myeloma* [2-methoxyestradiol]

Panzem NCD *investigational (orphan) for ovarian cancer* [2-methoxyestradiol]

papain USP *topical proteolytic enzyme for debridement of necrotic tissue*

papain & trypsin & chymotrypsin *investigational (orphan) enzyme combination adjunct to chemotherapy for multiple myeloma*

papain & urea & chlorophyllin *proteolytic enzyme for debridement of necrotic tissue; vulnerary; wound deodorant* 521 700 U/g•10%•0.5% topical

papaverine BAN *peripheral vasodilator; smooth muscle relaxant* [also: papaverine HCl]

papaverine HCl USP *peripheral vasodilator; smooth muscle relaxant for cerebral, myocardial, and peripheral ischemias; investigational (orphan) topical treatment for sexual dysfunction due to spinal cord injury* [also: papaverine] 150 mg oral; 30 mg/mL

papaveroline INN, BAN

papaya *(Carica papaya)* leaves, fruit, juice, and seeds *medicinal herb for aiding digestion, gas, insect bites, and intestinal worms*

Paplex Ultra topical solution ℞ *keratolytic* [salicylic acid in flexible collodion] 26%

papoose root *medicinal herb* [see: blue cohosh]

Pap-Urea ointment ℞ *proteolytic enzyme for debridement of necrotic tissue; vulnerary* [papain; urea] 830 000 IU/g•10% ⧈ bayberry

Par Glycerol elixir ℞ *expectorant* [iodinated glycerol] 60 mg/5 mL

para-aminobenzoate (PAB) [see: aminobenzoic acid]

Para-Aminobenzoic Acid tablets, powder OTC *water-soluble vitamin; "possibly effective" for scleroderma and other skin diseases and Peyronie disease* [aminobenzoic acid] 100, 500 mg; 120 g

para-aminobenzoic acid (PABA) [now: aminobenzoic acid]

para-aminohippurate (PAH) [see: aminohippuric acid]

para-aminohippurate sodium [see: aminohippurate sodium]

para-aminohippuric acid (PAHA) [see: aminohippuric acid]

para-aminosalicylate (PAS) [see: aminosalicylic acid]

para-aminosalicylic acid (PASA) [see: aminosalicylic acid]

Parabolan *brand name for trenbolone hexahydrobenzylcarbonate, a European veterinary anabolic steroid abused as a street drug*

parabromdylamine maleate [see: brompheniramine maleate]

Paracaine eye drops ℞ *topical anesthetic* [proparacaine HCl] 0.5% ⧈ Baricon; procaine; Puregon; pyrrocaine

paracetaldehyde [see: paraldehyde]

paracetamol INN, BAN *analgesic; antipyretic* [also: acetaminophen]

parachlorometaxylenol (PCMX) *topical antiseptic; broad-spectrum antibacterial*

parachlorophenol (PCP) USP *topical antibacterial*

parachlorophenol, camphorated USP *topical dental anti-infective*

paracodin [see: dihydrocodeine]

paraffin NF *stiffening agent* 🔄 Brovana; Preven; Privine; Profen II

paraffin, liquid [see: mineral oil]

paraffin, synthetic NF *stiffening agent*

Paraflex caplets ℞ *skeletal muscle relaxant* [chlorzoxazone] 250 mg

paraflutizide INN

Parafon Forte DSC caplets ℞ *skeletal muscle relaxant* [chlorzoxazone] 500 mg 🔄 Profen Forte DM

paraformaldehyde USP

ParaGard T 380A (intrauterine device) ℞ *T-shaped IUD contraceptive* [copper] 🔄 PerioGard; Procardia

Paraguay tea *medicinal herb* [see: yerba maté]

parahydrecin [now: isomerol]

Paral oral liquid, rectal liquid (discontinued 2008) ℞ *sedative; hypnotic* [paraldehyde] 🔄 barley; perilla; Prelu-2

paraldehyde USP *hypnotic; sedative; anticonvulsant* 1 g/mL oral or rectal

paramethadione USP, INN, BAN *anticonvulsant*

paramethasone INN *corticosteroid; anti-inflammatory* [also: paramethasone acetate] 🔄 perimetazine; promethazine

paramethasone acetate USAN, USP *corticosteroid; anti-inflammatory* [also: paramethasone]

para-nitrosulfathiazole NF [also: nitrosulfathiazole]

paranyline HCl USAN *anti-inflammatory* [also: renytoline]

parapenzolate bromide USAN, INN *anticholinergic*

Paraplatin injection, powder for IV injection (discontinued 2007) ℞ *alkylating antineoplastic for ovarian and other cancers* [carboplatin] 10 mg/mL; 50, 150, 450 mg

parapropamol INN

pararosaniline embonate INN *anti-schistosomal* [also: pararosaniline pamoate]

pararosaniline pamoate USAN *anti-schistosomal* [also: pararosaniline embonate]

parasympathomimetics *a class of agents that produce effects similar to those of the parasympathetic nervous system* [also called: cholinergic agonists]

Parathar powder for IV injection (discontinued 2004) ℞ *in vivo diagnostic aid for parathyroid-induced hypocalcemia* (orphan); *investigational* (orphan) *for idiopathic osteoporosis* [teriparatide acetate] 200 U

parathesin [see: benzocaine]

parathiazine INN

parathyroid USP *hormone*

parathyroid hormone (1-34), biosynthetic human [see: teriparatide]

parathyroid hormone (1-84), recombinant human *investigational (Phase III) agent to increase bone mineral content and density in postmenopausal osteoporosis*

paraxazone INN

parbendazole USAN, INN *anthelmintic* 🔄 propenidazole

parconazole INN *antifungal* [also: parconazole HCl] 🔄 pirquinozol

parconazole HCl USAN *antifungal* [also: parconazole]

Parcopa RapiTabs (orally disintegrating tablets) ℞ *dopamine precursor for Parkinson disease; decarboxylase inhibitor (levodopa potentiator)* [levodopa; carbidopa] 100•10, 100•25, 250•25 mg

parecoxib USAN, INN *COX-2 inhibitor; anti-inflammatory; analgesic*

parecoxib sodium USAN *COX-2 inhibitor; anti-inflammatory; analgesic*

Paredrine eye drops (discontinued 2006) ℞ *mydriatic* [hydroxyamphetamine hydrobromide] 1% 🔄 pyridarone

paregoric (PG) (a preparation of opium, anise oil, benzoic acid, camphor, alcohol, and glycerin) USP *antiperistaltic; narcotic analgesic; used in neonatal opioid withdrawal programs;*

sometimes abused as a street drug 2 mg opium/5 mL oral

Paremyd eye drops ℞ *mydriatic; weak cycloplegic* [hydroxyamphetamine hydrobromide; tropicamide] 1%• 0.25% ⊡ PerioMed; ProMod

parenabol [see: boldenone undecylenate]

Parepectolin concentrated oral liquid OTC *GI adsorbent; antidiarrheal* [attapulgite] 600 mg/15 mL

pareptide INN *antiparkinsonian* [also: pareptide sulfate]

pareptide sulfate USAN *antiparkinsonian* [also: pareptide]

parethoxycaine INN

parethoxycaine HCl [see: parethoxycaine]

Par-F tablets ℞ *vitamin/mineral/calcium/ iron supplement* [multiple vitamins & minerals; calcium; iron; folic acid] ± •250•60•1 mg

pargeverine INN

Pargluva tablets ℞ *antidiabetic to control blood glucose levels, lower triglycerides, and raise HDL* [muraglitazar] 5 mg

pargolol INN ⊡ pyrogallol

pargyline INN *antihypertensive* [also: pargyline HCl] ⊡ Percolone; piriqualone

pargyline HCl USAN, USP *antihypertensive* [also: pargyline]

paricalcitol USAN *fat-soluble vitamin; synthetic vitamin D analogue for hyperparathyroidism secondary to chronic kidney disease (CKD)*

paridocaine INN ⊡ piridocaine

Parlodel SnapTabs (scored tablets), capsules ℞ *dopamine agonist for Parkinson disease; lactation preventative; treatment for acromegaly, infertility, and hypogonadism* [bromocriptine mesylate] 2.5 mg; 5 mg

Par-Natal Plus 1 Improved tablets ℞ *vitamin/calcium/iron supplement* [multiple vitamins; calcium; iron; folic acid] ± •200•65•1 mg ⊡ Prenatal Plus

Parnate film-coated tablets ℞ *MAO inhibitor for major depression; also used for migraine prevention, social anxiety*

disorder (SAD), panic disorder, bipolar depression, and Alzheimer and Parkinson disease [tranylcypromine sulfate] 10 mg ⊡ burnet; Pronto

parodilol INN

parodyne [see: antipyrine]

paroleine [see: mineral oil]

paromomycin INN, BAN *aminoglycoside antibiotic; amebicide* [also: paromomycin sulfate]

Paromomycin *investigational (orphan) agent for visceral leishmaniasis* [aminosidine]

paromomycin sulfate USP *aminoglycoside antibiotic; amebicide for acute and chronic intestinal amebiasis; investigational (orphan) for cutaneous leishmaniasis* [also: paromomycin] 250 mg oral

paroxetine USAN, INN, BAN *selective serotonin reuptake inhibitor (SSRI) for depression, obsessive-compulsive disorder, and panic disorder*

paroxetine HCl *selective serotonin reuptake inhibitor (SSRI) for depression, obsessive-compulsive disorder, panic disorder, social anxiety disorder, generalized anxiety disorder, post-traumatic stress disorder, and premenstrual dysphoric disorder* 10, 12.5, 20, 25, 30, 37.5, 40 mg oral; 10 mg/5 mL oral

paroxetine mesylate *selective serotonin reuptake inhibitor (SSRI) for depression, obsessive-compulsive disorder, and panic disorder*

paroxyl [see: acetarsone]

paroxypropione INN

parpanit HCl [see: caramiphen HCl]

parsalmide INN

parsley (Petroselinum sativum) leaves and root *medicinal herb for amenorrhea, bladder infections, blood building and cleansing, body lice, colic, dysmenorrhea, flatulence, gallstones, inducing abortion, jaundice, nephritis, prostate disorder, and urinary retention* ⊡ Buro-Sol; ProSol

parsley fern *medicinal herb* [see: tansy]

parsnip, cow; wooly parsnip *medicinal herb* [see: masterwort]

Partaject (trademarked delivery device) *investigational (Phase II/III) intravenous delivery device*

Parthenocissus quinquefolia medicinal herb [see: American ivy]

partricin USAN, INN *antifungal; antiprotozoal*

partridge berry *medicinal herb* [see: squaw vine; wintergreen]

parvaquone INN, BAN ② Brevicon; porofocon A

Parvlex tablets OTC *hematinic* [ferrous fumarate; multiple B vitamins & minerals; vitamin C; folic acid] 100●±●50●0.1 mg

parvovirus B19 vaccine, recombinant *investigational (orphan) prevention of transient aplastic anemia due to sickle cell disease*

PAS (para-aminosalicylate) [see: aminosalicylic acid]

PASA (para-aminosalicylic acid) [see: aminosalicylic acid]

Paser delayed-release granules for oral solution ℞ *treatment for multidrug-resistant tuberculosis (MDR-TB) (orphan)* [aminosalicylic acid] 4 g/pkt.

pasiniazid INN

pasque flower (*Anemone patens*) plant *medicinal herb used as a diaphoretic, diuretic, and rubefacient; not generally regarded as safe and effective due to toxicity*

passion flower (*Passiflora incarnata*) plant *medicinal herb for asthma, bronchitis, eye infections, fever, inflamed hemorrhoids, insomnia, menopause, nervousness, pain related to neurasthenia, and attention-deficit disorder, nervousness, and excitability in children*

Pastilles (dosage form) *troches*

Pataday Drop-Tainers (eye drops) ℞ *once-daily antihistamine and mast cell stabilizer for allergic conjunctivitis* [olopatadine HCl] 0.2%

Patanase nasal spray ℞ *antihistamine and mast cell stabilizer for seasonal allergic rhinitis* [olopatadine HCl] 665 mcg/spray

Patanol Drop-Tainers (eye drops) ℞ *antihistamine and mast cell stabilizer for allergic conjunctivitis* [olopatadine HCl] 0.1% ② Botanol

PaTCO (prednisone, ara-C, thioguanine, cyclophosphamide, Oncovin) *chemotherapy protocol*

patience, garden *medicinal herb* [see: yellow dock]

patience dock *medicinal herb* [see: bistort]

pau d'arco (*Lapacho colorado; L. morado*) inner bark *medicinal herb for boils, blood cleansing, cancer, Candida albicans infections, chlorosis, diabetes, leukemia, skin wounds, syphilis, and pain*

Paullinia cupana; P. sorbilis *medicinal herb* [see: guarana]

paulomycin USAN, INN *antibacterial* ② bleomycin; peliomycin

Pausinystalia johimbe medicinal herb [see: yohimbe]

pauson *medicinal herb* [see: bloodroot]

Pavabid Plateau Caps (controlled-release capsules) (discontinued 2005) ℞ *peripheral vasodilator; smooth muscle relaxant for cerebral, myocardial, and peripheral ischemias* [papaverine HCl] 150 mg

Pavagen TD timed-release capsules ℞ *peripheral vasodilator; smooth muscle relaxant for cerebral, myocardial, and peripheral ischemias* [papaverine HCl] 150 mg

PAVe (procarbazine, Alkeran, Velban) *chemotherapy protocol*

Pavulon IM injection (discontinued 2004) ℞ *nondepolarizing neuromuscular blocking agent; muscle relaxant; adjunct to tracheal intubation for general anesthesia or mechanical ventilation* [pancuronium bromide] 1, 2 mg/mL ② bufylline

pawpaw (*Asimina triloba*) fruit *medicinal herb used as an antimicrobial and antineoplastic*

paxamate INN

Paxarel tablets (discontinued 2006) ℞ *anxiolytic; sedative* [acecarbromal] 250 mg

Paxene *investigational (Phase III, orphan) antineoplastic for AIDS-related Kaposi sarcoma* [paclitaxel]

Paxil film-coated tablets, oral suspension ℞ *selective serotonin reuptake inhibitor (SSRI) for depression, obsessive-compulsive disorder, panic disorder, social anxiety disorder, generalized anxiety disorder, and post-traumatic stress disorder* [paroxetine HCl] 10, 20, 30, 40 mg; 10 mg/5 mL ⚕ piquizil

Paxil CR enteric-coated controlled-release tablets ℞ *selective serotonin reuptake inhibitor (SSRI) for depression, panic disorder, premenstrual dysphoric disorder (PMDD), and social anxiety disorder (SAD)* [paroxetine HCl] 12.5, 25, 37.5 mg

pazelliptine INN

pazinaclone USAN *anxiolytic*

Pazo Hemorrhoid ointment OTC *temporary relief of hemorrhoidal symptoms; vasoconstrictor; antipruritic; counterirritant; astringent* [ephedrine sulfate; camphor; zinc oxide] 0.2%•2%•5%

Pazo Hemorrhoid suppositories OTC *temporary relief of hemorrhoidal symptoms; vasoconstrictor; astringent; emollient* [ephedrine sulfate; zinc oxide] 3.8•96.5 mg

pazoxide USAN, INN *antihypertensive*

PBM Allergy syrup ℞ *antitussive; antihistamine; decongestant* [dextromethorphan hydrobromide; brompheniramine maleate; pseudoephedrine HCl] 15•3•30 mg/5 mL

PBV (Platinol, bleomycin, vinblastine) *chemotherapy protocol*

PC (paclitaxel, carboplatin) *chemotherapy protocol for bladder cancer and non–small cell lung cancer (NSCLC)*

PC (paclitaxel, cisplatin) *chemotherapy protocol for non–small cell lung cancer (NSCLC)*

PC (phosphatidylcholine) [see: lecithin]

PC Tar shampoo OTC *antiseborrheic; antipsoriatic; antipruritic; antibacterial* [coal tar] 1% ⚕ beech tree

PCE Dispertabs (delayed-release tablets) ℞ *macrolide antibiotic* [erythromycin] 333, 500 mg

PCE (Platinol, cyclophosphamide, etoposide) *chemotherapy protocol*

PCE (polymer-coated erythromycin) [see: erythromycin]

PCM chewable tablets ℞ *decongestant; antihistamine; anticholinergic to dry mucosal secretions* [phenylephrine HCl; chlorpheniramine maleate; methscopolamine nitrate] 10•2• 1.25 mg

PCM Allergy extended-release tablets ℞ *decongestant; antihistamine; anticholinergic to dry mucosal secretions* [phenylephrine HCl; chlorpheniramine maleate; methscopolamine nitrate] 20•12•2.5 mg

PCMX (parachlorometaxylenol) [q.v.]

PCOs (procyanidolic oligomers) [q.v.]

PCP (parachlorophenol) [q.v.]

PCP (phenylcyclohexyl piperidine) *a powerful veterinary analgesic/anesthetic widely abused as a hallucinogenic street drug* [medically known as phencyclidine HCl]

PCV (pneumococcal vaccine) [q.v.]

PCV (procarbazine, CCNU, vincristine) *chemotherapy protocol for brain tumors*

PD-COF oral drops ℞ *antitussive; antihistamine; decongestant; for children 6–24 months* [dextromethorphan hydrobromide; chlorpheniramine maleate; phenylephrine HCl] 3•1• 3.5 mg/mL

PD-COF syrup ℞ *antitussive; antihistamine; decongestant* [dextromethorphan hydrobromide; chlorpheniramine maleate; phenylephrine HCl] 15•4•12.5 mg/5 mL

PDE III (phosphodiesterase III) inhibitors *a class of platelet aggregation inhibitors*

PDGA (pteroyldiglutamic acid)

PD-Hist D syrup, oral drops ℞ *decongestant; antihistamine; drops for children 6–24 months* [phenylephrine HCl; chlorpheniramine maleate] 12.5•4 mg/5 mL; 3.5•1 mg/mL ⑨ Bidhist

PDLA (phosphinicodilactic acid) [see: foscolic acid]

PE (paclitaxel, estramustine) *chemotherapy protocol for prostate cancer*

PE (phenylephrine) [q.v.]

PE (polyethylene) [q.v.]

pea, ground squirrel *medicinal herb* [see: twin leaf]

pea, turkey; wild turkey pea *medicinal herb* [see: turkey corn]

peach (*Prunus persica*) bark and leaves *medicinal herb for bladder disorders, chest congestion, chronic bronchitis, nausea, and water retention*

peanut oil NF *solvent* ⑨ Bentyl

PEB (Platinol, etoposide, bleomycin) *chemotherapy protocol*

pecazine INN, BAN ⑨ Biaxin; Bicozene

pecazine acetate [see: pecazine]

pecilocin INN, BAN ⑨ bizelesin

pecocycline INN

pectin USP *suspending agent; protectant; GI adsorbent*

pectorals *a class of agents that relieve disorders of the respiratory tract, such as expectorants*

Pedameth capsules, oral liquid (discontinued 2006) ℞ *urinary acidifier to control ammonia production* [racemethionine] 200 mg; 75 mg/5 mL ⑨ padimate

Pedia Relief Decongestant Plus Cough oral drops (discontinued 2007) OTC *antitussive; decongestant; for children 2–3 years* [dextromethorphan hydrobromide; pseudoephedrine HCl] 5•15 mg/1.6 mL

PediaCare Allergy Formula oral liquid OTC *antihistamine* [chlorpheniramine maleate] 1 mg/5 mL

PediaCare Children's Cold & Allergy oral liquid (discontinued 2007) OTC *decongestant; antihistamine*

[pseudoephedrine HCl; chlorpheniramine maleate] 30•2 mg/10 mL

PediaCare Children's Decongestant oral solution OTC *nasal decongestant* [phenylephrine HCl] 2.5 mg/5 mL

PediaCare Children's Long-Acting Cough freezer pops, oral solution OTC *antitussive for children 2–11 years* [dextromethorphan hydrobromide] 7.5 mg/pop; 7.5 mg/5 mL

PediaCare Children's Long-Acting Cough Plus Cold oral liquid (discontinued 2007) OTC *antitussive; decongestant; for children 2–11 years* [dextromethorphan hydrobromide; pseudoephedrine HCl] 7.5•15 mg/5 mL

PediaCare Children's Multi-Symptom Cold chewable tablets (discontinued 2007) OTC *antitussive; antihistamine; decongestant; for children 6–11 years* [dextromethorphan hydrobromide; chlorpheniramine maleate; pseudoephedrine HCl] 5•1•15 mg

PediaCare Children's NightRest Multi-Symptom Cold oral liquid OTC *decongestant; antihistamine; sleep aid; for children 6–11 years* [phenylephrine HCl; diphenhydramine HCl] 5•12.5 mg/5 mL

PediaCare Children's Nighttime Cough oral solution (discontinued 2007) OTC *antihistamine; antitussive; sleep aid* [diphenhydramine HCl] 12.5 mg/5 mL

PediaCare Cough-Cold; PediaCare Multi-Symptom Cold oral liquid (discontinued 2007) OTC *antitussive; antihistamine; decongestant; for children 6–11 years* [dextromethorphan hydrobromide; chlorpheniramine maleate; pseudoephedrine] 10•2•30 mg/10 mL

PediaCare Fever oral suspension, oral drops OTC *analgesic; antipyretic; nonsteroidal anti-inflammatory drug (NSAID) for minor aches and pains* [ibuprofen] 100 mg/5 mL; 40 mg/mL

PediaCare Infant Decongestant & Cough (PE) oral drops OTC *antitus-*

sive; decongestant; for children 2–5
years [dextromethorphan hydrobromide; phenylephrine HCl] 5•2.5
mg/1.6 mL

**PediaCare Infant Decongestant &
Cough (PSE)** oral drops OTC antitussive; decongestant; for children 2–5
years [dextromethorphan hydrobromide; pseudoephedrine HCl] 5•15
mg/1.6 mL

PediaCare Infant's Decongestant
oral drops OTC nasal decongestant
[pseudoephedrine HCl] 7.5 mg/0.8 mL

**PediaCare Infants' Long-Acting
Cough** oral drops OTC antitussive for
children 2–3 years [dextromethor-
phan hydrobromide] 3.75 mg/0.8 mL

**PediaCare NightRest Cough &
Cold** oral liquid (discontinued 2007)
OTC antitussive; antihistamine; decongestant; for children 6–11 years [dex-
tromethorphan hydrobromide; chlorpheniramine maleate; pseudoephedrine HCl] 15•2•30 mg/10 mL

Pediaflor drops R dental caries preventative [sodium fluoride] 1.1 mg/mL

Pediahist DM oral drops R antitussive; antihistamine; decongestant; for
children 1–18 months [dextromethor-
phan hydrobromide; brompheni-
amine maleate; pseudoephedrine
HCl] 4•1•15 mg/mL

Pediahist DM syrup R antitussive;
decongestant; antihistamine; expectorant [dextromethorphan hydrobromide; pseudoephedrine HCl; brompheniramine maleate; guaifenesin]
5•30•2•50/5 mL

Pedia-Lax chewable tablets OTC saline
laxative; antacid [magnesium hydrox-
ide] 400 mg

Pedialyte oral solution, freezer pops
OTC electrolyte replacement [sodium,
potassium, and chloride electrolytes]

Pediamist low-pressure nasal spray
OTC nasal moisturizer for children
[sodium chloride (saline solution)]

PediaPhyl D oral suspension R
decongestant; antihistamine [phenyl-

ephrine tannate; chlorpheniramine
tannate] 10•8 mg/5 mL

Pediapred oral solution R corticosteroid; anti-inflammatory [prednisolone
sodium phosphate] 6.7 mg/5 mL (5
mg/5 mL base)

Pediarix IM injection R active immunizing agent for diphtheria, tetanus,
pertussis, hepatitis B and D, and three
types of poliovirus [diphtheria & tetanus toxoids & acellular pertussis
(DTaP) vaccine; hepatitis B virus
vaccine; inactivated poliovirus vaccine Types 1, 2, and 3] 25 Lf•10 Lf•
25 mcg•10 mcg•40 DU•8 DU•32
DU per 0.5 mL dose

PediaSure; PediaSure with Fiber
ready-to-use oral liquid OTC total or
supplementary infant feeding

PediaTan oral suspension R antihistamine [chlorpheniramine tannate] 8
mg/5 mL

PediaTan D oral suspension R decongestant; antihistamine [phenylephrine
tannate; chlorpheniramine tannate]
10•8 mg/5 mL

Pediatex oral liquid R antihistamine
for allergic rhinitis [carbinoxamine
maleate] 1.67 mg/5 mL

Pediatex 12 oral suspension R antihistamine for allergic rhinitis [carbinoxa-
mine tannate] 3.2 mg/5 mL

Pediatex 12 D pediatric oral suspension (discontinued 2007) R decongestant; antihistamine [pseudoephed-
rine tannate; carbinoxamine tannate]
45.2•3.6 mg/5 mL

Pediatex HC syrup (discontinued
2007) R narcotic antitussive; antihistamine; decongestant [hydrocodone
bitartrate; chlorpheniramine maleate; pseudoephedrine HCl] 1.67•
2.5•17.5 mg/5 mL

Pediatex-CT chewable tablets R
decongestant; antihistamine; sleep aid
[phenylephrine HCl; diphenhydramine HCl] 5•12.5 mg/5 mL

Pediatex-D oral liquid (discontinued
2007) R decongestant; antihistamine

[pseudoephedrine HCl; carbinoxamine maleate] 12.5•1.67 mg/5 mL

Pediatex-DM oral liquid (discontinued 2007) ℞ *antitussive; antihistamine; decongestant* [dextromethorphan hydrobromide; carbinoxamine maleate; pseudoephedrine HCl] 15•2•15 mg/5 mL

Pediatric Cough & Cold Medicine oral liquid OTC *antitussive; antihistamine; decongestant; for children 6–11 years* [dextromethorphan hydrobromide; chlorpheniramine maleate; pseudoephedrine HCl] 10•2•30 mg/10 mL

Pediatric Decongestant and Cough oral drops (discontinued 2008) OTC *antitussive; decongestant; for children 2–5 years* [dextromethorphan hydrobromide; phenylephrine HCl] 2.5•7.5 mg/0.8 mL

Pediatric Electrolyte oral solution OTC *electrolyte replacement* [dextrose; multiple electrolytes] 1 L

pediatric VAC *chemotherapy protocol for pediatric sarcomas* [see: VAC pediatric]

Pediazole oral suspension ℞ *antibiotic* [erythromycin ethylsuccinate; sulfisoxazole acetyl] 200•600 mg/5 mL

Pedi-Boro Soak Paks powder packets OTC *astringent wet dressing (modified Burow solution)* [aluminum sulfate; calcium acetate]

pediculicides *a class of agents effective against head and pubic lice*

Pedi-Dri powder ℞ *antifungal* [nystatin] 100 000 U/g

Pediotic ear drop suspension ℞ *corticosteroidal anti-inflammatory; antibiotic* [hydrocortisone; neomycin sulfate; polymyxin B sulfate] 1%•5 mg•10 000 U per mL

Pediox pediatric chewable tablets (discontinued 2007) ℞ *decongestant; antihistamine* [pseudoephedrine HCl; chlorpheniramine maleate] 15•2 mg ⑨ Bidex-A

Pediox-S oral suspension ℞ *antihistamine* [chlorpheniramine maleate] 4 mg/5 mL

Pedi-Pro foot powder OTC *antifungal; anhidrotic* [benzalkonium chloride] 1%

Pedi-Vit-A Creme OTC *moisturizer; emollient* [vitamin A] 100 000 U/30 g

Pedotic otic suspension ℞ *corticosteroidal anti-inflammatory; antibiotic* [hydrocortisone; neomycin sulfate; polymyxin B sulfate] 1%•5 mg•10 000 U per mL

PedTE-Pak-4 IV injection ℞ *intravenous nutritional therapy* [multiple trace elements (metals)]

Pedtrace-4 IV injection ℞ *intravenous nutritional therapy* [multiple trace elements (metals)]

PedvaxHIB IM injection ℞ *vaccine for H. influenzae type b (HIB) infections in children 2–71 months* [Hemophilus b conjugate vaccine; Neisseria meningitidis OMPC] 7.5•125 mcg/dose

pefloxacin USAN, INN, BAN *antibacterial*

pefloxacin mesylate USAN *antibacterial*

PEG (polyethylene glycol) [q.v.]

pegacaristim USAN *megakaryocyte stimulating factor for thrombocytopenia*

PEG-ADA (polyethylene glycol–adenosine deaminase) [see: pegademase bovine]

pegademase INN *adenosine deaminase (ADA) replacement* [also: pegademase bovine]

pegademase bovine USAN *adenosine deaminase (ADA) replacement for severe combined immunodeficiency disease (orphan)* [also: pegademase]

PEG-adenosine deaminase (PEG-ADA) [see: pegademase bovine]

Peganone tablets ℞ *hydantoin anticonvulsant* [ethotoin] 250, 500 mg

pegaptanib sodium *pegylated VEGF (vascular endothelial growth factor) antagonist for neovascular (wet) age-related macular degeneration (AMD); also used for diabetic macular edema*

pegaspargase (PEG-L-asparaginase) USAN, INN *antineoplastic for acute lymphocytic leukemia (orphan) and acute lymphoblastic leukemia*

Pegasys subcu injection, prefilled syringes ℞ *immunomodulator for*

*chronic hepatitis B virus (HBV) and
chronic hepatitis C virus (HCV) infection; investigational (orphan) for renal
cell carcinoma and chronic myelogenous leukemia* [peginterferon alfa-2a]
180 mcg/mL

**PEG-ES (polyethylene glycol–elec-
trolyte solution)** [q.v.]

pegfilgrastim *recombinant human granulocyte colony-stimulating factor (G-
CSF) in polyethylene glycol (PEG);
hematopoietic stimulant for severe
chronic neutropenia following cancer
chemotherapy*

PEG-glucocerebrosidase *investigational (orphan) chronic enzyme replacement therapy for Gaucher disease*

peginterferon alfa-2a *immunomodulator for chronic hepatitis B virus (HBV)
and chronic hepatitis C virus (HCV)
infection; investigational (orphan) for
renal cell carcinoma and chronic myelogenous leukemia*

peginterferon alfa-2b *immunomodulator for chronic hepatitis C; investigational
(Phase III) for malignant melanoma
and chronic myelogenous leukemia*

PEG-interleukin-2 *investigational
(orphan) for primary immunodeficiencies associated with T-cell defects*

PEG-Intron *powder for subcu injection antiviral; long-acting formulation
of Intron A for chronic hepatitis C;
investigational (Phase III) for malignant melanoma and chronic myelogenous leukemia* [peginterferon alfa-2b]
100, 160, 240, 300 mcg/mL

peglicol 5 oleate USAN *emulsifying agent*

pegnartograstim USAN *immunostimulant adjunct to cancer chemotherapy*

pegorgotein USAN, INN *free-radical
scavenger*

pegoterate USAN, INN *suspending agent*

pegoxol 7 stearate USAN *emulsifying
agent*

**PEG-SOD (polyethylene glycol–
superoxide dismutase)** [see: pegor-
gotein]

**PEG-uricase (polyethylene glycol–
urate oxidase)** *investigational (Phase*

*III, orphan) agent for cancer-related
tumor lysis syndrome and hyperuricemia due to cancer or severe gout*

pegvisomant USAN *growth hormone
receptor antagonist for acromegaly
(orphan)*

pegylated [def.] *bound to polyethylene
glycol (PEG), an inactive solvent used
as a carrier for an active ingredient*

pegylated arginine deiminase [see:
arginine deiminase, pegylated]

pegylated doxorubicin [see: doxorubicin HCl, liposome-encapsulated]

pegylated interferon alfa-2b *investigational (Phase III) treatment for
malignant melanoma*

**pegylated megakaryocyte growth
factor** [see: megakaryocyte growth
and development factor, pegylated,
recombinant human]

pelanserin INN *antihypertensive; vasodilator; serotonin adrenergic blocker*
[also: pelanserin HCl]

pelanserin HCl USAN *antihypertensive;
vasodilator; serotonin adrenergic blocker*
[also: pelanserin]

peldesine USAN *purine nucleoside phos-
phorylase inhibitor for psoriasis; investigational (orphan) for cutaneous T-cell
lymphoma*

peliomycin USAN, INN *antineoplastic* ☒
bleomycin; paulomycin

pellants *a class of agents that purify or
cleanse the system, particularly the blood*
[also called: depurants; depuratives]

pelretin USAN, INN *antikeratinizing agent*

pelrinone INN *cardiotonic* [also: pelrinone HCl]

pelrinone HCl USAN *cardiotonic* [also:
pelrinone]

PemADD CT *chewable tablets (withdrawn from the market in 2005 due
to safety concerns)* ℞ *CNS stimulant
for attention-deficit/hyperactivity disorder (ADHD)* [pemoline] 37.5 mg

pemedolac USAN, INN *analgesic*

pemerid INN *antitussive* [also: pemerid
nitrate]

pemerid nitrate USAN *antitussive* [also:
pemerid]

pemetrexed disodium USAN *folic acid antagonist; inhibitor of thymidylate synthase, dihydrofolate reductase, and glycinamide ribonucleotide formyl transferase; antineoplastic for malignant pleural mesothelioma (orphan) and non–small cell lung cancer (NSCLC)*

pemirolast INN *ophthalmic antiallergic; mast cell stabilizer* [also: pemirolast potassium]

pemirolast potassium USAN *ophthalmic antiallergic; mast cell stabilizer* [also: pemirolast]

pemoline USAN, INN, BAN, JAN *CNS stimulant for attention-deficit/hyperactivity disorder (ADHD) and narcolepsy*

pempidine INN, BAN

penamecillin USAN, INN, BAN *antibacterial*

penbutolol INN, BAN *β-blocker for hypertension* [also: penbutolol sulfate]

penbutolol sulfate USAN *β-blocker for hypertension* [also: penbutolol]

penciclovir USAN, INN, BAN *topical antiviral for recurrent herpes labialis*

penciclovir sodium USAN *antiviral for herpes infections*

pendecamaine INN, BAN

pendiomide [see: azamethonium bromide]

Penecare cream, lotion OTC *moisturizer; emollient* [lactic acid] ☒ Benicar

Penecort cream, solution ℞ *corticosteroidal anti-inflammatory* [hydrocortisone] 1%

"penems" *brief term for a class of broad-spectrum antibiotics that include* **doripenem, fropenem, ertapenem, imipenem,** *and* **meropenem** [properly called: carbapenems]

PenFill (trademarked delivery form) *insulin injector refill cartridge* ☒ Panafil

penfluridol USAN, INN *antipsychotic*

penflutizide INN

pengitoxin INN

penicillamine USAN, USP, INN *metal chelating agent; antirheumatic*

penicillin aluminum

penicillin benzathine phenoxymethyl [now: penicillin V benzathine]

penicillin calcium USP

penicillin G benzathine USP *natural penicillin antibiotic* [also: benzathine benzylpenicillin; benzathine penicillin; benzylpenicillin benzathine]

penicillin G hydrabamine *natural penicillin antibiotic*

penicillin G potassium USP *natural penicillin antibiotic* [also: benzylpenicillin potassium] 1, 2, 3, 5, 10, 20 million U injection

penicillin G procaine USP *natural penicillin antibiotic* [also: procaine penicillin]

penicillin G redox [see: redox-penicillin G]

penicillin G sodium USP *natural penicillin antibiotic* [also: benzylpenicillin sodium] 5 000 000 U injection

penicillin hydrabamine phenoxymethyl [now: penicillin V hydrabamine]

penicillin N [see: adicillin]

penicillin O [see: almecillin]

penicillin O chloroprocaine

penicillin O potassium

penicillin O sodium

penicillin phenoxymethyl [now: penicillin V]

penicillin potassium G [see: penicillin G potassium]

penicillin potassium phenoxymethyl [now: penicillin V potassium]

penicillin V USAN, USP *natural penicillin antibiotic* [also: phenoxymethylpenicillin]

penicillin V benzathine USAN, USP *natural penicillin antibiotic*

penicillin V hydrabamine USAN, USP *natural penicillin antibiotic*

penicillin V potassium USAN, USP *natural penicillin antibiotic* 250, 500 mg oral

Penicillin VK tablets, powder for oral solution ℞ *natural penicillin antibiotic* [penicillin V potassium] 250, 500 mg; 125, 250 mg/5 mL

penicillin-152 potassium [see: phenethicillin potassium]

penicillinase INN, BAN

penicillinase-resistant penicillins *a subclass of penicillins (q.v.)*

penicillinphenyrazine [see: phenyracillin]

penicillins *a class of bactericidal antibiotics, divided into natural, penicillinase-resistant, aminopenicillin, and extended-spectrum penicillins, and effective against both gram-positive and gram-negative bacteria* [also called: "cillins"]

penidural [see: benzathine penicillin]

penimepicycline INN

penimocycline INN

PenInject (trademarked delivery form) *prefilled self-injection syringe*

penirolol INN

Pen-Kera cream OTC *moisturizer; emollient* 🔲 Benicar

Penlac Nail Lacquer topical solution ℞ *antifungal for onychomycosis* [ciclopirox] 8%

penmesterol INN

Pennsaid topical liquid *investigational (NDA filed) topical anti-inflammatory for osteoarthritis of the knee* [diclofenac sodium]

pennyroyal *(Hedeoma pulegeoides; Mentha pulegium) plant medicinal herb for childbirth pain, colds, colic, fever, gas, inducing abortion and menstruation, mouth sores, respiratory illnesses, and venomous bites; also used as an insect repellent; not generally regarded as safe and effective for ingestion due to toxicity* 🔲 Benuryl

penoctonium bromide INN

penprostene INN

penta tea *medicinal herb* [see: jiaogulan]

pentabamate USAN, INN *minor tranquilizer*

Pentacarinat IV or IM injection ℞ *antiprotozoal; treatment and prophylaxis of Pneumocystis pneumonia (PCP) (orphan)* [pentamidine isethionate] 300 mg

Pentacea *investigational (orphan) antineoplastic for small cell lung cancer*

Pentacel powder for IM injection ℞ *vaccine for diphtheria, pertussis, tetanus (DPT), polio, and* Haemophilus influenzae *type b* [diphtheria and tetanus toxoids and acellular pertussis, adsorbed; poliovirus, inactivated; Haemophilus b conjugate vaccine (DTaP-IPV/Hib)] 0.5 mL/dose

pentacosactride BAN [also: norleusactide]

pentacynium chloride INN

pentacyone chloride [see: pentacynium chloride]

pentaerithritol tetranicotinate [see: niceritrol]

pentaerithrityl tetranitrate INN *vasodilator* [also: pentaerythritol tetranitrate]

pentaerythritol tetranitrate (PETN) USP *coronary vasodilator; antianginal* [also: pentaerithrityl tetranitrate]

pentaerythritol trinitrate [see: pentrinitrol]

pentafilcon A USAN *hydrophilic contact lens material*

pentafluranol INN, BAN

pentagastrin USAN, INN, JAN *gastric secretion indicator*

pentagestrone INN

pentalamide INN, BAN

pentalyte USAN, USP, NF *electrolyte combination*

Pentam 300 IV or IM injection ℞ *antiprotozoal; treatment and prophylaxis of Pneumocystis pneumonia (PCP) (orphan)* [pentamidine isethionate] 300 mg

pentamethazene [see: azamethonium bromide]

pentamethonium bromide INN, BAN

pentamethylenetetrazol [see: pentylenetetrazol]

pentamidine INN, BAN

pentamidine isethionate *antiprotozoal; treatment and prophylaxis of Pneumocystis pneumonia (PCP) (orphan)* 300 mg injection

pentamin [see: azamethonium bromide]

pentamorphone USAN, INN *narcotic analgesic*

pentamoxane INN

pentamoxane HCl [see: pentamoxane]

pentamustine USAN *antineoplastic* [also: neptamustine]

pentanedial [see: glutaral]

pentanitrol [see: pentaerythritol tetranitrate]

pentaphonate

pentapiperide INN

pentapiperium methylsulfate USAN *anticholinergic* [also: pentapiperium metilsulfate]

pentapiperium metilsulfate INN *anticholinergic* [also: pentapiperium methylsulfate]

pentaquine INN [also: pentaquine phosphate] ⧄ Pontocaine

pentaquine phosphate USP [also: pentaquine]

Pentasa controlled-release capsules ℞ *anti-inflammatory for active ulcerative colitis, proctosigmoiditis, and proctitis* [mesalamine (5-aminosalicylic acid)] 250, 500 mg

pentasodium colistinmethanesulfonate [see: colistimethate sodium]

Pentaspan *investigational (orphan) leukapheresis adjunct to improve leukocyte yield* [pentastarch]

pentastarch USAN, BAN *red cell sedimenting agent; investigational (orphan) leukapheresis adjunct to improve leukocyte yield*

pentavalent gas gangrene antitoxin

pentazocine USAN, USP, INN, BAN *narcotic agonist-antagonist analgesic; also abused as a street drug*

pentazocine HCl USAN, USP *narcotic agonist-antagonist analgesic; also abused as a street drug*

pentazocine HCl & acetaminophen *narcotic analgesic* 25•650 mg oral

pentazocine lactate USAN, USP *narcotic agonist-antagonist analgesic for moderate to severe pain; adjunct to surgical anesthesia; also abused as a street drug*

pentazocine & naloxone HCl *narcotic agonist-antagonist analgesic; also abused as a street drug* 50•0.5 mg oral

pentetate calcium trisodium (Ca-DTPA) USAN *chelating agent for plutonium, americium, and curium; approved to treat contamination from radioactive materials (e.g., radiation sickness from "dirty bombs")* [also: calcium trisodium pentetate] 200 mg/mL (1000 mg/dose) injection

pentetate calcium trisodium Yb 169 USAN *radioactive agent*

pentetate disodium [see: pentetic acid, sodium salts]

pentetate indium disodium In 111 USAN *radiodiagnostic imaging agent for radionuclide cisternography*

pentetate monosodium [see: pentetic acid, sodium salts]

pentetate pentasodium [see: pentetic acid, sodium salts]

pentetate tetrasodium [see: pentetic acid, sodium salts]

pentetate trisodium [see: pentetic acid, sodium salts]

pentetate trisodium calcium [see: pentetate calcium trisodium]

pentetate zinc trisodium (Zn-DTPA) *chelating agent for plutonium, americium, and curium; approved to treat contamination from radioactive materials (e.g., radiation sickness from "dirty bombs") (orphan)* 200 mg/mL (1000 mg/dose) injection

pentethylcyclanone [see: cyclexanone]

pentetic acid USAN, BAN *diagnostic aid; investigational (orphan) chelating agent for radioactive plutonium, americium, or curium ingestion*

pentetic acid, sodium salts *diagnostic aid; investigational (orphan) chelating agent for radioactive plutonium, americium, or curium ingestion*

pentetrazol INN [also: pentylenetetrazol]

pentetreotide [see: indium In 111 pentetreotide]

penthanil diethylenetriamine pentaacetic acid (DTPA) [see: pentetic acid]

penthienate bromide NF

Penthrane liquid for vaporization ℞ *inhalation general anesthetic* [methoxyflurane]

penthrichloral INN, BAN

pentiapine INN *antipsychotic* [also: pentiapine maleate]

pentiapine maleate USAN *antipsychotic* [also: pentiapine]

penticide [see: chlorophenothane]

pentifylline INN, BAN

pentigetide USAN, INN *antiallergic*

pentisomicin USAN, INN *anti-infective*

pentisomide INN

pentizidone INN *antibacterial* [also: pentizidone sodium]

pentizidone sodium USAN *antibacterial* [also: pentizidone]

pentobarbital USP, INN *sedative; hypnotic; also abused as a street drug* [also: pentobarbitone; pentobarbital calcium]

pentobarbital calcium JAN *sedative; hypnotic; also abused as a street drug* [also: pentobarbital; pentobarbitone]

pentobarbital sodium USP, JAN *sedative; hypnotic; also abused as a street drug* [also: pentobarbitone sodium] 50 mg/mL injection

pentobarbitone BAN *sedative; hypnotic; also abused as a street drug* [also: pentobarbital]

pentobarbitone sodium BAN *sedative; hypnotic; also abused as a street drug* [also: pentobarbital sodium]

Pentolair eye drops ℞ *mydriatic; cycloplegic* [cyclopentolate HCl] 1%

pentolinium tartrate NF [also: pentolonium tartrate]

pentolonium tartrate INN [also: pentolinium tartrate]

pentolonum bitartrate [see: pentolinium tartrate]

pentomone USAN, INN *prostate growth inhibitor*

pentopril USAN, INN *antihypertensive; angiotensin-converting enzyme (ACE) inhibitor*

pentorex INN

pentosalen BAN

pentosan polysulfate sodium USAN, INN *urinary tract anti-inflammatory and analgesic for interstitial cystitis (orphan)* [also: pentosan polysulphate sodium]

pentosan polysulphate sodium BAN *urinary tract anti-inflammatory and analgesic* [also: pentosan polysulfate sodium]

Pentostam (available only from the Centers for Disease Control) ℞ *investigational anti-infective for leishmaniasis* [sodium stibogluconate]

pentostatin USAN, INN *antibiotic antineoplastic for hairy cell leukemia (orphan); investigational (orphan) for chronic lymphocytic leukemia and cutaneous and peripheral T-cell lymphomas; investigational (Phase III) for AIDS-related non-Hodgkin lymphoma* 10 mg/vial injection

Pentothal powder for IV injection ℞ *barbiturate general anesthetic* [thiopental sodium] 2%, 2.5% (20, 25 mg/mL)

pentoxifylline USAN, INN *peripheral vasodilator; hemorheologic agent* [also: oxpentifylline] 400 mg oral

pentoxiverine citrate [see: carbetapentane citrate]

pentoxyverine INN [also: carbetapentane citrate]

pentoxyverine citrate [see: carbetapentane citrate]

Pentrax shampoo OTC *antiseborrheic; antipsoriatic; antipruritic; antibacterial* [coal tar] 5%

pentrinitrol USAN, INN *coronary vasodilator*

***tert*-pentyl alcohol** [see: amylene hydrate]

6-pentyl-*m*-cresol [see: amylmetacresol]

pentylenetetrazol NF [also: pentetrazol]

pentymal [see: amobarbital]

Pen-Vee K tablets, powder for oral solution (discontinued 2002) ℞ *natural penicillin antibiotic* [penicillin V potassium] 250, 500 mg; 125, 250 mg/5 mL

peony (*Paeonia officinalis*) root (other parts are poisonous) *medicinal* *herb used as an antispasmodic, diuretic, and sedative*

Pepcid film-coated tablets, powder for oral suspension, IV injection, IV infusion ℞ *histamine H₂ antagonist for gastric and duodenal ulcers, gastroesophageal reflux disease (GERD), and gastric hypersecretory conditions* [famotidine] 20, 40 mg; 40 mg/5 mL; 10 mg/mL; 20 mg/50 mL

Pepcid AC ("acid controller") tablets, chewable tablets, gelcaps OTC *histamine H₂ antagonist for acid indigestion and heartburn* [famotidine] 10, 20 mg; 10 mg; 10 mg

Pepcid AC EZ Chews chewable tablets OTC *histamine H₂ antagonist for acid indigestion and heartburn* [famotidine] 20 mg

Pepcid Complete chewable tablets OTC *combination antacid and histamine H₂ antagonist for acid indigestion and heartburn* [calcium carbonate; magnesium hydroxide; famotidine] 800•165•10 mg

Pepcid RPD orally disintegrating tablets ℞ *histamine H₂ antagonist for gastric and duodenal ulcers, gastroesophageal reflux disease (GERD), and gastric hypersecretory conditions* [famotidine] 20, 40 mg

pepleomycin [see: peplomycin sulfate]

peplomycin INN *antineoplastic* [also: peplomycin sulfate]

peplomycin sulfate USAN *antineoplastic* [also: peplomycin]

pepper, African red; American red pepper; bird pepper; cayenne pepper; chili pepper; cockspur pepper; garden pepper; red pepper; Spanish pepper *medicinal herb* [see: cayenne]

pepper, Jamaica *medicinal herb* [see: allspice]

pepper, java; tailed pepper *medicinal herb* [see: cubeb]

pepper, water *medicinal herb* [see: knotweed]

pepper, wild *medicinal herb* [see: mezereon]

pepperidge bush *medicinal herb* [see: barberry]

peppermint NF *flavoring agent; perfume*

peppermint (Mentha piperita) leaves *medicinal herb for appetite stimulation, colds, colic, indigestion, fever, gas and heartburn, headache, shock, sore throat, and toothache*

peppermint oil NF *flavoring agent*

peppermint spirit USP *flavoring agent; perfume*

peppermint water NF *flavored vehicle*

pepsin *digestive aid*

pepstatin USAN, INN *pepsin enzyme inhibitor*

Peptamen ready-to-use oral liquid OTC *enteral nutritional therapy for GI impairment*

Peptic Relief chewable tablets, oral liquid OTC *antidiarrheal; antinauseant* [bismuth subsalicylate] 262 mg; 262 mg/15 mL

peptide YY (PYY) *endogenous peptides manufactured in the GI tract postprandially in proportion to the caloric content of a meal; subdivided into PYY 1-36 (PYY-I) and PYY 3-36 (PYY-II); exogenous administration of PYY-II is investigational for weight loss*

Peptinex; Peptinex DT oral liquid OTC *enteral nutritional treatment for patients with GI impairment* [whey protein–based] 8 oz./pkt.

Pepto Diarrhea Control oral solution OTC *antidiarrheal* [loperamide HCl] 1 mg/5 mL

Pepto-Bismol chewable tablets, caplets, oral liquid OTC *antidiarrheal; antinauseant* [bismuth subsalicylate] 262 mg; 262 mg; 262, 524 mg/15 mL

peraclopone INN

peradoxime INN

perafensine INN

peralopride INN

peramivir USAN *neuraminidase inhibitor for influenza A and B virus infections*

Peranex HC anorectal cream ℞ *local anesthetic and corticosteroidal anti-inflammatory for hemorrhoids* [lidocaine HCl; hydrocortisone acetate] 2%•2%

peraquinsin INN

perastine INN ⑨ prazitone; Prostin E2

peratizole INN, BAN

perbufylline INN

Perchloracap capsules (discontinued 2005) ℞ *radioimaging adjunct* [potassium perchlorate] 200 mg

Percocet tablets ℞ *narcotic analgesic; antipyretic* [oxycodone HCl; acetaminophen] 2.5•325, 5•325, 7.5•325, 7.5•500, 10•325, 10•650 mg ⑨ Pyrroxate

Percodan tablets ℞ *narcotic analgesic; antipyretic; also abused as a street drug* [oxycodone HCl; oxycodone terephthalate; aspirin] 4.5•0.38•325 mg

Percodan-Demi tablets (discontinued 2007) ℞ *narcotic analgesic; antipyretic; also abused as a street drug* [oxycodone HCl; oxycodone terephthalate; aspirin] 2.25•0.19•325 mg

Percogesic tablets OTC *antihistamine; sleep aid; analgesic; antipyretic* [phenyltoloxamine citrate; acetaminophen] 30•325 mg

Percogesic Extra Strength caplets OTC *antihistamine; sleep aid; analgesic; antipyretic* [diphenhydramine HCl; acetaminophen] 12.5•500 mg

Percolone tablets (discontinued 2005) ℞ *narcotic analgesic* [oxycodone HCl] 5 mg ⑨ piriqualone

Perdiem granules OTC *bulk laxative* [psyllium] 4.03 g/tsp. ⑨ Baridium; Prodium; Pyridium

Perdiem Overnight Relief granules OTC *bulk laxative; stimulant laxative* [psyllium; senna] 3.25•0.74 g/tsp.

perfilcon A USAN *hydrophilic contact lens material*

perflenapent USAN *ultrasound contrast medium*

perflexane USAN *ultrasound contrast medium*

perflisopent USAN *ultrasound contrast medium*

perfluamine INN, BAN

perflubron USAN, INN *oral MRI contrast medium; investigational (Phase III, orphan) treatment for acute respiratory distress syndrome (ARDS) in adults*

perflunafene INN, BAN

perflutren USAN *parenteral radiopaque contrast medium to enhance echocardiography*

perfomedil INN

Perforomist solution for inhalation ℞ *twice-daily bronchodilator for asthma, COPD, and emphysema* [formoterol fumarate] 20 mcg/2 mL dose

perfosfamide USAN *investigational (orphan) antineoplastic for the ex vivo treatment of autologous bone marrow in acute myelogenous/nonlymphocytic leukemia*

Pergamid *investigational (orphan) antineoplastic for the ex vivo treatment of autologous bone marrow in acute myelogenous/nonlymphocytic leukemia* [perfosfamide]

pergolide INN, BAN *dopamine agonist; antiparkinsonian; also used for restless legs syndrome (RLS)* [also: pergolide mesylate] ⑨ Baraclude

pergolide mesylate USAN *dopamine agonist; antiparkinsonian; also used for restless legs syndrome (RLS); investigational (orphan) for Tourette syndrome; removed from the market in 2007 due to safety concerns* [also: pergolide]

Pergonal powder for IM injection (discontinued 2005) ℞ *gonadotropin; follicle-stimulating hormone (FSH) and luteinizing hormone (LH) for the induction of ovulation in women and spermatogenesis in men; adjunct to assisted reproductive technologies (ART)* [menotropins] 75, 150 IU ⑨ proguanil

perhexiline INN *coronary vasodilator* [also: perhexiline maleate] ⑨ pyroxylin

perhexiline maleate USAN *coronary vasodilator* [also: perhexiline]

periciazine INN *phenothiazine antipsychotic* [also: pericyazine] ⑨ prazosin

PeriColace tablets OTC *stimulant laxative; stool softener* [sennosides; docusate sodium] 8.6•50 mg

pericyazine BAN *phenothiazine antipsy-chotic* [also: periciazine] ⚕ prazosin

Peridex mouth rinse ℞ *antimicrobial; gingivitis treatment; investigational (orphan) for oral mucositis in bone mar-row transplant patients* [chlorhexidine gluconate; alcohol 11.6%] 0.12%

Peridin-C tablets OTC *vitamin C sup-plement with bioflavonoids* [ascorbic acid; hesperidin] 200•200 mg

perilla (Perilla frutescens) plant *medicinal herb for asthma, inducing sweating, nausea, gastrointestinal spasms, and sunstroke* ⚕ barley; Paral; PPAR; Prelu-2

perimetazine INN

perindopril USAN, INN, BAN *angioten-sin-converting enzyme (ACE) inhibitor for hypertension*

perindopril erbumine USAN *angioten-sin-converting enzyme (ACE) inhibitor for hypertension and stable coronary artery disease (CAD)*

perindoprilat INN, BAN

PerioChip biodegradable polymer implant ℞ *antimicrobial adjunct to scaling and root planing procedures in periodontitis* [chlorhexidine gluconate] 2.5 mg ⚕ Parcopa

PerioGard mouth rinse ℞ *antimicro-bial; gingivitis treatment* [chlorhexidine gluconate; alcohol 11.6%] 0.12% ⚕ ParaGard T 380A; Procardia

PerioMed oral rinse ℞ *dental caries preventative* [stannous fluoride] 0.64% ⚕ Paremyd; ProMod

Periostat tablets ℞ *antibiotic for peri-odontal disease* [doxycycline hyclate] 20 mg ⚕ Pro-Stat 64

peripheral blood mononuclear cells *investigational (orphan) treatment for pancreatic cancer*

peripheral vasodilators *a class of car-diovascular drugs that cause dilation of the blood vessels*

Periploca sylvestris *medicinal herb* [see: gymnema]

perisoxal INN

peritoneal dialysis solution with 1.1% amino acids *investigational*

(orphan) nutritional supplement for continuous ambulatory peritoneal dialy-sis patients

periwinkle (Catharanthus roseus) plant *medicinal herb for cancer, dia-betes, diarrhea, insect stings, nervous-ness, ocular inflammation, and ulcers; not generally regarded as safe and effective for ingestion because of toxic-ity* ⚕ Bronchial

Perlane subcu injectable gel in 1 mL prefilled syringes ℞ *dermal filler for deep wrinkles and facial folds* [hyal-uronic acid] 20 mg/mL ⚕ Prelone; proline

perlapine USAN, INN *hypnotic*

Perles (dosage form) *soft gelatin capsule*

Perloxx tablets ℞ *narcotic analgesic; antipyretic* [oxycodone HCl; aceta-minophen] 2.5•300, 5•300, 7.5• 300, 10•300 mg ⚕ Pyrlex

permanganic acid, potassium salt [see: potassium permanganate]

Permapen Isoject (unit dose syringe) for deep IM injection ℞ *natural peni-cillin antibiotic* [penicillin G benza-thine] 1 200 000 U ⚕ prampine

Permax tablets (removed from the market in 2007 due to safety con-cerns) ℞ *dopamine agonist for Parkin-son disease; also used for restless legs syndrome (RLS); investigational (orphan) for Tourette syndrome* [per-golide mesylate] 0.05, 0.25, 1 mg

permethrin USAN, INN, BAN *ectoparasiti-cide for scabies and lice* 1%, 5% topical

Perna canaliculus *natural remedy* [see: New Zealand green-lipped mussel]

Pernox Scrub; Pernox Lathering Lotion OTC *antiseptic and keratolytic cleanser for acne* [sulfur; salicylic acid]

peroxide, dibenzoyl [see: benzoyl peroxide]

peroxisome proliferator–activated receptor (PPAR) agonists *a class of agents that increase insulin receptor sensitivity in type 2 diabetes; PPAR-alpha blockers are associated with lower triglyceride and higher HDL levels;*

PPAR-gamma blockers are associated with lower blood glucose levels

Peroxyl mouth rinse, oral gel OTC *cleansing of oral wounds* [hydrogen peroxide] 1.5%

perphenazine USP, INN *conventional (typical) phenothiazine antipsychotic for schizophrenia and psychotic disorders; treatment for nausea and vomiting* 2, 4, 8, 16 mg oral; 16 mg/5 mL oral

Persantine sugar-coated tablets ℞ *platelet aggregation inhibitor to prevent postoperative thromboembolic complications of cardiac valve replacement* [dipyridamole] 25, 50, 75 mg

Persantine IV injection ℞ *diagnostic aid for coronary artery function* [dipyridamole] 10 mg

Persea americana; P. gratissima medicinal herb [see: avocado]

Persian bark; Persian berries *medicinal herb* [see: buckthorn]

Persian walnut *medicinal herb* [see: English walnut]

persic oil NF *vehicle*

persilic acid INN

pertussis immune globulin USP *passive immunizing agent*

pertussis immune human globulin [now: pertussis immune globulin]

pertussis vaccine USP *active immunizing agent*

pertussis vaccine, acellular [see: diphtheria & tetanus toxoids & acellular pertussis (DTaP) vaccine, adsorbed]

pertussis vaccine, component (alternate name for acellular pertussis vaccine) [see: diphtheria & tetanus toxoids & acellular pertussis (DTaP) vaccine, adsorbed]

pertussis vaccine, whole-cell [see: diphtheria & tetanus toxoids & whole-cell pertussis (DTwP) vaccine, adsorbed]

pertussis vaccine adsorbed USP *active immunizing agent*

Peruvian balsam NF *topical protectant; rubefacient*

Peruvian balsam (*Myroxylon balsamum; M. pereirae*) oil *medicinal herb*

for edema, expelling worms, hemostasis, topical infections, and wound healing

Peruvian bark; yellow Peruvian bark *medicinal herb* [see: quinine]

Peruvian ginseng *medicinal herb* [see: maca]

Petasites hybridus medicinal herb [see: butterbur]

pethidine INN, BAN *narcotic analgesic; also abused as a street drug* [also: meperidine HCl] 🄑 Betadine

pethidine HCl [see: meperidine HCl]

PETN (pentaerythritol tetranitrate) [q.v.]

petrichloral INN

petrolatum USP *ointment base; emollient/protectant* [also: yellow petrolatum]

petrolatum, hydrophilic USP *absorbent ointment base; topical protectant*

petrolatum, liquid [see: mineral oil]

petrolatum, liquid emulsion [see: mineral oil emulsion]

petrolatum, white USP, JAN *oleaginous ointment base; topical protectant*

petrolatum gauze [see: gauze, petrolatum]

petroleum benzin [see: benzin, petroleum]

petroleum distillate inhalants *vapors from butane, toluene, acetone, benzene, gasoline, etc. which produce psychoactive effects, abused as street drugs* [see also: nitrous oxide; volatile nitrites]

petroleum jelly [see: petrolatum]

Petroselinum sativum medicinal herb [see: parsley]

Peumus boldus medicinal herb [see: boldo]

pexantel INN

Pexeva tablets ℞ *selective serotonin reuptake inhibitor (SSRI) for depression, obsessive-compulsive disorder, and panic disorder* [paroxetine mesylate] 10, 20, 30, 40 mg

pexiganan acetate USAN *broad-spectrum antibiotic*

PFA (phosphonoformic acid) [see: foscarnet sodium]

Pfaffia paniculata medicinal herb [see: suma]

Pfeiffer's Cold Sore lotion OTC *skin protectant; mild anesthetic; antipruritic; counterirritant; antiseptic* [gum benzoin; camphor; menthol; eucalyptol; alcohol 85%] 7% • 2 • 2 • 2

Pfizerpen powder for injection ℞ *natural penicillin antibiotic* [penicillin G potassium] 1, 5, 20 million U

PFL (Platinol, fluorouracil, leucovorin [rescue]) *chemotherapy protocol for head, neck, and gastric cancer*

PFT (L-phenylalanine mustard, fluorouracil, tamoxifen) *chemotherapy protocol*

PG (paregoric) [q.v.]

PG (prostaglandin) [q.v.]

PGA (pteroylglutamic acid) [see: folic acid]

PGE$_1$ (prostaglandin E$_1$) [now: alprostadil]

PGE$_2$ (prostaglandin E$_2$) [now: dinoprostone]

PGF$_{2\alpha}$ (prostaglandin F$_{2\alpha}$) [see: dinoprost]

PGF$_{2\alpha}$ (prostaglandin F$_{2\alpha}$) THAM [see: dinoprost tromethamine]

PGI$_2$ (prostaglandin I$_2$) [now: epoprostenol]

PGX (prostaglandin X) [now: epoprostenol]

PGxTest: Warfarin genetic test for professional use ℞ *measures levels of the VKORC1 and CYP2C9 genes to help determine the appropriate dosing regimen*

Phaenicia sericata natural treatment [see: maggots]

Phanatuss DM Cough syrup (discontinued 2007) OTC *antitussive; expectorant* [dextromethorphan hydrobromide; guaifenesin] 20 • 200 mg/10 mL

phanchinone [see: phanquinone; phanquone]

phanquinone INN [also: phanquone]

phanquone BAN [also: phanquinone] ② phenacaine

pharmaceutical glaze [see: glaze, pharmaceutical]

Pharmaflur; Pharmaflur df; Pharmaflur 1.1 chewable tablets ℞ *dental caries preventative* [sodium fluoride] 2.2 mg; 2.2 mg; 1.1 mg

Pharmalgen subcu or IM injection ℞ *venom sensitivity testing (subcu); venom desensitization therapy (IM)* [extracts of honeybee, yellow jacket, yellow hornet, white-faced hornet, mixed vespid, and wasp venom]

Pharmia regina natural treatment [see: maggots]

Phazyme tablets, softgels, oral drops OTC *antiflatulent* [simethicone] 60 mg; 180 mg; 40 mg/0.6 mL

Phazyme 95 tablets OTC *antiflatulent* [simethicone] 95 mg

Phazyme Quick Dissolve chewable tablets OTC *antiflatulent* [simethicone] 125 mg

phebutazine [see: febuverine]

phebutyrazine [see: febuverine]

phemfilcon A USAN *hydrophilic contact lens material*

Phenabid extended-release tablets ℞ *decongestant; antihistamine* [phenylephrine HCl; chlorpheniramine maleate] 20 • 8 mg

Phenabid DM timed-release caplets ℞ *antitussive; antihistamine; decongestant* [dextromethorphan hydrobromide; chlorpheniramine maleate; phenylephrine HCl] 30 • 8 • 20 mg

phenacaine INN [also: phenacaine HCl] ② phanquone

phenacaine HCl USP [also: phenacaine]

phenacemide USP, INN, BAN *anticonvulsant*

phenacetin USP, INN (*withdrawn from market*)

phenacon [see: fenaclon]

phenactropinium chloride INN, BAN

phenacyl 4-morpholineacetate [see: mobecarb]

N-phenacylhomatropinium chloride [see: phenactropinium chloride]

phenacylpivalate [see: pibecarb]

phenadoxone INN, BAN

Phenadoz suppositories ℞ *antihistamine; sedative; antiemetic; motion sick-*

ness relief [promethazine HCl] 12.5, 25 mg

phenaglycodol INN

phenamazoline INN

phenamazoline HCl [see: phenamazoline]

phenampromide INN

Phenapap tablets (discontinued 2007) OTC *decongestant; analgesic; antipyretic* [pseudoephedrine HCl; acetaminophen] 30•325 mg

Phenaphen with Codeine No. 3 & No. 4 capsules (discontinued 2004) ℞ *narcotic antitussive; analgesic; antipyretic* [codeine phosphate; acetaminophen] 30•325 mg; 60•325 mg

phenaphthazine *pH indicator*

phenarbutal [see: phetharbital]

phenarsone sulfoxylate INN

Phenaseptic throat spray OTC *antipruritic/counterirritant; mild local anesthetic* [phenol] 1.4%

PhenaVent dual-release capsules ℞ *decongestant; expectorant* [phenylephrine HCl (extended release); guaifenesin (immediate release)] 15•600 mg

PhenaVent D film-coated extended-release caplets ℞ *decongestant; expectorant* [phenylephrine HCl; guaifenesin] 40•1200 mg

PhenaVent LA dual-release capsules ℞ *decongestant; expectorant* [phenylephrine HCl (extended release); guaifenesin (immediate release)] 30•400 mg

PhenaVent LA film-coated caplets (discontinued 2007) ℞ *decongestant; expectorant* [phenylephrine HCl; guaifenesin] 30•600 mg

PhenaVent PED dual-release capsules ℞ *decongestant; expectorant* [phenylephrine HCl (extended release); guaifenesin (immediate release)] 7.5•200 mg

phenazocine INN

phenazocine hydrobromide [see: phenazocine]

phenazone INN, BAN *analgesic* [also: antipyrine] ② Fenesin; Vanocin

phenazopyridine INN, BAN *urinary tract analgesic for relief of pain, burning, urgency, and frequency due to mucosal irritation from surgery, catheterization, endoscopic procedures, or trauma; adjunct to antibacterial agents for urinary tract infection (UTI)* [also: phenazopyridine HCl]

phenazopyridine HCl USAN, USP *urinary tract analgesic for relief of pain, burning, urgency, and frequency due to mucosal irritation from surgery, catheterization, endoscopic procedures, or trauma; adjunct to antibacterial agents for urinary tract infection (UTI)* [also: phenazopyridine] 100, 200 mg oral

Phenazopyridine Plus tablets ℞ *urinary analgesic; antispasmodic; sedative* [phenazopyridine HCl; hyoscyamine hydrobromide; butabarbital] 150• 0.3•15 mg

phenbenicillin BAN [also: fenbenicillin]

phenbutazone sodium glycerate USAN *anti-inflammatory*

phenbutrazate BAN [also: fenbutrazate]

Phencarb GG syrup ℞ *antitussive; decongestant; expectorant* [carbetapentane citrate; phenylephrine HCl; guaifenesin] 20•10•100 mg/5 mL

phencarbamide USAN *anticholinergic* [also: fencarbamide]

phencyclidine INN *anesthetic* [also: phencyclidine HCl]

phencyclidine HCl USAN *anesthetic* [also: phencyclidine]

phendimetrazine INN *anorexiant* [also: phendimetrazine tartrate]

phendimetrazine tartrate USP *anorexiant; CNS stimulant* [also: phendimetrazine] 35, 105 mg oral

phenelzine INN, BAN *antidepressant; MAO inhibitor* [also: phenelzine sulfate]

phenelzine sulfate USP *MAO inhibitor for atypical, nonendogenous, or neurotic depression; also used for bulimia, post-traumatic stress disorders (PTSD), chronic migraine, and social anxiety disorder (SAD)* [also: phenelzine]

phenemal [see: phenobarbital]

Phenerbel·S tablets (discontinued 2008) Ŗ *GI/GU anticholinergic/anti-spasmodic; sedative; analgesic* [belladonna alkaloids; phenobarbital; ergotamine tartrate] 0.2•40•0.6 mg

Phenergan tablets, suppositories, injection Ŗ *antihistamine; sedative; antiemetic; motion sickness relief* [promethazine HCl] 12.5, 25, 50 mg; 12.5, 25 mg; 25, 50 mg/mL

Phenergan VC syrup (discontinued 2007) Ŗ *decongestant; antihistamine* [phenylephrine HCl; promethazine HCl; alcohol 7%] 5•6.25 mg/5 mL

pheneridine INN

phenethanol [see: phenylethyl alcohol]

phenethazine [see: fenethazine]

phenethicillin potassium USP [also: pheneticillin]

phenethyl alcohol BAN *antimicrobial agent* [also: phenylethyl alcohol]

N-phenethylanthranilic acid [see: enfenamic acid]

phenethylazocine bromide [see: phenazocine hydrobromide]

phenethylhydrazine sulfate [see: phenelzine sulfate]

pheneticillin INN [also: phenethicillin potassium]

pheneticillin potassium [see: phenethicillin potassium]

phenetsal [see: acetaminosalol]

pheneturide INN, BAN [also: acetylpheneturide]

Phenex-1 powder OTC *formula for infants with phenylketonuria*

Phenex-2 powder OTC *enteral nutritional therapy for phenylketonuria (PKU)*

Phenflu G tablets OTC *antitussive; decongestant; expectorant; analgesic; antipyretic* [dextromethorphan hydrobromide; phenylephrine HCl; guaifenesin; acetaminophen] 30•15•600•500 mg

phenformin INN, BAN *biguanide antidiabetic that decreases hepatic glucose production and increases cellular response to insulin* [also: phenformin HCl]

phenformin HCl USP *biguanide antidiabetic that decreases hepatic glucose*

production and increases cellular response to insulin (removed from the market by the FDA in 1977) [also: phenformin]

phenglutarimide INN, BAN

phenicarbazide INN

phenidiemal [see: phetharbital]

phenindamine INN *nonselective piperidine antihistamine* [also: phenindamine tartrate]

phenindamine tartrate USAN *nonselective piperidine antihistamine for allergic rhinitis* [also: phenindamine]

phenindione USP, INN *anticoagulant*

pheniodol sodium INN [also: iodoalphionic acid]

pheniprazine INN, BAN

pheniprazine HCl [see: pheniprazine]

pheniramine INN [also: pheniramine maleate] ⊉ fenharmane

pheniramine maleate USAN *antihistamine* [also: pheniramine]

pheniramine maleate & naphazoline HCl *topical ophthalmic antihistamine and decongestant* 0.3%•0.025% eye drops

phenisonone hydrobromide

phenmetraline HCl [see: phenmetrazine HCl]

phenmetrazine INN, BAN *anorexiant; CNS stimulant; also abused as a street drug* [also: phenmetrazine HCl]

phenmetrazine HCl USP *anorexiant; CNS stimulant; also abused as a street drug* [also: phenmetrazine]

phenobamate [see: febarbamate]

phenobarbital USP, INN, JAN *anticonvulsant; hypnotic; sedative; also abused as a street drug* [also: phenobarbitone] 15, 30, 60, 100 mg oral; 15, 20 mg/5 mL oral ⊉ vinbarbital

phenobarbital & belladonna alkaloids *gastrointestinal anticholinergic/antispasmodic; sedative* 16.2•0.13 mg oral

phenobarbital sodium USP, INN, JAN *anticonvulsant; hypnotic; sedative; also abused as a street drug* 30, 60, 65, 130 mg/mL injection ⊉ vinbarbital sodium

phenobarbitone BAN *anticonvulsant; hypnotic; sedative; also abused as a street drug* [also: phenobarbital] ② vinbarbitone

phenobutiodil INN

phenododecinium bromide [see: domiphen bromide]

phenol USP *topical antiseptic/antipruritic; local anesthetic; preservative* ② fennel; vanilla

phenol, liquefied USP *topical antipruritic*

phenol, sodium salt [see: phenolate sodium]

phenol red [see: phenolsulfonphthalein]

phenolate sodium USAN *disinfectant*

Phenolated Calamine lotion OTC *poison ivy treatment* [calamine; zinc oxide; phenol] 8%•8%•1%

phenolphthalein USP, INN *stimulant laxative* banned in all OTC laxatives in 1998

phenolphthalein, white [see: phenolphthalein]

phenolphthalein, yellow USP *stimulant laxative* banned in all OTC laxatives in 1998

phenolsulfonphthalein USP

phenolsulphonate sodium USP

phenomorphan INN, BAN

phenomycilline [see: penicillin V]

phenoperidine INN, BAN

phenopryldiasulfone sodium [see: solasulfone]

Phenoptic eye drops (discontinued 2006) ℞ *decongestant; vasoconstrictor; mydriatic* [phenylephrine HCl] 2.5%

Phenoptin *investigational (orphan) treatment for mild to moderate phenylketonuria* [phenylalanine ammonia lyase (PAL)]

phenosulfophthalein [see: phenolsulfonphthalein]

phenothiazine NF, INN *antipsychotic* ② fenethazine

phenothiazines *a class of dopamine receptor antagonists with antipsychotic, hypotensive, antiemetic, antispasmodic, and antihistaminic activity*

phenothrin INN, BAN

phenoxazoline HCl [see: fenoxazoline HCl]

phenoxybenzamine INN *antihypertensive* [also: phenoxybenzamine HCl]

phenoxybenzamine HCl USP *antihypertensive; pheochromocytomic agent* [also: phenoxybenzamine]

phenoxymethylpenicillin INN *natural penicillin antibiotic* [also: penicillin V]

phenoxypropazine BAN [also: fenoxypropazine]

phenoxypropylpenicillin [see: propicillin]

phenozolone [see: fenozolone]

phenprobamate INN, BAN

phenprocoumon USAN, USP, INN *anticoagulant*

phenprocumone [see: phenprocoumon]

phenpromethadrine [see: phenpromethamine]

phenpromethamine INN

phenpropamine citrate [see: alverine citrate]

phensuximide USP, INN, BAN *succinimide anticonvulsant*

phentermine USAN, INN *anorexiant; CNS stimulant; an adrenergic isomer of amphetamine*

phentermine HCl USP *anorexiant; CNS stimulant; water-soluble form for oral administration* 8, 15, 18.75, 30, 37.5 mg oral

phenthiazine [see: phenothiazine]

phentolamine INN, BAN *antihypertensive; pheochromocytomic agent* [also: phentolamine HCl]

phentolamine HCl USP *antihypertensive; pheochromocytomic agent* [also: phentolamine]

phentolamine mesilate INN, JAN *antiadrenergic; antihypertensive; pheochromocytomic agent* [also: phentolamine mesylate]

phentolamine mesylate USP *antihypertensive; α-adrenergic blocker; pheochromocytomic agent* [also: phentolamine mesilate] 5 mg injection

phentolamine methanesulfonate [now: phentolamine mesylate]

Phentrol 2; Phentrol 4; Phentrol 5 capsules ℞ *anorexiant; CNS stimulant* [phentermine HCl] 30 mg ⑤

fenoterol

phentydrone

Phenydex oral liquid (discontinued 2007) ℞ *antitussive; antihistamine; sleep aid; decongestant; expectorant* [dextromethorphan hydrobromide; pyrilamine maleate; phenylephrine HCl; guaifenesin] 20•25•10•200 mg/5 mL

Phenydex Pediatric oral liquid (discontinued 2007) ℞ *antitussive; decongestant; expectorant; for children 2–12 years* [dextromethorphan hydrobromide; phenylephrine HCl; guaifenesin] 5•2.5•50 mg/5 mL

phenyl aminosalicylate USAN, BAN *antibacterial; tuberculostatic* [also: fenamisal]

Phenyl Chlor-Tan Pediatric oral suspension ℞ *decongestant; antihistamine* [phenylephrine tannate; chlorpheniramine tannate] 5•4.5 mg/5 mL

phenyl salicylate NF *analgesic; not generally regarded as safe and effective as an antidiarrheal*

phenylalanine (L-phenylalanine) USAN, USP, INN *essential amino acid; symbols: Phe, F*

phenylalanine ammonia lyase (PAL) *investigational (orphan) treatment for mild to moderate phenylketonuria*

phenylalanine mustard (PAM) [see: melphalan]

L-phenylalanine mustard (L-PAM) [see: melphalan]

Phenylase *investigational (orphan) for hyperphenylalaninemia* [phenylalanine ammonia lyase (PAL)]

phenylazo diamino pyridine HCl [see: phenazopyridine HCl]

phenylbenzyl atropine [see: xenytropium bromide]

phenylbutazone USP, INN *antirheumatic; anti-inflammatory; antipyretic; analgesic*

phenylbutylpiperadines *a class of dopamine receptor antagonists with conventional (typical) antipsychotic activity* [also called: butyrophenones]

phenylbutyrate sodium [see: sodium phenylbutyrate]

2-phenylbutyrylurea [see: pheneturide; acetylphenetouride]

phenylcarbinol [see: benzyl alcohol]

phenylcinchoninic acid [now: cinchophen]

α-phenyl-*p*-cresol carbamate [see: diphenan]

phenylcyclohexyl piperidine (PCP) [see: PCP; phencyclidine HCl]

2-phenylcyclopentylamine HCl [see: cypenamine HCl]

phenyldimazone [see: normethadone]

phenylephrine (PE) INN, BAN *nasal decongestant; ocular vasoconstrictor; vasopressor for hypotensive or cardiac shock* [also: phenylephrine HCl]

phenylephrine bitartrate *bronchodilator; vasoconstrictor*

Phenylephrine CM extended-release caplets ℞ *decongestant; antihistamine; anticholinergic to dry mucosal secretions* [phenylephrine HCl; chlorpheniramine maleate; methscopolamine nitrate] 40•8•2.5 mg

phenylephrine HCl USP *nasal decongestant; ocular/otic vasoconstrictor; vasopressor for hypotensive or cardiac shock; investigational (orphan) treatment for fecal incontinence due to ileal pouch anal anastomosis* [also: phenylephrine] 0.25%, 0.5%, 1% nose drops or spray; 2.5%, 10% eye drops; 1% injection

phenylephrine HCl & chlorpheniramine maleate *decongestant; antihistamine* 20•4 mg oral; 12.5•4 mg/5 mL oral; 3.5•1 mg/mL oral

phenylephrine HCl & codeine phosphate & promethazine HCl *decongestant; narcotic antitussive; antihistamine* 5•10•6.25 mg/5 mL oral

phenylephrine HCl & guaifenesin *decongestant; expectorant* 15•600, 40•600, 25•900, 30•900, 30•1200 mg oral

phenylephrine HCl & promethazine HCl *decongestant; antihistamine* 5•6.25 mg/5 mL oral

phenylephrine tannate *nasal decongestant*

phenylephrine tannate & chlorpheniramine tannate & pyrilamine tannate *decongestant; antihistamine* 5•2•12.5 mg/5 mL oral

phenylethanol [see: phenylethyl alcohol]

phenylethyl alcohol USP *antimicrobial agent; preservative* [also: phenethyl alcohol]

phenylethylmalonylurea [see: phenobarbital]

Phenyl-Free oral liquid, powder for oral solution OTC *special diet for infants with phenylketonuria (PKU)*

Phenylgesic tablets (discontinued 2007) OTC *antihistamine; sleep aid; analgesic; antipyretic* [phenyltoloxamine citrate; acetaminophen] 30•325 mg

phenylindanedione [see: phenindione]

phenylmercuric acetate NF *antimicrobial agent; preservative*

phenylmercuric borate INN

phenylmercuric chloride NF

phenylmercuric nitrate NF *antimicrobial agent; preservative; topical antiseptic*

phenylone [see: antipyrine]

phenylpropanolamine (PPA) INN, BAN *vasoconstrictor; nasal decongestant; nonprescription diet aid (banned in all OTC products in 2001)* [also: phenylpropanolamine HCl]

phenylpropanolamine HCl USP *vasoconstrictor; nasal decongestant; nonprescription diet aid (banned in all OTC products in 2001)* [also: phenylpropanolamine]

phenylpropanolamine polistirex USAN *adrenergic; vasoconstrictor (banned in all OTC products in 2001)*

1-phenylsemicarbazide [see: phenicarbazide]

Phenyl-T oral suspension ℞ *nasal decongestant* [phenylephrine tannate] 7.5 mg/5 mL

phenylthilone [see: phenythilone]

phenyltoloxamine INN *antihistamine; sleep aid*

phenyltoloxamine citrate *antihistamine; sleep aid*

Phenyltoloxamine PE CPM oral liquid ℞ *antihistamine; sleep aid; decongestant* [phenyltoloxamine citrate; phenylephrine HCl; chlorpheniramine maleate] 7.5•5•2.5 mg/5 mL

phenyltriazines *a class of anticonvulsants*

phenyracillin INN

phenyramidol HCl USAN *analgesic; skeletal muscle relaxant* [also: fenyramidol]

Phenytek extended-release capsules ℞ *once-daily hydantoin anticonvulsant* [phenytoin sodium] 200, 300 mg

phenythilone INN ② fenethylline; Ventolin

phenytoin USAN, USP, INN, BAN *hydantoin anticonvulsant* 125 mg/5 mL oral ② Vantin

phenytoin redox [see: redox-phenytoin]

phenytoin sodium USP *hydantoin anticonvulsant* 30, 100 mg oral; 50 mg/mL injection

phetharbital INN

phezathion [see: fezatione]

Phicon cream OTC *anesthetic; emollient* [pramoxine HCl; vitamins A and E] 0.5%•7500 IU•2000 IU

Phicon F cream OTC *local anesthetic; antifungal* [pramoxine HCl; undecylenic acid] 0.05%•8%

Phillips' caplets OTC *antacid* [magnesium (as magnesium oxide)] 500 mg ② Folpace

Phillips' Chewable tablets OTC *antacid* [magnesium hydroxide] 311 mg

Phillips' Liqui-Gels OTC *laxative; stool softener* [docusate sodium] 100 mg

Phillips' Milk of Magnesia; Concentrated Phillips' Milk of Magnesia oral liquid OTC *antacid; saline laxative* [magnesium hydroxide] 400 mg/5 mL; 800 mg/5 mL

pHisoDerm; pHisoDerm for Baby topical liquid OTC *soap-free therapeutic skin cleanser*

pHisoDerm Cleansing Bar (discontinued 2004) OTC *therapeutic skin cleanser*

pHisoHex topical liquid R *bacteriostatic skin cleanser* [hexachlorophene] 3%

P-Hist syrup R *antitussive; antihistamine; sleep aid; decongestant* [dextromethorphan hydrobromide; pyrilamine maleate; dexchlorpheniramine maleate; phenylephrine HCl] 5•5•1.25•5 mg/5 mL ☑ Feocyte

P-Hist DM oral drops R *antitussive; antihistamine; decongestant* [dextromethorphan hydrobromide; brompheniramine maleate; pseudoephedrine HCl] 5•1•12 mg/mL ☑ Fosteum

Phlemex-PE; Phlemex Forte extended-release tablets R *antitussive; decongestant; expectorant* [dextromethorphan hydrobromide; phenylephrine HCl; guaifenesin] 20•20•800 mg; 30•30•1200 mg

phloropropiophenone [see: flopropione]

pholcodine INN

pholedrine INN, BAN

pholescutol [see: folescutol]

Phoradendron flavescens; P. serotinum; P. tomentosum medicinal herb [see: mistletoe]

PhosChol softgels, oral liquid concentrate OTC *natural lipotropic* [phosphatidylcholine] 565, 900 mg; 3 g/5 mL

phoscolic acid [see: foscolic acid]

Phos-Flur oral rinse R *dental caries preventative* [acidulated phosphate fluoride] 0.44 mg/mL

PhosLo tablets, capsules, gelcaps R *buffering agent for hyperphosphatemia in end-stage renal disease (orphan)* [calcium acetate] 667 mg; 333.3, 667 mg; 667 mg ☑ Feosol; VaZol

Phos-NaK powder for oral solution R *phosphorus/electrolyte supplement* [phosphorus; potassium; sodium] 250•280•160 mg/pkt.

phosphate salt of tricyclic nucleoside [now: triciribine phosphate]

phosphatidylcholine (PC) [see: lecithin]

phosphatidylserine (PS) *natural agent to improve neural function, maintain brain cell membrane integrity, and protect the brain against age-related functional deterioration*

phosphinic acid [see: hypophosphorous acid]

2,2'-phosphinicodilactic acid (PDLA) [see: foscolic acid]

Phosphocol P 32 suspension for intracavitary instillation, interstitial injection R *radiopharmaceutical antineoplastic* [chromic phosphate P 32] 10, 15 mCi

phosphocysteamine *investigational (orphan) for cystinosis*

phosphodiesterase III (PDE III) inhibitors *a class of platelet aggregation inhibitors*

Phospholine Iodide powder for eye drops R *antiglaucoma agent; irreversible cholinesterase inhibitor miotic* [echothiophate iodide] 0.125%

phosphonoformic acid (PFA) [see: foscarnet sodium]

phosphonomethoxypropyladenine (PMPA) [see: tenofovir]

phosphorated carbohydrate solution (hyperosmolar solution with phosphoric acid) *antiemetic for nausea associated with influenza, morning sickness, motion sickness, inhalation anesthesia, or food and drink indiscretions*

phosphoric acid NF *solvent; acidifying agent*

phosphoric acid, aluminum salt [see: aluminum phosphate gel]

phosphoric acid, calcium salt [see: calcium phosphate, dibasic]

phosphoric acid, chromium salt [see: chromic phosphate Cr 51 & P 32]

phosphoric acid, diammonium salt [see: ammonium phosphate]

phosphoric acid, dipotassium salt [see: potassium phosphate, dibasic]

phosphoric acid, disodium salt heptahydrate [see: sodium phosphate, dibasic]

phosphoric acid, disodium salt hydrate [see: sodium phosphate, dibasic]

phosphoric acid, magnesium salt [see: magnesium phosphate]

phosphoric acid, monopotassium salt [see: potassium phosphate, monobasic]

phosphoric acid, monosodium salt dihydrate [see: sodium phosphate, monobasic]

phosphoric acid, monosodium salt monohydrate [see: sodium phosphate, monobasic]

phosphorofluoridic acid, disodium salt [see: sodium monofluorophosphate]

phosphorothiolate antisense oligodeoxynucleotide, TGF(β)2-specific *investigational (orphan) for malignant glioma*

phosphorothiolate deoxyribose *investigational (orphan) agent for advanced malignant melanoma*

phosphorus *element (P)*

Phospho-soda [see: Fleet Phospho-soda]

phosphothiamine [see: monophosphothiamine]

Photofrin PDT powder for IV injection ℞ *laser light–activated antineoplastic for photodynamic therapy (PDT) of esophageal (orphan) and non–small cell lung cancers (NSCLC); used for ablation of high-grade dysplasia in Barrett esophagus patients; investigational (orphan) for bladder cancer* [porfimer sodium] 75 mg

phoxim INN, BAN

Phrenilin tablets ℞ *barbiturate sedative; analgesic; antipyretic* [butalbital; acetaminophen] 50•325 mg

Phrenilin Forte capsules ℞ *barbiturate sedative; analgesic; antipyretic* [butalbital; acetaminophen] 50•650 mg

Phrenilin with Caffeine and Codeine capsules ℞ *barbiturate sedative; narcotic antitussive; analgesic; antipyretic* [butalbital; codeine phosphate; acetaminophen; caffeine] 50• 30•325•40 mg

PHRT (procarbazine, hydroxyurea, radiotherapy) *chemotherapy protocol* ② Fortéo

phthalofyne USAN *veterinary anthelmintic* [also: ftalofyne]

phthalylsulfacetamide NF

phthalylsulfamethizole INN

phthalylsulfathiazole USP, INN

phylcardin [see: aminophylline]

phyllindon [see: aminophylline]

Phyllocontin controlled-release tablets (discontinued 2004) ℞ *antiasthmatic; bronchodilator* [aminophylline] 225 mg

phylloquinone [see: phytonadione]

Phylorinol mouthwash/gargle OTC *oral antiseptic; antipruritic/counterirritant; mild local anesthetic* [phenol] 0.6%

Phylorinol topical liquid OTC *antipruritic/counterirritant; mild local anesthetic; antiseptic; astringent; oral deodorant* [phenol; boric acid; strong iodine solution; chlorophyllin copper complex] 0.6%• ? • ? • ?

physic root *medicinal herb* [see: Culver root]

physiological irrigating solution *sterile irrigant for general washing and rinsing; not for injection*

Physiolyte topical liquid ℞ *sterile irrigant for general washing and rinsing* [physiological irrigating solution]

PhysioSol topical liquid ℞ *sterile irrigant* [physiological irrigating solution]

physostigmine USP, BAN *reversible cholinesterase inhibitor miotic for glaucoma*

physostigmine salicylate USP *cholinergic to reverse anticholinergic overdose; investigational (orphan) for Friedreich and other inherited ataxias* 1 mg/mL injection

physostigmine sulfate USP *ophthalmic cholinergic for glaucoma; miotic*

phytate persodium USAN *pharmaceutic aid*

phytate sodium USAN *calcium-chelating agent*

phytic acid [see: fytic acid]

Phytolacca americana; P. decandra; P. rigida medicinal herb [see: pokeweed]

phytomenadione (vitamin K₁) INN, BAN *fat-soluble vitamin; prothrombogenic* [also: phytonadione]

phytonadiol sodium diphosphate INN

phytonadione (vitamin K₁) USP, JAN *fat-soluble vitamin; prothrombogenic* [also: phytomenadione] 2 mg/mL injection

PIA (Platinol, ifosfamide, Adriamycin) chemotherapy protocol

pibecarb INN

piberaline INN ☑ piperylone

piboserod HCl USAN, BAN *selective serotonin 5-HT₄ receptor antagonist for irritable bowel syndrome*

pibrozelesin hydrobromide USAN *antineoplastic*

picafibrate INN

picartamide INN

Picea excelsa; P. mariana medicinal herb [see: spruce tree]

picenadol INN *analgesic* [also: picenadol HCl]

picenadol HCl USAN *analgesic* [also: picenadol]

picilorex INN

pick purse; pickpocket medicinal herb [see: shepherd's purse]

piclamilast USAN *phosphodiesterase type IV inhibitor for asthma*

piclonidine INN

piclopastine INN

picloxydine INN, BAN

picobenzide INN

picodralazine INN

picolamine INN ☑ Byclomine

piconol INN

picoperine INN

picoplatin investigational (Phase III) antineoplastic for small cell lung cancer

picoprazole INN

picotrin INN *keratolytic* [also: picotrin diolamine] ☑ buquiterine

picotrin diolamine USAN *keratolytic* [also: picotrin]

Picrasma excelsa medicinal herb [see: quassia]

picric acid [see: trinitrophenol]

picrotoxin NF

picumast INN, BAN

picumeterol INN, BAN *bronchodilator* [also: picumeterol fumarate]

picumeterol fumarate USAN *bronchodilator* [also: picumeterol]

pidolacetamol INN

pidolic acid INN

pifarnine USAN, INN *gastric antiulcerative*

pifenate INN, BAN

pifexole INN ☑ pivoxil

piflutixol INN

pifoxime INN

pigeonberry medicinal herb [see: pokeweed]

piketoprofen INN

Pilagan eye drops (discontinued 2004) ℞ *antiglaucoma agent; direct-acting miotic* [pilocarpine nitrate] 1%, 2%, 4% ☑ Bellacane; bulaquine; Polocaine

pildralazine INN

pilewort (Erechtites hieracifolia) plant medicinal herb used as an astringent and emetic

Pilocar eye drops ℞ *antiglaucoma agent; direct-acting miotic* [pilocarpine HCl] 0.5%, 1%, 2%, 3%, 4%, 6%

pilocarpine USP, BAN *antiglaucoma agent; ophthalmic cholinergic*

pilocarpine HCl USP *ophthalmic cholinergic; antiglaucoma; miotic; treatment of xerostomia and keratoconjunctivitis sicca due to radiotherapy or Sjögren syndrome (orphan); also for dry mouth* 0.5%, 1%, 2%, 4%, 6%, 8% eye drops; 5, 7.5 mg oral

pilocarpine nitrate USP *ophthalmic cholinergic; antiglaucoma; miotic*

Pilopine HS ophthalmic gel ℞ *antiglaucoma agent; direct-acting miotic* [pilocarpine HCl] 4%

Piloptic-½; Piloptic-1; Piloptic-2; Piloptic-3; Piloptic-4; Piloptic-6 eye drops ℞ *antiglaucoma agent; direct-acting miotic* [pilocarpine HCl] 0.5%; 1%; 2%; 3%; 4%; 6%

Pilopto-Carpine eye drops ℞ *antiglaucoma agent; direct-acting miotic* [pilocarpine HCl] 4%

Pilostat eye drops ℞ antiglaucoma agent; *direct-acting miotic* [pilocarpine HCl] 0.5%, 1%, 2%, 3%, 4%, 6%

Pilpak (trademarked packaging form) *patient compliance package*

Pima syrup ℞ *expectorant* [potassium iodide] 325 mg/5 mL

pimagedine HCl USAN *advanced glycosylation inhibitor for type 1 diabetes*

pimaricin JAN *ophthalmic antibacterial/ antifungal antibiotic* [also: natamycin]

pimavanserin *investigational (Phase III) treatment for Parkinson disease–related psychosis*

pimeclone INN

pimecrolimus USAN, INN *calcineurin inhibitor; immunomodulator for atopic dermatitis*

pimefylline INN ⚕ bamifylline

pimelautide INN

Pimenta dioica; P. officinalis medicinal herb [see: allspice]

pimetacin INN

pimethixene INN

pimetine INN *antihyperlipoproteinemic* [also: pimetine HCl]

pimetine HCl USAN *antihyperlipoproteinemic* [also: pimetine]

pimetixene [see: pimethixene]

pimetremide INN

pimeverine [see: pimetremide]

piminodine INN [also: piminodine esylate]

piminodine esylate NF [also: piminodine]

piminodine ethanesulfonate [see: piminodine esylate]

pimobendan USAN, INN *cardiotonic*

pimonidazole INN, BAN ⚕ bamnidazole

pimozide USAN, USP, INN, BAN, JAN *antispasmodic/antidyskinetic for Tourette syndrome; diphenylbutylpiperidine antipsychotic; neuroleptic*

pimpernel; small pimpernel *medicinal herb* [see: burnet]

pimpernel, blue *medicinal herb* [see: skullcap]

pimpernel, water *medicinal herb* [see: brooklime]

Pimpinella anisum medicinal herb [see: anise]

Pimpinella magna; P. saxifrage medicinal herb [see: burnet]

pinacidil USAN, INN *antihypertensive (approved in 1989, but not marketed by the manufacturer)*

pinadoline USAN, INN *analgesic* ⚕ binedaline

pinafide INN

pinaverium bromide INN *GI antispasmodic*

pinazepam INN

pincainide INN

pindolol USAN, USP, INN, BAN *β-blocker for hypertension; antianginal* 5, 10 mg oral

pine, Norway *medicinal herb* [see: spruce]

pine, prince's *medicinal herb* [see: pipsissewa]

pine bark extract *natural free radical scavenger for inflammatory collagen disease and peripheral vascular disease; contains 80%–85% procyanidolic oligomers (PCOs)*

pine needle oil NF

pine tar USP

pineapple (Ananas comosus) fruit *medicinal herb for constipation, jaundice, soft tissue inflammation, and topical wound debridement*

Pink Bismuth oral liquid OTC *antidiarrheal; antinauseant* [bismuth subsalicylate] 130, 262 mg/15 mL

pinolcaine INN

pinoxepin INN *antipsychotic* [also: pinoxepin HCl] ⚕ benaxibine

pinoxepin HCl USAN *antipsychotic* [also: pinoxepin]

Pin-Rid soft gel capsules, oral liquid OTC *anthelmintic for ascariasis (roundworm) and enterobiasis (pinworm)* [pyrantel pamoate] 180 mg; 50 mg/mL

Pinus palustris natural remedy [see: turpentine]

Pinus strobus medicinal herb [see: white pine]

Pin-X oral liquid, chewable tablets OTC *anthelmintic for ascariasis (roundworm)*

and enterobiasis (pinworm) [pyrantel pamoate] 144.1 mg/mL (50 mg/mL base); 720.5 mg (250 mg base) ⚕ Pain-X; Panokase

pioglitazone INN *thiazolidinedione (TZD) antidiabetic and peroxisome proliferator–activated receptor–gamma (PPARγ) agonist that increases cellular response to insulin without increasing insulin secretion* [also: pioglitazone HCl] ⚕ Baltussin

pioglitazone HCl USAN *thiazolidinedione (TZD) antidiabetic and peroxisome proliferator–activated receptor–gamma (PPARγ) agonist that increases cellular response to insulin without increasing insulin secretion* [also: pioglitazone]

pipacycline INN

pipamazine INN

pipamperone USAN, INN *antipsychotic*

pipaneperone [see: pipamperone]

pipazetate INN *antitussive* [also: pipazethate]

pipazethate USAN *antitussive* [also: pipazetate]

pipe plant; Dutchman's pipe; Indian pipe *medicinal herb* [see: fit root]

pipebuzone INN

pipecuronium bromide USAN, INN, BAN *nondepolarizing neuromuscular blocking agent; muscle relaxant; adjunct to general anesthesia*

pipemidic acid INN

pipenzolate bromide INN

pipenzolate methylbromide [see: pipenzolate bromide]

pipenzolone bromide [see: pipenzolate bromide]

pipequaline INN

Piper cubeba *medicinal herb* [see: cubeb]

Piper methysticum *medicinal herb* [see: kava kava]

piperacetazine USAN, USP, INN *antipsychotic*

piperacillin INN, BAN *extended-spectrum penicillin antibiotic* [also: piperacillin sodium]

piperacillin sodium USAN, USP, JAN *extended-spectrum penicillin antibiotic*

[also: piperacillin] 2, 3, 4, 40 g injection

piperamide INN *anthelmintic* [also: piperamide maleate]

piperamide maleate USAN *anthelmintic* [also: piperamide]

piperamine [see: bamipine]

piperazine USP *anthelmintic for enterobiasis (pinworm) and ascariasis (roundworm)*

piperazine calcium edetate INN *anthelmintic* [also: piperazine edetate calcium]

piperazine citrate USP *anthelmintic* 250 mg oral; 500 mg/mL oral

piperazine citrate hydrate [see: piperazine citrate]

piperazine edetate calcium USAN *anthelmintic* [also: piperazine calcium edetate]

piperazine estrone sulfate [now: estropipate]

piperazine hexahydrate [see: piperazine citrate]

piperazine phosphate

piperazine phosphate monohydrate [see: piperazine phosphate]

piperazine theophylline ethanoate [see: acefylline piperazine]

piperidine phosphate

piperidines *a class of antihistamines*

piperidolate INN [also: piperidolate HCl]

piperidolate HCl USP [also: piperidolate]

piperilate [see: pipethanate]

piperine USP *natural pepper extract that increases the absorption of various natural remedies* ⚕ Biobrane

piperocaine INN [also: piperocaine HCl]

piperocaine HCl USP [also: piperocaine]

piperonyl butoxide *pediculicide for lice*

piperoxan INN

piperphenidol HCl

piperylone INN ⚕ piberaline

pipethanate INN

pipobroman USAN, USP, INN *alkylating antineoplastic*

pipoctanone INN
pipofezine INN
piposulfan USAN, INN *antineoplastic*
pipotiazine INN *phenothiazine antipsychotic* [also: pipotiazine palmitate]
pipotiazine palmitate USAN *phenothiazine antipsychotic* [also: pipotiazine]
pipoxizine INN
pipoxolan INN *muscle relaxant* [also: pipoxolan HCl]
pipoxolan HCl USAN *muscle relaxant* [also: pipoxolan]
Pipracil powder for IV or IM injection (discontinued 2004) ℞ *extended-spectrum penicillin antibiotic* [piperacillin sodium] 2, 3, 4, 40 g/vial
pipradimadol INN
pipradrol INN [also: pipradrol HCl]
pipradrol HCl NF [also: pipradrol]
pipramadol INN
pipratecol INN
piprinhydrinate INN, BAN
piprocurarium iodide INN
piprofurol INN
piprozolin USAN, INN *choleretic*
pipsissewa (Chimaphila umbellata) plant *medicinal herb used as an astringent, diaphoretic, and diuretic*
piquindone INN *antipsychotic* [also: piquindone HCl]
piquindone HCl USAN *antipsychotic* [also: piquindone]
piquizil INN *bronchodilator* [also: piquizil HCl] ☑ Paxil
piquizil HCl USAN *bronchodilator* [also: piquizil]
piracetam USAN, INN, BAN *cognition adjuvant; investigational (orphan) for myoclonus*
pirandamine INN *antidepressant* [also: pirandamine HCl]
pirandamine HCl USAN *antidepressant* [also: pirandamine]
pirarubicin INN
piraxelate INN
pirazmonam INN *antimicrobial* [also: pirazmonam sodium]
pirazmonam sodium USAN *antimicrobial* [also: pirazmonam]

pirazofurin INN *antineoplastic* [also: pyrazofurin]
pirazolac USAN, INN, BAN *antirheumatic*
pirbenicillin INN *antibacterial* [also: pirbenicillin sodium]
pirbenicillin sodium USAN *antibacterial* [also: pirbenicillin]
pirbuterol INN *sympathomimetic bronchodilator* [also: pirbuterol acetate]
pirbuterol acetate USAN *sympathomimetic bronchodilator for asthma and bronchospasm* [also: pirbuterol]
pirbuterol HCl USAN *bronchodilator*
pirdonium bromide INN
pirenoxine INN
pirenperone USAN, INN, BAN *tranquilizer* ☑ bornaprine
pirenzepine INN, BAN *tricyclic benzodiazepine for peptic ulcers* [also: pirenzepine HCl] ☑ Principen
pirenzepine HCl USAN, JAN *tricyclic benzodiazepine for peptic ulcers* [also: pirenzepine]
pirepolol INN
piretanide USAN, INN *diuretic*
pirfenidone USAN, INN *analgesic; anti-inflammatory; antipyretic* ☑ pyrophendane
piribedil INN ☑ Prepidil
piribenzyl methylsulfate [see: bevonium metilsulfate]
piridicillin INN *antibacterial* [also: piridicillin sodium]
piridicillin sodium USAN *antibacterial* [also: piridicillin]
piridocaine INN ☑ paridocaine
piridocaine HCl [see: piridocaine]
piridoxilate INN, BAN
piridronate sodium USAN *calcium regulator*
piridronic acid INN
pirifibrate INN
pirinidazole INN
pirinitramide [see: piritramide]
pirinixic acid INN
pirinixil INN
piriprost USAN *antiasthmatic*
piriprost potassium USAN *antiasthmatic*
piriqualone INN ☑ Percolone
pirisudanol INN

piritramide INN, BAN

piritrexim INN *antiproliferative agent* [also: piritrexim isethionate]

piritrexim isethionate USAN *investigational (orphan) antiproliferative for* Pneumocystis, Toxoplasma gondii, *and* Mycobacterium avium-intracellulare *infections* [also: piritrexim]

pirlimycin HCl USAN *antibacterial*

pirlindole INN

pirmagrel USAN, INN *thromboxane synthetase inhibitor*

pirmenol INN *antiarrhythmic* [also: pirmenol HCl] ⊞ Prominol

pirmenol HCl USAN *antiarrhythmic* [also: pirmenol]

pirnabin INN *antiglaucoma agent* [also: pirnabine]

pirnabine USAN *antiglaucoma agent* [also: pirnabin]

piroctone USAN, INN *antiseborrheic*

piroctone olamine USAN *antiseborrheic*

pirodavir USAN, INN, BAN *antiviral*

pirogliride INN *antidiabetic* [also: pirogliride tartrate]

pirogliride tartrate USAN *antidiabetic* [also: pirogliride]

piroheptine INN

pirolate USAN, INN *antiasthmatic* ⊞ Prialt

pirolazamide USAN, INN *antiarrhythmic*

piromidic acid INN

piroxantrone INN *antineoplastic* [also: piroxantrone HCl]

piroxantrone HCl USAN *antineoplastic* [also: piroxantrone]

piroxicam USAN, USP, INN, BAN, JAN *analgesic; nonsteroidal anti-inflammatory drug (NSAID) for osteoarthritis and rheumatoid arthritis* 10, 20 mg oral

piroxicam β-cyclodextrin [see: piroxicam betadex]

piroxicam betadex USAN *analgesic; nonsteroidal anti-inflammatory drug (NSAID) for osteoarthritis and rheumatoid arthritis*

piroxicam cinnamate USAN *antiinflammatory*

piroxicam olamine USAN *analgesic; anti-inflammatory*

piroxicillin INN

piroximone USAN, INN, BAN *cardiotonic* ⊞ pyroxamine

pirozadil INN

pirprofen USAN, INN, BAN *anti-inflammatory*

pirquinozol USAN, INN *antiallergic* ⊞ parconazole

pirralkonium bromide INN

pirroksan [now: proroxan HCl]

pirsidomine USAN, INN *vasodilator*

pirtenidine INN *treatment for gingivitis* [also: pirtenidine HCl]

pirtenidine HCl USAN *treatment for gingivitis* [also: pirtenidine]

pistachio *medicinal herb* [see: witch hazel]

pitch tree, Canada; hemlock pitch tree *medicinal herb* [see: hemlock]

pitcher plant (Sarracenia purpurea) root *medicinal herb used as an astringent, diuretic, and stimulant*

pitenodil INN

Pitocin IV, IM injection ℞ *oxytocic for induction of labor, postpartum bleeding, and incomplete abortion* [oxytocin] 10 U/mL

pitofenone INN

pitrakinra *investigational oral leukotriene inhibitor for asthma*

Pitressin IM or subcu injection ℞ *pituitary antidiuretic hormone for diabetes insipidus or prevention of abdominal distention* [vasopressin] 20 U/mL ⊞ buterizine

pituitary, anterior

pituitary, posterior USP *antidiuretic hormone for postoperative ileus and surgical hemostasis*

pituxate INN

pivalate USAN, INN, BAN *combining name for radicals or groups*

pivampicillin INN *aminopenicillin antibiotic* [also: pivampicillin HCl]

pivampicillin HCl USAN *aminopenicillin antibiotic* [also: pivampicillin]

pivampicillin pamoate USAN *antibacterial*

pivampicillin probenate USAN *antibacterial*

pivenfrine INN

pivmecillinam INN, BAN *aminopenicillin antibiotic* [also: amdinocillin pivoxil; pivmecillinam HCl]

pivmecillinam HCl JAN *aminopenicillin antibiotic* [also: amdinocillin pivoxil; pivmecillinam]

pivopril USAN *antihypertensive*

pivoxazepam INN

pivoxetil USAN, INN *combining name for radicals or groups*

pivoxil USAN, INN *combining name for radicals or groups* ☑ pifexole

pivsulbactam BAN *β-lactamase inhibitor; penicillin/cephalosporin synergist* [also: sulbactam pivoxil]

pix pini [see: pine tar]

pixantrone *investigational (Phase III) treatment for relapsed, aggressive non-Hodgkin lymphoma*

pizotifen INN, BAN *anabolic; antidepressant; serotonin inhibitor (migraine specific)* [also: pizotyline]

pizotyline USAN *anabolic; antidepressant; serotonin inhibitor (migraine specific)* [also: pizotifen]

placebo *an inert substance with no therapeutic value* [also: obecalp]

placebo effect [L. I will please] *a perceived therapeutic effect from an inert substance* [compare to: nocebo effect]

Placidyl capsules (discontinued 2004) ℞ *hypnotic* [ethchlorvynol] 200, 500, 750 mg

plafibride INN

plague vaccine USP *active bacterin for plague* (Yersinia pestis)

Plan B tablets (in packs of 2) OTC ≥ 18 years; ℞ ≤ 17 years *emergency progestin-only postcoital contraceptive* [levonorgestrel] 0.75 mg

planadalin [see: carbromal]

Plantago lanceolata; P. major **and other species** *medicinal herb* [see: plantain]

Plantago ovata **(psyllium)** *medicinal herb* [see: plantain]

plantago seed USP *laxative*

plantain (*Plantago lanceolata; P. major* **and other species**) leaves and seeds *medicinal herb for bed-wetting, bladder infections, blood poisoning, constipation, diarrhea, diverticulitis, edema, hyperlipidemia, kidney disorders, neuralgia, snake bites, sores, and topical inflammation*

Plaquase powder for injection *investigational (orphan) for Peyronie disease* [collagenase]

Plaquenil film-coated tablets (discontinued 2008) ℞ *antimalarial; antirheumatic; lupus erythematosus suppressant* [hydroxychloroquine sulfate] 200 mg ☑ Belganyl

Plaretase 8000 tablets ℞ *porcine-derived digestive enzymes* [lipase; protease; amylase] 8000•30 000•30 000 USP units

Plasbumin-5; Plasbumin-25 IV infusion ℞ *blood volume expander for shock, burns, and hypoproteinemia* [human albumin] 5%; 25%

plasma, antihemophilic human USP

plasma concentrate factor IX [see: factor IX complex]

plasma expanders *a class of therapeutic blood modifiers used to increase the volume of circulating blood* [also called: blood volume expanders]

plasma protein fraction USP *blood volume supporter*

plasma protein fraction, human [now: plasma protein fraction]

plasma protein fractions *a class of therapeutic blood modifiers used to regulate the volume of circulating blood*

plasma thromboplastin component (PTC) [see: factor IX]

Plasma-Lyte A pH 7.4; Plasma-Lyte R; Plasma-Lyte 148 IV infusion ℞ *intravenous electrolyte therapy* [combined electrolyte solution]

Plasma-Lyte M (R; 56; 148) and 5% Dextrose IV infusion ℞ *intravenous nutritional/electrolyte therapy* [combined electrolyte solution; dextrose]

Plasmanate IV infusion ℞ *blood volume expander for shock due to burns, trauma, and surgery* [plasma protein fraction] 5%

Plasma-Plex IV infusion ℞ *blood volume expander for shock due to burns, trauma, and surgery* [plasma protein fraction] 5%

Plasmatein IV infusion ℞ *blood volume expander for shock due to burns, trauma, and surgery* [plasma protein fraction] 5%

plasmid DNA vector *investigational (orphan) genetic therapy for cystic fibrosis*

plasmin BAN [also: fibrinolysin, human]

Plateau Cap (trademarked dosage form) *controlled-release capsule*

platelet cofactor II [see: factor IX]

platelet concentrate USP *platelet replenisher*

Platinol-AQ IV injection (discontinued 2006) ℞ *alkylating antineoplastic for metastatic testicular tumors, metastatic ovarian tumors, and advanced bladder cancer* [cisplatin] 1 mg/mL

platinum *element (Pt)* ⬚ plutonium

cis-**platinum** [now: cisplatin]

cis-**platinum II** [now: cisplatin]

platinum diamminodichloride [see: cisplatin]

plaunotol INN

plauracin USAN, INN *veterinary growth stimulant* ⬚ belarizine

Plavix film-coated tablets ℞ *platelet aggregation inhibitor for stroke, myocardial infarction, peripheral artery disease, and acute coronary syndrome* [clopidogrel (as bisulfate)] 75, 300 mg

Plax mouthwash/gargle OTC *oral antiseptic* [sodium pyrophosphate; alcohol 8.7%] ⬚ Polycose

pleconaril USAN *investigational (NDA filed) viral replication inhibitor for treatment of viral respiratory infection and viral meningitis*

Plegisol solution ℞ *cardioplegic solution* [calcium chloride; magnesium chloride; potassium chloride; sodium chloride] 17.6•325.3•119.3•643 mg/100 mL

Plenaxis powder for IM injection ℞ *GnRH antagonist to suppress LH and FSH, leading to the cessation of testos-*terone production (medical castration, androgen ablation); treatment for prostate cancer [abarelix] 100 mg/vial

Plendil extended-release tablets ℞ *antihypertensive; calcium channel blocker* [felodipine] 2.5, 5, 10 mg ⬚ bolandiol

Pletal tablets ℞ *platelet aggregation inhibitor and vasodilator for intermittent claudication* [cilostazol] 50 mg ⬚ Bellatal

pleurisy root *(Asclepias tuberosa) medicinal herb for asthma, bronchitis, dysentery, emphysema, fever, pleurisy, and pneumonia*

pleuromulin INN

Plexion topical liquid, cleansing cloths ℞ *antibiotic and keratolytic for acne* [sulfacetamide sodium; sulfur] 10%•5%

Plexion SCT cream ℞ *antibiotic and keratolytic for acne* [sulfacetamide sodium; sulfur] 10%•5%

Plexion TS topical suspension ℞ *antibiotic and keratolytic for acne* [sulfacetamide sodium; sulfur] 10%•5%

Pliagel solution OTC *surfactant cleaning solution for soft contact lenses*

Pliaglis cream ℞ *anesthetic* [lidocaine; tetracaine] 7%•7%

plicamycin USAN, USP, INN *antibiotic antineoplastic for malignant testicular tumors*

plitidepsin *investigational (orphan) antineoplastic for multiple myeloma*

plomestane USAN *antineoplastic; aromatase inhibitor*

plum *(Prunus americana; P. domestica; P. spinosa) fruit and bark medicinal herb used as an anthelmintic, astringent, and laxative*

plutonium *element (Pu)* ⬚ platinum

pMDI (dosage form) *pressurized metered-dose inhaler*

PMMA (polymethylmethacrylate) [q.v.]

PMPA (phosphonomethoxypropyladenine) [see: tenofovir]

PMPA prodrug [see: tenofovir disoproxil fumarate]

P-MVAC (Platinol, methotrexate, vinblastine, Adriamycin, carboplatin) *chemotherapy protocol*

pneumococcal polysaccharide vaccine [see: pneumococcal vaccine, polyvalent]

pneumococcal vaccine, 7-valent (PCV7) *active bacterin for pneumococcal pneumonia; polysaccharide isolates of seven strains of* Streptococcus pneumoniae: *4, 6B, 9V, 14, 18C, 19F, and 23F*

pneumococcal vaccine, polyvalent *active bacterin for pneumococcal pneumonia (polysaccharide isolates of 23 strains of* Streptococcus pneumoniae*)*

Pneumopent *for inhalation investigational (orphan) prophylaxis of* Pneumocystis *pneumonia (PCP)* [pentamidine isethionate]

Pneumotussin caplets (discontinued 2007) ℞ *narcotic antitussive; expectorant* [hydrocodone bitartrate; guaifenesin] 2.5•300 mg ② niometacin

Pneumotussin 2.5 Cough syrup ℞ *narcotic antitussive; expectorant* [hydrocodone bitartrate; guaifenesin] 2.5•200 mg/5 mL

Pneumovax 23 subcu or IM injection ℞ *active immunization against 23 strains of* Streptococcus pneumoniae [pneumococcal vaccine, polyvalent] 25 mcg of each strain per 0.5 mL dose

pobilukast edamine USAN *antiasthmatic*

POC (procarbazine, Oncovin, CCNU) *chemotherapy protocol for pediatric brain tumors*

POCA (prednisone, Oncovin, cytarabine, Adriamycin) *chemotherapy protocol*

POCC (procarbazine, Oncovin, cyclophosphamide, CCNU) *chemotherapy protocol*

Pockethaler (trademarked delivery form) *nasal inhalation aerosol*

pod pepper *medicinal herb* [see: cayenne]

podilfen INN

Podocon-25 topical liquid ℞ *keratolytic for genital warts* [podophyllum resin] 25%

podofilox USAN *topical antimitotic for genital warts* [also: podophyllotoxin] 0.5% topical

Podofin topical liquid ℞ *keratolytic for genital warts* [podophyllum resin] 25%

podophyllin [see: podophyllum resin]

podophyllotoxin BAN *topical antimitotic* [also: podofilox]

podophyllotoxins *a class of mitotic-inhibiting antineoplastics derived from podophyllotoxin*

podophyllum USP *caustic; cytotoxic agent for genital warts*

Podophyllum peltatum *medicinal herb* [see: mandrake]

podophyllum resin USP *caustic; cytotoxic agent for genital warts*

poinsettia (Euphorbia pulcherrima; E. poinsettia; Poinsettia pulcherrima) *plant and sap medicinal herb for fever, pain relief, stimulating lactation, toothache, and warts; also used as an antibacterial and depilatory* ② boneset; Panacet 5/500

Point-Two oral rinse ℞ *dental caries preventative* [sodium fluoride; alcohol 6%] 0.2%

poison, dog *medicinal herb* [see: dog poison]

poison ash *medicinal herb* [see: fringe tree]

poison flag *medicinal herb* [see: blue flag]

poison hemlock (Conium maculatum) *plant medicinal herb that has been used for analgesia and sedation and as a method of execution; it is extremely poisonous*

poison ivy extract, alum precipitated USAN *ivy poisoning counteractant*

poison oak (Tocicodendron diversilobum) *extract medicinal herb used in homeopathic remedies for osteoarthritis*

poison oak extract USAN *antiallergic*

poke root (Phytolacca decandra) *medicinal herb* [see: pokeweed]

pokeweed (Phytolacca americana; P. decandra; P. rigida) *root and young* shoots *medicinal herb for arthritis, blood cleansing, bowel evacuation, dysmenorrhea, mucous membrane inflammation and discharge, mumps, pain, rheumatism, ringworm, scabies, syphilis, and tonsillitis; not generally regarded as safe and effective*

polacrilex [see: nicotine polacrilex]

polacrilin USAN, INN *pharmaceutic aid*

polacrilin potassium USAN, NF *tablet disintegrant*

Polaramine Expectorant pediatric oral liquid (discontinued 2007) ℞ *decongestant; antihistamine; expectorant* [pseudoephedrine sulfate; dexchlorpheniramine maleate; guaifenesin; alcohol 7.2%] 20•2•100 mg/5 mL

poldine methylsulfate USAN, USP *anticholinergic* [also: poldine metilsulfate]

poldine metilsulfate INN *anticholinergic* [also: poldine methylsulfate]

polecat weed *medicinal herb* [see: skunk cabbage]

policapram USAN, INN *tablet binder*

policosanol *natural supplement from sugar cane plants; enhanced extract of octacosanol (q.v.) used for hypercholesterolemia; therapeutic effects are similar to statin drugs but without side effects such as liver dysfunction and muscle atrophy*

policresulen INN

polidexide sulfate INN

polidocanol INN, JAN *polyethylene glycol monododecyl ether*

polifeprosan INN *pharmaceutic aid; implantable, biodegradable drug carrier* [also: polifeprosan 20]

polifeprosan 20 USAN *pharmaceutic aid; implantable, biodegradable drug carrier* [also: polifeprosan]

poligeenan USAN, INN *dispersing agent*

poliglecaprone 25 USAN *absorbable surgical suture material*

poliglecaprone 90 USAN *absorbable surgical suture coating*

poliglusam USAN *antihemorrhagic*

polignate sodium USAN *pepsin enzyme inhibitor*

polihexanide INN [also: polyhexanide]

poliomyelitis vaccine [now: poliovirus vaccine, inactivated]

poliovirus vaccine, enhanced inactivated (eIPV) *active immunizing agent for poliomyelitis*

poliovirus vaccine, inactivated (IPV) USP *active immunizing agent for poliomyelitis*

poliovirus vaccine, live oral (OPV) USP *active immunizing agent for poliomyelitis*

polipropene 25 USAN *tablet excipient*

polisaponin INN

politef INN *prosthetic aid* [also: polytef]

polixetonium chloride USAN, INN *preservative*

Polocaine injection ℞ *local anesthetic* [mepivacaine HCl] 1%, 2%, 3% 🔟 Bellacane; bulaquine; Pilagan

Polocaine MPF injection ℞ *local anesthetic* [mepivacaine HCl] 1%, 1.5%, 2%

Polocaine with levonordefrin injection ℞ *local anesthetic* [mepivacaine HCl; levonordefrin] 2%•1:20 000

polonium *element (Po)*

poloxalene USAN, INN, BAN *surfactant*

poloxamer USAN, NF, INN, BAN *ointment and suppository base; tablet binder*

poloxamer 124 USAN *surfactant; emulsifier; solubilizer; stabilizer*

poloxamer 188 USAN *surfactant; emulsifier; solubilizer; investigational (Phase III, orphan) for sickle cell crisis; investigational (orphan) for severe burns and vasospasm following cerebral aneurysm repair*

poloxamer 237 USAN *surfactant; emulsifier; solubilizer; stabilizer*

poloxamer 331 *investigational (orphan) for toxoplasmosis of AIDS*

poloxamer 338 USAN *surfactant; emulsifier; solubilizer; stabilizer*

poloxamer 407 USAN *surfactant; emulsifier; solubilizer; stabilizer*

Poly Hist DM oral liquid ℞ *antitussive; antihistamine; sleep aid; decongestant* [dextromethorphan hydrobromide; pyrilamine maleate; phenylephrine HCl] 15•12.5•7.5 mg/5 mL

Poly Hist HC oral liquid ℞ *narcotic antitussive; antihistamine; sleep aid; decongestant* [hydrocodone bitartrate; pyrilamine maleate; phenylephrine HCl] 3.5•12.5•7.5 mg/5 mL

poly I: poly C12U investigational (Phase III, orphan) *RNA synthesis inhibitor and immunomodulator for AIDS, renal cell carcinoma, metastatic melanoma, and chronic fatigue syndrome*

Poly Tan D oral suspension ℞ *decongestant; antihistamine; sleep aid* [phenylephrine tannate; dexbrompheniramine tannate; pyrilamine maleate] 25•4•3.5 mg/5 mL

Poly Tan DM oral suspension ℞ *antitussive; antihistamine; sleep aid; decongestant* [dextromethorphan tannate; dexbrompheniramine tannate; pyrilamine maleate; phenylephrine tannate] 30•4•3.5•25 mg/5 mL

polyamine-methylene resin

polyanhydroglucose [see: dextran]

polyanhydroglucuronic acid [see: dextran]

polybenzarsol INN

polybutester USAN *surgical suture material*

polybutilate USAN *surgical suture coating*

polycarbokane [see: polycarbophil]

polycarbophil USP, INN, BAN *bulk laxative; antidiarrheal*

Polycitra syrup ℞ *urinary alkalinizing agent* [potassium citrate; sodium citrate; citric acid] 550•500•334 mg/5 mL

Polycitra-K oral solution, crystals for oral solution ℞ *urinary alkalizing agent* [potassium citrate; citric acid] 1100•334 mg/5 mL; 3300•1002 mg/pkt.

Polycitra-LC solution ℞ *urinary alkalizing agent* [potassium citrate; sodium citrate; citric acid] 550•500•334 mg/5 mL

Polycose oral liquid, powder for oral liquid OTC *carbohydrate caloric supplement* [glucose polymers] ⊇ Plax

polydextrose USAN *food additive*

polydimethylsiloxane *surgical aid (retinal tamponade) for retinal detachment*

Polydine ointment, scrub, solution OTC *broad-spectrum antimicrobial* [povidone-iodine] ⊇ belladonna; Paladin

polydioxanone USAN *absorbable surgical suture material*

polyelectrolyte 211 [see: sodium alginate]

polyenes *a class of antifungals produced by a species of* Streptomyces *that damage fungal cell membranes* ⊇ Bell/ans

polyestradiol phosphate INN, BAN *estrogen; hormonal antineoplastic*

polyetadene INN *antacid* [also: polyethadene]

polyethadene USAN *antacid* [also: polyetadene]

polyethylene excipient NF *stiffening agent*

polyethylene glycol (PEG) NF *moisturizer/lubricant; ointment and suppository base; solvent*

polyethylene glycol *n* (*n* refers to the molecular weight: 300, 1000, etc.)

polyethylene glycol *n* **dioleate** (*n* refers to the molecular weight: 300, 1000, etc.)

polyethylene glycol 8 monostearate [see: polyoxyl 8 stearate]

polyethylene glycol 1000 monocetyl ether [see: cetomacrogol 1000]

polyethylene glycol 1540 NF

polyethylene glycol 3350 *laxative* 255, 527 g oral

polyethylene glycol 4000 USP [also: macrogol 4000]

polyethylene glycol 6000 USP

polyethylene glycol–electrolyte solution (PEG-ES) *pre-procedure bowel evacuant* [contains PEG 3350]

polyethylene glycol monoleyl ether [see: polyoxyl 10 oleyl ether]

polyethylene glycol monomethyl ether NF *excipient*

polyethylene glycol monostearate [see: polyoxyl 40 & 50 stearate]

polyethylene glycol–superoxide dismutase (PEG-SOD) [see: pegorgotein]

polyethylene glycol–urate oxidase; polyethylene glycol–uricase [see: PEG-uricase]

polyethylene oxide NF *suspending and viscosity agent; tablet binder*

polyferose USAN *hematinic*

Polygala senega medicinal herb [see: senega]

Polygam S/D freeze-dried powder for IV infusion (discontinued 2008) ℞ *passive immunizing agent for HIV, idiopathic thrombocytopenic purpura, and B-cell chronic lymphocytic leukemia* [immune globulin (IGIV), solvent/detergent treated] 90% (2.5, 5, 10 g/dose)

polygeline INN, BAN

polyglactin 370 USAN *absorbable surgical suture coating*

polyglactin 910 USAN *absorbable surgical suture material*

polyglycolic acid USAN, INN *surgical suture material*

polyglyconate USAN, BAN *absorbable surgical suture material*

Polygonatum multiflorum; P. odoratum medicinal herb [see: Solomon's seal]

Polygonum aviculare; P. hydropiper; P. persicaria; P. punctatum medicinal herb [see: knotweed]

Polygonum bistorta medicinal herb [see: bistort]

Polygonum multiflorum medicinal herb [see: fo-ti; ho-shou-wu]

PolyHeme *investigational (Phase III) hemoglobin–based red blood cell substitute* [human hemoglobin cross-linked with glutaral]

polyhexanide BAN [also: polihexanide]

Polyhist PD oral suspension ℞ *decongestant; antihistamine; sleep aid* [phenylephrine HCl; chlorpheniramine maleate; pyrilamine maleate] 7.5•2•12.5 mg/5 mL

Poly-Histine elixir ℞ *antihistamine for allergic and vasomotor rhinitis, allergic conjunctivitis, and mild urticaria; sleep aid* [pheniramine maleate; pyrilamine maleate; phenyltoloxamine citrate] 4•4•4 mg/5 mL

poly-ICLC *investigational (orphan) agent for orthopoxvirus infections and primary brain tumors* [polyinosinic-polycytidilic acid]

polyinosinic-polycytidilic acid *investigational (orphan) agent for orthopoxvirus infections and primary brain tumors*

poly-L-lactic acid *synthetic polymer for the correction of facial lipoatrophy due to HIV infections*

polyloxyl 8 stearate USAN *surfactant*

polymacon USAN *hydrophilic contact lens material*

polymanoacetate [now: acemannan]

polymeric oxygen [see: oxygen, polymeric]

polymetaphosphate P 32 USAN *radioactive agent*

polymethyl methacrylate (PMMA) *rigid hydrophobic polymer used for hard contact lenses*

polymixin E [see: colistin sulfate]

polymonine

polymyxin BAN *bactericidal antibiotic* [also: polymyxin B sulfate; polymyxin B]

polymyxin B INN *bactericidal antibiotic* [also: polymyxin B sulfate; polymyxin]

polymyxin B sulfate USP *bactericidal antibiotic* [also: polymyxin B; polymyxin] 500 000 U/vial eye drops or injection

polymyxin B sulfate & bacitracin zinc *topical antibiotic* 10 000•500 U/g ophthalmic

polymyxin B sulfate & bacitracin zinc & neomycin sulfate *topical antibiotic* 10 000 U•400 U•5 mg per g ophthalmic

polymyxin B sulfate & gramicidin & neomycin sulfate *topical antibiotic* 10 000 U•0.025 mg•1.75 mg per mL eye drops

polymyxin B sulfate & neomycin sulfate & dexamethasone *topical ophthalmic antibiotic and corticosteroidal anti-inflammatory* 10 000 U/mL•0.35%•0.1% eye drops

polymyxin B sulfate & neomycin sulfate & hydrocortisone *topical ophthalmic/otic antibiotic and corticosteroidal anti-inflammatory* 10 000 U/mL•0.35%•1% eye drops; 10 000 U/mL•5 mg/mL•1% ear drops

polymyxin B sulfate & trimethoprim sulfate *topical ophthalmic antibiotic* 10 000 U•1 mg per mL eye drops

polymyxin B$_1$ [see: polymyxin B]

polymyxin B$_2$ [see: polymyxin B]

polymyxin B$_3$ [see: polymyxin B]

polymyxin E [see: colistin sulfate]

polynoxylin INN, BAN

polyolprepolymer *topical base for gels and creams*

polyoxyethylene 20 sorbitan monolaurate [see: polysorbate 20]

polyoxyethylene 20 sorbitan monooleate [see: polysorbate 80]

polyoxyethylene 20 sorbitan monopalmitate [see: polysorbate 40]

polyoxyethylene 20 sorbitan monostearate [see: polysorbate 60]

polyoxyethylene 20 sorbitan trioleate [see: polysorbate 85]

polyoxyethylene 20 sorbitan tristearate [see: polysorbate 65]

polyoxyethylene 50 stearate [now: polyoxyl 50 stearate]

polyoxyethylene glycol 1000 monocetyl ether [see: cetomacrogol 1000]

polyoxyethylene nonyl phenol *surfactant/wetting agent*

polyoxyl 10 oleyl ether NF *surfactant*

polyoxyl 20 cetostearyl ether NF *surfactant*

polyoxyl 35 castor oil NF *emulsifying agent; surfactant*

polyoxyl 40 hydrogenated castor oil NF *emulsifying agent; surfactant*

polyoxyl 40 stearate USAN, NF *surfactant*

polyoxyl 50 stearate NF *surfactant; emulsifying agent*

polyoxypropylene 15 stearyl ether USAN *solvent*

polyphosphoric acid, sodium salt [see: sodium polyphosphate]

Polypodium vulgare medicinal herb [see: female fern]

Poly-Pred eye drop suspension ℞ *corticosteroidal anti-inflammatory; antibiotic* [prednisolone acetate; neomycin sulfate; polymyxin B sulfate] 0.5%•0.35%•10 000 U per mL

polypropylene glycol NF

polyribonucleotide [see: poly I: poly C12U]

polysaccharide-iron complex *hematinic; iron supplement* 150 mg Fe oral

Polysorb Hydrate cream OTC *moisturizer; emollient*

polysorbate 20 USAN, NF, INN *surfactant/wetting agent*

polysorbate 40 USAN, NF, INN *surfactant*

polysorbate 60 USAN, NF, INN *surfactant*

polysorbate 65 USAN, INN *surfactant*

polysorbate 80 USAN, NF, INN *surfactant/wetting agent; viscosity-increasing agent*

polysorbate 85 USAN, INN *surfactant*

Polysporin ointment OTC *antibiotic* [polymyxin B sulfate; bacitracin zinc] 10 000•500 U/g

Polysporin ophthalmic ointment (discontinued 2006) OTC *antibiotic* [polymyxin B sulfate; bacitracin zinc] 10 000•500 U/g

Polysporin topical powder (discontinued 2008) OTC *antibiotic* [polymyxin B sulfate; bacitracin zinc] 10 000•500 U/g

Polytabs-F pediatric chewable tablets ℞ *vitamin supplement; dental caries preventative* [multiple vitamins; fluoride; folic acid] ≐•1•0.3 mg

Polytar shampoo, soap OTC *antiseborrheic; antipsoriatic; antipruritic; antibacterial* [coal tar (solution includes pine tar and juniper tar)] 0.5% (4.5%); 0.5% (2.5%)

polytef USAN *prosthetic aid* [also: politef]

polytetrafluoroethylene (PTFE) [see: polytef]

polythiazide USAN, USP, INN *diuretic; antihypertensive*

Poly-Tussin HD syrup ℞ *narcotic antitussive; antihistamine; decongestant* [hydrocodone bitartrate; chlorpheniramine maleate; phenylephrine HCl] 6•2•5 mg/5 mL

Poly-Tussin XP oral liquid ℞ *narcotic antitussive; decongestant; expectorant* [hydrocodone bitartrate; phenylephrine HCl; guaifenesin] 5•10•200 mg/5 mL

polyurethane foam USAN *internal bone splint*

polyvalent Crotaline antivenin [see: antivenin (Crotalidae) polyvalent]

polyvalent gas gangrene antitoxin [see: gas gangrene antitoxin, pentavalent]

polyvidone INN *dispersing, suspending and viscosity-increasing agent* [also: povidone]

Poly-Vi-Flor drops ℞ *pediatric vitamin supplement and dental caries preventative* [multiple vitamins; sodium fluoride] ±•0.25, ±•0.5 mg/mL

Poly-Vi-Flor pediatric chewable tablets ℞ *vitamin supplement; dental caries preventative* [multiple vitamins; sodium fluoride; folic acid] ±•0.25•0.3, ±•0.5•0.3, ±•1•0.3 mg

Poly-Vi-Flor with Iron drops ℞ *pediatric vitamin/iron supplement and dental caries preventative* [multiple vitamins & minerals; sodium fluoride; iron] ±•0.25•10, ±•0.5•10 mg/mL

Poly-Vi-Flor with Iron pediatric chewable tablets ℞ *vitamin/iron supplement; dental caries preventative* [multiple vitamins & minerals; sodium fluoride; iron; folic acid] ±•0.25•12•0.3, ±•0.5•12•0.3, ±•1•12•0.3 mg

polyvinyl acetate phthalate NF *coating agent*

polyvinyl alcohol (PVA) USP *ophthalmic moisturizer; viscosity-increasing agent*

polyvinyl chloride, radiopaque *oral radiopaque contrast medium for severe constipation*

polyvinylpyrrolidone (PVP) [now: povidone]

Poly-Vi-Sol chewable tablets OTC *vitamin supplement* [multiple vitamins; folic acid] ±•0.3 mg

Poly-Vi-Sol drops OTC *vitamin supplement* [multiple vitamins]

Poly-Vi-Sol with Iron chewable tablets OTC *vitamin/iron supplement* [multiple vitamins; iron; folic acid] ±•12•0.3 mg

Poly-Vi-Sol with Iron drops OTC *vitamin/iron supplement* [multiple vitamins; iron] ±•10 mg/mL

Poly-Vitamin drops OTC *vitamin supplement* [multiple vitamins]

Polyvitamin Fluoride drops ℞ *pediatric vitamin supplement and dental caries preventative* [multiple vitamins; fluoride] ±•0.25, ±•0.5 mg/mL

Polyvitamin Fluoride pediatric chewable tablets ℞ *vitamin supplement; dental caries preventative* [multiple vitamins; fluoride; folic acid] ±•0.5•0.3, ±•1•0.3 mg

Polyvitamin Fluoride with Iron pediatric chewable tablets ℞ *vitamin/iron supplement; dental caries preventative* [multiple vitamins & minerals; fluoride; iron; folic acid] ±•1•12•0.3 mg

Poly-Vitamin with Iron drops OTC *vitamin/iron supplement* [multiple vitamins; iron] ±•10 mg/mL

Polyvitamin with Iron and Fluoride pediatric oral drops ℞ *vitamin/iron supplement; dental caries preventative* [multiple vitamins; iron; fluoride] ±•10•0.25 mg/mL

Polyvitamins with Fluoride and Iron pediatric chewable tablets (discontinued 2007) ℞ *vitamin/iron supplement; dental caries preventative* [multiple vitamins; fluoride; iron; folic acid] ±•0.5•12•0.3 mg

pomegranate *(Punica granatum)* seeds and fruit rind *medicinal herb used as an anthelmintic and astringent*

POMP (prednisone, Oncovin, methotrexate, Purinethol) *chemotherapy protocol* ⊡ BEMP; B-MOPP; BMP; BOMP

ponalrestat USAN, INN, BAN *aldose reductase inhibitor*

ponfibrate INN ☑ binifibrate

Ponstel capsules ℞ *analgesic; nonsteroidal anti-inflammatory drug (NSAID) for mild to moderate pain and primary dysmenorrhea* [mefenamic acid] 250 mg

Pontocaine cream (discontinued 2007) OTC *anesthetic* [tetracaine HCl] 1% ☑ pentaquine

Pontocaine ointment (discontinued 2007) OTC *anesthetic; antipruritic; counterirritant* [tetracaine; menthol] 0.5%•0.5% ☑ pentaquine

Pontocaine HCl injection, powder for injection ℞ *local anesthetic for spinal anesthesia* [tetracaine HCl] 0.2%, 0.3%, 1%; 20 mg

Pontocaine HCl Mono-Drop (eye drops) (discontinued 2006) ℞ *topical anesthetic* [tetracaine HCl] 0.5%

Pontocaine HCl oral solution (discontinued 2007) ℞ *mucous membrane anesthetic to abolish laryngeal and esophageal reflex* [tetracaine HCl; chlorobutanol] 2%•0.4%

poplar *(Populus tremuloides)* bark and buds *medicinal herb used as an antiperiodic, balsamic, febrifuge, and stomachic*

poplar, balsam *medicinal herb* [see: balm of Gilead]

poplar, black *medicinal herb* [see: black poplar]

Po-Pon-S sugar-coated tablets OTC *vitamin/mineral supplement* [multiple vitamins & minerals]

Populus balsamifera; P. candicans medicinal herb [see: balm of Gilead]

Populus nigra; P. tremula medicinal herb [see: black poplar]

Populus tremuloides medicinal herb [see: poplar]

poractant alfa BAN *porcine lung extract containing 90% phospholipids for emergency rescue and treatment of respiratory distress syndrome (RDS) in premature infants (orphan)*

porcine islet preparation, encapsulated *investigational (orphan) antidiabetic for type 1 patients on immunosuppression*

porfimer sodium USAN, INN *laser light–activated antineoplastic for photodynamic therapy (PDT) of esophageal (orphan) and non–small cell lung cancers; used for ablation of high-grade dysplasia in Barrett esophagus patients (orphan); investigational (orphan) for bladder cancer*

porfiromycin USAN, INN, BAN *antibacterial; investigational (Phase III, orphan) antineoplastic for head, neck, and cervical cancers*

Porites spp. natural material [see: coral]

porofocon A USAN *hydrophobic contact lens material* ☑ Brevicon; parvaquone

porofocon B USAN *hydrophobic contact lens material*

porphobilinogen deaminase, erythropoietic form, recombinant human *investigational (orphan) for prophylaxis of acute attacks of intermittent porphyria*

porphobilinogen deaminase, recombinant human *investigational (orphan) for treatment of acute attacks of intermittent porphyria*

Porphozyme *investigational (orphan) treatment for acute attacks of intermittent porphyria* [porphobilinogen deaminase, recombinant human]

Portagen powder OTC *enteral nutritional therapy* [lactose-free formula]

Portia film-coated tablets (in packs of 21 or 28) ℞ *monophasic oral contraceptive; emergency postcoital contraceptive* [levonorgestrel; ethinyl estradiol] 0.15 mg•30 mcg ☑ birch

porton asparaginase [see: erwinia L-asparaginase]

posaconazole USAN *broad-spectrum triazole antifungal for treatment of oropharyngeal candidiasis and prophylaxis of serious invasive fungal infections in immunocompromised patients; investigational (orphan) for zygomycosis*

posatirelin INN

posedrine [see: benzchlorpropamid]

poskine INN, BAN

Posoril *investigational (orphan) broadspectrum triazole antifungal for zygomycosis* [posaconazole]

posterior pituitary [see: pituitary, posterior]

Posture tablets OTC *calcium supplement* [calcium phosphate, tribasic] 600 mg Ca ☒ Bicitra

Posture-D film-coated tablets OTC *dietary supplement* [calcium phosphate, tribasic; vitamin D] 600 mg•125 IU

Potaba tablets, capsules, Envules (powder for oral solution) ℞ *watersoluble vitamin; "possibly effective" for scleroderma and other skin diseases and Peyronie disease* [aminobenzoate potassium] 500 mg; 500 mg; 2 g

Potasalan oral liquid ℞ *potassium supplement* [potassium chloride; alcohol 4%] 20 mEq K/15 mL

potash, sulfurated USP *source of sulfides*

potassic saline, lactated NF

potassium *element (K)*

potassium acetate USP *electrolyte replenisher* (10.2 mEq K/g) 2, 4 mEq/mL injection

potassium acid phosphate *urinary acidifier*

potassium alpha-phenoxyethyl penicillin [see: phenethicillin potassium]

potassium alum [see: alum, potassium]

potassium aminobenzoate [see: aminobenzoate potassium]

potassium aspartate [see: L-aspartate potassium]

potassium aspartate & magnesium aspartate USAN *nutrient*

potassium benzoate NF *preservative*

potassium benzyl penicillin [see: penicillin G potassium]

potassium bicarbonate USP *pH buffer; electrolyte replacement*

potassium bitartrate USAN

potassium borate *pH buffer*

potassium canrenoate JAN *aldosterone antagonist* [also: canrenoate potassium; canrenoic acid]

potassium carbonate USP *alkalizing agent*

potassium chloride (KCl) USP *electrolyte replenisher* (13.4 mEq K/g) 600, 750, 1500 mg oral; 20, 40 mEq/ 15 mL oral; 20 mEq/pkt oral; 2, 10, 20, 30, 40, 60, 90 mEq/mL injection

potassium chloride K 42 USAN *radioactive agent*

potassium citrate USP *electrolyte replacement; urinary alkalizer for nephrolithiasis and hypocitruria prevention* (orphan) 5, 10 mEq oral

potassium citrate & citric acid *investigational (orphan) agent for the dissolution and control of uric acid and cysteine calculi in the urinary tract*

potassium clavulanate & amoxicillin [see: amoxicillin]

potassium clavulanate & ticarcillin [see: ticarcillin disodium]

potassium dichloroisocyanurate [see: troclosene potassium]

potassium gamma hydroxybutyrate (KGHB) [see: gamma hydroxybutyrate (GHB)]

potassium glucaldrate USAN, INN *antacid*

potassium gluconate USP *electrolyte replenisher* 500, 595 mg oral; 20 mEq/15 mL oral

potassium guaiacolsulfonate USP *expectorant* [also: sulfogaiacol]

potassium hydroxide (KOH) NF *alkalizing agent*

potassium hydroxymethoxybenzenesulfonate hemihydrate [see: potassium guaiacolsulfonate]

potassium iodate *thyroid saturation agent to block the uptake of radioactive iodine after a nuclear accident or attack*

potassium iodide USP *antifungal; expectorant; dietary iodine supplement; thyroid agent; thyroid saturation agent to block the uptake of radioactive iodine after a nuclear accident or attack* (orphan) 1 g/mL oral

potassium mercuric iodide NF

potassium metabisulfite NF *antioxidant*

potassium metaphosphate NF *buffering agent*

potassium nitrate *tooth desensitizer*

potassium nitrazepate INN

potassium para-aminobenzoate (PAB) [see: aminobenzoate potassium]

potassium penicillin G [see: penicillin G potassium]

potassium perchlorate *radioimaging adjunct*

potassium permanganate USP *topical anti-infective*

potassium phosphate, dibasic (K_2HPO_4) USP *calcium regulator; phosphorus replacement; pH buffer* (11.5 mEq K/g)

potassium phosphate, monobasic (KH_2PO_4) NF *pH buffer; phosphorus replacement* (7.3 mEq K/g)

potassium sodium tartrate USP *laxative*

potassium sorbate NF *antimicrobial/ antiseptic*

potassium tetraborate *pH buffer*

potassium thiocyanate NF

potassium-sparing diuretics *a class of diuretic agents that interfere with sodium reabsorption, thus decreasing potassium secretion*

potato, wild; wild sweet potato vine *medicinal herb* [see: wild jalap]

Potentilla anserina; P. canadensis; P. reptans *medicinal herb* [see: cinquefoil]

Potentilla tormentilla *medicinal herb* [see: tormentil]

Povidine ointment, scrub, solution OTC *broad-spectrum antimicrobial* [povidone-iodine] 10%, 5%, 10%

povidone USAN, USP *dispersing, suspending, and viscosity-increasing agent* [also: polyvidone]

povidone I 125 USAN *radioactive agent*

povidone I 131 USAN *radioactive agent*

povidone-iodine USP, BAN *broad-spectrum antimicrobial* 10% topical

powdered cellulose [see: cellulose, powdered]

powdered ipecac [see: ipecac, powdered]

powdered opium [see: opium, powdered]

PowerMate tablets OTC *vitamin/mineral supplement* [multiple vitamins & minerals] ② buramate

PowerSleep tablets OTC *vitamin/mineral supplement; sleep aid* [multiple vitamins & minerals; 5-hydroxytryptophan; L-glutamine; melatonin; valerian] ±•250•25•0.25•75 mg

PowerVites tablets OTC *vitamin/mineral supplement* [multiple vitamins & minerals; folic acid; biotin] ±•150•25 mcg

PPA (phenylpropanolamine) [q.v.]

PPAR (peroxisome proliferator–activated receptor) agonists *a class of agents that increase insulin receptor sensitivity in type 2 diabetes; PPARα agonists are associated with lower triglyceride and higher HDL levels; PPARγ agonists are associated with lower blood glucose levels*

PPD (purified protein derivative [of tuberculin]) [see: tuberculin]

PPG-15 stearyl ether [now: polyoxypropylene 15 stearyl ether]

PPIs (proton pump inhibitors) [q.v.]

PR-1 vaccine *investigational (orphan) antineoplastic for myelodysplastic syndromes and acute or chronic myelogenous leukemia*

PR-122 (redox-phenytoin) *investigational (orphan) emergency rescue for grand mal status epilepticus*

PR-225 (redox-acyclovir) *investigational (orphan) treatment for AIDS-related herpes simplex infections*

PR-239 (redox penicillin G) *investigational (orphan) treatment for AIDS-related neurosyphilis*

PR-320 (molecusol & carbamazepine) *investigational (orphan) emergency rescue for grand mal status epilepticus*

practolol USAN, INN *antiadrenergic (β-receptor)*

Pradaxa ⓔ capsules (approved in the European Union) *direct thrombin inhibitor; investigational (Phase III)* oral anticoagulant for the prevention of deep vein thrombosis (DVT) or other venous thromboembolism (VTE) following total hip or total knee replacement surgery [dabigatran etexilate] 75, 110 mg

prajmalium bitartrate INN, BAN

pralidoxime chloride USAN, USP *cholinesterase reactivator for organophosphate poisoning and anticholinesterase overdose*

pralidoxime iodide USAN, INN *cholinesterase reactivator*

pralidoxime mesylate USAN *cholinesterase reactivator*

pralmorelin dihydrochloride USAN *growth hormone secretagogue*

PrameGel gel OTC *anesthetic; antipruritic; counterirritant* [pramoxine HCl; menthol] 1%•0.5%

Pramilet FA Filmtabs (film-coated tablets) ℞ *prenatal vitamin/mineral/calcium/iron supplement* [multiple vitamins & minerals; calcium; iron; folic acid] ≐•250•40•1 mg

pramipexole USAN, INN *dopamine agonist for Parkinson disease*

pramipexole dihydrochloride USAN *dopamine agonist for idiopathic Parkinson disease; treatment for primary restless legs syndrome (RLS)* 0.125, 0.25, 0.5, 1, 1.5 mg oral

pramiracetam INN *cognition adjuvant* [also: pramiracetam HCl]

pramiracetam HCl USAN *cognition adjuvant* [also: pramiracetam]

pramiracetam sulfate USAN *cognition adjuvant; investigational (orphan) to manage cognitive dysfunction and enhance antidepressant activity*

pramiverine INN, BAN

pramlintide USAN *antidiabetic for types 1 and 2 diabetes; synthetic amylin analogue that slows gastric emptying and decreases hepatic glucose production*

pramlintide acetate USAN *antidiabetic for types 1 and 2 diabetes; synthetic amylin analogue that slows gastric emptying and decreases hepatic glucose production*

pramocaine INN *topical anesthetic* [also: pramoxine HCl; pramoxine] 🔟

primaquine

pramocaine HCl [see: pramoxine HCl]

Pramosone cream, lotion, ointment ℞ *corticosteroidal anti-inflammatory; local anesthetic* [hydrocortisone acetate; pramoxine] 1%•1%, 2.5%•1%; 2.5%•1%; 2.5%•1% 🔟 bromazine; primycin; promazine; puromycin

pramoxine BAN *topical anesthetic* [also: pramoxine HCl; pramocaine] 🔟 bromhexine

Pramoxine HC anorectal aerosol foam, cream (discontinued 2007) ℞ *corticosteroidal anti-inflammatory; local anesthetic* [hydrocortisone acetate; pramoxine HCl] 1%•1%; 2.5%•1%

pramoxine HCl USP *topical anesthetic* [also: pramocaine; pramoxine]

prampine INN, BAN 🔟 Permapen

PrandiMet tablets ℞ *combination antidiabetic for type 2 diabetes that stimulates the release of insulin from the pancreas, decreases hepatic glucose production, and increases cellular response to insulin* [repaglinide; metformin] 1•500, 2•500 mg

Prandin tablets ℞ *meglitinide antidiabetic for type 2 diabetes that stimulates the release of insulin from the pancreas* [repaglinide] 0.5, 1, 2 mg

pranidipine INN 🔟 barnidipine

pranlukast INN, BAN *antiasthmatic*

pranolium chloride USAN, INN *antiarrhythmic*

pranoprofen INN

pranosal INN

praseodymium *element (Pr)*

prasterone INN *synthetic dehydroepiandrosterone (DHEA); investigational (NDA filed) agent to increase bone density in patients with systemic lupus erythematosus (SLE) on corticosteroid therapy*

prasugrel *investigational (NDA filed) oral adenosine phosphate inhibitor to block platelet aggregation in patients with acute coronary syndrome (ACS)*

Pravachol tablets ℞ HMG-CoA *reductase inhibitor for hyperlipidemia, hypertriglyceridemia, atherosclerosis, coronary procedures, and recurrent myocardial infarctions* [pravastatin sodium] 10, 20, 40, 80 mg

pravadoline INN *analgesic* [also: pravadoline maleate]

pravadoline maleate USAN *analgesic* [also: pravadoline]

pravastatin INN, BAN HMG-CoA *reductase inhibitor for hyperlipidemia, atherosclerosis, coronary procedures, and recurrent myocardial infarctions* [also: pravastatin sodium]

pravastatin sodium USAN, JAN HMG-CoA *reductase inhibitor for hyperlipidemia, atherosclerosis, coronary procedures, and recurrent myocardial infarctions* [also: pravastatin] 10, 20, 40, 80 mg oral

Pravigard PAC combo pack (1 tablet of each per dose) (discontinued 2006) ℞ *antihyperlipidemic; HMG-CoA reductase inhibitor; platelet aggregation inhibitor; analgesic; antipyretic* [pravastatin sodium; buffered aspirin] 20•81, 20•325, 40•81, 40•325, 80•81, 80•325 mg

Prax lotion, cream OTC *anesthetic* [pramoxine HCl] 1% ② Precose

praxadine INN

prazarelix acetate USAN *gonadotropin-releasing hormone (GnRH) antagonist for uterine fibroids, endometriosis, and prostate cancer*

prazepam USAN, USP, INN *sedative; anxiolytic* 5 mg oral

prazepine INN ② prozapine

praziquantel USAN, USP, INN, BAN *anthelmintic for schistosomiasis (flukes); investigational (orphan) for neurocysticercosis*

prazitone INN, BAN ② perastine; Prostin E2

prazocillin INN

prazosin INN, BAN *alpha₁-adrenergic blocker for hypertension* [also: prazosin HCl] ② periciazine

prazosin HCl USAN, USP, JAN *alpha₁-adrenergic blocker for hypertension* [also: prazosin] 1, 2, 5 mg oral

Pre-Attain oral liquid OTC *enteral nutritional therapy* [lactose-free formula] ② protein A

prebiotics *a class of natural foods, such as inulin and other fructo-oligosaccharides (FOS), that enhances or supports the growth of probiotic (beneficial) bacteria in the digestive system, thereby suppressing the growth of harmful bacteria* [compare to: probiotics]

PreCare Conceive film-coated tablets ℞ *pre-conception vitamin/mineral/calcium/iron supplement* [multiple vitamins & minerals; calcium; iron; folic acid] ≛•200•30•1 mg

PreCare Prenatal film-coated caplet ℞ *vitamin/mineral/calcium/iron supplement for pregnancy and lactation* [multiple vitamins & minerals; calcium; iron; folic acid] ≛•250•40•1 mg

precatory bean *(Abrus precatorius)* plant *medicinal herb for eye inflammation, hastening labor, and stimulating abortion; not generally regarded as safe and effective as it is highly toxic and ingestion may be fatal*

Precedex IV infusion ℞ *sedative for intubated and ventilated patients in an intensive care setting; premedication to anesthesia* [dexmedetomidine HCl] 100 mcg/mL

precipitated calcium carbonate JAN *antacid; dietary calcium supplement* [also: calcium carbonate]

precipitated chalk [see: calcium carbonate]

precipitated sulfur [see: sulfur, precipitated]

Precision High Nitrogen Diet powder OTC *enteral nutritional therapy* [lactose-free formula]

Precision LR Diet powder OTC *enteral nutritional therapy* [lactose-free formula]

preclamol INN

Precose tablets ℞ *antidiabetic agent for type 2 diabetes; alpha-glucosidase* *inhibitor that delays the digestion of dietary carbohydrates* [acarbose] 25, 50, 100 mg ⊇ Prax

Pred Mild; Pred Forte eye drop suspension ℞ *corticosteroidal anti-inflammatory* [prednisolone acetate] 0.12%; 1%

Predalone 50 IM injection (discontinued 2005) ℞ *corticosteroid; anti-inflammatory* [prednisolone acetate] 50 mg/mL ⊇ burodiline

Predcor-50 IM injection (discontinued 2008) ℞ *corticosteroid; anti-inflammatory* [prednisolone acetate] 50 mg/mL

Pred-G eye drop suspension ℞ *corticosteroidal anti-inflammatory; antibiotic* [prednisolone acetate; gentamicin sulfate] 1%•0.3%

Pred-G ophthalmic ointment ℞ *corticosteroidal anti-inflammatory; antibiotic* [prednisolone acetate; gentamicin sulfate; chlorobutanol] 0.6%•0.3%•0.5%

prednazate USAN, INN *anti-inflammatory*

prednazoline INN

prednicarbate USAN, INN *corticosteroid; anti-inflammatory* 0.1% topical

Prednicen-M tablets (discontinued 2008) ℞ *corticosteroid; anti-inflammatory; immunosuppressant* [prednisone] 5 mg

prednimustine USAN, INN *investigational (orphan) antineoplastic for malignant non-Hodgkin lymphomas*

Prednisol eye drops ℞ *corticosteroidal anti-inflammatory* [prednisolone sodium phosphate] 1%

Prednisol TBA intra-articular, intralesional, or soft tissue injection (discontinued 2008) ℞ *corticosteroid; anti-inflammatory* [prednisolone tebutate] 20 mg/mL

prednisolamate INN, BAN

prednisolone USP, INN *corticosteroidal anti-inflammatory* 5 mg oral; 15 mg/5 mL oral

prednisolone acetate USP, BAN *corticosteroidal anti-inflammatory* (base=90%) 1% eye drops

prednisolone hemisuccinate USP *corticosteroidal anti-inflammatory*

prednisolone sodium phosphate USP *corticosteroidal anti-inflammatory* (base=74%) 5, 10, 15, 20 mg/5 mL oral; 1% eye drops

prednisolone sodium succinate USP *corticosteroidal anti-inflammatory*

prednisolone steaglate INN, BAN *corticosteroidal anti-inflammatory*

prednisolone tebutate USP *corticosteroidal anti-inflammatory*

prednisone USP, INN *corticosteroidal anti-inflammatory; immunosuppressant* 1, 2.5, 5, 10, 20, 50 mg oral; 1, 5 mg/mL oral

prednival USAN *corticosteroidal anti-inflammatory*

prednylidene INN, BAN

prefenamate INN

PreferaOB tablets ℞ *prenatal vitamin/mineral/iron supplement* [multiple vitamins & minerals; folic acid; iron] ±•1•≐ mg

Prefest tablets (in packs of 30) ℞ *hormone replacement therapy for postmenopausal symptoms* [estradiol; norgestimate] 1•0 mg × 3 days; 1•0.09 mg × 3 days; repeat without interruption

Prefill (delivery form) *prefilled applicator* ⊇ Bravelle

Preflex Daily Cleaner Especially for Sensitive Eyes solution OTC *surfactant cleaning solution for soft contact lenses*

Prefrin Liquifilm eye drops (discontinued 2006) OTC *decongestant* [phenylephrine HCl] 0.12%

pregabalin USAN *gabamimetic anticonvulsant for partial-onset seizures and the management of fibromyalgia, diabetic peripheral neuropathy (DPN), and postherpetic neuralgia (PHN); investigational (Phase III) for generalized anxiety disorder (GAD)*

pregelatinized starch [see: starch, pregelatinized]

Pregestimil powder OTC *hypoallergenic infant food for severe malabsorption* *disorders* [enzymatically hydrolyzed protein formula]

pregnandiol JAN

pregneninolone [see: ethisterone]

pregnenolone INN *natural hormone precursor* [also: pregnenolone succinate]

pregnenolone succinate USAN *hormone precursor* [also: pregnenolone]

Pregnosis slide test for home use OTC *in vitro diagnostic aid; urine pregnancy test* [latex agglutination test]

Pregnyl powder for IM injection ℞ *a human-derived hormone used for prepubertal cryptorchidism or hypogonadism and to induce ovulation in anovulatory women* [chorionic gonadotropin] 1000 U/mL ☒ Pergonal; proguanil

Prehist sustained-release capsules ℞ *decongestant; antihistamine* [phenylephrine HCl; chlorpheniramine maleate] 20•8 mg

Pre-Hist-D sustained-release tablets ℞ *decongestant; antihistamine; anticholinergic to dry mucosal secretions* [phenylephrine HCl; chlorpheniramine maleate; methscopolamine nitrate] 20•8•2.5 mg

Prelone syrup ℞ *corticosteroid; antiinflammatory* [prednisolone; alcohol 5%] 15 mg/5 mL ☒ Perlane; proline

Prelu-2 timed-release capsules ℞ *anorexiant; CNS stimulant* [phendimetrazine tartrate] 105 mg ☒ Paral; perilla

premafloxacin USAN, INN *veterinary antibacterial*

Premarin tablets ℞ *a mixture of equine estrogens for the prevention and treatment of postmenopausal symptoms; palliative therapy for prostate and breast cancer* [conjugated estrogens] 0.3, 0.45, 0.625, 0.9, 1.25 mg ☒ Primorine

Premarin Intravenous IV or IM injection ℞ *a mixture of equine estrogens for the treatment of abnormal uterine bleeding due to hormonal imbalance* [conjugated estrogens] 25 mg/vial

Premarin Vaginal cream ℞ *a mixture of equine estrogens for postmenopausal atrophic vaginitis* [conjugated estrogens] 0.625 mg/g

premazepam INN, BAN ☒ bromazepam

PremesisRx tablets ℞ *prenatal vitamin/mineral supplement* [vitamins B$_6$ and B$_{12}$; folic acid; calcium carbonate] 75 mg•12 mcg•1 mg•200 mg

Premphase tablets (in packs of 28) ℞ *a mixture of equine and synthetic hormones; hormone replacement therapy for postmenopausal symptoms* [conjugated estrogens; medroxyprogesterone acetate] ☒ bromofos
Phase 1 (14 days): 0.625•0 mg;
Phase 2 (14 days): 0.625•5 mg

Prempro tablets (in packs of 28) ℞ *a mixture of equine and synthetic hormones; hormone replacement therapy for postmenopausal symptoms* [conjugated estrogens; medroxyprogesterone acetate] 0.3•1.5, 0.45•1.5, 0.625•2.5, 0.625•5 mg

Prēmsyn PMS caplets OTC *analgesic; antipyretic; diuretic; antihistamine; sleep aid* [acetaminophen; pamabrom; pyrilamine maleate] 500•25•15 mg

prenalterol INN, BAN *adrenergic* [also: prenalterol HCl]

prenalterol HCl USAN *adrenergic* [also: prenalterol]

Prenatabs RX film-coated tablets ℞ *vitamin/mineral/calcium/iron supplement* [multiple vitamins & minerals; calcium; iron; folic acid; biotin] ≛•200•29•1•0.03 mg

Prenatal 19 tablets, chewable tablets ℞ *vitamin/mineral/calcium/iron supplement* [multiple vitamins & minerals; calcium; iron; folic acid] ≛•200•29•1 mg ☒ pyrantel

Prenatal AD tablets ℞ *vitamin/mineral/calcium/iron supplement* [multiple vitamins & minerals; calcium; iron; folic acid] ≛•200•90•1 mg

Prenatal H.P. tablets ℞ *vitamin/calcium/iron supplement* [multiple vitamins; calcium; iron; folic acid] ≛• 50•30•0.8 mg

Prenatal Maternal tablets ℞ *vitamin/mineral/calcium/iron supplement* [multiple vitamins & minerals; calcium;

iron; folic acid; biotin] ≛•250•60•1•0.03 mg

Prenatal MR 90 delayed-release film-coated tablets ℞ *vitamin/calcium/iron supplement* [multiple vitamins; calcium; iron; folic acid] ≛•250•90•1 mg

Prenatal PC 40 film-coated caplets ℞ *vitamin/mineral/calcium/iron supplement* [multiple vitamins and minerals; calcium; iron; folic acid] ≛•250•40•1 mg

Prenatal Plus tablets ℞ *vitamin/calcium/iron supplement* [multiple vitamins; calcium; iron; folic acid] ≛•200•65•1 mg �ⓓ Par-Natal Plus

Prenatal Plus Improved tablets (discontinued 2007) ℞ *vitamin/calcium/iron supplement* [multiple vitamins; calcium; iron; folic acid] ≛•200•65•1 mg ⓓ Par-Natal Plus Improved

Prenatal Plus Iron tablets ℞ *vitamin/calcium/iron supplement* [multiple vitamins; calcium; iron; folic acid] ≛•200•27•1 mg ⓓ Par-Natal Plus

Prenatal Plus with Betacarotene tablets (discontinued 2004) ℞ *vitamin/calcium/iron supplement* [multiple vitamins; calcium; iron; folic acid] ≛•200•65•1 mg ⓓ Par-Natal Plus

Prenatal Rx; Prenatal Rx 1 tablets ℞ *vitamin/calcium/iron supplement* [multiple vitamins; calcium; iron; folic acid] ≛•175•29.5•1 mg

Prenatal Rx with Betacarotene tablets ℞ *vitamin/calcium/iron supplement* [multiple vitamins; calcium; iron; folic acid; biotin] ≛•200•60•1•0.03 mg

Prenatal with Folic Acid tablets OTC *vitamin/calcium/iron supplement* [multiple vitamins; calcium; iron; folic acid] ≛•200•60•0.8 mg

Prenatal Z delayed-release film-coated tablets ℞ *vitamin/calcium/iron supplement* [multiple vitamins; calcium; iron; folic acid] ≛•300•65•1 mg

Prenatal-1 + Iron tablets ℞ *vitamin/calcium/iron supplement* [multiple vitamins; calcium; iron; folic acid] ≛•200•65•1 mg

Prenatal-H capsules ℞ *vitamin/mineral/iron supplement* [multiple vitamins & minerals; iron; folic acid] ≛•106.5•1 mg ⓓ pyrantel

Prenatal-S tablets OTC *vitamin/calcium/iron supplement* [multiple vitamins; calcium; iron; folic acid] ≛•200•27•0.8 mg

Prenate Advance; Prenate 90 delayed-release film-coated tablets ℞ *prenatal vitamin/calcium/iron supplement* [multiple vitamins; calcium; iron; folic acid] ≛•200•90•1 mg; ≛•250•90•1 mg

Prenate DHA softgel ℞ *prenatal vitamin/calcium/iron/omega-3 supplement* [multiple vitamins; calcium; ferrous fumarate; folic acid; L-methylfolate; docosahexaenoic acid (DHA)] ≛•150•27•0.4•0.6•300 mg

Prenate GT delayed-release gel-coated tablets (discontinued 2004) ℞ *prenatal vitamin/calcium/iron supplement* [multiple vitamins; calcium; iron; folic acid] ≛•200•90•1 mg

Prenavite tablets OTC *vitamin/calcium/iron supplement* [multiple vitamins; calcium; iron; folic acid] ≛•200•60•0.8 mg

prenisteine INN

prenoverine INN

prenoxdiazine INN

prenylamine USAN, INN *coronary vasodilator*

Preos subcu injection *investigational (Phase III) recombinant human parathyroid hormone for postmenopausal osteoporosis in women*

Preparation H anorectal cream OTC *local anesthetic and astringent for temporary relief of hemorrhoidal symptoms* [pramoxine HCl; phenylephrine HCl; petrolatum; glycerin] 1%•0.25%•15%•14.4%

Preparation H anorectal ointment OTC *emollient and astringent for temporary relief of hemorrhoidal symptoms* [shark liver oil; phenylephrine HCl] 3%•0.25%

Preparation H cleansing tissues OTC *moisturizer and cleanser for external rectal/vaginal areas* [propylene glycol]

Preparation H rectal suppositories OTC *emollient for temporary relief of hemorrhoidal symptoms* [shark liver oil] 3%

Preparation H Cooling Gel OTC *emollient and astringent for temporary relief of hemorrhoidal symptoms* [phenylephrine HCl; hamamelis water (witch hazel); alcohol 7.5%] 0.25%•50%

prepared chalk [see: calcium carbonate]

Prepcat oral suspension ℞ *radiopaque contrast medium for gastrointestinal imaging* [barium sulfate] 1.5% ▣ Probec-T

Pre-Pen solution for dermal scratch test (discontinued 2006) ℞ *diagnostic aid for penicillin hypersensitivity* [benzylpenicilloyl polylysine] 0.25 mL ▣ propane

Pre-Pen/MDM solution for dermal scratch test *investigational (orphan) agent for penicillin hypersensitivity assessment* [benzylpenicillin]

Prepidil gel ℞ *prostaglandin for cervical ripening at term* [dinoprostone] 0.5 mg ▣ piribedil

PreserVision Lutein softgel OTC *vitamin/mineral supplement* [vitamins C and E; multiple minerals; lutein] 226 mg•200 IU• ± •5 mg

Prestara *investigational (NDA filed) agent to increase bone density in patients with systemic lupus erythematosus (SLE) on corticosteroid therapy* [prasterone]

pretamazium iodide INN, BAN

prethcamide

prethrombin [see: prothrombin complex, activated]

pretiadil INN

Pretts Diet-Aid chewable tablets OTC *diet aid* [sodium carboxymethylcellulose; alginic acid; sodium bicarbonate] 100•200•70 mg

Pretty Feet & Hands cream OTC *moisturizer; emollient*

Pretz solution OTC *nasal moisturizer* [sodium chloride (saline solution)] 0.6% ▣ Brite Eyes II; protease

Pretz Irrigating solution OTC *for postoperative irrigation* [sodium chloride (saline solution); glycerin; eriodictyon] 0.75%

Pretz Moisturizing nose drops OTC *nasal moisturizer* [sodium chloride (saline solution); glycerin; eriodictyon] 0.75%

Pretz-D nasal spray (discontinued 2006) OTC *nasal decongestant* [ephedrine sulfate] 0.25% ▣ Protuss-D

PretzPak ointment (discontinued 2004) OTC *antimicrobial postoperative nasal pack* [benzyl alcohol; polyethylene glycol; carboxymethylcellulose; urea; allantoin]

Prevacid delayed-release enteric-coated granules in capsules ℞ *proton pump inhibitor for gastric and duodenal ulcers, erosive esophagitis, gastroesophageal reflux disease (GERD), and other gastroesophageal disorders* [lansoprazole] 15, 30 mg

Prevacid delayed-release enteric-coated granules for oral suspension ℞ *proton pump inhibitor for gastric and duodenal ulcers, erosive esophagitis, gastroesophageal reflux disease (GERD), and other gastroesophageal disorders* [lansoprazole] 15, 30 mg

Prevacid I.V. powder for infusion ℞ *proton pump inhibitor for erosive esophagitis in hospitalized patients* [lansoprazole] 30 mg/vial

Prevacid NapraPAC 375; Prevacid NapraPAC 500 tablets + capsules in 7-day dose packs ℞ *nonsteroidal anti-inflammatory; proton pump inhibitor; treatment for gastric and duodenal ulcers* [naproxen (tablets); lansoprazole (capsules)] 375•15, 500•15 mg

Prevacid SoluTab (delayed-release enteric-coated granules in orally disintegrating tablets) ℞ *proton pump inhibitor for gastric and duodenal*

ulcers, erosive esophagitis, gastroesoph-ageal reflux disease (GERD), and other gastroesophageal disorders [lansopra-zole] 15, 30 mg

Prevalite powder for oral suspension ℞ cholesterol-lowering antihyperlipid-emic; treatment for pruritus due to par-tial biliary obstruction; also used as an antidote to Clostridium difficile and digitalis toxicity [cholestyramine resin] 4 g/dose

Prevelle Silk subcu injection in pre-filled syringes ℞ dermal filler for deep wrinkles and facial folds; topical anes-thetic [hyaluronic acid; lidocaine]

Preven kit (4 film-coated tablets + a pregnancy test) (discontinued 2008) ℞ (available OTC from pharmacists in some states) emergency postcoital contraceptive [levonorgestrel; ethinyl estradiol] 0.25•0.05 mg ⚕ Brovana; paraffin; Privine; Profen II

Prevent-X powder for oral solution OTC dietary supplement [multiple vitamins & minerals; multiple amino acids]

PreviDent dental gel for self-applica-tion ℞ caries preventative [sodium fluoride] 1.1%

PreviDent 5000 Plus dental cream for self-application ℞ caries preventa-tive [sodium fluoride] 1.1%

PreviDent Rinse oral solution ("swish and spit") ℞ dental caries preventative [sodium fluoride] 0.2%

Prevnar IM injection ℞ active immu-nization against seven strains of Strep-tococcus pneumoniae in infants and toddlers; investigational (Phase III) for adults over 50 years [pneumococcal vaccine, 7-valent] 2–4 mcg of each strain per 0.5 mL dose

Prevpac three-drug daily pack ℞ triple therapy for H. pylori: an antisecretory and two antibiotics [lansoprazole (cap-sules); clarithromycin (tablets); amoxicillin (capsules)] 2 × 30 mg; 2 × 500 mg; 4 × 500 mg

PreVue B. burgdorferi Antibody Detection Assay reagent kit for

professional use ℞ in vitro diagnostic aid for Lyme disease

Prexige Ⓒ Ⓔ (available in 30 coun-tries) investigational (Phase III) antiar-thritic for osteoarthritis; analgesic for acute pain; COX-2 inhibitor; nonste-roidal anti-inflammatory drug (NSAID) [lumiracoxib] 100 mg

prezatide copper acetate USAN, INN immunomodulator; investigational (Phase II) wound-healing gel for venous leg ulcers

Prezista film-coated tablets ℞ anti-retroviral protease inhibitor for HIV-1 infections [darunavir ethanolate] 300, 600 mg

Prialt intrathecal infusion ℞ calcium-channel blocker; non-narcotic analgesic for intractable pain of cancer or AIDS [ziconotide acetate] 25, 100 mcg/mL ⚕ pirolate

pribecaine INN

prickly ash (Xanthoxylum ameri-canum; X. fraxineum) bark medici-nal herb for fever, mouth sores, poor circulation, ulcers, and wounds

prickly juniper (Juniperus oxycedrus) medicinal herb [see: juniper]

prickly pear medicinal herb [see: nopal]

pride of China (Melia azedarach) root bark and fruit medicinal herb used as an anthelmintic, astringent, bit-ter tonic, emetic, emmenagogue, and purgative

pride weed medicinal herb [see: flea-bane; horseweed]

pridefine INN antidepressant [also: pri-define HCl] ⚕ proadifen

pridefine HCl USAN antidepressant [also: pridefine]

prideperone INN

pridinol INN

priest's crown medicinal herb [see: dandelion]

prifelone USAN, INN dermatologic anti-inflammatory ⚕ Prophyllin

prifinium bromide INN

Priftin film-coated tablets ℞ antibacte-rial for tuberculosis (orphan); investiga-tional (orphan) for AIDS-related Mycobacterium avium *complex* [rifapentine] 150 mg

prifuroline INN

priliximab USAN, INN *monoclonal antibody for organ transplants and autoimmune lymphoproliferative diseases; investigational (orphan) for multiple sclerosis*

prilocaine USAN, INN, BAN *topical/local anesthetic*

prilocaine HCl USAN, USP *topical/local anesthetic* [also: propitocaine HCl]

prilocaine & lidocaine *local anesthetic* 2.5%•2.5% topical

Prilosec delayed-release enteric-coated granules in capsules, delayed-release granules for oral suspension ℞ *proton pump inhibitor for gastric and duodenal ulcers, erosive esophagitis, GERD, and other gastroesophageal disorders* [omeprazole] 10, 20, 40 mg; 2.5, 10 mg/pkt

Prilosec OTC delayed-release tablets OTC *proton pump inhibitor for frequent heartburn* [omeprazole (as magnesium)] 20 mg (20.6 mg)

primachine phosphate [see: primaquine phosphate]

Primacor IV infusion ℞ *vasodilator for congestive heart failure* [milrinone lactate] 0.2 mg/mL

Primacor in 5% Dextrose IV infusion ℞ *vasodilator for congestive heart failure* [milrinone lactate; dextrose] 200 mcg/mL; 5%

primaperone INN

primaquine INN *antimalarial* [also: primaquine phosphate] ⑨ pramocaine

primaquine phosphate USP *used to treat malarial symptoms and prevent relapse; investigational (orphan) treatment adjunct to* Pneumocystis *pneumonia (PCP) infection* [also: primaquine] 26.3 mg oral

Primatene Asthma tablets OTC *bronchodilator; decongestant; expectorant* [ephedrine HCl; guaifenesin] 12.5•200 mg

Primatene Mist inhalation aerosol OTC *sympathomimetic bronchodilator;*

vasopressor for shock [epinephrine] 0.22 mg/spray

Primaxin I.M. powder for injection ℞ *carbapenem antibiotic* [imipenem; cilastatin sodium] 500•500 mg

Primaxin I.V. powder for injection ℞ *carbapenem antibiotic* [imipenem; cilastatin sodium] 250•250, 500•500 mg

primidolol USAN, INN *antihypertensive; antianginal; antiarrhythmic*

primidone USP, INN, BAN *anticonvulsant for grand mal, psychomotor, and focal epileptic seizures; also used for essential tremor and benign familial tremor* 50, 250 mg oral

Primorine (trademarked ingredient) *antioxidant; a proprietary blend of the nutritional supplements aminobenzoic acid, vitamin E, and alpha lipoic acid (ALA); also known as* **Benzamine** ⑨ Premarin

Primsol oral solution ℞ *antibiotic for otitis media in children and urinary tract infections in adults* [trimethoprim HCl] 50 mg/5 mL

primycin INN ⑨ bromazine; Pramosone; promazine; puromycin

prince's pine *medicinal herb* [see: pipsissewa]

Principen capsules, powder for oral suspension ℞ *aminopenicillin antibiotic* [ampicillin] 250, 500 mg; 125, 250 mg/5 mL ⑨ pirenzepine

Prinivil tablets ℞ *antihypertensive; angiotensin-converting enzyme (ACE) inhibitor; adjunctive treatment for congestive heart failure (CHF)* [lisinopril] 10, 20 mg

prinodolol [see: pindolol]

prinomastat USAN *matrix metalloprotease inhibitor*

prinomide INN *antirheumatic* [also: prinomide tromethamine]

prinomide tromethamine USAN *antirheumatic* [also: prinomide]

prinoxodan USAN, INN *cardiotonic*

Prinzide tablets ℞ *antihypertensive; angiotensin-converting enzyme (ACE) inhibitor; diuretic* [lisinopril; hydrochlorothiazide] 10•12.5, 20•12.5, 20•25 mg

pristinamycin INN, BAN

Pristiq tablets ℞ *once-daily selective serotonin and norepinephrine reuptake inhibitor (SSNRI) for major depressive disorder (MDD); investigational (NDA filed) for postmenopausal vasomotor symptoms; investigational (Phase III) for fibromyalgia and diabetic peripheral neuropathy* [desvenlafaxine (as succinate)] 50, 100 mg (76, 152 mg)

privet, Egyptian *medicinal herb* [see: henna (*Lawsonia*)]

Privigen IM injection ℞ *passive immunizing agent* [immune globulin (IGIV)] 10% (5, 10, 20 g/dose) ⍰ Brevicon; parvaquone; porofocon A

Privine nasal spray, nose drops OTC *nasal decongestant* [naphazoline HCl] 0.05% ⍰ Brovana; paraffin; Preven; Profen II

prizidilol INN, BAN *antihypertensive* [also: prizidilol HCl]

prizidilol HCl USAN *antihypertensive* [also: prizidilol]

PRO 542 *investigational (Phase I/II) recombinant fusion protein, antigen-binding agent, and HIV attachment inhibitor for HIV infection*

PRO 2000 *investigational (Phase II) antiviral and microbicide gel for HIV infection*

Pro Fem cream OTC *natural progesterone from soy; hormone replacement therapy; postmenopausal osteoporosis preventative* [progesterone USP (in a liposomal base)] 2.5%

Pro Skin capsules OTC *vitamin/zinc supplement* [vitamins A, B₅, C, and E; zinc] 6250 IU•10 mg•100 mg•100 IU•10 mg

Proact *investigational (Phase III) immunomodulator for sarcoma*

proadifen INN *non-specific synergist* [also: proadifen HCl] ⍰ pridefine

proadifen HCl USAN *non-specific synergist* [also: proadifen]

ProAir HFA inhalation aerosol with a CFC-free propellant ℞ *sympathomimetic bronchodilator* [albuterol sulfate] 90 mcg/dose

ProAmatine tablets ℞ *vasopressor for orthostatic hypotension (orphan); also used for urinary incontinence* [midodrine HCl] 2.5, 5, 10 mg

proanthocyanidins *natural free radical scavenger found in grape seed extract and pine bark extract* [also: procyanidolic oligomers (PCOs); procyanidins]

Pro-Banthīne tablets ℞ *GI antispasmodic; peptic ulcer treatment adjunct; antisecretory* [propantheline bromide] 7.5, 15 mg

probarbital sodium NF, INN

Probax gel OTC *relief from minor oral irritations* [propolis] 2%

Probec-T tablets OTC *vitamin supplement* [multiple B vitamins; vitamin C] ±•600 mg ⍰ Prepcat

probenecid USP, INN, BAN *uricosuric for gout* 500 mg oral

probicromil calcium USAN *prophylactic antiallergic* [also: ambicromil]

Pro-Bionate capsules, powder OTC *natural intestinal bacteria; probiotic; dietary supplement; fever blister treatment; not generally regarded as safe and effective as an antidiarrheal* [Lactobacillus acidophilus] 2 billion CFU; 2 billion CFU/g

probiotics *a class of natural bacteria, such as Lactobacillus acidophilus, that favorably alter the microflora balance in the digestive system; an abundance of probiotic bacteria inhibit the growth of harmful bacteria and promote good digestion* [compare to: prebiotics]

probucol USAN, USP, INN *antihyperlipidemic*

probutate USAN *combining name for radicals or groups* [also: buteprate]

procainamide INN *antiarrhythmic* [also: procainamide HCl]

procainamide HCl USP *antiarrhythmic* [also: procainamide] 250, 375, 500, 750, 1000 mg oral; 100, 500 mg/mL injection

procaine INN *injectable local anesthetic* [also: procaine borate] ⑨ Baricon; Paracaine; Puregon; pyrrocaine

procaine borate NF *injectable local anesthetic* [also: procaine]

procaine HCl USP *injectable local anesthetic; sometimes used as a treatment for the overall effects of aging such as alopecia, arthritis, cerebral atherosclerosis, hypertension, progressive dementia, and sexual dysfunction; investigational (Phase II) for HIV infections* 1%, 2%

procaine penicillin BAN *bactericidal antibiotic* [also: penicillin G procaine]

ProcalAmine IV infusion ℞ *peripheral parenteral nutrition* [multiple essential and nonessential amino acids; electrolytes]

Procanbid film-coated extended-release tablets ℞ *twice-daily antiarrhythmic* [procainamide HCl] 500, 1000 mg

procarbazine INN *antineoplastic* [also: procarbazine HCl]

procarbazine HCl USAN, USP *antineoplastic for Hodgkin disease; investigational (orphan) for malignant glioma; also used for other lymphomas, melanoma, brain tumors, and lung cancer* [also: procarbazine]

Procardia capsules ℞ *calcium channel blocker; vasodilator for angina with or without vasospasm; also used for anal fissures* [nifedipine] 10, 20 mg ⑨ ParaGard T 380A; PerioGard

Procardia XL film-coated sustained-release tablets ℞ *coronary vasodilator for angina with or without vasospasm; calcium channel blocker for hypertension; also used for anal fissures* [nifedipine] 30, 60, 90 mg

procaterol INN, BAN *bronchodilator* [also: procaterol HCl]

procaterol HCl USAN *bronchodilator* [also: procaterol]

Prochieve vaginal gel in prefilled applicators ℞ *natural progestin; hormone replacement for secondary amenorrhea; hormone supplementation for assisted reproductive technology (ART) treatments* [progesterone] 4%, 8% (45, 90 mg)

prochlorperazine USP, INN *conventional (typical) phenothiazine antipsychotic for schizophrenia; anxiolytic; antiemetic for nausea and vomiting; also used for acute treatment of migraine headaches* 2.5, 5, 25 mg suppositories; 5 mg/mL injection

prochlorperazine bimaleate *conventional (typical) phenothiazine antipsychotic for schizophrenia; anxiolytic; antiemetic for nausea and vomiting; also used for acute treatment of migraine headaches*

prochlorperazine edisylate USP *conventional (typical) phenothiazine antipsychotic for schizophrenia; anxiolytic; antiemetic for nausea and vomiting; also used for acute treatment of migraine headaches* 5 mg/mL injection

prochlorperazine ethanedisulfonate [see: prochlorperazine edisylate]

prochlorperazine maleate USP *conventional (typical) phenothiazine antipsychotic for schizophrenia; anxiolytic; antiemetic for nausea and vomiting; also used for acute treatment of migraine headaches* 5, 10, 25 mg oral

prochlorperazine mesylate *conventional (typical) phenothiazine antipsychotic for schizophrenia; anxiolytic; antiemetic for nausea and vomiting; also used for acute treatment of migraine headaches*

procinolol INN

procinonide USAN, INN *adrenocortical steroid*

proclonol USAN, INN *anthelmintic; antifungal*

procodazole INN

proconvertin [see: factor VII]

Procort cream, spray OTC *corticosteroidal anti-inflammatory* [hydrocortisone] 1%

Procrit IV or subcu injection ℞ *hematopoietic to stimulate RBC production for anemia of chronic renal failure, HIV, and chemotherapy (orphan) and to reduce the need for blood transfusions* *in surgery* [epoetin alfa] 2000, 3000, 4000, 10 000, 20 000, 40 000 U/mL

Proctocort anorectal cream, suppositories ℞ *corticosteroidal anti-inflammatory* [hydrocortisone] 1%; 30 mg

ProctoCream-HC 2.5% anorectal cream ℞ *corticosteroidal anti-inflammatory* [hydrocortisone acetate] 2.5%

ProctoFoam NS anorectal aerosol foam OTC *anesthetic* [pramoxine HCl] 1%

Proctofoam-HC anorectal aerosol foam ℞ *corticosteroidal anti-inflammatory; anesthetic* [hydrocortisone acetate; pramoxine HCl] 1%•1%

Pro-Cute lotion OTC *moisturizer; emollient* ⬛ Baro-cat

procyanidolic oligomers (PCOs) *natural free radical scavenger found in grape seed extract and pine bark extract* [also: proanthocyanidins; procyanidins]

ProCycle Gold tablets OTC *vitamin/mineral/iron supplement* [multiple vitamins & minerals; iron; folic acid; biotin] ≛•3•0.067• ²⁄ mg

procyclidine HCl USP *anticholinergic; antiparkinsonian; skeletal muscle relaxant* [also: procyclidine]

procymate INN

Procysteine *investigational (orphan) immunomodulator for adult respiratory distress syndrome and amyotrophic lateral sclerosis* [oxothiazolidine carboxylate]

prodeconium bromide INN

Proderm aerosol spray OTC *wound treatment for decubitus ulcers* [castor oil; Peruvian balsam] 650•72.5 mg/0.82 mL

prodilidine INN *analgesic* [also: prodilidine HCl]

prodilidine HCl USAN *analgesic* [also: prodilidine]

prodipine INN

Prodium tablets OTC *urinary tract analgesic for relief of pain, burning, urgency, and frequency due to mucosal irritation from surgery, catheterization, endoscopic procedures, or trauma; adjunct to antibacterial agents for urinary tract infec-* tion [phenazopyridine HCl] 95 mg ⬛ Baridium; Perdiem; Pyridium

prodolic acid USAN, INN *anti-inflammatory*

Prodose AAD (adaptive aerosol delivery) (trademarked delivery device) *oral inhalation solution dispenser*

pro-drugs *a class of agents which metabolize into a therapeutic or more potent form in the body*

profadol INN *analgesic* [also: profadol HCl]

profadol HCl USAN *analgesic* [also: profadol]

Profasi powder for IM injection ℞ *a human-derived hormone used for prepubertal cryptorchidism or hypogonadism and to induce ovulation in anovulatory women* [chorionic gonadotropin] 500, 1000 U/mL

Pro-Fast HS; Pro-Fast SR capsules ℞ *anorexiant; CNS stimulant* [phentermine HCl] 18.75 mg; 37.5 mg

Pro-Fast SA tablets ℞ *anorexiant; CNS stimulant* [phentermine HCl] 8 mg

Profen II; Profen Forte extended-release tablets (discontinued 2007) ℞ *decongestant; expectorant* [pseudoephedrine HCl; guaifenesin] 45•800 mg; 90•800 mg ⬛ Brovana; paraffin; Preven; Privine

Profen II DM extended-release caplets (discontinued 2007) ℞ *antitussive; decongestant; expectorant* [dextromethorphan hydrobromide; pseudoephedrine HCl; guaifenesin] 30•45•800 mg

Profen II DM oral liquid (discontinued 2004) ℞ *antitussive; decongestant; expectorant* [dextromethorphan hydrobromide; pseudoephedrine HCl; guaifenesin] 10•15•200 mg/5 mL

Profen Forte DM sustained-release caplets (discontinued 2007) ℞ *antitussive; decongestant; expectorant* [dextromethorphan hydrobromide; pseudoephedrine HCl; guaifenesin] 60•90•800 mg ⬛ Parafon Forte DSC

Profenal Drop-Tainers (eye drops) (discontinued 2006) ℞ *nonsteroidal anti-*

inflammatory drug (NSAID); intraoperative miosis inhibitor [suprofen] 1%

profenamine INN *antiparkinsonian* [also: ethopropazine HCl; ethopropazine]

profenamine HCl [see: ethopropazine HCl]

profexalone INN

Profiber oral liquid OTC *enteral nutritional therapy* [lactose-free formula]

Profilnine SD powder for IV injection ℞ *systemic hemostatic; antihemophilic for factor IX deficiency (hemophilia B; Christmas disease) (orphan)* [coagulation factor IX concentrate, solvent/detergent treated] 250, 500, 1000 U

proflavine INN [also: proflavine dihydrochloride]

proflavine dihydrochloride NF [also: proflavine]

proflavine sulfate NF

proflazepam INN

ProFree/GP Weekly Enzymatic Cleaner tablets OTC *enzymatic cleaner for rigid gas permeable contact lenses* [papain]

progabide USAN, INN *anticonvulsant; muscle relaxant*

Progestasert IUD ℞ *intrauterine contraceptive* [progesterone] 38 mg

progesterone USP, INN *natural progestin; intrauterine contraceptive; hormone replacement for secondary amenorrhea; hormone supplementation for assisted reproductive technology (ART) treatments; investigational (orphan) for in vitro fertilization and embryo transfer* 50 mg/mL injection

progestins *a class of sex hormones that cause a sloughing of the endometrial lining, also used as a hormonal antineoplastic*

proglumetacin INN

proglumide USAN, INN, BAN, JAN *anticholinergic*

Proglycem capsules, oral suspension ℞ *glucose-elevating agent for hyperinsulinemia due to pancreatic cancer* [diazoxide] 50 mg; 50 mg/mL

Prograf capsules, IV infusion ℞ *immunosuppressant for liver, kidney, and*

heart transplants; also used for rheumatoid arthritis and Crohn disease; investigational (orphan) for graft-versus-host disease [tacrolimus] 0.5, 1, 5 mg; 5 mg/mL

proguanil INN, BAN *antimalarial; dihydrofolate reductase inhibitor* [also: chloroguanide HCl] ⊡ Pergonal

proguanil HCl [see: chloroguanide HCl]

ProHance injection ℞ *radiopaque contrast media for head and neck imaging and to enhance MRIs of the brain, spine, and other CNS tissue* [gadoteridol] 279.3 mg/mL

proheptazine INN

Prohist DM oral drops ℞ *antitussive; antihistamine; decongestant; for children 2–11 years* [dextromethorphan hydrobromide; brompheniramine maleate; pseudoephedrine HCl] 5•1•12 mg/mL

proinsulin human USAN *antidiabetic*

Prolacria *investigational (NDA filed) treatment for dry eye* [diquafosol tetrasodium]

Prolastin powder for IV infusion ℞ *enzyme replacement therapy for hereditary alpha₁-proteinase inhibitor deficiency, which leads to progressive panacinar emphysema (orphan)* [alpha₁-proteinase inhibitor] ≥ 20 mg/mL (500, 1000 mg/vial)

Proleukin powder for IV infusion ℞ *antineoplastic for metastatic melanoma and renal cell carcinoma (orphan); investigational (Phase III, orphan) for immunodeficiency diseases and acute myelogenous leukemia (AML); investigational (Phase II) for non-Hodgkin lymphoma* [aldesleukin] 18 million IU/mL

Prolex DH oral liquid ℞ *narcotic antitussive; expectorant* [hydrocodone bitartrate; potassium guaiacolsulfonate] 4.5•300 mg/5 mL

proligestone INN

proline (L-proline) USAN, USP, INN *nonessential amino acid; symbols: Pro, P* ⊡ Perlane; Prelone

prolintane INN *antidepressant* [also: prolintane HCl]

prolintane HCl USAN *antidepressant* [also: prolintane]

Prolixin Decanoate subcu or IM injection (discontinued 2006) ℞ *conventional (typical) phenothiazine antipsychotic for schizophrenia and psychotic disorders; used for prolonged parenteral neuroleptic therapy* [fluphenazine decanoate] 25 mg/mL

prolonium iodide INN

Proloprim tablets ℞ *anti-infective; antibacterial* [trimethoprim] 100, 200 mg

ProMACE (prednisone, methotrexate [with leucovorin rescue], Adriamycin, cyclophosphamide, etoposide) *chemotherapy protocol for non-Hodgkin lymphoma*

ProMACE/cytaBOM (ProMACE [above], cytarabine, bleomycin, Oncovin, mitoxantrone) *chemotherapy protocol for non-Hodgkin lymphoma*

ProMACE/MOPP (full course of ProMACE, followed by MOPP) *chemotherapy protocol for non-Hodgkin lymphoma*

Promacet tablets ℞ *barbiturate sedative; analgesic; antipyretic* [butalbital; acetaminophen] 50•650 mg

Promacta (available in Europe as Revolade) *investigational (NDA filed) once-daily oral thrombopoietin (TPO) receptor agonist to increase platelet counts in idiopathic thrombocytopenic purpura (ITP)* [eltrombopag]

promazine INN *phenothiazine antipsychotic* [also: promazine HCl] ② bromazine; Pramosone; primycin; puromycin

promazine HCl USP *phenothiazine antipsychotic* [also: promazine]

Promega Pearls (softgels) OTC *dietary supplement* [omega-3 fatty acids; multiple vitamins & minerals] 600• ±, 1000• ± mg

promegestone INN

promelase INN

promestriene INN

Prometh VC Plain syrup ℞ *decongestant; antihistamine* [phenylephrine HCl; promethazine HCl; alcohol 7%] 5•6.25 mg/5 mL

Prometh VC with Codeine syrup (discontinued 2007) ℞ *narcotic antitussive; antihistamine; decongestant* [codeine phosphate; promethazine HCl; phenylephrine HCl; alcohol 7%] 10•6.25•5 mg/5 mL

Prometh with Codeine syrup (discontinued 2007) ℞ *narcotic antitussive; antihistamine* [codeine phosphate; promethazine HCl; alcohol 7%] 10•6.25 mg/5 mL

Prometh with Dextromethorphan syrup (discontinued 2007) ℞ *antitussive; antihistamine* [dextromethorphan hydrobromide; promethazine HCl; alcohol 7%] 15•6.25 mg/5 mL

promethazine INN *phenothiazine antihistamine; antiemetic; antidopaminergic; motion sickness relief* [also: promethazine HCl] ② paramethasone; perimetazine

promethazine HCl USP *phenothiazine antihistamine; antiemetic; antidopaminergic; motion sickness relief* [also: promethazine] 12.5, 25, 50 mg oral; 6.25 mg/5 mL oral; 12.5, 25, 50 mg suppositories; 25, 50 mg/mL injection

promethazine HCl & codeine phosphate *antihistamine; narcotic antitussive* 6.25•10 mg/5 mL oral

promethazine HCl & meperidine HCl *narcotic analgesic; sedative* 25•50 mg oral

promethazine HCl & phenylephrine HCl *antihistamine; decongestant* 6.25•5 mg/5 mL oral

promethazine HCl & phenylephrine HCl & codeine phosphate *antihistamine; decongestant; narcotic antitussive* 6.25•5•10 mg/5 mL oral

promethazine teoclate INN *phenothiazine antihistamine*

Promethazine VC syrup ℞ *decongestant; antihistamine* [phenylephrine HCl; promethazine HCl] 5•6.25 mg/5 mL

Promethazine VC with Codeine
syrup (discontinued 2007) ℞ *narcotic antitussive; antihistamine; decongestant* [codeine phosphate; promethazine HCl; phenylephrine HCl; alcohol 7%] 10•6.25•5 mg/5 mL

Promethazine with Dextromethorphan Cough syrup ℞ *antitussive; antihistamine* [dextromethorphan hydrobromide; promethazine HCl; alcohol 7%] 15•6.25 mg/5 mL

Promethegan suppositories ℞ *antihistamine; sedative; antiemetic; motion sickness relief* [promethazine HCl] 12.5, 25, 50 mg

promethestrol [see: methestrol]

promethium *element (Pm)*

Prometrium softgels ℞ *natural progestin for secondary amenorrhea and to prevent endometrial hyperplasia* [progesterone, micronized] 100, 200 mg

Prominol tablets ℞ *barbiturate sedative; analgesic; antipyretic* [butalbital; acetaminophen] 50•650 mg ⊘ pirmenol

Promit IV injection ℞ *monovalent hapten for prevention of dextran-induced anaphylactic reactions; investigational (orphan) for cystic fibrosis* [dextran 1] 150 mg/mL

ProMod powder OTC *oral protein supplement* [D-whey protein concentrate; soy lecithin] ⊘ Paremyd; PerioMed

promolate INN

promoxolane INN

prompt insulin zinc [see: insulin zinc, prompt]

Promycin *investigational (Phase III, orphan) antineoplastic for head, neck, and cervical cancers* [porfiromycin]

Pronemia Hematinic capsules ℞ *hematinic* [ferrous fumarate; cyanocobalamin; ascorbic acid; intrinsic factor concentrate; folic acid] 115 mg• 15 mcg•150 mg•75 mg•1 mg

Pronestyl tablets (discontinued 2008) ℞ *antiarrhythmic* [procainamide HCl] 375, 500 mg

pronetalol INN [also: pronethalol]

pronethalol BAN [also: pronetalol]

Pronto shampoo OTC *pediculicide for lice* [pyrethrins; piperonyl butoxide] 0.33%•4% ⊘ burnet; Parnate

Propac powder OTC *oral protein supplement* [whey protein; lactose] ⊘ Barobag; Boropak

Propacet 100 film-coated tablets ℞ *narcotic analgesic; antipyretic* [propoxyphene napsylate; acetaminophen] 100•650 mg

propacetamol INN

propafenone INN, BAN *antiarrhythmic* [also: propafenone HCl]

propafenone HCl USAN *antiarrhythmic* [also: propafenone] 150, 225, 300 mg oral

propamidine INN, BAN

propaminodiphen [see: pramiverine]

propane NF *aerosol propellant* ⊘ Pre-Pen

1,2-propanediol [see: propylene glycol]

propanidid USAN, INN *intravenous anesthetic*

propanocaine INN

propanoic acid, sodium salt hydrate [see: sodium propionate]

2-propanol [see: isopropyl alcohol]

2-propanone [see: acetone]

propantheline bromide USP, INN *GI antispasmodic; peptic ulcer adjunct* 15 mg oral

PROPApH Acne cream OTC *keratolytic for acne* [salicylic acid] 2%

PROPApH Astringent Cleanser topical liquid OTC *keratolytic for acne* [salicylic acid; alcohol 55%] 2%

PROPApH Cleansing; PROPApH Cleansing for Sensitive Skin; PROPApH Cleansing Maximum Strength pads OTC *keratolytic for acne* [salicylic acid] 0.5%; 0.5%; 2%

PROPApH Cleansing for Normal/ Combination Skin; PROPApH Cleansing for Oily Skin lotion OTC *keratolytic for acne* [salicylic acid] 0.5%

PROPApH Foaming Face Wash topical liquid ℞ *keratolytic cleanser for acne* [salicylic acid] 2%

PROPApH Peel-Off Acne Mask OTC *keratolytic for acne* [salicylic acid] 2%

proparacaine HCl USP *topical ophthalmic anesthetic* [also: proxymetacaine] 0.5% eye drops

proparacaine HCl & fluorescein sodium *topical ophthalmic anesthetic; corneal disclosing agent* 0.5%•0.25% eye drops

propatyl nitrate USAN *coronary vasodilator* [also: propatylnitrate]

propatylnitrate INN *coronary vasodilator* [also: propatyl nitrate]

propazolamide INN

Propecia film-coated tablets ℞ *androgen hormone inhibitor for androgenic alopecia in men* [finasteride] 1 mg

1-propene homopolymer [see: polipropene 25]

propenidazole INN ⊘ parbendazole

propentofylline INN

p-**propenylanisole** [see: anethole]

propenzolate HCl USAN *anticholinergic* [also: oxyclipine]

propericiazine [see: periciazine]

properidine INN, BAN

propetamide INN

propetandrol INN

prophenamine HCl [see: ethopropazine HCl]

Pro-Phree powder OTC *supplement to breast milk* [protein-free formula with vitamins & minerals]

Prophyllin ointment OTC *antifungal; vulnerary; wound deodorant* [sodium propionate; chlorophyll derivatives] 5%•0.0125% ⊘ prifelone

propicillin INN, BAN

propikacin USAN, INN *antibacterial*

Propimex-1 powder OTC *formula for infants with propionic or methylmalonicacidemia*

Propimex-2 powder OTC *enteral nutritional therapy for propionic or methylmalonic acidemia*

Propine eye drops ℞ *antiglaucoma agent* [dipivefrin HCl] 0.1% ⊘ Pre-Pen

propinetidine INN

propiodal [see: prolonium iodide]

propiolactone (β-propiolactone) USAN, INN *disinfectant*

propiomazine USAN, INN *preanesthetic sedative*

propiomazine HCl USP *sedative; analgesic adjunct*

propionic acid NF *antimicrobial; acidifying agent*

propionyl erythromycin lauryl sulfate [see: erythromycin estolate]

propipocaine INN

propiram INN, BAN *narcotic agonist-antagonist analgesic* [also: propiram fumarate] ⊘ pyrabrom

propiram fumarate USAN *narcotic agonist-antagonist analgesic* [also: propiram]

propisergide INN

propitocaine HCl JAN *topical/local anesthetic* [also: prilocaine HCl]

propiverine INN

propizepine INN

Proplex T powder for IV infusion ℞ *systemic hemostatic; antihemophilic to correct factor VII, factor VIII (hemophilia A), and factor IX (hemophilia B; Christmas disease) deficiencies* [coagulation factors II, VII, IX, and X, heat treated] 30 mL

propofol USAN, INN, BAN *rapid-acting general anesthetic* 1% injection

propolis *natural resin collected from the buds of certain trees by bees and used as an antibiotic, anti-inflammatory, antioxidant, antineoplastic, fungicide, immune system stimulant, and vulnerary* ⊘ Bayer Plus

propoxate INN

propoxycaine INN *local anesthetic* [also: propoxycaine HCl]

propoxycaine HCl USP *local anesthetic* [also: propoxycaine]

propoxyphene HCl USAN, USP *narcotic analgesic for mild to moderate pain* [also: dextropropoxyphene HCl] 65 mg oral

propoxyphene napsylate USAN, USP *narcotic analgesic for mild to moderate pain*

propoxyphene napsylate & acetaminophen *narcotic analgesic* 100•500, 100•650 mg oral

propranolol INN, BAN *antianginal; antiarrhythmic; antihypertensive; antiadrenergic (β-blocker); migraine preventative* [also: propranolol HCl]

propranolol HCl USAN, USP *antianginal; antiarrhythmic; antihypertensive; antiadrenergic (β-blocker); migraine preventative* [also: propranolol] 10, 20, 40, 60, 80, 90, 120, 160 mg oral; 4, 8 mg/mL oral; 1 mg/mL injection

propranolol HCl & hydrochlorothiazide *antihypertensive; antiadrenergic (β-blocker); diuretic* 40•25, 80•25 mg oral

Propranolol Intensol oral solution ℞ *antianginal; antiarrhythmic; antihypertensive; antiadrenergic (β-blocker); migraine preventative* [propranolol HCl] 80 mg/mL

propyl *p*-aminobenzoate [see: risocaine]

propyl docetrizoate INN, BAN

propyl gallate NF *antioxidant*

propyl *p*-hydroxybenzoate [see: propylparaben]

propyl *p*-hydroxybenzoate, sodium salt [see: propylparaben sodium]

N-propylajmalinium tartrate [see: prajmalinum bitartrate]

propylene carbonate NF *gelling agent*

propylene glycol USP *humectant; solvent; moisturizer/lubricant; suspending and viscosity-increasing agent*

propylene glycol alginate NF *suspending agent; viscosity-increasing agent*

propylene glycol diacetate NF *solvent*

propylene glycol ether of methylcellulose [see: hydroxypropyl methylcellulose]

propylene glycol monostearate NF *emulsifying agent*

propylhexedrine USP, INN, BAN *vasoconstrictor; nasal decongestant*

propyliodone USP, INN *radiopaque contrast medium (56.7% iodine)*

propylorvinol [see: etorphine]

propylparaben USAN, NF *antifungal agent; preservative*

propylparaben sodium USAN, NF *antimicrobial preservative*

2-propylpentanoic acid [see: valproic acid]

propylthiouracil (PTU) USP, INN *thyroid inhibitor* 50 mg oral

2-propylvaleramide [see: valpromide]

propylvaleric acid [see: valproic acid]

propyperone INN

propyphenazone INN, BAN

propyromazine bromide INN

Pro-Q foam OTC *skin protectant* [dimethicone; glycerin; parabens] ⚠ Berocca

ProQuad powder for subcu injection ℞ *measles, mumps, rubella, and varicella vaccine* [measles, mumps, rubella, and varicella virus vaccine, live attenuated] 0.5 mL/dose

proquamezine BAN [also: aminopromazine]

proquazone USAN, INN *anti-inflammatory*

Proquin XR film-coated extended-release tablets ℞ *broad-spectrum fluoroquinolone antibiotic* [ciprofloxacin] 500 mg

proquinolate USAN, INN *coccidiostat for poultry*

Pro-Red syrup ℞ *narcotic antitussive; antihistamine; sleep aid; decongestant* [hydrocodone bitartrate; pyrilamine maleate; phenylephrine HCl] 2•8.38•5 mg/5 mL

prorenoate potassium USAN, INN *aldosterone antagonist*

proroxan INN *antiadrenergic (α-receptor)* [also: proroxan HCl]

proroxan HCl USAN *antiadrenergic (α-receptor)* [also: proroxan]

Proscar film-coated tablets ℞ *androgen hormone inhibitor for benign prostatic hyperplasia (BPH); investigational for aggressive prostate tumors* [finasteride] 5 mg

proscillaridin USAN, INN *cardiotonic*

proscillaridin A [see: proscillaridin]

Prosed/DS sugar-coated tablets ℞ *urinary antibiotic; antiseptic; analgesic; antispasmodic* [methenamine; phenyl salicylate; methylene blue; benzoic acid; atropine sulfate; hyoscyamine

sulfate] 81.6•36.2•10.8•9•0.06•
0.06 mg

ProSight Lutein capsules OTC *dietary supplement* [calcium; vitamins C and E; zinc; copper (but no lutein)] 22 mg•60 mg•30 IU•15 mg•2 mg

ProSobee oral liquid, powder for oral liquid OTC *hypoallergenic infant food* [soy protein formula]

ProSobee LIPIL oral liquid, powder for oral liquid OTC *hypoallergenic infant food fortified with omega-3 fatty acids* [soy protein formula]

ProSol 20% IV infusion ℞ *total parenteral nutrition* [multiple essential and nonessential amino acids] 20 g ℞ Buro-Sol; parsley

ProSom tablets (discontinued 2007) ℞ *benzodiazepine sedative and hypnotic* [estazolam] 1, 2 mg

Prosorba Column for dialysis ℞ *treatment for rheumatoid arthritis* [protein A]

prospidium chloride INN

prostacyclin [now: epoprostenol]

prostaglandin agonists *a class of antiglaucoma agents that reduce intraocular pressure (IOP) by increasing the outflow of aqueous humor*

prostaglandin E_1 (PGE$_1$) [now: alprostadil]

prostaglandin E_1 enol ester *investigational (orphan) for advanced chronic critical limb ischemia*

prostaglandin E_2 (PGE$_2$) [see: dinoprostone]

prostaglandin $F_{2\alpha}$ (PGF$_{2\alpha}$) [see: dinoprost]

prostaglandin I_2 (PGI$_2$) [now: epoprostenol]

prostaglandin X (PGX) [now: epoprostenol]

prostaglandins *a class of agents that stimulate uterine contractions, used for abortions, cervical ripening, and postpartum hemorrhage*

prostalene USAN, INN *prostaglandin*

ProstaScint IV infusion *radiodiagnostic imaging agent for new or recurrent prostate cancer and its metastases* [cap-

romab pendetide, radiolabeled with indium In 111] 0.5 mg

Pro-Stat 64; Pro-Stat 101 oral liquid OTC *enteral nutritional therapy* [collagen hydrolysate formula] 500 g protein per 946 mL ℞ Periostat

Prostigmin subcu or IM injection ℞ *cholinergic urinary stimulant for postsurgical urinary retention; treatment for myasthenia gravis; antidote to neuromuscular blockers* [neostigmine methylsulfate] 1:1000 (1 mg/mL), 1:2000 (0.5 mg/mL), 1:4000 (0.25 mg/mL) (1:400 [2.5 mg/mL] is available in Canada)

Prostigmin tablets ℞ *myasthenia gravis treatment; antidote for neuromuscular blockers* [neostigmine bromide] 15 mg

Prostin E2 vaginal suppository ℞ *prostaglandin-type abortifacient* [dinoprostone] 20 mg ℞ perastine; prazitone

Prostin VR Pediatric IV injection ℞ *vasodilator; platelet aggregation inhibitor* [alprostadil] 500 mcg/mL

prosulpride INN

prosultiamine INN

ProSure oral liquid OTC *enteral nutritional therapy for cancer patients* 8 oz.

protactinium *element (Pa)*

protamine sulfate USP, INN *antidote to heparin overdose* [also: protamine sulphate] 10 mg/mL IV infusion

protamine sulphate BAN *antidote to heparin overdose* [also: protamine sulfate]

protamine zinc insulin (PZI) INN *antidiabetic* [also: insulin, protamine zinc; insulin zinc protamine]

protargin, mild [see: silver protein, mild]

protease *digestive enzyme (digests protein)* [100 IU/mg in pancrelipase; 25 IU/mg in pancreatin] ℞ Brite Eyes II; Pretz

protease inhibitors *a class of antivirals that block HIV replication*

proteasome inhibitors *a class of antineoplastics*

ProTech First Aid Stik topical liquid
OTC *analgesic; antiseptic* [lidocaine;
povidone-iodine] 2.5% • 10%

Protectol Medicated topical powder
OTC *antifungal* [calcium undecylen-
ate] 15%

Protegra softgels OTC *vitamin/mineral
supplement* [multiple vitamins &
minerals]

protein A *treatment for rheumatoid
arthritis* ⊉ Pre-Attain

protein C concentrate (human)
*thrombolytic; replacement therapy for
severe congenital protein C deficiency
in children and adults to prevent or
treat thrombosis, pulmonary emboli,
and purpura fulminans (orphan)*

protein hydrolysate USP *fluid and
nutrient replenisher*

α₁-proteinase inhibitor [see: alpha₁-
proteinase inhibitor]

Protenate IV infusion ℞ *blood volume
expander for shock due to burns,
trauma, and surgery* [plasma protein
fraction] 5%

proterguride INN

protheobromine INN

prothionamide BAN [also: protion-
amide]

prothipendyl INN

prothipendyl HCl [see: prothipendyl]

prothixene INN

prothrombin complex, activated BAN

ProTime test kit for home use OTC *in
vitro diagnostic aid for the management
of anticoagulation therapy*

protiofate INN

protionamide INN [also: prothion-
amide]

protirelin USAN, INN, BAN *prothyrotro-
pin; diagnostic aid for thyroid function;
investigational (orphan) for infant respiratory distress syndrome of prematurity and amyotrophic lateral sclerosis*

protizinic acid INN

protokylol HCl

proton pump inhibitors (PPIs) *a
class of gastric antisecretory agents that
inhibit the aTPase "proton pump"
within the gastric parietal cell* [also

called: aTPase inhibitors; substituted
benzimidazoles]

Protonix delayed-release tablets,
enteric-coated delayed-release granules for oral suspension ℞ *proton
pump inhibitor for erosive esophagitis
associated with gastroesophageal reflux
disease (GERD) and Zollinger-Ellison
syndrome* [pantoprazole sodium] 20,
40 mg; 40 mg/pkt

Protonix I.V. powder for infusion ℞
*proton pump inhibitor for erosive esophagitis associated with gastroesoph-
ageal reflux disease (GERD) and
Zollinger-Ellison syndrome* [pantopra-
zole sodium] 40 mg/vial

Protopam Chloride IV injection ℞
*antidote for organophosphate poisoning
and anticholinesterase overdose* [prali-
doxime chloride] 1 g

Protopic ointment ℞ *treatment for
moderate to severe atopic dermatitis;
also used for vitiligo and psoriasis*
[tacrolimus] 0.03%, 0.1%

Protostat tablets ℞ *antibiotic; antiprotozoal; amebicide* [metronidazole]
250, 500 mg

protoveratrine A

Protox *investigational (orphan) for toxoplasmosis of AIDS* [poloxamer 331]

protriptyline INN *tricyclic antidepressant* [also: protriptyline HCl]

protriptyline HCl USAN, USP *tricyclic
antidepressant* [also: protriptyline] 5,
10 mg oral

Protropin powder for subcu or IM
injection (discontinued 2005) ℞
*growth hormone for congenital growth
failure due to lack of endogenous growth
hormone (orphan); investigational
(orphan) for short stature due to Turner
syndrome* [somatrem] 5, 10 mg (15,
30 IU) per vial

Protuss oral liquid (discontinued 2005)
℞ *narcotic antitussive; expectorant*
[hydrocodone bitartrate; potassium
guaiacolsulfonate] 5 • 300 mg/5 mL
⊉ Pretz

Protuss DM sustained-release tablets
(discontinued 2004) ℞ *antitussive;*

decongestant; expectorant [dextromethorphan hydrobromide; pseudoephedrine HCl; guaifenesin] 30•60•600 mg

Protuss-D oral liquid (discontinued 2005) ℞ *narcotic antitussive; decongestant; expectorant* [hydrocodone bitartrate; pseudoephedrine HCl; potassium guaiacolsulfonate] 5•30•300 mg/5 mL ⧳ Pretz-D

prourokinase [see: saruplase]

Provenge *investigational (NDA filed) immunotherapy agent for hormone-refractory metastatic prostate cancer* [sipuleucel-T]

Proventil inhalation aerosol (discontinued 2008) ℞ *sympathomimetic bronchodilator* [albuterol] 90 mcg/dose

Proventil Repetabs (extended-release tablets) (discontinued 2004) ℞ *sympathomimetic bronchodilator* [albuterol sulfate] 4 mg

Proventil tablets, syrup, solution for inhalation ℞ *sympathomimetic bronchodilator* [albuterol sulfate] 2, 4 mg; 4 mg; 2 mg/5 mL; 0.5% (15 mg/3 mL)

Proventil HFA inhalation aerosol with a CFC-free propellant ℞ *sympathomimetic bronchodilator* [albuterol sulfate] 90 mcg/dose

Provera tablets ℞ *synthetic progestin for secondary amenorrhea, abnormal uterine bleeding, and endometrial hyperplasia* [medroxyprogesterone acetate] 2.5, 5, 10 mg

Provigil caplets ℞ *analeptic for excessive daytime sleepiness due to narcolepsy (orphan), obstructive sleep apnea, or shift work sleep disorder (SWSD); also used for fatigue associated with multiple sclerosis* [modafinil] 100, 200 mg ⧳ Pravachol

Proviron *brand name for mesterolone, an androgen abused with anabolic steroid street drugs*

ProVisc prefilled syringes ℞ *cohesive viscoelastic agent for ophthalmic surgery* [hyaluronate sodium] 0.55, 0.85 mL

provitamin A [see: beta carotene]

Provocholine powder for inhalation solution ℞ *bronchoconstrictor for in*

vivo pulmonary function challenge test [methacholine chloride] 100 mg/5 mL

proxazole USAN, INN *smooth muscle relaxant; analgesic; anti-inflammatory*

proxazole citrate USAN *smooth muscle relaxant; analgesic; anti-inflammatory*

proxetil INN *combining name for radicals or groups*

proxibarbal INN

proxibutene INN

proxicromil USAN, INN *antiallergic*

proxifezone INN

proxorphan INN *analgesic; antitussive* [also: proxorphan tartrate]

proxorphan tartrate USAN *analgesic; antitussive* [also: proxorphan]

proxymetacaine INN, BAN *topical ophthalmic anesthetic* [also: proparacaine HCl]

proxymetacaine HCl [see: proparacaine HCl]

proxyphylline INN, BAN

Prozac Pulvules (capsules), oral solution ℞ *selective serotonin reuptake inhibitor (SSRI) for major depressive disorder (MDD), obsessive-compulsive disorder (OCD), bulimia nervosa, premenstrual dysphoric disorder (PMDD), and panic disorder; investigational (orphan) for autism* [fluoxetine HCl] 10, 20, 40 mg; 20 mg/5 mL

Prozac tablets (discontinued 2008) ℞ *selective serotonin reuptake inhibitor (SSRI) for major depressive disorder (MDD), obsessive-compulsive disorder (OCD), bulimia nervosa, premenstrual dysphoric disorder (PMDD), and panic disorder; investigational (orphan) for autism* [fluoxetine HCl] 10 mg

Prozac Weekly enteric-coated delayed-release pellets in capsules ℞ *selective serotonin reuptake inhibitor (SSRI) for major depressive disorder (MDD), obsessive-compulsive disorder (OCD), and bulimia nervosa; once-weekly dosing for maintenance* [fluoxetine HCl] 90 mg

prozapine INN ⧳ prazepine

Prozine-50 IM injection ℞ *conventional (typical) antipsychotic* [promazine HCl] 50 mg/mL

prucalopride HCl USAN *prokinetic agent for severe constipation*

prucalopride succinate USAN *prokinetic agent for severe constipation*

Prudoxin cream ℞ *antihistamine; antipruritic* [doxepin HCl] 5% ⧠ pyridoxine

prulifloxacin *investigational (Phase III) antibiotic for traveler's diarrhea*

Prunella vulgaris medicinal herb [see: woundwort]

Prunus africana medicinal herb [see: pygeum]

Prunus americana; P. domestica; P. spinosa medicinal herb [see: plum]

Prunus amygdalus medicinal herb [see: almond]

Prunus armeniaca medicinal herb [see: apricot]

Prunus persica medicinal herb [see: peach]

Prunus serotina medicinal herb [see: wild black cherry]

Prunus virginiana medicinal herb [see: wild cherry]

Prussian blue [see: ferric hexacyanoferrate]

PSE (pseudoephedrine HCl) [q.v.]

PSE 120/MSC 2.5 sustained-release tablets ℞ *decongestant; anticholinergic to dry mucosal secretions* [pseudoephedrine HCl; methscopolamine nitrate] 120•2.5 mg

PSE 15/CPM 2 chewable tablets ℞ *decongestant; antihistamine* [pseudoephedrine HCl; chlorpheniramine maleate] 15•2 mg

PSE Brom DM syrup ℞ *antitussive; antihistamine; decongestant* [dextromethorphan hydrobromide; brompheniramine maleate; pseudoephedrine HCl] 30•4•60 mg/5 mL

PSE CPM chewable tablets ℞ *decongestant; antihistamine* [pseudoephedrine HCl; chlorpheniramine maleate] 15•2 mg

PSE-BPM oral liquid ℞ *decongestant; antihistamine* [pseudoephedrine HCl; brompheniramine maleate] 60•4 mg/5 mL

Pseudo Carb Pediatric oral liquid ℞ *decongestant; antihistamine* [pseudoephedrine HCl; carbinoxamine maleate] 12.5•2 mg/5 mL

Pseudo CM TR timed-release tablets (discontinued 2007) ℞ *decongestant; antihistamine; anticholinergic to dry mucosal secretions* [pseudoephedrine HCl; chlorpheniramine maleate; methscopolamine nitrate] 120•8•2.5 mg

Pseudo Cough oral liquid OTC *antitussive; decongestant; expectorant* [dextromethorphan hydrobromide; pseudoephedrine HCl; guaifenesin] 15•32•175 mg/5 mL

Pseudo-Carb DM Pediatric oral liquid ℞ *antitussive; antihistamine; decongestant; for adults and children ≥ 18 months* [dextromethorphan hydrobromide; carbinoxamine maleate; pseudoephedrine HCl] 15•3•12.5 mg/5 mL

pseudoephedrine INN, BAN *vasoconstrictor; nasal decongestant* [also: pseudoephedrine HCl]

pseudoephedrine HCl USAN, USP *vasoconstrictor; nasal decongestant* [also: pseudoephedrine] 30, 60 mg oral; 30 mg/5 mL oral

pseudoephedrine HCl & brompheniramine maleate *decongestant; antihistamine* 60•4 mg/5 mL oral

pseudoephedrine HCl & brompheniramine maleate & hydrocodone bitartrate *decongestant; antihistamine; narcotic antitussive* 30•3•2.5 mg/5 mL oral

pseudoephedrine HCl & carbinoxamine maleate *nasal decongestant; antihistamine* 60•4 mg/5 mL oral; 25•2 mg/mL oral

pseudoephedrine HCl & carbinoxamine maleate & hydrocodone bitartrate *nasal decongestant; antihistamine; antitussive* 30•2•5 mg/5 mL oral

pseudoephedrine HCl & chlorpheniramine maleate *decongestant;*

antihistamine 100•12, 120•8, 120•
12 mg oral

**pseudoephedrine HCl & dextro-
methorphan hydrobromide &
guaifenesin** *decongestant; antitussive; expectorant* 90•60•800 mg oral

**pseudoephedrine HCl & guaifene-
sin** *decongestant; expectorant* 45•800,
48•595, 50•1200, 60•500, 85•795,
90•800 mg oral

**pseudoephedrine HCl & triprolidine
HCl** *decongestant; antihistamine* 60•
2.5 mg/10 mL oral

pseudoephedrine polistirex USAN
nasal decongestant

pseudoephedrine sulfate USAN, USP
bronchodilator; nasal decongestant

pseudoephedrine tannate *bronchodilator; nasal decongestant*

**pseudoephedrine tannate & chlor-
pheniramine tannate** *decongestant;
antihistamine*

Pseudomonas aeruginosa **purified
extract** *investigational (orphan) agent
to increase platelet count in immune
thrombocytopenic purpura*

Pseudomonas **immune globulin** [see:
mucoid exopolysaccharide *Pseudomonas* hyperimmune globulin]

pseudomonic acid A [see: mupirocin]

Pseudovent dual-release capsules ℞
decongestant; expectorant [pseudo-
ephedrine HCl (extended release);
guaifenesin (immediate release)]
120•250 mg

Pseudovent-PED dual-release capsules
℞ *decongestant; expectorant* [pseudo-
ephedrine HCl (extended release);
guaifenesin (immediate release)]
60•300 mg

psilocin *a hallucinogenic street drug
closely related to psilocybin* 🔲 salicin;
Selsun; xylazine

psilocybin BAN *a hallucinogenic street
drug derived from the* Psilocybe mexi-
cana *mushroom* [also: psilocybine] 🔲
Soluspan

psilocybine INN *a hallucinogenic street
drug derived from the* Psilocybe mexi-

cana *mushroom* [also: psilocybin] 🔲
Soluspan

psoralens *a class of oral or topical skin
photosensitizing agents used with ultraviolet A light (320–400 nm wavelength)
for the treatment of severe recalcitrant
psoriasis*

Psor-a-set bar OTC *keratolytic skin
cleanser* [salicylic acid] 2%

Psorcon E cream, ointment ℞ *corticosteroidal anti-inflammatory* [diflora-
sone diacetate] 0.05%

Psoriatec cream ℞ (available OTC in
Canada as **Micanol**) *antipsoriatic*
[anthralin] 1% 🔲 Saratoga; Zyrtec

PsoriGel (discontinued 2006) OTC
antipsoriatic; antiseborrheic; antiseptic
[coal tar solution; alcohol 28.3%]
7.5% 🔲 Seroquel; Surgel

psyllium *(Plantago ovata) medicinal
herb* [see: plantain]

psyllium husk USP *bulk laxative* 🔲
Sulmasque

psyllium hydrocolloid *bulk laxative*

psyllium hydrophilic mucilloid *bulk
laxative*

psyllium seed [see: plantago seed]

P-Tann D oral suspension (discontinued 2008) ℞ *decongestant; antihistamine* [phenylephrine tannate; chlorpheniramine tannate] 10•8 mg/5 mL

P-Tanna 12 pediatric oral suspension
℞ *decongestant; antihistamine; sleep
aid* [phenylephrine tannate; pyrilamine tannate] 5•30 mg/5 mL 🔲
betony; biotin; Bitin; butane

**PTC (plasma thromboplastin com-
ponent)** [see: factor IX]

P.T.E.-4; P.T.E.-5 IV injection ℞
intravenous nutritional therapy [multi-
ple trace elements (metals)]

pterins *a class of investigational antineoplastics*

pteroyldiglutamic acid (PDGA)

pteroylglutamic acid (PGA) [see:
folic acid]

P-Tex oral suspension ℞ *antihistamine*
[brompheniramine tannate] 10 mg/5
mL

PTFE (polytetrafluoroethylene)
[see: polytef]

PTU (propylthiouracil) [q.v.]

Pt/VM (Platinol, VM-26) *chemotherapy protocol for pediatric neuroblastoma*

ptyalagogues *a class of agents that stimulate the secretion of saliva* [also called: sialagogues]

puccoon, yellow *medicinal herb* [see: goldenseal]

Pueraria lobata; P. thunbergiana *medicinal herb* [see: kudzu]

puffball *medicinal herb* [see: dandelion]

Pulexn DM syrup (discontinued 2007) ℞ *antitussive; expectorant* [dextromethorphan hydrobromide; guaifenesin] 20•200 mg/10 mL

Pulmicort Flexhaler (dry powder in a metered-dose inhaler) ℞ *corticosteroidal anti-inflammatory for chronic asthma* [budesonide] 80, 160 mcg/dose

Pulmicort Respules (single-dose ampule for inhalation) ℞ *corticosteroidal anti-inflammatory for chronic asthma in children* [budesonide] 0.25, 0.5, 1 mg

Pulmicort Turbuhaler (dry powder in a metered-dose inhaler) ℞ *corticosteroidal anti-inflammatory for chronic asthma* [budesonide] 160 mcg/dose

Pulmocare ready-to-use oral liquid OTC *enteral nutritional therapy for pulmonary problems*

Pulmonaria officinalis *medicinal herb* [see: lungwort]

pulmonary surfactant replacement, porcine [now: poractant alfa]

Pulmozyme solution for nebulization ℞ *reduces respiratory viscoelasticity of sputum in cystic fibrosis* (orphan) [dornase alfa] 1 mg/mL

pulse VAC (vincristine, Adriamycin, cyclophosphamide) *chemotherapy protocol for sarcomas* [also: VAC; VAC pulse]

PulsePak (trademarked packaging form) *one-week dosage pack*

Pulvule (trademarked dosage form) *bullet-shaped capsule*

Pulzium *investigational (NDA filed) antiarrhythmic for atrial fibrillation* [tedisamil]

pumice USP *dental abrasive*

pumitepa INN

Punctum Plug ℞ *blocks the puncta and canaliculus to eliminate tear loss in keratitis sicca* [silicone plug]

Punica granatum *medicinal herb* [see: pomegranate]

Puralube ophthalmic ointment OTC *ocular moisturizer/lubricant* [white petrolatum; mineral oil]

Puralube Tears eye drops OTC *moisturizer/lubricant* [polyvinyl alcohol; polyethylene glycol 400] 1%•1%

purgatives *a class of agents that cause vigorous evacuation of the bowels by increasing bulk, stimulating peristaltic action, etc.* [also called: cathartics]

Purge oral liquid OTC *stimulant laxative* [castor oil] 95% ☒ borage; Pro-Q

Puricase *investigational (Phase III, orphan) agent for hyperuricemia due to severe gout* [PEG-uricase]

purified cotton [see: cotton, purified]

purified protein derivative (PPD) of tuberculin [see: tuberculin]

purified rayon [see: rayon, purified]

purified siliceous earth [see: siliceous earth, purified]

purified water [see: water, purified]

H-purin-6-amine [see: adenine]

Purinethol tablets ℞ *antimetabolite antineoplastic for acute lymphocytic, lymphoblastic, myelogenous, and myelomonocytic leukemias* [mercaptopurine] 50 mg ☒ Prenatal; pyrantel

puromycin USAN, INN *antineoplastic; antiprotozoal (Trypanosoma)* ☒ Pramosone; primycin; promazine

puromycin HCl USAN *antineoplastic; antiprotozoal (Trypanosoma)*

purple angelica *medicinal herb* [see: angelica]

purple boneset *medicinal herb* [see: boneset]

purple cone flower *medicinal herb* [see: echinacea]

purple leptandra *medicinal herb* [see: Culver root]

Purpose Alpha Hydroxy Moisture lotion, cream OTC *moisturizer; emollient; exfoliant* [glycolic acid] 8%

Purpose Dry Skin cream OTC *moisturizer; emollient*

Purpose Soap bar OTC *therapeutic skin cleanser*

purshiana bark *medicinal herb* [see: cascara sagrada]

purslain, water *medicinal herb* [see: brooklime]

purvain *medicinal herb* [see: blue vervain]

pussywillow *medicinal herb* [see: willow]

PUVA *an acronym for psoralens (P) and ultraviolet A (UVA) light, used as a treatment for severe recalcitrant psoriasis* [see: psoralens; methoxsalen]

PVA (polyvinyl alcohol) [q.v.]

PVA (prednisone, vincristine, asparaginase) *chemotherapy protocol for acute lymphocytic leukemia (ALL)*

PVB (Platinol, vinblastine, bleomycin) *chemotherapy protocol for testicular cancer and adenocarcinoma*

PVC (polyvinyl chloride) [see: polyvinyl chloride, radiopaque]

PVDA (prednisone, vincristine, daunorubicin, asparaginase) *chemotherapy protocol for acute lymphocytic leukemia (ALL)*

PVP; PVP-16 (Platinol, VP-16) *chemotherapy protocol*

PVP (polyvinylpyrrolidone) [now: povidone]

PVS Basics ℞ *hydrophobic contact lens material* [paflufocon E]

P-V-Tussin caplets ℞ *narcotic antitussive; antihistamine* [hydrocodone bitartrate; pseudoephedrine HCl] 5•60 mg

P-V-Tussin syrup ℞ *narcotic antitussive; antihistamine; decongestant* [hydrocodone bitartrate; chlorpheniramine maleate; pseudoephedrine HCl; alcohol 5%] 2.5•2•30 mg/5 mL

Pycnanthemum virginianum medicinal herb [see: wild hyssop]

Pycnogenol OTC *natural free radical scavenger* [pine bark extract]

pygeum (Prunus africana; Pygeum africanum) bark *medicinal herb for prostate gland enlargement and urinary disorders* ⁇ BayGam; PCM

Pylera capsules ℞ *triple therapy for the eradication of H. pylori infections* [bismuth subcitrate potassium; metronidazole; tetracycline HCl] 140•125•125 mg

Pylori-Check test kit for professional use ℞ *in vivo diagnostic aid for H. pylori in the breath*

Pyloriset reagent kit for professional use ℞ *in vitro diagnostic aid for GI disorders*

pyrabrom USAN *antihistamine* ⁇ propiram

pyradone [see: aminopyrine]

pyrantel INN *anthelmintic for ascariasis (roundworm) and enterobiasis (pinworm)* [also: pyrantel pamoate] ⁇ Prenatal

pyrantel pamoate USAN, USP *anthelmintic for ascariasis (roundworm) and enterobiasis (pinworm)* (base=34.7%) [also: pyrantel]

pyrantel tartrate USAN *anthelmintic*

pyrathiazine HCl [see: parathiazine]

pyrazinamide (PZA) USP, INN, BAN *bactericidal; primary tuberculostatic* 500 mg oral

pyrazinecarboxamide [see: pyrazinamide]

pyrazofurin USAN *antineoplastic* [also: pirazofurin]

pyrazoline [see: antipyrine]

pyrazolopyrimidines *a class of sedative/hypnotics with rapid onset and short duration of action, used in the short-term treatment of insomnia*

pyrbenzindole [see: benzindopyrine HCl]

pyrbuterol HCl [see: pirbuterol HCl]

pyrethrins *a class of natural pesticides derived from pyrethrum flowers, especially Chrysanthemum cinerariaefolium and C. coccineum*

Pyrethrum parthenium *medicinal herb* [see: feverfew]

pyricarbate INN [also: pyridinol carbamate]

pyridarone INN ② Paredrine

Pyridiate tablets ℞ *urinary tract analgesic for relief of pain, burning, urgency, and frequency due to mucosal irritation from surgery, catheterization, endoscopic procedures, or trauma; adjunct to antibacterial agents for urinary tract infection* [phenazopyridine HCl] 100 mg

4-pyridinamine [see: fampridine]

2-pyridine aldoxime methylchloride (2-PAM) [see: pralidoxime chloride]

3-pyridine carboxamide [see: niacinamide; nicotinamide]

3-pyridinecarboxylic acid [see: niacin]

4-pyridinecarboxylic acid hydrazide [see: isoniazid]

3-pyridinecarboxylic acid methyl ester [see: methyl nicotinate]

3-pyridinemethanol [see: nicotinyl alcohol]

2-pyridinemethanol [see: piconol]

3-pyridinemethanol tartrate [see: nicotinyl tartrate]

pyridinol carbamate JAN [also: pyricarbate]

Pyridium tablets ℞ *urinary tract analgesic for relief of pain, burning, urgency, and frequency due to mucosal irritation from surgery, catheterization, endoscopic procedures, or trauma; adjunct to antibacterial agents for urinary tract infection* [phenazopyridine HCl] 100, 200 mg ② Baridium; Perdiem; Prodium

Pyridium Plus tablets ℞ *urinary analgesic; antispasmodic; sedative* [phenazopyridine HCl; hyoscyamine hydrobromide; butabarbital] 150•0.3•15 mg

pyridofylline INN

pyridostigmine bromide USP, INN *cholinergic/anticholinesterase muscle stimulant* 60 mg oral

pyridoxal-5′-phosphate [see: pyridoxine HCl]

pyridoxamine [see: pyridoxine HCl]

pyridoxine (vitamin B₆) INN *water-soluble vitamin; enzyme cofactor* [also: pyridoxine HCl] ② Prudoxin

pyridoxine HCl (vitamin B₆) USP *water-soluble vitamin; enzyme cofactor; treatment for vitamin B₆ deficiency; also used for hydrazine poisoning, premenstrual syndrome (PMS), oxalate kidney stones, pregnancy-related nausea and vomiting, and carpal tunnel syndrome* [also: pyridoxine] 50, 100, 250, 500 mg oral; 100 mg/mL injection

β-pyridylcarbinol [see: nicotinyl alcohol]

pyridylmethanol *me+* [see: nicotinyl alcohol]

pyrilamine maleate USP *anticholinergic; nonselective ethylenediamine antihistamine; sleep aid* [also: mepyramine]

pyrilamine tannate USP *anticholinergic; nonselective ethylenediamine antihistamine; sleep aid* [also: mepyramine]

pyrilamine tannate & phenylephrine tannate & chlorpheniramine tannate *antihistamine; decongestant* 12.5•5•2 mg/5 mL oral

pyrimethamine USP, INN *folic acid antagonist for malaria suppression and transmission control; toxoplasmosis treatment adjunct*

pyrimethamine & sulfadiazine *treatment for* Toxoplasma gondii *encephalitis (orphan)*

pyrimidinedione [see: uracil]

pyrimitate INN, BAN

pyrinoline USAN, INN *antiarrhythmic* ② bornelone

Pyrinyl Plus shampoo OTC *pediculicide for lice* [pyrethrins; piperonyl butoxide] 0.3%•4%

pyrithen [see: chlorothen citrate]

pyrithione sodium USAN *topical antimicrobial*

pyrithione zinc USAN, INN, BAN *topical antibacterial; antifungal; antiseborrheic*

pyrithyldione INN

pyritidium bromide INN

pyritinol INN, BAN

Pyrlex oral suspension ℞ *antihistamine; sleep aid* [pyrilamine tannate] 12 mg/ 5 mL 🔊 Perloxx

Pyrlex CB oral suspension ℞ *antitussive; antihistamine; sleep aid* [carbetapentane tannate; pyrilamine tannate] 22.5•12 mg/5 mL

pyrodifenium bromide [see: prifinium bromide]

pyrogallic acid [see: pyrogallol]

pyrogallol NF 🔊 pargolol

pyrophendane INN 🔊 pirfenidone

pyrophenindane [see: pyrophendane]

pyrovalerone INN *CNS stimulant* [also: pyrovalerone HCl]

pyrovalerone HCl USAN *CNS stimulant* [also: pyrovalerone]

pyroxamine INN *antihistamine* [also: pyroxamine maleate] 🔊 piroximone

pyroxamine maleate USAN *antihistamine* [also: pyroxamine]

pyroxylin USP, INN *pharmaceutic necessity for collodion* 🔊 perhexiline

pyrrobutamine phosphate USP

pyrrocaine USAN, INN *local anesthetic* 🔊 Baricon; Paracaine; procaine; Puregon

pyrrocaine HCl NF

pyrrolifene INN *analgesic* [also: pyrroliphene HCl]

pyrrolifene HCl [see: pyrroliphene HCl]

pyrroliphene HCl USAN *analgesic* [also: pyrrolifene]

pyrrolnitrin USAN, INN *antifungal*

pyrroxane [now: proroxan HCl]

Pyrroxate caplets OTC *decongestant; antihistamine; analgesic; antipyretic* [phenylephrine HCl; chlorpheniramine maleate; acetaminophen] 10• 4•650 mg 🔊 Percocet

Pyrus malus medicinal herb [see: apple]

pyruvate *investigational (orphan) for interstitial lung disease*

pyrvinium chloride INN

pyrvinium embonate [see: pyrvinium pamoate]

pyrvinium pamoate USP *anthelmintic* [also: viprynium embonate]

pytamine INN

PYtest reagent kit for professional use ℞ *in vitro diagnostic aid for* H. pylori *in the breath* [carbon C 14 urea] 1 mCi

PYY (peptide YY) [q.v.]

PZA (pyrazinamide) [q.v.]

PZI (protamine zinc insulin) [q.v.]

Qdall sustained-release capsules (discontinued 2007) ℞ *decongestant; antihistamine* [pseudoephedrine HCl; chlorpheniramine maleate] 100•12 mg

Qdall AR dual-release capsules ℞ *antihistamine* [chlorpheniramine maleate] 12 mg (2 mg immediate release; 10 mg sustained release)

Q-Pap tablets OTC *analgesic; antipyretic* [acetaminophen] 325, 500 mg 🔊 CABOP; CAP-BOP; CPOB; cubeb

Q-Pap, Children's oral liquid, oral suspension, elixir OTC *analgesic; antipyretic* [acetaminophen] 160 mg/5 mL

Q-Pap Infant Drops OTC *analgesic; antipyretic* [acetaminophen] 100 mg/mL

Q-Tapp elixir OTC *decongestant; antihistamine* [pseudoephedrine HCl; brompheniramine maleate] 30•2 mg/10 mL 🔊 CTAB; K-Tab

Q-Tapp DM Cold & Cough elixir OTC *antitussive; antihistamine; decongestant* [dextromethorphan hydrobromide; brompheniramine maleate; pseudoephedrine HCl] 10•2•30 mg/10 mL

QTest test stick for home use (discontinued 2004) OTC *in vitro diagnostic aid; urine pregnancy test* 🔊 Gets-It

QTest Ovulation test kit for professional use ℞ *in vitro diagnostic aid to predict ovulation time*

Q-Tussin CF oral liquid OTC *antitussive; decongestant; expectorant* [dextromethorphan hydrobromide; phenylephrine HCl; guaifenesin] 10•5•100 mg/5 mL

Quad Tann caplets (discontinued 2007) ℞ *antitussive; antihistamine; decongestant* [carbetapentane tannate; chlorpheniramine tannate; phenylephrine tannate; ephedrine tannate] 60•5•10•10 mg ☑ codeine; Kadian

Quad Tann Pediatric oral suspension ℞ *antitussive; antihistamine; decongestant* [carbetapentane tannate; chlorpheniramine tannate; phenylephrine tannate; ephedrine tannate] 30•4•5•5 mg/5 mL

quadazocine INN, BAN *opioid antagonist* [also: quadazocine mesylate]

quadazocine mesylate USAN *opioid antagonist* [also: quadazocine]

Quadra-Hist D; Quadra-Hist D Ped extended-release capsules (discontinued 2007) ℞ *decongestant; antihistamine; sleep aid* [pseudoephedrine HCl; phenyltoloxamine citrate; pyrilamine maleate; pheniramine maleate] 80•16•16•16 mg; 40•8•8•8 mg

Quadramet IV injection ℞ *radiopharmaceutical for treatment of bone pain from osteoblastic metastatic tumors* [samarium Sm 153 lexidronam] 1850 MBq/mL (50 mCi/mL)

quadrosilan INN

Quad-Tuss Tannate Pediatric oral suspension ℞ *antitussive; antihistamine; decongestant* [carbetapentane tannate; chlorpheniramine tannate; phenylephrine tannate; ephedrine tannate] 30•4•5•5 mg/5 mL

quaking aspen *medicinal herb* [see: poplar]

Qualaquin capsules ℞ *antimalarial for chloroquine-resistant falciparum malaria* [quinine sulfate] 324 mg ☑ Glaucon; Glyquin

Qual-Tussin oral drops ℞ *decongestant; antihistamine; expectorant; for children 2–24 months* [phenylephrine HCl; chlorpheniramine maleate; guaifenesin] 2•1•20 mg/mL

Qual-Tussin syrup (discontinued 2007) ℞ *antitussive; antihistamine; decongestant; expectorant* [dextromethorphan hydrobromide; chlorpheniramine maleate; phenylephrine HCl; guaifenesin] 15•4•20•200 mg/10 mL

Qual-Tussin DC syrup (discontinued 2007) ℞ *narcotic antitussive; decongestant; expectorant* [hydrocodone bitartrate; phenylephrine HCl; guaifenesin] 2.5•7.5•50 mg/5 mL

Quantaffirm reagent kit for professional use ℞ *in vitro diagnostic aid for mononucleosis*

Quasense film-coated tablets (in packs of 91) ℞ *extended-cycle (3 months) monophasic oral contraceptive* [levonorgestrel; ethinyl estradiol] 0.15 mg•30 mcg × 84 days; counters × 7 days

quassia *(Picrasma excelsa; Quassia amara)* bark *medicinal herb used as an anthelmintic, antimalarial, appetizer, digestive aid, febrifuge, insecticide, pediculicide, and tonic*

quatacaine INN ☑ ketocaine

quaternium-18 bentonite [see: bentoquatam]

quazepam USAN, INN *benzodiazepine sedative and hypnotic*

quazinone USAN, INN *cardiotonic*

quazodine USAN, INN *cardiotonic; bronchodilator*

quazolast USAN, INN *antiasthmatic; mediator release inhibitor*

Queen Anne's lace *medicinal herb* [see: carrot]

queen of the meadow *medicinal herb* [see: boneset; meadowsweet]

queen of the meadow *(Eupatorium purpureum)* leaves *medicinal herb for bursitis, gallstones, kidney infections and stones, neuralgias, rheumatism, ringworm, urinary disorders, and water retention*

Quelicin IV or IM injection ℞ *neuro-muscular blocker* [succinylcholine chloride] 20, 50, 100 mg/mL ⚕ Cleocin; Galzin; glycine

quercetin *natural flavonoid used to protect capillary walls; antioxidant; active flavonol of rutin* 50, 250 mg oral

Quercus alba *medicinal herb* [see: white oak]

Questran; Questran Light powder for oral suspension ℞ *cholesterol-lowering antihyperlipidemic; treatment for pruritus due to partial biliary obstruction; also used as an antidote to Clostridium difficile and digitalis toxicity* [cholestyramine resin] 4 g/dose

quetiapine fumarate USAN *novel (atypical) dibenzothiazepine antipsychotic for schizophrenia and both manic and depressive episodes of a bipolar disorder; investigational (NDA filed) for generalized anxiety disorder* (base=87%)

Quibron; Quibron-300 capsules (discontinued 2007) ℞ *antiasthmatic; bronchodilator; expectorant* [theophylline; guaifenesin] 150•90 mg; 300•180 mg ⚕ Gabarone; gepirone

Quibron-T Dividose (multiple-scored tablets) (discontinued 2006) ℞ *antiasthmatic; bronchodilator* [theophylline] 300 mg

Quibron-T/SR sustained-release Dividose (multiple-scored tablets) (discontinued 2006) ℞ *antiasthmatic; bronchodilator* [theophylline] 300 mg

Quick Care solutions OTC *two-step chemical disinfecting system for soft contact lenses* [hydrogen peroxide–based]

Quick Melts Children's Non-Aspirin, Quick Melts Jr. Strength Non-Aspirin orally disintegrating tablets OTC *analgesic; antipyretic* [acetaminophen] 80 mg; 160 mg

Quicklets (trademarked dosage form) *quickly dissolving tablets*

Quickscreen test kit for home use OTC *in vitro diagnostic aid for detection of multiple illicit drugs in the urine*

quick-set *medicinal herb* [see: hawthorn]

QuickVue H. pylori gII test kit for professional use ℞ *in vitro diagnostic aid for H. pylori in serum or plasma*

QuickVue Influenza Test for professional use ℞ *in vitro diagnostic aid for detection of influenza A and B from nasal excretions*

QuickVue Pregnancy Test cassettes for professional use ℞ *in vitro diagnostic aid; urine pregnancy test*

quifenadine INN

quiflapon sodium USAN *leukotriene biosynthesis inhibitor for asthma and inflammatory bowel disease*

quillaia (Quillaja saponaria) bark *medicinal herb for bronchitis and cough; also used topically for dandruff and scalp itchiness*

quillifoline INN

quilostigmine USAN *cholinesterase inhibitor for Alzheimer disease*

quinacainol INN

quinacillin INN, BAN

quinacrine HCl USP *antimalarial; anthelmintic for giardiasis and cestodiasis (tapeworm); investigational (orphan) to prevent the recurrence of pneumothorax in high-risk patients* [also: mepacrine]

quinalbarbitone sodium BAN *hypnotic; sedative* [also: secobarbital sodium]

quinaldine blue USAN *obstetric diagnostic aid*

quinambicide [see: clioquinol]

quinapril INN, BAN *antihypertensive; angiotensin-converting enzyme (ACE) inhibitor; adjunctive treatment for congestive heart failure (CHF)* [also: quinapril HCl]

quinapril HCl USAN *antihypertensive; angiotensin-converting enzyme (ACE) inhibitor; adjunctive treatment for congestive heart failure (CHF)* [also: quinapril] 5, 10, 20, 40 mg

quinapril HCl & hydrochlorothiazide *antihypertensive; angiotensin-converting enzyme (ACE) inhibitor; diuretic* 10•12.5, 20•12.5, 10•25, 20•25 mg oral

quinaprilat USAN, INN *antihypertensive; angiotensin-converting enzyme (ACE) inhibitor*

Quinaretic film-coated tablets ℞ *antihypertensive; angiotensin-converting enzyme (ACE) inhibitor; diuretic* [quinapril HCl; hydrochlorothiazide] 10•12.5, 20•12.5, 20•25 mg

quinazosin INN *antihypertensive* [also: quinazosin HCl]

quinazosin HCl USAN *antihypertensive* [also: quinazosin]

quinbolone USAN, INN *anabolic*

quincarbate INN

quindecamine INN *antibacterial* [also: quindecamine acetate]

quindecamine acetate USAN *antibacterial* [also: quindecamine]

quindonium bromide USAN, INN *antiarrhythmic*

quindoxin INN, BAN

quinelorane INN *antihypertensive; antiparkinsonian* [also: quinelorane HCl]

quinelorane HCl USAN *antihypertensive; antiparkinsonian* [also: quinelorane]

quinestradol INN, BAN

quinestrol USAN, USP, INN, BAN *estrogen replacement therapy for postmenopausal disorders*

quinetalate INN *smooth muscle relaxant* [also: quinetolate]

quinethazone USP, INN *diuretic; antihypertensive*

quinetolate USAN *smooth muscle relaxant* [also: quinetalate]

quinezamide INN

quinfamide USAN, INN *antiamebic*

quingestanol INN *progestin* [also: quingestanol acetate]

quingestanol acetate USAN *progestin* [also: quingestanol]

quingestrone USAN, INN *progestin*

Quinidex Extentabs (extended-release tablets) (discontinued 2004) ℞ *antiarrhythmic* [quinidine sulfate] 300 mg

quinidine NF, BAN *antiarrhythmic* ⍰ Candin

quinidine & dextromethorphan *investigational (NDA filed) dual-action glutamate inhibitor to treat involuntary emotional expression disorder (IEED)*

quinidine gluconate USP *antiarrhythmic; antimalarial* (base=62%) 324 mg oral; 80 mg/mL injection

quinidine sulfate USP *antiarrhythmic* (base=83%) 100, 200, 300 mg oral

quinine (*Cinchona calisaya; C. ledgeriana; C. succirubra*) NF, BAN bark *medicinal herb for cancer, fever, hemorrhoids, indigestion, inducing abortion, jaundice, malaria, mouth and throat diseases, parasites, stimulation of hair growth, and varicose veins*

quinine ascorbate USAN *smoking deterrent*

quinine biascorbate [now: quinine ascorbate]

quinine bisulfate NF

quinine dihydrochloride NF *anti-infective for pernicious malaria*

quinine ethylcarbonate NF

quinine glycerophosphate NF

quinine HCl NF

quinine hydrobromide NF

quinine hypophosphite NF

quinine monohydrobromide [see: quinine hydrobromide]

quinine monohydrochloride [see: quinine HCl]

quinine monosalicylate [see: quinine salicylate]

quinine phosphate NF

quinine phosphinate [see: quinine hypophosphite]

quinine salicylate NF

quinine sulfate USP *cinchona alkaloid; antimalarial for chloroquine-resistant falciparum malaria (orphan); also used for nocturnal leg cramps* 200, 260, 325 mg oral

quinine sulfate dihydrate [see: quinine sulfate]

quinine tannate USP

quinisocaine INN [also: dimethisoquin HCl; dimethisoquin] ⍰ guanisoquine

quinocide INN

8-quinolinol [see: oxyquinoline]

8-quinolinol benzoate [see: benzoxiquine]

quinolizidines *a class of antibiotics based on the quinolizidine (norlupinane) structure* [also called: norlupinanes]

quinolones [see: fluoroquinolones]

quinoxyl [see: chiniofon]

quinpirole INN *antihypertensive* [also: quinpirole HCl]

quinpirole HCl USAN *antihypertensive* [also: quinpirole]

quinprenaline INN *bronchodilator* [also: quinterenol sulfate]

quinprenaline sulfate [see: quinterenol sulfate]

Quinsana Plus powder OTC *antifungal* [tolnaftate] 1%

quinsy berry *medicinal herb* [see: currant]

Quintabs tablets OTC *vitamin supplement* [multiple vitamins; folic acid] ± •0.1 mg

Quintabs-M tablets OTC *vitamin/mineral/iron supplement* [multiple vitamins & minerals; iron; folic acid] ± •18•0.4 mg

quinterenol sulfate USAN *bronchodilator* [also: quinprenaline]

quintiofos INN, BAN

3-quinuclidinol benzoate [see: benzoclidine]

quinuclium bromide USAN, INN *antihypertensive*

quinupramine INN

quinupristin USAN, INN *streptogramin antibiotic; bacteriostatic to gram-positive infections*

quipazine INN *antidepressant; oxytocic* [also: quipazine maleate] ☑ Capsin; Cubicin; kebuzone

quipazine maleate USAN *antidepressant; oxytocic* [also: quipazine]

quisultazine INN

quisultidine [see: quisultazine]

Quixin eye drops ℞ *fluoroquinolone antibiotic for bacterial conjunctivitis* [levofloxacin] 0.5%

QV-Allergy syrup ℞ *decongestant; antihistamine; anticholinergic to dry mucosal secretions* [phenylephrine HCl; chlorpheniramine maleate; methscopolamine nitrate] 10•2•0.625 mg/5 mL

Qvar pressurized metered-dose inhaler (pMDI) with a CFC-free propellant ℞ *antiasthmatic* [beclomethasone dipropionate] 40, 80 mcg/puff

R

R & D Calcium Carbonate/600 *investigational (orphan) agent for hyperphosphatemia of end-stage renal disease* [calcium carbonate]

RA Lotion OTC *antiseptic, antifungal, and keratolytic for acne* [resorcinol; alcohol 43%] 3%

RabAvert IM injection ℞ *rabies vaccine for pre-exposure vaccination or post-exposure prophylaxis* [rabies vaccine, chick embryo cell] ≥ 2.5 IU/mL

rabeprazole INN *proton pump inhibitor for duodenal ulcers, erosive or ulcerative gastroesophageal reflux disease (GERD), and other gastroesophageal disorders* [also: rabeprazole sodium]

rabeprazole sodium USAN *proton pump inhibitor for duodenal ulcers, erosive or ulcerative gastroesophageal reflux disease (GERD), H. pylori infection, and other gastroesophageal disorders* [also: rabeprazole]

rabies immune globulin (RIG) USP *passive immunizing agent for use after rabies exposure*

rabies vaccine USP *rabies vaccine for pre-exposure vaccination or post-exposure prophylaxis; the virus is grown in either human diploid cells or chick embryo cells*

rabies vaccine, adsorbed (RVA) [see: rabies vaccine]

rabies vaccine, DCO (diploid cell origin) [see: rabies vaccine]

rabies vaccine, HDCV (human diploid cell vaccine) [see: rabies vaccine]

race ginger *medicinal herb* [see: ginger]

racecadotril [see: acetorphan]

racefemine INN

racefenicol INN *antibacterial* [also: racephenicol]

racemethadol [see: dimepheptanol]

racemethionine USAN, USP *urinary acidifier to control ammonia production* [also: methionine (the DL- form)]

racemethorphan INN, BAN

racemetirosine INN

racemic [def.] *A chemical compound with equal parts of (+) (formerly d- or dextro-) and (−) (formerly l- or levo-) enantiomers. Designated by the prefix (±) (formerly dl-).* [see also: isomer; enantiomer]

racemic amphetamine phosphate

racemic amphetamine sulfate [see: amphetamine sulfate]

racemic calcium pantothenate [see: calcium pantothenate, racemic]

racemoramide INN, BAN

racemorphan INN

racephedrine HCl USAN

racephenicol USAN *antibacterial* [also: racefenicol]

racepinefrine INN *sympathomimetic bronchodilator* [also: racepinephrine]

racepinephrine USP *sympathomimetic bronchodilator* [also: racepinefrine]

racepinephrine HCl USP *sympathomimetic bronchodilator*

raclopride INN, BAN

raclopride C 11 USAN *radiopharmaceutical*

racoonberry *medicinal herb* [see: mandrake]

ractopamine INN *veterinary growth stimulant* [also: ractopamine HCl]

ractopamine HCl USAN *veterinary growth stimulant* [also: ractopamine]

Radiesse subcu implant in prefilled syringes ℞ *collagen production stimulant for HIV-related facial lipoatrophy*

and moderate to severe facial wrinkles and folds [calcium hydroxylapatite] 0.3, 1.3 mL/syringe

radio-chromated serum albumin [see: albumin, chromated]

Radiogardase capsules ℞ *chelating agent for internal contamination with radioactive or nonradioactive cesium and/or thallium (orphan)* [ferric hexacyanoferrate (insoluble Prussian blue)] 500 mg

radio-iodinated I 125 serum albumin [see: albumin, iodinated]

radio-iodinated I 131 serum albumin [see: albumin, iodinated]

radiomerisoprol ^{197}**Hg** [see: merisoprol Hg 197]

radioselenomethionine ^{75}**Se** [see: selenomethionine Se 75]

radiotolpovidone I 131 INN *hypoalbuminemia test; radioactive agent* [also: tolpovidone I 131]

radish (Raphanus sativus) *root medicinal herb used as an antispasmodic, astringent, cholagogue, and diuretic*

radium *element (Ra)* ⧉ rhodium

radon *element (Rn)*

rafoxanide USAN, INN *anthelmintic*

ragged cup (Silphium perfoliatum) *root and gum medicinal herb used as an antispasmodic, diaphoretic, and stimulant*

ragwort *medicinal herb* [see: life root]

ralitoline USAN, INN *anticonvulsant*

Ralivia ER controlled-release tablets ℞ *once-daily central analgesic for moderate to severe pain* [tramadol HCl] 100, 200, 300 mg

Ralix extended-release tablets ℞ *decongestant; antihistamine; anticholinergic to dry mucosal secretions* [phenylephrine HCl; chlorpheniramine maleate; methscopolamine nitrate] 40•8•2.5 mg ⧉ RuLox

raloxifene INN *antiestrogen; selective estrogen receptor modulator (SERM) for the prevention for postmenopausal osteoporosis* [also: raloxifene HCl]

raloxifene HCl USAN *selective estrogen receptor modulator (SERM) for the*

*prevention and treatment of postmeno-
pausal osteoporosis; hormone antagonist for breast cancer* [also: raloxifene]

raltegravir (RGV) *integrase inhibitor
for drug-resistant HIV-1 infection*

raltitrexed USAN *antimetabolite antineoplastic; thymidylate synthase inhibitor*

raluridine USAN *antiviral*

rambufaside [see: meproscillarin]

ramciclane INN

ramelteon *melatonin MT$_1$ and MT$_2$
receptor agonist; hypnotic for insomnia
due to difficulty with sleep onset; investigational (Phase II) for circadian rhythm
sleep disorder*

ramifenazone INN

ramipril USAN, INN, BAN *antihypertensive; angiotensin-converting enzyme
(ACE) inhibitor; treatment for myocardial infarction (MI), congestive heart
failure (CHF), and stroke* 1.25, 2.5, 5,
10 mg oral

ramiprilat INN

ramixotidine INN

ramnodigin INN

ramoplanin USAN, INN *investigational
(Phase III) broad-spectrum glycolipo-
depsipeptide antibiotic for vancomycin-
resistant Enterococcus faecium
(VREF) and other vancomycin-resis-
tant enterococci (VRE)*

Ranamine (trademarked ingredient) *a
proprietary blend of vitamins B$_6$, B$_{12}$,
and folic acid* ⑨ RenAmin

Ranexa film-coated extended-release
tablets ℞ *antianginal for chronic stable
angina* [ranolazine HCl] 500, 1000
mg ⑨ Renax; Ryna-12X

ranibizumab *vascular endothelial
growth factor (VEGF-A) inhibitor for
neovascular (wet) age-related macular
degeneration (AMD)*

Raniclor chewable tablets ℞ *second-
generation cephalosporin antibiotic*
[cefaclor] 125, 187, 250, 375 mg

ranimustine INN

ranimycin USAN, INN *antibacterial*

ranitidine USAN, INN, BAN *histamine H$_2$
antagonist for gastric ulcers* 75, 150,
300 mg oral; 25 mg/mL injection

ranitidine bismuth citrate USAN *histamine H$_2$ antagonist for gastric ulcers
with H. pylori infection* [also: ranitidine bismutrex]

ranitidine bismutrex BAN *histamine
H$_2$ antagonist for gastric ulcers with H.
pylori infection* [also: ranitidine bismuth citrate]

ranitidine HCl USP, JAN *histamine H$_2$
antagonist for gastric ulcers* 75, 150,
300 mg oral; 15 mg/mL oral

ranolazine INN *antianginal* [also: ranolazine HCl]

ranolazine HCl USAN *antianginal for
chronic stable angina* [also: ranolazine]

ranpirnase USAN, INN *investigational
(Phase III) antineoplastic for unresectable malignant mesothelioma (UMM)
and small cell lung cancer (SCLC)*

*Ranunculus acris; R. bulbosus; R.
scleratus medicinal herb* [see: butter-
cup]

rapacuronium bromide USAN *neuromuscular blocker; adjunct to general
anesthesia*

Rapamune tablets, oral solution ℞
*immunosuppressant for renal trans-
plantation; investigational (Phase III)
for liver transplantation; also used for
psoriasis* [sirolimus] 1, 2 mg; 1 mg/mL

rapamycin [now: sirolimus]

Raphanus sativus medicinal herb [see:
radish]

Rapid Anthrax Test reagents for use
with **LightCycler** assay device ℞ *diagnostic aid for anthrax DNA in human
and environmental samples* [polymerase
chain reaction (PCR) test]

RapidVue test kit for home use OTC *in
vitro diagnostic aid; urine pregnancy test*

Rapimelt (trademarked dosage form)
orally disintegrating tablets

Rapinex (name changed to **Zegerid**
upon marketing release in 2004)

**Rapirun H. pylori Antibody Detec-
tion Kit** test kit for professional use
℞ *in vitro diagnostic aid for the detection
of anti-H. pylori IgG antibodies in urine*

RapiTabs (trademarked dosage form)
orally disintegrating tablets

Raptiva powder for subcu injection ℞ *immunosuppressant for plaque psoriasis* [efalizumab] 125 mg/dose

rasagiline INN *monoamine oxidase B (MAO-B) inhibitor for Parkinson disease*

rasagiline mesylate USAN *monoamine oxidase B (MAO-B) inhibitor for Parkinson disease*

rasburicase USAN, INN *antimetabolite antineoplastic for leukemia, lymphoma, and solid tumor malignancies (orphan)*

Rasilez (name changed to **Tektura** upon marketing release in 2007)

raspberry, ground *medicinal herb* [see: goldenseal]

raspberry, red; wild red raspberry *medicinal herb* [see: red raspberry]

raspberry [syrup] USP

rathyronine INN

rattleroot *medicinal herb* [see: black cohosh]

rattlesnake antivenin [see: antivenin (Crotalidae) polyvalent]

rattlesnake root *medicinal herb* [see: birthroot; black cohosh; senega]

rattleweed *medicinal herb* [see: black cohosh]

rauwolfia serpentina USP *antihypertensive; peripheral antiadrenergic; antipsychotic*

rauwolfia serpentina & bendroflumethiazide *antihypertensive; peripheral antiadrenergic; diuretic* 50•4 mg oral

Rauzide tablets (discontinued 2007) ℞ *antihypertensive; diuretic* [bendroflumethiazide; rauwolfia serpentina] 4•50 mg

rayon, purified USAN, USP *surgical aid*

Razadyne film-coated tablets, oral drops ℞ *acetylcholinesterase inhibitor to increase cognition in Alzheimer disease; investigational to block the effects of nerve gas agents sarin and soman* [galantamine hydrobromide] 4, 8, 12 mg; 4 mg/mL

Razadyne ER extended-release pellets in capsules ℞ *acetylcholinesterase inhibitor to increase cognition in Alzheimer disease; investigational to block* *the effects of nerve gas agents sarin and soman* [galantamine hydrobromide] 8, 16, 24 mg

razinodil INN

razobazam INN

razoxane INN, BAN

^{86}Rb [see: rubidium chloride Rb 86]

rBPI (bactericidal and permeability-increasing protein, recombinant) [q.v.]

rCD4 (recombinant CD4) [see: CD4, recombinant soluble human]

RCF oral liquid OTC *hypoallergenic infant formula* [soy protein formula, carbohydrate free]

RE2+30 syrup ℞ *antihistamine; decongestant* [chlorpheniramine maleate; pseudoephedrine HCl] 2•30 mg/5 mL

Reabilan; Reabilan HN ready-to-use oral liquid OTC *enteral nutritional therapy* [lactose-free formula]

reactrol [see: clemizole HCl]

rebamipide INN

Rebetol capsules, oral solution ℞ *nucleoside antiviral for chronic hepatitis C infections (orphan) and clinically stable HIV disease; also used for viral hemorrhagic fevers* [ribavirin] 200 mg; 40 mg/mL

Rebetron capsules + subcu or IM injection ℞ *combination treatment for chronic hepatitis C* [Rebetol (ribavirin capsules); Intron A (interferon alfa-2b injection)] 200 mg•3 million IU

Rebif prefilled syringes for subcu injection ℞ *immunomodulator for relapsing remitting multiple sclerosis (orphan); investigational (orphan) for malignant melanoma, metastatic renal cell carcinoma, T-cell lymphoma, and Kaposi sarcoma* [interferon beta-1a] 8.8, 22, 44 mcg (2.4, 6, 12 MIU)

reboxetine INN *fast-acting selective norepinephrine reuptake inhibitor for depression*

reboxetine mesilate INN, BAN *fast-acting selective norepinephrine reuptake inhibitor for depression* (base=76.5%) [also: reboxetine mesylate]

reboxetine mesylate USAN *fast-acting selective norepinephrine reuptake inhibitor for depression* (base=76.5%) [also: reboxetine mesilate]

recainam INN, BAN *antiarrhythmic* [also: recainam HCl]

recainam HCl USAN *antiarrhythmic* [also: recainam]

recainam tosylate USAN *antiarrhythmic*

recanescin [see: deserpidine]

Receptin *investigational (Phase II) antiviral for AIDS* [CD4, recombinant soluble human]

Reclast IV infusion ℞ *single-dose bisphosphonate bone resorption inhibitor for Paget disease of the bone; once-yearly treatment for postmenopausal osteoporosis* [zoledronic acid] 5 mg

reclazepam USAN, INN *sedative*

Reclipsen tablets (in packs of 28) ℞ *monophasic oral contraceptive* [desogestrel; ethinyl estradiol] 0.15 mg• 30 mcg × 21 days; counters × 7 days

Reclomide tablets ℞ *antiemetic for chemotherapy; antidopaminergic; peristaltic* [metoclopramide HCl] 10 mg

Recombigen HIV-1 LA Test reagent kit for professional use ℞ *in vitro diagnostic aid for HIV-1 antibodies in blood, serum, or plasma* [latex agglutination test]

recombinant factor VIII [see: antihemophilic factor, recombinant]

recombinant human activated protein C (rhAPC) [see: drotrecogan alfa]

recombinant human deoxyribonuclease (rhDNase) [see: dornase alfa]

recombinant human growth hormone (rhGH) [see: somatropin]

recombinant tissue plasminogen activator (rtPA; rt-PA) [see: alteplase]

Recombinate powder for IV injection ℞ *systemic hemostatic; antihemophilic for the prevention and control of bleeding in classical hemophilia (hemophilia A) and von Willebrand disease (orphan)* [antihemophilic factor concentrate, recombinant] 250, 500, 1000 IU

Recombivax HB adult IM injection, pediatric/adolescent IM injection, dialysis formulation ℞ *active immunizing agent for hepatitis B and D* [hepatitis B virus vaccine, inactvated, recombinant] 10 mcg/mL; 5 mcg/0.5 mL; 40 mcg/mL

Recomparin *investigational synthetic heparin*

Recothrom powder ℞ *topical hemostat for surgery* [thrombin, recombinant] 5000 IU

Rectacort rectal suppositories ℞ *corticosteroidal anti-inflammatory* [hydrocortisone acetate] 10%

Rectagene rectal suppositories OTC *temporary relief of hemorrhoidal symptoms* [live yeast cell derivative; shark liver oil] 2000 SRF U/oz.

Rectagene Medicated Rectal Balm ointment OTC *temporary relief of hemorrhoidal symptoms* [shark liver oil; phenyl mercuric nitrate; live yeast cell derivative] 3%•1:10 000•66.67 U/g

Rectolax suppositories OTC *stimulant laxative* [bisacodyl] 10 mg

red bay; red laurel *medicinal herb* [see: magnolia]

red bearberry *medicinal herb* [see: uva ursi]

red blood cells [see: blood cells, red]

red bush tea (Aspalathus contaminata; A. linearis; Borbonia pinifolia) leaves and stems *medicinal herb used as a free radical scavenger; investigational antineoplastic; investigational for preventing brain damage caused by aging*

red clover (Trifolium pratense) flower *medicinal herb for blood cleansing, bronchitis, cancer, clearing toxins, nervous disorders, and spasms*

Red Cross Toothache topical liquid OTC *oral analgesic* [eugenol] 85%

red currant (Ribes rubrum) *medicinal herb* [see: currant]

red elm *medicinal herb* [see: slippery elm]

red ferric oxide [see: ferric oxide, red]

red ink berries; red ink plant *medicinal herb* [see: pokeweed]

red laurel; red bay *medicinal herb* [see: magnolia]

red legs *medicinal herb* [see: bistort]

red mulberry (Morus rubra) *medicinal herb* [see: mulberry]

red oak (Quercus rubra) *medicinal herb* [see: white oak]

red paint root *medicinal herb* [see: bloodroot]

red pepper; African red pepper; American red pepper *medicinal herb* [see: cayenne]

red pimpernel (Anagallis arvensis) plant *medicinal herb used as a cholagogue, diaphoretic, diuretic, expectorant, nervine, purgative, and stimulant*

red puccoon *medicinal herb* [see: bloodroot]

red raspberry (Rubus idaeus; R. strigosus) leaves *medicinal herb for childbirth afterpains, diarrhea and other bowel disorders, fever, flu, morning sickness, menstrual disorders, mouth sores, nausea, and vomiting*

red root *medicinal herb* [see: bloodroot; danshen; New Jersey tea]

red sarsaparilla *medicinal herb* [see: sarsaparilla]

Red Throat Spray; Green Throat Spray OTC *mild mucous membrane anesthetic; antipruritic; counterirritant* [phenol] 1.4%

red veterinarian petrolatum (RVP) [see: petrolatum]

red weed *medicinal herb* [see: pokeweed]

redberry *medicinal herb* [see: ginseng]

Redi Vial (trademarked delivery form) *dual-compartment vial*

Rediject (trademarked delivery form) *prefilled disposable syringe*

Redipak (trademarked delivery form) *unit dose or unit-of-issue package*

RediTabs (trademarked dosage form) *rapidly disintegrating tablets*

Reditux IV infusion ℞ *monoclonal antibody for non-Hodgkin B-cell lymphoma and rheumatoid arthritis* [rituximab (biosimilar)] 10 mg/mL

redmond clay (montmorillonite) *natural remedy for bug bites and stings and other skin problems*

Redness Reliever eye drops OTC *decongestant; vasoconstrictor* [tetrahydrozoline HCl] 0.05%

Redur-PCM oral suspension ℞ *decongestant; antihistamine; anticholinergic to dry mucosal secretions* [phenylephrine tannate; chlorpheniramine tannate; methscopolamine nitrate] 10•2•1.5 mg/5 mL

Redutemp tablets (discontinued 2008) OTC *analgesic; antipyretic* [acetaminophen] 500 mg

Reese's Pinworm soft gel capsules, oral suspension OTC *anthelmintic for ascariasis (roundworm) and enterobiasis (pinworm)* [pyrantel pamoate] 180 mg; 50 mg/mL

ReFacto powder for IV injection ℞ *short-term anticoagulant for prophylaxis of spontaneous bleeding and for surgical procedures (orphan)* [antihemophilic factor, recombinant] 250, 500, 1000 IU

Refensen Plus Severe Strength Cough & Cold Medicine caplets (discontinued 2007) OTC *decongestant; expectorant* [pseudoephedrine HCl; guaifenesin] 60•400 mg

Refludan powder for IV injection *anticoagulant for heparin-associated thrombocytopenia (orphan)* [lepirudin] 50 mg ⚕ rofelodine

Refresh Classic eye drops OTC *moisturizer/lubricant* [polyvinyl alcohol] 1.4%

Refresh Dry Eye Therapy eye drops OTC *moisturizer/lubricant* [glycerin; polysorbate 80] 1%•1%

Refresh Eye Itch Relief eye drops OTC *antihistamine and mast cell stabilizer for allergic conjunctivitis* [ketotifen fumarate] 0.025%

Refresh Plus; Refresh Tears eye drops OTC *moisturizer/lubricant* [carboxymethylcellulose] 0.5%

Refresh P.M. ophthalmic ointment OTC *ocular moisturizer/lubricant* [white petrolatum; mineral oil; lanolin]

refrigerants *a class of agents that lower abnormal body heat (a term used in folk medicine)*

regadenoson *selective adenosine A_{2A} receptor agonist; coronary vasodilator to induce pharmacological stress for myocardial perfusion imaging*

Rēgain snack bar OTC *enteral nutritional therapy for impaired renal function* [multiple essential amino acids] 🔁 Rogaine

Regenecare HA gel OTC *anesthetic* [lidocaine] 2%

Regitine IV or IM injection (discontinued 2004) ℞ *antihypertensive for pheochromocytoma; α-blocker* [phentolamine mesylate] 5 mg/mL 🔁 Reactine; Roaccutane

Reglan syrup (discontinued 2004) ℞ *antiemetic for chemotherapy; antidopaminergic; peristaltic* [metoclopramide HCl] 5 mg/5 mL

Reglan tablets, IV infusion ℞ *antiemetic for chemotherapy and postoperative nausea and vomiting; GI stimulant for diabetic gastroparesis and symptomatic gastroesophageal reflux; also used as a radiosensitizer and to stimulate lactation* [metoclopramide HCl] 5, 10 mg; 5 mg/mL

regramostim USAN, INN *antineutropenic; hematopoietic stimulant; biologic response modifier; bone marrow stimulant*

Regranex gel ℞ *recombinant platelet-derived growth factor B for chronic diabetic foot ulcers* [becaplermin] 0.01%

Regroton tablets (discontinued 2007) ℞ *antihypertensive; diuretic* [chlorthalidone; reserpine] 50•0.25 mg

Regular Iletin II vials for subcu injection (discontinued 2005) OTC *antidiabetic* [insulin (pork)] 100 U/mL

regulator, female *medicinal herb* [see: life root]

Regulax SS capsules OTC *laxative; stool softener* [docusate sodium] 100 mg

Reguloid powder OTC *bulk laxative* [psyllium hydrophilic mucilloid] 3.4 g/tsp.

Rehydralyte oral solution OTC *electrolyte replacement* [sodium, potassium, and chloride electrolytes]

reishi mushrooms body and stem *medicinal herb for AIDS, allergies, fatigue, heart problems, and insomnia*

Rejuvenex cream OTC *antioxidant, moisturizer, and sunscreen for the face*

Rejuvex caplets OTC *natural/herbal supplement for the relief or postmenopausal symptoms* [multiple vitamins and minerals; phytoestrogens]

Relacon-DM NR oral liquid (discontinued 2007) ℞ *antitussive; decongestant; expectorant* [dextromethorphan hydrobromide; pseudoephedrine HCl; guaifenesin] 15•32•200 mg/5 mL

Relacon-HC; Relacon-HC NR oral liquid ℞ *narcotic antitussive; antihistamine; decongestant* [hydrocodone bitartrate; chlorpheniramine maleate; phenylephrine HCl] 3.5•2.5•10 mg/5 mL; 3.5•2.5•8 mg/5 mL

Relafen film-coated tablets (discontinued 2006) ℞ *analgesic; nonsteroidal anti-inflammatory drug (NSAID) for acute and chronic osteoarthritis and rheumatoid arthritis* [nabumetone] 500, 750 mg

Relagesic tablets (discontinued 2007) ℞ *analgesic; antipyretic; antihistamine; sleep aid* [acetaminophen; phenyltoloxamine citrate] 650•50 mg

Relamine tablets ℞ *nutritional supplement for osteoarthritis* [glucosamine; chondroitin; Primorine (q.v.)] 400•300•425 mg

Relasin DM oral liquid OTC *antitussive; decongestant; expectorant* [dextromethorphan hydrobromide; pseudoephedrine HCl; guaifenesin] 15•32•175 mg/5 mL

Relasin-HC oral liquid ℞ *narcotic antitussive; antihistamine; decongestant* [hydrocodone bitartrate; chlorpheniramine maleate; phenylephrine HCl] 3.25•2.5•8 mg/5 mL

relaxin, recombinant human *investigational (orphan) for progressive sys-*

temic sclerosis; investigational (Phase II/III) for scleroderma

Relcof PSE extended-release tablets ℞ decongestant; antihistamine; anticholinergic to dry mucosal secretions [pseudoephedrine HCl; chlorpheniramine maleate; methscopolamine nitrate] 120•8•2.5 mg

Release-Tabs (dosage form) timed-release tablets

Relenza Rotadisks (powder for oral inhalation, for use with a **Diskhaler** device) influenza neuraminidase inhibitor for the treatment of acute influenza types A and B [zanamivir] 5 mg

Reli On Ketone Test Strips reagent strips for home use OTC in vitro diagnostic aid for acetone (ketones) in the urine

Reliable Gentle Laxative delayed-release enteric-coated tablets, suppositories OTC stimulant laxative [bisacodyl] 5 mg; 10 mg

Relief eye drops OTC decongestant [phenylephrine HCl] 0.12%

Relistor subcu injection ℞ opioid receptor antagonist for opioid-induced constipation (orphan); investigational (NDA filed) for postoperative ileus [methylnaltrexone bromide] 12 mg/0.6 mL vial

relomycin USAN, INN antibacterial

Relora tablets, capsules OTC dietary supplement to relieve stress and anxiety by reducing cortisol levels and increasing DHEA levels; adjunct to weight reduction [Magnolia officinalis extract; Phellodendron amurense extract] 250 mg

Relpax film-coated tablets ℞ vascular serotonin 5-HT$_{1B/1D/1F}$ receptor agonist for the acute treatment of migraine [eletriptan hydrobromide] 24.2, 48.5 mg (20, 40 mg base)

Reluri extended-release caplets ℞ decongestant; expectorant [phenylephrine HCl; guaifenesin] 30•1200 mg

remacemide INN neuroprotective anticonvulsant [also: remacemide HCl]

remacemide HCl USAN neuroprotective anticonvulsant; investigational

(orphan) for Huntington disease [also: remacemide]

Reme Hist DM oral liquid ℞ antitussive; antihistamine; sleep aid; decongestant [dextromethorphan hydrobromide; pyrilamine maleate; phenylephrine HCl] 15•12.5•7.5 mg/5 mL

Remeron film-coated tablets ℞ tetracyclic antidepressant; serotonin 5-HT$_{1A}$ agonist [mirtazapine] 15, 30, 45 mg

Remeron SolTabs (orally disintegrating tablets) ℞ tetracyclic antidepressant; serotonin 5-HT$_{1A}$ agonist [mirtazapine] 15, 30, 45 mg

Remicade powder for IV infusion ℞ anti-inflammatory for severe and fistulizing Crohn disease (orphan), ulcerative colitis, rheumatoid and psoriatic arthritis, ankylosing spondylitis, and plaque psoriasis; also used for juvenile arthritis [infliximab] 100 mg

Remifemin Menopause tablets OTC natural remedy for postmenopausal symptoms [black cohosh (standardized extract)] 20 mg (1 mg triterpene glycosides)

remifentanil INN, BAN short-acting narcotic analgesic for general anesthesia [also: remifentanil HCl]

remifentanil HCl USAN short-acting narcotic analgesic for general anesthesia [also: remifentanil]

remikiren INN

Reminyl film-coated tablets, oral drops (name changed to **Razadyne** in 2005)

remiprostol USAN, INN antiulcerative

Remitogen investigational (orphan) agent for non-Hodgkin B-cell lymphoma [monoclonal antibody 1D10, humanized]

Remodulin continuous subcu or IV infusion ℞ prostacyclin analogue; peripheral vasodilator for pulmonary arterial hypertension (PAH; orphan) [treprostinil sodium] 1, 2.5, 5, 10 mg/mL

remoxipride USAN, INN, BAN antipsychotic

remoxipride HCl USAN antipsychotic

Remoxy gelcaps *investigational (NDA filed) abuse-resistant form of* **OxyContin** [oxycodone]

Remular-S tablets ℞ *skeletal muscle relaxant* [chlorzoxazone] 250 mg

Remune *investigational (Phase III) immunostimulant theraccine adjunct for HIV* [HIV-1 immunogen, gp120-depleted, inactivated]

Renacidin powder for solution ℞ *bladder and catheter irrigant for apatite or struvite calculi (orphan)* [citric acid; D-gluconic acid lactone; magnesium hydroxycarbonate] 6.602•0.198•3.177 g/100 mL

Renacidin Irrigation solution ℞ *bladder and catheter irrigant for apatite or struvite calculi (orphan)* [citric acid; glucono-delta-lactone; magnesium carbonate]

Renagel capsules (discontinued 2004) ℞ *phosphate-binding polymer for hyperphosphatemia of end-stage renal disease (ESRD)* [sevelamer HCl] 403 mg

Renagel film-coated tablets ℞ *phosphate-binding polymer for hyperphosphatemia in dialysis patients with chronic kidney disease (CKD); also used for hyperuricemia in dialysis patients* [sevelamer HCl] 400, 800 mg

RenAmin IV infusion ℞ *nutritional therapy for renal failure* [multiple essential and nonessential amino acids; electrolytes] ⚕ Ranamine

renanolone INN

Renax film-coated caplets ℞ *nutritional therapy for azotemia (uremia)* [multiple vitamins & minerals; folic acid; biotin] ±•2.5•0.3 mg ⚕ Ranexa; Ryna-12X

Renese-R tablets (discontinued 2007) ℞ *antihypertensive; diuretic* [polythiazide; reserpine] 2•0.25 mg

renin inhibitors *a class of antihypertensives that reduce the amount of serum angiotensin II by blocking the action of renin, an enzyme required to create its precursor, angiotensin I* [compare to: angiotensin-converting enzyme inhibitors; angiotensin II receptor antagonists]

rennet, cheese *medicinal herb* [see: bedstraw]

Reno-30 intracavitary instillation ℞ *radiopaque contrast medium for urological imaging* [diatrizoate meglumine (46.67% iodine)] 300 mg/mL (141 mg/mL)

RenoCal-76 injection ℞ *radiopaque contrast medium* [diatrizoate meglumine; diatrizoate sodium (48.7% total iodine)] 660•100 mg/mL (370 mg/mL)

Reno-Dip; Reno-60 injection ℞ *radiopaque contrast medium* [diatrizoate meglumine (46.67% iodine)] 300 mg/mL (141 mg/mL); 600 mg/mL (282 mg/mL)

Renografin-60 injection ℞ *radiopaque contrast medium* [diatrizoate meglumine; diatrizoate sodium (48.75% total iodine)] 520•80 mg/mL (292.5 mg/mL)

Renoquid tablets ℞ *broad-spectrum bacteriostatic* [sulfacytine] 250 mg

Renova cream ℞ *retinoid for photodamage, fine wrinkles, mottled hyperpigmentation, and roughness of facial skin* [tretinoin] 0.02%, 0.05%

rentiapril INN

ReNu solution OTC *rinsing/storage solution for soft contact lenses* [sodium chloride (preserved saline solution)]

ReNu Effervescent Enzymatic Cleaner; ReNu Thermal Enzymatic Cleaner tablets OTC *enzymatic cleaner for soft contact lenses* [subtilisin]

ReNu Multi-Purpose solution OTC *chemical disinfecting solution for soft contact lenses* [polyaminopropyl biguanide; EDTA] 0.00005%•0.01%

Renvela film-coated tablets ℞ *phosphate-binding polymer for hyperphosphatemia in dialysis patients with chronic kidney disease (CKD)* [sevelamer carbonate] 800 mg

renytoline INN *anti-inflammatory* [also: paranyline HCl]

renytoline HCl [see: paranyline HCl]

renzapride INN, BAN

ReoPro IV injection ℞ *platelet aggregation inhibitor for PTCA and acute arterial occlusive disorders* [abciximab] 2 mg/mL

repaglinide USAN *meglitinide antidiabetic for type 2 diabetes that stimulates the release of insulin from the pancreas* 0.5, 1, 2 mg oral

Repan tablets ℞ *barbiturate sedative; analgesic; antipyretic* [butalbital; acetaminophen; caffeine] 50•325•40 mg ⊡ Rheaban; Riopan

Repan CF caplets ℞ *barbiturate sedative; analgesic; antipyretic* [butalbital; acetaminophen] 50•650 mg

repertaxin *investigational (orphan) to prevent delayed graft function of solid organ transplants*

Repetab (trademarked dosage form) *extended-release tablet* ⊡ Ribatab; Robitab

repirinast USAN, INN *antiallergic; antiasthmatic*

Replagal *investigational (NDA filed, orphan) enzyme replacement therapy for Fabry disease* [agalsidase alfa]

Replens vaginal gel OTC *moisturizer/lubricant* [glycerin; mineral oil]

Replete ready-to-use oral liquid OTC *enteral nutritional therapy* [lactose-free formula]

Replicelle System and SC-1 Therapy Kit *investigational (orphan) peripheral stem cell replicator for patients receiving high-dose chemotherapy*

Repliva 21/7 film-coated tablets (in packs of 28) ℞ *hematinic* [ferrous bisglycinate chelate; ferrous fumarate; vitamin B_{12}; vitamin C; folic acid] 70•81•0.01•200•1 mg × 21 days; counters × 7 days

rEPO (recombinant erythropoietin) [see: epoetin alfa; epoetin beta]

repository corticotropin [see: corticotropin, repository]

Reprexain film-coated tablets ℞ *narcotic analgesic; antipyretic* [hydrocodone bitartrate; ibuprofen] 5•200 mg

repromicin USAN, INN *antibacterial*

Repronex powder or pellet for IM or subcu injection ℞ *gonadotropin; follicle-stimulating hormone (FSH) and luteinizing hormone (LH) for the induction of ovulation in women and spermatogenesis in men; adjunct to assisted reproductive technologies (ART)* [menotropins] 75, 150 FSH units + 75, 150 LH units

reproterol INN, BAN *bronchodilator* [also: reproterol HCl]

reproterol HCl USAN *bronchodilator* [also: reproterol]

Requip film-coated tablets ℞ *dopamine agonist for idiopathic Parkinson disease; treatment for primary restless legs syndrome (RLS)* [ropinirole HCl] 0.25, 0.5, 1, 2, 3, 4, 5 mg

Requip CR (controlled release) *investigational (NDA filed) dopamine agonist for restless legs syndrome (RLS)* [ropinirole HCl]

Requip XL film-coated extended-release tablets ℞ *once-daily dopamine agonist for idiopathic Parkinson disease* [ropinirole] 2, 3, 4, 8 mg

rescimetol INN

rescinnamine NF, INN, BAN *antihypertensive; rauwolfia derivative*

Rescon-DM oral liquid OTC *antitussive; antihistamine; decongestant* [dextromethorphan hydrobromide; chlorpheniramine maleate; pseudoephedrine HCl] 10•2•30 mg/5 mL

Rescon-GG oral liquid OTC *decongestant; expectorant* [phenylephrine HCl; guaifenesin] 10•200 mg/10 mL

Rescon-Jr. sustained-release caplets ℞ *decongestant; antihistamine* [phenylephrine HCl; chlorpheniramine maleate] 20•4 mg

Rescon-MX sustained-release tablets ℞ *decongestant; antihistamine; anticholinergic to dry mucosal secretions* [phenylephrine HCl; chlorpheniramine maleate; methscopolamine nitrate] 40•8•2.5

Rescriptor tablets ℞ *antiretroviral; nonnucleoside reverse transcriptase inhibi-*

tor (NNRTI) for HIV-1 infection [delavirdine mesylate] 100, 200 mg

Rescue Pak (trademarked delivery form) *unit dose package*

Rescula eye drops (discontinued 2005) ℞ *prostaglandin $F_{2\alpha}$ analogue for glaucoma and ocular hypertension* [unoprostone isopropyl] 0.15%

Resectisol solution ℞ *genitourinary irrigant* [mannitol] 5 g/100 mL

reserpine USP, INN *antihypertensive; peripheral antiadrenergic; rauwolfia derivative* 0.1, 0.25 mg oral

resibufogenin [see: bufogenin]

resiniferatoxin (RTX) *investigational (orphan) neuronal desensitizing agent for intractable pain at end-stage disease*

resocortol butyrate USAN *topical anti-inflammatory*

Resol oral solution OTC *electrolyte replacement* [sodium, potassium, chloride, calcium, magnesium, and phosphate electrolytes] ② rose oil

Resolve/GP solution OTC *cleaning solution for hard or rigid gas permeable contact lenses*

resorantel INN

resorcin [see: resorcinol]

resorcin acetate [see: resorcinol monoacetate]

resorcin brown NF

resorcinol USP *keratolytic; antifungal*

resorcinol monoacetate USP *antiseborrheic; keratolytic*

Resource; Resource Plus; Resource Diabetic; Resource Just for Kids ready-to-use oral liquid OTC *enteral nutritional therapy* [lactose-free formula]

ReSource Arginaid powder for oral liquid OTC *arginine-rich enteral nutritional therapy to speed recovery of pressure ulcers, burns, or surgery*

Resource Fruit Beverage ready-to-use oral liquid OTC *enteral nutritional therapy* [whey protein–based] 237 mL/pkt.

Respa A.R. tablets ℞ *decongestant; antihistamine; anticholinergic to dry mucosal secretions* [pseudoephedrine HCl; chlorpheniramine maleate; belladonna alkaloids (atropine, hyoscyamine, scopolamine)] 90•8•0.024 mg

Respa-1st sustained-release tablets ℞ *decongestant; expectorant* [pseudoephedrine HCl; guaifenesin] 58•600 mg

Respa-DM sustained-release tablets ℞ *antitussive; expectorant* [dextromethorphan hydrobromide; guaifenesin] 28•600 mg

Respa-GF sustained-release tablets (discontinued 2004) ℞ *expectorant* [guaifenesin] 600 mg

Respahist sustained-release capsules ℞ *decongestant; antihistamine* [pseudoephedrine HCl; brompheniramine maleate] 60•6 mg

Respaire-60 SR extended-release capsules ℞ *decongestant; expectorant* [pseudoephedrine HCl; guaifenesin] 60•200 mg

Respaire-120 SR dual-release capsules ℞ *decongestant; expectorant* [pseudoephedrine HCl (extended release); guaifenesin (immediate release)] 120•250 mg

Respalor ready-to-use oral liquid OTC *enteral nutritional therapy for pulmonary problems*

Respbid sustained-release tablets (discontinued 2004) ℞ *antiasthmatic; bronchodilator* [theophylline] 250, 500 mg

Resperal syrup ℞ *antitussive; antihistamine; sleep aid; decongestant* [dextromethorphan hydrobromide; pyrilamine maleate; dexchlorpheniramine maleate; phenylephrine HCl] 5•5•1.25•5 mg/5 mL

RespiGam IV infusion ℞ *preventative for respiratory syncytial virus (RSV) infections in high-risk infants (orphan)* [respiratory syncytial virus immune globulin (RSV-IG)] 2500 mg/dose (50 mg/mL)

Respihaler (trademarked delivery form) *oral inhalation aerosol*

RespiPak (trademarked packaging form) *tablets in daily compliance packaging*

Respiracult-Strep culture paddles for professional use ℞ *in vitro diagnostic test for Group A streptococci from throat and nasopharyngeal sources*

respiratory syncytial virus immune globulin (RSV-IG) *preventative for respiratory syncytial virus (RSV) infections in high-risk infants (orphan); investigational (orphan) treatment for RSV*

Respirgard II (trademarked delivery device) *nebulizer*

Respi-Tann chewable tablets, oral suspension ℞ *antitussive; decongestant* [carbetapentane tannate; pseudoephedrine tannate] 25•75 mg; 25•75 mg/5 mL

Respi-Tann G oral suspension ℞ *antitussive; expectorant* [carbetapentane citrate; guaifenesin] 7.5•200 mg/5 mL

Respi-Tann Pd oral suspension ℞ *antitussive; decongestant* [carbetapentane tannate; pseudoephedrine tannate] 15•60 mg/5 mL

Respules (trademarked delivery form) *single-dose ampule for inhalation*

Restasis eye drop emulsion ℞ *immunomodulator and anti-inflammatory to increase tear production in patients with Sjögren keratoconjunctivitis sicca (orphan)* [cyclosporine] 0.05%

restoratives *a class of agents that promote a restoration of strength and vigor (a term used in folk medicine)*

Restoril capsules ℞ *benzodiazepine sedative and hypnotic* [temazepam] 7.5, 15, 22.5, 30 mg

Restylane subcu injection in prefilled syringes ℞ *dermal filler for deep wrinkles and facial folds* [hyaluronic acid] 20 mg/mL

Retaane eye drop suspension *investigational (NDA filed) angiostatic steroid for neovascularization of the eye to preserve vision in patients with wet age-related macular degeneration* [anecortave acetate]

Re-Tann oral suspension ℞ *antitussive; decongestant* [carbetapentane tannate; pseudoephedrine tannate] 25•75 mg/5 mL ⑨ R-Tanna; rutin

retapamulin *topical pleuromutilin antibiotic for impetigo caused by* Staphylococcus aureus *and* Streptococcus pyogenes *infections*

Retavase powder for IV infusion ℞ *thrombolytic; tissue plasminogen activator (tPA) for acute myocardial infarction* [reteplase] 18.8 mg (10.8 IU)

retelliptine INN

reteplase USAN, INN *thrombolytic; tissue plasminogen activator (tPA) for acute myocardial infarction*

retigabine *investigational (Phase III) potassium channel opener for adjunctive treatment of partial-onset epilepsy in adults*

Retin-A cream, gel ℞ *keratolytic for acne* [tretinoin] 0.025%, 0.05%, 0.1% (0.01% available in Canada); 0.01%, 0.025%, 0.1% ⑨ R-Tanna; rutin

Retin-A topical liquid (discontinued 2006) ℞ *keratolytic for acne* [tretinoin] 0.05% ⑨ R-Tanna; rutin

Retin-A Micro gel ℞ *keratolytic for acne* [tretinoin] 0.04%, 0.1%

retinal epithelial cells transfected with plasmid vector expressing ciliary neurotropic growth factor *investigational (orphan) treatment for retinitis pigmentosa*

retinamide R-II *investigational (orphan) for myelodysplastic syndrome*

retinoic acid (all-*trans*-retinoic acid) [see: tretinoin]

9-*cis*-retinoic acid [see: alitretinoin]

13-*cis*-retinoic acid [see: isotretinoin]

retinoids *a class of antineoplastics chemically related to vitamin A*

Retinol cream OTC *moisturizer; emollient* [vitamin A] 100 000 IU

retinol INN, BAN *vitamin A₁*

Retinol-A cream OTC *moisturizer; emollient* [vitamin A palmitate] 10 000 IU/g

Retisert ocular implant ℞ *corticosteroidal anti-inflammatory for uveitis (orphan)* [fluocinolone acetonide] 0.59 mg

R-etodolac *investigational (orphan) treatment for chronic lymphocytic leukemia*

Retrovir film-coated tablets, capsules, syrup, IV injection ℞ *nucleoside antiviral for AIDS and AIDS-related complex (orphan), HIV infection, and to prevent maternal-fetal HIV transfer* [zidovudine] 300 mg; 100 mg; 50 mg/5 mL; 10 mg/mL

retroviral vector gamma-c cDNA [see: gamma-c cDNA, retroviral vector]

retroviral vector GC gene 1750 [see: glucocerebrosidase, recombinant retroviral vector]

retroviral vector glucocerebrosidase (GC) [see: glucocerebrosidase, recombinant retroviral vector]

Revaproxyn ⓔ (European name for U.S. product **Efaproxyn**)

Revatio film-coated tablets ℞ *phosphodiesterase type 5 (PDE5) inhibitor; selective vasodilator for pulmonary arterial hypertension (PAH)* [sildenafil citrate] 20 mg

Reveal Rapid HIV-1 Antibody Test kit for professional use ℞ *in vitro diagnostic aid for HIV-1 in blood*

revenast INN

reverse transcriptase (RT) inhibitors *a class of antiretroviral drugs that inhibit the activity of reverse transcriptase in viral cells, preventing cell replication; subdivided into nucleoside (purine- or pyrimidine-based) and nonnucleoside types* [reverse transcriptase is also known as DNA polymerase]

reversible proton pump inhibitors [see: proton pump inhibitors]

Reversol IV or IM injection ℞ *myasthenia gravis treatment; antidote to curare overdose* [edrophonium chloride] 10 mg/mL

Revex IV, IM, or subcu injection (discontinued 2008) ℞ *narcotic antagonist; antidote to opioid overdose; post-*

anesthesia "stir-up" [nalmefene] 0.1 mg/mL (postop), 1 mg/mL (antidote)

Rēv-Eyes powder for eye drops ℞ *miotic to reverse iatrogenic mydriasis* [dapiprazole HCl] 0.5% ⓡ Rivasa

ReVia film-coated tablets ℞ *narcotic antagonist for opiate dependence or overdose (orphan) and alcoholism; also used for eating disorders and postconcussional syndrome* [naltrexone HCl] 50 mg

Revimid *investigational (orphan) for multiple myeloma; investigational (Phase III) for malignant melanoma* [3-(4'-aminoisoindoline-1'-one)-1-piperidine-2,6-dione]

reviparin sodium *investigational (orphan) for deep vein thrombosis (DVT) in pediatric or pregnant patients*

Revlimid capsules ℞ *immunomodulator for multiple myeloma and transfusion-dependent anemia in patients with myelodysplastic syndrome (orphan)* [lenalidomide] 5, 10, 15, 25 mg

revospirone INN, BAN

Rexin-G IV injection *investigational (NDA filed, orphan) tumor-targeted gene therapy for pancreatic cancer*

Rexolate IM injection (discontinued 2006) ℞ *analgesic; antipyretic; anti-inflammatory; antirheumatic* [sodium thiosalicylate] 50 mg/mL

Reyataz capsules ℞ *antiviral; protease inhibitor for HIV-1 infection* [atazanavir (as sulfate)] 100, 150, 200, 300 mg

Rezamid lotion OTC *antiseptic, antifungal, and keratolytic for acne* [sulfur; resorcinol; alcohol] 5%•2%•28%

Rezipas *investigational (orphan) for ulcerative colitis* [aminosalicylic acid]

Rezonic *investigational (NDA filed) NK-1 receptor antagonist for the prevention of chemotherapy-induced nausea and vomiting* [casopitant]

rGCR (recombinant glucocerebrosidase) [see: glucocerebrosidase, recombinant retroviral vector]

rG-CSF (recombinant granulocyte colony-stimulating factor) [see: lenograstim]

R-Gel OTC *analgesic; counterirritant* [capsaicin] 0.025%

R-Gen elixir ℞ *expectorant* [iodinated glycerol] 60 mg/5 mL ② Rēgain; Rogaine

R-gene 10 IV injection ℞ *diagnostic aid for pituitary (growth hormone) function* [arginine HCl] 10% (950 mOsm/L) ② Rēgain; Rogaine

RGG0853, E1A lipid complex *investigational (orphan) for advanced ovarian cancer*

rGM-CSF; rhGM-CSF; rhuGM-CSF (granulocyte-macrophage colony-stimulating factor) [q.v.]

rgp160; rgp160 IIIB; rgp160 MN (recombinant glycoprotein) [see: AIDS vaccine]

RGV (raltegravir) [q.v.]

Rhamnus cathartica; R. frangula medicinal herb [see: buckthorn]

Rhamnus purshiana medicinal herb [see: cascara sagrada]

rhAPC (recombinant human activated protein C) [see: drotrecogan alfa]

(rhaTIII) recombinant human antithrombin III) [see: antithrombin III]

rhDNase (recombinant human deoxyribonuclease) [see: dornase alfa]

Rheaban caplets (discontinued 2004) OTC *antidiarrheal; GI adsorbent* [activated attapulgite] 750 mg ② Repan; Riopan

rhenium *element (Re)*

Rheomacrodex IV infusion ℞ *plasma volume expander for shock due to hemorrhage, burns, or surgery* [dextran 40] 10%

rheotran (45) [see: dextran 45]

rhetinic acid [see: enoxolone]

Rheum palmatum medicinal herb [see: rhubarb]

Rheumatex slide tests for professional use ℞ *in vitro diagnostic aid for rheumatoid factor in the blood*

rheumatism root *medicinal herb* [see: twin leaf; wild yam]

rheumatism weed *medicinal herb* [see: pipsissewa]

Rheumaton slide tests for professional use ℞ *in vitro diagnostic aid for rheumatoid factor in serum or synovial fluid*

Rheumatrex Dose Pack (tablets) ℞ *antimetabolite antineoplastic for leukemia; systemic antipsoriatic; antirheumatic for adult and juvenile rheumatoid arthritis (orphan)* [methotrexate] 2.5 mg

rhFSH (recombinant human follicle-stimulating hormone) [see: menotropins]

rhGAA (recombinant human glucosidase-alpha acid) [see: alglucosidase alfa]

rhGH (recombinant human growth hormone) [see: somatropin]

rhIGF-1 (recombinant human insulin-like growth factor-1) [now: mecasermin]

rhIL-1R; rhu IL-1R (recombinant human interleukin-1 receptor) [see: interleukin-1 receptor]

rhIL-11 (recombinant human interleukin-11) [see: oprelvekin]

rhIL-12 (recombinant human interleukin-12) [see: interleukin-12]

Rhinabid extended-release capsules (discontinued 2007) ℞ *decongestant; antihistamine* [phenylephrine HCl; brompheniramine maleate] 15•12 mg

Rhinabid PD extended-release pediatric capsules (discontinued 2007) ℞ *decongestant; antihistamine* [phenylephrine HCl; brompheniramine maleate] 7.5•6 mg

Rhinacon A extended-release caplets ℞ *decongestant; antihistamine; sleep aid* [phenylephrine HCl; chlorpheniramine maleate; phenyltoloxamine citrate] 20•4•40 mg

Rhinall nasal spray, nose drops OTC *decongestant* [phenylephrine HCl] 0.25% ② ronnel

Rhinaris Lubricating Mist nasal spray, nasal gel OTC *nasal moisturizer* [polyethylene glycol; propylene glycol] 15%•5%; 15%•20%

Rhinatate Pediatric oral suspension (discontinued 2007) ℞ *decongestant; antihistamine; sleep aid* [phenylephrine tannate; chlorpheniramine tannate; pyrilamine tannate] 5•2•12.5 mg/5 mL

Rhinatate-NF Pediatric oral suspension (discontinued 2007) ℞ *decongestant; antihistamine* [phenylephrine tannate; chlorpheniramine tannate] 5•4.5 mg/5 mL

Rhinocort nasal inhalation aerosol (discontinued 2004) ℞ *corticosteroidal anti-inflammatory for seasonal or perennial allergic rhinitis* [budesonide] 32 mcg/dose

Rhinocort Aqua nasal spray in a metered-dose pump ℞ *corticosteroidal anti-inflammatory for seasonal or perennial allergic rhinitis* [budesonide] 32 mcg/dose

Rh$_O$(D) immune globulin USP *passive immunizing agent for antenatal or postpartum prophylaxis of Rh hemolytic disease of the newborn; treatment for immune thrombocytopenic purpura (orphan)* [also see: globulin, immune]

Rh$_O$(D) immune human globulin [now: Rh$_O$(D) immune globulin]

rhodine [see: aspirin]

rhodium *element (Rh)* ⧗ radium

RhoGAM IM injection in prefilled syringes ℞ *immunizing agent for antenatal or postpartum prophylaxis of Rh hemolytic disease of the newborn* [Rh$_O$(D) immune globulin (gamma globulin)] 300 mcg

Rhophylac IV or IM injection in prefilled syringes ℞ *immunizing agent for antenatal or postpartum prophylaxis of Rh hemolytic disease of the newborn; treatment for immune thrombocytopenic purpura (orphan)* [Rh$_O$(D) immune globulin (gamma globulin)] 1500 IU (300 mcg)

rHSA (recombinant human serum albumin) [see: albumin, human]

rhubarb (*Rheum palmatum*) root *medicinal herb for colon and liver disorders*

rHuIFN-beta; rIFN-beta (recombinant [human] interferon beta) [see: interferon beta-1b, recombinant]

rhuMAb-E25 (monoclonal antibody E25, recombinant human) [now: omalizumab]

rhuMAb-VEGF (monoclonal antibody to vascular endothelial growth factor, recombinant human) [now: bevacizumab]

Rhus glabra medicinal herb [see: sumach]

Riba 3.0 SIA reagent kit for professional use ℞ *in vitro diagnostic aid for hepatitis C* [strip immunoblot assay (SIA)]

ribaminol USAN, INN *memory adjuvant*

RibaPak film-coated caplets (in 14 packs) ℞ *nucleoside antiviral for chronic hepatitis C infections (orphan) and clinically stable HIV disease; also used for viral hemorrhagic fevers* [ribavirin] 400 mg × 14, 600 mg × 14, 400 mg × 7 + 600 mg × 7

Ribasphere pellet-filled capsules, film-coated caplets ℞ *nucleoside antiviral for chronic hepatitis C infections (orphan) and clinically stable HIV disease; also used for viral hemorrhagic fevers* [ribavirin] 200 mg; 200, 400, 600 mg

Ribatab film-coated caplets ℞ *nucleoside antiviral for chronic hepatitis C infections (orphan) and clinically stable HIV disease; also used for viral hemorrhagic fevers* [ribavirin] 400, 600 mg ⧗ Repetab; Robitab

ribavirin USP, INN *nucleoside antiviral for severe lower respiratory tract infections, chronic hepatitis C infections (orphan), and stable HIV disease; investigational (orphan) for hemorrhagic fever with renal syndrome* [also: tribavirin] 200, 400, 500, 600 mg oral

Ribes nigrum; R. rubrum medicinal herb [see: currant]

ribgrass; ribwort medicinal herb [see: plantain]

riboflavin (vitamin B$_2$) USP, INN *water-soluble vitamin; enzyme cofactor* 50, 100 mg oral

riboflavin 5'-phosphate sodium USP *vitamin*

riboflavine [see: riboflavin]

Ribomustine ⓔᵁᴿ (European name for U.S. product **Treanda**)

riboprine USAN, INN *antineoplastic*

ribostamycin INN, BAN

riboxamide [see: tiazofurin]

ricainide [see: indecainide HCl]

rice bran oil (gamma oryzanol) extract *medicinal herb used as a hypolipidemic and to treat gastrointestinal and menopausal symptoms*

richweed *medicinal herb* [see: black cohosh; stone root]

RID shampoo, mousse (aerosol foam) OTC *pediculicide for lice* [pyrethrins; piperonyl butoxide] 0.33%•4%

RID Pure Alternative gel OTC *pediculicide for lice* [dimethicone] 100%

Rid-A-Pain oral gel OTC *mucous membrane anesthetic* [benzocaine] 10% ⑨ riodipine

Rid-A-Pain-HP cream OTC *analgesic; counterirritant* [capsaicin] 0.075%

Ridaura capsules ℞ *antirheumatic* [auranofin] 3 mg

ridazolol INN

RIDD (recombinant interleukin-2, dacarbazine, DDP) *chemotherapy protocol*

Ridenol elixir (discontinued 2008) OTC *analgesic; antipyretic* [acetaminophen] 80 mg/5 mL

ridogrel USAN, INN, BAN *thromboxane synthetase inhibitor*

rifabutin USAN, INN *antiviral; antibacterial; for prevention of* Mycobacterium avium *complex (MAC) in advanced HIV patients (orphan)*

Rifadin capsules, powder for IV injection ℞ *tuberculostatic (orphan)* [rifampin] 150, 300 mg; 600 mg

rifalazil USAN *rifampin derivative; investigational (orphan) for pulmonary tuberculosis; investigational (Phase II) for* Mycobacterium avium *complex*

Rifamate capsules ℞ *tuberculostatic* [rifampin; isoniazid] 300•150 mg

rifametane USAN, INN *antibacterial*

rifamexil USAN *antibacterial*

rifamide USAN, INN *antibacterial*

rifampicin INN, BAN, JAN *antibacterial* [also: rifampin]

rifampin USAN, USP *antibacterial; antituberculosis agent (orphan)* [also: rifampicin] 150, 300 mg oral; 600 mg injection

rifampin & isoniazid & pyrazinamide *short-course treatment of tuberculosis (orphan)*

rifamycin INN, BAN

rifamycin diethylamide [see: rifamide]

rifamycin M-14 [see: rifamide]

rifapentine USAN, INN, BAN *antibacterial for tuberculosis (orphan); investigational (orphan) for AIDS-related* Mycobacterium avium *complex (MAC)*

Rifater tablets ℞ *short-course treatment for tuberculosis (orphan)* [rifampin; isoniazid; pyrazinamide] 120•50•300 mg

rifaxidin [see: rifaximin]

rifaximin USAN, INN *broad-spectrum rifamycin antibiotic for traveler's diarrhea; investigational (orphan) for hepatic encephalopathy*

rIFN-A (recombinant interferon alfa) [see: interferon alfa-2a, recombinant]

rIFN-α2 (recombinant interferon alfa-2) [see: interferon alfa-2b, recombinant]

rIFN-beta; rHuIFN-beta (recombinant [human] interferon beta) [see: interferon beta-1a, recombinant]

rifomycin [see: rifamycin]

RIG (rabies immune globulin) [q.v.]

rilapine INN

rilmazafone INN

rilmenidine INN

rilonacept *immunosuppressant; interleukin-1 (IL-1) blocker for cryopyrin-associated periodic syndrome (CAPS), familial cold autoinflammatory syndrome (FCAS), and Muckle-Wells syndrome (MWS); investigational (Phase II) for chronic gout*

rilopirox INN

rilozarone INN

Rilutek film-coated tablets ℞ *neuro-protective agent for amyotrophic lateral sclerosis (ALS) (orphan); investigational (orphan) for Huntington disease* [riluzole] 50 mg

riluzole USAN, INN *neuroprotective agent for amyotrophic lateral sclerosis (ALS) (orphan); investigational (orphan) for Huntington disease*

Rimactane capsules ℞ *tuberculostatic* [rifampin] 300 mg

rimantadine INN *antiviral; prophylaxis and treatment for influenza A virus* [also: rimantadine HCl]

rimantadine HCl USAN *antiviral; prophylaxis and treatment for influenza A virus* [also: rimantadine] 100 mg oral

rimazolium metilsulfate INN

rimcazole INN *antipsychotic* [also: rimcazole HCl]

rimcazole HCl USAN *antipsychotic* [also: rimcazole]

rimexolone USAN, INN, BAN *topical ophthalmic corticosteroidal anti-inflammatory*

rimiterol INN *bronchodilator* [also: rimiterol hydrobromide]

rimiterol hydrobromide USAN *bronchodilator* [also: rimiterol]

rimonabant *investigational (NDA filed) selective cannabinoid CB_1 blocker for smoking cessation, weight loss, increasing HDL, increasing insulin sensitivity, and decreasing C-reactive protein (CRP)*

rimoprogin INN

Rimso-50 solution for bladder instillation ℞ *anti-inflammatory for symptomatic relief of interstitial cystitis* [dimethyl sulfoxide (DMSO)] 50% ☑ RMS

Rinade B.I.D. sustained-release capsules (discontinued 2004) ℞ *decongestant; antihistamine* [pseudoephedrine HCl; chlorpheniramine maleate] 120•8 mg

Rindal HD Plus syrup ℞ *narcotic antitussive; antihistamine; decongestant* [hydrocodone bitartrate; chlorpheniramine maleate; phenylephrine HCl] 3.5•2•7.5 mg/5 mL

Rindal HPD syrup ℞ *narcotic antitussive; antihistamine; sleep aid; decongestant* [hydrocodone bitartrate; diphenhydramine HCl; phenylephrine HCl] 2•12.5•7.5 mg/5 mL

Ringer injection USP *fluid and electrolyte replenisher* [also: compound solution of sodium chloride]

Ringer injection, lactated USP *fluid and electrolyte replenisher; systemic alkalizer* [also: compound solution of sodium lactate]

Ringer irrigation USP *irrigation solution*

Ringer irrigation, lactated *irrigation solution*

Ringer solution [now: Ringer irrigation]

Rinnovi Nail System topical stick ℞ *moisturizer; emollient; keratolytic* [urea] 50%

riodipine INN ☑ Rid-A-Pain

Riomet oral liquid ℞ *biguanide antidiabetic that decreases hepatic glucose production and increases cellular response to insulin* [metformin HCl] 500 mg/5 mL

Riopan oral suspension OTC *antacid* [magaldrate] 540 mg/5 mL ☑ Repan; Rheaban

Riopan Plus chewable tablets, oral suspension OTC *antacid; antiflatulent* [magaldrate; simethicone] 480•20, 1080•20 mg; 540•40, 1080•40 mg/5 mL

rioprostil USAN, INN *gastric antisecretory*

ripazepam USAN, INN *minor tranquilizer*

ripple grass *medicinal herb* [see: plantain]

Riquent *investigational (NDA filed, orphan) immunosuppressant for lupus-associated nephritis* [abetimus sodium]

risedronate sodium USAN *bisphosphonate bone resorption inhibitor for Paget disease and corticosteroid-induced or age-related osteoporosis in men and women*

rismorelin porcine USAN *growth stimulant for growth hormone deficiencies*

risocaine USAN, INN *local anesthetic*

risotilide HCl USAN *antiarrhythmic*

Risperdal tablets, M-Tabs (orally disintegrating tablets), oral drops ℞ *novel*

*(atypical) benzisoxazole antipsychotic
for schizophrenia, manic episodes of a
bipolar disorder, pediatric behavioral
problems, and autism; also used for
obsessive-compulsive disorder (OCD)
and Tourette syndrome* [risperidone]
0.25, 0.5, 1, 2, 3, 4 mg; 0.5, 1, 2, 3, 4
mg; 1 mg/mL

Risperdal Consta long-acting injection in prefilled syringes ℞ *novel
(atypical) benzisoxazole antipsychotic
for schizophrenia* [risperidone (encapsulated in polymer microspheres)]
12.5, 25, 37.5, 50 mg

risperidone USAN, INN, BAN *novel
(atypical) benzisoxazole antipsychotic
for schizophrenia, manic episodes of a
bipolar disorder, pediatric behavioral
problems, and autism; also used for
obsessive-compulsive disorder (OCD)
and Tourette syndrome* 0.25, 0.5, 1, 2,
3, 4 mg oral

ristianol INN, BAN *immunoregulator*
[also: ristianol phosphate]

ristianol phosphate USAN *immunoregulator* [also: ristianol]

ristocetin USP, INN, BAN

Ritalin tablets ℞ *CNS stimulant for
attention-deficit/hyperactivity disorder
(ADHD) and narcolepsy; also abused
as a street drug* [methylphenidate
HCl] 5, 10, 20 mg

Ritalin LA dual-release capsules (50%
immediate release, 50% delayed
release) ℞ *CNS stimulant for atten-
tion-deficit/hyperactivity disorder
(ADHD)* [methylphenidate HCl] 10,
20, 30, 40 mg

Ritalin SR sustained-release tablets ℞
*CNS stimulant for attention-deficit/
hyperactivity disorder (ADHD) and narcolepsy* [methylphenidate HCl] 20 mg

ritanserin USAN, INN, BAN *serotonin S$_2$
antagonist for various psychiatric illnesses and substance abuse*

ritiometan INN

ritodrine USAN, INN *smooth muscle
relaxant*

ritodrine HCl USAN, USP *smooth muscle relaxant; uterine relaxant to arrest
preterm labor* 10, 15 mg/mL injection

Ritodrine HCl in 5% Dextrose IV
infusion in 500 mL LifeCare bags
(discontinued 2006) ℞ *uterine relaxant to arrest preterm labor* [ritodrine
HCl; dextrose] 0.03%•5%

ritolukast USAN, INN *antiasthmatic;
leukotriene antagonist*

ritonavir USAN, INN *antiretroviral protease inhibitor for HIV infection*

ritropirronium bromide INN

ritrosulfan INN

Rituxan IV infusion ℞ *monoclonal
antibody for non-Hodgkin B-cell lymphoma (orphan) and rheumatoid arthritis (RA); investigational (orphan) for
chronic lymphocytic leukemia and
immune thrombocytopenic purpura;
investigational (Phase II) for MS; also
used for macroglobulinemia* [ritux-
imab] 10 mg/mL

rituximab USAN *monoclonal antibody
for non-Hodgkin B-cell lymphoma
(orphan) and rheumatoid arthritis (RA);
investigational (orphan) for chronic
lymphocytic leukemia and immune
thrombocytopenic purpura; also used
for macroglobulinemia*

rivaroxaban *factor Xa coagulation inhibitor; investigational (NDA filed) once-
daily oral antithrombotic for deep vein
thrombosis (DVT), venous thromboembolism (VTE), and stroke prevention*

rivastigmine USAN *acetylcholinesterase
inhibitor to increase cognition in Alzheimer and Parkinson disease*

rivastigmine tartrate *acetylcholinesterase inhibitor to increase cognition in
Alzheimer and Parkinson disease* 1.5,
3, 4.5, 6 mg oral

rivoglitazone USAN *antidiabetic for type
2 diabetes*

Rizaben *investigational (orphan) for
malignant glioma* [tranilast]

rizatriptan benzoate USAN *vascular
serotonin 5-HT$_{1B/1D}$ receptor agonist
for the acute treatment of migraine*

rizatriptan sulfate USAN *vascular serotonin 5-HT$_{1B/1D}$ receptor agonist for the acute treatment of migraine*

rizolipase INN

r-metHuLeptin [see: metreleptin]

RMP-7 (receptor-mediated permeabilizer) [see: lobradimil]

RMS suppositories ℞ *narcotic analgesic* [morphine sulfate] 5, 10, 20, 30 mg

rNPA (recombinant novel plasminogen activator) [see: novel plasminogen activator]

Roaccutane ⓔᵁᴿ gel (French name for U.S. product **Accutane**) ② Reactine

rob elder *medicinal herb* [see: elderberry]

Robafen CF oral liquid OTC *antitussive; decongestant; expectorant* [dextromethorphan hydrobromide; pseudoephedrine HCl; guaifenesin] 10•30•100 mg/5 mL

Robafen PE oral liquid (discontinued 2007) OTC *decongestant; expectorant* [pseudoephedrine HCl; guaifenesin] 60•200 mg/10 mL

RoBathol Bath Oil OTC *bath emollient*

Robaxin tablets, IV or IM injection ℞ *skeletal muscle relaxant* [methocarbamol] 500, 750 mg; 100 mg/mL

Robaxisal tablets (discontinued 2004) ℞ *skeletal muscle relaxant; analgesic; antipyretic* [methocarbamol; aspirin] 400•325 mg

robenidine INN *coccidiostat for poultry* [also: robenidine HCl]

robenidine HCl USAN *coccidiostat for poultry* [also: robenidine]

Robicap (trademarked dosage form) *capsule*

Robinul tablets, IV or IM injection ℞ *GI antispasmodic; anticholinergic; peptic ulcer treatment adjunct; antisecretory* [glycopyrrolate] 1 mg; 0.2 mg/5 mL

Robinul Forte tablets ℞ *GI antispasmodic; anticholinergic; peptic ulcer treatment adjunct; antisecretory* [glycopyrrolate] 2 mg

Robitab (trademarked dosage form) *tablet* ② Repetab; Ribatab

Robitussin oral liquid OTC *expectorant* [guaifenesin] 100 mg/5 mL

Robitussin Cold, Cold & Congestion caplets OTC *antitussive; decongestant; expectorant* [dextromethorphan hydrobromide; pseudoephedrine HCl; guaifenesin] 10•30•200 mg

Robitussin Cold, Cold & Cough softgels (discontinued 2007) OTC *antitussive; decongestant; expectorant* [dextromethorphan hydrobromide; pseudoephedrine HCl; guaifenesin] 10•30•200 mg

Robitussin Cold, Multi-Symptom Cold & Flu caplets, softgels (discontinued 2007) OTC *antitussive; decongestant; expectorant; analgesic; antipyretic* [dextromethorphan hydrobromide; pseudoephedrine HCl; guaifenesin; acetaminophen] 10•30•200•325 mg; 10•30•100•250 mg

Robitussin Cold, Sinus & Congestion caplets (discontinued 2007) OTC *decongestant; expectorant; analgesic; antipyretic* [pseudoephedrine HCl; guaifenesin; acetaminophen] 30•200•325 mg

Robitussin Cough oral liquid OTC *antitussive* [dextromethorphan hydrobromide; alcohol 1.4%] 15 mg/5 mL

Robitussin Cough, Cold & Flu Nighttime syrup OTC *antitussive; antihistamine; decongestant; analgesic; antipyretic* [dextromethorphan hydrobromide; chlorpheniramine maleate; phenylephrine HCl; acetaminophen] 10•2•5•320 mg/10 mL

Robitussin Cough & Allergy oral liquid OTC *antitussive; antihistamine; decongestant* [dextromethorphan hydrobromide; brompheniramine maleate; phenylephrine HCl] 10•2•5 mg/5 mL

Robitussin Cough & Cold infant oral drops (discontinued 2007) OTC *antitussive; decongestant; expectorant; for children 2–5 years* [dextromethorphan hydrobromide; pseudoephedrine HCl; guaifenesin] 5•15•100 mg/2.5 mL

Robitussin Cough & Cold; Robitussin Honey Cough & Cold; Robi-

tussin Pediatric Cough & Cold Formula oral liquid (discontinued 2007) OTC *antitussive; decongestant* [dextromethorphan hydrobromide; pseudoephedrine HCl] 30•60 mg/10 mL; 30•60 mg/15 mL; 7.5•15 mg/5 mL

Robitussin Cough & Congestion oral liquid OTC *antitussive; expectorant* [dextromethorphan hydrobromide; guaifenesin] 10•200 mg/5 mL

Robitussin Cough Drops (lozenges) OTC *mild anesthetic; antipruritic; counterirritant* [menthol] 7.4, 10 mg

Robitussin Cough Sugar-Free DM oral liquid OTC *antitussive; expectorant* [dextromethorphan hydrobromide; guaifenesin] 10•100 mg/5 mL

Robitussin CoughGels liquid-filled gelcaps OTC *antitussive* [dextromethorphan hydrobromide] 15 mg

Robitussin Flu oral liquid (discontinued 2007) OTC *antitussive; antihistamine; decongestant; analgesic; antipyretic* [dextromethorphan hydrobromide; chlorpheniramine maleate; pseudoephedrine HCl; acetaminophen] 20•4•60•640 mg/20 mL

Robitussin Honey Flu Multi-Symptom oral liquid (discontinued 2007) OTC *antitussive; decongestant; analgesic; antipyretic* [dextromethorphan hydrobromide; pseudoephedrine HCl; acetaminophen] 20•60•500 mg/15 mL

Robitussin Honey Flu Nighttime syrup for oral liquid (discontinued 2007) OTC *antitussive; antihistamine; decongestant; analgesic; antipyretic* [dextromethorphan hydrobromide; chlorpheniramine maleate; pseudoephedrine HCl; acetaminophen] 20•4•60•500 mg/pouch

Robitussin Honey Flu Non-Drowsy syrup for oral solution (discontinued 2007) OTC *antitussive; decongestant; analgesic; antipyretic* [dextromethorphan hydrobromide; pseudoephedrine HCl; acetaminophen] 20•60•500 mg/pouch

Robitussin Liquid Center Cough Drops (lozenges) OTC *mild anesthetic; antipruritic; counterirritant* [menthol] 10 mg

Robitussin Night Relief oral liquid (discontinued 2007) OTC *antitussive; antihistamine; sleep aid; decongestant; analgesic; antipyretic* [dextromethorphan hydrobromide; pyrilamine maleate; pseudoephedrine HCl; acetaminophen] 30•50•60•650 mg/30 mL

Robitussin PE Head and Chest Congestion oral liquid OTC *decongestant; expectorant* [phenylephrine HCl; guaifenesin] 10•200 mg/10 mL

Robitussin Pediatric Cough oral liquid OTC *antitussive* [dextromethorphan hydrobromide] 7.5 mg/5 mL

Robitussin Pediatric Cough & Cold Long-Acting oral liquid OTC *antitussive; antihistamine; for adults and children ≥ 6 years* [dextromethorphan hydrobromide; chlorpheniramine maleate] 15•2 mg/10 mL

Robitussin Pediatric Cough & Cold Nighttime oral liquid OTC *antitussive; antihistamine; decongestant; for adults and children ≥ 6 years* [dextromethorphan hydrobromide; chlorpheniramine maleate; phenylephrine HCl] 10•2•5 mg/10 mL

Robitussin Pediatric Cough/Cold CF oral drops OTC *antitussive; decongestant; expectorant; for children 2–5 years* [dextromethorphan hydrobromide; phenylephrine HCl; guaifenesin] 2•1•40 mg/mL

Robitussin PM Cough & Cold oral liquid (discontinued 2007) OTC *antitussive; antihistamine; decongestant* [dextromethorphan hydrobromide; chlorpheniramine maleate; pseudoephedrine HCl] 15•2•30 mg/10 mL

Robitussin Severe Congestion Liqui-Gels (liquid-filled softgels) (discontinued 2007) OTC *decongestant; expectorant* [pseudoephedrine HCl; guaifenesin] 30•200 mg

Robitussin Sugar Free Cough oral liquid (discontinued 2007) OTC *anti-*

tussive; expectorant [dextromethorphan hydrobromide; guaifenesin] 20•200 mg/10 mL

Robitussin-CF oral liquid (discontinued 2007) OTC *antitussive; decongestant; expectorant* [dextromethorphan hydrobromide; pseudoephedrine HCl; guaifenesin] 20•60•200 mg/10 mL

Robitussin-DM infants' oral drops (discontinued 2007) OTC *antitussive; expectorant; for children 2–5 years* [dextromethorphan hydrobromide; guaifenesin] 5•100 mg/2.5 mL

Robitussin-DM oral liquid OTC *antitussive; expectorant* [dextromethorphan hydrobromide; guaifenesin] 10•100 mg/5 mL

Robitussin-PE oral liquid (discontinued 2007) OTC *decongestant; expectorant* [pseudoephedrine HCl; guaifenesin; alcohol 1.4%] 60•200 mg/10 mL

Rocaltrol capsules, oral solution ℞ *vitamin D therapy for hypoparathyroidism and hypocalcemia due to chronic renal dialysis; also used to decrease the severity of psoriatic lesions* [calcitriol] 0.25, 0.5 mcg; 1 mcg/mL

rocastine INN *antihistamine* [also: rocastine HCl]

rocastine HCl USAN *antihistamine* [also: rocastine]

Rocephin powder or frozen premix for IV or IM injection ℞ *third-generation cephalosporin antibiotic* [ceftriaxone sodium] 0.25, 0.5, 1, 2, 10 g

rochelle salt [see: potassium sodium tartrate]

rociverine INN

rock brake; rock polypod *medicinal herb* [see: female fern]

rock elm *medicinal herb* [see: slippery elm]

rock parsley *medicinal herb* [see: parsley]

rock rose (Helianthemum canadense) plant *medicinal herb used as an astringent and tonic*

Rocky Mountain grape *medicinal herb* [see: Oregon grape]

Rocky Mountain spotted fever vaccine USP

rocuronium bromide USAN, INN, BAN *nondepolarizing neuromuscular blocking agent; muscle relaxant; adjunct to general anesthesia*

rodocaine USAN, INN *local anesthetic*

rodorubicin INN

rofecoxib *COX-2 inhibitor; nonsteroidal anti-inflammatory drug (NSAID) for osteoarthritis, rheumatoid arthritis, and primary dysmenorrhea; investigational (orphan) for juvenile rheumatoid arthritis* (withdrawn from the market in 2004 due to safety concerns)

rofelodine INN ⊘ Refludan

Roferon-A subcu or IM injection in prefilled syringes ℞ *immunostimulant for hairy cell leukemia, hepatitis C, Kaposi sarcoma (orphan), and chronic myelogenous leukemia (orphan); investigational (orphan) for malignant melanoma and esophageal, renal, colorectal, and other cancers* [interferon alfa-2a] 3, 6, 9 million IU

roflumilast *investigational (Phase III) agent for chronic obstructive pulmonary disease (COPD) and asthma*

roflurane USAN, INN *inhalation anesthetic*

Rogaine; Rogaine for Men; Rogaine for Women topical solution OTC *hair growth stimulant* [minoxidil] 2%; 2%, 5%; 2% ⊘ Rēgain

Rogaine Men's Extra Strength topical foam OTC *hair growth stimulant* [minoxidil] 5%

rogletimide USAN, INN, BAN *antineoplastic; aromatase inhibitor*

Rohypnol (banned in the U.S.) ℞ *sedative and hypnotic; smuggled into the U.S. as a street drug, commonly called "roofies" or "the date rape drug"* [flunitrazepam]

rokitamycin INN

Rolaids; Calcium Rich Rolaids chewable tablets OTC *antacid* [magnesium hydroxide; calcium carbonate] 110•550, 135•675 mg; 80•412 mg

Rolaids Multi-Symptom chewable tablets OTC *antacid; antiflatulent* [magnesium hydroxide; calcium carbonate; simethicone] 135•675•60 mg

Rolaids Plus Gas Relief chewable tablets OTC *antacid; antiflatulent* [calcium carbonate; simethicone] 1177•80 mg

Rolaids Softchews OTC *antacid; calcium supplement* [calcium carbonate] 1177 mg

Rolazar (name changed to **Alimta** upon marketing release in 2004)

roletamide USAN, INN *hypnotic*

rolgamidine USAN, INN, BAN *antidiarrheal*

rolicton [see: amisometradine]

rolicyclidine INN

rolicypram BAN *antidepressant* [also: rolicyprine]

rolicyprine USAN, INN *antidepressant* [also: rolicypram]

rolipram USAN, INN *tranquilizer*

rolitetracycline USAN, USP, INN *antibacterial*

rolitetracycline nitrate USAN *antibacterial*

rolodine USAN, INN *skeletal muscle relaxant*

rolofylline *investigational (Phase III) agent for acute heart failure*

rolziracetam INN, BAN

Roman camomile *medicinal herb* [see: chamomile]

Roman laurel *medicinal herb* [see: laurel]

romazarit USAN, INN, BAN *anti-inflammatory; antirheumatic*

Romazicon IV injection ℞ *benzodiazepine antagonist to reverse anesthesia or treat overdose* [flumazenil] 0.1 mg/mL

rometin [see: clioquinol]

romifenone INN

romifidine INN

Romilar AC oral liquid (discontinued 2007) ℞ *narcotic antitussive; expectorant* [codeine phosphate; guaifenesin] 20•200 mg/10 mL

romiplostim *oral thrombopoietin (TPO) receptor agonist to increase platelet production in immune thrombocytopenic purpura (ITP)*

romurtide INN

ronactolol INN

Rondamine-DM syrup (discontinued 2007) ℞ *antitussive; antihistamine; decongestant* [dextromethorphan hydrobromide; brompheniramine maleate; pseudoephedrine HCl] 15•4•60 mg/5 mL

Rondec syrup, oral drops ℞ *decongestant; antihistamine; drops for children 6–24 months* [phenylephrine HCl; chlorpheniramine maleate] 12.5•4 mg/5 mL; 3.5•1 mg/mL

Rondec tablets (discontinued 2007) ℞ *decongestant; antihistamine* [pseudoephedrine HCl; carbinoxamine maleate] 60•4 mg

Rondec-DM oral drops ℞ *antitussive; antihistamine; decongestant; for children 6–24 months* [dextromethorphan hydrobromide; carbinoxamine maleate; phenylephrine HCl] 3•1•3.5 mg/mL

Rondec-DM syrup (discontinued 2007) ℞ *antitussive; antihistamine; decongestant* [dextromethorphan hydrobromide; chlorpheniramine maleate; phenylephrine HCl] 15•4•12.5 mg/5 mL

Rondec-TR timed-release tablets (discontinued 2007) ℞ *decongestant; antihistamine* [pseudoephedrine HCl; carbinoxamine maleate] 120•8 mg

Rondex oral drops ℞ *decongestant; antihistamine; for children 6–24 months* [phenylephrine HCl; chlorpheniramine maleate] 3.5•1 mg/mL

Rondex-DM oral drops ℞ *antitussive; antihistamine; decongestant; for children 6–24 months* [dextromethorphan hydrobromide; carbinoxamine maleate; phenylephrine HCl] 3•1•3.5 mg/mL

ronidazole USAN, INN *antiprotozoal*

ronifibrate INN

ronipamil INN

ronnel USAN *systemic insecticide* [also: fenclofos; fenchlorphos] ② Rhinall

ropinirole INN, BAN *dopamine agonist for Parkinson disease; treatment for restless legs syndrome (RLS)* [also: ropinirole HCl]

ropinirole HCl USAN *dopamine agonist for idiopathic Parkinson disease; treatment for primary restless legs syndrome (RLS)* [also: ropinirole] 0.25, 0.5, 1, 2, 3, 4, 5 mg

ropitoin INN *antiarrhythmic* [also: ropitoin HCl]

ropitoin HCl USAN *antiarrhythmic* [also: ropitoin]

ropivacaine INN *long-acting injectable local anesthetic*

ropivacaine HCl *long-acting local or regional anesthetic for surgery; epidural block for cesarean section*

ropizine USAN, INN *anticonvulsant*

roquinimex USAN, INN *investigational (orphan) bone marrow transplant adjunct for leukemia*

Rosa acicularis; R. canina; R. rugosa **and other species** *medicinal herb* [see: rose]

Rosac cream ℞ *antibiotic and keratolytic for acne* [sulfacetamide sodium; sulfur] 10%•5%

Rosac Wash emulsion ℞ *antibiotic and keratolytic for acne* [sulfacetamide sodium; sulfur] 10%•1%

rosamicin [now: rosaramicin]

rosamicin butyrate [now: rosaramicin butyrate]

rosamicin propionate [now: rosaramicin propionate]

rosamicin sodium phosphate [now: rosaramicin sodium phosphate]

rosamicin stearate [now: rosaramicin stearate]

Rosanil cleanser ℞ *antibiotic and keratolytic for acne* [sulfacetamide sodium; sulfur] 10%•5%

rosaprostol INN

rosaramicin USAN, INN *antibacterial*

rosaramicin butyrate USAN *antibacterial*

rosaramicin propionate USAN *antibacterial*

rosaramicin sodium phosphate USAN *antibacterial*

rosaramicin stearate USAN *antibacterial*

rosary pea *medicinal herb* [see: precatory bean]

rose (*Rosa acicularis; R. canina; R. rugosa* **and other species**) *flowers and hips medicinal herb for blood cleansing, cancer, colds, flu, infections, and sore throat; also used as a diuretic, mild laxative, and source of vitamin C*

rose, sun *medicinal herb* [see: rock rose]

rose bengal *diagnostic aid for corneal injury and pathology* 1.3 mg/strip

rose bengal sodium (^{131}I) INN *hepatic function test; radioactive agent* [also: rose bengal sodium I 131]

rose bengal sodium I 125 USAN *radioactive agent*

rose bengal sodium I 131 USAN, USP *hepatic function test; radioactive agent* [also: rose bengal sodium (^{131}I)]

rose laurel *medicinal herb* [see: mountain laurel]

rose oil NF *perfume* ⚗ Resol

rose petal aqueous infusion *ocular emollient*

rose water, stronger NF *perfume*

rose water ointment USP *emollient; ointment base*

rosemary (*Rosmarinus officinalis*) leaves *medicinal herb for flatulence, gastrointestinal spasm, halitosis, heart tonic, inducing diaphoresis, migraine headache, promoting menstrual flow, stimulating abortion, and stomach disorders*

Rosets ophthalmic strips OTC *diagnostic aid for corneal injury and pathology* [rose bengal] 1.3 mg

rosiglitazone maleate USAN *thiazolidinedione (TZD) antidiabetic and peroxisome proliferator–activated receptor–gamma (PPARγ) agonist that increases cellular response to insulin without increasing insulin secretion*

rosin USP

rosoxacin USAN, INN *antibacterial* [also: acrosoxacin]

rostaporfin USAN *photosensitizer; investigational (orphan) to prevent access graft disease in hemodialysis patients*

rosterolone INN

Rosula gel ℞ *antibiotic and keratolytic for acne, rosacea, and seborrheic der-*

matitis [sulfacetamide sodium; sulfur; urea] 10%•5%•10% ⊡ Resol

Rosula Aqueous Cleanser; Rosula Clarifying Wash topical liquid ℞ *antibiotic and keratolytic for acne and rosacea* [sulfacetamide sodium; sulfur; urea] 10%•5%•10%; 10%•4%•10%

Rosula NS cleansing pads ℞ *treatment for acne and rosacea* [sulfacetamide sodium; urea] 10%•10%

rosuvastatin calcium USAN *HMG-CoA reductase inhibitor for hypercholesterolemia, mixed dyslipidemia, and hypertriglyceridemia; reduces atheroma (plaque build-up) in coronary arteries*

Rotacaps (trademarked dosage form) *encapsulated powder for inhalation*

Rotadisk (trademarked dosage form) *powder for inhalation* [used in a **Diskhaler** delivery device]

rotamicillin INN

Rotarix powder for oral suspension ℞ *immunization against rotavirus gastroenteritis in infants 6–24 weeks* [rotavirus vaccine, live attenuated] 1 mL/dose

RotaTeq oral suspension in single-dose tubes ℞ *live oral immunization against rotavirus gastroenteritis in infants 6–32 weeks* [rotavirus vaccine, live pentavalent (5 rotaviruses)] 2 mL/tube

rotavirus vaccine *live oral immunization against rotavirus gastroenteritis in infants 6–32 weeks*

rotigotine *dopamine D_2 agonist for early-stage Parkinson disease; investigational (NDA filed) for restless legs syndrome (RLS)*

rotoxamine USAN, INN *antihistamine*

rotoxamine tartrate NF

rotraxate INN

round-leaved plantain *medicinal herb* [see: plantain]

Rovamycine *macrolide antibiotic; investigational (orphan) treatment for chronic cryptosporidiosis in immunocompromised patients* [spiramycin]

rovelizumab USAN, INN *immunomodulator; cell adhesion inhibitor*

Rowasa enema ℞ *anti-inflammatory for active ulcerative colitis, proctosigmoiditis, and proctitis* [mesalamine (5-aminosalicylic acid)] 4 g/60 mL

Rowasa suppositories (discontinued 2008) ℞ *anti-inflammatory for active ulcerative colitis, proctosigmoiditis, and proctitis* [mesalamine (5-aminosalicylic acid)] 500 mg

roxadimate USAN, INN *sunscreen*

Roxanol; Roxanol T; Roxanol 100 oral concentrate ℞ *narcotic analgesic* [morphine sulfate] 20 mg/mL; 20 mg/mL; 100 mg/5 mL

roxarsone USAN, INN *antibacterial*

roxatidine INN, BAN *histamine H_2 antagonist for gastric and duodenal ulcers* [also: roxatidine acetate HCl]

roxatidine acetate HCl USAN *histamine H_2 antagonist for gastric and duodenal ulcers* [also: roxatidine]

roxibolone INN

Roxicet tablets, oral solution ℞ *narcotic analgesic; antipyretic* [oxycodone HCl; acetaminophen] 5•325 mg; 5•325 mg/5 mL

Roxicet 5/500 caplets ℞ *narcotic analgesic; antipyretic* [oxycodone HCl; acetaminophen] 5•500 mg

Roxicodone tablets, oral solution, Intensol (concentrated oral solution) ℞ *narcotic analgesic* [oxycodone HCl] 5, 15, 30 mg; 5 mg/5 mL; 20 mg/mL

roxifiban acetate USAN *antithrombotic; fibrinogen receptor antagonist*

Roxilox capsules ℞ *narcotic analgesic; antipyretic* [oxycodone HCl; acetaminophen] 5•500 mg

roxindole INN

Roxiprin tablets ℞ *narcotic analgesic; antipyretic* [oxycodone HCl; oxycodone terephthalate; aspirin] 4.5•0.38•325 mg

roxithromycin USAN, INN *macrolide antibiotic*

roxolonium metilsulfate INN

roxoperone INN

royal jelly *natural remedy for improving fertility and increasing longevity*

Rozerem film-coated tablets ℞ *hypnotic for insomnia due to difficulty with sleep onset* [ramelteon] 8 mg

rp24 [see: AIDS vaccine]

rPA; r-PA (recombinant plasmino-gen activator) *more properly called "recombinant tissue plasminogen activator" (rtPA)* [see: alteplase; anistreplase; lanoteplase; monteplase; reteplase; saruplase; tenecteplase]

R/S lotion OTC *antiseptic, antifungal, and keratolytic for acne* [sulfur; resorcinol; alcohol] 5%•2%•28%

rSP-C lung surfactant *investigational (orphan) for adult respiratory distress syndrome (ARDS)*

RSV-IG (respiratory syncytial virus immune globulin) [q.v.]

RT (reverse transcriptase) inhibitors [q.v.]

RTA 744 *investigational (orphan) anthracycline derivative for malignant gliomas*

R-Tanna caplets ℞ *decongestant; antihistamine* [phenylephrine tannate; chlorpheniramine tannate] 25•9 mg ⃝ Re-Tann; rutin

R-Tanna 12 oral suspension ℞ *decongestant; antihistamine; sleep aid* [phenylephrine tannate; pyrilamine tannate] 5•30 mg/5 mL ⃝ Re-Tann; rutin

R-Tanna S Pediatric oral suspension (discontinued 2007) ℞ *decongestant; antihistamine* [phenylephrine tannate; chlorpheniramine tannate] 5•4.5 mg/5 mL

R-Tannic-S A/D pediatric oral suspension (discontinued 2004) ℞ *decongestant; antihistamine; sleep aid* [phenylephrine tannate; pyrilamine tannate] 5•30 mg/5 mL

rtPA; rt-PA (recombinant tissue plasminogen activator) [see: alteplase; anistreplase; lanoteplase; monteplase; reteplase; saruplase; tenecteplase]

Rubazyme reagent kit for professional use ℞ *in vitro diagnostic aid for rubella virus IgG antibodies in serum* [enzyme immunoassay (EIA)]

rubbing alcohol [see: alcohol, rubbing]

rubbing isopropyl alcohol [see: isopropyl alcohol, rubbing]

rubefacients *a class of gentle local irritants that redden the skin by producing active or passive hyperemia*

rubella & mumps virus vaccine, live *active immunizing agent for rubella and mumps*

rubella virus vaccine, live USP *active immunizing agent for rubella*

rubeola vaccine [see: measles virus vaccine, live]

Rubex powder for IV injection (discontinued 2004) ℞ *anthracycline antibiotic antineoplastic* [doxorubicin HCl] 100 mg

rubidium *element (Rb)*

rubidium chloride Rb 82 USAN *radioactive diagnostic aid for cardiac disease*

rubidium chloride Rb 86 USAN *radioactive agent*

rubitecan USAN *topoisomerase I inhibitor; investigational (Phase III, orphan) for pancreatic cancer and pediatric HIV/AIDS infections*

ruboxistaurin *investigational (Phase III) protein kinase C beta (PKC-β) inhibitor for diabetic retinopathy*

Rubramin PC IM or subcu injection ℞ *hematinic; vitamin B₁₂ supplement* [cyanocobalamin] 100, 1000 mcg/mL

Rubus fructicosus; R. villosus *medicinal herb* [see: blackberry]

Rubus idaeus; R. strigosus *medicinal herb* [see: red raspberry]

rue (Ruta bracteosa; R. graveolens; R. montana) *plant medicinal herb for cramps, hypertension, hysteria, muscle strains, neuralgia, nervous disorders, sciatica, stimulation of abortion and menstruation, tendon strains, and trauma*

rufinamide USAN, INN *triazole anticonvulsant; investigational (NDA filed, orphan) adjunctive therapy for Lennox-Gastaut syndrome; investigational (NDA filed) for partial-onset seizures*

rufloxacin INN

rufocromomycin INN, BAN *antineoplastic* [also: streptonigrin]

Ru-lets M 500 film-coated tablets OTC *vitamin/mineral supplement* [multiple vitamins & minerals]

RuLox oral suspension oTc *antacid* [aluminum hydroxide; magnesium hydroxide] 225•200 mg/5 mL ⃞ Ralix

RuLox #1; RuLox #2 chewable tablets (discontinued 2004) oTc *antacid* [aluminum hydroxide; magnesium hydroxide] 200•200 mg; 400•400 mg ⃞ Ralix

RuLox Plus chewable tablets, oral suspension oTc *antacid; antiflatulent* [aluminum hydroxide; magnesium hydroxide; simethicone] 200•200•25 mg; 500•450•40 mg/5 mL

rum cherry *medicinal herb* [see: wild black cherry]

Rumex acetosa medicinal herb [see: sorrel]

Rumex crispus medicinal herb [see: yellow dock]

Rumex hymenosepalus medicinal herb [see: canaigre]

Rum-K oral liquid ℞ *potassium supplement* [potassium chloride] 30 mEq K/15 mL

ruplizumab USAN *treatment for immune thrombocytopenic purpura and systemic lupus erythematosus (SLE) (orphan); investigational (orphan) for hemophilia A and B and to prevent rejection of pancreatic islet cell and solid organ transplants*

Ruscus aculeatus medicinal herb [see: butcher's broom]

rush, sweet *medicinal herb* [see: calamus]

Ruta bracteosa; R. graveolens; R. montana medicinal herb [see: rue]

rutamycin USAN, INN *antifungal*

ruthenium *element (Ru)*

rutin NF *a bioflavonoid (q.v.)* [also: rutoside] ⃞ Re-Tann; R-Tanna

rutoside INN [also: rutin]

RVA (rabies vaccine, adsorbed) [see: rabies vaccine]

RVP (red veterinarian petrolatum) [see: petrolatum]

RxPak; ℞Pak (trademarked packaging form) *prescription package*

Ryna oral liquid (discontinued 2006) oTc *decongestant; antihistamine* [pseu-doephedrine HCl; chlorpheniramine maleate] 60•4 mg/10 mL

Ryna-12 caplets ℞ *decongestant; antihistamine; sleep aid* [phenylephrine tannate; pyrilamine tannate] 25•60 mg

Ryna-12 S oral suspension ℞ *decongestant; antihistamine; sleep aid* [phenylephrine tannate; pyrilamine tannate] 5•30 mg/5 mL

Ryna-12D S pediatric oral suspension (discontinued 2005) ℞ *antitussive; decongestant; antihistamine; sleep aid* [carbetapentane tannate; phenylephrine tannate; pyrilamine tannate] 30•5•30 mg/5 mL

Ryna-12X tablets, oral suspension ℞ *decongestant; antihistamine; sleep aid; expectorant* [phenylephrine tannate; pyrilamine tannate; guaifenesin] 25•60•200 mg; 5•30•100 mg/5 mL ⃞ Ranexa; Renax

Ryna-C oral liquid (discontinued 2005) ℞ *narcotic antitussive; antihistamine; decongestant* [codeine phosphate; chlorpheniramine maleate; pseudo-ephedrine HCl] 10•2•30 mg/5 mL

Rynatan caplets ℞ *decongestant; antihistamine* [phenylephrine tannate; chlorpheniramine tannate] 25•9 mg

Rynatan Pediatric chewable tablets, oral suspension ℞ *decongestant; antihistamine* [phenylephrine tannate; chlorpheniramine tannate] 5•4.5 mg; 5•4.5 mg/5 mL

Rynatan-12 S oral suspension ℞ *decongestant; antihistamine; sleep aid* [phenylephrine tannate; pyrilamine tannate] 5•30 mg/5 mL

Rynatuss caplets ℞ *antitussive; antihistamine; decongestant* [carbetapentane tannate; chlorpheniramine tannate; phenylephrine tannate; ephedrine tannate] 60•5•10•10 mg

Rynatuss Pediatric oral suspension ℞ *antitussive; antihistamine; decongestant* [carbetapentane tannate; chlorpheniramine tannate; phenylephrine tannate; ephedrine tannate] 30•4•5•5 mg/5 mL

Ryneze extended-release tablets (discontinued 2007) ℞ *antihistamine; anticholinergic to dry mucosal secretions* [chlorpheniramine maleate; methscopolamine nitrate] 8•2.5 mg

RY-T-12 oral suspension ℞ *decongestant; antihistamine; sleep aid* [phenyl-ephrine tannate; pyrilamine tannate] 5•30 mg/5 mL

Rythmol film-coated tablets ℞ *antiarrhythmic* [propafenone HCl] 150, 225, 300 mg

Rythmol SR extended-release capsules ℞ *antiarrhythmic* [propafenone HCl] 225, 325, 425 mg

S

S-2 solution for inhalation OTC *sympathomimetic bronchodilator; vasopressor for shock* [racepinephrine HCl] 2.25%

^{35}**S** [see: sodium sulfate S 35]

SA (salicylic acid) [q.v.]

SA (serum albumin) [see: albumin, human]

Sabatia angularis medicinal herb [see: American centaury]

sabcomeline HCl USAN *muscarinic receptor agonist for Alzheimer disease*

sabeluzole USAN, INN, BAN *anticonvulsant; antihypoxic*

Sabin vaccine [see: poliovirus vaccine, live oral]

Sabril ⒸⒶⓃ ⒺⓊⓇ (available in 40 foreign countries) *investigational (NDA filed, orphan) anticonvulsant for infantile spasms; investigational (Phase II) treatment for cocaine and methamphetamine addictions* [vigabatrin]

saccharated ferric oxide JAN *hematinic for iron-deficiency anemia in patients with chronic kidney disease* [also: iron sucrose]

saccharated iron; saccharated iron oxide [see: iron sucrose; saccharated ferric oxide]

saccharin NF *flavoring agent*

saccharin calcium USP *non-nutritive sweetener*

saccharin sodium USP *non-nutritive sweetener*

sacred bark medicinal herb [see: cascara sagrada]

sacrosidase USAN *enzyme replacement therapy for congenital sucrase-isomaltase deficiency* (orphan)

S-adenosyl-L-methionine (SAMe) *natural amino acid derivative used to treat depression and protect the liver from toxic overload; regenerates liver function and restores hepatic glutathione levels when taken with B vitamins; investigational (orphan) for AIDS-related myelopathy*

Saf-Clens spray OTC *wound cleanser*

Safe Tussin CD oral liquid OTC *antitussive; decongestant* [dextromethorphan hydrobromide; phenylephrine HCl] 15•2.5 mg/5 mL

Safe Tussin DM oral liquid OTC *antitussive; expectorant* [dextromethorphan hydrobromide; guaifenesin] 15•100 mg/5 mL

safflower (*Carthamus tinctorius*) flowers *medicinal herb for delirium, digestive disorders, fever, gout, inducing sweating, jaundice, liver disorders, lowering cholesterol, promoting expectoration, uric acid build-up, and urinary disorders*

safflower oil USP *oleaginous vehicle; essential fatty acid supplement*

saffron (*Crocus sativus*) flowers *medicinal herb for fever, gout, inducing sweating, measles, rheumatism, scarlet fever, and sedation; also used as an aphrodisiac and expectorant* ☒ Zofran; Zophren

saffron, American; bastard saffron *medicinal herb* [see: safflower]

safingol USAN *antipsoriatic; antineoplastic adjunct*

safingol HCl USAN *antipsoriatic; antineoplastic adjunct*

Saforis powder for oral liquid *investigational (NDA filed) agent for the prevention and treatment of oral mucositis* [glutamine]

safrole USP

sagackhomi *medicinal herb* [see: uva ursi]

sage (Salvia lavandulaefolia; S. lyrata; S. officinalis) leaves *medicinal herb for cough, diarrhea, dysmenorrhea, fever, gastritis, gum and mouth sores, memory improvement, nausea, nervous disorders, and sore throat*

SAHA (suberoylanilide hydroxamic acid) [see: vorinostat]

sailor's tobacco *medicinal herb* [see: mugwort]

St. Benedict thistle *medicinal herb* [see: blessed thistle]

St. James weed; St. James wort *medicinal herb* [see: shepherd's purse]

St. John's wort (Hypericum perforatum) plant *medicinal herb for AIDS, antiviral therapy, anxiety, bronchitis, cancer, childbirth afterpains, depression, gastritis, insomnia, and skin disorders*

St. Joseph Adult Chewable Aspirin chewable tablets OTC *analgesic; antipyretic; anti-inflammatory* [aspirin] 81 mg

St. Josephwort *medicinal herb* [see: basil]

Saizen powder for subcu or IM injection ℞ *growth hormone for children and adults with congenital or endogenous growth hormone deficiency (GHD), short bowel syndrome, or AIDS-wasting syndrome; for children with Turner syndrome, Prader-Willi syndrome, or renal-induced growth failure* [somatropin] 5, 8.8 mg (15, 26.4 IU) per vial ⚕ Susano; Zosyn

Saizen click.easy prefilled cartridge for subcu injection using a cool.click (needle-free injector) or one.click (disposable needle injector) pen ℞ *growth hormone for children and adults with congenital or endogenous growth*

hormone deficiency (GHD), short bowel syndrome, or AIDS-wasting syndrome; for children with Turner syndrome, Prader-Willi syndrome, or renal-induced growth failure* [somatropin] 8 mg (24 IU) per cartridge

SalAc topical liquid OTC *keratolytic cleanser for acne* [salicylic acid] 2% ⚕ Slow-K; Soyalac

salacetamide INN ⚕ cilostamide

salacetin [see: aspirin]

Sal-Acid plaster OTC *keratolytic* [salicylic acid in a collodion-like vehicle] 40%

Salactic Film topical liquid OTC *keratolytic* [salicylic acid in a collodion-like vehicle] 17%

salafibrate INN

Salagen film-coated tablets ℞ *treatment of xerostomia and keratoconjunctivitis sicca due to radiotherapy or Sjögren syndrome (orphan); also for dry mouth* [pilocarpine HCl] 5, 7.5 mg ⚕ Seloken; silicon; Solaquin; Xylocaine

salantel USAN, INN *veterinary anthelmintic* ⚕ zilantel

salazodine INN

Salazopyrin ⊕ (European name for U.S. product **Azulfidine**) ⚕ zalospirone

salazosulfadimidine INN [also: salazosulphadimidine]

salazosulfamide INN

salazosulfapyridine JAN *broad-spectrum bacteriostatic; anti-inflammatory for ulcerative colitis; antirheumatic* [also: sulfasalazine; sulphasalazine]

salazosulfathiazole INN

salazosulphadimidine BAN [also: salazosulfadimidine]

salbutamol INN, BAN *sympathomimetic bronchodilator* [also: albuterol]

salbutamol sulfate JAN *sympathomimetic bronchodilator* [also: albuterol sulfate]

salcatonin BAN *synthetic analogue of calcitonin (salmon); calcium regulator* [also: calcitonin salmon (synthesis)]

salcetogen [see: aspirin]

Sal-Clens Acne Cleanser gel OTC *keratolytic for acne* [salicylic acid] 2%

salcolex USAN, INN *analgesic; anti-inflammatory; antipyretic*

SalEst test kit for professional use ℞ *in vitro diagnostic aid for estriol levels in saliva, used to predict spontaneous pre-term labor and delivery*

saletamide INN *analgesic* [also: saleth-amide maleate]

saletamide maleate [see: salethamide maleate]

salethamide maleate USAN *analgesic* [also: saletamide]

saletin [see: aspirin]

Saleto tablets OTC *analgesic; antipyretic; anti-inflammatory* [acetaminophen; aspirin; salicylamide; caffeine] 115•210•65•16 mg ⌧ SLT; Zylet

Salex cream, lotion, shampoo ℞ *keratolytic for acne* [salicylic acid] 6% ⌧ Celexa; Cylex

Salflex film-coated tablets OTC *analgesic; antipyretic; anti-inflammatory; antirheumatic* [salsalate] 500, 750 mg ⌧ Sulfolax

salfluverine INN

salicain [now: salicyl alcohol]

salicin USP ⌧ psilocin; Selsun; xylazine

salicin willow *medicinal herb* [see: willow]

salicyl alcohol USAN *local anesthetic*

salicylamide USP *analgesic*

salicylanilide NF

salicylate meglumine USAN *antirheumatic; analgesic*

salicylates *a class of drugs that have analgesic, antipyretic, and anti-inflammatory effects*

salicylazosulfapyridine [now: sulfasalazine]

salicylic acid (SA) USP *keratolytic; antiseborrheic; antipsoriatic* 6% topical

salicylic acid, bimolecular ester [see: salsalate]

salicylic acid acetate [see: aspirin]

Salicylic Acid and Sulfur Soap bar OTC *antiseptic and keratolytic cleanser for acne* [salicylic acid; precipitated sulfur] 3%•10%

Salicylic Acid Cleansing bar OTC *medicated cleanser for acne* [salicylic acid] 2%

salicylic acid dihydrogen phosphate [see: fosfosal]

salicylsalicylic acid [see: salsalate]

saligenin [now: salicyl alcohol]

saligenol [now: salicyl alcohol]

salinazid INN, BAN

saline, lactated potassic [see: potassic saline, lactated]

saline laxatives *a subclass of laxatives that work by attracting and retaining water in the intestines to increase intraluminal pressure and cholecystokinin release* [see also: laxatives]

saline solution (SS) [also: normal saline]

SalineX nasal mist, nose drops OTC *nasal moisturizer* [sodium chloride (saline solution)] 0.4%

saliniazid [see: salinazid]

salinomycin INN, BAN

Saliva Substitute oral solution OTC *saliva substitute*

saliva substitutes *a class of oral moisturizers used to relieve dry mouth and throat (xerostomia) due to Sjögren syndrome, Bell palsy, surgery or radiation near the salivary glands, HIV/AIDS, lupus, diabetes, aging, or various medications*

Salivart throat spray OTC *saliva substitute*

Salix alba; S. caprea; S. nigra; S. purpurea *medicinal herb* [see: willow]

Salkera topical foam ℞ *keratolytic* [salicylic acid] 6%

salmaterol [see: salmeterol]

salmefamol INN, BAN

salmeterol USAN, INN, BAN *sympathomimetic bronchodilator*

salmeterol xinafoate USAN *adrenergic; sympathomimetic bronchodilator for asthma, bronchospasm, and chronic obstructive pulmonary disease (COPD)* (base=69%)

salmisteine INN

salmon calcitonin [see: salcatonin]

***Salmonella typhi* vaccine** [see: typhoid vaccine]

Salmonine subcu or IM injection (discontinued 2006) ℞ *calcium regulator for Paget disease (orphan), hypercalcemia, and postmenopausal osteoporosis* [calcitonin (salmon)] 200 IU/mL

salmotin [see: adicillin]

salnacedin USAN *topical anti-inflammatory*

Sal-Oil-T hair dressing ℞ *antipsoriatic; antiseborrheic; keratolytic* [coal tar; salicylic acid] 10%•6%

salol [see: phenyl salicylate]

Salonpas patch OTC *analgesic; mild anesthetic; counterirritant* [methyl salicylate; menthol] 10%•3%

Sal-Plant gel OTC *keratolytic* [salicylic acid in a collodion-like vehicle] 17% ▢ Sleepwell 2-nite

Salprofen (name changed to **NeoProfen** upon marketing release in 2006) ▢ zoliprofen

salprotoside INN

salsalate USAN, USP, INN, BAN *analgesic; antipyretic; anti-inflammatory; antirheumatic* 500, 750 mg oral

Salsitab film-coated tablets ℞ *analgesic; antipyretic; anti-inflammatory; antirheumatic* [salsalate] 500, 750 mg

salt [def.] *The inactive part of a compound, made by combining an acid with an alkali. In* naproxen sodium, *for example, the base is* naproxen *(an acid) and the salt is* sodium *(from sodium hydroxide, an alkali).* [compare to: base] ▢ SLT; Zylet

Sal-Tropine tablets ℞ *GI/GU antispasmodic; antiparkinsonian; anticholinergic "drying agent" for the respiratory tract; antidote to insecticide poisoning* [atropine sulfate] 0.4 mg ▢ sulotroban

Saluron tablets (discontinued 2008) ℞ *diuretic; antihypertensive* [hydroflumethiazide] 50 mg

Salutensin; Salutensin-Demi tablets (discontinued 2007) ℞ *antihypertensive* [hydroflumethiazide; reserpine] 50•0.125 mg; 25•0.125 mg

saluzide [see: opiniazide]

salvarsan [see: arsphenamine]

salverine INN

Salvia lavandulaefolia; S. lyrata; S. officinalis medicinal herb [see: sage]

Salvia miltiorrhiza medicinal herb [see: danshen]

samarium *element* (Sm)

samarium Sm 153 EDTMP (ethylenediaminetetramethylenephosphoric acid) [see: samarium Sm 153 lexidronam]

samarium Sm 153 lexidronam USAN *radiopharmaceutical for treatment of bone pain from osteoblastic metastatic tumors*

Sambucus canadensis; S. ebulus; S. nigra; S. racemosa medicinal herb [see: elder flower; elderberry]

SAMe (S-adenosyl-L-methionine) [q.v.]

Sanchi ginseng (Panax pseudoginseng) *medicinal herb* [see: ginseng]

Sanctura film-coated tablets ℞ *urinary antispasmodic for overactive bladder with urinary frequency, urgency, and incontinence* [trospium chloride] 20 mg

Sanctura XR extended-release capsules ℞ *urinary antispasmodic for overactive bladder with urinary frequency, urgency, and incontinence* [trospium chloride] 60 mg

Sancuso transdermal patch ℞ *antiemetic to prevent chemotherapy-induced nausea and vomiting (CINV)* [granisetron HCl] 34.3 mg ▢ Sina-12X; Xanax

sancycline USAN, INN *antibacterial*

sandalwood (Santalum album) oil *medicinal herb for headache, stomach ache, and urogenital disorders; also used topically as an antiseptic and astringent*

Sandimmune gelcaps, oral solution, IV injection ℞ *immunosuppressant for allogenic kidney, liver, and heart transplants (orphan)* [cyclosporine] 25, 100 mg; 100 mg/mL; 50 mg/mL ▢ xinidamine

Sandimmune ophthalmic ointment *investigational (orphan) for keratoconjunctivitis sicca, keratoplasty graft*

rejection, and corneal melting syndrome [cyclosporine] 2%

SandoPak (trademarked packaging form) *unit dose blister package*

Sandostatin subcu or IV injection ℞ *gastric antisecretory for acromegaly and severe diarrhea due to VIPomas and other tumors (orphan)* [octreotide acetate] 0.05, 0.1, 0.2, 0.5, 1 mg/mL

Sandostatin LAR Depot suspension for monthly IM injection ℞ *gastric antisecretory for acromegaly and severe diarrhea due to VIPomas and other tumors (orphan)* [octreotide] 10, 20, 30 mg/5 mL

sanfetrinem INN, BAN *antibacterial* [also: sanfetrinem sodium]

sanfetrinem cilexetil USAN *antibacterial*

sanfetrinem sodium USAN *antibacterial* [also: sanfetrinem]

SangCya oral solution (discontinued 2004) ℞ *immunosuppressive to prevent solid organ transplant rejection (orphan)* [cyclosporine; alcohol 10.5%] 100 mg/mL ⧉ Sina-12X; Xanax

Sanguinaria canadensis medicinal herb [see: bloodroot]

sanguinarine chloride [now: sanguinarium chloride]

sanguinarium chloride USAN, INN *antifungal; antimicrobial; anti-inflammatory*

sanicle (*Sanicula europea; S. marilandica*) root *medicinal herb used as an astringent, expectorant, discutient, depurative, nervine, and vulnerary* ⧉ Xenical

Sani-Pak (trademarked packaging form) *sanitary dispensing box* ⧉ Cinobac

Sani-Supp suppositories OTC *hyperosmolar laxative* [glycerin]

Santalum album medicinal herb [see: sandalwood]

santonin NF

Santyl ointment ℞ *enzyme for wound debridement* [collagenase] 250 U/g

Sanvar *antineoplastic; synthetic octapeptide analogue of somatostatin; investigational (Phase III, orphan) treatment for acute esophageal variceal bleeding*

secondary to portal hypertension; investigational (orphan) for acromegaly and carcinoid tumors [vapreotide acetate]

saperconazole USAN, INN, BAN *antifungal*

Saponaria officinalis medicinal herb [see: soapwort]

saprisartan INN, BAN *antihypertensive; angiotensin II receptor antagonist* [also: saprisartan potassium]

saprisartan potassium USAN *antihypertensive; angiotensin II receptor antagonist* [also: saprisartan]

sapropterin INN

sapropterin dihydrochloride *oral phenylalanine hydroxylase (PAH) enzyme for mild to moderate phenylketonuria (PKU)*

saquinavir USAN, INN, BAN *antiretroviral protease inhibitor for HIV infection* [also: saquinavir mesylate]

saquinavir mesylate USAN *antiretroviral protease inhibitor for HIV infection* [also: saquinavir]

Sarafem tablets, Pulvules (capsules) ℞ *selective serotonin reuptake inhibitor (SSRI) for premenstrual dysphoric disorder (PMDD)* [fluoxetine HCl] 10, 15, 20 mg; 10, 20 mg

sarafloxacin INN, BAN *anti-infective; DNA gyrase inhibitor* [also: sarafloxacin HCl]

sarafloxacin HCl USAN *anti-infective; DNA gyrase inhibitor* [also: sarafloxacin]

saralasin INN *antihypertensive* [also: saralasin acetate]

saralasin acetate USAN *antihypertensive* [also: saralasin]

Sarasar *investigational (Phase III) antineoplastic for lung cancer* [lonafarnib]

Saratoga ointment OTC *astringent; antiseptic; wound protectant* [zinc oxide; boric acid; eucalyptol] ⧉ Psoriatec; Zyrtec

sarcolysin INN

L-sarcolysin [see: melphalan]

Sardo Bath & Shower oil OTC *bath emollient*

Sardoettes towelettes OTC *moisturizer; emollient*

sargramostim USAN, INN, BAN *antineutropenic for bone marrow transplant and graft delay (orphan)*

sarmazenil INN

sarmoxicillin USAN, INN *antibacterial*

Sarmustine *investigational (orphan) for malignant glioma* [2-chloroethyl-3-sarcosinamide-1-nitrosourea]

Sarna Anti-Itch foam, lotion OTC *mild anesthetic; antipruritic; counterirritant* [camphor; menthol] 0.5%•0.5%

Sarna Sensitive Anti-Itch lotion OTC *anesthetic* [pramoxine HCl] 1%

Sarna Ultra cream OTC *anesthetic; antipruritic; counterirritant; emollient* [pramoxine HCl; menthol; petrolatum] 1%•0.5%•30%

saroten [see: amitriptyline]

Sarothamnus scoparius medicinal herb [see: broom]

sarpicillin USAN, INN *antibacterial*

Sarracenia purpurea medicinal herb [see: pitcher plant]

sarsaparilla (Smilax spp.) root *medicinal herb for blood cleansing (binding and expulsion of endotoxins), joint aches including arthritis and rheumatism, hormonal disorders, skin diseases including leprosy and psoriasis, and syphilis*

sarsasapogenin *investigational (orphan) agent for amyotrophic lateral sclerosis (ALS)*

saruplase INN *prourokinase (pro-UK)*

sassafras (Sassafras albidum; S. officinale) root and bark *medicinal herb for acne, blood cleansing, insect bites and stings, obesity, psoriasis, skin diseases, and water retention; not generally regarded as safe and effective and banned by the FDA as a carcinogen with other serious side effects*

sassafras, swamp *medicinal herb* [see: magnolia]

SAStid Soap bar OTC *antiseptic and keratolytic cleanser for acne* [sulfur; salicylic acid] 5%•3%

saterinone INN

satinflower *medicinal herb* [see: chickweed]

satoribine [now: isatoribine]

satranidazole INN

satraplatin USAN *investigational (Phase III) antineoplastic for hormone-refractory prostate cancer*

Satraplatin *investigational (Phase III) platinum agent for prostate cancer*

satumomab INN, BAN *radiodiagnostic monoclonal antibody for ovarian and colorectal carcinoma* [also: indium In 111 satumomab pendetide]

satumomab pendetide [see: indium In 111 satumomab pendetide]

Satureja hortensis medicinal herb [see: summer savory]

Satureja montana; S. obovata medicinal herb [see: winter savory]

savory *medicinal herb* [see: summer savory; winter savory]

savoxepin INN

Savvy vaginal gel *investigational (Phase I/II) microbicide and spermicide for HIV infection*

saw palmetto (Serenoa repens; S. serrulata) berries *medicinal herb for benign prostatic hypertrophy (BPH) and genitourinary, glandular, and reproductive disorders; also used to enlarge breasts, increase sperm production, promote weight gain, and enhance sexual vigor*

saxagliptin *DPP-4 inhibitor; investigational (Phase III) antidiabetic that enhances the function of the body's incretin system to increase insulin production in the pancreas and reduce glucose production in the liver*

saxifrage, burnet; European burnet saxifrage; small burnet saxifrage; small saxifrage *medicinal herb* [see: burnet]

saxifrax *medicinal herb* [see: sassafras]

SB-408075 *investigational (orphan) agent for pancreatic cancer*

SBR-Lipocream OTC *emollient for dry skin* [oil-in-water emulsion] 70% oil•30% water

SC (succinylcholine) [see: succinyl-choline chlorine]

scabicides *a class of agents effective against scabies*

scabwort *medicinal herb* [see: elecampane]

Scadan scalp lotion OTC *antiseptic; antiseborrheic* [myristyltrimethylammonium bromide; stearyl dimethyl benzyl ammonium chloride] 1%•0.1%

S-Caine Peel cream ℞ *anesthetic* [lidocaine; tetracaine] 7%•7%

Scalpicin topical liquid OTC *antiseborrheic* [salicylic acid] 3%

scaly dragon's claw *medicinal herb* [see: coral root]

scammony, wild *medicinal herb* [see: wild jalap]

scandium *element (Sc)*

Scar Cream OTC *to reduce the appearance of surgical scars; sunscreens* [octinoxate; octisalate] 7.5%•5%

scarlet bergamot *medicinal herb* [see: Oswego tea]

scarlet berry *medicinal herb* [see: bittersweet nightshade]

scarlet fever streptococcus toxin

scarlet red NF *promotes wound healing*

Scarlet Red Ointment Dressings medication-impregnated gauze ℞ *wound dressing; vulnerary* [scarlet red] 5%

scarlet sumach *medicinal herb* [see: sumach]

SCCS (simethicone-coated cellulose suspension) [see: SonoRx]

sCD4-PE40 [see: alvircept sudotox]

Sceletium tortuosum *medicinal herb* [see: kanna]

SCF (stem cell factor) [see: methionyl stem cell factor]

SCH-58500 *investigational (orphan) gene therapy for ovarian tumors*

SCH-530348 *investigational (Phase III) oral thrombin receptor antagonist for the prevention and treatment of atherosclerotic events in high-risk patients*

Schamberg lotion OTC *mild anesthetic; antipruritic; counterirritant; astringent;* emollient [menthol; phenol; zinc oxide] 0.25%•1.5%•8.25%

Schick test [see: diphtheria toxin for Schick test]

Schick test control USP *dermal reactivity indicator*

Schirmer Tear Test ophthalmic strips *diagnostic tear flow test aid*

schizandra (Schisandra arisanensis; S. chinensis; S. rubriflora; S. sphenanthera) berries *medicinal herb for cough, gastrointestinal disorders, increasing energy and mental alertness, nervous disorders, respiratory illnesses, and stress; also used as a liver protectant*

SCIG, IGSC (subcutaneous immune globulin) [see: globulin, immune]

Scleromate IV injection ℞ *sclerosing agent for varicose veins* [morrhuate sodium] 50 mg/mL

Sclerosol aerosol ℞ *treatment for malignant pleural effusion and pneumothorax via intrapleural thoracoscopy administration (orphan)* [talc, sterile]

Sclerosol *investigational (orphan) anti-inflammatory for the topical treatment for scleroderma* [dimethyl sulfoxide (DMSO)]

scoke *medicinal herb* [see: pokeweed]

Scopace tablets ℞ *GI antispasmodic; anticholinergic CNS depressant; motion sickness preventative* [scopolamine] 0.4 mg ⊡ ZE Caps

scopafungin USAN *antibacterial; antifungal*

Scope mouthwash OTC *oral antiseptic* [cetylpyridinium chloride]

scopolamine *oral/transdermal motion sickness preventative; post-surgical antiemetic*

scopolamine hydrobromide USP *GI antispasmodic; anticholinergic CNS depressant; motion sickness preventative; cycloplegic; mydriatic* [also: hyoscine hydrobromide] 0.3, 0.4, 0.86, 1 mg/mL injection

scopolamine methyl nitrate [see: methscopolamine nitrate]

scopolamine methylbromide [see: methscopolamine bromide]

Scott's Emulsion OTC *vitamin supplement* [vitamins A and D] 1250•100 IU/5 mL

Scot-Tussin Allergy Relief Formula Clear oral liquid OTC *antihistamine; sleep aid* [diphenhydramine HCl] 12.5 mg/5 mL

Scot-Tussin DM oral liquid OTC *antitussive; antihistamine* [dextromethorphan hydrobromide; chlorpheniramine maleate] 15•2 mg/5 mL

Scot-Tussin DM Cough Chasers lozenges OTC *antitussive* [dextromethorphan hydrobromide] 5 mg

Scot-Tussin Expectorant oral liquid OTC *expectorant* [guaifenesin] 100 mg/5 mL

Scot-Tussin Original 5-Action Cold Formula syrup, oral liquid OTC *decongestant; antihistamine; analgesic* [phenylephrine HCl; pheniramine maleate; sodium citrate; sodium salicylate; caffeine citrate] 4.2•13.3•83.3•83.3•25 mg

Scot-Tussin Senior Clear oral liquid OTC *antitussive; expectorant* [dextromethorphan hydrobromide; guaifenesin] 15•200 mg/5 mL

sCR1 (soluble complement receptor 1) [see: complement receptor type I, soluble recombinant human]

scrofula plant *medicinal herb* [see: figwort]

Scrophularia nodosa *medicinal herb* [see: figwort]

scullcap *medicinal herb* [see: skullcap]

Sculptra dermal injection ℞ *synthetic polymer for the correction of facial lipoatrophy due to HIV infections* [poly-L-lactic acid]

scuroforme [see: butyl aminobenzoate]

Scutellaria lateriflora *medicinal herb* [see: skullcap]

SD (streptodornase) [q.v.]

^{75}Se [see: selenomethionine Se 75]

sea girdles *medicinal herb* [see: kelp (*Laminaria*)]

Seale's Lotion Modified OTC *antiseptic and keratolytic for acne* [sulfur] 6.4%

sealroot; sealwort *medicinal herb* [see: Solomon's seal]

Sea-Omega 30; Sea-Omega 50 softgels OTC *dietary supplement* [omega-3 fatty acids] 1200 mg; 1000 mg ⑨ Simuc; sumach; Zomig

Seasonale film-coated tablets (in packs of 91) ℞ *extended-cycle (3 months) monophasic oral contraceptive* [levonorgestrel; ethinyl estradiol] 0.15 mg•30 mcg × 84 days; counters × 7 days

Seasonique film-coated tablets (in packs of 91) ℞ *extended-cycle (3 months) biphasic oral contraceptive* [levonorgestrel; ethinyl estradiol] Phase 1 (84 days): 0.15 mg•30 mcg; Phase 2 (7 days): 0•10 mcg

seawrack *medicinal herb* [see: kelp (*Fucus*)]

Seba-Nil Cleansing Mask scrub OTC *abrasive cleanser for acne*

Seba-Nil Oily Skin Cleanser topical liquid OTC *cleanser for acne* [alcohol; acetone]

Sebasorb lotion OTC *keratolytic for acne* [salicylic acid; attapulgite] 2%•10%

Sebazole gel (name changed to **Xolegel** upon marketing release in 2006)

Sebex shampoo OTC *antiseborrheic; keratolytic; antiseptic* [sulfur; salicylic acid] 2%•2%

Sebex-T shampoo OTC *antiseborrheic; antipsoriatic; keratolytic; antiseptic* [sulfur; salicylic acid; coal tar] 2%•2%•5%

Seb-Prev lotion ℞ *antibiotic; antiseborrheic* [sulfacetamide sodium] 10%

Seb-Prev Wash (soap) ℞ *antibiotic; antiseborrheic* [sulfacetamide sodium] 10%

Sebucare hair lotion (discontinued 2004) OTC *antiseborrheic; keratolytic* [salicylic acid; alcohol 61%] 1.8%

Sebulex with Conditioners shampoo OTC *antiseborrheic; keratolytic; antiseptic* [sulfur; salicylic acid] 2%•2%

secalciferol USAN, INN, BAN *calcium regulator; investigational (orphan) for familial hypophosphatemic rickets*

secbutabarbital sodium INN *sedative; hypnotic* [also: butabarbital sodium]

secbutobarbitone BAN *sedative; hypnotic* [also: butabarbital]

seclazone USAN, INN *anti-inflammatory; uricosuric* ⊡ cyclizine

secnidazole INN, BAN

secobarbital USP, INN *hypnotic; sedative*

secobarbital sodium USP, JAN *hypnotic; sedative; also abused as a street drug* [also: quinalbarbitone sodium] 100 mg oral; 50 mg/mL injection

Seconal Sodium Pulvules (capsules) ℞ *sedative; hypnotic; also abused as a street drug* [secobarbital sodium] 100 mg

secoverine INN

Secran oral liquid OTC *vitamin supplement* [vitamins B$_1$, B$_3$, and B$_{12}$; alcohol 17%] 10 mg•10 mg•25 mcg per 5 mL ⊡ Cycrin

SecreFlo powder for IV injection ℞ *diagnostic aid for pancreatic function* [secretin] 16 mcg/vial

secretin INN, BAN *diagnostic aid for pancreatic function*

secretin, synthetic human; secretin, synthetic porcine *investigational (orphan) diagnostic aid for pancreatic function*

secretory leukocyte protease inhibitor, recombinant *investigational (orphan) for bronchopulmonary dysplasia*

Sectral capsules ℞ *antihypertensive; antianginal; antiarrhythmic for premature ventricular contractions (PVCs); antiadrenergic (β-blocker)* [acebutolol HCl] 200, 400 mg

Secule (trademarked delivery form) *single-dose vial* ⊡ squill

securinine INN

sedaform [see: chlorobutanol]

Sedapap caplets ℞ *barbiturate sedative; analgesic; antipyretic* [butalbital; acetaminophen] 50•650 mg

sedatine [see: antipyrine]

sedatives *a class of soothing agents that reduce excitement, nervousness, distress, or irritation* [also called: calmatives]

sedecamycin USAN, INN *veterinary antibacterial*

sedeval [see: barbital]

sedge, sweet *medicinal herb* [see: calamus]

sedoxantrone trihydrochloride [now: ledoxantrone trihydrochloride]

seganserin INN, BAN

seglitide INN *antidiabetic* [also: seglitide acetate]

seglitide acetate USAN *antidiabetic* [also: seglitide]

selamectin USAN, INN *veterinary antiparasitic*

Select-A-Jet (trademarked delivery device) *syringe system*

selective estrogen receptor modulators (SERMs) *a class of osteoporosis prevention agents that reduce bone resorption and decrease overall bone turnover in postmenopausal women*

selective serotonin 5-HT$_3$ (hydroxytryptamine) blockers *a class of antiemetic and antinauseant agents used primarily after emetogenic cancer chemotherapy* [also called: 5-HT$_3$ receptor antagonists]

selective serotonin and norepinephrine reuptake inhibitors (SSNRIs) *a class of oral antidepressants that inhibit neuronal uptake of serotonin (5-HT) and norepinephrine, CNS neurotransmitters*

selective serotonin reuptake inhibitors (SSRIs) *a class of oral antidepressants that inhibit neuronal uptake of serotonin (5-HT), a CNS neurotransmitter*

selegiline INN, BAN *monoamine oxidase inhibitor (MAOI); dopaminergic antiparkinsonian; transdermal treatment for depression* [also: selegiline HCl]

selegiline HCl USAN *monoamine oxidase inhibitor (MAOI); dopaminergic for Parkinson disease (orphan); transdermal treatment for depression* [also: selegiline] 5 mg oral

selenious acid USP *dietary selenium supplement* (61% elemental selenium) 65.4 mcg/mL (40 mcg Se/mL) injection

selenium *element (Se)*

selenium dioxide, monohydrated
[see: selenious acid]

selenium sulfide USP *antiseborrheic; antipsoriatic; antifungal for tinea versicolor* 1%, 2.5% topical

selenomethionine (^{75}Se) INN *pancreas function test; radioactive agent* [also: selenomethionine Se 75]

selenomethionine Se 75 USAN, USP *pancreas function test; radioactive agent* [also: selenomethionine (^{75}Se)]

Sele-Pak IV injection ℞ *selenium supplement* [selenious acid (61% elemental selenium)] 65.4 mcg/mL (40 mcg Se/mL)

Selepen IV injection ℞ *selenium supplement* [selenious acid (61% elemental selenium)] 65.4 mcg/mL (40 mcg Se/mL)

Selfemra capsules ℞ *selective serotonin reuptake inhibitor (SSRI) for premenstrual dysphoric disorder (PMDD)* [fluoxetine HCl] 10, 20 mg

selfotel USAN *NMDA (N-methyl-D-aspartate) antagonist for treatment of stroke-induced impairment*

Seloken (foreign name for U.S. product **Lopressor**) ⊡ silicon; Solaquin; Xylocaine

Seloken ZOC (foreign name for U.S. product **Toprol XL**)

selprazine INN

Selsun lotion ℞ *antiseborrheic; antipsoriatic; antifungal for tinea versicolor* [selenium sulfide] 2.5% ⊡ psilocin; salicin; xylazine

Selsun Blue Medicated Treatment lotion/shampoo OTC *antiseborrheic; dandruff treatment* [selenium sulfide] 1%

Selsun Gold for Women lotion/shampoo (discontinued 2004) OTC *antiseborrheic; dandruff treatment* [selenium sulfide] 1%

Selzentry film-coated tablets ℞ *cellular chemokine receptor inhibitor; twice-daily antiretroviral for early-stage HIV infections* [maraviroc] 150, 300 mg

sematilide INN *antiarrhythmic* [also: sematilide HCl]

sematilide HCl USAN *antiarrhythmic* [also: sematilide]

semduramicin USAN, INN *coccidiostat*

semduramicin sodium USAN *coccidiostat*

Semicid vaginal suppositories OTC *spermicidal contraceptive* [nonoxynol 9] 100 mg

semisodium valproate BAN *anticonvulsant for complex partial seizures and simple or complex absence seizures; treatment for manic episodes of a bipolar disorder; migraine headache prophylaxis* [also: divalproex sodium; valproate semisodium]

semparatide acetate USAN *parathyroid hormone analogue to enhance fracture healing*

Semprex-D capsules ℞ *decongestant; antihistamine* [pseudoephedrine HCl; acrivastine] 60•8 mg

semustine USAN, INN *antineoplastic*

senecio, golden *medicinal herb* [see: life root]

Senecio aureus; S. jacoboea; S. vulgaris *medicinal herb* [see: life root]

senega (Polygala senega) root *medicinal herb used as an antitussive for asthma, chronic bronchitis, croup, lung congestion, and pneumonia* ⊡ Cena-K; zinc

Senexon tablets, oral liquid OTC *stimulant laxative* [sennosides] 8.6 mg; 8.8 mg/5 mL

Senilezol elixir ℞ *vitamin/iron supplement* [multiple B vitamins; ferric pyrophosphate] ≛•3.3 mg

senna USP *stimulant laxative* 176 mg/5 mL oral

senna (Cassia acutifolia; C. angustifolia; C. senna) leaves *medicinal herb for bowel evacuation before gastrointestinal procedures, constipation, edema, and expelling worms*

Senna Concentrate tablets OTC *stimulant laxative* [sennosides] 8.6 mg

Senna Plus tablets OTC *stimulant laxative; stool softener* [sennosides; docusate sodium] 8.6•50 mg

Senna Prompt capsules OTC *stimulant and bulk laxative combination* [sennosides; psyllium] 9•500 mg

Senna Smooth tablets OTC *stimulant laxative* [sennosides] 15 mg

Senna-Gen tablets OTC *stimulant laxative* [sennosides] 8.6 mg ☒ Sinequan; Zincon

Senna-S tablets OTC *stimulant laxative; stool softener* [sennosides; docusate sodium] 8.6•50 mg

sennosides USP *stimulant laxative*

Senokot tablets, granules, syrup OTC *stimulant laxative* [sennosides] 8.6 mg; 15 mg/5 mL; 8.8 mg/5 mL ☒ Cyanokit; Zincate

Senokot-S tablets OTC *stimulant laxative; stool softener* [sennosides; docusate sodium] 8.6•50 mg

SenokotXtra tablets OTC *stimulant laxative* [sennosides] 17 mg

Sensability kit OTC *breast self-examination aid*

Sensipar film-coated tablets ℞ *calcimimetic agent for hypercalcemia due to parathyroid carcinoma (orphan) and secondary hyperparathyroidism (SHPT) due to chronic kidney disease* [cinacalcet HCl] 33, 66, 99 mg (30, 60, 90 mg base)

Sensitive Eyes; Sensitive Eyes Plus solution OTC *rinsing/storage solution for soft contact lenses* [sodium chloride (preserved saline solution)]

Sensitive Eyes Daily Cleaner; Sensitive Eyes Saline/Cleaning Solution OTC *surfactant cleaning solution for soft contact lenses*

Sensitive Eyes Drops OTC *rewetting solution for soft contact lenses*

Sensitivity Protection Crest toothpaste OTC *tooth desensitizer; dental caries preventative* [potassium nitrate; sodium fluoride]

Sensodyne Cool Gel toothpaste OTC *tooth desensitizer; dental caries preventative* [potassium nitrate; sodium fluoride]

Sensodyne Fresh Mint toothpaste OTC *tooth desensitizer; dental caries preventative* [potassium nitrate; sodium monofluorophosphate]

Sensodyne-SC toothpaste OTC *tooth desensitizer* [strontium chloride hexahydrate] 10%

SensoGARD oral gel OTC *mucous membrane anesthetic* [benzocaine] 20%

Sensorcaine injection ℞ *local anesthetic* [bupivacaine HCl] 0.25%, 0.5%

Sensorcaine injection ℞ *local anesthetic* [bupivacaine HCl; epinephrine] 0.25%•1:200 000; 0.5%•1:200 000

Sensorcaine MPF injection ℞ *local anesthetic* [bupivacaine HCl] 0.25%, 0.5%, 0.75%

Sensorcaine MPF injection ℞ *local anesthetic* [bupivacaine HCl; epinephrine] 0.25%•1:200 000, 0.5%•1:200 000, 0.75%•1:200 000

Sensorcaine MPF Spinal injection ℞ *local anesthetic* [bupivacaine HCl] 0.75%

Sentinel test kit for professional use ℞ *urine test for HIV-1 antibodies*

sepazonium chloride USAN, INN *topical anti-infective*

seperidol HCl USAN *antipsychotic* [also: clofluperol]

Seprafilm hydrated gel film *to reduce the incidence, extent, and severity of postoperative adhesions* [hyaluronate sodium; carboxymethylcellulose]

seprilose USAN *antirheumatic*

seproxetine HCl USAN *antidepressant*

Septi-Soft solution ℞ *antiseptic; disinfectant* [triclosan] 0.25%

Septisol foam ℞ *bacteriostatic skin cleanser* [hexachlorophene; alcohol 56%] 0.23%

Septisol solution ℞ *antiseptic; disinfectant* [triclosan] 0.25%

Septocaine intraoral injection ℞ *local anesthetic for dentistry* [articaine HCl; epinephrine] 4%•1:100 000

septomonab [see: nebacumab]

Septopal polymethyl methacrylate (PMMA) beads on surgical wire *investigational (orphan) agent for chronic osteomyelitis* [gentamicin sulfate]

Septra tablets, oral suspension ℞ *anti-infective; antibacterial* [trimethoprim; sulfamethoxazole] 80•400 mg; 40•200 mg/5 mL

Septra DS tablets ℞ *anti-infective; antibacterial* [trimethoprim; sulfamethoxazole] 160•800 mg

Septra IV infusion (discontinued 2007) ℞ *anti-infective; antibacterial* [trimethoprim; sulfamethoxazole] 80•400 mg/5 mL

Sequels (trademarked dosage form) *sustained-release capsule or tablet* ② Cyclessa

sequential AC/paclitaxel (Adriamycin, cyclophosphamide; paclitaxel) *chemotherapy protocol for breast cancer*

sequential DOX → CMF (doxorubicin; cyclophosphamide, methotrexate, fluorouracil) *chemotherapy protocol for breast cancer*

sequifenadine INN

seractide INN *adrenocorticotropic hormone* [also: seractide acetate]

seractide acetate USAN *adrenocorticotropic hormone* [also: seractide]

Seradex-LA extended-release caplets ℞ *decongestant; antihistamine* [phenylephrine HCl; brompheniramine maleate] 19•6 mg

Ser-Ap-Es tablets (discontinued 2007) ℞ *antihypertensive; vasodilator; diuretic* [hydrochlorothiazide; reserpine; hydralazine HCl] 15•0.1•25 mg ② Surpass

seratrodast USAN, INN *anti-inflammatory; antiasthmatic; thromboxane receptor antagonist*

Serax capsules, tablets ℞ *benzodiazepine anxiolytic; sedative; alcohol withdrawal aid* [oxazepam] 10, 15, 30 mg; 15 mg

serazapine HCl USAN *anxiolytic*

Serc tablets ℞ *vasodilator; treatment for vertigo due to Meniere syndrome* [betahistine HCl] 24 mg

Serdolect ⓔⓤⓡ (available in Europe) *investigational (NDA filed) novel (atypical) antipsychotic; neuroleptic* [sertindole]

Sereine solution OTC *cleaning solution for hard contact lenses* [note: one of three different products with the same name] ② Ceron

Sereine solution OTC *wetting solution for hard contact lenses* [note: one of three different products with the same name] ② Ceron

Sereine solution OTC *wetting/soaking solution for hard contact lenses* [note: one of three different products with the same name] ② Ceron

Serenoa repens; S. serrulata *medicinal herb* [see: saw palmetto]

Serentil oral concentrate (discontinued 2004) ℞ *conventional (typical) phenothiazine antipsychotic for schizophrenia* [mesoridazine besylate] 25 mg/mL

Serentil tablets (discontinued 2004) ℞ *conventional (typical) phenothiazine antipsychotic for schizophrenia* [mesoridazine besylate] 10, 50 mg

Serevent oral metered dose inhaler (discontinued 2004) ℞ *twice-daily sympathomimetic bronchodilator for asthma and bronchospasm* [salmeterol xinafoate] 25 mcg/dose ② Survanta

Serevent Diskus oral inhalation powder ℞ *twice-daily sympathomimetic bronchodilator for asthma, bronchospasm, and chronic obstructive pulmonary disease (COPD)* [salmeterol xinafoate] 50 mcg/dose

serfibrate INN

sergliflozin *investigational (Phase III) sodium glucose uptake transporter 2 (SGLT-2) inhibitor for diabetes*

sergolexole INN *antimigraine* [also: sergolexole maleate]

sergolexole maleate USAN *antimigraine* [also: sergolexole]

serine (L-serine) USAN, USP, INN *nonessential amino acid; symbols: Ser, S* ② Ceron

L-serine diazoacetate [see: azaserine]

L-serine & L-leucine & L-tyrosine *investigational (orphan) for hepatocellular carcinoma*

84-L-serineplasminogen activator [see: monteplase]

sermetacin USAN, INN *anti-inflammatory*

sermorelin INN, BAN *diagnostic aid for pituitary function; treatment for growth hormone deficiency, anovulation, and AIDS-related weight loss* [also: sermorelin acetate]

sermorelin acetate USAN *diagnostic aid for pituitary function; treatment for growth hormone deficiency (orphan), anovulation (orphan), and AIDS-related weight loss (orphan)* [also: sermorelin]

SERMs (selective estrogen receptor modulators) [q.v.]

SeroJet (trademarked delivery device) *needle-free subcutaneous injector for Serostim*

Seromycin Pulvules (capsules) ℞ *tuberculostatic* [cycloserine] 250 mg
ⓓ cyromazine

Serophene tablets ℞ *ovulation stimulant* [clomiphene citrate] 50 mg

Seroquel film-coated tablets ℞ *novel (atypical) dibenzothiazepine antipsychotic for schizophrenia and both manic and depressive episodes of a bipolar disorder* [quetiapine fumarate] 25, 50, 100, 200, 300, 400 mg base

Seroquel XR extended-release film-coated caplets ℞ *novel (atypical) dibenzothiazepine antipsychotic for schizophrenia and both manic and depressive episodes of a bipolar disorder; investigational (NDA filed) for generalized anxiety disorder* [quetiapine] 50, 200, 300, 400 mg

Serostim powder for subcu injection ℞ *growth hormone for children and adults with congenital or endogenous growth hormone deficiency (GHD), short bowel syndrome, or AIDS-wasting syndrome; for children with Turner syndrome, Prader-Willi syndrome, or renal-induced growth failure* [somatropin] 4, 5, 6 mg (12, 15, 18 IU) per vial

Serostim prefilled one.click auto-injector syringe (discontinued 2008) ℞ *growth hormone for children and adults with congenital or endogenous growth hormone deficiency (GHD), short bowel syndrome, or AIDS-wasting syndrome;*

for children with Turner syndrome, Prader-Willi syndrome, or renal-induced growth failure [somatropin] 8.8 mg (26.4 IU) per syringe

Serostim LQ subcu injection cartridges (discontinued 2008) ℞ *growth hormone for children and adults with congenital or endogenous growth hormone deficiency (GHD), short bowel syndrome, or AIDS-wasting syndrome; for children with Turner syndrome, Prader-Willi syndrome, or renal-induced growth failure* [somatropin] 6 mg (18 IU) per 0.5 mL cartridge

serotonin (5-hydroxytriptamine$_1$; 5-HT$_1$) [see: selective serotonin reuptake inhibitors; vascular serotonin receptor antagonists]

Seroxat ⓔⓤⓡ (European name for U.S. product **Paxil**)

SERPACWA (Skin Exposure Reduction Paste Against Chemical Warfare Agents) cream ℞ *to delay absorption of chemical warfare agents through the skin when applied before exposure; used in conjunction with MOPP (Mission Oriented Protective Posture) gear* [polytef; perfluoroalkylpolyether]

serrapeptase INN

Serratia marcescens **extract (polyribosomes)** *investigational (orphan) for primary brain malignancies*

sertaconazole INN *topical antifungal*

sertaconazole nitrate *topical antifungal*

sertindole USAN, INN *investigational (NDA filed) novel (atypical) antipsychotic; neuroleptic*

Sertoli cells, porcine *investigational (orphan) intracerebral implant for stage 4 and 5 Parkinson disease (for co-implantation with fetal neural cells)*

sertraline INN, BAN *selective serotonin reuptake inhibitor (SSRI) for depression, obsessive-compulsive disorder (OCD), panic disorder, post-traumatic stress disorder (PTSD), premenstrual dysphoric disorder (PMDD), and social anxiety disorder (SAD)* [also: sertraline HCl]

sertraline HCl USAN *selective serotonin reuptake inhibitor (SSRI) for depression, obsessive-compulsive disorder (OCD), panic disorder, post-traumatic stress disorder (PTSD), premenstrual dysphoric disorder (PMDD), and social anxiety disorder* [also: sertraline] 25, 50, 100 mg; 20 mg/mL oral

serum albumin (SA) [see: albumin, human]

serum albumin, iodinated (^{125}I) human [see: albumin, iodinated I 125 serum]

serum albumin, iodinated (^{131}I) human [see: albumin, iodinated I 131 serum]

serum fibrinogen (SF) [see: fibrinogen, human]

serum globulin (SG) [see: globulin, immune]

serum gonadotrophin [see: gonadotrophin, serum]

serum gonadotropin [see: gonadotrophin, serum]

serum prothrombin conversion accelerator (SPCA) factor [see: factor VII]

Serutan granules OTC *bulk laxative* [psyllium] 2.5 g/tsp. ② Soriatane

Serzone tablets (withdrawn from the market in 2004 due to safety concerns) ℞ *antidepressant; selective serotonin and norepinephrine reuptake inhibitor (SSNRI)* [nefazodone HCl] 50, 100, 150, 200, 250 mg

sesame oil NF *solvent; oleaginous vehicle*

Sesame Street Complete chewable tablets OTC *vitamin/mineral/calcium/iron supplement* [multiple vitamins & minerals; calcium; iron; folic acid; biotin] ±•80•10•0.2•0.015 mg

Sesame Street Plus Extra C chewable tablets (discontinued 2004) OTC *vitamin supplement* [multiple vitamins; folic acid] ±•0.2 mg

Sesame Street Plus Iron chewable tablets OTC *vitamin/iron supplement* [multiple vitamins; iron; folic acid] ±•10•0.2 mg

setastine INN

setazindol INN

setiptiline INN

setoperone USAN, INN *antipsychotic*

setwall *medicinal herb* [see: valerian]

sevelamer carbonate *phosphate-binding polymer for hyperphosphatemia in dialysis patients with chronic kidney disease (CKD)*

sevelamer HCl USAN *phosphate-binding polymer for hyperphosphatemia in dialysis patients with chronic kidney disease (CKD); also used for hyperuricemia in dialysis patients*

7 + 3 protocol (cytarabine, daunorubicin) *chemotherapy protocol for acute myelocytic leukemia (AML)*

7 + 3 protocol (cytarabine, idarubicin) *chemotherapy protocol for acute myelocytic leukemia (AML)*

7 + 3 protocol (cytarabine, mitoxantrone) *chemotherapy protocol for acute myelocytic leukemia (AML)*

7 + 3 + 7 protocol (cytarabine, daunorubicin, etoposide) *chemotherapy protocol for acute myelocytic leukemia (AML)*

seven barks *medicinal herb* [see: hydrangea]

17 alpha-progesterone (17P) *naturally occurring progesterone; investigational (NDA filed) hormonal intervention to prevent preterm births*

17P (17 alpha-progesterone) [q.v.]

Severe Congestion Tussin softgels OTC *decongestant; expectorant* [pseudoephedrine HCl; guaifenesin] 30•200 mg

sevirumab USAN, INN *antiviral*

sevitropium mesilate INN

sevoflurane USAN, INN *inhalation general anesthetic*

sevopramide INN ② cefpiramide

sezolamide HCl USAN *carbonic anhydrase inhibitor*

SF (serum fibrinogen) [see: fibrinogen, human]

SFC lotion OTC *soap-free therapeutic skin cleanser*

sfericase INN ② Zephrex; Zovirax

SG (serum globulin) [see: globulin, immune]

SG (soluble gelatin) [see: gelatin]

shamrock, Indian *medicinal herb* [see: birthroot]

shamrock, water *medicinal herb* [see: buckbean]

shark cartilage (derived from *Sphyrna lewini, Squalus acanthias,* and other species) *natural remedy for cancer* [also: squalamine]

shark liver oil *emollient/protectant*

shavegrass *medicinal herb* [see: horsetail]

sheep laurel *medicinal herb* [see: mountain laurel]

Sheik Elite premedicated condom OTC *spermicidal/barrier contraceptive* [nonoxynol 9] 8%

shell flower *medicinal herb* [see: turtlebloom]

shellac NF *tablet coating agent* ⊡ Cholac

Shellgel intraocular injection ℞ *viscoelastic agent for ophthalmic surgery* [hyaluronate sodium] 12 mg/mL

Shepard's Cream Lotion; Shepard's Skin Cream OTC *moisturizer; emollient*

shepherd's club *medicinal herb* [see: mullein]

shepherd's heart *medicinal herb* [see: shepherd's purse]

shepherd's purse (*Capsella bursa-pastoris*) plant *medicinal herb for bleeding, ear disease, hypertension, painful menstruation, and urinary bleeding*

shigoka *medicinal herb* [see: eleuthero]

shiitake mushrooms (*Lentinula edodes; Tricholomopsis edodes*) stem and cap *medicinal herb for boosting the immune system, cancer, lowering cholesterol, and viral illnesses*

Shohl solution, modified (sodium citrate & citric acid) *urinary alkalizer; compounding agent*

short chain fatty acids *investigational (orphan) for left-sided ulcerative colitis and chronic radiation proctitis*

short-leaved buchu *medicinal herb* [see: buchu]

Shur-Clens solution OTC *wound cleanser* [poloxamer 188] 20%

Shur-Seal vaginal gel OTC *spermicidal contraceptive (for use with a diaphragm)* [nonoxynol 9] 2%

siagoside INN

sialagogues *a class of agents that stimulate the secretion of saliva* [also called: ptyalagogues]

Sibelium investigational (orphan) *vasodilator for alternating hemiplegia* [flunarizine HCl]

sibenadet HCl USAN *treatment for chronic obstructive pulmonary disease (COPD)*

Siberian ginseng (*Acanthopanax senticosus; Eleutherococcus senticosus*) an older (and incorrect) name for eleuthero; "Siberian ginseng" is not in the ginseng family [now: eleuthero; compare to: ginseng]

sibopirdine USAN *cognition enhancer for Alzheimer disease; nootropic*

sibrafiban USAN *platelet inhibitor; fibrinogen receptor antagonist; glycoprotein IIb/IIIa receptor antagonist*

sibutramine INN, BAN *anorexiant for the treatment of obesity; monoamine reuptake inhibitor antidepressant* [also: sibutramine HCl]

sibutramine HCl USAN *anorexiant for the treatment of obesity; monoamine reuptake inhibitor antidepressant* [also: sibutramine]

siccanin INN ⊡ zocainone

Sickledex test kit for professional use ℞ *in vitro diagnostic aid for hemoglobin S (sickle cell)*

sicklewort *medicinal herb* [see: woundwort]

side-flowering skullcap *medicinal herb* [see: skullcap]

SigPak (trademarked packaging form) *unit-of-use package*

Sigtab tablets OTC *vitamin supplement* [multiple vitamins; folic acid] ≛ •0.4 mg

Sigtab-M tablets OTC *vitamin/mineral/calcium/iron supplement* [multiple vitamins & minerals; calcium; iron;

folic acid; biotin] ≛•200•18•0.4•
0.045 mg

siguazodan INN, BAN

Silace syrup, oral liquid OTC *laxative;
stool softener* [docusate sodium] 60
mg/15 mL; 10 mg/mL ⊠ Cialis; xylose

Siladryl elixir OTC *antihistamine; sleep
aid* [diphenhydramine HCl] 12.5
mg/5 mL

Silafed syrup OTC *decongestant; antihistamine* [pseudoephedrine HCl; triprolidine HCl] 30•1.25 mg/5 mL

silafilcon A USAN *hydrophilic contact
lens material* ⊠ xylofilcon A

silafocon A USAN *hydrophobic contact
lens material*

silandrone USAN, INN *androgen*

Silapap, Children's oral liquid, elixir
OTC *analgesic; antipyretic* [acetamino-
phen] 160 mg/5 mL

Silapap, Infant's drops OTC *analgesic;
antipyretic* [acetaminophen] 100
mg/mL

Sildec oral drops ℞ *decongestant; antihistamine; for children 1–24 months*
[pseudoephedrine HCl; carbinoxamine maleate] 15•1 mg/mL

Sildec syrup ℞ *decongestant; antihistamine* [pseudoephedrine HCl; brompheniramine maleate] 45•4 mg/5 mL

Sildec-DM oral drops (discontinued
2007) ℞ *antitussive; antihistamine;
decongestant; for children 1–24 months*
[dextromethorphan hydrobromide;
carbinoxamine maleate; pseudoephedrine HCl] 4•1•15 mg/mL

Sildec-DM syrup ℞ *antitussive; antihistamine; decongestant* [dextromethor-
phan hydrobromide; brompheniramine maleate; pseudoephedrine
HCl] 15•4•45 mg/5 mL

sildenafil citrate USAN *phosphodiesterase type 5 (PDE5) inhibitor; selective
vasodilator for erectile dysfunction (ED)
and pulmonary arterial hypertension
(PAH)*

Silenor *investigational (NDA filed) low-
dose tricyclic antidepressant for the treatment of chronic insomnia* [doxepin
HCl]

Silfedrine, Children's oral liquid OTC
nasal decongestant [pseudoephedrine
HCl] 30 mg/5 mL

silibinin INN

silica, dental-type NF *pharmaceutic aid*

silica gel [now: silicon dioxide]

siliceous earth, purified NF *filtering
medium*

silicic acid, magnesium salt [see:
magnesium trisilicate]

silicon *element (Si)* ⊠ Seloken; silicone;
Solaquin; Xylocaine

silicon dioxide NF *dispersing and suspending agent*

silicon dioxide, colloidal NF *suspending agent; tablet and capsule diluent*

silicone ⊠ Seloken; silicon; Solaquin;
Xylocaine

Silicone No. 2 ointment OTC *skin protectant* [silicone; hydrophobic starch
derivative] 10%• ≛

silicone oil [see: polydimethylsiloxane]

silicristin INN

silidianin INN

silkweed *medicinal herb* [see: milkweed; pleurisy root]

silky swallow wort; Virginia silk
medicinal herb [see: milkweed]

silodosin *investigational (NDA filed)
alpha_{1a} adrenoceptor antagonist for
benign prostatic hyperplasia (BPH)*

silodrate USAN *antacid* [also: simaldrate]

Silphen Cough syrup (discontinued
2005) OTC *antihistamine; sleep aid;
antitussive* [diphenhydramine HCl;
alcohol 5%] 12.5 mg/5 mL

Silphen DM syrup OTC *antitussive*
[dextromethorphan hydrobromide;
alcohol 5%] 10 mg/5 mL

Silphium perfoliatum medicinal herb
[see: ragged cup]

Sil-Tex oral liquid ℞ *decongestant;
expectorant* [phenylephrine HCl;
guaifenesin] 7.5•100 mg/5 mL

Siltussin DAS oral liquid OTC *expectorant* [guaifenesin] 100 mg/5 mL

Siltussin DM oral liquid OTC *antitussive; expectorant* [dextromethorphan
hydrobromide; guaifenesin] 10•100
mg/5 mL

Siltussin SA oral liquid OTC *expectorant* [guaifenesin] 100 mg/5 mL

Silvadene cream ℞ *broad-spectrum bactericidal for adjunctive burn treatment* [silver sulfadiazine] 10 mg/g

silver *element (Ag)* ▣ sulphaurea

silver nitrate USP *ophthalmic neonatal anti-infective; strong caustic* 1% eye drops; 10%, 25%, 50%, 75% topical

silver nitrate, toughened USP *caustic*

silver protein, mild NF *ophthalmic antiseptic; ophthalmic surgical aid*

silver sulfadiazine (SSD) USAN, USP *broad-spectrum bactericidal; adjunct to burn therapy* [also: sulfadiazine silver]

silver sulfadiazine & cerium nitrate *investigational (orphan) for life-threatening burns*

silverweed; silver cinquefoil *medicinal herb* [see: cinquefoil]

Silybum marianum *medicinal herb* [see: milk thistle]

Simaal Gel 2 oral liquid (discontinued 2007) OTC *antacid; antiflatulent* [aluminum hydroxide; magnesium hydroxide; simethicone] 500•400•40 mg/5 mL

simaldrate INN *antacid* [also: silodrate]

Simcor film-coated, extended-release tablets ℞ *combination treatment for hypercholesterolemia and hypertriglyceridemia: HMG-CoA reductase inhibitor to lower LDL and total cholesterol plus niacin to raise HDL and lower triglycerides* [simvastatin; niacin] 20•500, 20•750, 20•1000 mg

Simdax ⓔ (available in several European countries) *investigational (Phase III) calcium sensitizer and vasodilator for decompensated heart failure* [levosimendan]

simethicone USAN, USP *antiflatulent; adjunct to gastrointestinal imaging* 80 mg oral; 40 mg/0.6 mL oral

simethicone-coated cellulose suspension (SCCS) [see: SonoRx]

simetride INN

simfibrate INN

Similac Advance with Iron ready-to-use oral liquid, powder for oral liquid OTC *infant formula fortified with omega-3 fatty acids*

Similac Human Milk Fortifier powder OTC *supplement to breast milk* 900 mg/pkt.

Similac Low Iron oral liquid, powder for oral liquid OTC *total or supplementary infant feeding*

Similac PM 60/40 Low-Iron oral liquid OTC *formula for infants predisposed to hypocalcemia* [whey formula with lowered mineral levels]

Similac with Iron oral liquid, powder for oral liquid OTC *total or supplementary infant feeding*

simple syrup [see: syrup]

Simpler's joy *medicinal herb* [see: blue vervain]

Simplet tablets (discontinued 2007) OTC *decongestant; antihistamine; analgesic; antipyretic* [pseudoephedrine HCl; chlorpheniramine maleate; acetaminophen] 60•4•650 mg ▣ Cymbalta

Simply Cough oral liquid OTC *antitussive* [dextromethorphan hydrobromide] 5 mg/5 mL

Simply Saline nasal spray OTC *nasal moisturizer* [sodium chloride (saline solution)]

Simply Sleep tablets OTC *antihistamine; sleep aid* [diphenhydramine HCl] 25 mg

Simply Stuffy tablets, oral liquid OTC *nasal decongestant* [pseudoephedrine HCl] 30 mg; 15 mg/5 mL

Simron Plus capsules OTC *vitamin/iron supplement* [multiple vitamins; ferrous gluconate; folic acid] ±•10•0.1 mg

simtrazene USAN, INN *antineoplastic*

Simuc; Simuc-GP extended-release tablets ℞ *decongestant; expectorant* [phenylephrine HCl; guaifenesin] 25•900 mg; 25•1200 mg ▣ Sea-Omega 30; sumach; Zomig

Simuc-HD elixir ℞ *narcotic antitussive; decongestant; expectorant* [hydrocodone bitartrate; phenylephrine HCl; guaifenesin] 2.5•10•225 mg/5 mL

Simulect powder for IV infusion *immunosuppressant; IL-2 receptor antagonist for the prevention of acute rejection of renal transplants (orphan)* [basiliximab] 20 mg

simvastatin USAN, INN, BAN *HMG-CoA reductase inhibitor for hyperlipidemia, hypertriglyceridemia, and coronary heart disease (CHD)* 5, 10, 20, 40, 80 mg oral

Sina-12X caplets, pediatric oral suspension Ṟ *decongestant; expectorant* [phenylephrine tannate; guaifenesin] 25•200 mg; 5•100 mg/5 mL ☒ Sancuso; Xanax

Sinapis alba medicinal herb [see: mustard]

sinapultide USAN *pulmonary surfactant for respiratory distress syndrome*

sincalide USAN, INN *choleretic; diagnostic aid for gallbladder function*

sinecatechins *a class of natural polyphenolic antioxidants; topical treatment for external genital and perianal warts (condyloma acuminatum) in immunocompromised adults* [also known as: kunecatechins]

sinefungin USAN, INN *antifungal*

Sinemet 10-100; Sinemet 25-100; Sinemet 25-250 tablets Ṟ *dopamine precursor for Parkinson disease; decarboxylase inhibitor (levodopa potentiator)* [levodopa; carbidopa] 100•10 mg; 100•25 mg; 250•25 mg

Sinemet CR sustained-release tablets Ṟ *dopamine precursor for Parkinson disease; decarboxylase inhibitor (levodopa potentiator)* [levodopa; carbidopa] 100•25, 200•50 mg

Sine-Off Cough/Cold; Sine-Off Multi Symptom Relief tablets OTC *antitussive; decongestant; expectorant; analgesic; antipyretic* [dextromethorphan hydrobromide; phenylephrine HCl; guaifenesin; acetaminophen] 15•5•200•325 mg

Sine-Off Night Time Formula Sinus, Cold, & Flu Medicine gelcaps (discontinued 2007) OTC *decongestant; antihistamine; sleep aid; analgesic; antipyretic* [pseudoephedrine HCl; diphenhydramine HCl; acetaminophen] 30•25•500 mg

Sine-Off No Drowsiness Formula caplets (discontinued 2007) OTC *decongestant; analgesic; antipyretic* [pseudoephedrine HCl; acetaminophen] 30•500 mg

Sine-Off Non-Drowsy tablets OTC *decongestant; analgesic; antipyretic* [phenylephrine HCl; acetaminophen] 5•500 mg

Sine-Off Sinus Medicine caplets (discontinued 2007) OTC *decongestant; antihistamine; analgesic; antipyretic* [pseudoephedrine HCl; chlorpheniramine maleate; acetaminophen] 30•2•500 mg

Sine-Off Sinus/Cold caplets OTC *decongestant; antihistamine; analgesic; antipyretic* [phenylephrine HCl; chlorpheniramine maleate; acetaminophen] 5•2•500 mg

Sinequan capsules Ṟ *tricyclic antidepressant; anxiolytic* [doxepin HCl] 10, 25, 50, 75, 100, 150 mg ☒ Zincon

Sinequan concentrate for oral solution (discontinued 2004) Ṟ *tricyclic antidepressant; anxiolytic* [doxepin HCl] 10 mg/mL ☒ Zincon

Sinex 12-Hour Long Acting; Sinex 12-Hour Ultra Fine Mist for Sinus Relief nasal spray OTC *nasal decongestant* [oxymetazoline HCl] 0.05%

Sinex Ultra Fine Mist nasal spray OTC *decongestant* [phenylephrine HCl] 0.5%

SingleJect (trademarked delivery form) *prefilled syringe*

Singlet for Adults tablets (discontinued 2007) OTC *decongestant; antihistamine; analgesic; antipyretic* [pseudoephedrine HCl; chlorpheniramine maleate; acetaminophen] 60•4•650 mg

Singulair film-coated tablets, chewable tablets, granules for oral solution Ṟ *leukotriene receptor inhibitor for allergic rhinitis, exercise-induced bronchoconstriction (EIB), and the prophylaxis and chronic treatment of*

asthma; also used for chronic urticaria and atopic dermatitis [montelukast sodium] 10 mg; 4, 5 mg; 4 mg/pkt.

Sinografin intracavitary instillation ℞ radiopaque contrast medium for gynecological imaging [diatrizoate meglumine; iodipamide meglumine (47.8% total iodine)] 727•268 mg/mL (380 mg/mL)

sinorphan [now: ecadotril]

sintropium bromide INN ② xenytropium bromide

Sinus Relief caplets (discontinued 2007) OTC decongestant; analgesic; antipyretic [pseudoephedrine HCl; acetaminophen] 30•500 mg

Sinustop capsules OTC nasal decongestant [pseudoephedrine HCl] 60 mg

Sinutab Non-Drying capsules OTC decongestant; expectorant [phenylephrine HCl; guaifenesin] 5•200 mg

Sinutab Sinus caplets OTC decongestant; analgesic; antipyretic [phenylephrine HCl; acetaminophen] 5•325 mg

Sinutab Sinus Allergy caplets OTC decongestant; antihistamine; analgesic; antipyretic [pseudoephedrine HCl; chlorpheniramine maleate; acetaminophen] 30•2•500 mg

Sinutab Sinus Without Drowsiness tablets, caplets (discontinued 2007) OTC decongestant; analgesic; antipyretic [pseudoephedrine HCl; acetaminophen] 30•325 mg; 30•500 mg

SINUtuss DM caplets ℞ antitussive; decongestant; expectorant [dextromethorphan hydrobromide; phenylephrine HCl; guaifenesin] 30•15•600 mg

SINUvent PE extended-release caplets ℞ decongestant; expectorant [phenylephrine HCl; guaifenesin] 15•600 mg

siplizumab investigational (orphan) monoclonal antibody for T-cell lymphomas

sipuleucel-T investigational (NDA filed) immunotherapy agent for hormone-refractory metastatic prostate cancer; recombinant fusion protein of prostatic acid phosphatase (PAP) linked to gran-

ulocyte-macrophage colony-stimulating factor (GM-CSF)

Sirdalud (foreign name for U.S. product **Zanaflex**)

sirolimus USAN immunosuppressant for renal transplantation; investigational (Phase III) for liver transplantation; also used for psoriasis

sisomicin USAN, INN antibacterial [also: sissomicin]

sisomicin sulfate USAN, USP antibacterial

sissomicin BAN antibacterial [also: sisomicin]

sitafloxacin USAN, INN antibacterial; DNA-gyrase inhibitor

sitagliptin phosphate dipeptidyl peptidase-4 (DPP-4) inhibitor; oral antidiabetic that enhances the function of the body's incretin system to increase insulin production in the pancreas and reduce glucose production in the liver

sitalidone INN

sitaxsentan sodium endothelin receptor antagonist (ERA) vasodilator; investigational (NDA filed, orphan) once-daily oral antihypertensive for pulmonary arterial hypertension (PAH)

sitofibrate INN

sitogluside USAN, INN antiprostatic hypertrophy

sitosterols NF

Sitrex extended-release caplets ℞ decongestant; expectorant [phenylephrine HCl; guaifenesin] 20•1200 mg ② storax

Sitrex PD oral liquid ℞ decongestant; expectorant [phenylephrine HCl; guaifenesin] 7.5•75 mg/5 mL

Sitzmarks capsules ℞ radiopaque contrast medium for severe constipation [polyvinyl chloride, radiopaque] 24 rings/capsule

666 Cold Preparation oral liquid (discontinued 2007) OTC antitussive; decongestant; analgesic; antipyretic [dextromethorphan hydrobromide; pseudoephedrine HCl; acetaminophen] 10•30•325 mg/15 mL

sizofiran INN

SK (streptokinase) [q.v.]

Skeeter Stik topical liquid OTC *anesthetic; antipruritic; counterirritant* [lidocaine; menthol] 4%•1%

Skelaxin tablets ℞ *skeletal muscle relaxant* [metaxalone] 800 mg

Skelid tablets ℞ *bisphosphonate bone resorption inhibitor for Paget disease; also used for osteoporosis* [tiludronate disodium] 240 mg

SK&F 110679 *investigational (orphan) long-term treatment for children with growth failure due to lack of endogenous growth hormone*

skin respiratory factor (SRF) *claimed to promote wound healing*

Skin Shield topical liquid OTC *skin protectant; local anesthetic* [dyclonine HCl; benzethonium chloride] 0.75%•0.2%

Skinoren ⒺⓊⓇ (German name for U.S. product **Azelex**)

skullcap *(Scutellaria lateriflora)* plant *medicinal herb for convulsions, epilepsy, fever, hypertension, infertility, insomnia, nervous disorders, rabies, and restlessness*

skunk cabbage *(Symplocarpus foetidus)* root *medicinal herb used as an antispasmodic, diuretic, emetic, expectorant, pectoral, stimulant, and sudorific*

skunk weed *medicinal herb* [see: skunk cabbage]

SL (sodium lactate) [q.v.]

Sleepinal capsules, soft gels OTC *antihistamine; sleep aid* [diphenhydramine HCl] 50 mg

Sleepwell 2-nite tablets OTC *antihistamine; sleep aid* [diphenhydramine HCl] 25 mg ⑨ Sal-Plant

Slidecase (packaging form) *patient compliance package for oral contraceptives* ⑨ Zeldox; Zoladex

slippery elm *(Ulmus fulva; U. rubra)* inner bark *medicinal herb for asthma, blackened or bruised eyes, boils, bronchitis, burns, cold sores, colitis, cough, diaper rash, diarrhea, indigestion, lung disorders, sore throat, and urinary tract inflammation*

slippery root *medicinal herb* [see: comfrey]

Slo-bid Gyrocaps (extended-release capsules) (discontinued 2008) ℞ *antiasthmatic; bronchodilator* [theophylline] 50, 75, 100, 125, 200, 300 mg

Slocaps (trademarked dosage form) *sustained-release capsules*

Slo-Niacin controlled-release tablets OTC *vitamin B₃ supplement; peripheral vasodilator; antihyperlipidemic* [niacin] 250, 500, 750 mg

Slo-phyllin Gyrocaps (extended-release capsules) (discontinued 2004) ℞ *antiasthmatic; bronchodilator* [theophylline] 60, 125, 250 mg ⑨ sulfalene

Slo-phyllin tablets, syrup (discontinued 2008) ℞ *antiasthmatic; bronchodilator* [theophylline] 100, 200 mg; 80 mg/15 mL ⑨ sulfalene

Slo-phyllin GG capsules, syrup (discontinued 2004) ℞ *antiasthmatic; bronchodilator; expectorant* [theophylline; guaifenesin] 150•90 mg; 150•90 mg/15 mL

Slo-Salt-K slow-release tablets OTC *electrolyte replacement; dehydration preventative* [sodium chloride; potassium chloride] 410•150 mg

slow channel blockers *a class of coronary vasodilators that inhibit cardiac muscle contraction and slow cardiac electrical conduction velocity* [also called: calcium channel blockers; calcium antagonists]

Slow Fe slow-release tablets OTC *hematinic; iron supplement* [ferrous sulfate, dried (source of iron)] 160 mg (50 mg) ⑨ Sulf-10

Slow Fe with Folic Acid slow-release tablets OTC *hematinic* [ferrous sulfate; folic acid] 50•0.4 mg

Slow-K controlled-release tablets (discontinued 2004) ℞ *potassium supplement* [potassium chloride] 600 mg (8 mEq K) ⑨ SalAc; shellac; Soyalac

Slow-Mag delayed-release enteric-coated tablets OTC *magnesium supplement* [magnesium chloride] 535 mg

Slow-Mag enteric-coated tablets OTC *magnesium supplement* [magnesium chloride hexahydrate] 64 mg Mg

Slow-Release Iron extended-release tablets OTC *hematinic; iron supplement* [ferrous fumarate, dried (source of iron)] 150 mg (50 mg)

SLT hair lotion (discontinued 2004) OTC *antiseborrheic; antipsoriatic; keratolytic; antiseptic* [coal tar; salicylic acid; lactic acid; alcohol 65%] 2%• 3%•5%

small burnet saxifrage *medicinal herb* [see: burnet]

small pimpernel *medicinal herb* [see: burnet]

small saxifrage *medicinal herb* [see: burnet]

smallpox vaccine USP *active immunizing agent*

SMART anti-tac; humanized anti-tac [now: daclizumab]

SmartMist (trademarked delivery device) *hand-held inhalation device*

smartweed; water smartweed *medicinal herb* [see: knotweed]

SMF (streptozocin, mitomycin, fluorouracil) *chemotherapy protocol for pancreatic cancer*

Smilax spp. *medicinal herb* [see: sarsaparilla]

smooth sumach *medicinal herb* [see: sumach]

SMX; SMZ (sulfamethoxazole) [q.v.]

SMZ-TMP (sulfamethoxazole & trimethoprim) [q.v.]

SN (streptonigrin) [q.v.]

snake bite *medicinal herb* [see: birthroot]

snake head *medicinal herb* [see: turtlebloom]

snake lily *medicinal herb* [see: blue flag]

snake weed *medicinal herb* [see: bistort; plantain]

snakebite antivenin [see: antivenin, Crotalidae & Micrurus fulvius]

snakeroot *medicinal herb* [see: echinacea]

snakeroot, black *medicinal herb* [see: black cohosh; sanicle]

snapping hazel *medicinal herb* [see: witch hazel]

SnapTab (trademarked dosage form) *scored tablet*

SnET2 (tin ethyl etiopurpurin) [see: rostaporfin]

Snooze Fast tablets OTC *antihistamine; sleep aid* [diphenhydramine HCl] 50 mg

Sno-Strips ophthalmic strips *diagnostic tear flow test aid*

snout, swine *medicinal herb* [see: dandelion]

snowball, wild *medicinal herb* [see: New Jersey tea]

snowdrop tree; snowflower *medicinal herb* [see: fringe tree]

Soac-Lens solution OTC *wetting/soaking solution for hard contact lenses*

soap, green USP *detergent*

soapwort (Saponaria officinalis) *plant and roots medicinal herb for acne, boils, eczema, poison ivy rash and psoriasis; also used in skin disinfectants and soaps* ⃞ Supprette

SOD (superoxide dismutase) [see: orgotein]

soda lime NF *carbon dioxide absorbent*

sodium *element (Na)*

sodium acetate USP *dialysis aid; electrolyte replenisher; pH buffer 2, 4 mEq/mL (16.4%, 32.8%) injection*

sodium acetate trihydrate [see: sodium acetate]

sodium acetrizoate INN, BAN [also: acetrizoate sodium]

sodium acetylsalicylate *analgesic*

sodium acid phosphate *urinary acidifier*

sodium alginate NF *suspending agent*

sodium aluminosilicate *investigational (orphan) for chronic hepatic encephalopathy*

sodium amidotrizoate INN *oral/rectal/parenteral radiopaque contrast medium (59.87% iodine)* [also: diatrizoate sodium; sodium diatrizoate]

sodium aminobenzoate [see: aminobenzoate sodium]

sodium amylopectin sulfate [see: sodium amylosulfate]

sodium amylosulfate USAN *enzyme inhibitor*

sodium anoxynaphthonate BAN *blood volume and cardiac output test* [also: anazolene sodium]

sodium antimony gluconate [see: sodium stibogluconate]

sodium antimonylgluconate BAN

sodium apolate INN, BAN *anticoagulant* [also: lyapolate sodium]

sodium arsenate, exsiccated NF

sodium arsenate As 74 USAN *radioactive agent*

sodium ascorbate (vitamin C) USP, INN *water-soluble vitamin; antiscorbutic*

sodium aurothiomalate INN *antirheumatic* [also: gold sodium thiomalate]

sodium aurotiosulfate INN [also: gold sodium thiosulfate]

sodium azodisalicylate [now: olsalazine sodium]

sodium benzoate USAN, NF, JAN *adjunctive therapy (rescue agent) to prevent and treat hyperammonemia due to urea cycle enzymopathy; antifungal agent; preservative*

sodium benzoate & caffeine *analeptic for respiratory depression due to an overdose of CNS depressants* 250 mg/ mL injection

sodium benzoate & sodium phenylacetate *adjunctive therapy (rescue agent) to prevent and treat hyperammonemia due to urea cycle enzymopathy (orphan)*

sodium benzyl penicillin [see: penicillin G sodium]

sodium bicarbonate USP *electrolyte replenisher; systemic alkalizer; antacid* 325, 600, 650 mg oral; 0.5, 0.6, 0.9, 1 mEq/mL (4.2%, 5%, 7.5%, 8.4%) injection

sodium biphosphate *urinary acidifier; pH buffer*

sodium bisulfite NF *antioxidant*

sodium bitionolate INN *topical antiinfective* [also: bithionolate sodium]

sodium borate NF *alkalizing agent; antipruritic; bacteriostatic agent in cold creams, eye washes, and mouth rinses*

sodium borocaptate (^{10}B) INN *antineoplastic; radioactive agent* [also: borocaptate sodium B 10]

sodium cacodylate NF

sodium calcium edetate INN *heavy metal chelating agent* [also: edetate calcium disodium; sodium calciumedetate; calcium disodium edetate]

sodium calciumedetate BAN *heavy metal chelating agent* [also: edetate calcium disodium; sodium calcium edetate; calcium disodium edetate]

sodium caprylate *antifungal*

sodium carbonate NF *alkalizing agent*

sodium chloride (NaCl) USP *ophthalmic hypertonic; electrolyte replacement; abortifacient* [sterile isotonic solution] 650, 1000, 2250 mg oral; 0.45%, 0.9%, 3%, 5%, 14.6%, 23.4% injection/diluent

0.45% sodium chloride (½ normal saline; ½ NS) *electrolyte replacement*

0.9% sodium chloride (normal saline; NS) *electrolyte replacement* [also: saline solution]

sodium chloride, compound solution of INN *fluid and electrolyte replenisher* [also: Ringer's injection]

sodium chloride Na 22 USAN *radioactive agent*

sodium chondroitin sulfate [see: chondroitin sulfate sodium]

sodium chromate (^{51}Cr) INN *blood volume test; radioactive agent* [also: sodium chromate Cr 51]

sodium chromate Cr 51 USAN *blood volume test; radioactive agent* [also: sodium chromate (^{51}Cr)]

sodium citrate USP *systemic alkalizer; pH buffer; antacid; investigational (orphan) adjunct to leukapheresis procedures*

sodium citrate & citric acid *urinary alkalinizing agent* 500•334 mg/5 mL oral

sodium colistin methanesulfonate [see: colistimethate sodium]

sodium cromoglycate [see: cromolyn sodium]

sodium cyclamate NF, INN

sodium cyclohexanesulfamate [see: sodium cyclamate]

sodium dehydroacetate NF antimicrobial preservative

sodium dehydrocholate INN [also: dehydrocholate sodium]

sodium denyl [see: phenytoin sodium]

sodium diatrizoate BAN oral/rectal/parenteral radiopaque contrast medium (59.87% iodine) [also: diatrizoate sodium; sodium amidotrizoate]

sodium dibunate INN, BAN

sodium dichloroacetate (sodium DCA) USAN pyruvate dehydrogenase activator; investigational (orphan) for severe head trauma, lactic acidosis, homozygous familial hypercholesterolemia, and monochloroacetic acid poisoning

sodium diethyldithiocarbamate [see: ditiocarb sodium]

sodium diiodomethanesulfonate [see: dimethiodal sodium]

sodium dioctyl sulfosuccinate INN stool softener; surfactant [also: docusate sodium]

sodium diphenylhydantoin [see: phenytoin sodium]

sodium diprotrizoate INN, BAN [also: diprotrizoate sodium]

Sodium Edecrin [see: Edecrin Sodium]

sodium edetate [see: edetate sodium]

sodium estrone sulfate estrogen replacement therapy for postmenopausal disorders 0.625, 1.25, 2.5, 5 mg oral

sodium etasulfate INN detergent [also: sodium ethasulfate]

sodium ethasulfate USAN detergent [also: sodium etasulfate]

sodium feredetate INN [also: sodium ironedetate]

sodium ferric gluconate hematinic for iron deficiency due to chronic hemodialysis with epoetin therapy

sodium fluoride USP fluoride replacement therapy; dental caries preventative (45% fluoride) 1.1, 2.2 mg oral; 0.125, 0.5 mg/mL oral

sodium fluoride F 18 USP

sodium fluoride & phosphoric acid USP dental caries prophylactic

sodium formaldehyde sulfoxylate NF preservative

sodium gamma hydroxybutyrate (NaGHB) [see: gamma hydroxybutyrate (GHB); sodium oxybate]

sodium gammahydroxyburate [see: sodium oxybate]

sodium gentisate INN

sodium glucaspaldrate INN, BAN

sodium gluconate USP electrolyte replenisher

sodium glucosulfone USP

sodium glutamate

sodium glycerophosphate NF

sodium glycocholate [see: bile salts]

sodium gualenate INN [also: azulene sulfonate sodium]

sodium hyaluronate [see: hyaluronate sodium]

sodium hydroxide NF alkalizing agent

sodium hydroxybenzenesulfonate [see: phenolsulphonate sodium]

sodium 4-hydroxybutyrate [see: sodium oxybate]

sodium hypochlorite USP, JAN disinfectant; bleach; used for utensils and equipment

sodium hypochlorite, diluted NF [also: antiformin, dental]

sodium hypophosphite NF

sodium iodide USP dietary iodine supplement (85% elemental iodine)

sodium iodide (^{123}I) JAN thyroid function test; radioactive agent [also: sodium iodide I 123]

sodium iodide (^{125}I) INN thyroid function test; radioactive agent [also: sodium iodide I 125]

sodium iodide (^{131}I) JAN radioactive antineoplastic for thyroid carcinoma; thyroid inhibitor for hyperthyroidism [also: sodium iodide I 131]

sodium iodide I 123 USP diagnostic aid for thyroid function; radioactive agent [also: sodium iodide (^{123}I)] 3.7, 7.4 MBq oral

sodium iodide I 125 USAN, USP *thyroid function test; radioactive agent* [also: sodium iodide (^{125}I)]

sodium iodide I 131 USAN, USP, INN *radioactive antineoplastic for thyroid carcinoma; thyroid inhibitor for hyperthyroidism* [also: sodium iodide (^{131}I)] 0.75–100, 3.5–150 mCi oral

sodium iodohippurate (^{131}I) INN, JAN *renal function test; radioactive agent* [also: iodohippurate sodium I 131]

sodium iodomethanesulfonate [see: methiodal sodium]

sodium iopodate JAN *oral radiopaque contrast medium for cholecystography (61.4% iodine)* [also: ipodate sodium; sodium ipodate]

sodium iotalamate (^{125}I) INN *radioactive agent* [also: iothalamate sodium I 125]

sodium iotalamate (^{131}I) INN *radioactive agent* [also: iothalamate sodium I 131]

sodium iothalamate BAN *parenteral radiopaque contrast medium (59.9% iodine)* [also: iothalamate sodium]

sodium ioxaglate BAN *radiopaque contrast medium* [also: ioxaglate sodium]

sodium ipodate INN, BAN *oral radiopaque contrast medium for cholecystography (61.4% iodine)* [also: ipodate sodium; sodium iopodate]

sodium ironedetate BAN [also: sodium feredetate]

sodium lactate (SL) USP *electrolyte replenisher* 167 mEq/L (1/6 molar) injection

sodium lactate, compound solution of INN *electrolyte and fluid replenisher; systemic alkalizer* [also: Ringer's injection, lactated]

sodium lauryl sulfate NF *surfactant/ wetting agent* [also: laurilsulfate]

sodium lignosulfonate [see: polignate sodium]

sodium metabisulfite NF *antioxidant*

sodium metrizoate INN *radiopaque contrast medium* [also: metrizoate sodium]

sodium monododecyl sulfate [see: sodium lauryl sulfate]

sodium monofluorophosphate USP *dental caries prophylactic*

sodium monomercaptoundecahydro-closo-dodecaborate *investigational (orphan) for boron neutron capture therapy (BNCT) for glioblastoma multiforme*

sodium morrhuate INN *sclerosing agent* [also: morrhuate sodium]

sodium nitrite USP *adjunct to cyanide detoxification; also used for hydrogen sulfide poisoning* 30 mg/mL injection

sodium nitrite & sodium thiosulfate & amyl nitrite [inhalant] *emergency treatment of cyanide poisoning* 300 mg•12.5 g•0.3 mL kit

sodium nitroferricyanide [see: sodium nitroprusside]

sodium nitroferricyanide dihydrate [see: sodium nitroprusside]

sodium nitroprusside USP *emergency antihypertensive; vasodilator; investigational (orphan) for the prevention and treatment of cerebral vasospasm following subarachnoid hemorrhage* 50 mg/ dose injection

sodium noramidopyrine methanesulfonate [see: dipyrone]

sodium oxybate USAN *adjunct to anesthesia; CNS depressant for narcolepsy (orphan), cataplexy, sleep paralysis, and hypnagogic hallucinations; also used for fibromyalgia and fatigue* [also known as: gamma hydroxybutyrate (GHB)]

sodium oxychlorosene [see: oxychlorosene sodium]

sodium paratoluenesulfan chloramide [see: chloramine-T]

sodium PCA; Na PCA (sodium pyrrolidone carboxylic acid) [q.v.]

sodium penicillin G [see: penicillin G sodium]

sodium pentosan polysulfate [see: pentosan polysulfate sodium]

sodium perborate *topical antiseptic/ germicidal*

sodium perborate monohydrate USAN *topical antiseptic/germicidal*

sodium pertechnetate Tc 99m USAN, USP *radioactive agent*

sodium phenolate [see: phenolate sodium]

sodium phenylacetate USAN *adjunctive therapy (rescue agent) to prevent and treat hyperammonemia due to urea cycle enzymopathy*

sodium phenylacetate & sodium benzoate *adjunctive therapy (rescue agent) to prevent and treat hyperammonemia due to urea cycle enzymopathy (orphan)*

sodium phenylbutyrate USAN *antihyperammonemic for urea cycle disorders (orphan); investigational (orphan) for malignant glioma and various sickling disorders*

sodium phosphate (^{32}P) INN *antineoplastic; antipolycythemic; neoplasm test* [also: sodium phosphate P 32]

sodium phosphate, dibasic (Na$_2$HPO$_4$) USP *saline laxative; phosphorus replacement; pH buffer*

sodium phosphate, monobasic (NaH$_2$PO$_4$) USP *saline laxative; phosphorus replacement; pH buffer*

sodium phosphate P 32 USAN, USP *antipolycythemic; radiopharmaceutical antineoplastic for various leukemias and skeletal metastases* [also: sodium phosphate (^{32}P)] 0.67 mCi/mL

sodium picofosfate INN

sodium picosulfate INN

sodium polyphosphate USAN *pharmaceutic aid*

sodium polystyrene sulfonate USP *potassium-removing ion-exchange resin for hyperkalemia 15 g/60 mL oral*

sodium 1,3-propanedisulfonate *investigational (orphan) for secondary amyloidosis*

sodium propionate NF *preservative; antifungal*

sodium propionate hydrate [see: sodium propionate]

sodium 2-propylvalerate [see: valproate sodium]

sodium psylliate NF

sodium pyrophosphate USAN *pharmaceutic aid*

sodium pyrrolidone carboxylic acid (sodium PCA; Na PCA) *natural skin moisturizing factor; humectant*

sodium pyruvate *investigational (orphan) for cystic fibrosis*

sodium radiochromate [see: sodium chromate Cr 51]

sodium rhodanate [see: thiocyanate sodium]

sodium salicylate (SS) USP *analgesic; antipyretic; anti-inflammatory; antirheumatic* 325, 650 mg oral

sodium starch glycolate NF *tablet excipient*

sodium stearate NF *emulsifying and stiffening agent*

sodium stearyl fumarate NF *tablet and capsule lubricant*

sodium stibocaptate INN [also: stibocaptate]

sodium stibogluconate INN, BAN *investigational antiparasitic for leishmaniasis and trypanosomiasis*

Sodium Sulamyd eye drops, ophthalmic ointment ℞ *antibiotic* [sulfacetamide sodium] 10%, 30%; 10%

sodium sulfacetamide [see: sulfacetamide sodium]

sodium sulfate USP *calcium regulator*

sodium sulfate S 35 USAN *radioactive agent*

sodium sulfocyanate [see: thiocyanate sodium]

sodium taurocholate [see: bile salts]

sodium tetradecyl (STD) sulfate INN *sclerosing agent for varicose veins; investigational (orphan) for bleeding esophageal varices*

sodium thiomalate, gold [see: gold sodium thiomalate]

sodium thiosalicylate *analgesic; antipyretic; anti-inflammatory; antirheumatic* 50 mg/mL injection

sodium thiosulfate USP *antidote to cyanide poisoning; antiseptic; antifungal; also used for cisplatin-induced nephrotoxicity in adults; investigational (orphan) for platinum-induced toxicity* *in pediatric patients* 10%, 25% (100, 250 mg/mL) injection

sodium thiosulfate, gold [see: gold sodium thiosulfate]

sodium thiosulfate pentahydrate [see: sodium thiosulfate]

sodium thiosulfate & sodium nitrite & amyl nitrite [inhalant] *emergency treatment of cyanide poisoning* 12.5 g•300 mg•0.3 mL kit

sodium timerfonate INN *topical antiinfective* [also: thimerfonate sodium]

sodium trimetaphosphate USAN *pharmaceutic aid*

sodium tyropanoate INN *oral radiopaque contrast medium for cholecystography (57.4% iodine)* [also: tyropanoate sodium]

sodium valproate [see: valproate sodium]

Sodol Compound tablets ℞ *skeletal muscle relaxant; analgesic; antipyretic* [carisoprodol; aspirin] 200•325 mg

sofalcone INN

Sofenol 5 lotion (discontinued 2004) OTC *moisturizer; emollient*

Sof-lax softgels OTC *laxative; stool softener* [docusate sodium] 100 mg

Soft Mate Comfort Drops for Sensitive Eyes OTC *rewetting solution for soft contact lenses*

Soft Mate Consept solution + aerosol spray OTC *two-step chemical disinfecting system for soft contact lenses* [hydrogen peroxide–based]

Soft Mate Disinfecting for Sensitive Eyes solution OTC *chemical disinfecting solution for soft contact lenses* [EDTA; chlorhexidine gluconate] 0.1%•0.005%

Soft Mate Hands Off Daily Cleaner solution OTC *surfactant cleaning solution for soft contact lenses*

soft pine *medicinal herb* [see: white pine]

Soft Sense lotion OTC *moisturizer; emollient*

Softabs (trademarked dosage form) *chewable tablets*

softgels (dosage form) *soft gelatin capsules*

SoftWear solution OTC *rinsing/storage solution for soft contact lenses* [sodium chloride (preserved saline solution)]

Sojourn liquid for vaporization ℞ *inhalation general anesthetic* [sevoflurane]

Solagé topical solution ℞ *depigmenting agent for solar lentigines* [mequinol; tretinoin; alcohol 77.8%] 2%•0.01% ☒ SalAc; Slow-K; Soyalac

Solanum dulcamara medicinal herb [see: bittersweet nightshade]

solapsone BAN [also: solasulfone]

Solaquin cream OTC *hyperpigmentation bleaching agent* [hydroquinone in a sunscreen base] 2% ☒ Seloken; silicon; Xylocaine

Solaquin Forte cream, gel ℞ *hyperpigmentation bleaching agent* [hydroquinone (in a sunscreen base)] 4%

Solaraze gel ℞ *treatment for actinic keratosis (AK)* [diclofenac sodium] 3%

Solarcaine aerosol spray, lotion OTC *anesthetic; antiseptic* [benzocaine; triclosan] 20%•0.13%

Solarcaine Aloe Extra Burn Relief cream, gel, topical spray OTC *anesthetic* [lidocaine] 0.5%

Solarcaine Medicated First Aid Spray OTC *anesthetic; antiseptic* [benzocaine; triclosan] 20%•0.13%

solasulfone INN [also: solapsone]

soldier's woundwort *medicinal herb* [see: yarrow]

Solfoton tablets, capsules ℞ *long-acting barbiturate sedative, hypnotic, and anticonvulsant* [phenobarbital] 16 mg

Solganal IM injection ℞ *antirheumatic* [aurothioglucose] 50 mg/mL

Solia tablets (in packs of 28) ℞ *monophasic oral contraceptive* [desogestrel; ethinyl estradiol] 0.15 mg•30 mcg × 21 days; counters × 7 days

Solidago nemoralis; S. odora; S. virgaurea medicinal herb [see: goldenrod]

solifenacin succinate *selective muscarinic M_3 receptor antagonist; urinary antispasmodic for overactive bladder with urinary incontinence, urgency, and frequency*

Soliris IV infusion ℞ *monoclonal antibody; antihemolytic for paroxysmal nocturnal hemoglobinuria (PNH; orphan); investigational (orphan) for idiopathic membranous glomerular nephropathy* [eculizumab] 10 mg/mL (300 mg/vial)

Solodyn film-coated extended-release tablets ℞ *tetracycline antibiotic for severe acne* [minocycline HCl] 45, 90, 135 mg

Solomon's seal *(Polygonatum multiflorum; P. odoratum)* root *medicinal herb used as an astringent, demulcent, emetic, and expectorant*

SoloStar (trademarked insulin delivery device) *prefilled subcu injector for* **Lantus**

Solotuss oral suspension ℞ *antitussive* [carbetapentane tannate] 30 mg/5 mL

solpecainol INN

SolTabs (trademarked dosage form) *orally disintegrating tablets*

Soltamox oral solution ℞ *antiestrogen antineoplastic for the treatment of breast cancer and the reduction of breast cancer incidence in high-risk women* [tamoxifen citrate] 10 mg/5 mL

Soltice Quick-Rub ointment OTC *analgesic; counterirritant* [methyl salicylate; camphor] 5.1%•5.1%

soluble complement receptor [see: complement receptor type I, soluble recombinant human]

soluble ferric pyrophosphate [see: ferric pyrophosphate, soluble]

soluble gelatin (SG) [see: gelatin]

Soluble T4 *investigational (orphan) treatment for AIDS* [CD4 human truncated 369 AA polypeptide]

Solu-Cortef powder for IV or IM injection ℞ *corticosteroid; anti-inflammatory* [hydrocortisone sodium succinate] 100, 250, 500, 1000 mg/vial

Solu-Medrol powder for IV or IM injection ℞ *corticosteroid; anti-inflammatory; immunosuppressant* [methylprednisolone sodium succinate] 40, 125, 500, 1000, 2000 mg/vial

Solumol OTC *ointment base*

Solurex intra-articular, intralesional, soft tissue, or IM injection (discontinued 2006) ℞ *corticosteroid; anti-inflammatory* [dexamethasone sodium phosphate] 4 mg/mL

Solurex LA intralesional, intra-articular, soft tissue, or IM injection (discontinued 2006) ℞ *corticosteroid; anti-inflammatory* [dexamethasone acetate] 8 mg/mL

Soluspan (trademarked dosage form) *injectable suspension* ℞ psilocybin

Soluvite C.T. pediatric chewable tablets ℞ *vitamin supplement; dental caries preventative* [multiple vitamins; fluoride; folic acid] ≛•1•0.3 mg

Soluvite-f pediatric oral drops (discontinued 2006) ℞ *vitamin supplement; dental caries preventative* [vitamins A, C, and D; fluoride] 1500 IU•35 mg•400 IU•0.25 mg per 0.6 mL

Solvent-G OTC *liquid base*

Solvet (trademarked dosage form) *soluble tablet* ℞ Zoloft

solypertine INN *antiadrenergic* [also: solypertine tartrate]

solypertine tartrate USAN *antiadrenergic* [also: solypertine]

Solzira extended-release tablets *investigational (NDA filed) treatment for moderate-to-severe restless legs syndrome (RLS)* [gabapentin enacarbil]

Soma tablets ℞ *skeletal muscle relaxant* [carisoprodol] 250, 350 mg

Soma Compound tablets (discontinued 2008) ℞ *skeletal muscle relaxant; analgesic; antipyretic* [carisoprodol; aspirin] 200•325 mg

Soma Compound with Codeine tablets (discontinued 2008) ℞ *skeletal muscle relaxant; narcotic antitussive; analgesic; antipyretic* [carisoprodol; aspirin; codeine phosphate] 200•325•16 mg

somagrebove USAN *veterinary galactopoietic agent*

somalapor USAN, INN, BAN *porcine growth hormone*

somantadine INN *antiviral* [also: somantadine HCl]

somantadine HCl USAN *antiviral* [also: somantadine]

SomatoKine *investigational (orphan) treatment for growth hormone insensitivity syndrome (Laron syndrome) and extreme insulin-resistance syndromes (type A, type B, Rabson-Mendenhall syndrome, leprechaunism)* [mecasermin rinfabate]

somatomedin-C [see: mecasermin]

somatorelin INN *growth hormone-releasing factor (GH-RF)*

somatostatin (SS) INN, BAN *growth hormone-release inhibiting factor; investigational (orphan) for cutaneous gastrointestinal fistulas and bleeding esophageal varices*

somatostatin analogue, multi-ligand *investigational (orphan) for functional gastroenteropancreatic neuroendocrine tumors (insulinoma, gastrinoma, somatostatinoma, GRFoma, VIPoma, and glucagonoma)*

SomatoTher *investigational (orphan) radiotherapeutic agent for somatostatin receptor–positive neuroendocrine tumors* [indium In 111 pentetreotide]

somatotropin, human [see: somatropin]

Somatrel *investigational (orphan) diagnostic aid for pituitary release of growth hormone* [NG-29 (code name — generic name not yet assigned)]

somatrem USAN, INN, BAN *growth hormone for congenital growth failure due to lack of endogenous growth hormone (orphan); investigational (orphan) for short stature due to Turner syndrome*

somatropin USAN, INN, BAN, JAN *growth hormone for children and adults with congenital or endogenous growth hormone deficiency (GHD), short bowel syndrome, or AIDS-wasting syndrome; for children with Turner syndrome, Prader-Willi syndrome, or renal-induced growth failure* [also: human growth hormone]

Somatuline Depot subcu injection in prefilled syringes *reduces endogenous growth hormone (GH) and insulin growth factor-1 (IGF-1) levels to treat acromegaly (orphan)* [lanreotide (as acetate)] 60, 90, 120 mg (79.8, 116.4, 155.5 mg)

Somavert subcu injection ℞ *growth hormone receptor antagonist for acromegaly (orphan)* [pegvisomant] 10, 15, 20 mg/dose

somavubove USAN, INN *veterinary galactopoietic agent*

somenopor USAN *porcine growth hormone*

sometribove USAN, INN, BAN *veterinary growth stimulant*

sometripor USAN, INN, BAN *veterinary growth stimulant*

somfasepor USAN *veterinary growth stimulant*

somidobove USAN, INN *synthetic bovine growth hormone*

Sominex tablets, caplets OTC *antihistamine; sleep aid* [diphenhydramine HCl] 25 mg; 50 mg

Sominex Pain Relief tablets OTC *antihistamine; sleep aid; analgesic; antipyretic* [diphenhydramine HCl; acetaminophen] 25•500 mg

Somnote capsules ℞ *nonbarbiturate sedative and hypnotic; also abused as a street drug* [chloral hydrate] 500 mg

Sonata capsules ℞ *rapid-onset, short-duration hypnotic for the short-term treatment of insomnia* [zaleplon] 5, 10 mg

sonepiprazole mesylate USAN *dopamine D_4 antagonist; antipsychotic*

SonoRx oral suspension ℞ *ultrasound imaging agent to reduce gas shadowing* [simethicone-coated cellulose] 7.5 mg/mL

Soothaderm lotion OTC *anesthetic; antihistamine; emollient* [pyrilamine maleate; benzocaine; zinc oxide] 2.07•2.08•41.35 mg/mL

Soothe eye drops OTC *moisturizer/lubricant* [polysorbate 80] 0.4%

Soothe & Cool cream OTC *diaper rash treatment* [zinc oxide; dimethicone] 5%•5%

Soothe XP eye drops OTC *moisturizer/ lubricant* [mineral oil; light mineral oil] 4.5%•1% ⍰ Zotex-PE

sopecainol [see: solpecainol]

sopitazine INN

sopromidine INN

soproxil USAN *combining name for radicals or groups* [also: disoproxil]

soquinolol INN

sorafenib tosylate *multikinase inhibitor; antineoplastic for advanced renal cell carcinoma (orphan) and hepatocellular carcinoma* (base=73%)

sorb apple *medicinal herb* [see: mountain ash]

sorbic acid NF *antimicrobial agent; preservative*

sorbide nitrate [see: isosorbide dinitrate]

sorbimacrogol laurate 300 [see: polysorbate 20]

sorbimacrogol oleate 300 [see: polysorbate 80]

sorbimacrogol palmitate 300 [see: polysorbate 40]

sorbimacrogol stearate [see: polysorbate 60]

sorbimacrogol tristearate 300 [see: polysorbate 65]

sorbinicate INN

sorbinil USAN, INN, BAN *aldose reductase enzyme inhibitor*

sorbitan laurate INN *surfactant* [also: sorbitan monolaurate]

sorbitan monolaurate USAN, NF *surfactant* [also: sorbitan laurate]

sorbitan monooleate USAN, NF *surfactant* [also: sorbitan oleate]

sorbitan monopalmitate USAN, NF *surfactant* [also: sorbitan palmitate]

sorbitan monostearate USAN, NF *surfactant* [also: sorbitan stearate]

sorbitan oleate INN *surfactant* [also: sorbitan monooleate]

sorbitan palmitate INN *surfactant* [also: sorbitan monopalmitate]

sorbitan sesquioleate USAN, INN *surfactant*

sorbitan stearate INN *surfactant* [also: sorbitan monostearate]

sorbitan trioleate USAN, INN *surfactant*

sorbitan tristearate USAN, INN *surfactant*

sorbitol NF *flavoring agent; tablet excipient; urologic irrigant* 3%, 3.3%

sorbitol (solution) USP *flavoring agent; urologic irrigant* 70%

Sorbitrate sublingual tablets (discontinued 2004) ℞ *antianginal; vasodilator* [isosorbide dinitrate] 2.5, 5 mg

Sorbitrate tablets, chewable tablets (discontinued 2005) ℞ *antianginal; vasodilator* [isosorbide dinitrate] 5, 10, 20, 30, 40 mg; 5, 10 mg

Sorbsan pads *absorbent dressing for wet wounds* [calcium alginate fiber] ⍰ zorubicin

Sorbus americana; S. aucuparia *medicinal herb* [see: mountain ash]

Soriatane capsules ℞ *systemic antipsoriatic* [acitretin] 10, 25 mg ⍰ Serutan

sorivudine USAN, INN, BAN *investigational (NDA filed) antiviral for herpes zoster (orphan) and varicella zoster infections in immunocompromised patients*

sornidipine INN

sorrel (Rumex acetosa) plant *medicinal herb used as an antiscorbutic, astringent, diuretic, laxative, refrigerant, and vermifuge* ⍰ Xiral

sorrel, common; mountain sorrel; white sorrel *medicinal herb* [see: wood sorrel]

sorrel, Jamaica *medicinal herb* [see: hibiscus]

Sortis ⓔ (European name for the U.S. product **Lipitor**)

sotalol INN, BAN *antiarrhythmic; antiadrenergic (β-receptor)* [also: sotalol HCl]

sotalol HCl USAN *antiarrhythmic (β-blocker) for ventricular arrhythmias (orphan)* [also: sotalol] 80, 120, 160, 240 mg oral

Sotalol HCl AF tablets ℞ *antiarrhythmic (β-blocker) for atrial fibrillation or atrial flutter* [sotalol HCl] 80, 120, 160 mg

soterenol INN *adrenergic; bronchodilator* [also: soterenol HCl] ⍰ cioteronel; citronella; SteriNail

soterenol HCl USAN *adrenergic; bronchodilator* [also: soterenol]

Sotradecol IV injection, Dosette (unit-of-use injection) ℞ *sclerosing agent for varicose veins; investigational (orphan) for bleeding esophageal varices* [sodium tetradecyl sulfate] 10, 30 mg/mL

Sotret softgels ℞ *keratolytic for severe recalcitrant cystic acne* [isotretinoin] 10, 20, 30, 40 mg

sour dock *medicinal herb* [see: yellow dock]

sourberry; sowberry *medicinal herb* [see: barberry]

sourgrass *medicinal herb* [see: sorrel]

Southern ginseng *medicinal herb* [see: jiaogulan]

Soviet gramicidin [see: gramicidin S]

sowberry; sourberry *medicinal herb* [see: barberry]

soy; soya; soybean (Glycine max) *medicinal herb and food crop; isoflavone compounds provide phytoestrogens to alleviate menopausal symptoms, including osteoporosis, and provide antineoplastic, cardiovascular, and gastrointestinal benefits*

Soyalac; I-Soyalac oral liquid, powder for oral liquid OTC *hypoallergenic infant food* [soy protein formula] ⚕ SalAc; Slow-K

soybean oil USP *pharmaceutic necessity*

spaglumic acid INN

Span C tablets OTC *vitamin C supplement with bioflavonoids* [ascorbic acid and rose hips; citrus bioflavonoids] 200•300 mg

Spancap No. 1 sustained-release capsules ℞ *CNS stimulant* [dextroamphetamine sulfate] 15 mg

Spancaps (dosage form) *timed-release capsules*

Spanidin *investigational (orphan) immunosuppressant for acute renal graft rejection* [gusperimus]

Spanish chestnut *medicinal herb* [see: horse chestnut]

Spanish pepper *medicinal herb* [see: cayenne]

Spansule (trademarked dosage form) *sustained-release capsule*

sparfloxacin (SPFX) USAN, INN, BAN *broad-spectrum fluoroquinolone antibiotic* ⚕ ciprofloxacin

sparfosate sodium USAN *antineoplastic* [also: sparfosic acid]

sparfosic acid INN *antineoplastic* [also: sparfosate sodium]

Sparkles effervescent granules OTC *antacid; antiflatulent; aid in endoscopic examination* [sodium bicarbonate; citric acid; simethicone] 2000• 1500• ≟ mg/dose

Sparlon tablets *investigational (NDA filed) treatment for attention-deficit/ hyperactivity disorder in children and adolescents 6–17 years* [modafinil]

sparsomycin USAN, INN *antineoplastic*

Spartaject (trademarked delivery device) *investigational (Phase II/III) intravenous injector*

Spartaject Busulfan *investigational (orphan) alkylating antineoplastic for neoplastic meningitis and primary brain malignancies* [busulfan]

sparteine INN *oxytocic* [also: sparteine sulfate] ⚕ Ceprotin

sparteine sulfate USAN *oxytocic* [also: sparteine]

Spasmolin tablets ℞ *GI antispasmodic; anticholinergic; sedative* [atropine sulfate; scopolamine hydrobromide; hyoscyamine hydrobromide; phenobarbital] 0.0194•0.0065•0.1037•16.2 mg

SPCA (serum prothrombin conversion accelerator) factor [see: factor VII]

spearmint NF

spearmint (Mentha spicata) leaves *medicinal herb for colds, colic, flu, gas, nausea, and vomiting*

spearmint oil NF

Spec-T lozenges OTC *mucous membrane anesthetic* [benzocaine] 10 mg

Spectazole cream ℞ *antifungal* [econazole nitrate] 1%

spectinomycin INN *antibiotic* [also: spectinomycin HCl]

spectinomycin HCl USAN, USP *antibiotic for gonorrhea* [also: spectinomycin]

Spectracef film-coated tablets ℞ *broad-spectrum cephalosporin antibiotic* [cefditoren pivoxil] 200 mg

Spectrocin Plus ointment (discontinued 2005) OTC *antibiotic; local anesthetic* [polymyxin B sulfate; neomycin sulfate; bacitracin zinc; pramoxine HCl] 10 000 U•3.5 mg•500 U•10 mg per g

Spectro-Jel topical liquid OTC *soap-free therapeutic skin cleanser*

speedwell (Veronica officinalis) flowering plant *medicinal herb used as a diuretic, expectorant, and stomachic*

speedwell, tall *medicinal herb* [see: Culver root]

spenbolic [see: methandriol]

spermaceti, synthetic [see: cetyl esters wax]

spermicides *a class of topical contraceptive agents that kill sperm*

SPFX (sparfloxacin) [q.v.]

Spheramine *investigational (Phase II, orphan) dopamine-producing brain implants for stage 3 and 4 Parkinson disease* [human retinal pigment epithelial (RPE) cells on spherical cell-coated microcarriers (CCM)]

Spherulin intradermal injection ℞ *diagnostic aid for coccidioidomycosis* [coccidioidin] 1:100, 1:10

spiceberry *medicinal herb* [see: wintergreen]

spiclamine INN

spiclomazine INN

spicy wintergreen *medicinal herb* [see: wintergreen]

spider bite antivenin [see: antivenin (Latrodectus mactans)]

spignet *medicinal herb* [see: spikenard]

spikenard (Aralia racemosa) root *medicinal herb for asthma, childbirth, cough, and rheumatism*

spindle tree *medicinal herb* [see: wahoo]

spiperone USAN, INN *antipsychotic*

spiradoline INN *analgesic* [also: spiradoline mesylate]

spiradoline mesylate USAN *analgesic* [also: spiradoline]

spiramide INN

spiramycin USAN, INN, BAN *macrolide antibiotic; investigational (orphan) treatment for chronic cryptosporidiosis in immunocompromised patients* [also: acetylspiramycin]

spirapril INN, BAN *antihypertensive; angiotensin-converting enzyme (ACE) inhibitor* [also: spirapril HCl]

spirapril HCl USAN *antihypertensive; angiotensin-converting enzyme (ACE) inhibitor* [also: spirapril]

spiraprilat USAN, INN *antihypertensive; angiotensin-converting enzyme (ACE) inhibitor*

spirazine INN ⊡ Sprayzoin

spirazine HCl [see: spirazine]

spirendolol INN

spirgetine INN

spirilene INN, BAN ⊡ Supprelin

spirit of nitrous ether [see: ethyl nitrite]

Spiriva powder in capsules for inhalation (used with **HandiHaler** device) ℞ *once-daily bronchodilator for emphysema and chronic obstructive pulmonary disease (COPD)* [tiotropium bromide] 18 mcg/dose ⊡ Cipro I.V.

spirobarbital sodium

spirofylline INN

spirogermanium INN, BAN *antineoplastic* [also: spirogermanium HCl]

spirogermanium HCl USAN *antineoplastic* [also: spirogermanium]

spirohydantoin mustard [now: spiromustine]

spiromustine USAN, INN *antineoplastic*

spironolactone USP, INN, BAN, JAN *antihypertensive; potassium-sparing diuretic; aldosterone antagonist* 25, 50, 100 mg oral

spiroplatin USAN, INN, BAN *antineoplastic*

spirorenone INN

spirotriazine HCl [see: spirazine]

spiroxamide [see: spiroxatrine]

spiroxasone USAN, INN *diuretic*

spiroxatrine INN

spiroxepin INN

spirulina (Spirulina pratensis) plant *medicinal herb for chronic disease, enhancing antibody production, lowering serum lipids and triglycerides, and reducing gastric secretory activity; also used as a blood builder and food supplement* ⊕ Supprelin

spizofurone INN

spoonwood *medicinal herb* [see: linden tree]

Sporanox capsules, PulsePak, IV infusion ℞ *systemic triazole antifungal* [itraconazole] 100 mg; 100 mg × 28; 10 mg/mL

Sporanox oral solution ("swish and swallow") ℞ *antifungal for esophageal and oropharyngeal candidiasis* [itraconazole] 10 mg/mL

Sporidin-G *investigational (orphan) treatment of cryptosporidiosis-induced diarrhea in immunocompromised patients* [Cryptosporidium parvum bovine colostrum IgG concentrate]

Sports Spray OTC *analgesic; mild anesthetic; antipruritic; counterirritant; antiseptic* [methyl salicylate; menthol; camphor; alcohol 58%] 3.5%•10%•5%

Sportscreme OTC *analgesic* [trolamine salicylate] 10%

Sportscreme Ice gel OTC *analgesic; mild anesthetic; antipruritic; counterirritant* [trolamine; menthol] ≟•2%

spotted alder *medicinal herb* [see: witch hazel]

spotted comfrey *medicinal herb* [see: lungwort]

spotted cranesbill *medicinal herb* [see: alum root]

spotted geranium *medicinal herb* [see: alum root]

spotted hemlock; spotted cowbane; spotted parsley *medicinal herb* [see: poison hemlock]

spotted lungwort *medicinal herb* [see: lungwort]

spotted thistle *medicinal herb* [see: blessed thistle]

spp. plural of *species*

SPP100 *investigational (Phase III) renin antagonist for hypertension*

SPPG (sulfated polysaccharide peptidoglycan) [see: tecogalan sodium]

Sprayzoin spray OTC *skin protectant; antiseptic* [benzoin; ethyl alcohol] ⊕ spirazine

spring wintergreen *medicinal herb* [see: wintergreen]

Sprinkle Caps (trademarked dosage form) *powder*

Sprintec tablets (in packs of 28) ℞ *monophasic oral contraceptive* [norgestimate; ethinyl estradiol] 0.25 mg•35 mcg × 21 days; counters × 7 days

sprodiamide USAN *heart and CNS imaging aid for MRI*

spruce (Picea excelsa; P. mariana) young shoots *medicinal herb used as a calmative, diaphoretic, expectorant, and pectoral*

spruce, Norway *medicinal herb* [see: spruce]

spruce, weeping *medicinal herb* [see: hemlock]

Sprycel film-coated tablets ℞ *antineoplastic for chronic myeloid leukemia (CML) and acute lymphoblastic leukemia in patients expressing the Philadelphia chromosome (Ph+ ALL)* [dasatinib] 20, 50, 70, 100 mg

SPS oral suspension ℞ *potassium-removing agent for hyperkalemia* [sodium polystyrene sulfonate] 15 g/60 mL

spurge laurel; spurge olive *medicinal herb* [see: mezereon]

squalamine lactate *natural remedy; shark cartilage derivative; investigational (orphan) angiogenesis inhibitor for ovarian cancer* [also: shark cartilage]

squalane NF *oleaginous vehicle*

square, carpenter's *medicinal herb* [see: figwort]

squaw balm; squaw mint *medicinal herb* [see: pennyroyal]

squaw root *medicinal herb* [see: black cohosh; blue cohosh]

squaw tea *medicinal herb* [see: ephedra]

squaw vine (Mitchella repens) plant *medicinal herb for easing childbirth,*

Stahist 659

lactation, and menstruation and for uterine disorders

squaw weed *medicinal herb* [see: life root]

squawberry *medicinal herb* [see: squaw vine]

squill (Urginea indica; U. maritima; U. scilla) *bulb medicinal herb for edema and inducing emesis and expectoration; also used as a rat poison* ⬚ Secule

squirrel pea, ground *medicinal herb* [see: twin leaf]

⁸⁵Sr [see: strontium chloride Sr 85]

⁸⁵Sr [see: strontium nitrate Sr 85]

⁸⁵Sr [see: strontium Sr 85]

SRF (skin respiratory factor) [q.v.]

Sronyx film-coated tablets (in packs of 28) ℞ *monophasic oral contraceptive* [levonorgestrel; ethinyl estradiol] 0.1 mg•20 mcg × 21 days; counters × 7 days

SS (saline solution)

SS (sodium salicylate) [q.v.]

SS (somatostatin) [q.v.]

SSD (silver sulfadiazine) [q.v.]

SSD; SSD AF cream ℞ *broad-spectrum bactericidal for adjunctive burn treatment* [silver sulfadiazine] 10 mg/g

SSKI oral solution ℞ *expectorant* [potassium iodide] 1 g/mL

SSNRIs (selective serotonin and norepinephrine reuptake inhibitors) [q.v.]

SSRIs (selective serotonin reuptake inhibitors) [q.v.]

S.S.S. High Potency Vitamin Tablets OTC *vitamin/mineral/iron supplement* [multiple vitamins & minerals; iron; biotin] ±•27•0.0225 mg

S.S.S. Vitamin and Mineral Complex oral liquid OTC *vitamin/mineral/iron supplement* [multiple vitamins & minerals; iron; biotin; alcohol 6.6%] ±•3•0.1 mg

S.T. 37 topical solution OTC *antiseptic* [hexylresorcinol] 0.1%

S-T Cort lotion ℞ *corticosteroidal anti-inflammatory* [hydrocortisone] 0.5% ⬚ Cetacort

S-T Forte 2 oral liquid (discontinued 2007) ℞ *narcotic antitussive; antihistamine* [hydrocodone bitartrate; chlorpheniramine maleate] 2.5•2 mg/5 mL

ST1-RTA immunotoxin (SR 44163) *investigational (orphan) for graft vs. host disease and B-chronic lymphocytic leukemia*

Staarvisc intraocular injection ℞ *viscoelastic agent for ophthalmic surgery* [hyaluronate sodium]

stable factor [see: factor VII]

Staccato (trademarked delivery device) *investigational (Phase III) single-dose oral inhaler, currently being tested with* **loxapine** *for acute agitation associated with schizophrenia*

Stachys officinalis *medicinal herb* [see: betony]

Stadol IV or IM injection ℞ *narcotic agonist-antagonist analgesic* [butorphanol tartrate] 1, 2 mg/mL ⬚ cetiedil

Stadol NS nasal spray (discontinued 2004) ℞ *narcotic agonist-antagonist analgesic; antimigraine agent* [butorphanol tartrate] 10 mg/mL

staff vine *medicinal herb* [see: bittersweet nightshade]

Staflex caplets ℞ *analgesic; antipyretic; antihistamine; sleep aid* [acetaminophen; phenyltoloxamine citrate] 500•55 mg

Stagesic capsules ℞ *narcotic analgesic; antipyretic* [hydrocodone bitartrate; acetaminophen] 5•500 mg ⬚ Zotex-G

staggerweed *medicinal herb* [see: turkey corn]

staghorn *medicinal herb* [see: club moss]

Stahist sustained-release tablets ℞ *decongestant; antihistamine; anticholinergic to dry mucosal secretions* [phenylephrine HCl; pseudoephedrine HCl; chlorpheniramine maleate; hyoscyamine sulfate; atropine sulfate; scopolamine hydrobromide] 25•40•8•0.19•0.04•0.01 mg

Stalevo 50; Stalevo 100; Stalevo 150; Stalevo 200 tablets ℞ *multimodal treatment for Parkinson disease: dopamine precursor + decarboxylase inhibitor (levodopa potentiator) + COMT (catechol-O-methyltransferase) inhibitor* [levodopa; carbidopa; entacapone] 50•12.5•200 mg; 100•25•200 mg; 150•37.5•200 mg; 200•50•200 mg

stallimycin INN *antibacterial* [also: stallimycin HCl]

stallimycin HCl USAN *antibacterial* [also: stallimycin]

Stamoist E caplets ℞ *decongestant; expectorant* [pseudoephedrine HCl; guaifenesin] 45•600 mg

Stanback Headache Powder OTC *analgesic; antipyretic; anti-inflammatory* [aspirin; salicylamide; caffeine] 650•200•32 mg/pkt.

standard VAC *chemotherapy protocol for sarcomas* [see: VAC standard]

Stanford V (mechlorethamine, doxorubicin, vinblastine, vincristine, bleomycin, etoposide, prednisone) *chemotherapy protocol for Hodgkin lymphoma*

stannous chloride USAN *pharmaceutic aid*

stannous fluoride USP *dental caries prophylactic* 0.4%, 0.63% topical oral

stannous pyrophosphate USAN *skeletal imaging aid*

stannous sulfur colloid USAN *bone, liver and spleen imaging aid*

stannsoporfin USAN *bilirubin inhibitor*

stanolone BAN *anabolic steroid; investigational (orphan) for AIDS-wasting syndrome* [also: androstanolone]

stanozolol USAN, USP, INN, BAN *androgen; anabolic steroid for hereditary angioedema*

StaphVAX *investigational (Phase III) vaccine against* Staphylococcus aureus *infection of end-stage renal disease*

Staphylococcus aureus immune globulin, human *investigational (orphan) prophylaxis against* S. aureus *infections in low birthweight neonates*

star anise *(Illicium anisatum; I. verum)* seeds *medicinal herb used as a carminative, stimulant, and stomachic; also added to other herbal medications to improve digestibility and taste*

star chickweed; starweed *medicinal herb* [see: chickweed]

star grass *(Aletris farinosa)* root and rhizome *medicinal herb for diarrhea, dysmenorrhea and menstrual discomfort, gas and colonic cramps, and rheumatism*

star root *medicinal herb* [see: star grass]

starch NF *dusting powder; pharmaceutic aid* ☑ Cytra-K

starch, pregelatinized NF *tablet excipient*

starch, topical USP *dusting powder*

starch carboxymethyl ether, sodium salt [see: sodium starch glycolate]

starch glycerite NF

starch 2-hydroxyethyl ether [see: hetastarch; pentastarch]

Starlix tablets ℞ *meglitinide antidiabetic for type 2 diabetes that stimulates the release of insulin from the pancreas* [nateglinide] 60, 120 mg ☑ Citralax

Star-Otic ear drops OTC *antibacterial; antifungal; antiseptic; astringent* [acetic acid; aluminum acetate; boric acid]

Starsis (Japanese name for U.S. product **Starlix**)

Starvisc [see: Staarvisc]

starwort; mealy starwort *medicinal herb* [see: chickweed; star grass]

Stat-Crit electrode device for professional use ℞ *in vitro diagnostic aid for hemoglobin/hematocrit measurement*

STaTdose (trademarked delivery form) *prefilled syringes for self-administration*

Staticin topical solution (discontinued 2004) ℞ *antibiotic for acne* [erythromycin; alcohol 55%] 1.5%

"statins" *brief term for a class of antihyperlipidemics that include atorvastatin, cerivastatin, fluvastatin, lovastatin, pravastatin, rosuvastatin, and simvastatin* [properly called: HMG-CoA reductase inhibitors]

statolon USAN *antiviral* [also: vistatolon]

Stat-One gel (discontinued 2004) OTC *antiseptic* [hydrogen peroxide] 3%

Stat-One gel (discontinued 2004) OTC *antiseptic* [isopropyl alcohol] 70%

Stat-Pak (trademarked packaging form) *unit-dose package*

Statuss Green oral liquid ℞ *narcotic antitussive; antihistamine; sleep aid; decongestant* [hydrocodone bitartrate; chlorpheniramine maleate; pyrilamine maleate; phenylephrine HCl; pseudoephedrine HCl] 2.5•2•3.3• 5•3.3 mg/5 mL

staunch, blood *medicinal herb* [see: fleabane; horseweed]

stavudine USAN, INN *nucleoside reverse transcriptase inhibitor; antiviral for HIV-1 infections*

stavudine & lamivudine *combination nucleoside reverse transcriptase inhibitor (NRTI) for HIV and AIDS* 30• 150, 40•15 mg oral

stavudine & nevirapine & lamivudine *combination nucleoside reverse transcriptase inhibitor (NRTI) and non-nucleoside reverse transcriptase inhibitor (NNRTI) for HIV and AIDS* 6•50•30, 12•100•60, 30•200•150, 40•200•150 mg oral

Stavzor delayed-release softgels ℞ *anticonvulsant for complex partial seizures and simple or complex absence seizures; treatment for manic episodes of a bipolar disorder; migraine prophylactic* [valproic acid] 125, 250, 500 mg

Stay Awake tablets OTC *CNS stimulant; analeptic* [caffeine] 200 mg ② Zoto-HC

Stay-Wet 3; Stay-Wet 4 solution OTC *disinfecting/wetting/soaking solution for rigid gas permeable contact lenses*

STD (sodium tetradecyl sulfate) [q.v.]

steaglate INN *combining name for radicals or groups*

STEAM (streptonigrin, thioguanine, cyclophosphamide, actinomycin, mitomycin) *chemotherapy protocol*

stearethate 40 [see: polyoxyl 40 stearate]

stearic acid NF *emulsion adjunct; tablet and capsule lubricant* ② citric acid

stearyl alcohol NF *emulsion adjunct*

stearyl dimethyl benzyl ammonium chloride

stearylsulfamide INN

steffimycin USAN, INN *antibacterial; antiviral*

Stellaria media medicinal herb [see: chickweed]

stem and progenitor cells derived from ex vivo allogenic umbilical cord blood *investigational (orphan) hematopoietic support for patients on high-dose therapy for hematologic malignancies*

stem cell factor (SCF) [see: methionyl stem cell factor]

stem cells, T-cell depleted, derived from peripheral blood stem cells *investigational (orphan) for chronic granulomatous disease*

StemEx *investigational (orphan) hematopoietic support for patients on high-dose therapy for hematologic malignancies* [stem and progenitor cells derived from ex vivo allogenic umbilical cord blood]

Stemgen ⒸⒶⓃ powder for subcu injection (available in Canada) *investigational (NDA filed) recombinant human stem cell factor; hematopoietic growth factor; adjunct to myelosuppressive and myeloablative therapy* [ancestim] 187.5 mg/vial

stenbolone INN *anabolic steroid; also abused as a street drug* [also: stenbolone acetate]

stenbolone acetate USAN *anabolic steroid; also abused as a street drug* [also: stenbolone]

Stenorol *investigational (orphan) antiprotozoal for scleroderma* [halofuginone hydrobromide]

stepronin INN

Sterapred; Sterapred DS tablets, Unipak (dispensing pack) ℞ *corticosteroid; anti-inflammatory* [prednisone] 5 mg; 10 mg

Sterculia tragacantha; S. urens; S. villosa medicinal herb [see: karaya gum]

stercuronium iodide INN

Sterecyt *investigational (orphan) antineoplastic for malignant non-Hodgkin lymphomas* [prednimustine]

Steri-Dose (trademarked delivery form) *prefilled disposable syringe*

SteriNail topical solution OTC *antifungal* [undecylenic acid; tolnaftate] ≛ • ≛ ☐ cioteronel; citronella; soterenol

Steritalc *investigational (orphan) treatment for malignant pleural effusion and pneumothorax* [talc, sterile]

Steri-Vial (trademarked delivery form) *ampule*

Sterules (trademarked dosage form) *solution for nebulization*

stevaladil INN

stevia (*Stevia rebaudiana*) leaves *medicinal herb used as a non-caloric sugar substitute; also used for diabetes, food cravings, hypertension, obesity, and tobacco cravings*

stibamine glucoside INN, BAN

stibocaptate BAN [also: sodium stibocaptate]

stibophen NF

stibosamine INN

stickwort; sticklewort *medicinal herb* [see: agrimony]

stigmata maidis (corn silk) *medicinal herb* [see: Indian corn]

stilbamidine isethionate [see: stilbamidine isetionate]

stilbamidine isetionate INN

stilbazium iodide USAN, INN *anthelmintic*

stilbestroform [see: diethylstilbestrol]

stilbestrol [see: diethylstilbestrol]

stilbestronate [see: diethylstilbestrol dipropionate]

stilboestroform [see: diethylstilbestrol]

stilboestrol BAN *estrogen* [also: diethylstilbestrol]

stilboestrol DP [see: diethylstilbestrol dipropionate]

stillingia (*Stillingia ligustina*) root *medicinal herb for acne, eczema, and other skin disorders, blood cleansing,* liver disorders, respiratory illnesses, and syphilis

Stilnoct; Stilnox ⓔ (European name for U.S. product **Ambien**)

stilonium iodide USAN, INN *antispasmodic*

stilronate [see: diethylstilbestrol dipropionate]

Stimate metered-dose nasal spray ℞ *posterior pituitary hormone for hemophilia A and von Willebrand disease (orphan)* [desmopressin acetate] 150 mcg (600 IU)/dose

stimulant laxatives *a subclass of laxatives that work by direct action on the intestinal mucosa and nerve plexus to increase peristaltic action* [see also: laxatives]

stimulants *a class of agents that excite the activity of physiological processes*

Stimuvax *investigational (Phase III) antineoplastic vaccine against MUC-1 for the treatment of non–small cell lung cancer* [BLP-25 liposome vaccine]

Sting-Eze topical solution concentrate OTC *anesthetic; antihistamine; antipruritic; antiseptic* [benzocaine; diphenhydramine HCl; camphor; phenol; eucalyptol]

stinging nettle *medicinal herb* [see: nettle]

Sting-Kill swabs, wipes OTC *anesthetic; antipruritic; counterirritant* [benzocaine; menthol; isopropyl alcohol 15%] 20%•1%

stingless nettle *medicinal herb* [see: blind nettle]

stinking nightshade *medicinal herb* [see: henbane]

stirimazole INN, BAN

stiripentol USAN, INN *anticonvulsant*

stirocainide INN

stirofos USAN *veterinary insecticide*

stitchwort *medicinal herb* [see: chickweed]

Stocrin ⓔ (foreign name for the U.S. product **Sustiva**)

stomachics *a class of agents that promote the functional activity of the stomach*

stone root *(Collinsonia canadensis)* roots and leaves *medicinal herb used as a diuretic and vulnerary*

Stool Softener capsules OTC *laxative; stool softener* [docusate sodium] 100, 250 mg

Stool Softener; Stool Softener DC capsules OTC *laxative; stool softener* [docusate calcium] 240 mg

stool-softening laxatives *a subclass of laxatives that work by increasing the amount of fat and water in the stool to ease its movement through the intestines* [see also: laxatives]

Stop gel ℞ *dental caries preventative* [stannous fluoride] 0.4%

storax USP ⊘ Sitrex

storax *(Liquidambar orientalis; L. styraciflua)* leaves and gum *medicinal herb for diarrhea, inducing expectoration, parasitic infections, promoting sweating and diuresis, skin sores and wounds, and sore throat* ⊘ Sitrex

Storzfen eye drops ℞ *decongestant; vasoconstrictor; mydriatic* [phenylephrine HCl] 2.5%

Storzine 2 eye drops ℞ *antiglaucoma agent; direct-acting miotic* [pilocarpine HCl] 2% ⊘ cetirizine

Storz-N-D eye drops ℞ *corticosteroidal anti-inflammatory; antibiotic* [dexamethasone sodium phosphate; neomycin sulfate] 0.1%•0.35%

Storz-N-P-D eye drop suspension ℞ *corticosteroidal anti-inflammatory; antibiotic* [dexamethasone; neomycin sulfate; polymyxin B sulfate] 0.1%•0.35%•10 000 U/mL

Storz-Sulf eye drops ℞ *antibiotic* [sulfacetamide sodium] 10%

stramonium [see: jimsonweed]

Strattera capsules ℞ *non-stimulant treatment for attention-deficit/hyperactivity disorder (ADHD); investigational (orphan) for Tourette syndrome* [atomoxetine HCl] 10, 18, 25, 40, 60, 80, 100 mg

strawberry *(Fragaria vesca)* leaves *medicinal herb for blood cleansing, diarrhea, eczema, intestinal disorders,* preventing miscarriage, and stomach cleansing

strawberry bush; strawberry tree *medicinal herb* [see: wahoo]

Strep Detect slide tests for professional use ℞ *in vitro diagnostic aid for streptococcal antigens in throat swabs*

Streptase powder for IV or intracoronary infusion ℞ *thrombolytic enzyme for lysis of thrombi and catheter clearance* [streptokinase] 250 000, 750 000, 1 500 000 IU

streptococcus immune globulin, group B *investigational (orphan) for neonatal group B streptococcal infection*

Streptococcus sp. [see also: lactic acid bacteria]

streptodornase (SD) INN, BAN

streptoduocin USP

streptogramins *a class of antibiotics, isolated from Streptomyces pristinaespirales, used for gram-positive infections*

streptokinase (SK) INN *thrombolytic enzymes for myocardial infarction, thrombosis or embolism*

streptomycin INN, BAN *aminoglycoside antibiotic; primary tuberculostatic* [also: streptomycin sulfate]

streptomycin sulfate USP *aminoglycoside antibiotic; primary tuberculostatic* [also: streptomycin] 1 g injection

Streptonase-B test kit for professional use ℞ *in vitro diagnostic test for DNAse-B streptococcal antigens in serum*

streptoniazid INN *antibacterial* [also: streptonicozid]

streptonicozid USAN *antibacterial* [also: streptoniazid]

streptonigrin (SN) USAN *antineoplastic* [also: rufocromomycin]

streptovarycin INN

streptozocin USAN, INN *nitrosourea-type alkylating antineoplastic for metastatic islet cell carcinoma of the pancreas*

streptozotocin [see: streptozocin]

Streptozyme slide tests for professional use ℞ *in vitro diagnostic test for streptococcal extracellular antigens in blood, plasma, and serum*

Stress 600 with Zinc tablets OTC *vitamin/mineral supplement* [multiple vitamins & minerals; folic acid; biotin] ± • 400 • 45 mcg

Stress B Complex tablets OTC *vitamin/mineral supplement* [multiple vitamins & minerals; folic acid; biotin] ± • 400 • 45 mcg

Stress B Complex with Vitamin C timed-release tablets OTC *vitamin/mineral supplement* [multiple B vitamins; vitamin C; zinc] ± • 300 • 15 mg

Stress Formula 600 tablets OTC *vitamin supplement* [multiple vitamins; folic acid; biotin] ± • 400 • 45 mcg

Stress Formula Vitamins capsules, tablets OTC *vitamin supplement* [multiple vitamins; folic acid; biotin] ± • 400 • 45 mcg

Stress Formula with Iron film-coated tablets OTC *vitamin/iron supplement* [multiple B vitamins; vitamins C and E; ferrous fumarate; folic acid; biotin] ± • 500 mg • 30 IU • 27 mg • 0.4 mg • 45 mcg

Stress Formula with Zinc tablets OTC *vitamin/iron supplement* [multiple B vitamins; vitamins C and E; multiple minerals; folic acid; biotin] ± • 500 mg • 30 IU • ± • 0.4 mg • 45 mcg

Stresstabs tablets OTC *vitamin supplement* [multiple vitamins; folic acid; biotin] ± • 400 • 45 mcg

Stresstabs + Iron film-coated tablets OTC *vitamin/iron supplement* [multiple B vitamins; vitamins C and E; ferrous fumarate; folic acid; biotin] ± • 500 mg • 30 IU • 18 mg • 0.4 mg • 45 mcg

Stresstabs + Zinc film-coated tablets OTC *vitamin/mineral supplement* [multiple vitamins & minerals; folic acid; biotin] ± • 400 • 45 mcg

Stresstein powder OTC *enteral nutritional therapy for moderate to severe stress or trauma* [multiple branched chain amino acids]

Striant mucoadhesive buccal tablets R *androgen for hypogonadism or testosterone deficiency in men; hormone replacement therapy (HRT) for postandropausal symptoms* [testosterone] 30 mg

Stri-Dex pads OTC *keratolytic cleanser for acne* [salicylic acid; alcohol] 0.5% • 28%, 2% • 44%, 2% • 54%

Stri-Dex Cleansing bar OTC *medicated cleanser for acne* [triclosan] 1%

Stri-Dex Clear gel OTC *keratolytic cleanser for acne* [salicylic acid; alcohol] 2% • 9.3%

Stri-Dex Face Wash solution OTC *medicated cleanser for acne* [triclosan] 1%

strinoline INN

striped alder *medicinal herb* [see: winterberry; witch hazel]

Stromectol tablets R *anthelmintic for strongyloidiasis and onchocerciasis* [ivermectin] 3, 6 mg

strong ammonia solution [see: ammonia solution, strong]

Strong Iodine solution, tincture R *antiseptic* [iodine; potassium iodide] 5% • 10%; 7% • 5%

stronger rose water [see: rose water, stronger]

StrongStart caplets R *vitamin/mineral/calcium/iron supplement; stool softener* [multiple vitamins & minerals; calcium; iron; folic acid; docusate sodium] ± • 200 • 29 • 1 • 25 mg

StrongStart chewable tablets R *vitamin/mineral/calcium/iron supplement* [multiple vitamins & minerals; calcium; iron; folic acid] ± • 200 • 29 • 1 mg

strontium *element* (Sr)

strontium chloride *topical anti-irritant*

strontium chloride Sr 85 USAN *radioactive agent*

strontium chloride Sr 89 USAN *radioactive agent; analgesic for metastatic bone pain*

strontium nitrate Sr 85 USAN *radioactive agent*

strontium salicylate NF

strontium Sr 85 USP

Strovite tablets R *vitamin supplement* [multiple B vitamins; vitamin C; folic acid] ± • 500 • 0.5 mg

Strovite Advance; Strovite Forte; Strovite Plus caplets R *geriatric*

vitamin/mineral therapy [multiple vitamins & minerals; folic acid; biotin] ✠•1000•100 mcg; ✠•1000• 150 mcg; ✠•800•150 mcg

structum *natural remedy* [see: chondroitin sulfate]

strychnine NF *an extremely poisonous CNS stimulant; occasionally abused as a street drug in combination with LSD*

strychnine glycerophosphate NF

strychnine nitrate NF

strychnine phosphate NF

strychnine sulfate NF

strychnine valerate NF

Stuart Formula tablets OTC *vitamin/ mineral/iron supplement* [multiple vitamins & minerals; iron; folic acid] ✠•18•0.1 mg

Stuart Prenatal tablets OTC *vitamin/ calcium/iron supplement* [multiple vitamins; calcium; iron; folic acid] ✠•200•28•0.8 mg

StuartNatal Plus 3 tablets ℞ *vitamin/ calcium/iron supplement* [multiple vitamins; calcium; iron; folic acid] ✠•200•28•1 mg

stugeron [see: cinnarizine]

stutgin [see: cinnarizine]

Stye ophthalmic ointment OTC *emollient* [white petrolatum; mineral oil] 58%•32%

styptics *a class of hemostatic agents that stop bleeding of the skin by astringent action* [see also: astringents; hemostatics]

Stypto-Caine topical solution OTC *styptic to the stop bleeding of minor cuts* [aluminum chloride; tetracaine HCl; oxyquinoline sulfate] 250•2.5•1 mg/g

styramate INN

styronate resins

SU-5416 *investigational (Phase II/III) angiogenesis inhibitor for AIDS-related Kaposi sarcoma*

subathizone INN ② sopitazine

subendazole INN

suberoylanilide hydroxamic acid (SAHA) [see: vorinostat]

Sublimaze IV or IM injection ℞ *narcotic analgesic for breakthrough pain in cancer patients; adjunct to anesthesia* [fentanyl citrate] 50 mcg/mL

sublimed sulfur [see: sulfur, sublimed]

Sublingual B Total drops OTC *vitamin supplement* [multiple B vitamins; vitamin C] ✠•60 mg/mL

Suboxone sublingual tablets ℞ *narcotic agonist-antagonist analgesic for outpatient maintenance of opiate dependence (orphan)* [buprenorphine HCl; naloxone HCl] 2•0.5, 8•2 mg

substance F [see: demecolcine]

substituted benzimidazoles *a class of gastric antisecretory agents that inhibit the aTPase "proton pump" within the gastric parietal cell* [also called: proton pump inhibitors; aTPase inhibitors]

Subutex sublingual tablets ℞ *narcotic agonist-antagonist analgesic for inpatient treatment of opiate dependence (orphan)* [buprenorphine HCl] 2, 8 mg

Suby G solution; Suby solution G (citric acid, magnesium oxide, sodium carbonate) *urologic irrigant to dissolve phosphatic calculi*

succimer USAN, INN, BAN *heavy metal chelating agent for lead poisoning (orphan); investigational (orphan) for mercury poisoning and cysteine kidney stones*

succinchlorimide NF

succinimides *a class of anticonvulsants*

succinylcholine chloride USP *neuromuscular blocker; muscle relaxant; anesthesia adjunct* [also: suxamethonium chloride] 20 mg/mL injection

succinyldapsone [see: succisulfone]

succinylsulfathiazole USP

succisulfone INN

succory *medicinal herb* [see: chicory]

Succus Cineraria Maritima eye drops ℞ *natural treatment for optic opacity caused by cataract* [senecio compositae; hamamelis water (witch hazel); boric acid]

suclofenide INN, BAN

Sucraid oral solution ℞ *enzyme replacement therapy for congenital sucrase-isomaltase deficiency (orphan)* [sacrosidase] 8500 IU/mL

sucralfate USAN, INN, BAN *cytoprotective agent for gastric ulcers; investigational (orphan) for oral mucositis and stomatitis following cancer radiation or chemotherapy* 1 g oral; 1 g/10 mL oral

sucralose BAN

sucralox INN, BAN

Sucrets throat spray OTC *antipruritic/counterirritant; mild local anesthetic* [dyclonine HCl] 0.1%

Sucrets Children's Formula; Sucrets Maximum Strength Sore Throat lozenges OTC *mucous membrane anesthetic* [dyclonine HCl] 1.2 mg; 3 mg

Sucrets Complete lozenges OTC *mucous membrane anesthetic* [dyclonine HCl; menthol] 3•6 mg

Sucrets Defense Kid's Formula lozenges OTC *vitamin/mineral supplement* [vitamin C; zinc; glutathione] 3.9•0.93•20 mg

Sucrets DM Cough Formula; Sucrets DM Cough Suppressant lozenges OTC *antitussive* [dextromethorphan hydrobromide] 10 mg

Sucrets Herbal lozenges OTC *mild anesthetic; antipruritic; counterirritant* [menthol; pectin] 50•60 mg

Sucrets Original Formula Sore Throat (Cherry) lozenges OTC *mucous membrane anesthetic* [dyclonine HCl] 2 mg

Sucrets Original Formula Sore Throat (Mint) lozenges OTC *antiseptic* [hexylresorcinol] 2.4 mg

sucrose NF *flavoring agent; tablet excipient* ℞ Xigris

sucrose octaacetate NF *alcohol denaturant*

sucrosofate potassium USAN *antiulcerative*

Sudafed tablets OTC *nasal decongestant* [pseudoephedrine HCl] 30, 60 mg

Sudafed, Children's chewable tablets OTC *nasal decongestant* [pseudoephedrine HCl] 15 mg

Sudafed, Children's Non-Drowsy oral liquid OTC *nasal decongestant* [pseudoephedrine HCl] 15 mg/5 mL

Sudafed Children's Non-Drowsy Cold & Cough oral liquid OTC *antitussive; decongestant* [dextromethorphan hydrobromide; pseudoephedrine HCl] 5•15 mg/5 mL

Sudafed Cold & Allergy tablets (name changed to **Sudafed Sinus & Allergy** in 2006)

Sudafed Multi-Symptom Cold & Cough liquid caps (discontinued 2007) OTC *antitussive; decongestant; expectorant; analgesic; antipyretic* [dextromethorphan hydrobromide; pseudoephedrine HCl; guaifenesin; acetaminophen] 10•30•100•250 mg

Sudafed Non-Drowsy tablets OTC *nasal decongestant* [pseudoephedrine HCl] 30 mg

Sudafed Non-Drowsy 12 Hour Long Acting extended-release caplets OTC *nasal decongestant* [pseudoephedrine HCl] 120 mg

Sudafed Non-Drowsy 24 Hour Long Acting dual-release tablets OTC *nasal decongestant* [pseudoephedrine HCl] 240 mg (60 mg immediate release, 180 mg extended release)

Sudafed Non-Drowsy Non-Drying Sinus liquid-filled capsules (discontinued 2007) OTC *decongestant; expectorant* [pseudoephedrine HCl; guaifenesin] 30•120 mg

Sudafed Non-Drowsy Severe Cold Formula caplets (discontinued 2007) OTC *antitussive; decongestant; analgesic; antipyretic* [dextromethorphan hydrobromide; pseudoephedrine HCl; acetaminophen] 15•30•500 mg

Sudafed PE tablets OTC *nasal decongestant* [phenylephrine HCl] 10 mg

Sudafed PE Multi-Symptom Cold and Cough caplets OTC *antitussive; decongestant; expectorant; analgesic; antipyretic* [dextromethorphan hydrobromide; phenylephrine HCl; guaifenesin; acetaminophen] 10•5•100•325 mg

Sudafed PE Multi-Symptom Severe Cold caplets OTC *decongestant; antihistamine; sleep aid; analgesic; antipy-*

retic [phenylephrine HCl; diphenhydramine HCl; acetaminophen] 5•12.5•325 mg

Sudafed PE Nighttime Cold caplets OTC *decongestant; antihistamine; sleep aid; analgesic; antipyretic* [phenylephrine HCl; diphenhydramine HCl; acetaminophen] 5•25•325 mg

Sudafed PE Nighttime Nasal Decongestant tablets OTC *decongestant; antihistamine; sleep aid* [phenylephrine HCl; diphenhydramine HCl] 10•25 mg

Sudafed PE Non-Drying Sinus caplets OTC *decongestant; expectorant* [phenylephrine HCl; guaifenesin] 5•200 mg

Sudafed PE Quick-Dissolve orally disintegrating film OTC *nasal decongestant* [phenylephrine HCl] 10 mg

Sudafed PE Sinus & Allergy tablets OTC *decongestant; antihistamine* [phenylephrine HCl; chlorpheniramine maleate] 10•4 mg

Sudafed PE Sinus Headache caplets OTC *decongestant; analgesic; antipyretic* [phenylephrine HCl; acetaminophen] 5•325 mg

Sudafed Sinus & Allergy tablets OTC *decongestant; antihistamine* [pseudoephedrine HCl; chlorpheniramine maleate] 60•4 mg

Sudafed Sinus & Cold Non-Drowsy Liqui-Caps (liquid-filled gelcaps) OTC *decongestant; analgesic; antipyretic* [pseudoephedrine HCl; acetaminophen] 30•325 mg

Sudafed Sinus Headache Non-Drowsy tablets, caplets (discontinued 2007) OTC *decongestant; analgesic; antipyretic* [pseudoephedrine HCl; acetaminophen] 30•500 mg

Sudafed Sinus Nighttime tablets (discontinued 2007) OTC *decongestant; antihistamine* [pseudoephedrine HCl; triprolidine HCl] 60•2.5 mg

Sudafed Sinus Nighttime Plus Pain Relief caplets OTC *decongestant; antihistamine; sleep aid; analgesic; antipyretic* [pseudoephedrine HCl; diphenhydramine HCl; acetaminophen] 30•25•500 mg

Sudal 60/500 sustained-release caplets (discontinued 2006) ℞ *decongestant; expectorant* [pseudoephedrine HCl; guaifenesin] 60•500 mg ☒ Xodol

Sudal-12 chewable tablets, extended-release oral suspension (discontinued 2007) ℞ *decongestant; antihistamine* [pseudoephedrine polistirex; chlorpheniramine polistirex] 30•4 mg; 30•6 mg/5 mL ☒ Xodol

Sudal-12 Tannate chewable tablets ℞ *decongestant; antihistamine* [pseudoephedrine HCl; chlorpheniramine maleate] 30•4 mg

Sudal-DM sustained-release tablets (discontinued 2007) ℞ *antitussive; expectorant* [dextromethorphan hydrobromide; guaifenesin] 30•500 mg

Sudatuss-2 DF oral liquid (discontinued 2007) ℞ *narcotic antitussive; decongestant; expectorant* [codeine phosphate; pseudoephedrine HCl; guaifenesin; alcohol 1.4%] 10•30•100 mg/5 mL

Sudex dual-release caplets ℞ *decongestant; expectorant* [phenylephrine HCl; guaifenesin] 20•600 mg (5•200 mg immediate release; 15•400 mg extended release) ☒ Cedax; ciadox; Cidex

sudexanox INN

sudismase INN

Sudodrin tablets (discontinued 2007) OTC *nasal decongestant* [pseudoephedrine HCl] 30 mg

SudoGest tablets OTC *decongestant* [pseudoephedrine HCl] 60 mg

SudoGest Children's Syrup OTC *antitussive; decongestant* [dextromethorphan hydrobromide; pseudoephedrine HCl] 5•15 mg/5 mL

SudoGest Cold & Allergy tablets OTC *decongestant; antihistamine* [pseudoephedrine HCl; chlorpheniramine maleate] 60•4 mg

SudoGest Sinus tablets (discontinued 2007) OTC *decongestant; analgesic;*

antipyretic [pseudoephedrine HCl; acetaminophen] 30•500 mg

sudorifics *a class of agents that promote profuse perspiration* [also called: diaphoretics]

sudoxicam USAN, INN *anti-inflammatory*

Sufenta IV injection or infusion ℞ *narcotic analgesic for general or epidural anesthesia* [sufentanil citrate] 50 mcg/mL

sufentanil USAN, INN, BAN *narcotic analgesic; investigational (Phase III) for cancer-related pain*

sufentanil citrate USAN *narcotic analgesic for general or epidural anesthesia* 50 mcg/mL

sufosfamide INN

sufotidine USAN, INN, BAN *antagonist to histamine H_2 receptors*

sugammadex *investigational (NDA filed) selective relaxation binding agent (SRBA) to reverse the effects of strong muscle relaxants, used for postanesthesia "stir-up"*

sugar, compressible NF *flavoring agent; tablet excipient*

sugar, confectioner's NF *flavoring agent; tablet excipient*

sugar, invert (50% dextrose & 50% fructose) USP *fluid and nutrient replenisher; caloric replacement*

sugar spheres NF *solid carrier vehicle*

sulamserod HCl USAN *selective 5-HT_4 receptor antagonist; antiarrhythmic; treatment for urge incontinence*

Sulamyd [see: Sodium Sulamyd]

Sular extended-release film-coated tablets ℞ *calcium channel blocker for hypertension* [nisoldipine] 8.5, 17, 25.5, 34 mg ⁂ celery; Xolair

sulazepam USAN, INN *minor tranquilizer* ⁂ zolazepam

sulbactam INN, BAN *β-lactamase inhibitor; penicillin/cephalosporin synergist*

sulbactam benzathine USAN *β-lactamase inhibitor; penicillin/cephalosporin synergist*

sulbactam pivoxil USAN *β-lactamase inhibitor; penicillin/cephalosporin synergist* [also: pivsulbactam]

sulbactam sodium USAN, USP *β-lactamase inhibitor; penicillin/cephalosporin synergist*

sulbenicillin INN

sulbenox USAN, INN *veterinary growth stimulant*

sulbentine INN

sulbutiamine INN [also: bisibutiamine]

sulclamide INN

sulconazole INN, BAN *antifungal* [also: sulconazole nitrate]

sulconazole nitrate USAN, USP *topical antifungal* [also: sulconazole]

sulergine [see: disulergine]

sulesomab USAN *monoclonal antibody; diagnostic aid for infectious lesions* [also: technetium Tc 99m sulesomab]

Sulf-10 eye drops ℞ *antibiotic* [sulfacetamide sodium] 10% ⁂ Slow Fe

sulfabenz USAN, INN *antibacterial; coccidiostat for poultry*

sulfabenzamide USAN, USP, INN *bacteriostatic antibiotic*

sulfabromomethazine sodium NF

sulfacarbamide INN [also: sulphaurea]

sulfacecole INN

sulfacetamide USP, INN *bacteriostatic antibiotic*

sulfacetamide sodium USP *bacteriostatic antibiotic* 10%, 30% eye drops; 10% topical

Sulfacet-R lotion ℞ *antibiotic; keratolytic for acne* [sulfacetamide sodium; sulfur] 10%•5%

sulfachlorpyridazine INN

sulfachrysoidine INN

sulfacitine INN *antibacterial* [also: sulfacytine]

sulfaclomide INN

sulfaclorazole INN

sulfaclozine INN

sulfacombin [see: sulfadiazine]

sulfacytine USAN *broad-spectrum bacteriostatic* [also: sulfacitine]

sulfadiasulfone sodium INN *antibacterial; leprostatic* [also: acetosulfone sodium]

sulfadiazine USP, INN, JAN *broad-spectrum sulfonamide bacteriostatic* [also: sulphadiazine] 500 mg oral

sulfadiazine & pyrimethamine *oral* Toxoplasma gondii *encephalitis treatment (orphan)*

sulfadiazine silver JAN *broad-spectrum bactericidal; adjunct to burn therapy* [also: silver sulfadiazine]

sulfadiazine sodium USP, INN *antibacterial* [also: sulphadiazine sodium]

sulfadicramide INN

sulfadicrolamide [see: sulfadicramide]

sulfadimethoxine NF [also: sulphadimethoxine]

sulfadimidine INN, BAN *antibacterial* [also: sulfamethazine]

sulfadoxine USAN, USP *bacteriostatic; antimalarial adjunct*

sulfaethidole NF, INN [also: sulphaethidole]

sulfafurazole INN *broad-spectrum sulfonamide bacteriostatic* [also: sulfisoxazole; sulphafurazole]

sulfaguanidine NF, INN

sulfaguanole INN

sulfaisodimidine [see: sulfisomidine]

sulfalene USAN, INN *antibacterial* [also: sulfametopyrazine] ⃞ Slo-phyllin

sulfaloxic acid INN [also: sulphaloxic acid]

sulfamates *a class of broad-spectrum anticonvulsants*

sulfamazone INN

sulfamerazine USP, INN *broad-spectrum bacteriostatic*

sulfamerazine sodium NF, INN

sulfameter USAN *antibacterial* [also: sulfametoxydiazine; sulfamethoxydiazine]

sulfamethazine USP *broad-spectrum bacteriostatic* [also: sulfadimidine]

sulfamethizole USP, INN, JAN *broad-spectrum sulfonamide bacteriostatic* [also: sulphamethizole]

sulfamethoxazole (SMX; SMZ) USAN, USP, INN, JAN *broad-spectrum sulfonamide antibiotic* [also: sulphamethoxazole; acetylsulfamethoxazole; sulfamethoxazole sodium]

sulfamethoxazole sodium JAN *broad-spectrum sulfonamide antibiotic* [also: sulfamethoxazole; sulphamethoxazole; acetylsulfamethoxazole]

sulfamethoxydiazine BAN *antibacterial* [also: sulfameter; sulfametoxydiazine]

sulfamethoxypyridazine USP, INN [also: sulphamethoxypyridazine]

sulfamethoxypyridazine acetyl

sulfametin [see: sulfameter]

sulfametomidine INN

sulfametopyrazine BAN *antibacterial* [also: sulfalene]

sulfametoxydiazine INN *antibacterial* [also: sulfameter; sulfamethoxydiazine]

sulfametrole INN, BAN

sulfamidothiodiazol [see: glybuzole]

sulfamonomethoxine USAN, INN, BAN *antibacterial*

sulfamoxole USAN, INN *antibacterial* [also: sulphamoxole]

p-**sulfamoylbenzoic acid** [see: carzenide]

4′-sulfamoylsuccinanilic acid [see: sulfasuccinamide]

Sulfamylon cream ℞ *broad-spectrum bacteriostatic for second- and third-degree burns* [mafenide acetate] 85 mg/g

Sulfamylon powder for topical solution ℞ *broad-spectrum bacteriostatic to prevent meshed autograft loss on second- and third-degree burns (orphan)* [mafenide acetate] 5%

sulfanilamide NF, INN *broad-spectrum sulfonamide antibiotic* 15% topical

sulfanilanilide [see: sulfabenz]

sulfanilate zinc USAN *antibacterial*

N-sulfanilylacetamide [see: sulfacetamide]

N-sulfanilylacetamide monosodium salt monohydrate [see: sulfacetamide sodium]

N-*p*-sulfanilylphenylglycine sodium [see: acediasulfone sodium]

N-sulfanilylstearamide [see: stearylsulfamide]

4′-sulfanilylsuccinanilic acid [see: succisulfone]

sulfanilylurea [see: sulfacarbamide]

sulfanitran USAN, INN, BAN *antibacterial; coccidiostat for poultry*

sulfaperin INN

sulfaphenazole INN [also: sulphaphenazole]

sulfaphtalythiazol [see: phthalysulfa-thiazole]

sulfaproxyline INN [also: sulpha-proxyline]

sulfapyrazole INN, BAN *antibacterial* [also: sulfazamet]

sulfapyridine USP, INN *investigational (orphan) dermatitis herpetiformis suppressant* [also: sulphapyridine]

sulfapyridine sodium NF

sulfaquinoxaline INN, BAN

sulfarsphenamine NF, INN

sulfasalazine USAN, USP, INN *broad-spectrum bacteriostatic; anti-inflammatory for ulcerative colitis, rheumatoid arthritis (RA), and juvenile rheumatoid arthritis (JRA); also used for ankylosing spondylitis, Crohn disease, and regional enteritis* [also: sulphasalazine; salazosulfapyridine] 500 mg oral

sulfasomizole USAN, INN *antibacterial* [also: sulphasomizole]

sulfastearyl [see: stearylsulfamide]

sulfasuccinamide INN

sulfasymazine INN

sulfated polysaccharide peptidoglycan (SPPG) [see: tecogalan sodium]

sulfathiazole USP, INN *bacteriostatic antibiotic* [also: sulphathiazole]

sulfathiazole sodium NF

sulfathiocarbamide [see: sulfathiourea]

sulfathiourea INN

sulfatolamide INN

Sulfatrim oral suspension ℞ *anti-infective; antibacterial* [trimethoprim; sulfamethoxazole] 40•200 mg/5 mL

sulfatroxazole INN

sulfatrozole INN

sulfazamet USAN *antibacterial* [also: sulfapyrazole]

sulfinalol INN *antihypertensive* [also: sulfinalol HCl]

sulfinalol HCl USAN *antihypertensive* [also: sulfinalol]

sulfinpyrazone USP, INN *uricosuric for gout* [also: sulphinpyrazone] 100, 200 mg oral

sulfiram INN [also: monosulfiram]

sulfisomidine [also: sulphasomidine]

sulfisoxazole USP, JAN *broad-spectrum sulfonamide antibiotic* [also: sulfafurazole; sulphafurazole] 500 mg oral

sulfisoxazole acetyl USP *broad-spectrum sulfonamide antibiotic*

sulfisoxazole diolamine USAN, USP *broad-spectrum sulfonamide antibiotic*

Sulfoam shampoo OTC *antiseborrheic; keratolytic; antiseptic* [sulfur] 2%

sulfobenzylpenicillin [see: sulbenicillin]

sulfobromophthalein sodium USP *hepatic function test*

sulfobromphthalein sodium [see: sulfobromophthalein sodium]

sulfocon B USAN *hydrophobic contact lens material*

sulfogaiacol INN *expectorant* [also: potassium guaiacolsulfonate]

Sulfoil topical liquid (discontinued 2004) OTC *soap-free therapeutic skin cleanser* [sulfonated castor oil]

Sulfolax soft gels OTC *laxative; stool softener* [docusate calcium] 240 mg �ê Salflex

sulfomyxin USAN, INN *antibacterial* [also: sulphomyxin sodium]

sulfonal [see: sulfonmethane]

sulfonamides *a class of broad-spectrum bacteriostatic antibiotics effective against both gram-positive and gram-negative organisms*

sulfonated hydrogenated castor oil [see: hydroxystearin sulfate]

sulfonethylmethane NF

sulfonmethane NF

sulfonterol INN *bronchodilator* [also: sulfonterol HCl]

sulfonterol HCl USAN *bronchodilator* [also: sulfonterol]

sulfonylureas *a class of antidiabetic agents that stimulate insulin production in the pancreas*

Sulforcin lotion OTC *antiseptic, antifungal, and keratolytic for acne* [sulfur; resorcinol; alcohol] 5%•2%•11.65%

sulforidazine INN

sulfosalicylic acid

sulfoxone sodium USP *antibacterial; leprostatic* [also: aldesulfone sodium]

Sulfoxyl Regular; Sulfoxyl Strong
lotion ℞ *antiseptic and keratolytic for
acne* [benzoyl peroxide; sulfur] 5%•
2%; 10%•5%

sulfur *element (S)* [see: sulfur, precipitated; sulfur, sublimed]

sulfur, precipitated USP *scabicide; topical antibacterial; topical exfoliant*

sulfur, sublimed USP *scabicide; topical
antibacterial; topical exfoliant*

sulfur dioxide NF *antioxidant*

sulfur hexafluoride (SF₆) USAN *ultrasound imaging agent*

Sulfur Soap bar OTC *antiseptic and keratolytic cleanser for acne* [precipitated
sulfur] 10%

sulfurated lime solution [see: lime,
sulfurated]

sulfurated potash [see: potash, sulfu-
rated]

sulfuric acid NF *acidifying agent*

**sulfuric acid, aluminum ammonium
salt, dodecahydrate** [see: alum,
ammonium]

**sulfuric acid, aluminum potassium
salt, dodecahydrate** [see: alum,
potassium]

**sulfuric acid, aluminum salt,
hydrate** [see: aluminum sulfate]

sulfuric acid, barium salt [see: barium sulfate]

sulfuric acid, calcium salt [see: calcium sulfate]

**sulfuric acid, copper salt pentahy-
drate** [see: cupric sulfate]

**sulfuric acid, disodium salt decahy-
drate** [see: sodium sulfate]

sulfuric acid, magnesium salt [see:
magnesium sulfate]

sulfuric acid, manganese salt [see:
manganese sulfate]

sulfuric acid, zinc salt hydrate [see:
zinc sulfate]

sulfurous acid, monosodium salt
[see: sodium bisulfite]

sulglicotide INN [also: sulglycotide]

sulglycotide BAN [also: sulglicotide]

sulicrinat INN

sulindac USAN, USP, INN, BAN *nonsteroidal anti-inflammatory drug*

*(NSAID) for osteoarthritis, rheumatoid
arthritis, ankylosing spondylitis, acute
bursitis/tendinitis, and other inflammatory conditions* 150, 200 mg oral

sulisatin INN ☒ Celestone

sulisobenzone USAN, INN *ultraviolet
screen*

sulmarin USAN, INN *hemostatic*

Sulmasque mask OTC *antiseptic and
keratolytic for acne* [sulfur] 6.4% ☒
psyllium husk

sulmazole INN

sulmepride INN

sulnidazole USAN, INN *antiprotozoal
(Trichomonas)*

sulocarbilate INN

suloctidil USAN, INN, BAN *peripheral
vasodilator*

sulodexide INN *investigational (Phase
III) glycosaminoglycan for diabetic
nephropathy*

sulofenur USAN, INN *antineoplastic*

sulopenem USAN, INN *antibacterial*

sulosemide INN

sulotroban USAN, INN, BAN *treatment
for glomerulonephritis* ☒ Sal-Tropine

suloxifen INN *bronchodilator* [also:
suloxifen oxalate]

suloxifen oxalate USAN *bronchodilator*
[also: suloxifen]

sulphabutin [see: busulfan]

sulphadiazine BAN *broad-spectrum
bacteriostatic* [also: sulfadiazine]

sulphadiazine sodium BAN *antibacterial* [also: sulfadiazine sodium]

sulphadimethoxine BAN [also: sulfa-
dimethoxine]

sulphaethidole BAN [also: sulfaethidole]

sulphafurazole BAN *broad-spectrum
sulfonamide bacteriostatic* [also: sulfisoxazole; sulfafurazole]

sulphaloxic acid BAN [also: sulfaloxic
acid]

sulphamethizole BAN *broad-spectrum
sulfonamide bacteriostatic* [also: sulfa-
methizole]

sulphamethoxazole BAN *broad-spectrum sulfonamide bacteriostatic* [also:
sulfamethoxazole; acetylsulfamethoxazole; sulfamethoxazole sodium]

sulphamethoxypyridazine BAN [also: sulfamethoxypyridazine]

sulphamoxole BAN *antibacterial* [also: sulfamoxole]

sulphan blue BAN *lymphangiography aid* [also: isosulfan blue]

sulphaphenazole BAN [also: sulfaphenazole]

sulphaproxyline BAN [also: sulfaproxyline]

sulphapyridine BAN *dermatitis herpetiformis suppressant* [also: sulfapyridine]

sulphasalazine BAN *broad-spectrum bacteriostatic; antirheumatic; antiinflammatory for ulcerative colitis* [also: sulfasalazine; salazosulfapyridine]

sulphasomidine BAN [also: sulfisomidine]

sulphasomizole BAN *antibacterial* [also: sulfasomizole]

sulphathiazole BAN *antibacterial* [also: sulfathiazole]

sulphaurea BAN [also: sulfacarbamide] ⑨ silver

sulphinpyrazone BAN *uricosuric for gout* [also: sulfinpyrazone]

sulphocarbolate sodium [see: phenolsulphonate sodium]

Sulpho-Lac cream, soap OTC *antiseptic and keratolytic for acne* [sulfur] 5% ⑨ Salofalk

Sulpho-Lac Acne Medication cream OTC *antiseptic and keratolytic for acne* [sulfur; zinc sulfate] 5%•27%

sulphomyxin sodium BAN *antibacterial* [also: sulfomyxin]

sulphonal [see: sulfonmethane]

sulpiride USAN, INN *antidepressant*

sulprosal INN

sulprostone USAN, INN *prostaglandin*

sultamicillin USAN, INN, BAN *antibacterial*

sulthiame USAN *anticonvulsant* [also: sultiame]

sultiame INN *anticonvulsant* [also: sulthiame]

sultopride INN

sultosilic acid INN

sultroponium INN

sulukast USAN, INN *antiasthmatic; leukotriene antagonist*

sulverapride INN

suma (Pfaffia paniculata) bark and root *medicinal herb for circulatory disorders, chronic disease, fatigue, hormone regulation, immune system stimulation, lowering cholesterol levels, and stress; also used as a tonic*

Sumacal powder OTC *carbohydrate caloric supplement* [glucose polymers]

sumacetamol INN, BAN

sumach (Rhus glabra) bark, leaves, and berries *medicinal herb used as an antiseptic, astringent, diaphoretic, diuretic, emmenagogue, febrifuge, and refrigerant* ⑨ Sea-Omega 30; Simuc; Zomig

sumarotene USAN, INN *keratolytic*

sumatriptan INN, BAN *vascular serotonin 5-HT$_1$ receptor agonist for the acute treatment of migraine headaches* [also: sumatriptan succinate]

sumatriptan succinate USAN *vascular serotonin 5-HT$_1$ receptor agonist for the acute treatment of migraine and cluster headaches* (base=71.4%) [also: sumatriptan]

sumetizide INN

summer savory (Calamintha hortensis; Satureja hortensis) leaves and stems *medicinal herb for diarrhea, nausea, promoting expectoration, relieving gas and flatulence, and stimulation of menstruation; also used as an aphrodisiac*

Summer's Eve Anti-Itch vaginal gel OTC *anesthetic* [pramoxine HCl] 1%

Summer's Eve Disposable Douche vaginal solution OTC *antifungal; cleanser and deodorizer; acidity modifier* [sodium benzoate; citric acid]

Summer's Eve Disposable Douche; Summer's Eve Disposable Douche Extra Cleansing vaginal solution OTC *acidity modifier; cleanser and deodorizer* [vinegar (acetic acid)]

Summer's Eve Feminine Bath topical liquid OTC *external perivaginal cleanser*

Summer's Eve Feminine Powder OTC *vaginal moisture absorbent; antiseptic* [cornstarch; benzethonium chloride]

Summer's Eve Feminine Wash topical liquid, wipes OTC *external perivaginal cleanser*

Summer's Eve Medicated Disposable Douche vaginal solution OTC *antiseptic/germicidal cleanser and deodorizer* [povidone-iodine] 0.3%

Summer's Eve Post-Menstrual Disposable Douche vaginal solution OTC *cleanser and deodorizer; acidity modifier* [monosodium phosphate; disodium phosphate]

Summit Extra Strength coated caplets OTC *analgesic; antipyretic; anti-inflammatory* [acetaminophen; aspirin; caffeine] 250•250•65 mg

Sumycin syrup ℞ *broad-spectrum antibiotic* [tetracycline HCl] 125 mg/5 mL

Sumycin '250'; Sumycin '500' capsules, tablets ℞ *broad-spectrum antibiotic* [tetracycline HCl] 250 mg; 500 mg

sun rose *medicinal herb* [see: rock rose]

sunagrel INN

suncillin INN *antibacterial* [also: suncillin sodium]

suncillin sodium USAN *antibacterial* [also: suncillin]

sunepitron HCl USAN *anxiolytic; antidepressant*

sunitinib malate *receptor tyrosine kinase (RTK) inhibitor antineoplastic for gastrointestinal stromal tumor (GIST) and metastatic renal cell carcinoma*

SunKist Multivitamins Complete, Children's chewable tablets OTC *vitamin/mineral/iron supplement* [multiple vitamins & minerals; iron; folic acid; biotin] ± •18 mg•400 mcg•40 mcg

SunKist Multivitamins + Extra C chewable tablets OTC *vitamin supplement* [multiple vitamins; folic acid] ± •0.3 mg

SunKist Multivitamins + Iron, Children's chewable tablets (discontinued 2004) OTC *vitamin/iron supplement* [multiple vitamins; iron; folic acid] ± •15•0.3 mg

SunKist Vitamin C chewable tablets OTC *vitamin C supplement* [ascorbic acid and sodium ascorbate] 60, 250, 500 mg

Supartz intra-articular injection in prefilled syringes ℞ *viscoelastic lubricant and "shock absorber" for osteoarthritis and TMJ syndrome* [hyaluronate sodium] 25 mg/2.5 mL

Super 2 Daily softgels OTC *vitamin/mineral supplement* [multiple vitamins & minerals; fish oil concentrate; lecithin; phosphatidyl choline; bioflavonoids; lutein] ± •385•30•25•12.5•0.025 mg

Super CalciCaps tablets OTC *dietary supplement* [dibasic calcium phosphate; calcium gluconate; calcium carbonate; vitamin D] 400 mg (Ca)•42 mg (P)•133 IU

Super CalciCaps M-Z tablets OTC *dietary supplement* [vitamins A and D; multiple minerals] 1667 mg•133 IU• ±

Super Calcium '1200' softgels OTC *dietary supplement* [calcium; vitamin D] 600 mg•200 IU

Super Carnosine capsules OTC *anti-aging supplement; glycation inhibitor* [carnosine] 500 mg

Super D Perles (capsules) OTC *vitamin supplement* [vitamins A and D] 10 000•400 IU

Super Flavons; Super Flavons-300 tablets (discontinued 2007) OTC *dietary supplement* [mixed bioflavonoids] 300 mg

Super Hi Potency tablets OTC *vitamin/mineral supplement* [multiple vitamins & minerals; folic acid; biotin] ± •0.4 mg•0.075 mg

Super Ivy-Dry lotion OTC *poison ivy treatment* [zinc acetate; benzyl alcohol; isopropanol] 2%•10%•35%

Super MiraForte with Chrysin capsules OTC *natural supplement to increase free testosterone levels in men* [chrysin; muira puama; maca; nettle;

ginger; piperine; zinc] 375•212.5•
80•70.5•12.5•3.75•3.75 mg

Super Quints-50 tablets OTC *vitamin
supplement* [multiple B vitamins;
folic acid; biotin] ±•400•50 mcg

Superdophilus powder OTC *natural
intestinal bacteria; probiotic; dietary
supplement; fever blister treatment; not
generally regarded as safe and effective
as an antidiarrheal* [Lactobacillus acido-
philus] 2 billion CFU/g

SuperEPA 1200; SuperEPA 2000
softgels OTC *dietary supplement*
[omega-3 fatty acids] 1200 mg; 1000
mg ⓡ X-Prep

superoxide dismutase (SOD) [see:
orgotein]

Superplex-T tablets OTC *vitamin supplement* [multiple B vitamins; vitamin C] ±•500 mg

Supervent *investigational (orphan) surfactant for cystic fibrosis* [tyloxapol]

supidimide INN

Suplena ready-to-use oral liquid OTC
*enteral nutritional therapy for renal fail-
ure* [multiple essential amino acids]

Supprelin subcu injection (discontinued 2004) ℞ *LHRH agonist for treatment of central precocious puberty
(orphan)* [histrelin acetate] 120, 300,
600 mcg/0.6 mL ⓡ spirilene

Supprelin-LA once-yearly subcu
implant ℞ *LHRH agonist for central
precocious puberty (orphan)* [histrelin
acetate] 50 mg

Supprette (trademarked dosage form)
suppository ⓡ soapwort

Suprane liquid for vaporization ℞
inhalation general anesthetic [desflu-
rane] ⓡ Syprine

Suprax film-coated tablets ℞ *third-generation cephalosporin antibiotic*
[cefixime] 400 mg ⓡ Zyprexa

Suprax powder for oral suspension ℞
third-generation cephalosporin antibiotic
[cefixime] 100, 200 mg/5 mL ⓡ
Zyprexa

suproclone USAN, INN *sedative*

suprofen USAN, INN, BAN *ocular nonsteroidal anti-inflammatory drug
(NSAID); antimiotic*

Supule (trademarked dosage form)
suppository

suramin hexasodium USAN *investigational (NDA filed, orphan) growth factor antagonist for prostate cancer*

suramin sodium USP, BAN *antiparasitic
for African trypanosomiasis and onchocerciasis*

Surbex Filmtabs (film-coated tablets)
OTC *vitamin supplement* [multiple B
vitamins] ⓡ Cerebyx

Surbex 750 with Iron Filmtabs (film-
coated tablets) OTC *vitamin/iron supplement* [multiple B vitamins; vitamins C and E; ferrous sulfate, dried;
folic acid] ±•750 mg•30 IU•27
mg•0.4 mg

Surbex 750 with Zinc Filmtabs
(film-coated tablets) OTC *vitamin/zinc
supplement* [multiple vitamins; zinc
sulfate; folic acid] ±•22.5•0.4 mg

Surbex-T; Surbex with C Filmtabs
(film-coated tablets) OTC *vitamin
supplement* [multiple B vitamins;
vitamin C] ±•500 mg; ±•250 mg

Surbu-Gen-T film-coated tablets OTC
vitamin supplement [multiple B vitamins; vitamin C] ±•500 mg

Sure Cell Chlamydia Test reagent
kit for professional use ℞ *in vitro
diagnostic aid for* Chlamydia trachomatis [monoclonal antibody-based
enzyme-linked immunosorbent assay]

Sure Cell Herpes (HSV) Test reagent
kit for professional use ℞ *in vitro
diagnostic aid for herpes simplex virus
in genital, rectal, oral, or dermal swabs*
[monoclonal antibody-based enzyme-
linked immunosorbent assay (ELISA)]

Sure Cell Pregnancy test kit for professional use ℞ *in vitro diagnostic aid;
urine pregnancy test* [monoclonal/
polyclonal antibody ELISA test]

Sure Cell Streptococci test kit for
professional use ℞ *in vitro diagnostic
aid for Group A streptococcal antigens*

in blood and throat swabs [enzyme-linked immunosorbent assay (ELISA)]

SureLac chewable tablets OTC *digestive aid for lactose intolerance* [lactase enzyme] 3000 U

surface active extract of saline lavage of bovine lungs [see: beractant]

surfactant, human amniotic fluid derived *investigational (orphan) agent for the prevention and treatment of respiratory distress syndrome (RDS) in premature infants*

surfactant laxatives *a subclass of laxatives that work by increasing the amount of fat and water in the stool to ease its movement through the intestines* [more commonly called stool softeners]

surfactant TA [see: beractant]

surfactant TA, modified bovine lung surfactant extract [see: beractant]

Surfak Liquigels (capsules) OTC *laxative; stool softener* [docusate calcium] 240 mg

Surfaxin *investigational (NDA filed, orphan) KL4 pulmonary surfactant for acute respiratory distress syndrome (ARDS) and meconium aspiration syndrome (MAS)* [lucinactant]

surfilcon A USAN *hydrophilic contact lens material*

Surfol Post-Immersion Bath Oil OTC *bath emollient*

surfomer USAN, INN *hypolipidemic*

Surgel vaginal gel OTC *moisturizer/lubricant* [propylene glycol; glycerin] ⊘ PsoriGel; Seroquel

surgibone USAN *internal bone splint*

surgical catgut [see: suture, absorbable surgical]

surgical gut [see: suture, absorbable surgical]

Surgicel strips, Nu-knit pads ℞ *topical hemostat for surgery* [cellulose, oxidized]

suricainide INN *antiarrhythmic* [also: suricainide maleate]

suricainide maleate USAN, INN *antiarrhythmic* [also: suricainide]

suriclone INN, BAN

Surinam wood *medicinal herb* [see: quassia]

suritozole USAN, INN *antidepressant*

Surmontil capsules ℞ *tricyclic antidepressant* [trimipramine maleate] 25, 50, 100 mg

suronacrine INN *cholinesterase inhibitor* [also: suronacrine maleate]

suronacrine maleate USAN *cholinesterase inhibitor* [also: suronacrine]

Surpass chewing gum OTC *antacid; calcium supplement* [calcium carbonate] 300, 450 mg ⊘ Ser-Ap-Es

Survanta suspension for intratracheal instillation ℞ *pulmonary surfactant for neonatal respiratory distress syndrome or respiratory failure (orphan)* [beractant] 25 mg/mL ⊘ Serevent

Susano elixir (discontinued 2008) ℞ *GI/GU anticholinergic/antispasmodic; sedative* [atropine sulfate; scopolamine hydrobromide; hyoscyamine hydrobromide; phenobarbital] 0.0194•0.0065•0.1037•16.2 mg/5 mL ⊘ Saizen; Zosyn

Sustacal powder OTC *enteral nutritional therapy* [milk-based formula]

Sustacal pudding OTC *enteral nutritional therapy* [milk-based formula]

Sustacal ready-to-use oral liquid OTC *enteral nutritional therapy* [lactose-free formula]

Sustacal Basic; Sustacal Plus ready-to-use oral liquid OTC *enteral nutritional therapy* [lactose-free formula]

Sustagen powder OTC *enteral nutritional therapy* [milk-based formula] ⊘ Cystagon

Sustain tablets ℞ *electrolyte replacement; dehydration preventative* [sodium chloride; potassium chloride; calcium carbonate] 220•15•18 mg ⊘ cystine; Systane

Sustaire timed-release tablets (discontinued 2004) ℞ *antiasthmatic; bronchodilator* [theophylline] 100, 300 mg ⊘ Zestra

Sustiva capsules, film-coated caplets ℞ *antiviral non-nucleoside reverse transcriptase inhibitor (NNRTI) for*

HIV infection [efavirenz] 50, 200 mg; 600 mg

Sutent capsules ℞ *receptor tyrosine kinase (RTK) inhibitor antineoplastic for gastrointestinal stromal tumor (GIST) and metastatic renal cell carcinoma; investigational (Phase III) for lung, breast, and colorectal cancers* [sunitinib malate] 12.5, 25, 50 mg

sutilains USAN, USP, INN, BAN *topical proteolytic enzymes for necrotic tissue debridement*

sutoprofen [see: suprofen]

suture, absorbable surgical USP *surgical aid*

suture, nonabsorbable surgical USP *surgical aid*

Su-Tuss DM oral liquid ℞ *antitussive; expectorant* [dextromethorphan hydrobromide; guaifenesin; alcohol 5%] 20•200 mg/5 mL

Su-Tuss HD elixir ℞ *narcotic antitussive; decongestant; expectorant* [hydrocodone bitartrate; pseudoephedrine HCl; guaifenesin] 2.5•30•100 mg/5 mL

suxamethone [see: succinylcholine chloride]

suxamethonium chloride INN, BAN *neuromuscular blocking agent* [also: succinylcholine chloride]

suxemerid INN *antitussive* [also: suxemerid sulfate]

suxemerid sulfate USAN *antitussive* [also: suxemerid]

suxethonium chloride INN

suxibuzone INN

swallow wort, orange *medicinal herb* [see: pleurisy root]

swallow wort, silky *medicinal herb* [see: milkweed]

swamp cabbage *medicinal herb* [see: skunk cabbage]

swamp laurel; swamp sassafras *medicinal herb* [see: magnolia]

sweet, mountain *medicinal herb* [see: New Jersey tea]

sweet, winter *medicinal herb* [see: marjoram]

sweet anise; sweet chervil *medicinal herb* [see: sweet cicely]

sweet balm *medicinal herb* [see: lemon balm]

sweet basil *medicinal herb* [see: basil]

sweet bay *medicinal herb* [see: laurel]

sweet birch *medicinal herb* [see: birch]

sweet birch oil [see: methyl salicylate]

sweet cicely (Osmorhiza longistylis) root *medicinal herb used as a carminative, expectorant, and stomachic*

sweet clover *medicinal herb* [see: melilot]

sweet dock *medicinal herb* [see: bistort]

sweet elder *medicinal herb* [see: elderberry]

sweet elm *medicinal herb* [see: slippery elm]

sweet fennel *medicinal herb* [see: fennel]

sweet flag *medicinal herb* [see: calamus]

sweet grass *medicinal herb* [see: calamus]

sweet leaf *medicinal herb* [see: stevia]

sweet magnolia *medicinal herb* [see: magnolia]

sweet marjoram *medicinal herb* [see: marjoram]

sweet myrtle *medicinal herb* [see: calamus]

sweet orange peel tincture [see: orange peel tincture, sweet]

sweet potato vine, wild *medicinal herb* [see: wild jalap]

sweet root *medicinal herb* [see: calamus]

sweet rush *medicinal herb* [see: calamus]

sweet sedge *medicinal herb* [see: calamus]

sweet spirit of nitre [see: ethyl nitrite]

sweet vernal grass (Anthoxanthum odoratum) *natural flavoring banned by the FDA as it is not generally regarded as safe and effective*

sweet violet *medicinal herb* [see: violet]

sweet water lily; sweet-scented water lily *medicinal herb* [see: white pond lily]

sweet weed *medicinal herb* [see: marsh mallow]

sweet woodruff (Asperula odorata; Galium odoratum) plant *medicinal herb for diuresis, inducing expectoration, liver disorders, promoting wound* *healing, relieving gastrointestinal spasms, and sedation*

sweet-scented pond lily; sweet-scented water lily *medicinal herb* [see: white pond lily]

sweetwood *medicinal herb* [see: licorice]

Swim-Ear ear drops OTC *antiseptic* [isopropyl alcohol] 95% ℞ Zemaira; Zymar

swine snout *medicinal herb* [see: dandelion]

Syllact powder OTC *bulk laxative* [psyllium husks] 3.3 g/tsp.

Symax Duotab dual-release caplets (33% immediate release, 67% extended-release) ℞ *GI/GU antispasmodic; antiparkinsonian; anticholinergic "drying agent" for allergic rhinitis and hyperhidrosis* [hyoscyamine sulfate] 0.375 mg

Symax FasTab (orally disintegrating tablets) ℞ *GI/GU antispasmodic; antiparkinsonian; anticholinergic "drying agent" for allergic rhinitis and hyperhidrosis* [hyoscyamine sulfate] 0.125 mg

Symax-SL sublingual tablets ℞ *GI/GU antispasmodic; antiparkinsonian; anticholinergic "drying agent" for allergic rhinitis and hyperhidrosis* [hyoscyamine sulfate] 0.125 mg

Symax-SR sustained-release caplets ℞ *GI/GU antispasmodic; antiparkinsonian; anticholinergic "drying agent" for allergic rhinitis and hyperhidrosis* [hyoscyamine sulfate] 0.375 mg

Symbicort inhalation aerosol in a metered-dose inhaler ℞ *corticosteroidal anti-inflammatory and bronchodilator combination for chronic asthma* [budesonide; formoterol fumarate dihydrate] 80•4.5, 160•4.5 mcg/dose

Symbyax capsules ℞ *antipsychotic plus selective serotonin reuptake inhibitor (SSRI) for depressive episodes of a bipolar disorder* [olanzapine; fluoxetine HCl] 3•25, 6•25, 6•50, 12•25, 12•50 mg

symclosene USAN, INN *topical anti-infective*

symetine INN *antiamebic* [also: symetine HCl]

symetine HCl USAN *antiamebic* [also: symetine]

Symlin subcu injection ℞ *antidiabetic for types 1 and 2 diabetes; synthetic amylin analogue that slows gastric emptying and decreases hepatic glucose production* [pramlintide acetate] 0.6, 1 mg/mL

SymlinPen 60; SymlinPen 120 self-injectors prefilled with **Symlin** ℞ *antidiabetic for types 1 and 2 diabetes; synthetic amylin analogue that slows gastric emptying and decreases hepatic glucose production* [pramlintide acetate] 15, 30, 45, 60 mcg/dose; 60, 120 mcg/dose

Symmetrel tablets, syrup ℞ *antiviral for influenza A infections; dopaminergic antiparkinson agent* [amantadine HCl] 100 mg; 50 mg/5 mL ℞ cimaterol; xamoterol

sympatholytics *a class of cardiovascular drugs that block the passage of impulses through the sympathetic nervous system* [also called: antiadrenergics]

sympathomimetics *a class of bronchodilators that relax the bronchial muscles, reducing bronchospasm; a class of cardiac agents that increase myocardial contractility, causing a vasopressor effect to counteract shock (inadequate tissue perfusion)* [also called: adrenergic agonists]

Symphytum officinale; S. tuberosum medicinal herb [see: comfrey]

Symplocarpus foetidus medicinal herb [see: skunk cabbage]

Synacort cream ℞ *corticosteroidal anti-inflammatory* [hydrocortisone] 1%, 2.5%

Synagis IM injection, powder for IM injection ℞ *monoclonal antibody for prophylaxis of respiratory syncytial virus (RSV) in infants* [palivizumab] 100 mg/mL; 50, 100 mg/vial ℞ Sancuso; Sina-12X; Xanax

Synalar cream, ointment, topical solution ℞ *corticosteroidal anti-inflamma-*

tory [fluocinolone acetonide] 0.01, 0.25%; 0.025%; 0.01%

Synalar-HP cream (discontinued 2006) ℞ *corticosteroidal anti-inflammatory* [fluocinolone acetonide] 0.2%

Synalgos-DC capsules ℞ *narcotic analgesic; antipyretic* [dihydrocodeine bitartrate; aspirin; caffeine] 16•356.4•30 mg

Synarel nasal spray ℞ *gonadotropin-releasing hormone for central precocious puberty (orphan) and endometriosis* [nafarelin acetate] 2 mg/mL (200 mcg/spray)

SynBiotics-3 capsules OTC *natural intestinal bacteria; probiotic; dietary supplement* [Bifidobacterium longum; Lactobacillus rhamnosus A; L. plantarum; Saccharomyces boulardii] 4.5 billion CFU

Synemol cream ℞ *corticosteroidal anti-inflammatory* [fluocinolone acetonide] 0.025%

Synera transdermal patch ℞ *local anesthetic* [lidocaine; tetracaine] 70•70 mg

Synercid powder for IV infusion ℞ *semi-synthetic streptogramin antibiotic for life-threatening infections* [quinupristin; dalfopristin] 150•350 mg/10 mL

synestrin [see: diethylstilbestrol]

synnematin B [see: adicillin]

Synophylate-GG syrup (discontinued 2007) ℞ *antiasthmatic; bronchodilator; expectorant* [theophylline; guaifenesin; alcohol 10%] 150•100 mg/15 mL

Synsorb Cd *investigational (Phase III) antidiarrheal for AIDS-related diarrhea due to* Clostridium difficile *infection*

Synsorb Pk *investigational (Phase III, orphan)* E. coli *neutralizer for traveler's diarrhea and hemolytic uremic syndrome (HUS)* [8-methoxycarbonyloctyl oligosaccharides]

Syntest D.S.; Syntest H.S. film-coated caplets (discontinued 2008) ℞ *estrogen/androgen hormone replacement for postmenopausal symptoms*

[esterified estrogens; methyltestosterone] 1.25•2.5 mg; 0.625•1.25 mg

synthestrin [see: diethylstilbestrol]

synthetic conjugated estrogens [see: estrogens, synthetic conjugated (A and B)]

synthetic lung surfactant [see: colfosceril palmitate]

synthetic monosaccharides *a class of investigational synthetic carbohydrates with immunomodulatory and anti-inflammatory effects being evaluated for the treatment of rheumatic arthritis*

synthetic paraffin [see: paraffin, synthetic]

synthetic spermaceti [now: cetyl esters wax]

synthoestrin [see: diethylstilbestrol]

Synthroid tablets, powder for injection ℞ *synthetic thyroid hormone (T_4 fraction only)* [levothyroxine sodium] 25, 50, 75, 88, 100, 112, 125, 137, 150, 175, 200, 300 mcg; 200, 500 mcg

synvinolin [now: simvastatin]

Synvisc intra-articular injection in prefilled syringes ℞ *viscoelastic lubricant and "shock absorber" for osteoarthritis and TMJ syndrome* [hylan G-F 20] 16 mg/2 mL syringe

Syprine capsules ℞ *copper chelating agent for Wilson disease (orphan)* [trientine HCl] 250 mg ② Suprane

syrosingopine NF, INN, BAN

syrup NF *flavoring agent*

syrupus cerasi [see: cherry juice]

Syrvite oral liquid OTC *vitamin supplement* [multiple vitamins] ② Cerovite

Systane eye drops OTC *moisturizer/lubricant* [polyethylene glycol 400; polypropylene glycol] 0.4%•0.3% ② cystine; Sustain

Syzygium aromaticum medicinal herb [see: cloves]

Syzygium claviflorum medicinal herb for diarrhea and bleeding disorders

(S)-zopiclone [see: esopiclone]

T-2 protocol (dactinomycin, doxorubicin, vincristine, cyclophosphamide, radiation) *chemotherapy protocol*

T₃ (liothyronine sodium) [q.v.]

T₄ (levothyroxine sodium) [q.v.]

T4 endonuclease V (T4N5), liposome encapsulated *investigational (orphan) for prevent cutaneous neoplasms in xeroderma pigmentosum*

T-10 protocol (methotrexate, doxorubicin, cisplatin, bleomycin, cyclophosphamide, dactinomycin) *chemotherapy protocol*

T-67 *investigational (Phase III) tubulin antagonist for liver cancer*

T-1249 *investigational (Phase I/II) fusion inhibitor for HIV infection*

Tab-A-Vite tablets OTC *vitamin supplement* [multiple vitamins; folic acid] ≜•0.4 mg

Tab-A-Vite + Iron tablets OTC *vitamin/iron supplement* [multiple vitamins; iron; folic acid] ≜•18•0.4 mg

Tabebuia avellanedae; T. impetiginosa *medicinal herb* [see: pau d'arco]

Tabernanthe iboga *street drug* [see: iboga]

tabilautide INN

Tabloid (trademarked dosage form) *tablet with raised lettering*

Tabloid tablets ℞ *antimetabolite antineoplastic for acute nonlymphocytic leukemias (ANLL); also used for psoriasis, ulcerative colitis, and Crohn disease* [thioguanine] 40 mg

Tabules (dosage form) *tablets*

Tac-3 IM, intra-articular, intrabursal, intradermal injection (discontinued 2008) ℞ *corticosteroid; anti-inflammatory* [triamcinolone acetonide] 3 mg/mL

Tac-40 suspension for injection (discontinued 2008) ℞ *corticosteroid; anti-inflammatory* [triamcinolone acetonide] 40 mg/mL

taclamine INN *minor tranquilizer* [also: taclamine HCl]

taclamine HCl USAN *minor tranquilizer* [also: taclamine]

Taclonex ointment ℞ *antipsoriatic; steroidal anti-inflammatory for plaque psoriasis* [calcipotriene; betamethasone dipropionate] 0.005%•0.064%

Taclonex Scalp topical suspension ℞ *antipsoriatic; steroidal anti-inflammatory for plaque psoriasis* [calcipotriene; betamethasone dipropionate] 0.005%•0.064%

tacmahac *medicinal herb* [see: balm of Gilead]

tacrine INN, BAN *reversible cholinesterase inhibitor; cognition adjuvant for Alzheimer dementia* [also: tacrine HCl]

tacrine HCl USAN *reversible cholinesterase inhibitor; cognition adjuvant for Alzheimer dementia* [also: tacrine]

tacrolimus USAN, INN *topical treatment for moderate to severe atopic dermatitis; systemic immunosuppressant for liver, kidney, and heart transplants; also used for rheumatoid arthritis and Crohn disease; investigational (orphan) for graft-versus-host disease*

TAD (thioguanine, ara-C, daunorubicin) *chemotherapy protocol for acute myelocytic leukemia (AML)* [also: DaT; DCT]

tadalafil *phosphodiesterase type 5 (PDE5) inhibitor; selective vasodilator for erectile dysfunction (ED); investigational (Phase III) for pulmonary arterial hypertension; investigational (Phase II) for benign prostatic hyperplasia*

taeniacides *a class of agents that destroy tapeworms* [see also: anthelmintics; vermicides; vermifuges]

Tagamet film-coated tablets ℞ *histamine H₂ antagonist for gastric and duodenal ulcers and gastric hypersecretory conditions* [cimetidine] 300, 400, 800 mg

Tagamet oral liquid, IV or IM injection, premixed injection (discontinued 2005) ℞ *histamine H₂ antagonist for gastric and duodenal ulcers and gastric hypersecretory conditions* [cimetidine HCl] 300 mg/5 mL; 300 mg/2 mL; 300 mg/vial

Tagamet HB film-coated tablets, oral suspension (discontinued 2005) OTC *histamine H$_2$ antagonist for episodic heartburn and acid indigestion* [cimetidine] 100 mg; 200 mg

Tagamet HB 200 film-coated tablets OTC *histamine H$_2$ antagonist for episodic heartburn and acid indigestion* [cimetidine] 200 mg

taglutimide INN

taheebo *medicinal herb* [see: pau d'arco]

TA-HPV *investigational (orphan) vaccine for cervical cancer* [human papillomavirus (HPV) recombinant vaccine]

tail, colt's; cow's tail; horse tail; mare's tail *medicinal herb* [see: fleabane; horseweed]

tail, lion's *medicinal herb* [see: motherwort]

tailed cubebs; tailed pepper *medicinal herb* [see: cubeb]

TAK-603 *investigational (orphan) for Crohn disease*

Talacen caplets ℞ *narcotic agonist-antagonist analgesic; antipyretic* [pentazocine HCl; acetaminophen] 25•650 mg ☒ tylosin

talampicillin INN *antibacterial* [also: talampicillin HCl]

talampicillin HCl USAN *antibacterial* [also: talampicillin]

talastine INN

talbutal USP, INN *barbiturate sedative; hypnotic*

talc USP, JAN *dusting powder; tablet and capsule lubricant*

talc, sterile aerosol *treatment for malignant pleural effusion and pneumothorax via intrapleural thoracoscopy administration (orphan)*

taleranol USAN, INN *gonadotropin enzyme inhibitor*

talinolol INN

talipexole INN

talisomycin USAN, INN *antineoplastic*

tall speedwell *medicinal herb* [see: Culver root]

tall veronica *medicinal herb* [see: Culver root]

tallimustine INN *antineoplastic*

tallow shrub *medicinal herb* [see: bayberry]

tallysomycin A [now: talisomycin]

talmetacin USAN, INN *analgesic; anti-inflammatory; antipyretic*

talmetoprim INN

talnetant HCl USAN *NK$_3$ receptor antagonist for urinary frequency, urgency, and incontinence*

talniflumate USAN, INN *anti-inflammatory; analgesic*

talopram INN *catecholamine potentiator* [also: talopram HCl]

talopram HCl USAN *catecholamine potentiator* [also: talopram]

talosalate USAN, INN *analgesic; anti-inflammatory*

Taloxa Ⓔᵁᴿ (foreign name for the U.S. product **Felbatol**) ☒ Tylox

taloximine INN, BAN

talsaclidine INN

talsaclidine fumarate USAN *muscarinic M$_1$ agonist for Alzheimer disease*

talsupram INN

taltibride [see: metibride]

taltrimide INN

taludipine [see: teludipine]

taludipine HCl [see: teludipine HCl]

Talwin IV, IM, or subcu injection, Carpuject (prefilled syringes) ℞ *narcotic agonist-antagonist analgesic for moderate to severe pain; adjunct to surgical anesthesia; also abused as a street drug* [pentazocine lactate] 30 mg/mL; 60 mg

Talwin Compound caplets ℞ *narcotic agonist-antagonist analgesic; antipyretic; also abused as a street drug* [pentazocine HCl; aspirin] 12.5•325 mg

Talwin NX tablets ℞ *narcotic agonist-antagonist analgesic; also abused as a street drug* [pentazocine HCl; naloxone HCl] 50•0.5 mg

tamarind (*Tamarindus indica*) fruit and leaves *medicinal herb used as an anthelmintic, laxative, and refrigerant*

tamatinib fosdium *investigational (Phase III) treatment for autoimmune disorders, including rheumatoid arthritis (RA) and idiopathic thrombocytopenic purpura (ITP)*

Tambocor tablets ℞ *antiarrhythmic* [flecainide acetate] 50, 100, 150 mg

tameridone USAN, INN, BAN *veterinary sedative*

tameticillin INN

tametraline INN *antidepressant* [also: tametraline HCl]

tametraline HCl USAN *antidepressant* [also: tametraline]

Tamiflu capsules, powder for oral suspension ℞ *antiviral for the prophylaxis and treatment of influenza A and B infections* [oseltamivir phosphate] 30, 45, 75 mg; 12 mg/mL

tamitinol INN

tamoxifen INN, BAN *antiestrogen antineoplastic for breast cancer* [also: tamoxifen citrate]

tamoxifen citrate USAN, USP, JAN *antiestrogen antineoplastic for the treatment of breast cancer and the reduction of breast cancer incidence in high-risk women* (base=65.8%) [also: tamoxifen] 10, 20 mg oral

tamoxifen & DTIC *chemotherapy protocol for malignant melanoma*

tamoxifen & epirubicin *chemotherapy protocol for breast cancer*

tampramine INN *antidepressant* [also: tampramine fumarate]

tampramine fumarate USAN *antidepressant* [also: tampramine]

Tamp-R-Tel (trademarked packaging form) *tamper-evident cartridge-needle unit*

tamsulosin INN *alpha₁-adrenergic blocker for benign prostatic hyperplasia (BPH)* [also: tamsulosin HCl]

tamsulosin HCl USAN, JAN *alpha₁-adrenergic blocker for benign prostatic hyperplasia (BPH); also used as adjunctive therapy for ureteral stones* [also: tamsulosin]

Tanac gel OTC *oral anesthetic; vulnerary* [dyclonine HCl; allantoin] 1%•0.5% ⚕ Ten-K; Ting; Twin-K

Tanac topical liquid OTC *mucous membrane anesthetic; antiseptic* [benzocaine; benzalkonium chloride] 10%•0.12% ⚕ Ten-K; Ting; Twin-K

Tanac Dual Core stick OTC *mucous membrane anesthetic; antiseptic; astringent* [benzocaine; benzalkonium chloride; tannic acid] 7.5%•0.12%•6%

Tanacetum parthenium medicinal herb [see: feverfew]

Tanacetum vulgare medicinal herb [see: tansy]

TanaCof A12 oral suspension (discontinued 2007) ℞ *decongestant; antihistamine; sleep aid* [phenylephrine tannate; chlorpheniramine tannate; pyrilamine tannate] 30•12•75 mg/30 mL

TanaCof-DM oral suspension (discontinued 2007) ℞ *antitussive; antihistamine; decongestant* [dextromethorphan tannate; dexchlorpheniramine tannate; pseudoephedrine tannate] 50•5•150 mg/10 mL

Tanafed DMX oral suspension (discontinued 2007) ℞ *antitussive; antihistamine; decongestant* [dextromethorphan tannate; dexchlorpheniramine tannate; pseudoephedrine tannate] 50•5•150 mg/10 mL

Tanafed DP oral suspension (discontinued 2007) ℞ *decongestant; antihistamine* [pseudoephedrine tannate; dexchlorpheniramine tannate] 150•9 mg/10 mL

TanaHist PD oral suspension ℞ *antihistamine* [chlorpheniramine tannate] 2 mg/mL

tanaproget *investigational (Phase III) oral progesterone receptor antagonist contraceptive that inhibits ovulation*

Tanate DMP-DEX oral liquid (discontinued 2007) ℞ *antitussive; antihistamine; decongestant* [dextromethorphan tannate; dexchlorpheniramine tannate; pseudoephedrine tannate] 50•5•150 mg/10 mL

Tanavan oral suspension (discontinued 2007) ℞ *decongestant; antihistamine; sleep aid* [phenylephrine tannate; pyrilamine tannate] 12.5•30 mg/5 mL

tandamine INN *antidepressant* [also: tandamine HCl]

tandamine HCl USAN *antidepressant* [also: tandamine]

Tandem capsules ℞ *hematinic* [iron (as ferrous fumarate; polysaccharide-iron complex)] 106 (162; 115.2) mg

Tandem DHA capsules ℞ *vitamin/iron supplement; omega-3 supplement* [vitamins B₆ & C; folic acid; iron; docosahexaenoic acid (DHA); eicosapentaenoic acid (EPA)] 25•20•1•30• 215.2•53.46 mg

Tandem F capsules ℞ *hematinic* [iron (as ferrous fumarate; polysaccharide-iron complex); folic acid] 106 (162; 115.2)•1 mg

Tandem OB; Tandem Plus capsules ℞ *vitamin/mineral/iron supplement* [multiple vitamins & minerals; iron; folic acid] ±•106•1 mg

tandospirone INN, BAN *anxiolytic* [also: tandospirone citrate]

tandospirone citrate USAN *anxiolytic* [also: tandospirone]

TanDur DM oral suspension ℞ *antitussive; antihistamine; decongestant* [dextromethorphan tannate; dexchlorpheniramine tannate; pseudoephedrine tannate] 27.5•3•50 mg/ 5 mL

taniplon INN

Tannate 12 S oral suspension ℞ *antitussive; antihistamine* [carbetapentane tannate; chlorpheniramine tannate] 30•4 mg/5 mL

Tannate-12D S oral suspension ℞ *antitussive; antihistamine; sleep aid; decongestant* [carbetapentane tannate; pyrilamine tannate; phenylephrine tannate] 30•30•5 mg/5 mL

Tannate DMP-DEX oral suspension ℞ *antitussive; antihistamine; decongestant* [dextromethorphan tannate; dexchlorpheniramine tannate; pseu-

doephedrine tannate] 25•2.5•75 mg/5 mL

Tannate-V-DM oral suspension ℞ *antitussive; antihistamine; sleep aid; decongestant* [dextromethorphan tannate; pyrilamine tannate; phenylephrine tannate] 25•30•12.5 mg/5 mL

tannic acid USP, JAN *astringent; topical mucosal protectant* ② tung seed

tannic acid acetate [see: acetyltannic acid]

Tannic-12 caplets ℞ *antitussive; antihistamine* [carbetapentane tannate; chlorpheniramine tannate] 60•5 mg ② Ten-K; Ting; Twin-K

Tannic-12 oral suspension (discontinued 2007) ℞ *antitussive; antihistamine; decongestant* [carbetapentane tannate; chlorpheniramine tannate; phenylephrine tannate] 30•4•5 mg/5 mL ② Ten-K; Ting; Twin-K

Tannic-12 S oral suspension ℞ *antitussive; antihistamine* [carbetapentane tannate; chlorpheniramine tannate] 30•4 mg/5 mL ② TNKase; tonics

Tannihist-12 D oral suspension ℞ *antitussive; antihistamine; sleep aid; decongestant* [carbetapentane tannate; pyrilamine tannate; phenylephrine tannate] 30•30•5 mg/5 mL

tannin [see: tannic acid]

tannyl acetate [see: acetyltannic acid]

tansy (Chrysanthemum vulgare; Tanacetum vulgare) leaves and seeds *medicinal herb for inducing diaphoresis, promoting wound healing, relieving spasms, stimulating menstruation, and treating worm infections*

tantalum *element (Ta)*

Tantum *investigational (orphan) radioprotectant for oral mucosa following radiation therapy for head and neck cancer* [benzydamine HCl]

Tao capsules (discontinued 2004) ℞ *macrolide antibiotic* [troleandomycin] 250 mg

taoryi edisylate [see: caramiphen edisylate]

Tapanol tablets, caplets, gelcaps (discontinued 2007) OTC *analgesic; anti-*

pyretic [acetaminophen] 325, 500 mg; 500 mg; 500 mg

Tapazole tablets ℞ *thyroid inhibitor* [methimazole] 5, 10 mg

tape, adhesive USP *surgical aid*

tapentadol HCl *investigational (NDA filed) central analgesic for moderate to severe pain*

Taperpak (trademarked packaging form) *corticosteroid packaging to taper off the dosage*

taprostene INN

tar [see: coal tar]

tarweed *medicinal herb* [see: yerba santa]

Tarabine PFS subcu, intrathecal, or IV injection ℞ *antimetabolite antineoplastic for various leukemias* [cytarabine] 20 mg/mL

taranabant *investigational (Phase III) selective cannabinoid CB₁ blocker for weight loss*

Taraphilic ointment OTC *antipsoriatic; antiseborrheic* [coal tar] 1%

Taraxacum officinale *medicinal herb* [see: dandelion]

Tarceva film-coated tablets ℞ *antineoplastic for advanced or metastatic non–small cell lung cancer (NSCLC) and pancreatic cancer; investigational (Phase III) for breast cancer; investigational (orphan) for malignant gliomas* [erlotinib HCl] 25, 100, 150 mg

tarenflurbil *investigational (Phase III) amyloid-β-42–blocking agent to delay the progression of mild Alzheimer disease*

targeted monoclonal antibody vehicles (T-MAVs) *a class of agents that deliver a cytotoxic drug or radioactivity directly to the targeted tissue, usually a cancerous tumor; T-MAVs are not therapeutic per se, but transport the therapeutic agent (effector molecule) to a specific site*

Targretin capsules, gel ℞ *synthetic retinoid analogue antineoplastic for cutaneous T-cell lymphoma (orphan); investigational (Phase III) for lung cancer* [bexarotene] 75 mg; 1%

tariquidar *investigational (Phase III) p-glycoprotein pump inhibitor for lung cancer*

Tarka film-coated dual-release tablets ℞ *once-daily antihypertensive; angiotensin-converting enzyme (ACE) inhibitor; calcium channel blocker* [trandolapril (immediate release); verapamil HCl (extended release)] 2•180, 1•240, 2•240, 4•240 mg ⍰ Touro CC; Tri-K

Tarlene hair lotion OTC *antiseborrheic; antipsoriatic; keratolytic* [salicylic acid; coal tar] 2.5%•2% ⍰ Trilone

tarragon (Artemisia dracunculus) flowering plant *medicinal herb used as a diuretic, emmenagogue, hypnotic, and stomachic* ⍰ Torecan; Trocaine

Tarsum shampoo OTC *antipsoriatic; antiseborrheic; keratolytic* [coal tar; salicylic acid] 10%•5% ⍰ Trizyme

tartar emetic [see: antimony potassium tartrate]

tartaric acid NF *buffering agent*

Tasigna capsules ℞ *kinase inhibitor antineoplastic for Philadelphia chromosome–positive chronic myeloid leukemia (CML)* [nilotinib (as HCl)] 200 mg ⍰ tisoquone; Tussigon; Tyzine

tasimelteon *investigational (Phase III) melatonin agonist to treat insomnia and circadian rhythm sleep disorders*

Tasmar film-coated tablets ℞ *COMT (catechol-O-methyltransferase) inhibitor for Parkinson disease* [tolcapone] 100, 200 mg

tasosartan USAN, INN *antihypertensive; angiotensin II receptor antagonist*

tasuldine INN

TaT antagonist *investigational (Phase I/II) antiviral for HIV infection*

taurine INN [also: aminoethylsulfonic acid]

taurocholate sodium [see: sodium taurocholate]

taurolidine INN, BAN *antitoxin*

tauromustine INN *antineoplastic* ⍰ trimustine

tauroselcholic acid INN, BAN

taurultam INN, BAN

Tavist Allergy tablets OTC *antihistamine for allergic rhinitis and urticaria* [clemastine fumarate] 1.34 mg

Tavist Allergy/Sinus/Headache caplets (discontinued 2007) OTC *decongestant; antihistamine; analgesic; antipyretic* [pseudoephedrine HCl; clemastine fumarate; acetaminophen] 30•0.335•500 mg

Tavist ND tablets OTC *nonsedating antihistamine for allergic rhinitis; also used for chronic idiopathic urticaria* [loratadine] 10 mg

Tavist Sinus caplets (discontinued 2007) OTC *decongestant; analgesic; antipyretic* [pseudoephedrine HCl; acetaminophen] 30•500 mg

tavocept *investigational (Phase III) agent to prevent or mitigate chemotherapy-associated neuropathy*

Tavocept *investigational (Phase III) neuroprotectant for paclitaxel and cisplatin therapy for non–small cell lung cancer*

taxanes; taxoids *a class of antineoplastics that inhibits cancer cell mitosis by disrupting the cells' microtubular network*

Taxol IV infusion ℞ *antineoplastic for AIDS-related Kaposi sarcoma (orphan), breast and ovarian cancers, and non–small cell lung cancer (NSCLC)* [paclitaxel] 6 mg/mL

Taxoprexin *investigational (orphan) taxane for hormone-refractory prostate cancer, pancreatic cancer, malignant melanoma, and adenocarcinoma of the GI tract; investigational (Phase III) for breast cancer* [docosahexaenoic acid (DHA); paclitaxel]

Taxotere IV infusion ℞ *antineoplastic for advanced or metastatic breast, prostate, stomach, head, neck, and non–small cell lung cancer (NSCLC); also used for ovarian, esophageal, and other cancers; analogue to paclitaxel* [docetaxel] 20, 80 mg/vial

Taxus bacatta and other species *medicinal herb* [see: yew]

tazadolene INN *analgesic* [also: tazadolene succinate]

tazadolene succinate USAN *analgesic* [also: tazadolene]

tazanolast INN

tazarotene USAN, INN *retinoid prodrug; topical keratolytic for acne and psoriasis; adjuvant treatment for facial wrinkles, hyper- and hypopigmentation, and benign lentigines*

tazasubrate INN, BAN

tazeprofen INN

Tazicef powder or frozen premix for IV or IM injection ℞ *third-generation cephalosporin antibiotic* [ceftazidime] 1, 2, 6 g

Tazidime powder for IV or IM injection ℞ *third-generation cephalosporin antibiotic* [ceftazidime] 1, 2, 6 g ☑ Tuss-DM

tazifylline INN *antihistamine* [also: tazifylline HCl]

tazifylline HCl USAN *antihistamine* [also: tazifylline]

taziprinone INN

tazobactam USAN, INN, BAN *β-lactamase inhibitor; penicillin synergist*

tazobactam sodium USAN *β-lactamase inhibitor; penicillin synergist*

Tazocin ⓔ (European name for U.S. product **Zosyn**)

tazofelone USAN

tazolol INN *cardiotonic* [also: tazolol HCl]

tazolol HCl USAN *cardiotonic* [also: tazolol]

tazomeline citrate USAN *cholinergic agonist for Alzheimer disease*

Tazorac cream, gel ℞ *retinoid pro-drug; keratolytic for acne and psoriasis* [tazarotene] 0.05%, 0.1%

Taztia XT extended-release capsules ℞ *antihypertensive; calcium channel blocker* [diltiazem HCl] 120, 180, 240, 300, 360 mg

TBC-3B *investigational (Phase I) vaccine for AIDS*

TBZ (thiabendazole) [q.v.]

TC (thioguanine, cytarabine) *chemotherapy protocol*

3TC [now: lamivudine]

⁹⁹ᵐTc [see: macrosalb (⁹⁹ᵐTc)]

^{99m}Tc [see: sodium pertechnetate Tc 99m]

^{99m}Tc [see: technetium Tc 99m albumin]

^{99m}Tc [see: technetium Tc 99m albumin aggregated]

^{99m}Tc [see: technetium Tc 99m albumin colloid]

^{99m}Tc [see: technetium Tc 99m albumin microaggregated]

^{99m}Tc [see: technetium Tc 99m antimony trisulfide colloid]

^{99m}Tc [see: technetium Tc 99m biciromab]

^{99m}Tc [see: technetium Tc 99m bicisate]

^{99m}Tc [see: technetium Tc 99m disofenin]

^{99m}Tc [see: technetium Tc 99m etidronate]

^{99m}Tc [see: technetium Tc 99m exametazine]

^{99m}Tc [see: technetium Tc 99m ferpentetate]

^{99m}Tc [see: technetium Tc 99m furifosmin]

^{99m}Tc [see: technetium Tc 99m gluceptate]

^{99m}Tc [see: technetium Tc 99m lidofenin]

^{99m}Tc [see: technetium Tc 99m mebrofenin]

^{99m}Tc [see: technetium Tc 99m medronate]

^{99m}Tc [see: technetium Tc 99m medronate disodium]

^{99m}Tc [see: technetium Tc 99m mertiatide]

^{99m}Tc [see: technetium Tc 99m oxidronate]

^{99m}Tc [see: technetium Tc 99m pentetate]

^{99m}Tc [see: technetium Tc 99m pentetate calcium trisodium]

^{99m}Tc [see: technetium Tc 99m (pyro- & trimeta-) phosphates]

^{99m}Tc [see: technetium Tc 99m pyrophosphate]

^{99m}Tc [see: technetium Tc 99m red blood cells]

^{99m}Tc [see: technetium Tc 99m sestamibi]

^{99m}Tc [see: technetium Tc 99m siboroxime]

^{99m}Tc [see: technetium Tc 99m succimer]

^{99m}Tc [see: technetium Tc 99m sulfur colloid]

^{99m}Tc [see: technetium Tc 99m teboroxime]

^{99m}Tc [see: technetium Tc 99m tetrofosmin]

^{99m}Tc [see: technetium Tc 99m tiatide]

TCC (trichlorocarbanilide) [see: triclocarban]

T-cell depleted stem cells derived from peripheral blood stem cells *investigational (orphan) for chronic granulomatous disease*

T-cell receptor (TCR) ligand, recombinant *investigational (orphan) for multiple sclerosis*

T-cells cultured with anti-CD3 and IL-2, expressing herpes simplex 1 virus-thymidine kinase (HSV-TK) *investigational (orphan) immunotherapy for allogenic hematopoietic stem cell transplantation*

TCF (Taxol, cisplatin, fluorouracil) *chemotherapy protocol for esophageal cancer*

TCI Ovulation Tester test kit for home use OTC *in vitro diagnostic aid to predict ovulation time from a saliva sample*

TCR (T-cell receptor) ligand [q.v.]

TD; Td (tetanus & diphtheria [toxoids]) the designation TD (or DT) denotes the pediatric vaccine; Td denotes the adult vaccine [see: diphtheria & tetanus toxoids, adsorbed]

Tdap (tetanus, diphtheria, acellular pertussis) vaccine Tdap (tetanus predominant) is the booster vaccine used in adults and children $\geq$ 10 years; compare to Dtap [see: diphtheria & tetanus toxoids & acellular pertussis (DTaP; Dtap; Tdap) vaccine]

tea, Canada; mountain tea; redberry tea *medicinal herb* [see: wintergreen]

tea tree oil *(Melaleuca alternifolia)*
*medicinal herb for acne, boils, burns,
Candida infections, cold sores, joint
pain, skin disorders, staphylococcal and
streptococcal infections, and sunburn;
also used as a douche for trichomonal
cervicitis and vaginal candidiasis*

**TEAB (tetraethylammonium bro-
mide)** [see: tetrylammonium bro-
mide]

teaberry oil [see: methyl salicylate]

**TEAC (tetraethylammonium chlo-
ride)** [q.v.]

teamster's tea *medicinal herb* [see:
ephedra]

TearGard *eye drops* OTC *moisturizer/
lubricant* [hydroxyethylcellulose] ⊠
terguride

Teargen *eye drops* OTC *moisturizer/
lubricant* [polyvinyl alcohol] ⊠ tarragon; Torecan; Trocaine; Trugene

Tearisol *eye drops* OTC *moisturizer/
lubricant* [hydroxypropyl methylcel-
lulose] 0.5% ⊠ Terazol 3

Tears Again *eye drops* OTC *moisturizer/
lubricant* [hydroxypropyl methylcel-
lulose] 0.3% ⊠ triazaquone

**Tears Naturale; Tears Naturale II;
Tears Naturale Free** *eye drops* OTC
moisturizer/lubricant [hydroxypropyl
methylcellulose] 0.3%

Tears Naturale Forte *eye drops* OTC
moisturizer/lubricant [hydroxypropyl
methylcellulose; glycerin] 0.3%•0.2%

Tears Plus *eye drops* OTC *moisturizer/
lubricant* [polyvinyl alcohol] 1.4%

Tears Renewed *eye drops* OTC *mois-
turizer/lubricant* [hydroxypropyl
methylcellulose] 0.3%

Tears Renewed *ophthalmic ointment*
OTC *ocular moisturizer/lubricant*
[white petrolatum; mineral oil]

TearSaver Punctum Plugs ℞ *blocks
the puncta and canaliculus to eliminate
tear loss in keratitis sicca* [silicone plug]

Tebamide *suppositories, pediatric suppositories* (removed from the market
in 2007 due to lack of efficacy) ℞
*anticholinergic; post-surgical antiemetic;
local anesthetic* [trimethobenzamide

HCl; benzocaine] 200 mg•2%; 100
mg•2%

tebatizole INN

tebethion [see: thioacetazone; thiacet-
azone]

tebufelone USAN, INN *analgesic; anti-
inflammatory*

tebuquine USAN, INN *antimalarial*

tebutate USAN, INN *combining name for
radicals or groups*

**TEC (thiotepa, etoposide, carbo-
platin)** *chemotherapy protocol*

tecadenoson *investigational (Phase III)
agent for paroxysmal supraventricular
tachycardia (PSVT)*

teceleukin USAN, INN, BAN *immunostimulant; investigational (orphan) for
metastatic renal cell carcinoma and
metastatic malignant melanoma*

technetium *element (Tc)*

**technetium (^{99m}Tc) dimercaptosuc-
cinic acid** JAN *diagnostic aid for renal
function testing* [also: technetium Tc
99m succimer]

**technetium (^{99m}Tc) human serum
albumin** JAN *radioactive agent*

**technetium (^{99m}Tc) labeled macro-
aggregated human albumin** JAN
[also: macrosalb (^{99m}Tc)]

**technetium (^{99m}Tc) methylenedi-
phosphonate** JAN *radioactive diagnostic aid for skeletal imaging* [also:
technetium Tc 99m medronate]

technetium (^{99m}Tc) phytate JAN
radioactive agent

technetium Tc 99m albumin USP
radioactive agent

**technetium Tc 99m albumin aggre-
gated** USAN, USP *radioactive diagnostic aid for lung imaging*

**technetium Tc 99m albumin col-
loid** USAN, USP *radioactive agent*

**technetium Tc 99m albumin micro-
aggregated** USAN *radioactive agent*

**technetium Tc 99m antimony trisul-
fide colloid** USAN *radioactive agent*

technetium Tc 99m apcitide *radiopharmaceutical diagnostic aid for acute
venous thrombosis*

technetium Tc 99m arcitumomab USAN *radiopharmaceutical diagnostic aid for recurrent or metastatic thyroid and colorectal cancers*

technetium Tc 99m bectumomab *monoclonal antibody IgG$_{2a}$ to B cell, murine; investigational (Phase III, orphan) diagnostic aid for non-Hodgkin B-cell lymphoma, AIDS-related lymphomas, and other acute and chronic B-cell leukemias* [also: bectumomab]

technetium Tc 99m biciromab *radioactive diagnostic aid for deep vein thrombosis*

technetium Tc 99m bicisate USAN, INN, BAN *radioactive diagnostic aid for brain imaging*

technetium Tc 99m disofenin USP *radioactive diagnostic aid for hepatobiliary function testing*

technetium Tc 99m DMSA (dimercaptosuccinic acid) [see: technetium Tc 99m succimer]

technetium Tc 99m DTPA (diethylenetriaminepentaacetic acid) [see: technetium Tc 99m pentetate]

technetium Tc 99m etidronate USP *radioactive agent*

technetium Tc 99m exametazine USAN *radioactive agent*

technetium Tc 99m ferpentetate USP *radioactive agent*

technetium Tc 99m furifosmin USAN, INN *radioactive agent; diagnostic aid for cardiac disease*

technetium Tc 99m gluceptate USP *radioactive agent*

technetium Tc 99m HSA (human serum albumin) [see: technetium Tc 99m albumin]

technetium Tc 99m iron ascorbate pentetic acid complex [now: technetium Tc 99m ferpentetate]

technetium Tc 99m lidofenin USAN, USP *radioactive agent*

technetium Tc 99m MAA (microaggregated albumin) [see: technetium Tc 99m albumin aggregated]

technetium Tc 99m MDP (methylenediphosphonate) [see: technetium Tc 99m medronate]

technetium Tc 99m mebrofenin USAN, USP *radioactive hepatobiliary imaging agent for cholescintigraphy* 100 mCi in 45 mg injection

technetium Tc 99m medronate USP *radioactive diagnostic aid for skeletal imaging* [also: technetium (^{99m}Tc) methylenediphosphonate]

technetium Tc 99m medronate disodium USAN *radioactive agent*

technetium Tc 99m mertiatide USAN *radioactive diagnostic aid for renal function testing*

technetium Tc 99m oxidronate USP *radioactive diagnostic aid for skeletal imaging*

technetium Tc 99m pentetate USP *radioactive agent* [also: human serum albumin diethylenetriaminepentaacetic acid technetium (^{99m}Tc)]

technetium Tc 99m pentetate calcium trisodium USAN *radioactive agent*

technetium Tc 99m pentetate sodium [now: technetium Tc 99m pentetate]

technetium Tc 99m pterotetramide *investigational (orphan) radiodiagnostic aid for ovarian carcinoma*

technetium Tc 99m (pyro- and trimeta-) phosphates USP *radioactive agent*

technetium Tc 99m pyrophosphate USP, JAN *radioactive agent*

technetium Tc 99m red blood cells USAN *radioactive agent*

technetium Tc 99m rh-Annexin V *investigational (orphan) radiodiagnostic aid to assess the rejection status of heart and lung transplants*

technetium Tc 99m sestamibi USAN, INN, BAN *radioactive/radiopaque diagnostic aid for cardiac perfusion imaging and mammography*

technetium Tc 99m siboroxime USAN, INN *radioactive diagnostic aid for brain imaging*

technetium Tc 99m sodium gluceptate [now: technetium Tc 99m gluceptate]

technetium Tc 99m succimer USP *diagnostic aid for renal function testing* [also: technetium (^{99m}Tc) dimercaptosuccinic acid]

technetium Tc 99m sulesomab *monoclonal antibody; diagnostic aid for infectious lesions* [also: sulesomab]

technetium Tc 99m sulfur colloid (TSC) USAN, USP *radioactive agent*

technetium Tc 99m teboroxime USAN, INN, BAN *radioactive/radiopaque diagnostic aid for cardiac perfusion imaging*

technetium Tc 99m tetrofosmin *radioactive agent for cardiovascular imaging*

technetium Tc 99m tiatide BAN

technetium Tc 99m TSC (technetium sulfur colloid) [see: technetium Tc 99m sulfur colloid]

technetium Tc 99m-labeled CEA scan [see: arcitumomab]

Techni-Care surgical scrub ℞ *broadspectrum microbicide* [chloroxylenol] 3%

Technosphere (trademarked delivery device) *investigational (Phase III) oral inhalation device*

teclothiazide INN, BAN

teclozan USAN, INN *antiamebic*

Tecnu Outdoor Skin Cleanser lotion OTC *for the removal of toxic oils from poison ivy, oak, or sumac; use before or as soon as rash appears; can also be used to clean clothing and equipment* [deodorized mineral spirits; propylene glycol; fatty acid soap]

tecogalan sodium USAN *antiangiogenic antineoplastic*

Teczem film-coated extended-release tablets (discontinued 2007) ℞ *antihypertensive; angiotensin-converting enzyme (ACE) inhibitor; calcium channel blocker* [diltiazem maleate; enalapril maleate] 180•5 mg

tedisamil INN *investigational (NDA filed) antiarrhythmic for atrial fibrillation*

Tedrigen tablets (discontinued 2007) OTC *antiasthmatic; bronchodilator; decongestant; sedative* [theophylline; ephedrine HCl; phenobarbital] 120•22.5•7.5 mg

teduglutide *investigational (Phase III) glucagon-like peptide 2 (GLP-2) analogue for short bowel syndrome*

tefazoline INN ⑨ tofisoline

tefenperate INN

tefludazine INN

teflurane USAN, INN *inhalation anesthetic*

teflutixol INN

tegafur USAN, INN, BAN *antineoplastic; prodrug of fluorouracil*

tegaserod USAN *selective serotonin 5-HT_4 receptor antagonist for irritable bowel syndrome (IBS)*

tegaserod maleate *selective serotonin 5-HT_4 receptor antagonist for irritable bowel syndrome (IBS) with chronic constipation in women and chronic idiopathic constipation in all*

Tegretol chewable tablets, caplets, oral suspension ℞ *iminostilbene anticonvulsant; analgesic for trigeminal neuralgia; also used for restless legs syndrome (RLS), alcohol withdrawal, and postherpetic neuralgia* [carbamazepine] 100 mg; 200 mg; 100 mg/5 mL

Tegretol-XR extended-release filmcoated tablets ℞ *twice-daily anticonvulsant; analgesic for trigeminal neuralgia; also used for restless legs syndrome (RLS), alcohol withdrawal, and postherpetic neuralgia* [carbamazepine] 100, 200, 400 mg

Tegrin-HC ointment OTC *corticosteroidal anti-inflammatory* [hydrocortisone] 1%

teholamine [see: aminophylline]

TEIB (triethyleneiminobenzoquinone) [see: triaziquone]

teicoplanin USAN, INN, BAN *glycopeptide antibiotic*

teicoplanin A$_{2-1}$, A$_{2-2}$, A$_{2-3}$, A$_{2-4}$, A$_{2-5}$, and A$_{3-1}$ *components of teicoplanin*

Tekturna tablets ℞ *once-daily direct renin inhibitor for hypertension* [aliskiren hemifumarate] 150, 300 mg

Tekturna HCT film-coated tablets ℞ *combination direct renin inhibitor and diuretic for hypertension* [aliskiren hemifumarate; hydrochlorothiazide] 150•12.5, 150•25, 300•12.5, 300•25 mg

Teladar cream ℞ *corticosteroidal anti-inflammatory* [betamethasone dipropionate] 0.05%

telaprevir *investigational (Phase III) hepatitis C virus (HCV) protease inhibitor for the treatment of HCV infections*

telavancin *investigational (NDA filed) injectable antibiotic for drug-resistant gram-positive bacteria*

telbermin USAN *angiogenic growth factor; vascular endothelial growth factor, recombinant human (rhVEGF); investigational (Phase II, orphan) for peripheral vascular disease and coronary artery disease*

telbivudine *oral nucleoside reverse-transcriptase inhibitor (NRTI) for chronic hepatitis B virus (HBV) infection in adults* 🔲 tolpovidone I 131

telcagepant *investigational (Phase III) calcitonin gene-related peptide (CGRP) receptor antagonist for migraine headaches*

Telcyta *investigational (Phase III) antineoplastic for non–small cell lung cancers*

Tel-E-Amp (trademarked delivery form) *unit dose ampule*

Tel-E-Dose (trademarked packaging form) *unit dose package*

Tel-E-Ject (trademarked delivery form) *prefilled disposable syringe*

telenzepine INN

Tel-E-Pack (trademarked packaging form) *packaging system*

Telepaque tablets (discontinued 2006) ℞ *radiopaque contrast medium for cholecystography* [iopanoic acid (66.68% iodine)] 500 mg (333.4 mg)

Tel-E-Vial (trademarked packaging form) *unit dose vial*

telinavir USAN *antiviral; HIV protease inhibitor*

telithromycin *broad-spectrum ketolide antibiotic for community-acquired pneumonia (CAP); approval to treat other types of respiratory tract infections was withdrawn by the FDA in 2007*

tellurium *element (Te)*

telmisartan USAN *antihypertensive; angiotensin II receptor antagonist*

teloxantrone INN *antineoplastic* [also: teloxantrone HCl]

teloxantrone HCl USAN *antineoplastic* [also: teloxantrone]

teludipine INN, BAN *antihypertensive; calcium channel antagonist* [also: teludipine HCl]

teludipine HCl USAN *antihypertensive; calcium channel antagonist* [also: teludipine]

Telzir 🇪🇺 (European name for the U.S. product **Lexiva**)

temafloxacin INN, BAN *antibacterial; microbial DNA topoisomerase inhibitor* [also: temafloxacin HCl]

temafloxacin HCl USAN *antibacterial; microbial DNA topoisomerase inhibitor* [also: temafloxacin]

temarotene INN

tematropium methylsulfate USAN *anticholinergic* [also: tematropium metilsulfate]

tematropium metilsulfate INN *anticholinergic* [also: tematropium methylsulfate]

temazepam USAN, INN *benzodiazepine sedative and hypnotic* 15, 30 mg oral

Tembid (trademarked dosage form) *sustained-action capsule*

temefos USAN, INN *veterinary ectoparasiticide*

temelastine USAN, INN, BAN *antihistamine*

temocapril HCl USAN *antihypertensive*

temocillin USAN, INN, BAN *antibacterial*

temocillin sodium *investigational (orphan) antibiotic for pulmonary Burkholderia cepacia infections*

Temodar capsules ℞ *alkylating antineoplastic for refractory anaplastic astrocytoma (AA), recurrent glioblastoma multiforme (GBM), and malignant glioma* *(orphan); investigational (NDA filed, orphan) for advanced metastatic melanoma* [temozolomide] 5, 20, 100, 140, 180, 250 mg

temodox USAN, INN *veterinary growth stimulant*

temoporfin USAN, INN, BAN *photosensitizer for photodynamic cancer therapy; investigational (NDA filed, orphan) palliative treatment for head and neck cancer*

Temovate ointment, gel, cream, scalp application ℞ *corticosteroidal anti-inflammatory* [clobetasol propionate] 0.05%

Temovate Emollient cream ℞ *corticosteroidal anti-inflammatory* [clobetasol propionate in an emollient base] 0.05%

temozolomide INN, BAN *alkylating antineoplastic for refractory anaplastic astrocytoma (AA), recurrent glioblastoma multiforme (GBM), and malignant glioma (orphan); investigational (NDA filed, orphan) for advanced metastatic melanoma*

TEMP (tamoxifen, etoposide, mitoxantrone, Platinol) *chemotherapy protocol*

Temp Tab tablets OTC *electrolyte replacement* [sodium, potassium, and chloride electrolytes] 180•15•287 mg

Tempo chewable tablets OTC *antacid; antiflatulent* [aluminum hydroxide; magnesium hydroxide; calcium carbonate; simethicone] 133•81•414•20 mg

Tempra 1 oral drops (discontinued 2008) OTC *analgesic; antipyretic* [acetaminophen] 100 mg/mL

Tempra 2 syrup (discontinued 2008) OTC *analgesic; antipyretic* [acetaminophen] 160 mg/5 mL

Tempra 3 chewable tablets (discontinued 2008) OTC *analgesic; antipyretic* [acetaminophen] 80, 160 mg

Tempra Quicklets (quickly dissolving tablets) (discontinued 2008) OTC *analgesic; antipyretic* [acetaminophen] 80, 160 mg

Tempule (trademarked dosage form) *timed-release capsule or tablet*

temsirolimus *antineoplastic for renal cell carcinoma (orphan); investigational (NDA filed) for metastatic breast cancer and mantle cell lymphoma; investigational (Phase II) immunosuppressant for rheumatoid arthritis and multiple sclerosis*

temurtide USAN, INN, BAN *vaccine adjuvant*

10 Benzagel; 5 Benzagel gel ℞ *keratolytic for acne* [benzoyl peroxide] 10%; 5%

10% LMD IV injection ℞ *plasma volume expander for shock due to hemorrhage, burns, or surgery* [dextran 40] 10%

tenamfetamine INN

Tencet capsules ℞ *barbiturate sedative; analgesic; antipyretic* [butalbital; acetaminophen; caffeine] 50•325•40 mg

Tencon capsules (discontinued 2004) ℞ *barbiturate sedative; analgesic; antipyretic* [butalbital; acetaminophen] 50•650 mg

tendamistat INN

tenecteplase USAN *genetically engineered mutation of tissue plasminogen activator (tPA); thrombolytic/fibrinolytic for acute myocardial infarction (AMI)*

Tenex tablets ℞ *antihypertensive; antiadrenergic; investigational (NDA filed) treatment for attention-deficit/hyperactivity disorder; investigational (orphan) for fragile X syndrome* [guanfacine HCl] 1, 2 mg

tenidap USAN, INN *anti-inflammatory for osteoarthritis and rheumatoid arthritis; cytokine inhibitor*

tenidap sodium USAN *anti-inflammatory for osteoarthritis and rheumatoid arthritis*

tenilapine INN

teniloxazine INN

tenilsetam INN

teniposide USAN, INN, BAN *antineoplastic for refractory childhood acute lymphocytic leukemia (orphan)*

Ten-K controlled-release tablets ℞ *potassium supplement* [potassium chloride] 750 mg (10 mEq K) ⊡ Tanac; Ting; Twin-K

tenoate INN *combining name for radicals or groups*

tenocyclidine INN

tenofovir USAN *antiviral; nucleotide reverse transcriptase inhibitor (NRTI) for HIV-1 infection*

tenofovir disoproxil fumarate (tenofovir DF) *oral antiviral; nucleotide reverse transcriptase inhibitor (NRTI) for HIV-1 and chronic hepatitis B infections* (base=82%)

tenonitrozole INN

Tenoretic 50; Tenoretic 100 tablets ℞ *antihypertensive; β-blocker; diuretic* [chlorthalidone; atenolol] 25•50 mg; 25•100 mg

Tenormin IV injection (discontinued 2008) ℞ *antianginal; antihypertensive; β-blocker* [atenolol] 5 mg/10 mL

Tenormin tablets ℞ *antianginal; antihypertensive; β-blocker* [atenolol] 25, 50, 100 mg

tenoxicam USAN, INN, BAN *anti-inflammatory*

Tensilon IV or IM injection ℞ *myasthenia gravis treatment; antidote to curare overdose* [edrophonium chloride] 10 mg/mL ⊡ tinazoline; Tonsaline

Ten-Tab (trademarked dosage form) *controlled-release tablet*

Tenuate tablets, Dospan (controlled-release tablets) (discontinued 2006) ℞ *anorexiant; CNS stimulant* [diethylpropion HCl] 25 mg; 75 mg

tenylidone INN

teoclate INN *combining name for radicals or groups* [also: theoclate]

teopranitol INN

teoprolol INN

tepirindole INN

teplizumab *investigational (Phase II/III) to slow the progression of type 1 diabetes*

tepoxalin USAN, INN *antipsoriatic*

teprenone INN ⊡ tiopronin; toborinone

teprosilate INN *combining name for radicals or groups*

teprotide USAN, INN *antihypertensive; angiotensin-converting enzyme (ACE) inhibitor*

Tequin film-coated tablets, powder for oral suspension, IV infusion (discontinued 2006) ℞ *broad-spectrum fluoroquinolone antibiotic* [gatifloxacin] 200, 400 mg; 200 mg/5 mL; 200, 400 mg/vial ⊡ Ticon; Tigan

Tera-Gel shampoo OTC *antiseborrheic; antipsoriatic; antipruritic; antibacterial* [coal tar] 0.5% ⊡ Trocal

Terak with Polymyxin B Sulfate ophthalmic ointment ℞ *antibiotic* [oxytetracycline HCl; polymyxin B sulfate] 5 mg•10 000 U per g

Terazol 3 vaginal suppositories, vaginal cream in prefilled applicator ℞ *antifungal* [terconazole] 80 mg; 0.8% ⊡ Tearisol

Terazol 7 vaginal cream in prefilled applicator ℞ *antifungal* [terconazole] 0.4% ⊡ Tearisol

terazosin INN, BAN *alpha$_1$-adrenergic blocker for hypertension and benign prostatic hyperplasia (BPH)* [also: terazosin HCl]

terazosin HCl USAN *alpha$_1$-adrenergic blocker for hypertension and benign prostatic hyperplasia (BPH)* [also: terazosin] 1, 2, 5, 10 mg oral

terbinafine USAN, INN, BAN *systemic allylamine antifungal* [also: terbinafine HCl]

terbinafine HCl JAN *allylamine antifungal* [also: terbinafine] 250 mg oral; 1% topical

terbium *element (Tb)*

terbogrel USAN *platelet aggregation inhibitor*

terbucromil INN

terbufibrol INN

terbuficin INN

terbuprol INN

terbutaline INN, BAN *sympathomimetic bronchodilator for asthma and bronchospasm* [also: terbutaline sulfate]

terbutaline sulfate USAN, USP *sympathomimetic bronchodilator for asthma and bronchospasm; also used as a* *tocolytic to stop preterm labor* [also: terbutaline] 2.5, 5 mg oral; 1 mg/mL injection

terciprazine INN

terconazole USAN, INN, BAN *topical antifungal* 0.4%, 0.8%, 80 mg vaginal

terfenadine USAN, USP, INN, JAN *piperidine antihistamine*

terflavoxate INN

terfluranol INN

terguride INN *dopamine agonist* ☑ Tear-Gard

teriparatide USAN, INN *human parathyroid hormone, recombinant; osteoporosis treatment that stimulates new bone formation* (orphan); *diagnostic aid for parathyroid-induced hypocalcemia* (orphan); *investigational* (orphan) *for hypoparathyroidism*

teriparatide acetate USAN, JAN *diagnostic aid for parathyroid-induced hypocalcemia* (orphan)

terizidone INN ☑ trazodone

terlakiren USAN *antihypertensive; renin inhibitor*

terlipressin INN, BAN *synthetic vasopressin derivative; investigational (NDA filed, orphan) hormone for bleeding esophageal varices and to improve renal function in patients with hepatorenal syndrome (HRS)*

ternidazole INN

terodiline INN, BAN, JAN *coronary vasodilator* [also: terodiline HCl]

terodiline HCl USAN *coronary vasodilator* [also: terodiline]

terofenamate INN

teroxalene INN *antischistosomal* [also: teroxalene HCl] ☑ trixolane

teroxalene HCl USAN *antischistosomal* [also: teroxalene]

teroxirone USAN, INN *antineoplastic*

terpin hydrate USP (*disapproved for use as an expectorant in 1991*)

terpinol [see: terpin hydrate]

terrafungine [see: oxytetracycline]

Terramycin IM or IV injection (discontinued 2007) ℞ *broad-spectrum tetracycline antibiotic* [oxytetracy-cline; lidocaine] 100 mg•2%, 250 mg•2% per 2 mL dose ☑ Trimo-San

Terramycin with Polymyxin B ophthalmic ointment ℞ *ophthalmic antibiotic* [oxytetracycline HCl; polymyxin B sulfate] 5 mg•10 000 U per g

Terrell liquid for vaporization ℞ *inhalation general anesthetic* [isoflurane] ☑ Touro LA

Tersaseptic shampoo/cleanser OTC *soap-free therapeutic cleanser*

Tersi Foam topical foam OTC *antiseborrheic; dandruff treatment* [selenium sulfide] 2.5%

tertatolol INN, BAN

tertiary amyl alcohol [see: amylene hydrate]

***tert*-pentyl alcohol** [see: amylene hydrate]

tesaglitazar *investigational (Phase III) peroxisome proliferator–activated receptor (PPAR)-alpha and -gamma agonist for type 2 diabetes*

tesamorelin *investigational (Phase III) for HIV-associated lipodystrophy*

tesicam USAN, INN *anti-inflammatory*

tesimide USAN, INN *anti-inflammatory*

Teslac tablets (discontinued 2008) ℞ *adjunctive hormonal chemotherapy for advanced postmenopausal breast carcinoma* [testolactone] 50 mg

Teslascan IV injection ℞ *radiopaque contrast agent to enhance MRIs of the liver* [mangafodipir trisodium] 37.9 mg/mL (50 mcmol/mL)

tesmilifene HCl USAN *antihistamine; chemopotentiator for adjunctive treatment of malignant tumors*

TESPA (triethylenethiophosphoramide) [see: thiotepa]

Tessalon Perles (capsules) ℞ *antitussive* [benzonatate] 100, 200 mg ☑ tiosalan

Test Pack kit for professional use ℞ *in vitro diagnostic aid for Group A streptococcal antigens in throat swabs* [enzyme immunoassay]

Testim gel ℞ *androgen for hypogonadism or testosterone deficiency in men; hormone replacement therapy (HRT) for*

postandropausal symptoms [testosterone; alcohol 74%] 1% (50 mg/pkt.)

Testoderm; Testoderm with Adhesive transdermal patch (for scrotal area) (discontinued 2005) ℞ *androgen for hypogonadism or testosterone deficiency in men; hormone replacement therapy for postandropausal symptoms* [testosterone] 4, 6 mg/day (10, 15 mg total)

testolactone USAN, USP, INN *antineoplastic; androgen hormone*

Testopel pellets for subcu implantation ℞ *androgen for hypogonadism or testosterone deficiency in men; hormone replacement therapy (HRT) for postandropausal symptoms* [testosterone] 75 mg

testosterone USP, INN, BAN *natural androgen for hypogonadism or testosterone deficiency in men; hormone replacement therapy (HRT) for postandropausal symptoms; investigational (Phase II, orphan) for AIDS-wasting syndrome and delay of growth and puberty in boys*

Testosterone Aqueous IM injection ℞ *androgen for hypogonadism or testosterone deficiency in men, delayed puberty in boys, and androgen-responsive metastatic cancers in women; testosterone replacement therapy for postandropausal symptoms* [testosterone] 25, 50, 100 mg/mL

testosterone cyclopentanepropionate [see: testosterone cypionate]

testosterone cyclopentylpropionate [see: testosterone cypionate]

testosterone cypionate USP *parenteral natural androgen for hypogonadism or testosterone deficiency in men; hormone replacement therapy (HRT) for postandropausal symptoms; sometimes abused as a street drug* 100, 200 mg/mL (in oil) injection

testosterone enanthate USP *parenteral natural androgen for testosterone deficiency in men, delayed puberty in boys, and metastatic breast cancer in women; hormone replacement therapy (HRT)*

for postandropausal symptoms; sometimes abused as a street drug 200 mg/mL (in oil) injection

testosterone heptanoate [see: testosterone enanthate]

testosterone ketolaurate USAN, INN *androgen*

testosterone 3-oxododecanoate [see: testosterone ketolaurate]

testosterone phenylacetate USAN *androgen*

testosterone propionate USP *parenteral androgen for hypogonadism or testosterone deficiency in men; hormone replacement therapy (HRT) for postandropausal symptoms; investigational (orphan) topical treatment for vulvar dystrophies* 100 mg/mL injection

testosterone undecanoate *investigational (Phase III) parenteral natural androgen for testosterone deficiency in men*

TestPack [see: Abbott TestPack]

Testred capsules ℞ *synthetic androgen for hypogonadism or testosterone deficiency in men, delayed puberty in boys, and metastatic breast cancer in women; hormone replacement therapy (HRT) for postandropausal symptoms; also abused as a street drug* [methyltestosterone] 10 mg

tetanus antitoxin USP *passive immunizing agent*

tetanus & gas gangrene antitoxins NF

tetanus & gas gangrene polyvalent antitoxin [see: tetanus & gas gangrene antitoxins]

tetanus immune globulin (TIG) USP *passive immunizing agent*

tetanus immune human globulin [now: tetanus immune globulin]

tetanus toxoid USP *active immunizing agent*

tetanus toxoid, adsorbed USP *active immunizing agent*

tetanus toxoid & diphtheria toxoid & acellular pertussis (TDaP; Tdap) vaccine *active immunizing agent for tetanus, diphtheria, and per-*

tussis; vaccine booster for adolescents 10–18 years

Tetcaine eye drops ℞ *topical anesthetic* [tetracaine HCl] 0.5%

tetiothalein sodium [see: iodophthalein sodium]

tetnicoran [see: nicofurate]

tetrabarbital INN

tetrabenazine INN, BAN *selective dopamine depletor for chorea associated with Huntington disease (orphan)*

TetraBriks (trademarked delivery form) *ready-to-use liquid containers*

tetracaine USP, INN *topical/local anesthetic* [also: amethocaine]

tetracaine HCl USP, JAN *ophthalmological local anesthetic; injectable local anesthetic for spinal anesthesia* [also: amethocaine HCl] 0.5% eye drops

tetrachlorodecaoxide *investigational (Phase III) immunomodulator and growth factor for HIV and AIDS*

tetrachloroethylene USP

tetrachloromethane [see: carbon tetrachloride]

tetracosactide INN *adrenocorticotropic hormone* [also: cosyntropin; tetracosactrin]

tetracosactrin BAN *adrenocorticotropic hormone* [also: cosyntropin; tetracosactide]

tetracyclics *a class of antidepressants which enhance noradrenergic and serotonergic activity by blocking norepinephrine or serotonin uptake*

tetracycline USP, INN, BAN *bacteriostatic antibiotic; antirickettsial*

tetracycline HCl USP *bacteriostatic antibiotic; antirickettsial* 250, 500 mg oral

tetracycline phosphate complex USP, BAN *antibacterial*

tetracyclines *a class of bacteriostatic, antimicrobial antibiotics*

tetradecanoic acid, methylethyl ester [see: isopropyl myristate]

tetradonium bromide INN

tetraethylammonium bromide (TEAB) [see: tetrylammonium bromide]

tetraethylammonium chloride (TEAC)

tetraethylthiuram disulfide [see: disulfiram]

tetrafilcon A USAN *hydrophilic contact lens material*

Tetra-Formula lozenges OTC *antitussive; mucous membrane anesthetic* [dextromethorphan hydrobromide; benzocaine] 10•15 mg

tetraglycine hydroperiodide *source of iodine for disinfecting water*

tetrahydroacridinamine (THA) [see: tacrine HCl]

tetrahydroaminoacridine (THA) [see: tacrine HCl]

tetrahydrobiopterin *investigational (orphan) for hyperphenylalaninemia*

tetrahydrocannabinol (THC), delta-9 *a psychoactive derivative of the Cannabis sativa (marijuana) plant; approved in Canada as an analgesic for pain associated with cancer and multiple sclerosis* [also: dronabinol]

tetrahydrolipstatin [see: orlistat]

tetrahydrozoline BAN *vasoconstrictor; nasal decongestant; topical ophthalmic decongestant* [also: tetrhydrozoline HCl; tetryzoline]

tetrahydrozoline HCl USP *vasoconstrictor; nasal decongestant; topical ophthalmic decongestant* [also: tetryzoline; tetrahydrozoline] 0.05% eye drops

tetraiodophenolphthalein sodium [see: iodophthalein sodium]

tetraiodothyroacetic acid *investigational (orphan) for the suppression of thyroid-stimulating hormone (TSH) in patients with thyroid cancer*

tetrallobarbital [see: butalbital]

tetramal [see: tetrabarbital]

tetrameprozine [see: aminopromazine]

tetramethrin INN

tetramethylene dimethanesulfonate [see: busulfan]

tetramisole INN *anthelmintic* [also: tetramisole HCl]

tetramisole HCl USAN *anthelmintic* [also: tetramisole]

tetranitrol [see: erythrityl tetranitrate]

tetrantoin

TetraPaks (trademarked delivery form) *ready-to-use open system containers*

Tetrasine; Tetrasine Extra eye drops (discontinued 2006) OTC *decongestant; vasoconstrictor* [tetrahydrozoline HCl] 0.05%

tetrasodium ethylenediaminetetraacetate [see: edetate sodium]

tetrasodium pyrophosphate [see: sodium pyrophosphate]

tetrazepam INN

tetrazolast INN *antiallergic; antiasthmatic* [also: tetrazolast meglumine]

tetrazolast meglumine USAN *antiallergic; antiasthmatic* [also: tetrazolast]

tetridamine INN *analgesic; anti-inflammatory* [also: tetrydamine]

tetriprofen INN

tetrofosmin USAN, INN, BAN *diagnostic aid*

tetronasin INN, BAN *veterinary growth promoter* [also: tetronasin sodium; tetronasin 5930]

tetronasin 5930 INN *veterinary growth promoter* [also: tetronasin sodium; tetronasin]

tetronasin sodium USAN *veterinary growth promoter* [also: tetronasin; tetronasin 5930]

tetroquinone USAN, INN *systemic keratolytic*

tetroxoprim USAN, INN *antibacterial*

tetrydamine USAN *analgesic; anti-inflammatory* [also: tetridamine]

tetrylammonium bromide INN

tetryzoline INN *vasoconstrictor; nasal decongestant; topical ocular decongestant* [also: tetrahydrozoline HCl; tetrahydrozoline]

tetryzoline HCl [see: tetrahydrozoline HCl]

Tetterine ointment ℞ *antifungal for tinea pedis, tinea cruris, and tinea corporis* [miconazole nitrate] 2%

tetterwort *medicinal herb* [see: bloodroot; celandine]

Teveten film-coated caplets *antihypertensive; angiotensin II receptor antagonist* [eprosartan mesylate] 600 mg

Teveten HCT film-coated caplets ℞ *antihypertensive; angiotensin II receptor antagonist; diuretic* [eprosartan mesylate; hydrochlorothiazide] 600•12.5 mg

Tev-Tropin powder for subcu injection ℞ *growth hormone for children and adults with congenital or endogenous growth hormone deficiency (GHD), short bowel syndrome, or AIDS-wasting syndrome; for children with Turner syndrome, Prader-Willi syndrome, or renal-induced growth failure* [somatropin] 5 mg (15 IU) per vial

Texacort topical solution ℞ *corticosteroidal anti-inflammatory* [hydrocortisone] 2.5%

texacromil INN

tezacitabine USAN *antineoplastic for colon and rectal cancers; investigational (orphan) for adenocarcinoma of the esophagus and stomach*

6-TG (6-thioguanine) [see: thioguanine]

TG (thyroglobulin) [q.v.]

T-Gen suppositories, pediatric suppositories (removed from the market in 2007 due to lack of efficacy) ℞ *anticholinergic; post-surgical antiemetic; local anesthetic* [trimethobenzamide HCl; benzocaine] 200 mg•2%; 100 mg•2% ⚠ Tequin; Ticon; Tigan

T-Gesic capsules ℞ *narcotic analgesic; antipyretic* [hydrocodone bitartrate; acetaminophen] 5•500 mg

αTGI (α-triglycidyl isocyanurate) [see: teroxirone]

TH (theophylline) [q.v.]

TH (thyroid hormone) [see: levothyroxine sodium]

THA (tetrahydroaminoacridine or tetrahydroacridinamine) [see: tacrine HCl]

thalidomide USAN, INN, BAN *immunomodulator for erythema nodosum leprosum (ENL; orphan) and multiple myeloma (orphan); investigational (orphan) for aphthous ulcers, graft vs. host disease, AIDS-wasting syndrome,*

Crohn disease, mycobacterial infections, and various cancers

Thalitone tablets ℞ *antihypertensive; diuretic* [chlorthalidone] 15 mg

thallium *element (Tl)* ⧠ thulium

thallous chloride Tl 201 USAN, USP *radiopaque contrast medium; radioactive agent*

Thalomid capsules ℞ *immunomodulator for erythema nodosum leprosum (ENL; orphan) and multiple myeloma (orphan); investigational (orphan) for aphthous ulcers, graft vs. host disease, AIDS-wasting syndrome, Crohn disease, mycobacterial infections, and various cancers* [thalidomide] 50, 100, 200 mg

Tham IV infusion ℞ *systemic alkalizer; corrects acidosis associated with cardiac bypass surgery or cardiac arrest* [tromethamine] 18 g/500 mL (150 mEq/500 mL)

thaumatin BAN

THC (tetrahydrocannabinol) [q.v.]

THC (thiocarbanidin)

theanine (L-theanine) *natural extract of green tea that produces calming and relaxing effects without drowsiness; effective in controlling PMS symptoms; increases brain levels of the neurotransmitters GABA and dopamine, which increase alpha brain wave activity*

thebacon INN, BAN ⧠ tebuquine

theine [see: caffeine]

Thelin *endothelin receptor antagonist (ERA) vasodilator; investigational (NDA filed) once-daily oral antihypertensive for pulmonary arterial hypertension (PAH)* [sitaxsentan sodium]

thenalidine INN ⧠ tenylidone

thenium closilate INN *veterinary anthelmintic* [also: thenium closylate]

thenium closylate USAN *veterinary anthelmintic* [also: thenium closilate]

thenyldiamine INN

thenylpyramine HCl [see: methapyrilene HCl]

Theo-24 extended-release capsules ℞ *antiasthmatic; bronchodilator* [theophylline] 100, 200, 300, 400 mg

Theobid Duracaps (sustained-release capsules) (discontinued 2004) ℞ *antiasthmatic; bronchodilator* [theophylline] 260 mg

theobromine NF

theobromine calcium salicylate NF

theobromine sodium acetate NF

theobromine sodium salicylate NF

Theobromo cacao medicinal herb [see: cocoa]

Theochron extended-release tablets ℞ *antiasthmatic; bronchodilator* [theophylline] 100, 200, 300, 450 mg ⧠ tacrine

theoclate BAN *combining name for radicals or groups* [also: teoclate]

Theoclear L.A. extended-release capsules (discontinued 2004) ℞ *antiasthmatic; bronchodilator* [theophylline] 130, 260 mg

Theoclear-80 oral solution (discontinued 2004) ℞ *antiasthmatic; bronchodilator* [theophylline] 80 mg/15 mL

theodrenaline INN, BAN

Theodrine tablets (discontinued 2007) OTC *antiasthmatic; bronchodilator; decongestant* [theophylline; ephedrine HCl] 120•22.5 mg

theofibrate USAN *antihyperlipoproteinemic* [also: etofylline clofibrate]

Theolair oral liquid (discontinued 2004) ℞ *antiasthmatic; bronchodilator* [theophylline] 80 mg/15 mL

Theolair tablets (discontinued 2008) ℞ *antiasthmatic; bronchodilator* [theophylline] 125 mg

Theolair-SR sustained-release tablets (discontinued 2008) ℞ *antiasthmatic; bronchodilator* [theophylline] 200, 250, 300, 500 mg

Theolate oral liquid (discontinued 2007) ℞ *antiasthmatic; bronchodilator; expectorant* [theophylline; guaifenesin] 150•90 mg/15 mL ⧠ Twilite

Theomax DF pediatric syrup (discontinued 2007) ℞ *antiasthmatic; bronchodilator; decongestant; antihistamine* [theophylline; ephedrine sulfate; hydroxyzine HCl; alcohol 5%] 97.5•18.75•7.5 mg/15 mL

theophyldine [see: aminophylline]

theophyllamine [see: aminophylline]

Theophyllin KI elixir (discontinued 2007) ℞ *antiasthmatic; bronchodilator; expectorant* [theophylline; potassium iodide] 80•130 mg/15 mL

theophylline (TH) USP, BAN *bronchodilator* 100, 125, 200, 300, 450 mg oral; 0.8, 1.6, 2, 3.2, 4 mg/mL injection

theophylline aminoisobutanol [see: ambuphylline]

theophylline calcium salicylate *bronchodilator*

theophylline ethylenediamine [now: aminophylline]

theophylline monohydrate [see: theophylline]

theophylline olamine USP

theophylline sodium acetate NF

theophylline sodium glycinate USP *smooth muscle relaxant*

Theo-Sav controlled-release tablets (discontinued 2004) ℞ *antiasthmatic; bronchodilator* [theophylline] 100, 200, 300 mg

Theovent timed-release capsules (discontinued 2004) ℞ *antiasthmatic; bronchodilator* [theophylline] 125, 250 mg ⊡ thiophanate

Theo-X controlled-release tablets (discontinued 2004) ℞ *antiasthmatic; bronchodilator* [theophylline] 100, 200, 300 mg ⊡ Tucks

Thera Hematinic tablets OTC *hematinic; vitamin supplement* [ferrous fumarate; multiple vitamins; folic acid] 66.7•±•0.33 mg

Thera Multi-Vitamin oral liquid OTC *vitamin supplement* [multiple vitamins]

Therabid tablets OTC *vitamin supplement* [multiple vitamins] ⊡ Tripedia

Therac lotion (discontinued 2004) OTC *antiseptic and keratolytic for acne* [colloidal sulfur] 10% ⊡ Tarka; Touro CC; Tri-K

theraccines *a class of vaccines with therapeutic action, usually used to help prevent the spread of cancer*

TheraCLEC-Total *investigational (orphan) for pancreatic insufficiency* [digestive enzymes (amylase; lipase; protease)]

TheraCys powder for intravesical instillation ℞ *antineoplastic for urinary bladder cancer* [BCG vaccine, live] 81 mg (1.8–19.2 × 10⁸ CFU)

TheraDerm transdermal patch *investigational (Phase II, orphan) for AIDS-wasting syndrome* [testosterone]

Therafectin *investigational (NDA filed) synthetic monosaccharide anti-inflammatory for rheumatoid arthritis* [amiprilose HCl]

TheraFlu Cold & Cough powder for oral solution OTC *antitussive; antihistamine; decongestant* [dextromethorphan hydrobromide; pheniramine maleate; phenylephrine HCl] 20•20•20 mg/pkt.

TheraFlu Cold & Sore Throat powder for oral solution OTC *decongestant; antihistamine; analgesic; antipyretic* [phenylephrine HCl; pheniramine maleate; acetaminophen] 10•20•325 mg/pkt.

TheraFlu Daytime Severe Cold powder for oral solution OTC *decongestant; analgesic; antipyretic* [phenylephrine HCl; acetaminophen] 10•650 mg/pkt.

TheraFlu Flu, Cold & Cough Night Time; TheraFlu Flu, Cold & Cough, and Sore Throat; TheraFlu Severe Cold & Cough; TheraFlu Severe Cold & Congestion powder for oral solution (discontinued 2007) OTC *antitussive; antihistamine; decongestant; analgesic; antipyretic* [dextromethorphan hydrobromide; chlorpheniramine maleate; pseudoephedrine HCl; acetaminophen] 20•4•60•1000 mg/pkt.

TheraFlu Flu & Chest Congestion powder for oral solution OTC *expectorant; analgesic; antipyretic* [guaifenesin; acetaminophen] 400•1000 mg

TheraFlu Flu & Chest Congestion Non-Drowsy; TheraFlu Flu, Cold & Cough powder for oral solution (discontinued 2007) OTC *antitussive;*

decongestant; expectorant; analgesic; antipyretic [dextromethorphan hydrobromide; pseudoephedrine HCl; guaifenesin; acetaminophen] 30•60•400•1000 mg/pkt

TheraFlu Flu & Cold Medicine for Sore Throat powder for oral solution (discontinued 2007) oTc decongestant; antihistamine; analgesic [pseudoephedrine HCl; chlorpheniramine maleate; acetaminophen] 60•4•1000 mg/pkt.

TheraFlu Flu & Cold Medicine Original Formula powder for oral solution (discontinued 2006) oTc decongestant; antihistamine; analgesic; antipyretic [pseudoephedrine HCl; chlorpheniramine maleate; acetaminophen] 60•4•650 mg/pkt.

TheraFlu Flu & Cough Night Time powder for oral solution (discontinued 2005) oTc antitussive; antihistamine; decongestant; analgesic; antipyretic [dextromethorphan hydrobromide; chlorpheniramine maleate; pseudoephedrine HCl; acetaminophen] 20•4•60•1000 mg/pkt.

TheraFlu Flu & Sore Throat powder for oral solution oTc decongestant; antihistamine; analgesic; antipyretic [phenylephrine HCl; pheniramine maleate; acetaminophen] 10•20•650 mg/pkt.

TheraFlu Flu & Sore Throat; TheraFlu Flu & Sore Throat Night Time powder for oral solution (discontinued 2006) oTc decongestant; antihistamine; analgesic [pseudoephedrine HCl; chlorpheniramine maleate; acetaminophen] 60•4•1000 mg/pkt.

TheraFlu Nighttime Severe Cold caplets oTc antitussive; decongestant; antihistamine; decongestant; analgesic; antipyretic [dextromethorphan hydrobromide; chlorpheniramine maleate; phenylephrine HCl; acetaminophen] 10•2•5•325 mg

TheraFlu Nighttime Severe Cold powder for oral solution oTc decongestant; antihistamine; analgesic; anti-

pyretic [phenylephrine HCl; pheniramine maleate; acetaminophen] 10•20•650 mg/pkt.

TheraFlu Non-Drowsy Flu, Cold & Cough; Theraflu Severe Cold Non-Drowsy; TheraFlu Severe Cold & Congestion Non-Drowsy powder for oral solution (discontinued 2007) oTc antitussive; decongestant; analgesic; antipyretic [dextromethorphan hydrobromide; pseudoephedrine HCl; acetaminophen] 30•60•1000 mg/pkt.

TheraFlu Severe Cold caplets (discontinued 2007) oTc antitussive; decongestant; antihistamine; decongestant; analgesic; antipyretic [dextromethorphan hydrobromide; chlorpheniramine maleate; pseudoephedrine HCl; acetaminophen] 15•2•30•500 mg

TheraFlu Severe Cold Non-Drowsy caplets, powder for oral solution (discontinued 2007) oTc antitussive; decongestant; analgesic; antipyretic [dextromethorphan hydrobromide; pseudoephedrine HCl; acetaminophen] 15•30•500 mg; 30•60•1000 mg/pkt.

Theraflu Thin Strips Daytime Cough & Cold orally disintegrating film oTc antitussive; decongestant [dextromethorphan hydrobromide; phenylephrine HCl] 20•10 mg

TheraFlu Thin Strips Long Acting Cough orally disintegrating film oTc antitussive [dextromethorphan hydrobromide] 15 mg

TheraFlu Thin Strips Multi Symptom orally disintegrating film (discontinued 2007) oTc antitussive; antihistamine; sleep aid [diphenhydramine HCl] 25 mg

Theraflu Thin Strips Nighttime Cold & Cough orally disintegrating film oTc decongestant; antihistamine; sleep aid [phenylephrine HCl; diphenhydramine HCl] 10•25 mg

TheraFlu Vapor Stick; TheraFlu Vapor Stick Cough & Muscle

Aches (discontinued 2007) OTC *mild anesthetic; antipruritic; counterirritant* [camphor; menthol] 4.8%•2.6%

Thera-Flur; Thera-Flur-N gel for self-application ℞ *dental caries preventative* [sodium fluoride] 1.1%

Thera-Gesic cream OTC *analgesic; mild anesthetic; antipruritic; counterirritant* [methyl salicylate; menthol] 15%•≛

Theragran caplets OTC *vitamin supplement* [multiple vitamins; folic acid; biotin] ≛•400•30 mcg

Theragran oral liquid OTC *vitamin supplement* [multiple vitamins]

Theragran AntiOxidant softgels OTC *vitamin/mineral supplement* [vitamins A, C, and E; multiple minerals] 5000 IU•250 mg•200 IU•≛

Theragran Stress Formula tablets OTC *vitamin/iron supplement* [multiple B vitamins; vitamins C and E; ferrous fumarate; folic acid; biotin] ≛•600 mg•30 IU•27 mg•0.4 mg•45 mcg

Theragran-M caplets (discontinued 2005) OTC *vitamin/mineral/calcium/iron supplement* [multiple vitamins & minerals; calcium; iron; folic acid; biotin] ≛•40•27•0.4•0.03 mg

Theragyn *investigational (Phase III, orphan) adjunctive treatment for ovarian cancer* [monoclonal antibody to polymorphic epithelial mucin, murine]

Thera-Hist Cold & Allergy pediatric syrup (discontinued 2007) OTC *decongestant; antihistamine* [pseudoephedrine HCl; chlorpheniramine maleate] 30•2 mg/10 mL

Thera-Hist Cold & Cough syrup (discontinued 2007) OTC *antitussive; antihistamine; decongestant* [dextromethorphan hydrobromide; chlorpheniramine maleate; pseudoephedrine HCl] 10•2•30 mg/10 mL

Thera-Hist Expectorant Chest Congestion pediatric oral liquid (discontinued 2007) OTC *decongestant; expectorant* [pseudoephedrine HCl; guaifenesin] 15•50 mg/5 mL

Thera-Ject (trademarked delivery form) *prefilled disposable syringe*

Thera-M tablets OTC *vitamin/mineral/iron supplement* [multiple vitamins & minerals; iron; folic acid; biotin] ≛• 27 mg•0.4 mg•35 mcg ⚠ thiram; thorium; Triam-A

TheraPatch patch OTC *analgesic; mild anesthetic; antipruritic; counterirritant* [methyl salicylate; menthol; camphor]

TheraPatch Cold Sore transmucosal patch OTC *mucous membrane anesthetic; antipruritic; counterirritant; emollient* [lidocaine; camphor; aloe vera; eucalyptus oil] 4%•0.5%•≛•≛

TheraPatch Vapor Patch for Kids Cough Suppressant (discontinued 2007) OTC *mild anesthetic; antipruritic; counterirritant* [camphor; menthol] 4.7%•2.6%

Therapeutic tablets OTC *vitamin supplement* [multiple vitamins; folic acid; biotin] ≛•400•30 mcg

Therapeutic B with C capsules (discontinued 2008) OTC *vitamin supplement* [multiple B vitamins; vitamin C] ≛•300 mg

Therapeutic Bath lotion, oil OTC *moisturizer; emollient*

Therapeutic Mineral Ice; Therapeutic Mineral Ice Exercise Formula gel OTC *mild anesthetic; antipruritic; counterirritant* [menthol] 2%; 4%

Therapeutic-H tablets OTC *hematinic; vitamin supplement* [ferrous fumarate; multiple vitamins; folic acid] 66.7• ≛•0.33 mg

Therapeutic-M tablets OTC *vitamin/mineral/iron supplement* [multiple vitamins & minerals; iron; folic acid; biotin] ≛•27 mg•0.4 mg•30 mcg

Therapy Ice gel OTC *mild anesthetic; antipruritic; counterirritant* [menthol] 2%

Theraseed (name changed to **BrachySeed Pd-103** upon marketing release in 2004)

TheraTears ophthalmic gel OTC *ocular moisturizer/lubricant* [carboxymethylcellulose sodium] 1%

Theratope-STn *investigational (Phase III) theraccine for adenocarcinoma*

Theravee tablets OTC *vitamin supplement* [multiple vitamins; folic acid; biotin] ≗•400•15 mcg ⊠ Thrive

Theravee Hematinic tablets OTC *hematinic; vitamin supplement* [ferrous fumarate; multiple vitamins; folic acid] 66.7•≗•0.33 mg

Theravee-M tablets OTC *vitamin/mineral/iron supplement* [multiple vitamins & minerals; iron; folic acid; biotin] ≗•27 mg•0.4 mg•15 mcg

Theravim tablets OTC *vitamin supplement* [multiple vitamins; folic acid; biotin] ≗•400•35 mcg

Theravim-M tablets OTC *vitamin/mineral/iron supplement* [multiple vitamins & minerals; iron; folic acid; biotin] ≗•27 mg•0.4 mg•30 mcg

Theravite oral liquid OTC *vitamin supplement* [multiple vitamins]

Therems tablets OTC *vitamin supplement* [multiple vitamins; folic acid; biotin] ≗•400•15 mcg

Therems-M tablets OTC *vitamin/mineral/iron supplement* [multiple vitamins & minerals; iron; folic acid; biotin] ≗•27 mg•0.4 mg•30 mcg

Therevac-Plus disposable enema OTC *hyperosmotic laxative; stool softener; local anesthetic* [glycerin; docusate sodium; benzocaine] 275•283•20 mg

Therevac-SB disposable enema OTC *hyperosmotic laxative; stool softener* [glycerin; docusate sodium] 275•283 mg

Thermazene cream ℞ *broad-spectrum bactericidal for adjunctive burn treatment* [silver sulfadiazine] 10 mg/g ⊠ Terramycin; Trimo-San

ThexForte caplets OTC *vitamin supplement* [multiple B vitamins; vitamin C] ≗•500 mg

THF (thymic humoral factor) [q.v.]

thiabendazole (TBZ) USAN, USP *anthelmintic for strongyloidiasis (threadworm), larva migrans, and trichinosis* [also: tiabendazole]

thiabutazide [see: buthiazide]

thiacetarsamide sodium INN

thiacetazone BAN [also: thioacetazone]

thialbarbital INN [also: thialbarbitone]

thialbarbitone BAN [also: thialbarbital]

thialisobumal sodium [see: buthalital sodium]

thiamazole INN *thyroid inhibitor* [also: methimazole] ⊠ Timecelle

thiambutosine INN, BAN

Thiamilate enteric-coated tablets OTC *vitamin B_1 supplement* [thiamine HCl] 20 mg

thiamine (vitamin B_1) INN *water-soluble vitamin; enzyme cofactor* [also: thiamine HCl; compare: benfotiamine]

thiamine HCl (vitamin B_1) USP *water-soluble vitamin; enzyme cofactor* [also: thiamine; compare: benfotiamine] 50, 100, 250 mg oral; 100 mg/mL injection

thiamine mononitrate USP *vitamin B_1; enzyme cofactor*

thiamine propyl disulfide [see: prosultiamine]

thiaminogen *medicinal herb* [see: rice bran oil]

thiamiprine USAN *antineoplastic* [also: tiamiprine] ⊠ timiperone

thiamphenicol USAN, INN, BAN *antibacterial*

thiamylal USP *barbiturate general anesthetic* ⊠ timolol

thiamylal sodium USP, JAN *barbiturate general anesthetic*

thiazesim HCl USAN *antidepressant* [also: tiazesim]

thiazides *a class of diuretic agents that increase urinary excretion of sodium and chloride in approximately equal amounts* ⊠ Tussi-12D S; TZDs

thiazinamium chloride USAN *antiallergic*

thiazinamium metilsulfate INN

4-thiazolidinecarboxylic acid [see: timonacic]

thiazolidinediones (TZDs) *a class of antidiabetic agents that increase cellular response to insulin without increasing insulin secretion*

thiazolsulfone [see: thiazosulfone]

thiazosulfone INN

thiazothielite [see: antienite]

thiazothienol [see: antazonite]

thienamycins *a class of antibiotics*

thienobenzodiazepines *a class of novel (atypical) antipsychotic agents*

thiethylperazine USAN, INN *antiemetic; antidopaminergic*

thiethylperazine malate USP *antiemetic; antipsychotic*

thiethylperazine maleate USAN, USP *antiemetic for postoperative nausea and vomiting*

thihexinol methylbromide NF, INN

thimbleberry *medicinal herb* [see: blackberry]

thimerfonate sodium USAN *topical anti-infective* [also: sodium timerfonate]

thimerosal USP *topical anti-infective; preservative (49% mercury)* [also: thiomersal] 1:1000 topical

thioacetazone INN [also: thiacetazone]

thiocarbanidin (THC)

thiocarlide BAN [also: tiocarlide]

thiocolchicine glycoside [see: thiocolchicoside]

thiocolchicoside INN

thioctan; thioctacid; thioctic acid *natural antioxidant* [see: alpha lipoic acid]

thiocyanate sodium NF

thiodiglycol INN

thiodiphenylamine [see: phenothiazine]

thiofuradene INN

thioguanine (6-TG) USAN, USP *antimetabolite antineoplastic for acute nonlymphocytic leukemias (ANLL); also used for psoriasis, ulcerative colitis, and Crohn disease* [also: tioguanine]

thiohexallymal [see: thialbarbital]

thiohexamide INN

Thiola *sugar-coated tablets* ℞ *prevention of cystine nephrolithiasis in homozygous cystinuria (orphan)* [tiopronin] 100 mg

thiomebumal sodium [see: thiopental sodium]

thiomersal INN, BAN *topical anti-infective; preservative* [also: thimerosal]

thiomesterone BAN [also: tiomesterone]

thiomicid [see: thioacetazone; thiacetazone]

thioparamizone [see: thioacetazone; thiacetazone]

thiopental sodium USP, INN, JAN *barbiturate general anesthetic; anticonvulsant* [also: thiopentone sodium] 2%, 2.5% (20, 25 mg/mL) injection

thiopentone sodium BAN *general anesthetic; anticonvulsant* [also: thiopental sodium]

thiophanate BAN ⧉ Theovent

thiophosphoramide [see: thiotepa]

Thioplex *powder for IV, intracavitary, or intravesical injection* ℞ *alkylating antineoplastic for lymphomas and carcinoma of the breast, ovary, or bladder* [thiotepa] 15 mg

thiopropazate INN [also: thiopropazate HCl]

thiopropazate HCl NF [also: thiopropazate]

thioproperazine INN, BAN *phenothiazine antipsychotic* [also: thioproperazine mesylate]

thioproperazine mesylate *phenothiazine antipsychotic* [also: thioproperazine]

thioproperazine methanesulfonate [see: thioproperazine mesylate]

thioridazine USAN, USP, INN *conventional (typical) phenothiazine antipsychotic for schizophrenia; sedative*

thioridazine HCl USP *conventional (typical) phenothiazine antipsychotic for schizophrenia; sedative; also used for agitation or psychosis due to Alzheimer or other dementias* 10, 15, 25, 50, 100, 150, 200 mg oral

thiosalan USAN *disinfectant* [also: tiosalan] ⧉ Tessalon

thiosulfuric acid, disodium salt pentahydrate [see: sodium thiosulfate]

thiotepa USP, INN, BAN, JAN *alkylating antineoplastic for lymphomas and carcinoma of the breast, ovary, or bladder* 15, 30 mg/vial injection

thiotetrabarbital INN

thiothixene USAN, USP, BAN *conventional (typical) thioxanthene antipsy-*

chotic for schizophrenia [also: tiotix-ene] 1, 2, 5, 10 mg oral

thiothixene HCl USAN, USP *conventional (typical) thioxanthene antipsychotic for schizophrenia*

thiouracil 🔁 Tearisol; Terazol 3

thiourea *antioxidant*

thioxanthenes *a class of dopamine receptor antagonists with conventional (typical) antipsychotic activity*

thioxolone BAN [also: tioxolone]

thiphenamil HCl USAN *smooth muscle relaxant* [also: tifenamil]

thiphencillin potassium USAN *antibacterial* [also: tifencillin]

thiram USAN, INN *antifungal* 🔁 Thera-M; thorium; Triam-A

thistle, bitter; holy thistle; Saint Benedict thistle; spotted thistle *medicinal herb* [see: blessed thistle]

thistle, carline; ground thistle *medicinal herb* [see: carline thistle]

thonzonium bromide USAN, USP *detergent; surface-active agent* [also: tonzonium bromide]

thonzylamine HCl USAN, INN

Thorazine tablets, IV or IM injection, suppositories (discontinued 2008) ℞ *conventional antipsychotic for schizophrenia, manic episodes of a bipolar disorder, pediatric hyperactivity, and severe pediatric behavioral problems; treatment for acute intermittent porphyria, nausea/vomiting, and intractable hiccoughs* [chlorpromazine] 25, 50, 100, 200 mg; 25 mg/mL; 100 mg 🔁 Trisan; tyrosine

thorium *element (Th)* 🔁 Thera-M; thiram; Triam-A

thorn, Egyptian *medicinal herb* [see: acacia]

thorn-apple *medicinal herb* [see: hawthorn; jimsonweed]

thousand-leaf; thousand seal *medicinal herb* [see: yarrow]

thozalinone USAN *antidepressant* [also: tozalinone]

THQ (tetrahydroxybenzoquinone) [see: tetroquinone]

THR (trishydroxyethyl rutin) [see: troxerutin]

3 in 1 Toothache Relief topical liquid, gum, oral lotion/gel OTC *mucous membrane anesthetic* [benzocaine]

three-leaved nightshade *medicinal herb* [see: birthroot]

3TC [now: lamivudine]

threonine (L-threonine) USAN, USP, INN *essential amino acid; symbols: Thr, T; investigational (orphan) for familial spastic paraparesis and amyotrophic lateral sclerosis* 500 mg oral

Threostat *investigational (orphan) for familial spastic paraparesis and amyotrophic lateral sclerosis* [L-threonine]

Thrive chewing gum OTC *smoking cessation aid for the relief of nicotine withdrawal symptoms* [nicotine polacrilex] 2, 4 mg 🔁 Theravee

Throat Discs lozenges OTC *analgesic; counterirritant* [capsicum; peppermint oil]

throatwort *medicinal herb* [see: figwort; foxglove]

Thrombate III powder for IV infusion ℞ *for thrombosis and pulmonary emboli due to congenital aT-III deficiency (orphan)* [antithrombin III] 500, 1000 IU

thrombin USP, INN *topical hemostat*

Thrombinar powder ℞ *topical hemostat for surgery* [thrombin] 1000, 5000, 50 000 IU

Thrombin-JMI powder (discontinued 2004) ℞ *topical hemostat for surgery* [thrombin] 10 000, 20 000, 50 000 IU

thrombinogen (prothrombin)

Thrombogen powder (discontinued 2008) ℞ *topical hemostat for surgery* [thrombin] 1000, 5000, 10 000, 20 000 IU

thrombolytics *a class of enzymes that dissolve blood clots, used emergently to treat stroke, pulmonary embolus, and myocardial infarct*

thromboplastin USP

thrombopoietin, recombinant human *investigational (orphan)* adjunct to hematopoietic stem cell transplantation

Thrombostat powder ℞ *topical hemostat for surgery* [thrombin] 5000, 10 000, 20 000 IU

throw-wort *medicinal herb* [see: motherwort]

thulium *element (Tm)* ▣ thallium

thunder god vine (Tripterygium wilfordii) *plant medicinal herb for abscesses, autoimmune diseases, boils, fever, inflammation, tumors, and viruses; also used as an insecticide to kill maggots or larvae and as a rat and bird poison* [also: triptolide]

thymalfasin USAN *vaccine enhancer for hepatitis C, cancer, and infectious diseases; investigational (Phase III, orphan) for chronic active hepatitis B; investigational (orphan) for DiGeorge syndrome with immune defects and hepatocellular carcinoma; investigational (Phase II) for AIDS*

thyme (Thymus serpyllum; T. vulgaris) *plant medicinal herb for acute bronchitis, colic, digestive disorders, gas, gout, headache, laryngitis, lung congestion, sciatica, and throat disorders*

thymic tissue for transplantation, cultured, partially T-cell depleted *investigational (orphan) agent for primary immune deficiency due to athymia associated with DiGeorge syndrome*

thymidylate synthase (TS) inhibitors *a class of folate-based antineoplastics*

Thymitaq *thymidylate synthase inhibitor that disrupts DNA replication; investigational (Phase III, orphan) for inoperable primary liver cancer* [nolatrexed dihydrochloride]

thymocartin INN

thymoctonan INN *antiviral*

Thymoglobulin powder for IV infusion ℞ *passive immunizing agent to prevent allograft rejection of renal transplants (orphan); investigational (orphan) for myelodysplastic syndrome (MDS); also used for other transplants and aplastic anemia* [antithymocyte globulin, rabbit] 25 mg

thymol NF *stabilizer; topical antiseptic*

thymol iodide NF

thymopentin USAN, INN, BAN *immunoregulator; investigational (Phase III) for asymptomatic HIV infection*

thymopoietin 32-36 [now: thymopentin]

thymosin alpha-1 [now: thymalfasin]

thymosin beta-4 *investigational (orphan) for epidermolysis bullosa*

thymostimulin INN *immunomodulator*

thymotrinan INN

thymoxamine BAN [also: moxisylyte]

thymoxamine HCl *investigational (orphan) to reverse phenylephrine-induced mydriasis in patients at risk for acute angle-closure glaucoma*

Thymus serpyllum; T. vulgaris *medicinal herb* [see: thyme]

Thyro-Block tablets ℞ *thyroid-blocking therapy* [potassium iodide] 130 mg

thyrocalcitonin [see: calcitonin]

Thyrogen powder for IM injection ℞ *recombinant human thyroid-stimulating hormone (rhTSH); diagnostic aid for thyroid cancer (orphan); adjunctive treatment for thyroid cancer (orphan)* [thyrotropin alfa] 1.1 mg ▣ tarragon; Torecan; Trocaine

thyroglobulin (TG) USAN, USP, INN *thyroid hormone for hypothyroidism or thyroid cancer*

thyroid USP *natural thyroid hormone (a 4:1 mixture of T_4 and T_3)* 32.5, 65, 130, 195 mg oral ▣ Triad

thyroid hormone (TH) [see: levothyroxine sodium]

thyroid-stimulating hormone (TSH) [see: thyrotropin]

Thyrolar tablets ℞ *synthetic thyroid hormone (a 4:1 mixture of T_4 and T_3)* [liotrix] 15, 30, 60, 120, 180 mg

thyromedan HCl USAN *thyromimetic* [also: tyromedan]

thyropropic acid INN

ThyroShield oral solution OTC *thyroid saturation agent to block the uptake of radioactive iodine after a nuclear accident or attack (orphan)* [potassium iodide] 65 mg/mL

Thyro-Tabs tablets ℞ *synthetic thyroid hormone (T_4 fraction only)* [levothyroxine sodium] 25, 50, 75, 88, 100, 112, 125, 150, 175, 200, 300 mcg

thyrotrophic hormone [see: thyrotrophin]

thyrotrophin INN *thyroid-stimulating hormone* [also: thyrotropin]

thyrotropin *thyroid-stimulating hormone; in vivo diagnostic aid for thyroid function* [also: thyrotrophin]

thyrotropin alfa USAN *recombinant human thyroid-stimulating hormone (rhTSH); diagnostic aid for thyroid cancer (orphan); adjunctive treatment for thyroid cancer (orphan)*

thyrotropin-releasing hormone (TRH) [see: protirelin]

thyroxine BAN *synthetic thyroid hormone (T_4 fraction only)* [also: levothyroxine sodium]

D-thyroxine [see: dextrothyroxine sodium]

L-thyroxine [see: levothyroxine sodium]

thyroxine I 125 USAN *radioactive agent*

thyroxine I 131 USAN *radioactive agent*

tiabendazole INN *anthelmintic* [also: thiabendazole]

tiacrilast USAN, INN *antiallergic*

tiacrilast sodium USAN *antiallergic*

tiadenol INN

tiafibrate INN

tiagabine INN *anticonvulsant; adjunctive treatment for partial seizures*

tiagabine HCl USAN *anticonvulsant; adjunctive treatment for partial seizures*

tiamenidine USAN, INN *antihypertensive*

tiamenidine HCl USAN *antihypertensive*

tiametonium iodide INN

tiamiprine INN *antineoplastic* [also: thiamiprine]

tiamizide INN *diuretic; antihypertensive* [also: diapamide]

tiamulin USAN, INN *veterinary antibacterial*

tiamulin fumarate USAN *veterinary antibacterial*

tianafac INN

tianeptine INN

tiapamil INN, BAN *antagonist to calcium* [also: tiapamil HCl]

tiapamil HCl USAN *antagonist to calcium* [also: tiapamil]

tiapirinol INN

tiapride INN *investigational (orphan) for Tourette syndrome*

tiaprofenic acid INN *nonsteroidal anti-inflammatory drug (NSAID)*

tiaprost INN

tiaramide INN, BAN *antiasthmatic* [also: tiaramide HCl]

tiaramide HCl USAN *antiasthmatic* [also: tiaramide]

Tiazac extended-release capsules ℞ *antihypertensive; antianginal; antiarrhythmic; calcium channel blocker* [diltiazem HCl] 120, 180, 240, 300, 360, 420 mg

tiazesim INN *antidepressant* [also: thiazesim HCl]

tiazesim HCl [see: thiazesim HCl]

tiazofurin USAN *investigational (Phase II/III, orphan) antineoplastic for chronic myelogenous leukemia* [also: tiazofurine]

tiazofurine INN *antineoplastic* [also: tiazofurin]

tiazuril USAN, INN *coccidiostat for poultry*

tibalosin INN

Tibamine LA sustained-release tablets ℞ *decongestant; antihistamine* [pseudoephedrine HCl; chlorpheniramine maleate] 120•12 mg

tibenelast sodium USAN *antiasthmatic; bronchodilator*

tibenzate INN

tibezonium iodide INN

tibolone USAN, INN, BAN *investigational (NDA filed) synthetic steroid for osteoporosis and other postmenopausal symptoms*

tibric acid USAN, INN *antihyperlipoproteinemic*

tibrofan USAN, INN *disinfectant*

ticabesone INN *corticosteroid; anti-inflammatory* [also: ticabesone propionate]

ticabesone propionate USAN *corticosteroid; anti-inflammatory* [also: ticabesone]

Ticar powder for IV or IM injection ℞ *extended-spectrum penicillin antibiotic* [ticarcillin disodium] 3 g/vial

ticarbodine USAN, INN *anthelmintic*

ticarcillin INN *extended-spectrum penicillin antibiotic* [also: ticarcillin disodium]

ticarcillin cresyl sodium USAN *extended-spectrum penicillin antibiotic*

ticarcillin disodium USAN, USP *extended-spectrum penicillin antibiotic* [also: ticarcillin]

Tice BCG powder for intravesical instillation ℞ *antineoplastic for urinary bladder cancer* [BCG vaccine, Tice strain] 50 mg (1–8 × 10⁸ CFU)

Tice BCG vaccine [see: BCG vaccine]

tickweed *medicinal herb* [see: pennyroyal]

ticlatone USAN, INN *antibacterial; antifungal*

Ticlid film-coated tablets ℞ *platelet aggregation inhibitor for stroke* [ticlopidine HCl] 250 mg

ticlopidine INN, BAN *platelet aggregation inhibitor* [also: ticlopidine HCl]

ticlopidine HCl USAN *platelet aggregation inhibitor for stroke* [also: ticlopidine] 250 mg oral

ticolubant USAN *leukotriene B₄ receptor antagonist for psoriasis*

Ticon IM injection (discontinued 2005) ℞ *anticholinergic; post-surgical antiemetic* [trimethobenzamide HCl] 100 mg/mL ☒ Tequin; Tigan

ticrynafen USAN *diuretic; uricosuric; antihypertensive* [also: tienilic acid]

Tidefen DM extended-release caplets ℞ *antitussive; decongestant; expectorant* [dextromethorphan hydrobromide; pseudoephedrine HCl; guaifenesin] 60•90•800 mg

tidembersat USAN *antimigraine*

tidiacic INN

tiemonium iodide INN, BAN

tienilic acid INN *diuretic; uricosuric; antihypertensive* [also: ticrynafen]

tienocarbine INN

tienopramine INN

tienoxolol INN

tifacogin USAN *anticoagulant; lipoprotein-associated coagulation inhibitor (LACI); recombinant tissue factor pathway inhibitor*

tifemoxone INN

tifenamil INN *smooth muscle relaxant* [also: thiphenamil HCl]

tifenamil HCl [see: thiphenamil HCl]

tifencillin INN *antibacterial* [also: thiphencillin potassium]

tifencillin potassium [see: thiphencillin potassium]

tiflamizole INN

tiflorex INN

tifluadom INN

tiflucarbine INN

Tifolar (name changed to **Alimta** upon marketing release in 2004)

tiformin INN [also: tyformin]

tifurac INN *analgesic* [also: tifurac sodium]

tifurac sodium USAN *analgesic* [also: tifurac]

TIG (tetanus immune globulin) [q.v.]

Tigan capsules, IM injection ℞ *anticholinergic; post-surgical antiemetic* [trimethobenzamide HCl] 300 mg; 100 mg/mL ☒ Tequin; Ticon

Tigan suppositories, pediatric suppositories (removed from the market in 2007 due to lack of efficacy) ℞ *anticholinergic; post-surgical antiemetic; local anesthetic* [trimethobenzamide HCl; benzocaine] 200 mg•2%; 100 mg•2% ☒ Tequin; Ticon

tigecycline *broad-spectrum glycylcycline antibiotic for intra-abdominal and complicated skin structure infections and methicillin-resistant* Staphylococcus aureus *(MRSA); investigational (Phase III) for pneumonia*

tigemonam INN *antimicrobial* [also: tigemonam dicholine]

tigemonam dicholine USAN *antimicrobial* [also: tigemonam]

tigestol USAN, INN *progestin*

tigloidine INN, BAN

tiglylpseudotropine [see: tigloidine]

tiglyltropeine [see: tropigline]

Tikosyn capsules ℞ *antiarrhythmic; potassium channel blocker* [dofetilide] 125, 250, 500 mcg ⊡ toquizine

tilactase INN *digestive enzyme*

Tilad ⓔⓤⓡ (Spanish name for U.S. product **Tilade**)

Tilade oral inhalation aerosol (discontinued 2008) ℞ *respiratory antiinflammatory; mast cell stabilizer; antiasthmatic; bronchodilator* [nedocromil sodium] 1.75 mg/dose

tilarginine acetate *investigational (Phase III) nitric oxide inhibitor for the treatment of cardiogenic shock*

tilbroquinol INN

tiletamine INN *anesthetic; anticonvulsant* [also: tiletamine HCl]

tiletamine HCl USAN *anesthetic; anticonvulsant* [also: tiletamine]

Tilia americana; T. cordata; T. europaea; T. platyphyllos **medicinal herb** [see: linden tree]

Tilia Fe tablets (in packs of 28) ℞ *triphasic oral contraceptive; iron supplement* [norethindrone acetate; ethinyl estradiol; ferrous fumarate]
Phase 1 (5 days): 1•0.02•75 mg;
Phase 2 (7 days): 1•0.03•75 mg;
Phase 3 (9 days): 1•0.035•75 mg;
Counters (7 days): 0•0•75 mg

tilidate HCl BAN *analgesic* [also: tilidine HCl; tilidine]

tilidine INN *analgesic* [also: tilidine HCl; tilidate HCl]

tilidine HCl USAN *analgesic* [also: tilidine; tilidate HCl]

tiliquinol INN

tilisolol INN

tilmicosin USAN, INN, BAN *veterinary antibacterial*

tilmicosin phosphate USAN *veterinary antibacterial*

tilomisole USAN, INN *immunoregulator*

tilorone INN *antiviral* [also: tilorone HCl]

tilorone HCl USAN *antiviral* [also: tilorone]

tilozepine INN

tilsuprost INN

Tiltab (trademarked dosage form) *filmcoated tablets*

tiludronate disodium USAN *bisphosphonate bone resorption inhibitor for Paget disease; also used for osteoporosis*

tiludronic acid INN

timcodar dimesylate USAN *antineoplastic adjunct to prevent emergence of multidrug-resistant tumors*

Timecap (trademarked dosage form) *sustained-release capsule*

Timecelle (trademarked dosage form) *timed-release capsule*

timefurone USAN, INN *antiatherosclerotic*

timegadine INN

Time-Hist sustained-release capsules (discontinued 2007) ℞ *decongestant; antihistamine* [pseudoephedrine HCl; chlorpheniramine maleate] 120•8 mg

Time-Hist QD extended-release tablets ℞ *decongestant; antihistamine; anticholinergic to dry mucosal secretions* [pseudoephedrine HCl; chlorpheniramine maleate; methscopolamine bromide] 120•6•2.5 mg

timelotem INN

Timentin powder or frozen premix for IV infusion ℞ *extended-spectrum penicillin antibiotic plus synergist* [ticarcillin disodium; clavulanate potassium] 3•0.1 g

timepidium bromide INN

Timespan (trademarked dosage form) *timed-release tablets*

Timesules (dosage form) *sustainedrelease capsules*

timiperone INN

timobesone INN *topical adrenocortical steroid* [also: timobesone acetate]

timobesone acetate USAN *topical adrenocortical steroid* [also: timobesone]

timofibrate INN

Timolide 10-25 tablets ℞ *antihypertensive; β-blocker; diuretic* [timolol maleate; hydrochlorothiazide] 10•25 mg

timolol USAN, INN, BAN *topical antiglaucoma agent (β-blocker)*

timolol hemihydrate *topical antiglaucoma agent (β-blocker)*

timolol maleate USAN, USP *antianginal; antihypertensive; antiadrenergic (β-receptor); topical antiglaucoma agent; migraine prophylaxis* 5, 10, 20 mg oral; 0.25%, 0.5% eye drops

timonacic INN

timoprazole INN

Timoptic Ocumeter (eye drops), Ocu-dose (single-use eye drop dispenser) ℞ *antiglaucoma agent (β-blocker)* [timolol maleate] 0.25%, 0.5%

Timoptic-XE gel-forming Ocumeter (eye drops) ℞ *once-daily antiglaucoma agent (β-blocker)* [timolol maleate] 0.25%, 0.5%

Timunox *investigational (Phase III) immunomodulator for asymptomatic HIV infection* [thymopentin]

tin *element (Sn)*

tin chloride dihydrate [see: stannous chloride]

tin ethyl etiopurpurin (SnET2) [see: rostaporfin]

tin fluoride [see: stannous fluoride]

tinabinol USAN, INN *antihypertensive*

Tinactin cream, powder, spray powder, spray liquid, topical solution OTC *antifungal* [tolnaftate] 1%

Tinactin for Jock Itch cream, spray powder OTC *antifungal* [tolnaftate] 1%

tinazoline INN ☑ Tensilon; Tonsaline

TinBen tincture OTC *skin protectant; antiseptic* [benzoin; alcohol 75–83%]

Tincture of Green Soap topical liquid OTC *antiseptic cleanser* [green soap; alcohol 28–32%]

Tindamax film-coated tablets ℞ *antiprotozoal/amebicide for amebiasis (orphan), giardiasis (orphan), trichomoniasis, and bacterial vaginosis* [tinidazole] 250, 500 mg

Ting cream OTC *antifungal* [tolnaftate] 1% ☑ Tanac; Ten-K; Twin-K

Ting spray powder OTC *antifungal for tinea pedis, tinea cruris, and tinea corporis* [miconazole nitrate] 2% ☑ Tanac; Ten-K; Twin-K

tinidazole USAN, INN *antiprotozoal/amebicide for amebiasis (orphan), giar-diasis (orphan), trichomoniasis, and bacterial vaginosis*

tinisulpride INN

tinofedrine INN

tinoridine INN

Tinver lotion ℞ *antifungal; keratolytic; antipruritic; anesthetic* [sodium thiosulfate; salicylic acid; alcohol 10%] 25%•1%

tinzaparin sodium USAN, INN, BAN *a low molecular weight heparin–type anticoagulant and antithrombotic for the prevention and treatment of deep vein thrombosis (DVT)*

tiocarlide INN [also: thiocarlide]

tioclomarol INN

tioconazole USAN, USP, INN, BAN, JAN *topical antifungal*

tioctilate INN

tiodazosin USAN, INN *antihypertensive*

tiodonium chloride USAN, INN *antibacterial*

tiofacic [see: stepronin]

tioguanine INN *antineoplastic* [also: thioguanine]

tiomergine INN

tiomesterone INN [also: thiomesterone]

tioperidone INN *antipsychotic* [also: tioperidone HCl] ☑ tipredane

tioperidone HCl USAN *antipsychotic* [also: tioperidone]

tiopinac USAN, INN *anti-inflammatory; analgesic; antipyretic*

tiopronin INN *prevention of cystine nephrolithiasis in homozygous cystinuria (orphan)* ☑ teprenone; toborinone

tiopropamine INN

tiosalan INN *disinfectant* [also: thiosalan] ☑ Tessalon

tiosinamine [see: allylthiourea]

tiospirone INN *antipsychotic* [also: tiospirone HCl] ☑ tisopurine; tizabrin

tiospirone HCl USAN *antipsychotic* [also: tiospirone]

tiotidine USAN, INN *antagonist to histamine H_2 receptors*

tiotixene INN *conventional (typical) thioxanthene antipsychotic for schizophrenia* [also: thiothixene]

tiotropium bromide *long-acting anti-cholinergic bronchodilator for emphysema and chronic obstructive pulmonary disease (COPD)*

tioxacin INN

tioxamast INN

tioxaprofen INN

tioxidazole USAN, INN *anthelmintic*

tioxolone INN [also: thioxolone]

TIP (Taxol, isosfamide [with mesna rescue], Platinol) *chemotherapy protocol for head, neck, and esophageal cancers*

tipentosin INN, BAN *antihypertensive* [also: tipentosin HCl]

tipentosin HCl USAN *antihypertensive* [also: tipentosin]

tipepidine INN

tipetropium bromide INN

tipifarnib USAN *investigational (NDA filed, orphan) antineoplastic for acute myeloid leukemia (AML)*

tipindole INN

tipranavir disodium USAN *antiviral; HIV-1 protease inhibitor*

tipredane USAN, INN, BAN *topical adrenocortical steroid* ② tioperidone

tiprenolol INN *antiadrenergic (β-receptor)* [also: tiprenolol HCl]

tiprenolol HCl USAN *antiadrenergic (β-receptor)* [also: tiprenolol]

tiprinast INN *antiallergic* [also: tiprinast meglumine]

tiprinast meglumine USAN *antiallergic* [also: tiprinast]

tipropidil INN *vasodilator* [also: tipropidil HCl]

tipropidil HCl USAN *vasodilator* [also: tipropidil]

tiprostanide INN, BAN

tiprotimod INN

tiqueside USAN, INN *antihyperlipidemic*

tiquinamide INN *gastric anticholinergic* [also: tiquinamide HCl]

tiquinamide HCl USAN *gastric anticholinergic* [also: tiquinamide]

tiquizium bromide INN

tirapazamine USAN, INN *antineoplastic; investigational (Phase III, orphan) for head, neck, and lung cancers*

tiratricol INN *investigational (orphan) for suppression of thyroid-stimulating hormone (TSH) for thyroid cancer*

tirilazad INN, BAN *antioxidant; lipid peroxidation inhibitor; 21-aminosteroid (lazaroid)* [also: tirilizad mesylate]

tirilazad mesylate USAN *antioxidant; lipid peroxidation inhibitor; 21-aminosteroid (lazaroid)* [also: tirilazad]

tirofiban HCl USAN *glycoprotein (GP) IIb/IIIa receptor antagonist; platelet aggregation inhibitor for acute coronary syndrome, unstable angina, myocardial infarction, and cardiac surgery*

tiropramide INN

Tirosint *capsules* ℞ *synthetic thyroid hormone (T_4 fraction only)* [levothyroxine sodium] 13 mcg

tisilfocon A USAN *hydrophobic contact lens material*

Tisit *topical liquid, gel, shampoo* OTC *pediculicide for lice* [pyrethrins; piperonyl butoxide] 0.3%•2%; 0.3%•3%; 0.3%•4%

tisocromide INN

TiSol *throat irrigation solution* OTC *antiseptic; mild anesthetic; antipruritic; counterirritant* [benzyl alcohol; menthol] 1%•0.04% ② Tussall

tisopurine INN ② tiospirone; tizabrin

tisoquone INN ② Tussigon

tissue factor [see: thromboplastin]

tissue plasminogen activator (tPA; t-PA) [see: alteplase]

Tis-U-Sol *solution* ℞ *sterile irrigant for general washing and rinsing* [physiological irrigating solution]

TIT (methotrexate, cytarabine, hydrocortisone) *chemotherapy protocol for CNS prophylaxis of pediatric acute lymphocytic leukemia; intrathecal (IT) administration*

Titan *solution* OTC *cleaning solution for hard contact lenses*

titanium *element (Ti)*

titanium dioxide USP *topical protectant; astringent*

titanium oxide [see: titanium dioxide]

Titradose (trademarked dosage form) *scored tablet*

Titralac chewable tablets OTC *antacid* [calcium carbonate] 420, 750 mg

Titralac Plus chewable tablets, oral liquid OTC *antacid; antiflatulent* [calcium carbonate; simethicone] 420•21 mg; 500•20 mg/5 mL

tivanidazole INN

tivazine [see: piperazine citrate]

tixadil INN

tixanox USAN *antiallergic* [also: tixanoxum]

tixanoxum INN *antiallergic* [also: tixanox]

tixocortol INN *topical anti-inflammatory* [also: tixocortol pivalate]

tixocortol pivalate USAN *topical anti-inflammatory* [also: tixocortol]

tizabrin INN 🔄 tiospirone; tisopurine

tizanidine INN, BAN *central* α_2 *agonist; skeletal muscle relaxant; antispasmodic* [also: tizanidine HCl]

tizanidine HCl USAN, JAN *central* α_2 *agonist; skeletal muscle relaxant; antispasmodic for multiple sclerosis and spinal cord injury (orphan)* [also: tizanidine] 2, 4 mg oral

tizolemide INN

tizoprolic acid INN

²⁰¹Tl [see: thallous chloride Tl 201]

T-lymphotrophic virus antigens [see: human T-lymphotropic virus type III (HTLV-III) gp-160 antigens]

T-MAVs (targeted monoclonal antibody vehicles) [q.v.]

TMB (trimedoxime bromide) [q.v.]

TMC125 *investigational (Phase III) non-nucleoside reverse transcriptase inhibitor (NNRTI) antiviral for HIV and AIDS in treatment-experienced patients*

TMG (trimethylglycine) [q.v.]

TMP (trimethoprim) [q.v.]

TMP-SMZ (trimethoprim & sulfamethoxazole) [q.v.]

TNF (tumor necrosis factor) [q.v.]

TNKase powder for IV injection R *thrombolytic/fibrinolytic for the treatment of acute myocardial infarction (AMI)* [tenecteplase] 50 mg/vial 🔄 Tannic-12 S; tonics

TNK-tPA *a genetically engineered mutation of tissue plasminogen activator (tPA); "TNK" refers to the three specific sites of genetic modification* [see: tenecteplase]

TOAP (thioguanine, Oncovin, [cytosine] arabinoside, prednisone) *chemotherapy protocol*

tobacco *dried leaves of the* Nicotiana tabacum *plant; sedative narcotic; emetic; diuretic; heart depressant; antispasmodic* [see also: nicotine] 🔄 Topic

tobacco, British *medicinal herb* [see: coltsfoot]

tobacco, Indian; wild tobacco *medicinal herb* [see: lobelia]

tobacco, sailor's *medicinal herb* [see: mugwort]

tobacco wood *medicinal herb* [see: witch hazel]

TOBI solution for inhalation R *antibiotic for* Pseudomonas aeruginosa *lung infections in cystic fibrosis patients (orphan)* [tobramycin] 300 mg/5 mL

toborinone USAN *cardiotonic* 🔄 teprenone; tiopronin

TobraDex eye drop suspension R *corticosteroidal anti-inflammatory; antibiotic* [dexamethasone; tobramycin] 0.1%•0.3%

TobraDex ophthalmic ointment R *corticosteroidal anti-inflammatory; antibiotic* [dexamethasone; tobramycin; chlorobutanol] 0.1%•0.3%•0.5%

tobramycin USAN, USP, INN, BAN *aminoglycoside antibiotic; inhalant for* Pseudomonas aeruginosa *lung infections in cystic fibrosis patients (orphan)* 0.3% eye drops

Tobramycin in 0.9% Sodium Chloride IV or IM injection R *aminoglycoside antibiotic* [tobramycin sulfate] 0.8, 1.2 mg/mL (60, 80 mg/dose)

tobramycin sulfate USP *aminoglycoside antibiotic* 10, 40 mg/mL injection

Tobrex Drop-Tainers (eye drops), ophthalmic ointment R *aminoglycoside antibiotic* [tobramycin] 0.3%; 3 mg/g

tobuterol INN

tocainide USAN, INN, BAN *antiarrhythmic*

tocainide HCl USP *antiarrhythmic*

tocamphyl USAN, INN *choleretic*

Tocicodendron diversilobum *medicinal herb* [see: poison oak]

tocilizumab *humanized monoclonal antibody to interleukin-6 receptors; investigational (Phase III) for moderate to severe rheumatoid arthritis*

tocladesine USAN *immunomodulator; antineoplastic*

tocofenoxate INN

tocofersolan INN *dietary vitamin E supplement* [also: tocophersolan]

tocofibrate INN

tocolytics *a class of drugs used to inhibit uterine contractions; often administered in an attempt to arrest preterm labor*

tocopherol, *d*-alpha [see: vitamin E]

tocopherol, *dl*-alpha [see: vitamin E]

tocopherols, mixed [see: vitamin E]

tocopherols excipient NF *antioxidant*

tocophersolan USAN *dietary vitamin E supplement; investigational (orphan) for vitamin E deficiency due to prolonged cholestatic hepatobiliary disease* [also: tocofersolan]

tocopheryl acetate, *d*-alpha [see: vitamin E]

tocopheryl acetate, *dl*-alpha [see: vitamin E]

tocopheryl acid succinate, *d*-alpha [see: vitamin E]

tocopheryl acid succinate, *dl*-alpha [see: vitamin E]

tocopheryl polyethylene glycol succinate (TPGS) [see: tocophersolan]

tocosol paclitaxel [see: paclitaxel tocosol]

Today *vaginal sponge* OTC *spermicidal/ barrier contraceptive* [nonoxynol 9] 1 g

todralazine INN, BAN

tofenacin INN *anticholinergic* [also: tofenacin HCl]

tofenacin HCl USAN *anticholinergic* [also: tofenacin]

tofesilate INN *combining name for radicals or groups*

tofetridine INN

tofisoline ⍰ tefazoline

tofisopam INN

Tofranil *sugar-coated tablets* ℞ *tricyclic antidepressant; treatment for childhood enuresis* [imipramine HCl] 10, 25, 50 mg

Tofranil-PM *capsules* ℞ *tricyclic antidepressant* [imipramine pamoate] 75, 100, 125, 150 mg

tolamolol USAN, INN *vasodilator; antiarrhythmic; antiadrenergic (β-receptor)*

tolazamide USAN, USP, INN, BAN *sulfonylurea antidiabetic that stimulates insulin secretion in the pancreas* 100, 250, 500 mg oral

tolazoline INN *antiadrenergic; peripheral vasodilator for hypertension* [also: tolazoline HCl]

tolazoline HCl USP *antiadrenergic; peripheral vasodilator for neonatal persistent pulmonary hypertension* [also: tolazoline]

tolboxane INN

tolbutamide USP, INN, BAN *sulfonylurea antidiabetic that stimulates insulin secretion in the pancreas* 500 mg oral

tolbutamide sodium USP *in vivo diagnostic aid for pancreatic islet cell adenoma*

tolcapone USAN, INN COMT (*catechol-O-methyltransferase*) *inhibitor for Parkinson disease*

tolciclate USAN, INN *antifungal*

tolclotide [see: disulfamide]

toldimfos INN, BAN

Tolectin 200; Tolectin 600 *tablets* (discontinued 2006) ℞ *analgesic; nonsteroidal anti-inflammatory drug (NSAID) for osteoarthritis, rheumatoid arthritis, and juvenile rheumatoid arthritis* [tolmetin sodium] 200 mg; 600 mg

Tolectin DS *capsules* (discontinued 2006) ℞ *analgesic; nonsteroidal anti-inflammatory drug (NSAID) for osteoarthritis, rheumatoid arthritis, and juvenile rheumatoid arthritis* [tolmetin sodium] 400 mg

Tolerex *powder* OTC *enteral nutritional therapy* [lactose-free formula]

tolevamer *investigational (Phase III) polymer therapy for Clostridium difficile-associated diarrhea*

tolfamide USAN, INN *urease enzyme inhibitor*

tolfenamic acid INN, BAN

Tolfrinic film-coated tablets OTC *hematinic* [ferrous fumarate; cyanocobalamin; ascorbic acid] 200 mg•25 mcg•100 mg

tolgabide USAN, INN, BAN *anticonvulsant*

tolhexamide [see: glycyclamide]

tolimidone USAN, INN *antiulcerative*

Tolinase tablets (discontinued 2006) ℞ *sulfonylurea antidiabetic that stimulates insulin secretion in the pancreas* [tolazamide] 250 mg

tolindate USAN, INN *antifungal*

toliodium chloride USAN, INN *veterinary food additive*

toliprolol INN

tolmesoxide INN

tolmetin USAN, INN *analgesic; nonsteroidal anti-inflammatory drug (NSAID) for osteoarthritis, rheumatoid arthritis, and juvenile rheumatoid arthritis*

tolmetin sodium USAN, USP *analgesic; nonsteroidal anti-inflammatory drug (NSAID) for osteoarthritis, rheumatoid arthritis, and juvenile rheumatoid arthritis* 200, 400, 600 mg oral

tolnaftate USAN, USP, INN, BAN *antifungal* 1% topical

tolnapersine INN

tolnidamine INN

toloconium metilsulfate INN

tolofocon A USAN *hydrophobic contact lens material*

tolonidine INN

tolonium chloride INN *blue dye used in histology; diagnostic aid for oral cancer*

toloxatone INN

toloxichloral [see: toloxychlorinol]

toloxychlorinol INN

tolpadol INN

tolpentamide INN, BAN

tolperisone INN, BAN

tolpiprazole INN, BAN

tolpovidone I 131 USAN *hypoalbuminemia test; radioactive agent* [also: radiotolpovidone I 131] ☒ telbivudine

tolpronine INN, BAN

tolpropamine INN, BAN

tolpyrramide USAN, INN *antidiabetic*

tolquinzole INN

tolrestat USAN, INN, BAN *aldose reductase inhibitor*

tolterodine USAN *anticholinergic; muscarinic receptor antagonist for urinary frequency, urgency, and incontinence*

tolterodine tartrate USAN *anticholinergic; muscarinic receptor antagonist for urinary frequency, urgency, and incontinence*

toltrazuril USAN, INN, BAN *veterinary coccidiostat*

tolu balsam USP *pharmaceutic aid*

p-**toluenesulfone dichloramine** [see: dichloramine T]

tolufazepam INN

toluidine blue O [see: tolonium chloride]

toluidine blue O chloride [see: tolonium chloride]

Tolu-Sed DM oral liquid (discontinued 2007) OTC *antitussive; expectorant* [dextromethorphan hydrobromide; guaifenesin; alcohol 10%] 10•100 mg/5 mL

tolvaptan *investigational (NDA filed) selective vasopressin V₂–receptor antagonist for heart failure and hyponatremia*

tolycaine INN, BAN

tomelukast USAN, INN *antiasthmatic; leukotriene antagonist*

Tomocat concentrated rectal suspension ℞ *radiopaque contrast medium for gastrointestinal imaging* [barium sulfate] 5%

tomoglumide INN

tomoxetine INN *antidepressant* [also: tomoxetine HCl]

tomoxetine HCl USAN *antidepressant* [also: tomoxetine]

tomoxiprole INN

Tom's of Maine Natural Cough & Cold Rub Cough Suppressant vaporizing ointment (discontinued 2007) OTC *mild anesthetic; antipruritic; counterirritant* [menthol; camphor] 4.8%•2.6%

tonazocine INN *analgesic* [also: tonazocine mesylate]

tonazocine mesylate USAN *analgesic*
[also: tonazocine]

tongue grass *medicinal herb* [see:
chickweed]

tonics *a class of agents that restore normal tone to tissue and strengthen or
invigorate organs (a term used in folk
medicine)* ⊠ Tannic-12 S; TNKase

tonka bean *(Dipteryx odorata; D.
oppositifolia)* fruit and seed *medicinal
herb for cramps, nausea, and schistosomiasis*

Tonocard film-coated tablets (discontinued 2004) ℞ *antiarrhythmic*
[tocainide HCl] 400, 600 mg

Tonopaque powder for oral/rectal suspension ℞ *radiopaque contrast medium
for gastrointestinal imaging* [barium
sulfate] 95%

Tonsaline mouthwash OTC *oral antiseptic*
[alcohol 4%] ⊠ Tensilon; tinazoline

tonzonium bromide INN *detergent;
surface-active agent* [also: thonzonium
bromide]

tooth, lion's *medicinal herb* [see: dan-
delion]

Toothache oral gel OTC *mucous membrane anesthetic* [benzocaine]

toothache bush; toothache tree
medicinal herb [see: prickly ash]

**Top Care Flu, Cold, & Cough
Medicine Night Time** powder for
oral solution (discontinued 2007)
OTC *antitussive; antihistamine; decongestant; analgesic; antipyretic* [dextro-
methorphan hydrobromide; chlorpheniramine maleate; pseudoephedrine HCl; acetaminophen] 20•4•
60•1000 mg/pkt.

**Top Care Multi-Symptom Pain
Relief Cold** caplets (discontinued
2007) OTC *antitussive; decongestant;
analgesic; antipyretic* [dextromethor-
phan hydrobromide; pseudoephedrine
HCl; acetaminophen] 15•30•325 mg

**Top Care Multi-Symptom Pain
Relief Cold** caplets (discontinued
2007) OTC *antitussive; antihistamine;*

decongestant; analgesic; antipyretic
[dextromethorphan hydrobromide;
chlorpheniramine maleate; pseudoephedrine HCl; acetaminophen]
15•2•30•325 mg

**Top Care Nite Time Multi-Symp-
tom Cold/Flu Relief** LiquiCaps
(liquid-filled gelcaps) (discontinued
2007) OTC *antitussive; antihistamine;
sleep aid; decongestant; analgesic; antipyretic* [dextromethorphan hydrobromide; doxylamine succinate; pseudoephedrine HCl; acetaminophen]
10•6.25•30•250 mg

**Top Care Soothing Cough & Head
Congestion Relief D** oral liquid
(discontinued 2007) OTC *antitussive;
decongestant* [dextromethorphan
hydrobromide; pseudoephedrine
HCl; alcohol 5%] 30•60 mg/15 mL

Topamax coated tablets, sprinkle caps
℞ *broad-spectrum sulfamate anticonvulsant for Lennox-Gastaut syndrome
(orphan) and partial-onset and generalized tonic-clonic seizures; migraine
headache preventative; also used for a
variety of psychiatric disorders* [topira-
mate] 25, 50, 100, 200 mg; 15, 25 mg

Topic gel OTC *mild anesthetic; antipruritic; counterirritant; antiseptic* [benzyl
alcohol; camphor; menthol; alcohol
30%] 5%• ≟ • ≟ ⊠ tobacco

topical starch [see: starch, topical]

TopiCare (trademarked ingredient)
*topical polyolprepolymer base for
creams and gels*

Topicort ointment, cream, gel ℞ *corticosteroidal anti-inflammatory* [desoxi-
metasone] 0.25%; 0.25%; 0.05%

Topicort LP cream ℞ *corticosteroidal
anti-inflammatory* [desoximetasone]
0.05%

topiramate USAN, INN, BAN *broad-
spectrum sulfamate anticonvulsant for
Lennox-Gastaut syndrome (orphan)
and partial-onset and generalized tonic-
clonic seizures; migraine headache preventative; also used for a variety of psychiatric disorders* 25, 100, 200 mg oral

topo/CTX (topotecan, cyclophos-phamide [with mesna rescue]) *chemotherapy protocol for pediatric bone and soft tissue sarcomas*

topoisomerase I inhibitors *a class of hormonal antineoplastics that prevent DNA replication of tumors by inhibiting the re-ligation of naturally occurring single-strand breaks*

Toposar IV injection ℞ *antineoplastic for testicular and small cell lung cancers* [etoposide; alcohol 30.5%] 20 mg/mL

topotecan INN, BAN *topoisomerase I inhibitor; antineoplastic for ovarian, cervical, and small cell lung cancers* [also: topotecan HCl]

topotecan HCl USAN *topoisomerase I inhibitor; antineoplastic for ovarian, cervical, and small cell lung cancers; investigational (Phase II) for AIDS-related progressive multifocal leukoencephalopathy (PML)* [also: topotecan]

toprilidine INN

Toprol-XL film-coated extended-release tablets ℞ *antihypertensive; long-term antianginal; antiadrenergic (β-blocker)* [metoprolol succinate] 25, 50, 100, 200 mg

topterone USAN, INN *antiandrogen*

TOPV (trivalent oral poliovirus vaccine) [see: poliovirus vaccine, live oral]

toquizine USAN, INN *anticholinergic* ② Tikosyn

Toradol film-coated tablets, Tubex (prefilled syringes) for IM or IV injection (discontinued 2006) ℞ *analgesic; nonsteroidal anti-inflammatory drug (NSAID) for moderately severe acute pain* [ketorolac tromethamine] 10 mg; 15, 30 mg/mL ② Tridal

toralizumab *investigational (orphan) for immune thrombocytopenic purpura*

torasemide INN, BAN *antihypertensive; loop diuretic* [also: torsemide]

torbafylline INN

torcetrapib *investigational (Phase III) antihyperlipidemic; cholesterol ester transfer protein (CETP) inhibitor that raises HDL cholesterol*

Torecan IM injection (discontinued 2008) ℞ *antiemetic for postoperative nausea and vomiting* [thiethylperazine maleate] 5 mg/mL ② tarragon; Trocaine

Torecan tablets (discontinued 2004) ℞ *antiemetic for postoperative nausea and vomiting* [thiethylperazine maleate] 10 mg ② tarragon; Trocaine

toremifene INN, BAN *antiestrogen; antineoplastic* [also: toremifene citrate]

toremifene citrate USAN *selective estrogen receptor modulator (SERM); antiestrogen antineoplastic for metastatic breast cancer in postmenopausal women (orphan); investigational (orphan) for desmoid tumors; investigational (Phase III) adjunctive treatment of advanced prostate cancer* [also: toremifene]

toripristone INN

Torisel IV infusion ℞ *antineoplastic for renal cell carcinoma (orphan); investigational (NDA filed) for metastatic breast cancer and mantle cell lymphoma; investigational (Phase II) immunosuppressant for rheumatoid arthritis and multiple sclerosis* [temsirolimus] 25 mg/mL

tormentil (Potentilla tormentilla; Tormentilla erecta) root *medicinal herb used as an antiphlogistic, antiseptic, astringent, and hemostatic*

Tornalate solution for inhalation ℞ *sympathomimetic bronchodilator* [bitolterol mesylate] 0.2%

torsemide USAN *antihypertensive; loop diuretic* [also: torasemide] 5, 10, 20, 100 mg oral; 10 mg/mL injection

tosactide INN [also: octacosactrin]

tosifen USAN, INN *antianginal*

tosilate INN *combining name for radicals or groups* [also: tosylate]

tositumomab *monoclonal antibody to non-Hodgkin lymphoma (orphan)* [see also: iodine I 131 tositumomab]

tosufloxacin USAN, INN *antibacterial*

tosulur INN ② Tussall-ER

tosylate USAN, BAN *combining name for radicals or groups* [also: tosilate]

tosylchloramide sodium INN [also: chloramine-T]

Total solution OTC *cleaning/soaking/wetting solution for hard contact lenses*

Total Formula; Total Formula-2 tablets OTC *vitamin/mineral/iron supplement* [multiple vitamins & minerals; iron; folic acid; biotin] ±•20•0.4•0.3 mg

Total Formula-3 without Iron tablets OTC *vitamin/mineral supplement* [multiple vitamins & minerals; folic acid; biotin] ±•0.4•0.3 mg

Totect powder for IV infusion ℞ *cytoprotectant for anthracycline extravasation during chemotherapy* [dexrazoxane HCl] 589 mg (500 mg base)

touch-me-not; pale touch-me-not *medicinal herb* [see: celandine; jewelweed; eleuthero]

toughened silver nitrate [see: silver nitrate, toughened]

Touro Allergy tablets, sustained-release capsules ℞ *decongestant; antihistamine* [pseudoephedrine HCl; brompheniramine maleate] 45•6 mg; 60•5.75 mg

Touro CC sustained-release caplets (discontinued 2007) ℞ *antitussive; decongestant; expectorant* [dextromethorphan hydrobromide; pseudoephedrine HCl; guaifenesin] 30•60•575 mg ℞ Tarka; Tri-K

Touro CC-LD sustained-release caplets ℞ *antitussive; decongestant; expectorant* [dextromethorphan hydrobromide; pseudoephedrine HCl; guaifenesin] 30•25•575 mg ℞ Triglide

Touro DM sustained-release tablets ℞ *antitussive; expectorant* [dextromethorphan hydrobromide; guaifenesin] 30•575 mg

Touro Ex sustained-release caplets (discontinued 2004) ℞ *expectorant* [guaifenesin] 575 mg ℞ Tyrex-2

Touro HC extended-release caplets (discontinued 2007) ℞ *narcotic antitussive; expectorant* [hydrocodone

bitartrate; guaifenesin] 5•575 mg ℞ Tarka; Tri-K

Touro LA sustained-release caplets ℞ *decongestant; expectorant* [pseudoephedrine HCl; guaifenesin] 120•525 mg ℞ Terrell

Tovalt ODT (orally disintegrating tablets) ℞ *imidazopyridine sedative and hypnotic for the short-term treatment of insomnia* [zolpidem tartrate] 5, 10 mg

Toviaz ⓔⓤⓡ (available in Europe) *investigational (NDA filed) muscarinic receptor antagonist for overactive bladder* [fesoterodine]

toxoids *a class of drugs used for active immunization that produce endogenous antibodies to toxins*

toywort *medicinal herb* [see: shepherd's purse]

tozalinone INN *antidepressant* [also: thozalinone]

tPA; t-PA (tissue plasminogen activator) [see: alteplase; anistreplase; lanoteplase; monteplase; reteplase; saruplase; tenecteplase]

TPCH (thioguanine, procarbazine, CCNU, hydroxyurea) *chemotherapy protocol* ℞ tobacco; Topic

TPDCV (thioguanine, procarbazine, DCD, CCNU, vincristine) *chemotherapy protocol*

TPGS (tocopheryl polyethylene glycol succinate) [see: tocophersolan]

T-Phyl timed-release tablets (discontinued 2008) ℞ *antiasthmatic; bronchodilator* [theophylline] 200 mg

TPM Test kit for professional use ℞ *in vitro diagnostic aid for* Toxoplasma gondii *antibodies in serum* [indirect hemagglutination test]

TPN Electrolytes; TPN Electrolytes II; TPN Electrolytes III IV admixture ℞ *intravenous electrolyte therapy* [combined electrolyte solution]

trabectedin [see: ecteinascidin]

traboxopine INN

Trac Tabs 2X tablets (discontinued 2006) ℞ *urinary antibiotic; analgesic; antispasmodic; acidifier* [methen-

amine; phenyl salicylate; atropine
sulfate; hyoscyamine sulfate; benzoic
acid; methylene blue] 120•30•
0.06•0.03•7.5•6 mg

tracazolate USAN, INN, BAN *sedative*

Trace Metals Additive in 0.9% NaCl
IV injection (name changed to **4
Trace Elements** in 2005)

Tracleer film-coated tablets ℞ *endothelin receptor antagonist (ERA) for
pulmonary arterial hypertension
(orphan); also used to prevent digital
ulcers in systemic sclerosis* [bosentan]
62.5, 125 mg

Tracrium IV infusion ℞ *nondepolarizing
neuromuscular blocker; adjunct to anesthesia* [atracurium besylate] 10 mg/mL

trafermin USAN *fibroblast growth factor*

tragacanth NF *suspending agent*

tralonide USAN, INN *corticosteroid; anti-
inflammatory*

tramadol INN *central analgesic for moderate to severe pain* [also: tramadol HCl]

Tramadol ER extended-release tablets
℞ *central analgesic for moderate to
severe chronic pain* [tramadol] 100,
200, 300 mg

tramadol HCl USAN *central analgesic
for moderate to severe pain; also used
for premature ejaculation; investigational (orphan) for HIV-associated neuropathy* [also: tramadol] 50 mg oral

tramadol HCl & acetaminophen
central analgesic for acute pain 37.5•
325 mg oral

Tramadol ODT (orally disintegrating
tablets) ℞ *central analgesic for moderate to severe pain* [tramadol] 50 mg

tramazoline INN *adrenergic* [also: tramazoline HCl]

tramazoline HCl USAN *adrenergic*
[also: tramazoline]

tramiprosate *investigational (Phase III)
amyloid-beta antagonist to reduce
plaque formation in Alzheimer disease*

Trandate film-coated tablets, IV injection ℞ *antihypertensive; antiadrenergic
(α- and β-blocker)* [labetalol HCl]
100, 200, 300 mg; 5 mg/mL

trandolapril INN, BAN *antihypertensive;
angiotensin-converting enzyme (ACE)
inhibitor; treatment for congestive heart
failure (CHF)* 1, 2, 4 mg oral

trandolaprilat INN

tranexamic acid USAN, INN, BAN *systemic hemostatic; surgical adjunct for
patients with congenital coagulopathies
(orphan); investigational (orphan) for
hereditary angioneurotic edema*

tranilast USAN, INN *antiasthmatic; investigational (orphan) for malignant glioma*

**trans AMCHA (*trans*-aminomethyl
cyclohexanecarboxylic acid)** [see:
tranexamic acid]

transcainide USAN, INN *antiarrhythmic*

transclomiphene [now: zuclomiphene]

Transderm Scōp transdermal patch ℞
*motion sickness preventative; post-sur-
gical antiemetic* [scopolamine] 1.5 mg
(1 mg dose over 3 days)

Transderm-Nitro transdermal patch
(discontinued 2005) ℞ *coronary
vasodilator; antianginal* [nitroglycerin]
0.1, 0.2, 0.4, 0.6, 0.8 mg/hr. (12.5,
25, 50, 75, 100 mg total)

transferrin, human *investigational
(orphan) treatment for malignant
tumors of the central nervous system,
conjugated with a diphtheria* CRM_{107}
(*q.v.*) *carrier*

transforming growth factor beta 2
*investigational (orphan) growth stimu-
lator for full-thickness macular holes*

TransMID *investigational (orphan)
treatment for malignant tumors of the
central nervous system* [human transferrin; diphtheria CRM_{107} conjugate]

***trans*-π-oxocamphor** JAN *topical anti-
pruritic; mild local anesthetic; counterirritant* [also: camphor]

***trans*-retinoic acid** [see: tretinoin]

**Trans-Ver-Sal Adult-Patch; Trans-
Ver-Sal Pedia-Patch; Trans-Ver-
Sal Plantar-Patch** patch OTC *kera-
tolytic* [salicylic acid] 15%

trantelinium bromide INN

Tranxene T-tabs ("T"-imprinted tablets) ℞ *benzodiazepine anxiolytic;
minor tranquilizer; alcohol withdrawal*

aid; anticonvulsant adjunct [clorazepate dipotassium] 3.75, 7.5, 15 mg

Tranxene-SD; Tranxene-SD Half Strength extended-release tablets ℞ *benzodiazepine anxiolytic; minor tranquilizer; alcohol withdrawal aid; anticonvulsant adjunct* [clorazepate dipotassium] 22.5 mg; 11.25 mg

tranylcypromine INN, BAN *antidepressant; MAO inhibitor* [also: tranylcypromine sulfate]

tranylcypromine sulfate USP MAO *inhibitor for major depression; also used for migraine prevention, social anxiety disorder (SAD), panic disorder, bipolar depression, and Alzheimer and Parkinson disease* [also: tranylcypromine] 10 mg oral

trapencaine INN

trapidil INN

trapymin [see: trapidil]

trastuzumab *monoclonal antibody to human epidermal growth factor receptor 2 (HER2) protein; antineoplastic for metastatic HER2-overexpressing breast cancer; investigational (orphan) for pancreatic cancer*

trastuzumab & paclitaxel *chemotherapy protocol for breast cancer*

Trasylol IV infusion ℞ *systemic hemostatic for coronary artery bypass graft (CABG) surgery (orphan)* [aprotinin] 10 000 KIU/mL (kallikrein inhibitor units)

TraumaCal ready-to-use oral liquid OTC *enteral nutritional therapy for moderate to severe stress or trauma* [multiple branched chain amino acids]

Travasol 2.75% in 5% (10%, 25%) Dextrose; Travasol 4.25% in 5% (10%, 25%) Dextrose IV infusion ℞ *total parenteral nutrition; peripheral parenteral nutrition* [multiple essential and nonessential amino acids; dextrose]

Travasol 3.5% (5.5%, 8.5%) with Electrolytes IV infusion ℞ *total parenteral nutrition (all except 3.5%); peripheral parenteral nutrition (all)* [multiple essential and nonessential amino acids; electrolytes] ② Triphasil

Travasol 5.5% (8.5%, 10%) IV infusion ℞ *total parenteral nutrition; peripheral parenteral nutrition* [multiple essential and nonessential amino acids] ② Triphasil

Travasorb HN; Travasorb MCT; Travasorb STD powder OTC *enteral nutritional therapy* [lactose-free formula]

Travatan; Travatan Z Drop-Tainers (eye drops) ℞ *prostaglandin $F_{2\alpha}$ analogue for glaucoma and ocular hypertension* [travoprost] 0.004%

traveler's joy *medicinal herb* [see: blue vervain; woodbine]

5% Travert and Electrolyte No. 2; 10% Travert and Electrolyte No. 2 IV infusion ℞ *intravenous nutritional/electrolyte therapy* [combined electrolyte solution; invert sugar (50% dextrose + 50% fructose)]

travoprost USAN *topical prostaglandin $F_{2\alpha}$ analogue for glaucoma and ocular hypertension*

traxanox INN

traxoprodil mesylate USAN *selective NMDA receptor antagonist for traumatic brain injury*

Traypak (trademarked packaging form) *multivial carton*

trazitiline INN ② trestolone

trazium esilate INN

trazodone INN *triazolopyridine antidepressant; serotonin uptake inhibitor; also used for aggressive behavior, alcoholism, panic disorder, agoraphobia, and cocaine withdrawal* [also: trazodone HCl] ② terizidone

trazodone HCl USAN *triazolopyridine antidepressant; serotonin uptake inhibitor; also used for aggressive behavior, alcoholism, panic disorder, agoraphobia, and cocaine withdrawal* [also: trazodone] 50, 100, 150, 300 mg oral

trazolopride INN

Treanda powder for IV infusion ℞ *alkylating antineoplastic for chronic lymphocytic leukemia (orphan); investi-*

gational (NDA filed, orphan) for non-Hodgkin lymphoma [bendamustine HCl] 100 mg/vial

trebenzomine INN *antidepressant* [also: trebenzomine HCl]

trebenzomine HCl USAN *antidepressant* [also: trebenzomine]

trecadrine INN

Trecator film-coated tablets ℞ *tuberculostatic* [ethionamide] 250 mg

trecetilide fumarate USAN *antiarrhythmic*

trecovirsen sodium USAN *antisense antiviral for HIV and AIDS*

Tredaptive Ⓔ (European name for the investigational U.S. product **Cordaptive**)

trefentanil HCl USAN *analgesic*

trefoil, bean; bitter trefoil; marsh trefoil *medicinal herb* [see: buckbean]

Trellium Plus tablets ℞ *urinary analgesic; antispasmodic; sedative* [phenazopyridine HCl; hyoscyamine hydrobromide; butabarbital] 150•0.3•15 mg

treloxinate USAN, INN *antihyperlipoproteinemic*

Trelstar Depot IM injection (once monthly) ℞ *gonadotropin-releasing hormone (GnRH) antineoplastic for palliative treatment of advanced prostate cancer; investigational (orphan) for palliative treatment of advanced ovarian cancer* [triptorelin pamoate] 3.75 mg

Trelstar LA IM injection (three-month depot) ℞ *gonadotropin-releasing hormone (GnRH) antineoplastic for palliative treatment of advanced prostate cancer; investigational (orphan) for palliative treatment of advanced ovarian cancer* [triptorelin pamoate] 11.25 mg

tremacamra USAN *antiviral; inhibits viral attachment to host cells*

trembling poplar; trembling tree *medicinal herb* [see: poplar]

trenbolone INN, BAN *veterinary anabolic steroid, also abused as a street drug* [also: trenbolone acetate]

trenbolone acetate USAN *veterinary anabolic steroid, also abused as a street drug* [also: trenbolone]

trenbolone hexahydrobenzylcarbonate *veterinary anabolic steroid, also abused as a street drug*

trengestone INN

trenizine INN

Trental film-coated controlled-release tablets ℞ *peripheral vasodilator to improve blood microcirculation in intermittent claudication* [pentoxifylline] 400 mg

treosulfan INN, BAN *investigational (orphan) for ovarian cancer*

trepibutone INN

trepipam INN *sedative* [also: trepipam maleate]

trepipam maleate USAN *sedative* [also: trepipam]

trepirium iodide INN

treprostinil sodium *prostacyclin analogue; peripheral vasodilator for pulmonary arterial hypertension (orphan)*

treptilamine INN

trequinsin INN

trestolone INN *antineoplastic; androgen* [also: trestolone acetate] Ⓓ trazitiline

trestolone acetate USAN *antineoplastic; androgen* [also: trestolone]

tretamine INN, BAN [also: triethylenemelamine]

trethinium tosilate INN

trethocanic acid INN

trethocanoic acid [see: trethocanic acid]

tretinoin USAN, USP, INN, BAN *first generation retinoid; topical keratolytic for acne; treatment for acute promyelocytic leukemia (APL; orphan); investigational (orphan) for other leukemias and ophthalmic squamous metaplasia* 0.01%, 0.025%, 0.05%, 0.1% topical; 10 mg oral

Tretin-X cream, gel ℞ *keratolytic for acne* [tretinoin] 0.025%, 0.05%, 0.1%; 0.01%, 0.025%

tretoquinol INN

Trexall film-coated tablets ℞ *antimetabolite antineoplastic for leukemia;*

systemic antipsoriatic; antirheumatic for adult and juvenile rheumatoid arthritis [methotrexate] 5, 7.5, 10, 15 mg ☒ Tricosal

Treximet tablets ℞ combination 5-HT$_{1B/1D}$ agonist and nonsteroidal anti-inflammatory drug (NSAID) for the acute treatment of migraine headaches [sumatriptan; naproxen sodium] 85•500 mg

TRH (thyrotropin-releasing hormone) [see: protirelin]

Tri Vit with Fluoride pediatric oral drops (discontinued 2007) ℞ vitamin supplement; dental caries preventative [vitamins A, C, and D; fluoride] 1500 IU•35 mg•400 IU•0.25 mg, 1500 IU•35 mg•400 IU•0.5 mg per mL

TRIAC (triiodothyroacetic acid) [q.v.]

Triacana investigational (orphan) for suppression of thyroid-stimulating hormone (TSH) for thyroid cancer; used with levothyroxine sodium [tiratricol]

Triacet cream ℞ corticosteroidal anti-inflammatory [triamcinolone acetonide] 0.1% ☒ Trycet

triacetin USP, INN antifungal

triacetyloleandomycin BAN macrolide antibiotic [also: troleandomycin]

Triacin-C Cough syrup (discontinued 2007) ℞ narcotic antitussive; antihistamine; decongestant [codeine phosphate; triprolidine HCl; pseudoephedrine HCl; alcohol 4.3%] 20•2.5•60 mg/10 mL

triaconazole [now: terconazole]

Triacting oral liquid OTC decongestant; expectorant; for children 2–12 years [pseudoephedrine HCl; guaifenesin] 15•50 mg/5 mL

Triacting Cold & Allergy pediatric oral liquid (discontinued 2007) OTC decongestant; antihistamine [pseudoephedrine HCl; chlorpheniramine maleate] 30•2 mg/10 mL

Tri-Acting Cold & Allergy pediatric syrup (discontinued 2007) OTC decongestant; antihistamine [pseudoephedrine HCl; chlorpheniramine maleate] 30•2 mg/10 mL

Tri-Acting Cold & Cough syrup (discontinued 2007) OTC antitussive; antihistamine; decongestant; for children 6–11 years [dextromethorphan hydrobromide; chlorpheniramine maleate; pseudoephedrine HCl] 10•2•30 mg/10 mL

Triad capsules ℞ barbiturate sedative; analgesic; antipyretic [butalbital; acetaminophen; caffeine] 50•325•40 mg

triafungin USAN, INN antifungal

Trial AG (Anti-Gas) tablets OTC antacid; antiflatulent [aluminum hydroxide; magnesium hydroxide; simethicone] 200•200•25 mg

Trial Antacid tablets OTC antacid; calcium supplement [calcium carbonate] 420 mg

Triam Forte IM injection (discontinued 2006) ℞ corticosteroid; anti-inflammatory [triamcinolone diacetate] 40 mg/mL

Triam-A IM, intra-articular, intrabursal, intradermal injection (discontinued 2008) ℞ corticosteroid; anti-inflammatory [triamcinolone acetonide] 40 mg/mL

triamcinolone USP, INN, BAN, JAN corticosteroid

triamcinolone acetonide USP, JAN topical corticosteroidal anti-inflammatory; oral inhalation aerosol for chronic asthma; nasal aerosol for allergic rhinitis 0.025%, 0.1%, 0.5% topical; 40 mg/mL injection

triamcinolone acetonide sodium phosphate USAN corticosteroid

triamcinolone benetonide INN corticosteroid

triamcinolone diacetate USP, JAN corticosteroid

triamcinolone furetonide INN corticosteroid

triamcinolone hexacetonide USAN, USP, INN, BAN corticosteroidal anti-inflammatory

Triaminic Allerchews orally disintegrating tablets OTC nonsedating antihistamine for allergic rhinitis [loratadine] 10 mg

Triaminic Allergy, Sinus, & Head-ache Softchews (pediatric chewable tablets) (discontinued 2007) OTC *decongestant; analgesic; antipyretic* [pseudoephedrine HCl; acetaminophen] 15•150 mg

Triaminic Allergy Congestion Softchews (chewable tablets), pediatric oral liquid OTC *nasal decongestant* [pseudoephedrine HCl] 15 mg; 15 mg/5 mL

Triaminic AM Non-Drowsy Cough & Decongestant oral liquid (discontinued 2007) OTC *antitussive; decongestant; for children 2–11 years* [dextromethorphan hydrobromide; pseudoephedrine HCl] 7.5•15 mg/5 mL

Triaminic Chest & Nasal Congestion oral liquid OTC *decongestant; expectorant; for children 2–12 years* [phenylephrine HCl; guaifenesin] 2.5•50 mg/5 mL

Triaminic Children's Thin Strips Daytime Cold & Cough orally disintegrating film OTC *antitussive; decongestant* [dextromethorphan hydrobromide; phenylephrine HCl] 5•2.5 mg

Triaminic Children's Thin Strips Night Time Cold & Cough orally disintegrating film OTC *decongestant; antihistamine; sleep aid* [phenylephrine HCl; diphenhydramine HCl] 5•12.5 mg

Triaminic Cold & Allergy oral liquid OTC *decongestant; antihistamine; for children 6–11 years* [phenylephrine HCl; chlorpheniramine maleate] 5•2 mg/10 mL

Triaminic Cold & Cough oral liquid (discontinued 2007) OTC *antitussive; antihistamine; decongestant; for children 6–11 years* [dextromethorphan hydrobromide; chlorpheniramine maleate; pseudoephedrine HCl] 10•2•30 mg/10 mL

Triaminic Cold & Cough Softchews (discontinued 2007) OTC *antitussive; antihistamine; decongestant* [dextromethorphan hydrobromide; chlorpheniramine maleate; pseudoephedrine HCl] 5•1•15 mg

Triaminic Cold & Cough Thin Strips (orally disintegrating film) OTC *antitussive; decongestant* [dextromethorphan; phenylephrine HCl] 5•2.5 mg

Triaminic Cold & Sore Throat Softchews; Triaminic Throat Pain & Cough Softchews (discontinued 2007) OTC *antitussive; decongestant; analgesic; antipyretic; for children 2–11 years* [dextromethorphan hydrobromide; pseudoephedrine HCl; acetaminophen] 5•15•160 mg

Triaminic Cough oral liquid (discontinued 2007) OTC *antitussive; decongestant; for children 2–11 years* [dextromethorphan hydrobromide; pseudoephedrine HCl] 7.5•15 mg/5 mL

Triaminic Cough & Runny Nose orally disintegrating film OTC *antihistamine; sleep aid* [diphenhydramine HCl] 12.5 mg

Triaminic Cough & Sore Throat softchews, oral liquid OTC *antitussive; analgesic; antipyretic; for children 2–11 years* [dextromethorphan hydrobromide; acetaminophen] 5•160 mg; 5•160 mg/5 mL

Triaminic Daytime Cold & Cough pediatric oral liquid OTC *antitussive; decongestant; for children 2–11 years* [dextromethorphan; phenylephrine HCl] 5•2.5 mg

Triaminic Decongestant pediatric oral drops OTC *decongestant* [pseudoephedrine HCl] 7.5 mg/0.8 mL

Triaminic Flu, Cough, & Fever oral liquid OTC *antitussive; antihistamine; analgesic; antipyretic; for children 6–11 years* [dextromethorphan hydrobromide; chlorpheniramine maleate; acetaminophen] 15•2•320 mg/10 mL

Triaminic Infant Decongestant Plus Cough Thin Strips orally disintegrating film OTC *antitussive; decongestant; for children 2–3 years*

[dextromethorphan; phenylephrine HCl] 1.83•1.25 mg

Triaminic Infant Thin Strips (orally disintegrating film) OTC *decongestant* [phenylephrine HCl] 1.25 mg

Triaminic Long Acting Cough oral liquid OTC *antitussive* [dextromethorphan hydrobromide] 7.5 mg/5 mL

Triaminic MultiSymptom orally disintegrating film OTC *antihistamine; sleep aid* [diphenhydramine HCl] 25 mg

Triaminic Night Time Cold & Cough oral liquid OTC *decongestant; antihistamine; sleep aid; for children 6–11 years* [phenylephrine HCl; diphenhydramine HCl] 5•12.5 mg/10 mL

Triaminic Softchews (pediatric chewable tablets) (discontinued 2007) OTC *decongestant; antihistamine* [pseudoephedrine HCl; chlorpheniramine maleate] 15•1 mg

Triaminic Sore Throat Spray OTC *mild mucous membrane anesthetic; antipruritic; counterirritant* [phenol] 0.5%

Triaminic Thin Strips Cold orally disintegrating film OTC *decongestant* [phenylephrine HCl] 2.5 mg

Triaminic Thin Strips Cough & Runny Nose orally disintegrating film (discontinued 2007) OTC *antitussive; antihistamine; sleep aid* [diphenhydramine HCl] 12.5 mg

Triaminic Thin Strips Long Acting Cough orally disintegrating film OTC *antitussive* [dextromethorphan hydrobromide] 7.5 mg

Triaminic Throat Pain & Cough Softchews; Triaminic Cold & Sore Throat Softchews (discontinued 2007) OTC *antitussive; decongestant; analgesic; antipyretic* [dextromethorphan hydrobromide; pseudoephedrine HCl; acetaminophen] 5•15•160 mg

Triaminic Vapor Patch for Cough (withdrawn from the market in 2006 due to safety concerns) OTC *mild anesthetic; antipruritic; counterirritant* [camphor; menthol] 4.7%•2.6%

Triaminicin Cold, Allergy, Sinus Medicine tablets (discontinued 2007) OTC *decongestant; antihistamine; analgesic; antipyretic* [pseudoephedrine HCl; chlorpheniramine maleate; acetaminophen] 60•4•650 mg

Triamolone 40 IM injection ℞ *corticosteroid; anti-inflammatory* [triamcinolone diacetate] 40 mg/mL

Triamonide 40 IM, intra-articular, intrabursal, intradermal injection (discontinued 2008) ℞ *corticosteroid; anti-inflammatory* [triamcinolone acetonide] 40 mg/mL

triampyzine INN *anticholinergic* [also: triampyzine sulfate]

triampyzine sulfate USAN *anticholinergic* [also: triampyzine]

triamterene USAN, USP, INN, BAN, JAN *antihypertensive; potassium-sparing diuretic*

triamterene & hydrochlorothiazide *antihypertensive; potassium-sparing diuretic* 37.5•25 mg oral

trianisestrol [see: chlorotrianisene]

Triant-HC oral liquid ℞ *narcotic antitussive; antihistamine; decongestant* [hydrocodone bitartrate; chlorpheniramine maleate; phenylephrine HCl] 1.67•2•5 mg/5 mL

Triavil tablets (discontinued 2004) ℞ *conventional (typical) phenothiazine antipsychotic for schizophrenia and psychotic disorders; antidepressant* [perphenazine; amitriptyline HCl] 2•10 mg; 2•25 mg; 4•10 mg; 4•25 mg

Tri-A-Vite F pediatric oral drops ℞ *vitamin supplement; dental caries preventative* [vitamins A, C, and D; fluoride] 1500 IU•35 mg•400 IU•0.5 mg per mL

Triaz lotion ℞ *keratolytic for acne* [benzoyl peroxide] 3%, 6%, 10%

triaziquone INN, BAN ② Tears Again

triazolam USAN, USP, INN *benzodiazepine sedative and hypnotic* 0.125, 0.25 mg oral

Triban; Pediatric Triban suppositories (removed from the market in 2007 due to lack of efficacy) ℞ *anticholiner-*

gic; *post-surgical antiemetic; local anesthetic* [trimethobenzamide HCl; benzocaine] 200 mg•2%; 100 mg•2%

tribasic calcium phosphate [see: calcium phosphate, tribasic]

tribavirin BAN *antiviral for severe lower respiratory tract infections* [also: ribavirin]

tribendilol INN

tribenoside USAN, INN *sclerosing agent*

Tri-Biozene ointment OTC *antibiotic; local anesthetic* [polymyxin B sulfate; neomycin sulfate; bacitracin zinc; pramoxine HCl] 10 000 U•3.5 mg• 500 U•10 mg per g ☑ Trobicin

tribromoethanol NF

tribromomethane [see: bromoform]

tribromsalan USAN, INN *disinfectant*

tribuzone INN ☑ Trobicin

tricalcium phosphate [see: calcium phosphate, tribasic]

tricarbocyanine dye [see: indocyanine green]

tricetamide USAN *sedative*

Trichinella extract USP

Tri-Chlor topical liquid Ŗ *cauterant; keratolytic* [trichloroacetic acid] 80% ☑ Tracleer

trichlorethoxyphosphamide [see: defosfamide]

trichlorfon USP *veterinary anthelmintic; investigational (NDA filed) acetylcholinesterase inhibitor for Alzheimer dementia* [also: metrifonate; metriphonate]

trichlorisobutylalcohol [see: chlorobutanol]

trichlormethiazide USP, INN *diuretic; antihypertensive*

trichlormethine INN [also: trimustine]

trichloroacetic acid USP *strong keratolytic/cauterant*

trichlorocarbanilide (TCC) [see: triclocarban]

trichloroethylene NF, INN

trichlorofluoromethane [see: trichloromonofluoromethane]

trichlorofon [see: metrifonate]

trichloromonofluoromethane NF *aerosol propellant; topical anesthetic*

trichlorphon [see: metrifonate]

Tricholomopsis edodes medicinal herb [see: shiitake mushrooms]

trichorad [see: acinitrazole]

Trichosanthes kirilowii medicinal herb [see: Chinese cucumber]

Trichotine Douche solution OTC *antiseptic/germicidal; vaginal cleanser and deodorizer; acidity modifier* [sodium borate]

Trichotine Douche vaginal powder OTC *antiseptic/germicidal cleanser and deodorizer* [sodium perborate]

triciribine INN *antineoplastic* [also: triciribine phosphate]

triciribine phosphate USAN *antineoplastic* [also: triciribine]

tricitrates (sodium citrate, potassium citrate, and citric acid) USP *systemic alkalizer; urinary alkalizer; antiurolithic*

triclabendazole INN

triclacetamol INN

triclazate INN

triclobisonium chloride NF, INN

triclocarban USAN, INN *disinfectant; antiseptic*

triclodazol INN

triclofenate INN *combining name for radicals or groups*

triclofenol piperazine USAN, INN *anthelmintic*

triclofos INN *hypnotic; sedative* [also: triclofos sodium]

triclofos sodium USAN *hypnotic; sedative* [also: triclofos]

triclofylline INN

triclonide USAN, INN *anti-inflammatory*

triclosan USAN, INN, BAN *disinfectant/antiseptic*

Tricodene Cough and Cold oral liquid (discontinued 2007) Ŗ *narcotic antitussive; antihistamine; sleep aid* [codeine phosphate; pyrilamine maleate] 16.4•25 mg/10 mL

Tricodene Sugar Free Cough & Cold oral liquid OTC *antitussive; antihistamine* [dextromethorphan hydrobromide; chlorpheniramine maleate] 10•2 mg/5 mL

Tricof syrup (discontinued 2007) Ŗ *narcotic antitussive; antihistamine;*

decongestant [dihydrocodeine bitartrate; chlorpheniramine maleate; pseudoephedrine HCl] 7.5•2•15 mg/5 mL

Tricof EXP syrup (discontinued 2007) ℞ *narcotic antitussive; decongestant; expectorant* [dihydrocodeine bitartrate; pseudoephedrine HCl; guaifenesin] 7.5•15•100 mg/5 mL

Tricof PD syrup (discontinued 2007) ℞ *narcotic antitussive; antihistamine; decongestant* [dihydrocodeine bitartrate; chlorpheniramine maleate; phenylephrine HCl] 3•2•7.5 mg/5 mL

TriCor tablets ℞ *antihyperlipidemic for primary hypercholesterolemia, hypertriglyceridemia, and mixed dyslipidemia; also used for hyperuricemia* [fenofibrate] 48, 145 mg

tricosactide INN

Tricosal film-coated tablets ℞ *analgesic; antipyretic; antirheumatic* [choline magnesium trisalicylate] 500, 750, 1000 mg ⊡ Trexall

tricyclamol chloride INN

Tri-Cyclen [see: Ortho Tri-Cyclen]

tricyclics *a class of antidepressants that inhibit reuptake of amines, norepinephrine, and serotonin*

Tridal syrup (discontinued 2007) ℞ *narcotic antitussive; decongestant; expectorant* [codeine phosphate; phenylephrine HCl; guaifenesin] 10•4•125 mg/5 mL ⊡ Toradol

Tridal HD oral liquid (discontinued 2007) ℞ *narcotic antitussive; antihistamine; decongestant* [hydrocodone bitartrate; chlorpheniramine maleate; phenylephrine HCl] 4•4•15 mg/10 mL

Tridal HD Plus syrup (discontinued 2007) ℞ *narcotic antitussive; antihistamine; decongestant* [hydrocodone bitartrate; chlorpheniramine maleate; phenylephrine HCl] 7•4•15 mg/10 mL

Triderm cream ℞ *corticosteroidal anti-inflammatory* [triamcinolone acetonide] 0.1%

Tridesilon cream, ointment ℞ *corticosteroidal anti-inflammatory* [desonide] 0.05%

Tridesilon Otic [see: Otic Tridesilon]

tridihexethyl chloride USP *peptic ulcer treatment adjunct*

tridihexethyl iodide INN

Tridil IV infusion (discontinued 2004) ℞ *antianginal; vasodilator; perioperative antihypertensive; treatment for congestive heart failure with myocardial infarction* [nitroglycerin] 0.5, 5 mg/mL ⊡ Toradol

Tridione capsules, Dulcets (chewable tablets) (discontinued 2004) ℞ *anticonvulsant for absence (petit mal) seizures* [trimethadione] 300 mg; 150 mg

tridolgosir HCl USAN *chemoprotectant for solid tumor chemotherapy*

Tridrate Bowel Cleansing System oral solution + 3 tablets + 1 suppository OTC *pre-procedure bowel evacuant* [magnesium citrate (solution); bisacodyl (tablets and suppository)] 300 mL; 5 mg; 10 mg

trientine INN *copper chelating agent* [also: trientine HCl; trientine dihydrochloride]

trientine dihydrochloride BAN *copper chelating agent* [also: trientine HCl; trientine]

trientine HCl USAN, USP *copper chelating agent for Wilson disease (orphan)* [also: trientine; trientine dihydrochloride]

Triesence intravitreal injection ℞ *corticosteroid; anti-inflammatory* [triamcinolone acetonide] 40 mg/mL

triest; triestrogen [see: estriol]

triethanolamine [now: trolamine]

triethyl citrate NF *plasticizer*

triethyleneiminobenzoquinone (TEIB) [see: triaziquone]

triethylenemelamine NF [also: tretamine]

triethylenethiophosphoramide (TSPA; TESPA) [see: thiotepa]

Tri-Fed X oral suspension ℞ *antitussive; antihistamine; decongestant* [dextromethorphan tannate; dexchlorpheniramine tannate; pseudoephedrine tannate] 25•2.5•75 mg/5 mL

trifenagrel USAN, INN *antithrombotic*

trifezolac INN

triflocin USAN, INN *diuretic*

Tri-Flor-Vite with Fluoride pediatric oral drops ℞ *vitamin supplement; dental caries preventative* [vitamins A, C, and D; fluoride] 1500 IU•35 mg•400 IU•0.25 mg per mL

triflubazam USAN, INN *minor tranquilizer*

triflumidate USAN, INN *anti-inflammatory*

trifluomeprazine INN, BAN

trifluoperazine INN *conventional (typical) phenothiazine antipsychotic for schizophrenia; anxiolytic for nonpsychotic anxiety* [also: trifluoperazine HCl]

trifluoperazine HCl USP *conventional (typical) phenothiazine antipsychotic for schizophrenia; anxiolytic for nonpsychotic anxiety* [also: trifluoperazine] 1, 2, 5, 10 mg oral

trifluorothymidine [see: trifluridine]

trifluperidol USAN, INN *antipsychotic*

triflupromazine USP, INN *phenothiazine antipsychotic; antiemetic*

triflupromazine HCl USP *phenothiazine antipsychotic; antiemetic*

trifluridine USAN, INN *ophthalmic antiviral* 1% eye drops

triflusal INN

triflutate USAN, INN *combining name for radicals or groups*

Trifolium pratense medicinal herb [see: red clover]

trigevolol INN

Triglide tablets ℞ *antihyperlipidemic for primary hypercholesterolemia, hypertriglyceridemia, and mixed dyslipidemia; also used for hyperuricemia* [fenofibrate] 50, 160 mg ② Touro CC-LD

α-triglycidyl isocyanurate (αTGI) [see: teroxirone]

Trigonella foenum-graecum medicinal herb [see: fenugreek]

TriHemic 600 film-coated tablets ℞ *hematinic* [ferrous fumarate; cyanocobalamin; ascorbic acid; vitamin E; intrinsic factor concentrate; docusate sodium; folic acid] 115 mg•25 mcg•600 mg•30 IU•75 mg•50 mg•1 mg

Trihexy-2; Trihexy-5 tablets ℞ *anticholinergic; antiparkinsonian* [trihexyphenidyl HCl] 2 mg; 5 mg

trihexyphenidyl INN *anticholinergic; antiparkinsonian* [also: trihexyphenidyl HCl; benzhexol]

trihexyphenidyl HCl USP *anticholinergic; antiparkinsonian* [also: trihexyphenidyl; benzhexol] 2, 5 mg oral; 2 mg/5 mL oral

TriHIBit IM injection ℞ *active immunizing agent for diphtheria, tetanus, pertussis, and Haemophilus influenzae type b* [diphtheria & tetanus toxoids & acellular pertussis (DTaP) vaccine; Hemophilus B conjugate vaccine] supplied as separate 0.5 mL vials of Tripedia (q.v.) and ActHib (q.v.)

Tri-Hydroserpine tablets (discontinued 2007) ℞ *antihypertensive; vasodilator; diuretic* [hydrochlorothiazide; reserpine; hydralazine HCl] 15•0.1•25 mg

3,5,3′-triiodothyroacetate *investigational (orphan) for thyroid carcinoma*

triiodothyroacetic acid (TRIAC) *thyroid hormone analogue*

triiodothyronine sodium, levo [see: liothyronine sodium]

Tri-K oral liquid ℞ *potassium supplement* [potassium acetate; potassium bicarbonate; potassium citrate] 45 mEq K/15 mL ② Tarka; Touro CC

trikates USP *electrolyte replenisher*

Tri-Kort IM, intra-articular, intrabursal, or intradermal injection (discontinued 2008) ℞ *corticosteroid; anti-inflammatory* [triamcinolone acetonide] 40 mg/mL

TriLegest Fe tablets (in packs of 28) ℞ *triphasic oral contraceptive; iron supplement* [norethindrone acetate; ethinyl estradiol; ferrous fumarate] Phase 1 (5 days): 1•0.02•75 mg; Phase 2 (7 days): 1•0.03•75 mg; Phase 3 (9 days): 1•0.035•75 mg; Counters (7 days): 0•0•75 mg

Trileptal film-coated tablets, oral suspension ℞ *anticonvulsant for partial seizures in adults or children; also used for bipolar disorder and diabetic neuropathy* [oxcarbazepine] 150, 300, 600 mg; 300 mg/5 mL

triletide INN

Tri-Levlen film-coated tablets (in Slidecases of 28) (discontinued 2008) ℞ *triphasic oral contraceptive; emergency postcoital contraceptive* [levonorgestrel; ethinyl estradiol]
Phase 1 (6 days): 0.5 mg•30 mcg;
Phase 2 (5 days): 0.75 mg•40 mcg;
Phase 3 (10 days): 0.125 mg•30 mcg

Trilisate tablets, oral liquid (discontinued 2004) ℞ *analgesic; antipyretic; anti-inflammatory; antirheumatic* [choline salicylate; magnesium salicylate] 750, 1000 mg; 500 mg/5 mL

trilithium citrate tetrahydrate [see: lithium citrate]

Trillium erectum; T. grandiflorum; T. pendulum medicinal herb [see: birthroot]

Trilog IM, intra-articular, intrabursal, intradermal injection (discontinued 2008) ℞ *corticosteroid; anti-inflammatory* [triamcinolone acetonide] 40 mg/mL

Trilone IM injection (discontinued 2006) ℞ *corticosteroid; anti-inflammatory* [triamcinolone diacetate] 40 mg/mL ☒ Tarlene

trilostane USAN, INN, BAN *adrenocortical suppressant; antisteroidal antineoplastic*

Tri-Luma cream ℞ *short-term treatment for melasma of the face* [hydroquinone; fluocinolone acetonide; tretinoin] 4%•0.01%•0.05%

TriLyte powder for oral solution ℞ *pre-procedure bowel evacuant* [PEG 3350; sodium bicarbonate; sodium chloride; potassium chloride] 420•5.72•11.2•1.48 g/4 L bottle

Trimazide suppositories, pediatric suppositories (removed from the market in 2007 due to lack of efficacy) ℞ *anticholinergic; post-surgical antiemetic* [trimethobenzamide HCl] 200 mg; 100 mg

trimazosin INN, BAN *antihypertensive* [also: trimazosin HCl]

trimazosin HCl USAN *antihypertensive* [also: trimazosin]

trimebutine INN GI *antispasmodic*

trimecaine INN

trimedoxime bromide INN

trimegestone USAN *progestin for postmenopausal hormone deficiency*

trimeperidine INN, BAN

trimeprazine BAN *phenothiazine antihistamine; antipruritic* [also: trimeprazine tartrate; alimemazine; alimemazine tartrate]

trimeprazine tartrate USP *phenothiazine antihistamine; antipruritic* [also: alimemazine; trimeprazine; alimemazine tartrate]

trimeproprimine [see: trimipramine]

trimetamide INN

trimetaphan camsilate INN *antihypertensive* [also: trimethaphan camsylate; trimetaphan camsylate]

trimetaphan camsylate BAN *antihypertensive* [also: trimethaphan camsylate; trimetaphan camsilate]

trimetazidine INN, BAN

trimethadione USP, INN *oxazolidinedione anticonvulsant for absence (petit mal) seizures* [also: troxidone]

trimethamide [see: trimetamide]

trimethaphan camphorsulfonate [see: trimethaphan camsylate]

trimethaphan camsylate USP *emergency antihypertensive* [also: trimetaphan camsilate; trimetaphan camsylate]

trimethidinium methosulfate NF, INN

trimethobenzamide INN *anticholinergic; post-surgical antiemetic* [also: trimethobenzamide HCl]

trimethobenzamide HCl USP *anticholinergic; post-surgical antiemetic; suppositories removed from the market in 2007 due to lack of efficacy* [also: trimethobenzamide] 300 mg oral; 100 mg/mL injection

trimethoprim (TMP) USAN, USP, INN, BAN *antibacterial antibiotic* 100, 200 mg oral

trimethoprim sulfate USAN *antibiotic*

trimethoprim sulfate & polymyxin B sulfate *topical ophthalmic antibiotic* 1 mg•10 000 U per mL eye drops

trimethoquinol [see: tretoquinol]

trimethylammonium chloride carbamate [see: bethanechol chloride]

3,3,5-trimethylcyclohexyl salicylate [see: homosalate]

trimethylene [see: cyclopropane]

trimethylglycine (TMG) *natural methylation agent used to prevent cardiovascular disease by lowering homocysteine levels, to boost neurological function by remyelinating nerve cells, and to slow cellular aging by protecting DNA; precursor to SAMe (q.v.)*

trimethyltetradecylammonium bromide [see: tetradonium bromide]

trimetozine USAN, INN *sedative*

trimetrexate USAN, INN, BAN *antimetabolic antineoplastic; systemic antiprotozoal*

trimetrexate glucuronate USAN *antiprotozoal for AIDS-related Pneumocystis pneumonia (PCP) (orphan); investigational (orphan) antineoplastic for multiple cancers*

trimexiline INN

trimipramine USAN, INN *tricyclic antidepressant*

trimipramine maleate USAN *tricyclic antidepressant*

trimolide [see: trimetozine]

trimopam maleate [now: trepipam maleate]

trimoprostil USAN, INN *gastric antisecretory*

Trimo-San vaginal jelly OTC *antiseptic; astringent* [oxyquinoline sulfate; boric acid; sodium borate] 0.025%•1%•0.7% ⊡ Terramycin

Trimox chewable tablets, capsules, powder for oral suspension (discontinued 2008) ℞ *aminopenicillin antibiotic* [amoxicillin] 125, 250 mg; 250, 500 mg; 250 mg/5 mL ⊡ Tyromex

Trimox powder for oral suspension ℞ *aminopenicillin antibiotic* [amoxicillin] 125 mg/5 mL ⊡ Tyromex-1

trimoxamine INN *antihypertensive* [also: trimoxamine HCl]

trimoxamine HCl USAN *antihypertensive* [also: trimoxamine]

Trimpex tablets ℞ *anti-infective; antibacterial* [trimethoprim] 100 mg

trimustine BAN [also: trichlormethine] ⊡ tauromustine

Trinalin Repetabs (sustained-release tablets) (discontinued 2006) ℞ *decongestant; antihistamine* [pseudoephedrine sulfate; azatadine maleate] 120•1 mg ⊡ Tronolane

Trinam reservoir delivery device *investigational (Phase II, orphan) gene-based therapy for neointimal hyperplasia disease* [vascular endothelial growth factor (VEGF)]

Trinate tablets ℞ *vitamin/mineral/calcium/iron supplement* [multiple vitamins & minerals; calcium; iron; folic acid] ≛•200•28•1 mg

trinecol (pullus) USAN *collagen derivative for treatment of rheumatoid arthritis*

TriNessa tablets (in packs of 28) ℞ *triphasic oral contraceptive* [norgestimate; ethinyl estradiol]
Phase 1 (7 days): 0.18 mg•35 mcg;
Phase 2 (7 days): 0,215 mg•35 mcg;
Phase 3 (7 days): 0.25 mg•35 mcg

trinitrin [see: nitroglycerin]

trinitrophenol NF

Tri-Norinyl tablets (in Wallettes of 28) ℞ *triphasic oral contraceptive* [norethindrone; ethinyl estradiol]
Phase 1 (7 days): 0.5 mg•35 mcg;
Phase 2 (9 days): 1 mg•35 mcg;
Phase 3 (5 days): 0.5 mg•35 mcg

Trinsicon capsules ℞ *hematinic* [ferrous fumarate; cyanocobalamin; ascorbic acid; intrinsic factor concentrate; folic acid] 110 mg•15 mcg•75 mg•240 mg•0.5 mg

2',3',5'-tri-o-acetyluridine *investigational (orphan) treatment for mitochondrial disease*

triolein I 125 USAN *radioactive agent* 🔘 Tarlene

triolein I 131 USAN *radioactive agent* 🔘 Tarlene

trional [see: sulfonethylmethane]

Trionate caplets ℞ *antitussive; antihistamine* [carbetapentane tannate; chlorpheniramine tannate] 60•5 mg

Triostat IV injection ℞ *synthetic thyroid hormone (T₃ fraction only) for myxedema coma or precoma (orphan)* [liothyronine sodium] 10 mcg/mL

Triotann Pediatric oral suspension ℞ *decongestant; antihistamine; sleep aid* [phenylephrine tannate; chlorpheniramine tannate; pyrilamine tannate] 5•2•12.5 mg/5 mL

Triotann-S Pediatric oral suspension (discontinued 2007) ℞ *decongestant; antihistamine; sleep aid* [phenylephrine tannate; chlorpheniramine tannate; pyrilamine tannate] 5•2•12.5 mg/5 mL

Tri-Otic ear drops (discontinued 2008) ℞ *corticosteroidal anti-inflammatory; anesthetic; antiseptic* [hydrocortisone; pramoxine HCl; chloroxylenol] 10•10•1 mg/mL

trioxifene INN *antiestrogen* [also: trioxifene mesylate]

trioxifene mesylate USAN *antiestrogen* [also: trioxifene]

trioxsalen USAN, USP *systemic psoralens for repigmentation of idiopathic vitiligo; also used to enhance pigmentation and increase tolerance to sunlight* [also: trioxysalen]

trioxyethylrutin [see: troxerutin]

trioxymethylene [see: paraformaldehyde]

trioxysalen INN *systemic psoralens for repigmentation of idiopathic vitiligo; also used to enhance pigmentation and increase tolerance to sunlight* [also: trioxsalen]

tripamide USAN, INN *antihypertensive; diuretic*

triparanol INN *(withdrawn from market)*

Tripedia IM injection ℞ *active immunizing agent for diphtheria, tetanus,* and pertussis; *Dtap (diphtheria predominant) vaccine used in the initial immunization series of infants and children 6 weeks to 6 years* [diphtheria toxoid; tetanus toxoid; pertussis antigens] 6.7 LfU•5 LfU•46.8 mcg per 0.5 mL dose

tripelennamine INN *ethylenediamine antihistamine* [also: tripelennamine citrate]

tripelennamine citrate USP *ethylenediamine antihistamine* [also: tripelennamine]

tripelennamine HCl USP *ethylenediamine antihistamine*

Triphasil tablets (in packs of 21 or 28) ℞ *triphasic oral contraceptive; emergency postcoital contraceptive* [levonorgestrel; ethinyl estradiol] 🔘 Travasol
Phase 1 (6 days): 0.5 mg•30 mcg;
Phase 2 (5 days): 0.75 mg•40 mcg;
Phase 3 (10 days): 0.125 mg•30 mcg

Triple Antibiotic ointment OTC *antibiotic* [polymyxin B sulfate; neomycin sulfate; bacitracin] 5000 U•3.5 mg•400 U per g

Triple Paste AF ointment OTC *antifungal* [miconazole nitrate] 2%

triple sulfa (sulfathiazole, sulfacetamide, and sulfabenzamide) [q.v.]

Triple Tannate Pediatric oral suspension ℞ *decongestant; antihistamine; sleep aid* [phenylephrine tannate; chlorpheniramine tannate; pyrilamine tannate] 5•2•12.5 mg/5 mL

Triple Vitamin ADC with Fluoride pediatric oral drops ℞ *vitamin supplement; dental caries preventative* [vitamins A, C, and D; fluoride] 1500 IU•35 mg•400 IU•0.5 mg per mL

Triplex AD oral liquid ℞ *decongestant; antihistamine; sleep aid* [phenylephrine HCl; chlorpheniramine maleate; pyrilamine maleate] 7.5•2•12.5 mg/5 mL

Triplex DM oral liquid ℞ *antitussive; antihistamine; sleep aid; decongestant* [dextromethorphan hydrobromide; pyrilamine maleate; phenylephrine HCl] 15•12.5•7.5 mg/5 mL

Tripohist D oral liquid ℞ *decongestant; antihistamine* [pseudoephedrine HCl; triprolidine HCl] 45•1.25 mg/5 mL

tripotassium citrate monohydrate [see: potassium citrate]

Tri-Previfem tablets (in packs of 28) ℞ *triphasic oral contraceptive* [norgestimate; ethinyl estradiol]
Phase 1 (7 days): 0.18 mg•35 mcg;
Phase 2 (7 days): 0.215 mg•35 mcg;
Phase 3 (7 days): 0.25 mg•35 mcg

triproamylin [see: pramlintide]

triprolidine INN *antihistamine* [also: triprolidine HCl]

triprolidine HCl USP *antihistamine* [also: triprolidine] 1.25 mg/5 mL oral

triprolidine HCl & pseudoephedrine HCl *antihistamine; decongestant* 2.5•60 mg/10 mL oral

Tripterygium wilfordii medicinal herb [see: thunder god vine]

Triptone long-acting caplets OTC *antinauseant; antiemetic; antivertigo; motion sickness preventative* [dimenhydrinate] 50 mg

triptorelin USAN, INN *gonadotropin-releasing hormone (GnRH) antineoplastic*

triptorelin pamoate *gonadotropin-releasing hormone (GnRH) antineoplastic for palliative treatment of advanced prostate cancer; investigational (orphan) for palliative treatment of advanced ovarian cancer*

trisaccharides A and B *investigational (orphan) for newborn hemolytic disease and ABO blood incompatibility of organ or bone marrow transplants*

Trisenox injection ℞ *antineoplastic for acute promyelocytic leukemia (orphan); investigational (orphan) for other leukemias, multiple myeloma, myelodysplastic syndromes, liver cancer, and malignant glioma* [arsenic trioxide] 10 mg/10 mL

trisodium calcium DTPA [see: pentetate calcium trisodium]

trisodium citrate [see: sodium citrate]

trisodium citrate dihydrate [see: sodium citrate]

trisodium hydrogen ethylenediaminetetraacetate [see: edetate trisodium]

trisodium zinc DTPA [see: pentetate zinc trisodium]

Trispec PSE oral liquid (discontinued 2007) ℞ *antitussive; decongestant; expectorant* [dextromethorphan hydrobromide; pseudoephedrine HCl; guaifenesin] 15•30•25 mg/5 mL

Tri-Sprintec tablets (in packs of 28) ℞ *triphasic oral contraceptive* [norgestimate; ethinyl estradiol]
Phase 1 (7 days): 0.18 mg•35 mcg;
Phase 2 (7 days): 0.215 mg•35 mcg;
Phase 3 (7 days): 0.25 mg•35 mcg

Tri-Statin II cream ℞ *corticosteroidal anti-inflammatory; antifungal* [triamcinolone acetonide; nystatin] 0.1%• 100 000 U per g

Tristoject IM injection (discontinued 2006) ℞ *corticosteroid; anti-inflammatory* [triamcinolone diacetate] 40 mg/mL

trisulfapyrimidines USP (a mixture of sulfadiazine, sulfamerazine, and sulfamethazine) *broad-spectrum bacteriostatic*

Tri-Super Flavons 1000 tablets OTC *dietary supplement* [mixed bioflavonoids] 1000 mg

Tritec film-coated tablets (discontinued 2004) ℞ *histamine H_2 antagonist for duodenal ulcers with H. pylori infection* [ranitidine bismuth citrate] 400 mg

tritheon [see: acinitrazole]

tritiated water USAN *radioactive agent*

Triticum repens medicinal herb [see: couch grass]

tritiozine INN

tritoqualine INN

TriTuss syrup ℞ *antitussive; decongestant; expectorant* [dextromethorphan hydrobromide; phenylephrine HCl; guaifenesin] 25•12.5•175 mg/5 mL

Trituss-A oral drops (discontinued 2007) ℞ *antitussive; antihistamine; decongestant; for children 3–24 months* [dextromethorphan hydrobromide;

carbinoxamine maleate; phenylephrine HCl] 4•1•2 mg/mL

TriTuss-ER extended-release caplets ℞ *antitussive; decongestant; expectorant* [dextromethorphan hydrobromide; phenylephrine HCl; guaifenesin] 30•10•600 mg

Tritussin syrup (discontinued 2007) ℞ *narcotic antitussive; antihistamine; decongestant* [hydrocodone bitartrate; chlorpheniramine maleate; phenylephrine HCl] 10•4•10 mg/10 mL

Trivagizole 3 vaginal cream OTC *antifungal for yeast infections* [clotrimazole] 2%

trivalent oral poliovirus vaccine (TOPV) [see: poliovirus vaccine, live oral]

Trivaris gel suspension for ocular, IM, or intra-articular injection ℞ *corticosteroidal anti-inflammatory* [triamcinolone acetonide] 80 mg/mL

Tri-Vi-Flor pediatric chewable tablets, pediatric oral drops ℞ *vitamin supplement; dental caries preventative* [vitamins A, C, and D; sodium fluoride] 2500 IU•60 mg•400 IU•1 mg; 1500 IU•35 mg•400 IU•0.25 mg, 1500 IU•35 mg•400 IU•0.5 mg per mL

Tri-Vi-Flor with Iron pediatric oral drops ℞ *vitamin/iron supplement; dental caries preventative* [vitamins A, C, and D; iron; sodium fluoride] 1500 IU•35 mg•400 IU•0.25 mg per mL

Tri-Vi-Sol pediatric oral drops OTC *vitamin supplement* [vitamins A, C, and D] 1500 IU•35 mg•400 IU per mL ⌧ Travasol 3.5%

Tri-Vi-Sol with Iron drops OTC *vitamin/iron supplement* [vitamins A, C, and D; ferrous sulfate] 1500 IU•35 mg•400 IU•10 mg per mL

Trivitamin Fluoride pediatric chewable tablets, pediatric oral drops ℞ *vitamin supplement; dental caries preventative* [vitamins A, C, and D; fluoride] 2500 IU•60 mg•400 IU•1 mg; 1500 IU•35 mg•400 IU•0.25 mg, 1500 IU•35 mg•400 IU•0.5 mg per mL

Tri-Vitamin Infants' Drops OTC *vitamin supplement* [vitamins A, C, and D] 1500 IU•35 mg•400 IU per mL

Tri-Vitamin with Fluoride pediatric oral drops ℞ *vitamin supplement; dental caries preventative* [vitamins A, C, and D; fluoride] 1500 IU•35 mg•400 IU•0.5 mg per mL

Trivora tablets (in packs of 28) ℞ *triphasic oral contraceptive* [levonorgestrel; ethinyl estradiol]
Phase 1 (6 days): 0.5 mg•30 mcg;
Phase 2 (5 days): 0.75 mg•40 mcg;
Phase 3 (10 days): 0.125 mg•30 mcg

trixolane INN ⌧ teroxalene

Trizivir film-coated caplets ℞ *antiretroviral nucleoside reverse transcriptase inhibitor (NRTI) for HIV infection* [abacavir sulfate; zidovudine; lamivudine] 300•300•150 mg

trizoxime INN

Trizyme (trademarked ingredient) *digestive enzymes* [amylolytic, proteolytic, and cellulolytic enzymes (amylase; protease; cellulase)] ⌧ Tarsum

Trobicin powder for IM injection ℞ *antibiotic for gonorrhea* [spectinomycin HCl] 400 mg/mL ⌧ Tri-Biozene

Trocaine lozenges OTC *mucous membrane anesthetic* [benzocaine] 10 mg ⌧ tarragon; Torecan

Trocal lozenges OTC *antitussive* [dextromethorphan hydrobromide] 7.5 mg

trocimine INN

troclosene potassium USAN, INN *topical anti-infective*

trofosfamide INN

troglitazone USAN, INN *thiazolidinedione (TZD) antidiabetic and peroxisome proliferator–activated receptor–gamma (PPARγ) agonist that increases cellular response to insulin without increasing insulin secretion*

trolamine USAN, NF *alkalizing agent; analgesic*

trolamine polypeptide oleate-condensate *cerumenolytic to emulsify and disperse ear wax*

trolamine salicylate *topical analgesic*

troleandomycin USAN, USP *macrolide antibiotic; investigational (orphan) for severe asthma* [also: triacetyloleandomycin]

trolnitrate INN

trolnitrate phosphate [see: trolnitrate]

tromantadine INN

trometamol INN, BAN *systemic alkalizer; corrects acidosis associated with cardiac bypass surgery or cardiac arrest* [also: tromethamine]

tromethamine USAN, USP *systemic alkalizer; corrects acidosis associated with cardiac bypass surgery or cardiac arrest* [also: trometamol]

Tronolane anorectal cream OTC *local anesthetic; astringent; emollient* [pramoxine HCl; zinc oxide] 1%•5% ⧉ Trinalin

Tronolane rectal suppositories OTC *astringent* [phenylephrine HCl] 0.25% ⧉ Trinalin

Tronothane HCl cream OTC *anesthetic* [pramoxine HCl] 1% ⧉ trientine HCl

tropabazate INN

Tropaeolum majus medicinal herb [see: Indian cress]

tropanserin INN, BAN *migraine-specific serotonin receptor antagonist* [also: tropanserin HCl]

tropanserin HCl USAN *migraine-specific serotonin receptor antagonist* [also: tropanserin]

tropapride INN

tropatepine INN

tropenziline bromide INN

TrophAmine 6%; TrophAmine 10% IV infusion ℞ *total parenteral nutrition; peripheral parenteral nutrition* [multiple essential and nonessential amino acids]

Trophite + Iron oral liquid OTC *hematinic* [ferric pyrophosphate; vitamins B_1 and B_{12}] 60 mg•30 mg•75 mcg per 15 mL

trophosphamide [see: trofosfamide]

Tropicacyl eye drops ℞ *cycloplegic; mydriatic* [tropicamide] 0.5%, 1%

tropicamide USAN, USP, INN *ophthalmic anticholinergic; cycloplegic; short-acting mydriatic*

tropigline INN, BAN

tropirine INN

tropisetron INN, BAN *antiemetic*

Tropi-Storz eye drops ℞ *cycloplegic; mydriatic* [tropicamide] 0.5%, 1%

tropodifene INN

troquidazole INN

trospectomycin INN, BAN *broad-spectrum aminocyclitol antibiotic* [also: trospectomycin sulfate]

trospectomycin sulfate USAN *broad-spectrum aminocyclitol antibiotic* [also: trospectomycin]

trospium chloride INN *muscarinic receptor antagonist; urinary antispasmodic for overactive bladder with urinary frequency, urgency, and incontinence*

trovafloxacin mesylate USAN *broad-spectrum fluoroquinolone antibiotic*

Trovan film-coated tablets ℞ *broad-spectrum fluoroquinolone antibiotic* [trovafloxacin mesylate] 100, 200 mg

Trovan IV infusion ℞ *broad-spectrum fluoroquinolone antibiotic* [alatrofloxacin mesylate] 5 mg/mL

Trovan/Zithromax Compliance Pak ℞ *single-dose antibiotic treatment for sexually transmitted diseases* [**Trovan** (trovafloxacin mesylate); **Zithromax** (azithromycin)] 100 mg tablet; 1 g pkt. of powder for oral suspension

TroVax *investigational (Phase III) immunotherapeutic for advanced or metastatic renal cell carcinoma (RCC)*

troxacitabine USAN, INN *antineoplastic for various leukemias and solid tumors; investigational (orphan) for acute myeloid leukemia*

Troxatyl *investigational (orphan) antineoplastic for acute myeloid leukemia* [troxacitabine]

troxerutin INN, BAN *vitamin P_4*

troxidone BAN *anticonvulsant* [also: trimethadione]

troxipide INN

troxolamide INN

troxonium tosilate INN [also: troxonium tosylate]

troxonium tosylate BAN [also: troxonium tosilate]

troxundate INN *combining name for radicals or groups*

troxypyrrolium tosilate INN [also: troxypyrrolium tosylate]

troxypyrrolium tosylate BAN [also: troxypyrrolium tosilate]

true ivy *medicinal herb* [see: English ivy]

T.R.U.E. Test patch *diagnostic aid for contact dermatitis* [skin test antigens (23 different) plus 1 negative control]

Trugene genetic testing system for professional use ℞ *in vitro diagnostic aid for HIV mutations that cause resistance to anti-AIDS drugs; used to determine which treatment regimen is most effective in individual patients* ⚠ tarragon; Teargen; Torecan; Trocaine

Truphylline suppositories (discontinued 2006) ℞ *antiasthmatic; bronchodilator* [aminophylline] 250, 500 mg

Trusopt eye drops ℞ *carbonic anhydrase inhibitor for glaucoma* [dorzolamide HCl] 2%

Truvada film-coated caplets ℞ *once-daily nucleoside reverse transcriptase inhibitor (NRTI) antiviral combination for HIV infections* [emtricitabine; tenofovir disoproxil fumarate] 200•300 mg

truxicurium iodide INN

truxipicurium iodide INN

Trycet film-coated caplets ℞ *narcotic analgesic; antipyretic* [propoxyphene napsylate; acetaminophen] 100•325 mg ⚠ Triacet

trypaflavine [see: acriflavine HCl]

trypan blue *surgical aid for staining the anterior capsule of the lens*

tryparsamide USP, INN

trypsin, crystallized USP *topical proteolytic enzyme; necrotic tissue debridement*

tryptizol [see: amitriptyline]

tryptizol HCl [see: amitriptyline HCl]

tryptophan (L-tryptophan) USAN, USP, INN *essential amino acid; seroto-*

nin precursor (The FDA has banned all OTC tryptophan supplements.)

TSC (technetium sulfur colloid) [see: technetium Tc 99m sulfur colloid]

T/Scalp topical liquid OTC *corticosteroidal anti-inflammatory* [hydrocortisone] 1%

TSH (thyroid-stimulating hormone) [see: thyrotropin]

TSPA (triethylenethiophosphoramide) [see: thiotepa]

TST (tuberculin skin test) [see: tuberculin]

T-Stat topical solution, medicated pads (discontinued 2004) ℞ *antibiotic for acne* [erythromycin; alcohol 71.2%] 2% ⚠ Tusstat

Tsuga canadensis *medicinal herb* [see: hemlock]

T-Tabs (trademarked dosage form) *tablets with a "T" imprint*

tuaminoheptane USP, INN *adrenergic; vasoconstrictor*

tuaminoheptane sulfate USP

tuberculin USP *tuberculosis skin test*

tuberculin, crude [see: tuberculin]

tuberculin, old (OT) [see: tuberculin]

tuberculin purified protein derivative (PPD) [see: tuberculin]

tuberculosis vaccine [see: BCG vaccine]

Tubersol intradermal injection ℞ *tuberculosis skin test* [tuberculin purified protein derivative] 5 U/0.1 mL

Tubex (trademarked delivery device) *cartridge-needle unit*

tubocurarine chloride USP, INN, BAN *neuromuscular blocker; muscle relaxant* 3 mg (20 U)/mL injection

tubocurarine chloride HCl pentahydrate [see: tubocurarine chloride]

tubulozole INN *antineoplastic; microtubule inhibitor* [also: tubulozole HCl]

tubulozole HCl USAN, INN *antineoplastic; microtubule inhibitor* [also: tubulozole]

tucaresol INN, BAN *investigational (Phase II) immunopotentiator for HIV infection*

Tucks anorectal ointment OTC *cortico-steroidal anti-inflammatory* [hydrocortisone acetate] [note: one of two different products with the same name] 1%

Tucks anorectal ointment OTC *local anesthetic; astringent* [pramoxine HCl; zinc oxide] [note: one of two different products with the same name] 1%•12.5%

Tucks rectal suppositories OTC *emollient* [topical starch] 51%

Tucks; Tucks Take-Alongs cleansing pads OTC *moisturizer and cleanser for the perineal area; astringent* [witch hazel; glycerin] 50%•10%

Tucks Clear gel OTC *emollient; astringent* [hamamelis water (witch hazel); glycerin] 50%•10%

tuclazepam INN

Tuinal Pulvules (capsules) ℞ *sedative; hypnotic; also abused as a street drug* [amobarbital sodium; secobarbital sodium] 50•50, 100•100 mg

tulobuterol INN, BAN, JAN [also: tulobuterol HCl]

tulobuterol HCl JAN [also: tulobuterol]

tulopafant INN

tumeric root *medicinal herb* [see: goldenseal]

tumor necrosis factor-binding protein I and II *investigational (orphan) for symptomatic AIDS patients*

Tums; Tums E-X; Tums Ultra; Tums Calcium for Life PMS chewable tablets OTC *antacid; calcium supplement* [calcium carbonate] 500 mg (200 mg Ca); 750 mg (300 mg Ca); 1 g (400 mg Ca); 750 mg (300 mg Ca)

Tums Calcium for Life Bone Health chewable tablets (discontinued 2006) OTC *antacid; calcium supplement* [calcium carbonate] 1250 mg (500 mg Ca)

Tums Smooth Dissolve (orally disintegrating tablets) OTC *antacid; calcium supplement* [calcium carbonate] 750 mg (300 mg Ca)

tung seed (*Aleurites cordata; A. moluccana*) seed and oil *medicinal herb for asthma, bowel evacuation, and*

tumors; not generally regarded as safe and effective as it is highly toxic ⚕ tannic acid

tungsten *element* (W)

Turbinaire (trademarked dosage form) *nasal inhalation aerosol*

Turbuhaler (trademarked delivery form) *dry powder in a metered-dose inhaler*

turkey corn (*Corydalis formosa*) root *medicinal herb used as an antisyphilitic, bitter tonic, and diuretic*

turkey pea; wild turkey pea *medicinal herb* [see: turkey corn]

turmeric (*Curcuma domestica; C. longa*) rhizomes *medicinal herb for flatulence, hemorrhage, hepatitis and jaundice, topical analgesia, and ringworm*

Turnera aphrodisiaca; T. diffusa; T. microphylla *medicinal herb* [see: damiana]

turosteride INN

turpentine (*Pinus palustris*) gum *natural treatment for colds, cough, and toothache; also used topically as a counterirritant for muscle pain and rheumatic disorders*

turtlebloom (*Chelone glabra*) leaves *medicinal herb used as an anthelmintic, aperient, cholagogue, and detergent*

Tusana-D oral liquid ℞ *narcotic antitussive; antihistamine; decongestant* [hydrocodone bitartrate; chlorpheniramine maleate; phenylephrine HCl] 6•2•12 mg/5 mL

Tusdec-DM oral liquid ℞ *antitussive; antihistamine; decongestant* [dextromethorphan hydrobromide; brompheniramine maleate; phenylephrine HCl] 15•2•7.5 mg/5 mL

Tusdec-HC oral liquid ℞ *narcotic antitussive; decongestant* [hydrocodone bitartrate; phenylephrine HCl] 3.75•7.5 mg/5 mL

Tusnel; Tusnel Pediatric oral liquid ℞ *antitussive; decongestant; expectorant* [dextromethorphan hydrobromide; pseudoephedrine HCl; guaifenesin] 15•30•200 mg/5 mL; 5•15•50 mg/5 mL

Tusnel C syrup ℞ *narcotic antitussive; decongestant; expectorant* [codeine phosphate; pseudoephedrine HCl; guaifenesin; alcohol 1.9%] 10•30•100 mg/5 mL

Tusnel-HC oral liquid ℞ *narcotic antitussive; antihistamine; decongestant* [hydrocodone bitartrate; brompheniramine maleate; phenylephrine HCl] 2.5•4•7.5 mg/5 mL

Tussafed syrup (discontinued 2007) ℞ *antitussive; antihistamine; decongestant* [dextromethorphan hydrobromide; carbinoxamine maleate; pseudoephedrine HCl] 15•4•60 mg/5 mL

Tussafed Ex syrup (discontinued 2007) ℞ *antitussive; decongestant; expectorant* [dextromethorphan hydrobromide; phenylephrine HCl; guaifenesin] 30•10•200 mg/5 mL

Tussafed HC; Tussafed HCG syrup ℞ *narcotic antitussive; decongestant; expectorant* [hydrocodone bitartrate; phenylephrine HCl; guaifenesin] 2.5•7.5•50 mg/5 mL; 2.5•6•150 mg/5 mL

Tussafed LA sustained-release caplets (discontinued 2007) ℞ *antitussive; decongestant; expectorant* [dextromethorphan hydrobromide; pseudoephedrine HCl; guaifenesin] 30•60•600 mg

Tussall syrup ℞ *antitussive; antihistamine; decongestant* [dextromethorphan hydrobromide; dexbrompheniramine maleate; phenylephrine HCl] 20•2•10 mg/5 mL ② TiSol

Tussall-ER extended-release caplets ℞ *antitussive; antihistamine; decongestant* [dextromethorphan hydrobromide; dexbrompheniramine maleate; phenylephrine HCl] 30•6•20 mg ② tosulur

Tussbid extended-release capsules ℞ *decongestant; expectorant* [phenylephrine HCl; guaifenesin] 15•400 mg

Tussbid PD extended-release capsules ℞ *decongestant; expectorant* [phenylephrine HCl; guaifenesin] 7.5•200 mg

Tuss-DM tablets (discontinued 2006) OTC *antitussive; expectorant* [dextromethorphan hydrobromide; guaifenesin] 10•200 mg ② Tazidime

Tussend caplets (discontinued 2007) ℞ *narcotic antitussive; antihistamine; decongestant* [hydrocodone bitartrate; chlorpheniramine maleate; pseudoephedrine HCl] 5•4•60 mg

Tussend syrup (discontinued 2007) ℞ *narcotic antitussive; antihistamine; decongestant* [hydrocodone bitartrate; chlorpheniramine maleate; pseudoephedrine HCl; alcohol 5%] 5•4•60 mg/10 mL

Tussex Cough syrup (discontinued 2005) OTC *antitussive; decongestant; expectorant* [dextromethorphan hydrobromide; phenylephrine HCl; guaifenesin] 10•5•100 mg/5 mL

Tussi-12 caplets ℞ *antitussive; antihistamine* [carbetapentane tannate; chlorpheniramine tannate] 60•5 mg

Tussi-12 D caplets ℞ *antitussive; decongestant; antihistamine; sleep aid* [carbetapentane tannate; phenylephrine tannate; pyrilamine tannate] 60•40•10 mg

Tussi-12 S oral suspension ℞ *antitussive; antihistamine* [carbetapentane tannate; chlorpheniramine tannate] 30•4 mg/5 mL

Tussi-12D S oral suspension ℞ *antitussive; antihistamine; sleep aid; decongestant* [carbetapentane tannate; pyrilamine tannate; phenylephrine tannate] 30•30•5 mg/5 mL ② TZDs

Tussi-bid sustained-release caplets ℞ *antitussive; expectorant* [dextromethorphan hydrobromide; guaifenesin] 60•1200 mg

Tussiden DM oral liquid ℞ *antitussive; expectorant* [dextromethorphan hydrobromide; guaifenesin] 10•100 mg/5 mL

Tussigon tablets ℞ *narcotic antitussive; anticholinergic* [hydrocodone bitartrate; homatropine methylbromide] 5•1.5 mg ② tisoquone

Tussilago farfara medicinal herb [see: coltsfoot]

TussiNaTE syrup (discontinued 2007) R narcotic antitussive; antihistamine; sleep aid; decongestant [hydrocodone bitartrate; diphenhydramine HCl; phenylephrine HCl] 7•25•10 mg/10 mL

Tussionex Pennkinetic extended-release oral suspension R narcotic antitussive; antihistamine [hydrocodone polistirex; chlorpheniramine polistirex] 10•8 mg/5 mL

Tussi-Organidin DM NR; Tussi-Organidin DM-S NR oral liquid ("S" includes an oral syringe) R antitussive; expectorant [dextromethorphan hydrobromide; guaifenesin] 10•300 mg/5 mL

Tussi-Organidin NR; Tussi-Organidin-S NR oral liquid ("S" includes an oral syringe) R narcotic antitussive; expectorant [codeine phosphate; guaifenesin] 10•300 mg/5 mL

Tussi-Pres; Tussi-Pres Pediatric oral liquid R antitussive; decongestant; expectorant [dextromethorphan hydrobromide; phenylephrine HCl; guaifenesin] 15•5•200 mg/5 mL; 5•2.5•75 mg/5 mL

Tussirex syrup, oral liquid R narcotic antitussive; decongestant; antihistamine; expectorant; analgesic [codeine phosphate; phenylephrine HCl; pheniramine maleate; sodium citrate; sodium salicylate; caffeine citrate] 10•4.17•13.33•83.3•83.33•25 mg/5 mL

Tussizone-12 RF caplets, oral suspension R antitussive; antihistamine [carbetapentane tannate; chlorpheniramine tannate] 60•5 mg; 30•4 mg/5 mL

Tusso DM dual-release caplets R antitussive; decongestant; expectorant [dextromethorphan hydrobromide; phenylephrine HCl; guaifenesin] 23 mg (65% extended release)•9 mg (100% extended release)•600 mg (67% extended release) ⊚ Tazidime

Tusso HC caplets R narcotic antitussive; expectorant [hydrocodone bitartrate; guaifenesin] 10•1200 mg ⊚ Tyzeka

Tusso XR oral suspension R antitussive; decongestant; expectorant [dextromethorphan hydrobromide; phenylephrine HCl; guaifenesin] 20•10•100 mg/5 mL

Tussplex syrup R narcotic antitussive; decongestant; antihistamine; sleep aid [hydrocodone bitartrate; phenylephrine HCl; pyrilamine maleate] 6•5•12 mg/5 mL

Tuss-Tan tablets, pediatric oral suspension (discontinued 2005) R antitussive; decongestant; antihistamine [carbetapentane tannate; phenylephrine tannate; ephedrine tannate; chlorpheniramine tannate] 60•10•10•5 mg; 30•5•5•4 mg/5 mL

Tusstat syrup R antihistamine; sleep aid [diphenhydramine HCl; alcohol 5%] 12.5 mg/5 mL ⊚ T-Stat

tuvatidine INN

tuvirumab USAN, INN investigational (orphan) prophylaxis of hepatitis B reinfection following liver transplants

T-Vites tablets OTC vitamin/mineral supplement [multiple vitamins & minerals; biotin] ±•30 mcg

12 Hour nasal spray OTC nasal decongestant [oxymetazoline HCl] 0.05%

Twelve Resin-K tablets OTC vitamin B_{12} supplement [cyanocobalamin on resin] 1000 mcg

20/20 eye drops OTC decongestant; vasoconstrictor; moisturizer/lubricant [naphazoline HCl; glycerin] 0.012%•0.2% ⊚ tenoate

Twice-A-Day 12-Hour nasal spray OTC nasal decongestant [oxymetazoline HCl] 0.05%

Twilite caplets OTC antihistamine; sleep aid [diphenhydramine HCl] 50 mg

twin leaf (Jeffersonia diphylla) root medicinal herb used as an antirheumatic, antispasmodic, antisyphilitic, diuretic, emetic, and expectorant

Twinject prefilled auto-injector (2 doses per unit) R sympathomimetic broncho-

dilator for bronchial asthma, bronchospasm, and COPD; vasopressor for
shock [epinephrine HCl] 0.15, 0.3 mg

Twin-K oral liquid ℞ potassium supplement [potassium gluconate; potassium citrate] 20 mEq K/15 mL 🄰
Tanac; Ten-K; Ting

Twinrix IM injection ℞ immunizing
agent for hepatitis A, B, and D in adults
[hepatitis A vaccine, inactivated;
hepatitis B virus vaccine, recombi-
nant] 720 EL.U.•20 mcg per mL

TwoCal HN ready-to-use oral liquid
OTC enteral nutritional therapy [lac-
tose-free formula]

tybamate USAN, NF, INN, BAN minor
tranquilizer

tyformin BAN [also: tiformin]

Tygacil powder for IV infusion ℞
broad-spectrum glycylcycline antibiotic
for intra-abdominal and complicated
skin structure infections and methicillin-
resistant Staphylococcus aureus
(MRSA); investigational (Phase III) for
pneumonia [tigecycline] 50 mg/vial

Tykerb film-coated tablets ℞ tyrosine
kinase inhibitor; once-daily antineoplastic for advanced or metastatic breast
cancer; investigational for kidney, head,
and neck cancers [lapatinib ditosylate]
250 mg

tylcalsin [see: calcium acetylsalicylate]

tylemalum [see: carbubarb]

Tylenol gelcaps (discontinued 2008)
OTC analgesic; antipyretic [acetamino-
phen] 500 mg

Tylenol tablets, caplets, oral liquid OTC
analgesic; antipyretic [acetaminophen]
325 mg; 500 mg; 166.6 mg/5 mL

Tylenol, Children's chewable tablets
(discontinued 2008) OTC analgesic;
antipyretic [acetaminophen] 80 mg

Tylenol, Children's oral suspension
OTC analgesic; antipyretic [acetamino-
phen] 160 mg/5 mL

Tylenol 8 Hour extended-release caplets OTC analgesic; antipyretic [aceta-
minophen] 650 mg

Tylenol 8 Hour extended-release geltabs (discontinued 2008) OTC analge-

sic; antipyretic [acetaminophen] 650
mg

Tylenol Allergy Multi-Symptom
caplets, gelcaps OTC decongestant;
antihistamine; analgesic; antipyretic
[phenylephrine HCl; chlorpheniramine maleate; acetaminophen] 5•
2•325 mg

**Tylenol Allergy Multi-Symptom
Convenience Pack** caplets OTC
decongestant; analgesic; antipyretic;
antihistamine; sleep aid added PM
[phenylephrine HCl; acetaminophen; chlorpheniramine maleate
(AM); diphenhydramine HCl (PM)]
5•325•2 mg AM; 5•325•25 mg PM

**Tylenol Allergy Multi-Symptom
Night-time** caplets OTC decongestant; antihistamine; sleep aid; analgesic; antipyretic [phenylephrine HCl;
diphenhydramine HCl; acetamino-
phen] 5•25•325 mg

Tylenol Arthritis Pain extended-
release caplets, extended-release geltabs OTC analgesic; antipyretic [aceta-
minophen] 650 mg

Tylenol Chest Congestion caplets,
oral liquid OTC expectorant; analgesic;
antipyretic [guaifenesin; acetamino-
phen] 200•325 mg; 400•1000 mg/
30 mL

Tylenol Children's Cold chewable
tablets, oral liquid (discontinued
2007) OTC decongestant; antihistamine; analgesic; antipyretic [pseudo-
ephedrine HCl; chlorpheniramine
maleate; acetaminophen] 7.5•0.5•
80 mg; 30•2•320 mg/10 mL

Tylenol Children's Cold Plus Cough
chewable tablets, oral suspension
(discontinued 2007) OTC antitussive;
antihistamine; decongestant; analgesic;
antipyretic; for children 6–11 years
[dextromethorphan hydrobromide;
chlorpheniramine maleate; pseudoephedrine HCl; acetaminophen]
2.5•0.5•7.5•80 mg; 5•1•15•160
mg/5 mL

Tylenol Children's Meltaways orally disintegrating tablets OTC *analgesic; antipyretic* [acetaminophen] 80 mg

Tylenol Children's Plus Cold oral suspension (discontinued 2007) OTC *decongestant; analgesic; antipyretic* [pseudoephedrine HCl; acetaminophen] 15•160 mg/5 mL

Tylenol Cold, Children's pediatric chewable tablets, oral liquid OTC *decongestant; antihistamine; analgesic; antipyretic* [pseudoephedrine HCl; chlorpheniramine maleate; acetaminophen] 7.5•0.5•80 mg; 15•1•160 mg/5 mL

Tylenol Cold Complete Formula caplets (discontinued 2007) OTC *antitussive; antihistamine; decongestant; analgesic; antipyretic* [dextromethorphan hydrobromide; chlorpheniramine maleate; pseudoephedrine HCl; acetaminophen] 15•2•30•325 mg

Tylenol Cold & Flu Severe oral liquid (discontinued 2007) OTC *antitussive; decongestant; analgesic; antipyretic; antihistamine/sleep aid added* PM [dextromethorphan hydrobromide; pseudoephedrine HCl; acetaminophen; doxylamine succinate (PM)] 30•60•1000 mg/30 mL AM; 30•60•1000•12.6 mg PM

Tylenol Cold Head Congestion Daytime gelcaps OTC *antitussive; decongestant; analgesic; antipyretic* [dextromethorphan hydrobromide; phenylephrine HCl; acetaminophen] 10•5•325 mg

Tylenol Cold Head Congestion Daytime Cool Burst; Tylenol Cold Multi-Symptom Daytime Cool Burst caplets OTC *antitussive; decongestant; analgesic; antipyretic* [dextromethorphan hydrobromide; phenylephrine HCl; acetaminophen] 10•5•325 mg

Tylenol Cold Head Congestion Nighttime Cool Burst; Tylenol Cold Multi-Symptom Nighttime Cool Burst caplets OTC *antitussive; antihistamine; decongestant; analgesic; antipyretic* [dextromethorphan hydrobromide; chlorpheniramine maleate; phenylephrine HCl; acetaminophen] 10•2•5•325 mg

Tylenol Cold Multi-Symptom Daytime Citrus Burst oral liquid OTC *antitussive; decongestant; analgesic; antipyretic* [dextromethorphan hydrobromide; phenylephrine HCl; acetaminophen] 20•10•650 mg/30 mL

Tylenol Cold Multi-Symptom Nighttime Cool Burst oral liquid OTC *antitussive; antihistamine; sleep aid; decongestant; analgesic; antipyretic* [dextromethorphan hydrobromide; doxylamine succinate; phenylephrine HCl; acetaminophen] 20•12.5•10•650 mg/30 mL

Tylenol Cold Non-Drowsy Formula caplets, gelcaps (discontinued 2007) OTC *antitussive; decongestant; analgesic; antipyretic* [dextromethorphan hydrobromide; pseudoephedrine HCl; acetaminophen] 15•30•325 mg

Tylenol Cold Severe Congestion caplets OTC *antitussive; decongestant; expectorant; analgesic; antipyretic* [dextromethorphan hydrobromide; pseudoephedrine HCl; guaifenesin; acetaminophen] 15•30•200•325 mg

Tylenol Cough & Sore Throat Daytime oral liquid OTC *antitussive; analgesic; antipyretic* [dextromethorphan hydrobromide; acetaminophen] 30•1000 mg/30 mL

Tylenol Cough & Sore Throat Nighttime oral liquid OTC *antitussive; antihistamine; sleep aid; analgesic; antipyretic* [dextromethorphan hydrobromide; doxylamine succinate; acetaminophen] 30•12.5•1000 mg/30 mL

Tylenol Extra Strength for Arthritis Pain tablets (discontinued 2008) OTC *analgesic; antipyretic* [acetaminophen] 500 mg

Tylenol EZ Tabs tablets OTC *analgesic; antipyretic* [acetaminophen] 500 mg

Tylenol Flu; Tylenol Flu Night Time
gelcaps (discontinued 2007) OTC
*decongestant; antihistamine; sleep aid;
analgesic; antipyretic* [pseudoephed-
rine HCl; diphenhydramine HCl;
acetaminophen] 30•25•500 mg

Tylenol Flu Night Time oral liquid
(discontinued 2007) OTC *antitussive;
antihistamine; sleep aid; decongestant;
analgesic; antipyretic* [dextromethor-
phan hydrobromide; doxylamine
succinate; pseudoephedrine HCl;
acetaminophen] 30•12.6•60•1000
mg/30 mL

Tylenol Flu Non-Drowsy gelcaps
(discontinued 2007) OTC *antitussive;
decongestant; analgesic; antipyretic*
[dextromethorphan hydrobromide;
pseudoephedrine HCl; acetamino-
phen] 15•30•500 mg

Tylenol GoTabs chewable tablets OTC
analgesic; antipyretic [acetaminophen]
500 mg

Tylenol Infants' Drops solution OTC
analgesic; antipyretic [acetaminophen]
100 mg/mL

Tylenol Infants' Drops Plus Cold
OTC *decongestant; analgesic; antipyretic* [phenylephrine HCl; acetamin-
ophen] 2.5•160 mg/1.6 mL

Tylenol Jr. Meltaways orally disintegrating tablets OTC *analgesic; antipyretic* [acetaminophen] 160 mg

Tylenol Junior Strength chewable
tablets (discontinued 2008) OTC
analgesic; antipyretic [acetaminophen]
160 mg

**Tylenol Multi-Symptom Menstrual
Relief, Women's** caplets OTC *analgesic; antipyretic; diuretic* [acetamino-
phen; pamabrom] 500•25 mg

Tylenol No. 2, No. 3, and No. 4
[see: Tylenol with Codeine]

Tylenol Plus Children's Cold oral
suspension OTC *decongestant; antihistamine; analgesic; antipyretic; for children 6–11 years* [phenylephrine HCl;
chlorpheniramine maleate; aceta-
minophen] 5•2•320 mg/10 mL

**Tylenol Plus Children's Cough &
Runny Nose** oral suspension OTC
*antitussive; antihistamine; analgesic;
antipyretic; for children 6–11 years*
[dextromethorphan hydrobromide;
chlorpheniramine maleate; aceta-
minophen] 10•2•320 mg/10 mL

**Tylenol Plus Children's Cough &
Sore Throat** oral suspension OTC
*antitussive; analgesic; antipyretic; for
children 2–11 years* [dextromethor-
phan hydrobromide; acetamino-
phen] 5•160 mg/5 mL

**Tylenol Plus Children's Flu; Tylenol
Plus Children's Multi-Symptom
Cold** oral suspension OTC *antitussive;
antihistamine; decongestant; analgesic;
antipyretic; for children 6–11 years*
[dextromethorphan hydrobromide;
chlorpheniramine maleate; phenylephrine HCl; acetaminophen] 15•
2•30•320 mg/10 mL

**Tylenol Plus Infants' Cold & Cough
Concentrated Drops** OTC *antitussive; decongestant; analgesic; antipyretic;
for children 2–3 years* [dextromethor-
phan hydrobromide; phenylephrine
HCl; acetaminophen] 5•2.5•160
mg/1.6 mL

Tylenol PM tablets, caplets, gelcaps
OTC *analgesic; antipyretic; antihistamine; sleep aid* [acetaminophen;
diphenhydramine HCl] 500•25 mg

Tylenol Rapid Release Gels OTC
analgesic; antipyretic [acetaminophen]
500 mg

Tylenol Severe Allergy caplets OTC
*antihistamine; sleep aid; analgesic;
antipyretic* [diphenhydramine HCl;
acetaminophen] 12.5•500 mg

**Tylenol Sinus Congestion & Pain
Nighttime** caplets OTC *decongestant;
antihistamine; analgesic; antipyretic*
[phenylephrine HCl; chlorpheniramine maleate; acetaminophen] 5•
2•325 mg

**Tylenol Sinus Congestion & Pain
Severe Daytime** caplets OTC *decongestant; expectorant; analgesic; antipy-*

retic [phenylephrine HCl; guaifenesin; acetaminophen] 5•200•325 mg

Tylenol Sinus Night Time caplets (discontinued 2007) OTC *decongestant; antihistamine; sleep aid; analgesic; antipyretic* [pseudoephedrine HCl; doxylamine succinate; acetaminophen] 30•6.25•500 mg

Tylenol Sinus Non-Drowsy caplets, geltabs, gelcaps OTC *decongestant; analgesic; antipyretic* [pseudoephedrine HCl; acetaminophen] 30•500 mg

Tylenol Sinus Severe Congestion caplets OTC *decongestant; expectorant; analgesic; antipyretic* [pseudoephedrine HCl; guaifenesin; acetaminophen] 30•200•325 mg

Tylenol Sore Throat Daytime oral liquid OTC *analgesic; antipyretic* [acetaminophen] 166.6 mg/5 mL

Tylenol Sore Throat Nighttime oral liquid OTC *antihistamine; sleep aid; analgesic; antipyretic* [diphenhydramine HCl; acetaminophen] 48• 1000 mg/30 mL

Tylenol with Codeine elixir ℞ *narcotic antitussive; analgesic; antipyretic* [codeine phosphate; acetaminophen] 12•120 mg/5 mL

Tylenol with Codeine No. 2, No. 3, and No. 4 tablets ℞ *narcotic antitussive; analgesic; antipyretic; sometimes abused as a street drug* [codeine phosphate; acetaminophen] 15•300 mg; 30•300 mg; 60•300 mg

Tylenol with Flavor Creator, Children's oral suspension OTC *analgesic; antipyretic* [acetaminophen] 160 mg/ 5 mL

tylosin INN, BAN ☒ Talacen

Tylox capsules ℞ *narcotic analgesic; antipyretic* [oxycodone HCl; acetaminophen] 5•500 mg ☒ Taloxa

tyloxapol USAN, USP, INN, BAN *detergent; wetting agent; cleaner/lubricant for artificial eyes; investigational (orphan) surfactant for cystic fibrosis*

Tympagesic ear drops (discontinued 2006) ℞ *anesthetic; analgesic; vaso-*

constrictor [benzocaine; antipyrine; phenylephrine HCl] 5%•5%•0.25%

Typhim Vi IM injection ℞ *typhoid vaccine for adults and children over 2 years* [typhoid vaccine (Ty-2), Vi polysaccharide] 25 mcg/0.5 mL dose

typhoid vaccine USP *active bacterin for typhoid fever (Salmonella typhi Ty21a, attenuated)*

Typhoid Vaccine (AKD) subcu injection by jet injectors only ℞ *typhoid vaccine for military use only* [typhoid vaccine (Ty-2), acetone-killed and dried] 8 U/mL

typhoid Vi capsular polysaccharide vaccine *active bacterin for typhoid fever (Salmonella typhi Ty-2, inactivated)*

typhus vaccine USP

"typical" antipsychotics [see: conventional antipsychotics]

Tyrex-2 powder OTC *enteral nutritional therapy for tyrosinemia type II* ☒ Touro Ex

tyromedan INN *thyromimetic* [also: thyromedan HCl]

tyromedan HCl [see: thyromedan HCl]

Tyromex-1 powder OTC *formula for infants with tyrosinemia type I* ☒ Trimox

tyropanoate sodium USAN, USP *oral radiopaque contrast medium for cholecystography (57.4% iodine)* [also: sodium tyropanoate]

tyrosine (L-tyrosine) USAN, USP, INN *nonessential amino acid; symbols: Tyr, Y* ☒ Trisan

L-tyrosine & L-serine & L-leucine *investigational (orphan) for hepatocellular carcinoma*

Tyrosum Cleanser topical liquid, packets OTC *cleanser for acne* [isopropanol; acetone] 50%•10%

tyrothricin USP, INN *antibacterial*

Tysabri IV infusion (withdrawn from the market in 2005, reintroduced in 2006) ℞ *humanized monoclonal antibody (huMAb) anti-inflammatory for treatment of multiple sclerosis and Crohn disease; investigational (Phase*

III) for rheumatoid arthritis [natalizumab] 300 mg

Tyzeka film-coated tablets ℞ *once-daily nucleoside reverse-transcriptase inhibitor (NRTI) for chronic hepatitis B virus (HBV) infection in adults* [telbivudine] 600 mg ⊡ Tusso HC

Tyzine nasal spray, nose drops, pediatric nose drops ℞ *nasal decongestant* [tetrahydrozoline HCl] 0.1%; 0.1%; 0.05% ⊡ Tasigna

TZDs (thiazolidinediones) *a class of antidiabetic agents that increase cellular response to insulin without increasing insulin secretion* ⊡ Tussi-12D S

UAA sugar-coated tablets ℞ *urinary antibiotic; analgesic; antispasmodic; acidifier* [methenamine; phenyl salicylate; atropine sulfate; methylene blue; hyoscyamine sulfate; benzoic acid] 40.8•18.1•0.03•5.4•0.03•4.5 mg

UAD Otic ear drop suspension (discontinued 2006) ℞ *corticosteroidal anti-inflammatory; antibiotic* [hydrocortisone; neomycin sulfate; polymyxin B sulfate] 1%•5 mg•10 000 U per mL

ubenimex INN

ubidecarenone USAN, INN

Ubi-Q-Gel; Ubi-Q-Nol *natural enzyme cofactor; investigational (orphan) for Huntington disease, pediatric CHF, and mitochondrial cytopathies* [coenzyme Q10]

ubiquinol; ubiquinone [see: coenzyme Q10]

ubisindine INN

Ucephan oral solution ℞ *adjunctive therapy (rescue agent) to prevent and treat hyperammonemia due to urea cycle enzymopathy (orphan)* [sodium benzoate; sodium phenylacetate] 10•10 g/100 mL ⊡ Acephen; Asaphen

UCG Beta Slide Monoclonal II slide tests for professional use ℞ *in vitro diagnostic aid; urine pregnancy test*

UCG Slide tests for professional use ℞ *in vitro diagnostic aid; urine pregnancy test* [latex agglutination test]

U-Cort cream ℞ *corticosteroidal anti-inflammatory* [hydrocortisone acetate] 1%

UDIP (trademarked packaging form) *unit-dose identification package* ⊡ ADOAP; EDAP

Udo's Choice Oil oral liquid OTC *a blend of natural seed oils that supply a balance of essential fatty acids* [omega-3 oils; omega-6 oils; omega-9 oils; medium-chain triglycerides] 6.4•3.2•3•0.231 g/15 mL

Uendex *investigational (orphan) inhalant for cystic fibrosis* [dextran sulfate]

ufenamate INN

ufiprazole INN

U-Ject (trademarked delivery form) *prefilled disposable syringe*

Ulcerease mouth rinse OTC *mild mucous membrane anesthetic; antipruritic; counterirritant* [phenol] 0.6%

uldazepam USAN, INN *sedative*

ulinastatin INN

Ulmus fulva; U. rubra *medicinal herb* [see: slippery elm]

ulobetasol INN *topical corticosteroidal anti-inflammatory* [also: halobetasol propionate]

Ultane liquid for vaporization ℞ *inhalation general anesthetic* [sevoflurane]

Ultiva powder for IV infusion ℞ *short-acting narcotic analgesic for general anesthesia* [remifentanil HCl] 1, 2, 5 mg/vial

Ultra Derm lotion, bath oil (discontinued 2004) OTC *moisturizer; emollient*

Ultra KLB6 tablets OTC *dietary supplement* [vitamin B$_6$; multiple food supplements] 16.7• $\pm$ mg

Ultra Mide 25 lotion OTC *moisturizer; emollient; keratolytic* [urea] 25%

Ultra Tears eye drops OTC *moisturizer/lubricant* [hydroxypropyl methylcellulose] 1%

Ultra Vent (trademarked delivery device) *jet nebulizer*

Ultra Vita Time tablets OTC *dietary supplement* [multiple vitamins & minerals; multiple food products; iron; folic acid; biotin] $\pm$ •6•0.4•1 mg

UltraBrom extended-release capsules ℞ *decongestant; antihistamine* [pseudoephedrine HCl; brompheniramine maleate] 120•12 mg

UltraBrom PD extended-release pediatric capsules (discontinued 2007) ℞ *decongestant; antihistamine* [pseudoephedrine HCl; brompheniramine maleate] 60•6 mg

Ultracal oral liquid OTC *enteral nutritional therapy* [lactose-free formula]

Ultra-Care solution + tablets OTC *two-step chemical disinfecting system for soft contact lenses* [hydrogen peroxide–based]

Ultracet film-coated caplets ℞ *central analgesic for acute pain; antipyretic* [tramadol HCl; acetaminophen] 37.5•325 mg

Ultra-Freeda; Ultra Freeda, Iron Free tablets OTC *geriatric vitamin/mineral supplement* [multiple vitamins & minerals; folic acid; biotin] $\pm$ •270•100 mcg

UltraJect prefilled syringe ℞ *narcotic analgesic* [morphine sulfate]

Ultralan oral liquid OTC *enteral nutritional therapy* [lactose-free formula]

Ultralytic 2 topical foam ℞ *moisturizer; emollient; keratolytic* [urea; ammonium lactate] 20%•12%

Ultram film-coated caplets ℞ *central analgesic for moderate to severe pain; also used for premature ejaculation* [tramadol HCl] 50 mg

Ultram ER extended-release tablets ℞ *central analgesic for moderate to severe pain; also used for premature ejaculation* [tramadol HCl] 100, 200, 300 mg

UltraMide 25 lotion OTC *moisturizer; emollient* [urea] 25%

Ultra-NatalCare tablets ℞ *vitamin/mineral/iron supplement for pregnancy and lactation* [multiple vitamins & minerals; carbonyl iron; folic acid] $\pm$ •90 mg iron•1 mg

Ultrase; Ultrase MT 12; Ultrase MT 18; Ultrase MT 20 capsules containing enteric-coated microspheres ℞ *porcine-derived digestive enzymes* [lipase; protease; amylase] 4500• 25 000•20 000; 12 000•39 000• 39 000; 18 000•58 500•58 500; 20 000•65 000•65 000 USP units

Ultravate ointment, cream ℞ *corticosteroidal anti-inflammatory* [halobetasol propionate] 0.05%

Ultravist 150; Ultravist 240; Ultravist 300; Ultravist 370 IV injection ℞ *radiopaque contrast medium for imaging of the head, heart, peripheral vascular system, and genitourinary tract* [iopromide (39% iodine)] 311.7 mg/mL (150 mg/mL); 498.72 mg/mL (240 mg/mL); 623.4 mg/mL (300 mg/mL); 768.86 mg/mL (370 mg/mL)

Ultrazyme Enzymatic Cleaner effervescent tablets OTC *enzymatic cleaner for soft contact lenses* [subtilisin A]

Ultrex gel in unit-dose packs OTC *hydrogel wound dressing* [acemannan]

Umecta emulsion, topical suspension, aerosol ℞ *moisturizer; emollient; keratolytic* [urea] 40%

Umecta 40% nail film, topical suspension ℞ *moisturizer; emollient; keratolytic* [urea] 40%

Umecta PD emulsion, topical suspension ℞ *moisturizer; emollient; keratolytic* [urea] 40%

umespirone INN

uña de gato *medicinal herb* [see: cat's claw]

UN-Aspirin caplets OTC *analgesic; antipyretic* [acetaminophen] 500 mg

Unasyn powder for IV or IM injection ℞ *aminopenicillin antibiotic plus synergist* [ampicillin sodium; sulbactam sodium] 1•0.5, 2•1, 10•5 g 🔲 Anacin; Enzone; inosine

Uncaria guianensis; U. tomentosa medicinal herb [see: cat's claw]

10-undecenoic acid [see: undecylenic acid]

10-undecenoic acid, calcium salt [see: calcium undecylenate]

undecoylium chloride-iodine

undecylenic acid USP *antifungal*

unfractionated heparin [see: heparin, unfractionated]

Unguentine cream OTC *anesthetic; antifungal* [benzocaine; resorcinol] 5%•2%

Unguentine ointment OTC *minor burn treatment* [phenol; zinc oxide; eucalyptus oil] 1%• 🔲 • 🔲

Unguentine Plus cream OTC *anesthetic; antiseptic; antipruritic; counter-irritant* [lidocaine HCl; chloroxylenol; phenol] 2%•2%•0.5%

Uni-Ace drops (discontinued 2008) OTC *analgesic; antipyretic* [acetaminophen] 100 mg/mL 🔲 anise

Uni-Amp (trademarked delivery form) *single-dose ampule*

Unibase OTC *ointment base*

Unicap capsules, tablets OTC *vitamin supplement* [multiple vitamins; folic acid] 🔲 •0.4 mg

Unicap Jr. chewable tablets OTC *vitamin supplement* [multiple vitamins; folic acid] 🔲 •0.4 mg

Unicap M; Unicap T tablets OTC *vitamin/mineral/iron supplement* [multiple vitamins & minerals; iron; folic acid] 🔲 •18•0.4 mg

Unicap Plus Iron tablets OTC *vitamin/ iron supplement* [multiple vitamins; iron; folic acid] 🔲 •22.5•0.4 mg

Unicap Sr. tablets OTC *vitamin/mineral/ iron supplement* [multiple vitamins & minerals; iron; folic acid] 🔲 •10•0.4 mg

Unicomplex T & M tablets OTC *vitamin/mineral/iron supplement* [multiple vitamins & minerals; iron; folic acid] 🔲 •18•0.4 mg

Unifed oral liquid OTC *nasal decongestant* [pseudoephedrine HCl] 30 mg/5 mL 🔲 INFeD

Unifiber powder OTC *bulk laxative* [cellulose powder]

unifocon A USAN *hydrophobic contact lens material*

Unimatic (trademarked delivery form) *prefilled disposable syringe*

Uni-nest (trademarked delivery form) *ampule*

Unipak (packaging form) *dispensing pack*

Uniphyl timed-release tablets ℞ *antiasthmatic; bronchodilator* [theophylline] 400, 600 mg

Uniquin (foreign name for U.S. product **Maxaquin**)

Uniretic tablets ℞ *antihypertensive; angiotensin-converting enzyme (ACE) inhibitor; diuretic* [moexipril HCl; hydrochlorothiazide] 7.5•12.5, 15• 12.5, 15•25 mg

Uni-Rx (trademarked packaging form) *unit-dose containers and packages*

Unisert (trademarked dosage form) *suppository*

Unisol; Unisol 4 solution OTC *rinsing/ storage solution for soft contact lenses* [sodium chloride (saline solution)] 🔲 anise oil; Anusol; Enisyl; Enseal

Unisol Plus aerosol solution OTC *rinsing/storage solution for soft contact lenses* [sodium chloride (saline solution)]

Unisom Nighttime Sleep-Aid tablets OTC *antihistamine; sleep aid* [doxylamine succinate] 25 mg

Unisom SleepGels (capsules) OTC *antihistamine; sleep aid* [diphenhydramine HCl] 50 mg

Unisom with Pain Relief tablets OTC *antihistamine; sleep aid; analgesic; antipyretic* [diphenhydramine citrate; acetaminophen] 50•650 mg

Unistep hCG test kit for professional use ℞ *in vitro diagnostic aid; urine pregnancy test*

Uni-Tex 120/10 ER extended-release capsules (discontinued 2006) ℞ *decongestant; antihistamine* [pseudoephedrine HCl; brompheniramine maleate] 120•10 mg ⧆ Entex ER

Unithroid Direct tablets ℞ *synthetic thyroid hormone (T₄ fraction only)* [levothyroxine sodium] 25, 50, 75, 88, 100, 112, 125, 150, 175, 200, 300 mcg

Univasc tablets ℞ *antihypertensive; angiotensin-converting enzyme (ACE) inhibitor* [moexipril HCl] 7.5, 15 mg

Univial (trademarked packaging form) *single-dose vials*

Unna's boot [see: Dome-Paste bandage]

unoprostone isopropyl *topical prostaglandin F₂ₐ analogue for glaucoma and ocular hypertension*

Uracid capsules ℞ *urinary acidifier to control ammonia production* [racemethionine] 200 mg ⧆ Urised

uracil USAN *antineoplastic potentiator for tegafur (not available separately; combined with tegafur in a 1:4 ratio)* ⧆ Eryzole; Orasol

uracil mustard USAN, USP *nitrogen mustard–type alkylating antineoplastic* [also: uramustine]

uradal [see: carbromal]

uralenic acid [see: enoxolone]

uramustine INN, BAN *nitrogen mustard–type alkylating antineoplastic* [also: uracil mustard]

uranin [see: fluorescein sodium]

uranium *element (U)*

urapidil INN, BAN

urate oxidase, recombinant *investigational (orphan) for prevention of chemotherapy-induced hyperuricemia*

urea USP *osmotic diuretic; keratolytic; emollient* 35%, 40%, 50% topical

Urea Nail Gel ℞ *for the removal of dystrophic nails* [urea] 50%

urea peroxide [see: carbamide peroxide]

Ureacin-10 lotion OTC *moisturizer; emollient; keratolytic* [urea] 10% ⧆ AeroZoin; Orasone

Ureacin-20 cream OTC *moisturizer; emollient; keratolytic* [urea] 20% ⧆ AeroZoin; Orasone

Ureaphil IV infusion ℞ *osmotic diuretic* [urea] 40 g/150 mL ⧆ Oruvail

Urecholine tablets ℞ *cholinergic urinary stimulant for postsurgical and postpartum urinary retention* [bethanechol chloride] 5, 10, 25, 50 mg

uredepa USAN, INN *antineoplastic*

uredofos USAN, INN *veterinary anthelmintic*

urefibrate INN

***p*-ureidobenzenearsonic acid** [see: carbarsone]

Urelle sugar-coated tablets ℞ *urinary antibiotic; antiseptic; analgesic; antispasmodic* [methenamine; sodium phosphate; phenyl salicylate; methylene blue; hyoscyamine sulfate] 81•40.8•32.4•10.8•0.12 mg

urethan NF [also: urethane] ⧆ Uritin

urethane INN, BAN [also: urethan] ⧆ Uritin

urethane polymers [see: polyurethane foam]

Uretron D/S sugar-coated tablets ℞ *urinary antibiotic; antiseptic; analgesic; antispasmodic* [methenamine; sodium biphosphate; phenyl salicylate; methylene blue; hyoscyamine sulfate] 120•40.8•36.2•10.8•0.12 mg

Urex tablets ℞ *urinary antibiotic* [methenamine hippurate] 1 g ⧆ Eurax

Urginea indica; U. maritima; U. scilla *medicinal herb* [see: squill]

Uricult culture paddles for professional use ℞ *in vitro diagnostic aid for nitrate, uropathogens, or bacteria in the urine*

uridine 5′-triphosphate *investigational (Phase I/II, orphan) for cystic fibrosis and primary ciliary dyskinesia*

Uridon Modified sugar-coated tablets (discontinued 2007) ℞ *urinary antibiotic; analgesic; antispasmodic; acidifier* [methenamine; phenyl salicylate; atropine sulfate; methylene blue; hyoscyamine sulfate; benzoic acid] 40.8•18.1•0.03•5.4•0.03•4.5 mg

Urief (available in Japan) *investigational (NDA filed) alpha$_{1a}$ adrenoceptor antagonist for benign prostatic hyperplasia (BPH)* [silodosin]

Urimar-T tablets ℞ *urinary antibiotic; antiseptic; analgesic; antispasmodic* [methenamine; sodium biphosphate; phenyl salicylate; methylene blue; hyoscyamine sulfate] 120•40.8•36.2•10.8•0.12 mg

Urimax film-coated delayed-release tablets ℞ *urinary antibiotic; analgesic; antispasmodic; acidifier* [methenamine; phenyl salicylate; methylene blue; hyoscyamine sulfate; sodium biphosphate] 81.6•36.2•10.8•0.12•40.8 mg

Urinary Antiseptic No. 2 tablets ℞ *urinary antibiotic; analgesic; antispasmodic; acidifier* [methenamine; phenyl salicylate; atropine sulfate; methylene blue; hyoscyamine sulfate; benzoic acid] 40.8•18.1•0.03•5.4•0.03•4.5 mg

Urised sugar-coated tablets (discontinued 2008) ℞ *urinary antibiotic; analgesic; antispasmodic; acidifier* [methenamine; phenyl salicylate; atropine sulfate; methylene blue; hyoscyamine sulfate; benzoic acid] 40.8•18.1•0.03•5.4•0.03•4.5 mg ▣ Uracid

Urisedamine tablets ℞ *urinary antibiotic; antispasmodic* [methenamine mandelate; hyoscyamine] 500•0.15 mg

Uriseptic film-coated tablets ℞ *urinary antibiotic; antiseptic; analgesic; antispasmodic* [methenamine; phenyl salicylate; methylene blue; benzoic acid; atropine sulfate; hyoscyamine sulfate] 40.8•18.1•5.4•4.5•0.03•0.03 mg

Urispas film-coated tablets ℞ *urinary antispasmodic* [flavoxate HCl] 100 mg (200 mg available in Canada)

Uristat tablets ℞ *urinary analgesic* [phenazopyridine HCl] 95 mg

Uristix; Uristix 4 reagent strips *in vitro diagnostic aid for multiple urine products*

UriSym capsules (discontinued 2008) ℞ *urinary antibiotic; antiseptic; analgesic; antispasmodic* [methenamine; sodium biphosphate; phenyl salicylate; methylene blue; hyoscyamine sulfate] 100•40.8•40•10.8•0.12 mg

Uritact DS caplets ℞ *urinary antibiotic; analgesic; antispasmodic; acidifier* [methenamine; phenyl salicylate; atropine sulfate; methylene blue; hyoscyamine sulfate; benzoic acid] 81.6•36.2•0.06•10.8•0.06•9 mg

Uritin tablets ℞ *urinary antibiotic; analgesic; antispasmodic; acidifier* [methenamine; phenyl salicylate; atropine sulfate; methylene blue; hyoscyamine sulfate; benzoic acid] 40.8•18.1•0.03•5.4•0.03•4.5 mg

Uro Blue sugar-coated tablets ℞ *urinary antibiotic; antiseptic; analgesic; antispasmodic* [methenamine; sodium biphosphate; phenyl salicylate; methylene blue; hyoscyamine sulfate] 120•40.8•36.2•10.8•0.12 mg

urocidin *investigational (Phase III) mycobacterial cell wall complex (MCC) for bladder cancer*

Urocit-K tablets ℞ *urinary alkalizer for nephrolithiasis and hypocitruria prevention (orphan)* [potassium citrate] 5, 10 mEq K

urofollitrophin BAN *follicle-stimulating hormone (FSH)* [also: urofollitropin]

urofollitropin USAN, INN *follicle-stimulating hormone (FSH); ovulation stimulant for polycystic ovary disease (orphan) and assisted reproductive technologies (ART); investigational (orphan) for spermatogenesis in hormone-deficient males* [also: urofollitrophin]

urogastrone *investigational (orphan) to accelerate corneal regeneration following corneal transplant surgery*

Urogesic tablets ℞ *urinary tract analgesic for relief of pain, burning, urgency, and frequency due to mucosal irritation from surgery, catheterization, endoscopic procedures, or trauma; adjunct to antibacterial agents for urinary tract infection (UTI)* [phenazopyridine HCl] 100 mg ▣ Argesic

Urogesic Blue sugar-coated tablets ℞ *urinary antibiotic; antiseptic; analgesic; antispasmodic* [methenamine; sodium biphosphate; phenyl salicylate; methylene blue; hyoscyamine sulfate] 81.6•40.8•36.2•10.8•0.12 mg

urokinase USAN, INN, BAN, JAN *plasminogen activator; thrombolytic enzyme*

urokinase alfa USAN *plasminogen activator; thrombolytic enzyme*

Uro-KP-Neutral film-coated caplets ℞ *urinary acidifier; phosphorus supplement* [sodium phosphate; potassium phosphate; monobasic sodium phosphate] 250 mg P

Urolene Blue tablets ℞ *urinary antiinfective and antiseptic; antidote to cyanide poisoning* [methylene blue] 65 mg

Uro-Mag capsules OTC *antacid; magnesium supplement* [magnesium oxide] 140 mg (84.5 mg Mg)

uronal [see: barbital]

Uro-Phosphate film-coated tablets ℞ *urinary antibiotic; acidifier* [methenamine; sodium biphosphate] 300•434.78 mg

Uroqid-Acid No. 2 film-coated tablets ℞ *urinary antibiotic; acidifier* [methenamine mandelate; sodium acid phosphate] 500•500 mg

Urotrol ⓔ (Spanish name for the U.S. product **Detrol**) ⓩ Aerotrol

Uroxatral extended-release tablets ℞ *α₁-adrenergic blocker for benign prostatic hyperplasia (BPH)* [alfuzosin HCl] 10 mg

Urso 250; Urso Forte tablets ℞ *naturally occurring bile acid for primary biliary cirrhosis (orphan)* [ursodiol] 250 mg; 500 mg ⓩ Aerius; Ear-Eze; Oracea; OROS

Ursocarb *naturally occurring bile acid; investigational (orphan) for pruritus due to Alagille syndrome* [ursodiol]

ursodeoxycholic acid INN, BAN *naturally occurring bile acid; anticholelithogenic* [also: ursodiol]

ursodiol USAN *naturally occurring bile acid for primary biliary cirrhosis (orphan); gallstone preventative and dissolving agent; investigational (orphan) for pruritus due to Alagille syndrome* [also: ursodeoxycholic acid] 300 mg oral

ursulcholic acid INN

Urtica dioica; U. urens *medicinal herb* [see: nettle]

ustekinumab *investigational (NDA filed) tumor necrosis factor (TNF) blocker for psoriasis*

UTI Relief tablets ℞ *urinary tract analgesic for relief of pain, burning, urgency, and frequency due to mucosal irritation from surgery, catheterization, endoscopic procedures, or trauma; adjunct to antibacterial agents for urinary tract infection (UTI)* [phenazopyridine HCl] 97.2 mg

Utira-C tablets ℞ *urinary antibiotic; antiseptic; analgesic; antispasmodic* [methenamine; sodium phosphate; phenyl salicylate; methylene blue; hyoscyamine sulfate] 81.6•40.8•36.2•10.8•0.12 mg

uva ursi (Arbutus uva ursi; Arctostaphylos uva ursi) *leaves medicinal herb for bladder and kidney infections, Bright disease, constipation, diabetes, gonorrhea, nephritis, spleen disorders, urethritis, and uterine ulcerations*

Uvadex extracorporeal solution (leukocytes are collected, photoactivated with the UVAR Photopheresis System, then reinfused) ℞ *palliative treatment for cutaneous T-cell lymphoma (CTCL); investigational (orphan) treatment of diffuse systemic sclerosis and to prevent rejection of cardiac allografts* [methoxsalen] 20 mcg/mL

Uvidem *investigational (Phase II) theraccine (therapeutic vaccine) for melanoma* [melanoma vaccine]

VA (vincristine, actinomycin D) *chemotherapy protocol*

VAAP (vincristine, asparaginase, Adriamycin, prednisone) *chemotherapy protocol*

VAB; VAB-I (vinblastine, actinomycin D, bleomycin) *chemotherapy protocol*

VAB-II (vinblastine, actinomycin D, bleomycin, cisplatin) *chemotherapy protocol*

VAB-III (vinblastine, actinomycin D, bleomycin, cisplatin, chlorambucil, cyclophosphamide) *chemotherapy protocol*

VAB-V (vinblastine, actinomycin D, bleomycin, cyclophosphamide, cisplatin) *chemotherapy protocol*

VAB-6 (vinblastine, actinomycin D, bleomycin, cyclophosphamide, cisplatin) *chemotherapy protocol for testicular cancer*

VABCD (vinblastine, Adriamycin, bleomycin, CCNU, DTIC) *chemotherapy protocol*

VAC (vincristine, Adriamycin, cisplatin) *chemotherapy protocol*

VAC (vincristine, Adriamycin, cyclophosphamide) *chemotherapy protocol for small cell lung cancer (SCLC)* [also: CAV]

VAC pediatric (vincristine, actinomycin D, cyclophosphamide) *chemotherapy protocol for pediatric sarcomas*

VAC pulse; VAC standard (vincristine, actinomycin D, cyclophosphamide) *chemotherapy protocol for sarcomas*

VACA (vincristine, actinomycin D, cyclophosphamide, Adriamycin) *chemotherapy protocol*

VACAD (vincristine, actinomycin D, cyclophosphamide, Adriamycin, dacarbazine) *chemotherapy protocol*

VACAdr (vincristine, actinomycin D, cyclophosphamide, Adriamycin) *chemotherapy protocol for pediatric bone and soft tissue sarcomas*

vaccines *a class of drugs used for active immunization that consist of antigens that induce the endogenous production of antibodies*

vaccinia immune globulin (VIG) USP *passive immunizing agent; treatment for severe complications arising from smallpox vaccination (orphan)*

vaccinia immune human globulin [now: vaccinia immune globulin]

vaccinia virus, recombinant [now: human papillomavirus, recombinant]

Vaccinium edule; V. erythrocarpum; V. macrocarpon; V. oxycoccos; V. vitis *medicinal herb* [see: cranberry]

Vaccinium myrtillus *medicinal herb* [see: bilberry]

VACP (VePesid, Adriamycin, cyclophosphamide, Platinol) *chemotherapy protocol* 🔼 FCAP; FCP; VCAP; VCP; VOCAP

VAD (vincristine, Adriamycin, dactinomycin) *chemotherapy protocol for pediatric Wilms tumor*

VAD (vincristine, Adriamycin, dexamethasone) *chemotherapy protocol for multiple myeloma and acute lymphocytic leukemia (ALL)*

Vademin-Z capsules OTC *vitamin/mineral supplement* [multiple vitamins & minerals]

vadocaine INN

VAdrC (vincristine, Adriamycin, cyclophosphamide) *chemotherapy protocol*

VAD/V (vincristine, Adriamycin, dexamethasone, verapamil) *chemotherapy protocol*

VAFAC (vincristine, amethopterin, fluorouracil, Adriamycin, cyclophosphamide) *chemotherapy protocol* 🔼 FUVAC

Vagifem film-coated vaginal tablets ℞ *synthetic estrogen for postmenopausal atrophic vaginitis* [estradiol (as hemihydrate)] 25 (25.8) mcg

Vagi-Gard; Vagi-Gard Advanced Sensitive Formula vaginal cream OTC *anesthetic; keratolytic; antifungal* [benzocaine; resorcinol] 20%•3%; 5%•2%

Vaginex vaginal cream OTC *antihistamine* [tripelennamine HCl]

Vagisec Douche vaginal solution Ŗ *cleanser and deodorizer*

Vagisec Plus vaginal suppositories Ŗ *antiseptic* [aminacrine HCl] 6 mg

Vagisil vaginal cream OTC *anesthetic; keratolytic; antifungal* [benzocaine; resorcinol] 5%•2% ⍰ Vexol

Vagisil vaginal powder OTC *moisture absorbent* [cornstarch; aloe] ⍰ Vexol

Vagisil wipes OTC *local anesthetic* [pramoxine HCl] 1% ⍰ Vexol

Vagistat-1 vaginal ointment in prefilled applicator OTC *antifungal* [tioconazole] 6.5%

Vagistat-3 Combination Pack vaginal inserts + cream OTC *antifungal* [miconazole nitrate] 200 mg + 2%

VAI (vincristine, actinomycin D, ifosfamide) *chemotherapy protocol*

valaciclovir INN *oral antiviral for herpes simplex virus types 1 and 2 (HSV-1, cold sores; HSV-2, genital herpes) and herpes zoster (shingles) infections; suppressive therapy for recurrent outbreaks* [also: valacyclovir HCl]

valacyclovir HCl USAN *oral antiviral for herpes simplex virus types 1 and 2 (HSV-1, cold sores; HSV-2, genital herpes) and herpes zoster (shingles) infections; suppressive therapy for recurrent outbreaks* [also: valaciclovir]

valconazole INN ⍰ fluconazole

Valcyte tablets Ŗ *nucleoside analogue antiviral for AIDS-related cytomegalovirus (CMV) retinitis; CMV prevention in organ transplants* [valganciclovir HCl] 450 mg

valdecoxib USAN *COX-2 inhibitor; nonsteroidal anti-inflammatory drug (NSAID) for osteoarthritis (OA), rheumatoid arthritis (RA), and primary dysmenorrhea (withdrawn from the market in 2005 due to safety concerns)*

valdetamide INN

valdipromide INN

Valdoxan *investigational (Phase III) oral treatment for major depressive disorder (MDD)* [agomelatine]

valepotriate [see: valtrate]

valerian (Valeriana officinalis) root *medicinal herb for convulsions, hypertension, hysteria, hypochondria, nervousness, pain, and sedation* ⍰ Florone; fluorine

valerian, false *medicinal herb* [see: life root]

valethamate bromide NF

valganciclovir HCl USAN *nucleoside analogue antiviral for AIDS-related cytomegalovirus (CMV) retinitis; CMV prevention in organ transplants; oral prodrug of ganciclovir* 450 mg oral

valine (L-valine) USAN, USP, INN, JAN *essential amino acid; symbols: Val, V*

valine & isoleucine & leucine *investigational (orphan) for hyperphenylalaninemia*

Valisone ointment, cream, lotion Ŗ *corticosteroidal anti-inflammatory* [betamethasone valerate] 0.1% ⍰ Fluzone

Valisone Reduced Strength cream Ŗ *corticosteroidal anti-inflammatory* [betamethasone valerate] 0.01%

Valium tablets Ŗ *benzodiazepine sedative; anxiolytic; skeletal muscle relaxant; anticonvulsant; alcohol withdrawal aid; also abused as a street drug* [diazepam] 2, 5, 10 mg

valnoctamide USAN, INN *tranquilizer*

valofane INN ⍰ Voluven

valomaciclovir stearate USAN *DNA polymerase inhibitor; antiviral for herpes zoster infections*

Valorin tablets OTC *analgesic; antipyretic* [acetaminophen] 325, 500 mg ⍰ Florone; fluorine

valperinol INN

valproate pivoxil INN

valproate semisodium INN *anticonvulsant for complex partial seizures and simple or complex absence seizures; treatment for manic episodes of a bipolar disorder; migraine headache prophy-*

laxis [also: divalproex sodium; semi-sodium valproate]

valproate sodium USAN *anticonvulsant for complex partial seizures and simple or complex absence seizures; valproic acid derivative* 500 mg injection

valproic acid USAN, USP, INN, BAN *anticonvulsant for complex partial seizures and simple or complex absence seizures* 125, 250, 500 mg oral; 250 mg/5 mL oral

valpromide INN ⍰ fluperamide

valrubicin USAN *investigational (NDA filed, orphan) anthracycline antibiotic antineoplastic for bladder cancer*

valsartan USAN, INN *angiotensin II receptor antagonist for hypertension, heart failure, or myocardial infarction*

valspodar USAN, INN *cyclosporine-derived P-glycoprotein (P-gp) inhibitor*

Valstar *intravesical solution investigational (NDA filed, orphan) anthracycline antibiotic antineoplastic for bladder cancer* [valrubicin] 40 mg/mL

valtrate INN

Valtrex *film-coated caplets* ℞ *antiviral for herpes simplex virus types 1 and 2 (HSV-1, cold sores; HSV-2, genital herpes) and herpes zoster (shingles) infections; suppressive therapy for recurrent outbreaks* [valacyclovir HCl] 500, 1000 mg

VAM (vinblastine, Adriamycin, mitomycin) *chemotherapy protocol*

VAM (VP-16-213, Adriamycin, methotrexate) *chemotherapy protocol*

VAMP (vincristine, actinomycin, methotrexate, prednisone) *chemotherapy protocol* ⍰ VM-26PP; VMP

VAMP (vincristine, Adriamycin, methylprednisolone) *chemotherapy protocol* ⍰ VM-26PP; VMP

VAMP (vincristine, amethopterin, mercaptopurine, prednisone) *chemotherapy protocol* ⍰ VM-26PP; VMP

vanadium *element (V)*

Vanamide *cream* ℞ *keratolytic for the removal of dystrophic nails* [urea] 40% ⍰ fenimide

Vancenase Pockethaler (nasal inhalation aerosol) (discontinued 2004) ℞ *corticosteroidal anti-inflammatory for seasonal or perennial rhinitis* [beclomethasone dipropionate] 42 mcg/dose

Vancenase AQ *nasal spray* (discontinued 2004) ℞ *corticosteroidal anti-inflammatory for seasonal or perennial rhinitis* [beclomethasone dipropionate] 0.084% (100 mcg/dose)

Vancocin Pulvules (capsules), powder for oral solution, powder for IV or IM injection ℞ *tricyclic glycopeptide antibiotic* [vancomycin HCl] 125, 250 mg; 1, 10 g; 0.5, 1, 10 g ⍰ fenquizone

Vancoled powder for IV or IM injection ℞ *tricyclic glycopeptide antibiotic* [vancomycin HCl] 0.5, 1, 5 g

vancomycin INN, BAN *tricyclic glycopeptide antibiotic* [also: vancomycin HCl]

vancomycin HCl USP *tricyclic glycopeptide antibiotic* [also: vancomycin] 1 g oral; 0.5, 1, 5, 10 g/vial injection

Vandazole *vaginal gel* ℞ *antibacterial for bacterial vaginosis* [metronidazole] 0.75% ⍰ fenadiazole

vandetanib *investigational (Phase III) oral antineoplastic for advanced or metastatic non–small cell lung cancer*

vaneprim INN

Vanex HD *oral liquid* (discontinued 2007) ℞ *narcotic antitussive; antihistamine; decongestant* [hydrocodone bitartrate; chlorpheniramine maleate; phenylephrine HCl] 3.4•4•10 mg/10 mL

Vanicream OTC *cream base*

vanilla NF *flavoring agent* ⍰ fennel; phenol

vanilla (Vanilla fragrans; V. planifolia; V. tahitensis) *bean medicinal herb for CNS stimulation, fever, and flatulence; also used as an aphrodisiac* ⍰ fennel; phenol

vanillin NF *flavoring agent*

N-vanillylnonamide [see: nonivamide]

N-vanillyloleamide [see: olvanil]

Vaniqa *cream* ℞ *hair growth inhibitor for unwanted facial hair on women* [eflornithine HCl] 13.9% ☒ Finac; FNC; Fung-O

vanitiolide INN

Vanocin lotion ℞ *antibiotic and keratolytic for acne* [sulfacetamide sodium; sulfur] 10%•5% ☒ Fenesin; phenazone

Vanos cream ℞ *corticosteroidal anti-inflammatory* [fluocinonide] 0.1% ☒ Finacea; Phenazo

Vanoxide-HC lotion ℞ *keratolytic and corticosteroidal anti-inflammatory for acne* [benzoyl peroxide; hydrocortisone] 5%•0.5%

Vanquish caplets OTC *analgesic; antipyretic; anti-inflammatory* [acetaminophen; aspirin (buffered with magnesium hydroxide and aluminum hydroxide); caffeine] 194•227•(50•25)•33 mg

Vantas once-yearly subcu implant ℞ *LHRH agonist for palliative treatment of advanced prostate cancer* [histrelin acetate] 50 mg

Vanticon ⓔ (German name for U.S. product **Accolate**)

Vantin film-coated tablets ℞ *broad-spectrum third-generation cephalosporin antibiotic* [cefpodoxime proxetil] 100, 200 mg ☒ phenytoin

Vantin granules for suspension (discontinued 2008) ℞ *broad-spectrum third-generation cephalosporin antibiotic* [cefpodoxime proxetil] 50, 100 mg/5 mL ☒ phenytoin

vanyldisulfamide INN

VAP (vinblastine, actinomycin D, Platinol) *chemotherapy protocol*

VAP (vincristine, Adriamycin, prednisone) *chemotherapy protocol*

VAP (vincristine, Adriamycin, procarbazine) *chemotherapy protocol*

VAP (vincristine, asparaginase, prednisone) *chemotherapy protocol*

vapiprost INN, BAN *antagonist to thromboxane* A_2 [also: vapiprost HCl]

vapiprost HCl USAN *antagonist to thromboxane* A_2 [also: vapiprost]

Vapor Lemon Sucrets lozenges (discontinued 2008) OTC *mucous membrane anesthetic* [dyclonine HCl] 2 mg

Vaporole (trademarked delivery form) *crushable ampule for inhalation*

vapreotide USAN *antineoplastic; synthetic octapeptide analogue of somatostatin*

vapreotide acetate *antineoplastic; synthetic octapeptide analogue of somatostatin; investigational (Phase III, orphan) treatment for acute esophageal variceal bleeding due to portal hypertension; investigational (orphan) for GI and pancreatic fistulas, acromegaly, and carcinoid tumors*

Vaprisol IV infusion ℞ *arginine vasopressin antagonist; diuretic for euvolemic and hypervolemic hyponatremia in hospitalized patients; treatment for syndrome of inappropriate antidiuretic hormone (SIADH)* [conivaptan HCl] 20 mg ☒ fuprazole

Vaqta adult IM injection, pediatric/adolescent IM injection ℞ *immunization against hepatitis A virus (HAV)* [hepatitis A vaccine, inactivated] 50 U/mL; 25 U/0.5 mL

vardenafil HCl USAN *phosphodiesterase type 5 (PDE5) inhibitor; selective vasodilator for erectile dysfunction (ED)*

varenicline tartrate *nicotine receptor agonist/antagonist; a non-nicotine smoking cessation aid; also used to reduce alcohol cravings*

varicella virus vaccine *live, attenuated vaccine for chickenpox*

varicella-zoster immune globulin (VZIG) USP *passive immunizing agent* 10%–18% (125 U/2.5 mL)

varicella-zoster virus vaccine, live *vaccine for adults* $\geq$ 60 *years to prevent herpes zoster infections; investigational for post-herpetic neuralgia and shingles-associated pain*

Varivax powder for subcu injection ℞ *vaccine for chickenpox* [varicella virus vaccine, live attenuated] 1350 PFU/0.5 mL

Varoniscastrum virgincum medicinal herb [see: Culver root]

vascular endothelial growth factor (VEGF) *investigational (Phase II, orphan) gene-based therapy for neointimal hyperplasia disease*

vascular serotonin 5-HT₁ receptor agonists *a class of antimigraine agents that constrict cranial blood vessels and inhibit the release of inflammatory neuropeptides*

Vaseretic 5-12.5; Vaseretic 10-25 tablets ℞ *antihypertensive; angiotensin-converting enzyme (ACE) inhibitor; diuretic* [enalapril maleate; hydrochlorothiazide] 5●12.5 mg; 10●25 mg

vasoactive intestinal polypeptide (VIP) *investigational (orphan) for acute esophageal food impaction, pulmonary arterial hypertension, and acute respiratory distress syndrome (ARDS)*

Vasocidin eye drops ℞ *corticosteroidal anti-inflammatory; antibiotic* [prednisolone sodium phosphate; sulfacetamide sodium] 0.25%●10%

VasoClear eye drops (discontinued 2006) oTc *decongestant; moisturizer/lubricant* [naphazoline HCl; polyvinyl alcohol; polyethylene glycol 400] 0.02%●0.25%●1%

VasoClear A eye drops oTc *decongestant; astringent* [naphazoline HCl; zinc sulfate] 0.02%●0.25%

Vasocon Regular eye drops (discontinued 2006) ℞ *decongestant; vasoconstrictor* [naphazoline HCl] 0.1%

Vasocon-A eye drops ℞ *decongestant; antihistamine* [naphazoline HCl; antazoline phosphate] 0.05%●0.5% ⑫ Visken

vasoconstrictors *a class of cardiovascular drugs that narrow the blood vessels*

Vasodilan tablets ℞ *peripheral vasodilator* [isoxsuprine HCl] 10, 20 mg

vasodilators *a class of cardiovascular drugs that dilate the blood vessels*

vasopressin (VP) USP, INN *pituitary antidiuretic hormone for diabetes insipidus or prevention of abdominal distention* 20 U/mL injection

vasopressin tannate USP *pituitary antidiuretic hormone for diabetes insipidus or prevention of abdominal distention*

vasopressors *a class of posterior pituitary hormones that raise blood pressure by causing contraction of capillaries and arterioles; a class of sympathomimetic agents that raise blood pressure by increasing myocardial contractility* [also called: vasopressins]

Vasoprost *investigational (orphan) prostaglandin for severe peripheral arterial occlusive disease* [alprostadil]

Vasosulf eye drops ℞ *antibiotic; decongestant* [sulfacetamide sodium; phenylephrine HCl] 15%●0.125%

Vasotan Tannate oral suspension ℞ *antitussive; antihistamine; decongestant* [carbetapentane tannate; brompheniramine tannate; phenylephrine tannate] 50●12●2 mg/5 mL

Vasotate HC ear drops ℞ *corticosteroidal anti-inflammatory; antiseptic* [hydrocortisone; acetic acid] 1%●2%

Vasotec tablets ℞ *antihypertensive; angiotensin-converting enzyme (ACE) inhibitor; treatment for congestive heart failure (CHF)* [enalapril maleate] 2.5, 5, 10, 20 mg ⑫ Fastic

VaT (vinblastine, Adriamycin, thiotepa) *chemotherapy protocol*

vatalanib *investigational (Phase III) tyrosine kinase inhibitor for cervical cancer*

VaTD; VaT-D (vincristine, ara-C, thioguanine, daunorubicin) *chemotherapy protocol*

VaTH (vinblastine, Adriamycin, thiotepa, Halotestin) *chemotherapy protocol for breast cancer*

Vatronol [see: Vicks Vatronol]

VAV (VP-16-213, Adriamycin, vincristine) *chemotherapy protocol*

VaxSyn HIV-1 *investigational (orphan) antiviral (therapeutic, Phase II) and vaccine (preventative, Phase I) for HIV and AIDS* [gp160 antigens]

VaZol oral liquid ℞ *antihistamine* [brompheniramine tannate] 2 mg/5 mL ⑫ Feosol; PhosLo

VaZol-D oral liquid ℞ *decongestant; antihistamine* [phenylephrine HCl; brompheniramine maleate] 7.5•4 mg/5 mL

Vazotab chewable tablets ℞ *decongestant; antihistamine* [phenylephrine HCl; brompheniramine maleate] 15•6 mg

Vazotuss HC Tannate oral suspension ℞ *narcotic antitussive; antihistamine; decongestant* [hydrocodone tannate; chlorpheniramine tannate; phenylephrine tannate] 10•12•20 mg/5 mL

VB (vinblastine, bleomycin) *chemotherapy protocol*

VBA (vincristine, BCNU, Adriamycin) *chemotherapy protocol*

VBAP (vincristine, BCNU, Adriamycin, prednisone) *chemotherapy protocol for multiple myeloma* ☑ VBP

VBC (VePesid, BCNU, cyclophosphamide) *chemotherapy protocol*

VBC (vinblastine, bleomycin, cisplatin) *chemotherapy protocol*

VBCMP (vincristine, BCNU, cyclophosphamide, melphalan, prednisone) *chemotherapy protocol for multiple myeloma*

VBD (vinblastine, bleomycin, DDP) *chemotherapy protocol*

VBM (vincristine, bleomycin, methotrexate) *chemotherapy protocol*

VBMCP (vincristine, BCNU, melphalan, cyclophosphamide, prednisone) *chemotherapy protocol*

VBMF (vincristine, bleomycin, methotrexate, fluorouracil) *chemotherapy protocol*

VBP (vinblastine, bleomycin, Platinol) *chemotherapy protocol*

VC (VePesid, carboplatin) *chemotherapy protocol*

VC (vincristine) [q.v.]

VC (vinorelbine, cisplatin) *chemotherapy protocol for non–small cell lung cancer (NSCLC)*

VCAP (vincristine, cyclophosphamide, Adriamycin, prednisone) *chemotherapy protocol for multiple myeloma* ☑ FCAP; FCP; VACP; VCP; VOCAP*

V-CAP III (VP-16-213, cyclophosphamide, Adriamycin, Platinol) *chemotherapy protocol* ☑ FCAP; FCP; VACP; VCP; VOCAP

VCF (vaginal contraceptive film) OTC *spermicidal contraceptive* [nonoxynol 9] 28%

VCF (vincristine, cyclophosphamide, fluorouracil) *chemotherapy protocol*

VCMP (vincristine, cyclophosphamide, melphalan, prednisone) *chemotherapy protocol for multiple myeloma* [also: VMCP]

VCP (vincristine, cyclophosphamide, prednisone) *chemotherapy protocol*

VCR (vincristine) [q.v.]

VD (vinorelbine, doxorubicin) *chemotherapy protocol for breast cancer*

V-Dec-M sustained-release tablets (discontinued 2007) ℞ *decongestant; expectorant* [pseudoephedrine HCl; guaifenesin] 120•500 mg

VDP (vincristine, daunorubicin, prednisone) *chemotherapy protocol*

VEC-162 *investigational (Phase III) melatonin receptor agonist to treat circadian rhythm sleep disorders (CRSD) and improve persistent sleep*

Vectibix IV infusion ℞ *monoclonal antibody antineoplastic for metastatic colorectal cancer* [panitumumab] 20 mg/mL

vecuronium bromide USAN, INN, BAN *nondepolarizing neuromuscular blocker; muscle relaxant; adjunct to anesthesia* 10, 20 mg injection

Veetids film-coated tablets, powder for oral solution ℞ *natural penicillin antibiotic* [penicillin V potassium] 250, 500 mg; 125, 250 mg/5 mL

vegetable oil, hydrogenated NF *tablet and capsule lubricant*

vegetable tallow; vegetable wax *medicinal herb* [see: bayberry]

VEGF (vascular endothelial growth factor) [see: telbermin]

Vehicle/N; Vehicle/N Mild OTC
lotion base

VeIP (Velban, ifosfamide [with mesna rescue], Platinol) *chemotherapy protocol for genitourinary and testicular cancer*

Velac (name changed to **Ziana** upon marketing release in 2006) ② FLAC

Velban powder for IV injection ℞ *antineoplastic for lung, breast, and testicular cancers, lymphomas, sarcomas, and neuroblastoma* [vinblastine sulfate] 10 mg/vial ② filipin; fleabane

Velcade powder for IV injection ℞ *proteasome inhibitor; antineoplastic for multiple myeloma (orphan) and mantle cell (non-Hodgkin) lymphoma; also used for myelomatous pleural effusion* [bortezomib] 3.5 mg/vial

Veldona low-dose oral lozenges *investigational (orphan) immunostimulant for oral human papillomavirus (HPV) warts in HIV-infected patients* [interferon alfa]

Velivet tablets (in packs of 28) ℞ *triphasic oral contraceptive; emergency postcoital contraceptive* [desogestrel; ethinyl estradiol] ② Folvite
Phase 1 (7 days): 0.1 mg•25 mcg;
Phase 2 (7 days): 0.125 mg•25 mcg;
Phase 3 (7 days): 0.15 mg•25 mcg;
Counters (7 days)

velnacrine INN, BAN *cholinesterase inhibitor* [also: velnacrine maleate]

velnacrine maleate USAN *cholinesterase inhibitor for Alzheimer disease* [also: velnacrine]

Velosef capsules, oral suspension (discontinued 2006) ℞ *first-generation cephalosporin antibiotic* [cephradine] 250, 500 mg; 125, 250 mg/5 mL

Velosef powder for IV or IM injection (discontinued 2004) ℞ *first-generation cephalosporin antibiotic* [cephradine] 250, 500, 1000, 2000 mg

Velosulin BR vials for subcu injection (discontinued 2005) OTC *antidiabetic* [human insulin (rDNA)] 100 U/mL

Velvachol OTC *cream base*

Venice turpentine *medicinal herb* [see: larch]

venlafaxine INN, BAN *antidepressant; anxiolytic; selective serotonin and norepinephrine reuptake inhibitor (SSNRI)* [also: venlafaxine HCl]

venlafaxine HCl USAN *antidepressant; anxiolytic; selective serotonin and norepinephrine reuptake inhibitor (SSNRI) for major depressive disorder (MDD), generalized anxiety disorder (GAD), social anxiety disorder (SAD), and panic disorder* [also: venlafaxine] 25, 37.5, 50, 75, 100, 150, 225 mg oral

Venofer IV injection ℞ *hematinic for iron deficiency in patients with non-dialysis-dependent chronic kidney disease (NDD-CKD), hemodialysis-dependent chronic kidney disease (HDD-CKD), and peritoneal dialysis-dependent chronic kidney disease (PDD-CKD)* [iron sucrose] 20 mg Fe/mL (100 mg Fe/vial)

Venoglobulin-S powder for IV infusion (discontinued 2005) ℞ *passive immunizing agent for HIV and idiopathic thrombocytopenic purpura (ITP)* [immune globulin, solvent/detergent treated] 5%, 10%

Venomil subcu or IM injection ℞ *venom sensitivity testing (subcu); venom desensitization therapy (IM)* [extracts of honeybee, yellow jacket, yellow hornet, white-faced hornet, mixed vespid, and wasp venom] ② fenamole

Ventavis solution for inhalation in single-dose ampules, for use with an adaptive aerosol delivery (AAD) system ℞ *prostacyclin analogue for pulmonary arterial hypertension (PAH) (orphan); investigational (orphan) intravenous treatment for thrombocytopenia and Raynaud phenomenon associated with systemic sclerosis* [iloprost] 10, 20 mcg

Venticute *investigational (orphan) for adult respiratory distress syndrome (ARDS)* [rSP-C lung surfactant]

Ventolin HFA inhalation aerosol with a CFC-free propellant ℞ *sympathomimetic bronchodilator* [albuterol] 90 mcg/dose

VePesid IV injection, capsules ℞ *anti-neoplastic for testicular and small cell lung cancers* [etoposide] 20 mg/mL; 50 mg

veradoline INN *analgesic* [also: veradoline HCl]

veradoline HCl USAN *analgesic* [also: veradoline]

veralipride INN

Veramyst nasal spray in a metered-dose pump ℞ *once-daily corticosteroidal anti-inflammatory for seasonal or perennial allergic rhinitis* [fluticasone furoate] 27.5 mcg/dose

verapamil USAN, INN, BAN *coronary vasodilator; calcium channel blocker*

verapamil HCl USAN, USP *antianginal; antiarrhythmic; antihypertensive; calcium channel blocker* 40, 80, 100, 120, 180, 200, 240, 300, 360 mg oral; 2.5 mg/mL injection

Veratrum **species** *medicinal herb* [see: hellebore]

veratrylidene-isoniazid [see: verazide]

verazide INN, BAN

Verazinc capsules OTC *zinc supplement* [zinc sulfate] 220 mg

Verbascum nigrum; V. phlomoides; V. thapsiforme; V. thapsus *medicinal herb* [see: mullein]

Verbena hastata *medicinal herb* [see: blue vervain]

Verdeso foam ℞ *corticosteroidal anti-inflammatory* [desonide] 0.05%

Veregen ointment ℞ *topical treatment for external genital and perianal warts (condyloma acuminatum) in immunocompromised adults* [sinecatechins] 15% ☒ Fergon

Verelan sustained-release capsules ℞ *antihypertensive; antianginal; antiarrhythmic; calcium channel blocker* [verapamil HCl] 120, 180, 240, 360 mg ☒ Furalan; Virilon

Verelan PM delayed-onset, extended-release capsules ℞ *antihypertensive; calcium channel blocker* [verapamil HCl] 100, 200, 300 mg

Vergon capsules (discontinued 2005) OTC *anticholinergic; antihistamine; anti-vertigo agent; motion sickness preventative* [meclizine HCl] 30 mg ☒ Fergon

Veridate (trademarked packaging form) *patient compliance package for oral contraceptives*

verilopam INN *analgesic* [also: verilopam HCl]

verilopam HCl USAN *analgesic* [also: verilopam]

verlukast USAN, INN *bronchodilator; antiasthmatic*

Verluma technetium Tc 99 prep kit ℞ *monoclonal antibody imaging agent for small cell lung cancer* [nofetumomab merpentan]

vermicides; vermifuges *a class of drugs effective against parasitic infections* [also called: anthelmintics]

Vermox chewable tablets ℞ *anthelmintic for trichuriasis, enterobiasis, ascariasis, and uncinariasis* [mebendazole] 100 mg

vernakalant *investigational (NDA filed) selective ion channel blocker for the acute conversion of atrial fibrillation*

verofylline USAN, INN *bronchodilator; antiasthmatic* ☒ furafylline

veronal [see: barbital]

veronal sodium [see: barbital sodium]

Veronate *investigational (orphan) agent to reduce or prevent staphylococci-induced nosocomial bacteremia in very low birthweight infants* [INH-A00021 (code name—generic name not yet assigned)]

veronica, tall *medicinal herb* [see: Culver root]

Veronica beccabunga *medicinal herb* [see: brooklime]

Veronica officinalis *medicinal herb* [see: speedwell]

Versa Alcohol Base; Versa Aqua Base; Versa PLO20 OTC *gel base*

Versa HRT Base Botanical; Versa HRT Base Heavy; Versa HRT Base Natural; Versa LipoBase Heavy; Versa LipoBase Regular; Versa VaniBase OTC *cream base*

Versacaps sustained-release capsules (discontinued 2007) ℞ *decongestant;*

expectorant [pseudoephedrine HCl; guaifenesin] 60•300 mg

Versed IV or IM injection, Tel-E-Ject syringes, pediatric syrup ℞ *short-acting benzodiazepine general anesthetic adjunct for preoperative sedation* [midazolam HCl] 1, 5 mg/mL; 2 mg/mL

versetamide USAN *stabilizer; carrier agent for gadoversetamide*

Versiclear lotion ℞ *antifungal; keratolytic; antipruritic; anesthetic* [sodium thiosulfate; salicylic acid; alcohol 10%] 25%•1%

verteporfin USAN *light-activated treatment for subfoveal choroidal neovascularization (CNV) due to age-related macular degeneration (AMD), pathologic myopia, or ocular histoplasmosis*

vervain *medicinal herb* [see: blue vervain]

Vesanoid capsules ℞ *antineoplastic for acute promyelocytic leukemia (orphan)* [tretinoin] 10 mg

vesicants *a class of agents that cause blisters*

VESIcare film-coated tablets ℞ *once-daily urinary antispasmodic for overactive bladder with urinary incontinence, urgency, and frequency* [solifenacin succinate] 5, 10 mg

vesnarinone USAN, INN *cardiotonic; inotropic for congestive heart failure*

vesperal [see: barbital]

vetrabutine INN, BAN

Vexol eye drop suspension ℞ *corticosteroidal anti-inflammatory* [rimexolone] 1%

Vfend film-coated tablets, powder for oral suspension, powder for IV injection ℞ *triazole antifungal for invasive aspergillosis, candidemia of the skin and internal organs, esophageal candidiasis, and other serious fungal infections* [voriconazole] 50, 200 mg; 40 mg/mL; 200 mg/vial

Viactiv chewable tablets OTC *calcium supplement* [calcium carbonate; vitamin D; vitamin K] 1.25 g•100 IU•40 mcg ⑫ Factive

Viadur DUROS (once-yearly subcu implant) ℞ *antihormonal antineoplastic for the palliative treatment of advanced prostate cancer* [leuprolide acetate] 72 mg (120 mcg/day)

Viaflex (trademarked packaging form) *ready-to-use IV bag*

Viagra film-coated tablets ℞ *phosphodiesterase type 5 (PDE5) inhibitor; selective vasodilator for erectile dysfunction (ED)* [sildenafil citrate] 25, 50, 100 mg

Viaject subcu injection *investigational (Phase III) fast-acting insulin for diabetes*

Vianain *investigational (orphan) proteolytic enzymes for debridement of severe burns* [ananain; comosain; bromelains]

vibesate

Vibramycin capsules ℞ *tetracycline antibiotic* [doxycycline hyclate] 100 mg

Vibramycin powder for oral suspension ℞ *tetracycline antibiotic* [doxycycline monohydrate] 25 mg/5 mL

Vibramycin syrup ℞ *tetracycline antibiotic* [doxycycline calcium] 50 mg/5 mL

Vibra-Tabs film-coated tablets ℞ *tetracycline antibiotic* [doxycycline hyclate] 100 mg

Viburnum opulus medicinal herb [see: cramp bark]

VIC (VePesid, ifosfamide [with mesna rescue], carboplatin) *chemotherapy protocol for non–small cell lung cancer (NSCLC)* [also: CVI]

VIC (vinblastine, ifosfamide, CCNU) *chemotherapy protocol*

Vicam injection ℞ *parenteral vitamin therapy* [multiple B vitamins; vitamin C] ≐•50 mg/mL ⑫ FAC-M

Vicks Cough Drops; Vicks Menthol Cough Drops OTC *mild anesthetic; antipruritic; counterirritant* [menthol] 10 mg; 8.4 mg

Vicks Cough Silencers lozenges (discontinued 2005) OTC *antitussive; mucous membrane anesthetic* [dextromethorphan hydrobromide; benzocaine] 2.5•1 mg

Vicks DayQuil products [see: DayQuil]

Vicks Formula 44 products [see: Formula 44]

Vicks NyQuil products [see: NyQuil]

Vicks Sinex products [see: Sinex]

Vicks Vapor inhaler OTC *nasal decongestant* [levmetamfetamine] 50 mg

Vicks VapoRub cream OTC *mild anesthetic; antipruritic; counterirritant; antiseptic* [camphor; menthol; eucalyptus oil] 5.2%•2.8%•1.2%

Vicks VapoRub vaporizing ointment OTC *mild anesthetic; antipruritic; counterirritant; antiseptic* [camphor; menthol; eucalyptus oil] 4.8%•2.6%•1.2%

Vicks Vitamin C Drops (lozenges) OTC *vitamin C supplement* [ascorbic acid and sodium ascorbate] 25 mg

Vicodin; Vicodin ES; Vicodin HP tablets ℞ *narcotic analgesic; antipyretic* [hydrocodone bitartrate; acetaminophen] 5•500 mg; 7.5•750 mg; 10•660 mg

Vicodin Tuss syrup (discontinued 2005) ℞ *narcotic antitussive; expectorant* [hydrocodone bitartrate; guaifenesin] 5•100 mg/5 mL

Vicon Forte capsules ℞ *vitamin/mineral supplement* [multiple vitamins & minerals; folic acid] ±•1 mg

Vicon Plus capsules OTC *vitamin/mineral supplement* [multiple vitamins & minerals]

Vicon-C capsules OTC *vitamin/mineral supplement* [multiple B vitamins & minerals; vitamin C] ±•300 mg

Vicoprofen film-coated tablets ℞ *narcotic analgesic & antitussive; antipyretic* [hydrocodone bitartrate; ibuprofen] 7.5•200 mg

vicotrope [see: cosyntropin]

vicriviroc *cellular chemokine receptor 5 (CCR5) inhibitor; investigational (Phase III) antiretroviral for HIV infections*

vidarabine USAN, USP, INN, BAN *antiviral*

vidarabine monohydrate [see: vidarabine]

vidarabine phosphate USAN *antiviral*

vidarabine sodium phosphate USAN *antiviral*

Vi-Daylin ADC drops OTC *vitamin supplement* [vitamins A, C, and D] 1500 IU•35 mg•400 IU per mL

Vi-Daylin ADC Vitamins + Iron drops OTC *vitamin/iron supplement* [vitamins A, C, and D; ferrous gluconate] 1500 IU•35 mg•400 IU•10 mg per mL

Vi-Daylin Multivitamin oral liquid, drops OTC *vitamin supplement* [multiple vitamins]

Vi-Daylin Multivitamin + Iron oral liquid, drops OTC *vitamin/iron supplement* [multiple vitamins; ferrous gluconate] ±•10 mg/5 mL; ±•10 mg/mL

Vi-Daylin/F ADC pediatric oral drops ℞ *vitamin supplement; dental caries preventative* [vitamins A, C, and D; sodium fluoride] 1500 IU•35 mg•400 IU•0.25 mg per mL

Vi-Daylin/F ADC + Iron pediatric oral drops ℞ *vitamin/iron supplement; dental caries preventative* [vitamins A, C, and D; sodium fluoride; ferrous sulfate] 1500 IU•35 mg•400 IU•0.25 mg•10 mg per mL

Vi-Daylin/F Multivitamin drops ℞ *pediatric vitamin supplement and dental caries preventative* [multiple vitamins; sodium fluoride] ±•0.25 mg/mL

Vi-Daylin/F Multivitamin pediatric chewable tablets (discontinued 2004) ℞ *vitamin supplement; dental caries preventative* [multiple vitamins; sodium fluoride; folic acid] ±•1•0.3 mg

Vi-Daylin/F Multivitamin + Iron pediatric chewable tablets ℞ *vitamin/iron supplement; dental caries preventative* [multiple vitamins; sodium fluoride; ferrous sulfate; folic acid] ±•1•12•0.3 mg

Vi-Daylin/F Multivitamin + Iron pediatric oral drops ℞ *vitamin/iron supplement; dental caries preventative* [multiple vitamins; sodium fluoride; ferrous sulfate] ±•0.25•10 mg/mL

Vidaza suspension for subcu injection or IV infusion ℞ *demethylating antineoplastic for myelodysplastic syndrome (orphan); also used for acute lymphocytic leukemia and acute myelogenous leukemia* [azacitidine] 100 mg/vial

Videx chewable/dispersible tablets, powder for oral solution, powder for pediatric oral solution ℞ *antiviral for advanced HIV infection* [didanosine] 25, 50, 100, 200 mg; 100, 250 mg/pkt.; 2, 4 g/bottle

Videx EC delayed-release capsules with enteric-coated beads ℞ *antiviral for advanced HIV infection* [didanosine] 200, 250, 500 mg

VIE (vincristine, ifosfamide, etoposide) *chemotherapy protocol*

vifilcon A USAN *hydrophilic contact lens material*

vifilcon B USAN *hydrophilic contact lens material*

Vi-Flor [see: Poly-Vi-Flor; Tri-Vi-Flor]

VIG (vaccinia immune globulin) [q.v.]

vigabatrin USAN, INN, BAN *investigational (NDA filed, orphan) anticonvulsant for infantile spasms; investigational (Phase II) treatment for cocaine and methamphetamine addictions*

Vigamox eye drops ℞ *broad-spectrum fluoroquinolone antibiotic* [moxifloxacin HCl] 0.5%

Vigomar Forte tablets OTC *vitamin/mineral/iron supplement* [multiple vitamins & minerals; iron] ≛•12 mg

Vigortol oral liquid OTC *geriatric vitamin/mineral supplement* [multiple B vitamins & minerals; alcohol 18%]

VIL *investigational (orphan) for hyperphenylalaninemia* [valine; isoleucine; leucine]

vilazodone *investigational (Phase III) selective serotonin reuptake inhibitor (SSRI) and partial 5-HT_{1A} agonist for depression and other mood disorders*

vildagliptin *investigational (NDA filed) dipeptidyl peptidase-4 (DPP-4) inhibitor oral antidiabetic that enhances the function of the body's incretin system to* *increase insulin production in the pancreas and reduce glucose production in the liver*

viloxazine INN, BAN *bicyclic antidepressant* [also: viloxazine HCl] ⊡ Flexzan

viloxazine HCl USAN *investigational (orphan) bicyclic antidepressant for cataplexy and narcolepsy* [also: viloxazine]

Viminate oral liquid OTC *geriatric vitamin/mineral supplement* [multiple B vitamins & minerals]

viminol INN

Vimpat ⓔⓤⓡ tablets, syrup, IV injection (available in Europe) *investigational (Phase III) adjunctive therapy for adults with uncontrolled partial seizures* [lacosamide]

vinafocon A USAN *hydrophobic contact lens material*

Vinate Good Start Prenatal Formula chewable tablets ℞ *prenatal vitamin/mineral/calcium/iron supplement* [multiple vitamins & minerals; calcium; iron; folic acid] ≛•200•29•1 mg

Vinate GT tablets ℞ *prenatal vitamin/mineral/calcium/iron supplement; stool softener* [multiple vitamins & minerals; calcium; iron; folic acid; biotin; docusate sodium] ≛•200•90•1•0.03•50 mg

vinbarbital NF, INN [also: vinbarbitone] ⊡ phenobarbital

vinbarbital sodium NF ⊡ phenobarbital sodium

vinbarbitone BAN [also: vinbarbital] ⊡ phenobarbitone

vinblastine INN *vinca alkaloid antineoplastic* [also: vinblastine sulfate]

vinblastine sulfate USAN, USP *vinca alkaloid antineoplastic* [also: vinblastine] 10 mg/vial, 1 mg/mL injection

vinblastine sulfate & estramustine *chemotherapy protocol for prostate cancer*

vinburnine INN

vinca alkaloids *a class of natural antineoplastics*

Vinca major; V. minor *medicinal herb* [see: periwinkle]

vincaleukoblastine sulfate [see: vin-blastine sulfate]

vincamine INN, BAN

vincanol INN

vincantenate [see: vinconate]

vincantril INN

Vincasar PFS IV injection ℞ *antineo-plastic* [vincristine sulfate] 1 mg/mL

vincofos USAN, INN *anthelmintic*

vinconate INN

vincristine (VC; VCR) INN *antineo-plastic* [also: vincristine sulfate]

vincristine sulfate USAN, USP *antineo-plastic* [also: vincristine] 1 mg/mL injection

vindeburnol INN

vindesine USAN, INN, BAN *synthetic vinca alkaloid antineoplastic* ⍰ Fun-duscein-10

vindesine sulfate USAN, JAN *investiga-tional (NDA filed) synthetic vinca alkaloid antineoplastic for leukemia, melanoma, breast and lung cancers*

vinegar [see: acetic acid]

vinepidine INN *antineoplastic* [also: vinepidine sulfate]

vinepidine sulfate USAN *antineoplastic* [also: vinepidine]

vinformide INN

vinglycinate INN *antineoplastic* [also: vinglycinate sulfate]

vinglycinate sulfate USAN *antineo-plastic* [also: vinglycinate]

vinleurosine INN *antineoplastic* [also: vinleurosine sulfate]

vinleurosine sulfate USAN *antineo-plastic* [also: vinleurosine]

vinmegallate INN

vinorelbine INN *antineoplastic* [also: vinorelbine tartrate]

vinorelbine & cisplatin *chemotherapy protocol for cervical cancer and non–small cell lung cancer (NSCLC)*

vinorelbine & doxorubicin *chemo-therapy protocol for breast cancer*

vinorelbine & gemcitabine *chemo-therapy protocol for non–small cell lung cancer (NSCLC)*

vinorelbine & paclitaxel *chemother-apy protocol for breast cancer*

vinorelbine tartrate USAN *antineoplas-tic* [also: vinorelbine] 10 mg/mL injection

vinpocetine USAN, INN *natural deriva-tive of vincamine, an extract of the periwinkle plant; increases aTP levels in the brain, which increases memory and mental function by increasing the neuronal firing rate; also increases serotonin levels in the brain*

vinpoline INN

vinrosidine INN *antineoplastic* [also: vinrosidine sulfate]

vinrosidine sulfate USAN *antineoplas-tic* [also: vinrosidine]

vintiamol INN

vintoperol INN

vintriptol INN

vinyl alcohol polymer [see: polyvinyl alcohol]

vinyl ether USP

vinyl gamma-aminobutyric acid [see: vigabatrin]

vinylbital INN [also: vinylbitone]

vinylbitone BAN [also: vinylbital]

vinylestrenolone [see: norgesterone]

vinymal [see: vinylbital]

vinyzene [see: bromchlorenone]

vinzolidine INN *antineoplastic* [also: vinzolidine sulfate]

vinzolidine sulfate USAN *antineoplas-tic* [also: vinzolidine]

Viogen-C capsules OTC *vitamin/mineral supplement* [multiple B vitamins & minerals; vitamin C] ± • 300 mg ⍰ Vicon-C

Viokase powder ℞ *porcine-derived digestive enzymes* [lipase; protease; amylase] 16 800 • 70 000 • 70 000 USP units per ¼ tsp.

Viokase 8; Viokase 16 tablets ℞ *por-cine-derived digestive enzymes* [lipase; protease; amylase] 8000 • 30 000 • 30 000 USP units; 16 000 • 60 000 • 60 000 USP units

Viola odorata *medicinal herb* [see: violet]

Viola tricolor *medicinal herb* [see: pansy]

violet (Viola odorata) *flowers and leaves medicinal herb for asthma, bronchitis,* cancer, colds, cough, sinus congestion, tumors, and ulcers ⚕ Fleet

violet, garden medicinal herb [see: pansy]

violetbloom medicinal herb [see: bittersweet nightshade]

viomycin INN [also: viomycin sulfate]

viomycin sulfate USP [also: viomycin]

viosterol in oil [see: ergocalciferol]

Vioxx tablets, oral suspension (withdrawn from the market in 2004 due to safety concerns) ℞ COX-2 inhibitor; nonsteroidal anti-inflammatory drug (NSAID) for osteoarthritis, rheumatoid arthritis, and primary dysmenorrhea; investigational (orphan) for juvenile rheumatoid arthritis [rofecoxib] 12.5, 25, 50 mg; 12.5, 25 mg/5 mL

VIP (vasoactive intestinal polypeptide) [q.v.]

VIP (VePesid, ifosfamide [with mesna rescue], Platinol) chemotherapy protocol for genitourinary cancers, testicular cancer, small cell lung cancer (SCLC), and non–small cell lung cancer (NSCLC)

VIP (vinblastine, ifosfamide [with mesna rescue], Platinol) chemotherapy protocol

VIP-B (VP-16, ifosfamide, Platinol, bleomycin) chemotherapy protocol

Viprinex ⓒ subcu injection, IV infusion (approved in Canada) anticoagulant for deep vein thrombosis (DVT) and severe chronic peripheral circulatory disorders; investigational (orphan) for cardiopulmonary bypass in heparin-intolerant patients [ancrod] 70 IU/mL

viprostol USAN, INN, BAN hypotensive; vasodilator

viprynium embonate BAN anthelmintic [also: pyrvinium pamoate]

Vi-Q-Tuss syrup (discontinued 2007) ℞ narcotic antitussive; expectorant [hydrocodone bitartrate; guaifenesin] 5•100 mg/5 mL

viqualine INN ⚕ Focalin

viquidil INN

Vira-A ophthalmic ointment (discontinued 2004) ℞ antiviral for acute keratoconjunctivitis and recurrent epithelial keratitis due to herpes simplex virus infection [vidarabine] 3%

Viracept film-coated tablets, powder for oral solution ℞ antiretroviral; protease inhibitor for HIV-1 infection [nelfinavir mesylate] 250, 650 mg; 50 mg/g

Viramune tablets, oral suspension ℞ antiviral non-nucleoside reverse transcriptase inhibitor (NNRTI) for HIV-1 infections [nevirapine] 200 mg; 50 mg/5 mL ⚕ FreAmine; furomine

ViraTan-DM B.I.D. chewable tablets, oral suspension ℞ antitussive; antihistamine; sleep aid; decongestant [dextromethorphan tannate; pyrilamine tannate; phenylephrine tannate] 25•30•25 mg; 12•30•12.5 mg/5 mL

Viravan-DM oral suspension, chewable tablets (discontinued 2007) ℞ antitussive; antihistamine; sleep aid; decongestant; for children 2–12 years [dextromethorphan tannate; pyrilamine tannate; phenylephrine tannate] 25•30•12.5 mg/5 mL; 25•30•25 mg

Viravan-S oral suspension (discontinued 2006) ℞ decongestant; antihistamine; sleep aid [phenylephrine tannate; pyrilamine tannate] 12.5•30 mg/5 mL

Viravan-T chewable tablets (discontinued 2007) ℞ decongestant; antihistamine; sleep aid [phenylephrine tannate; pyrilamine tannate] 25•30 mg

Virazole powder for inhalation aerosol ℞ nucleoside antiviral for severe lower respiratory tract infections caused by respiratory syncytial virus (RSV); investigational (orphan) for hemorrhagic fever with renal syndrome [ribavirin] 6 g/vial (20 mg/mL reconstituted)

Viread film-coated tablets ℞ antiviral; nucleotide reverse transcriptase inhibitor (NRTI) for HIV-1 and chronic hepatitis B infections [tenofovir disoproxil fumarate] 300 mg

Virginia mountain mint; Virginia thyme medicinal herb [see: wild hyssop]

Virginia silk *medicinal herb* [see: milk-weed]

virginiamycin USAN, INN *antibacterial; veterinary food additive*

virginiamycin factor M₁ [see: virginiamycin]

virginiamycin factor S [see: virginiamycin]

virgin's bower *medicinal herb* [see: woodbine]

viridofulvin USAN, INN *antifungal*

Virilon capsules ℞ *synthetic androgen for hypogonadism or testosterone deficiency in men, delayed puberty in boys, and metastatic breast cancer in women; hormone replacement therapy (HRT) for postandropausal symptoms; also abused as a street drug* [methyltestosterone] 10 mg ⊡ Furalan; Verelan

Virilon IM injection (discontinued 2006) ℞ *androgen for hypogonadism or testosterone deficiency in men, delayed puberty in boys, and metastatic breast cancer in women; hormone replacement therapy for postandropausal symptoms; also abused as a street drug* [methyltestosterone] 200 mg/mL ⊡ Furalan; Verelan

Virogen Herpes slide test for professional use ℞ *in vitro diagnostic aid for herpes simplex virus antigen in lesions or cell cultures* [latex agglutination test]

Virogen Rotatest slide test for professional use ℞ *in vitro diagnostic aid for fecal rotavirus* [latex agglutination test]

Viroptic Drop-Dose (eye drops) ℞ *antiviral for keratoconjunctivitis and epithelial keratitis due to herpes simplex virus infection* [trifluridine] 1%

viroxime USAN, INN *antiviral*

viroxime component A [see: zinviroxime]

viroxime component B [see: enviroxime]

Viroxyn oral gel OTC *germicide for cold sores/fever blisters* [benzalkonium chloride; isopropyl alcohol] 0.13%•70% ⊡ Furoxone

Virulizin *investigational (Phase III) macrophage activator for AIDS-related lymphomas and Kaposi sarcoma; investigational (Phase III, orphan) for pancreatic cancer*

Viscoat prefilled syringes ℞ *viscoelastic agent for ophthalmic surgery* [hyaluronate sodium; chondroitin sulfate sodium] 30•40 mg/mL

Viscum album *medicinal herb* [see: mistletoe]

Visicol tablets ℞ *saline laxative; preprocedure bowel evacuant* [sodium phosphate (monobasic and dibasic)] 1.5 g (1.102•0.398 g) ⊡ FazaClo

visilizumab USAN *monoclonal antibody to CD3; investigational immunosuppressant for organ transplants, autoimmune diseases, and other T lymphocyte disorders*

visiluzumab [now: visilizumab]

Visine eye drops OTC *decongestant; vasoconstrictor* [tetrahydrozoline HCl] 0.05% ⊡ Fuzeon; Vusion

Visine Advanced Relief eye drops (discontinued 2006) OTC *decongestant; vasoconstrictor; moisturizer/lubricant* [tetrahydrozoline HCl; polyethylene glycol 400; povidone] 0.05%•1%•1%

Visine Allergy Relief eye drops OTC *decongestant; astringent* [tetrahydrozoline HCl; zinc sulfate] 0.05%•0.25%

Visine L.R. eye drops OTC *decongestant; vasoconstrictor* [oxymetazoline HCl] 0.025%

Visine Moisturizing eye drops (discontinued 2006) OTC *decongestant; vasoconstrictor; moisturizer/lubricant* [tetrahydrozoline HCl; polyethylene glycol 400] 0.05%•1%

Visine Pure Tears; Visine Tears; Visine Tears Preservative Free eye drops OTC *moisturizer/lubricant* [polyethylene glycol 400; glycerin; hypromellose] 1%•0.2%•0.2%

Visine-A eye drops OTC *decongestant; vasoconstrictor* [naphazoline HCl; pheniramine maleate] 0.025%•0.3% ⊡ Fuzeon; Vusion

Vision (trademarked delivery device) *needle-free insulin injection system* ⊡ Fuzeon; Vusion

Vision Care Enzymatic Cleaner tablets OTC *enzymatic cleaner for soft contact lenses* [pork pancreatin]

Vision Clear eye drops (discontinued 2008) OTC *decongestant; vasoconstrictor* [tetrahydrozoline HCl] 0.05%

VisionBlue ophthalmic injection in prefilled syringes ℞ *surgical aid for staining the anterior capsule of the lens* [trypan blue] 0.06% in 0.5 mL syringes

Visipak (trademarked packaging form) *reverse-numbered package* ⊡ Faspak

Visipaque 270; Visipaque 320 intra-arterial or IV injection ℞ *radiopaque contrast medium for CT, x-ray, and visceral digital subtraction angiography* [iodixanol (49.1% iodine)] 550 mg/mL (270 mg/mL); 652 mg/mL (320 mg/mL) ⊡ Faspak

Visken tablets ℞ *β-blocker for hypertension; antianginal* [pindolol] 5, 10 mg ⊡ Vasocon-A

visnadine INN, BAN

visnafylline INN

Vi-Sol [see: Poly-Vi-Sol; Tri-Vi-Sol]

Visonex film-coated, extended-release tablets ℞ *decongestant; expectorant* [phenylephrine HCl; guaifenesin] 30•900 mg

Vistaril capsules, oral suspension ℞ *anxiolytic; minor tranquilizer; antihistamine for allergic pruritus* [hydroxyzine pamoate] 25, 50, 100 mg; 25 mg/5 mL ⊡ Fostril

Vistaril deep IM injection ℞ *anxiolytic; antiemetic; antihistamine for allergic pruritus; adjunct to preoperative or prepartum analgesia* [hydroxyzine HCl] 25 mg/mL ⊡ Fostril

vistatolon INN *antiviral* [also: statolon]

Vistide IV infusion ℞ *nucleoside antiviral for AIDS-related cytomegalovirus (CMV) retinitis* [cidofovir] 75 mg/mL

Visual-Eyes ophthalmic solution OTC *extraocular irrigating solution* [sterile isotonic solution]

Visudyne powder for IV infusion ℞ *treatment for subfoveal choroidal neovascularization (CNV) due to age-related macular degeneration (AMD), pathologic myopia, or ocular histoplasmosis; activated with the Opal Photoactivator laser* [verteporfin] 2 mg/mL (15 mg/vial) ⊡ Fucidin

Vita-bee with C Captabs (capsule-shaped tablets) OTC *vitamin supplement* [multiple B vitamins; vitamin C] ± •300 mg

Vita-Bob softgel capsules OTC *vitamin supplement* [multiple vitamins; folic acid] ± •0.4 mg

Vita-C crystals for oral liquid OTC *vitamin C supplement* [ascorbic acid] 4 g/tsp.

Vitafol syrup ℞ *hematinic* [ferric pyrophosphate; multiple B vitamins; folic acid] 90• ± •0.75 mg/15 mL

Vitafol; Vitafol-PN film-coated caplets ℞ *hematinic; vitamin supplement* [ferrous fumarate; multiple vitamins; folic acid] 65 mg• ± •1 mg

Vita-Kid chewable wafers OTC *vitamin supplement* [multiple vitamins; folic acid] ± •0.3 mg

Vital B-50 timed-release tablets OTC *vitamin supplement* [multiple B vitamins; folic acid; biotin] ± •100•50 mcg

Vital High Nitrogen powder OTC *enteral nutritional therapy* [lactose-free formula] 79 g

Vitalets chewable tablets OTC *vitamin/mineral/iron supplement* [multiple vitamins & minerals; iron; biotin] ± •10 mg•25 mcg

Vitalize SF oral liquid OTC *hematinic* [ferric pyrophosphate; multiple B vitamins; lysine] 66• ± •300 mg/15 mL

vitamin A USP *fat-soluble vitamin; antixerophthalmic; topical emollient; essential for vision, dental development, growth, cortisone synthesis, epithelial tissue differentiation, embryonic development, reproduction, and mucous membrane maintenance* 10 000, 15 000, 25 000 IU oral

vitamin A acid [see: tretinoin]

vitamin A palmitate

vitamin A₁ [see: retinol]

Vitamin B Complex 100 injection ℞ *parenteral vitamin therapy* [multiple B vitamins]

vitamin B₁ [see: thiamine HCl]

vitamin B₁ mononitrate [see: thiamine mononitrate]

vitamin B₂ [see: riboflavin]

vitamin B₃ [see: niacin; niacinamide; nicotinamide; nicotinic acid]

vitamin B₅ [see: calcium pantothenate; pantothenic acid]

vitamin B₆ [see: pyridoxine HCl]

vitamin B₈ [see: adenosine phosphate]

vitamin B₁₂ [see: cyanocobalamin; hydroxocobalamin]

vitamin B₁₅ [see: dimethylglycine HCl]

vitamin Bₑ [see: folic acid]

vitamin Bₜ [see: carnitine]

vitamin C [see: ascorbic acid; calcium ascorbate; sodium ascorbate]

vitamin D *a family of fat-soluble vitamins consisting of ergocalciferol (vitamin D₂) and cholecalciferol (vitamin D₃), that is converted to calcitriol (the active form) in the body; considered a non-endogenous hormone* [see also: calcifediol; dihydrotachysterol; doxercalciferol; paricalcitol]

vitamin D₁ [see: dihydrotachysterol]

vitamin D₂ [see: ergocalciferol]

vitamin D₃ [see: cholecalciferol]

vitamin E USP *fat-soluble vitamin; antioxidant; platelet aggregation inhibitor; topical emollient; also used for reducing the toxic effects of oxygen therapy in premature infants, for preeclampsia, and for various cardiac and autoimmune conditions* [note relative potencies at alpha tocopherol, et seq.] 100, 200, 400, 500, 800, 1000 IU oral; 15 IU/30 mL oral

Vitamin E with Mixed Tocopherols tablets OTC *vitamin supplement* [vitamin E] 100, 200, 400 IU

vitamin E-TPGS (tocopheryl polyethylene glycol succinate) [see: tocophersolan]

vitamin G [see: riboflavin]

vitamin H [see: biotin]

vitamin K₁ [see: phytonadione]

vitamin K₂ [see: menaquinone]

vitamin K₃ [see: menadione]

vitamin K₄ [see: menadiol sodium diphosphate]

vitamin M [see: folic acid]

vitamin P [see: bioflavonoids]

vitamin P₄ [see: troxerutin]

Vitamin-Mineral Supplement oral liquid OTC *vitamin/mineral supplement* [multiple B vitamins & minerals; alcohol 18%]

Vitaneed oral liquid OTC *enteral nutritional therapy* [lactose-free formula]

Vita-Plus E softgels OTC *vitamin supplement* [vitamin E (as *d*-alpha tocopheryl acetate)] 400 IU

Vita-Plus G softgel capsules OTC *geriatric vitamin/mineral supplement* [multiple vitamins & minerals]

Vita-Plus H softgel capsules OTC *vitamin/mineral/iron supplement* [multiple vitamins & minerals; iron] ≟•13.4 mg

Vita-PMS; Vita-PMS Plus tablets OTC *vitamin/mineral supplement; digestive enzymes* [multiple vitamins & minerals; folic acid; biotin; amylase; protease; lipase; betaine acid HCl] ≟•0.33 mg•10.4 mcg•2500 U• 2500 U•200 U•16.7 mg

Vitarex tablets OTC *vitamin/mineral/ iron supplement* [multiple vitamins & minerals; iron] ≟•15 mg

Vite E cream OTC *emollient* [vitamin E] 50 mg/g

Vitec cream OTC *emollient* [vitamin E]

Vitelle Irospan capsules OTC *hematinic; vitamin/iron supplement* [ferrous sulfate, dried (source of iron); ascorbic acid] 200 (65)•150 mg

Vitelle Irospan timed-release tablets (discontinued 2005) OTC *hematinic; vitamin/iron supplement* [ferrous sulfate, dried (source of iron); ascorbic acid] 200 (65)•150 mg

Vitelle Lurline PMS tablets OTC *analgesic; antipyretic; diuretic; vitamin B₆* [acetaminophen; pamabrom; pyridoxine HCl] 500•25•50 mg

Vitelle Nesentials tablets OTC *vitamin/mineral supplement* [multiple vitamins & minerals]

Vitelle Nestabs OTC tablets OTC *prenatal vitamin/calcium/iron supplement* [multiple vitamins; calcium; iron; folic acid] ≜•200•29•0.8 mg

Vitelle Nestrex tablets OTC *vitamin B_6 supplement* [pyridoxine HCl] 25 mg

vitellin *natural remedy* [see: lecithin]

Vitex agnus-castus medicinal herb [see: chaste tree]

Vitis coigetiae; V. vinifera medicinal herb [see: grape seed]

Vitrase powder for injection, solution for injection ℞ *adjuvant to increase the absorption and dispersion of injected drugs, hypodermoclysis, and subcutaneous urography; investigational (NDA filed) agent to clear vitreous hemorrhage; also used for diabetic retinopathy* [hyaluronidase (ovine)] 6200 U; 200 U/mL

Vitrasert intraocular implant (5–8 months' duration) ℞ *antiviral for AIDS-related CMV retinitis (orphan)* [ganciclovir] 4.5 mg

Vitravene intravitreal injection (discontinued 2006) ℞ *ophthalmic antiviral for AIDS-related CMV retinitis* [fomivirsen sodium] 6.6 mg/mL

Vitron-C tablets OTC *hematinic; vitamin/iron supplement* [ferrous fumarate (source of iron); ascorbic acid] 200 (66)•125 mg

Vitussin syrup ℞ *narcotic antitussive; expectorant* [hydrocodone bitartrate; guaifenesin] 5•100 mg/5 mL

Vivactil film-coated tablets ℞ *tricyclic antidepressant* [protriptyline HCl] 5, 10 mg

Viva-Drops eye drops OTC *moisturizer/lubricant*

Vivaglobin subcu injection ℞ *passive immunizing agent for primary immune deficiency (PID) (orphan)* [immune globulin (IGSC)] 160 mg/mL (0.48, 1.6, 3.2 g/dose)

Vivarin tablets OTC *CNS stimulant; analeptic* [caffeine] 200 mg

Vivelle; Vivelle-Dot transdermal patch ℞ *estrogen replacement therapy for the treatment of postmenopausal symptoms and prevention of postmenopausal osteoporosis* [estradiol] 37.5, 50, 75, 100 mcg/day; 25, 37.5, 50, 75, 100 mcg/day

Viviant *second-generation selective estrogen receptor modulator (SERM); investigational (NDA filed) for the prevention and treatment of postmenopausal osteoporosis* [bazedoxifene]

Vivitrol extended-release IM injection ℞ *once monthly narcotic agonist for the treatment of alcoholism and opiate addiction (orphan)* [naltrexone HCl] 380 mg

Vivonex T.E.N. powder OTC *enteral nutritional therapy* [lactose-free formula]

Vivotif Berna enteric-coated capsules ℞ *typhoid fever vaccine* [typhoid vaccine (Ty21a), live attenuated] 2–6 × 10^9 viable CFU + 5–50 × 10^9 nonviable cells

Vi-Zac capsules OTC *vitamin/zinc supplement* [vitamins A, C, and E; zinc] 5000 IU•500 mg•50 mg•18 mg

VLP (vincristine, L-asparaginase, prednisone) *chemotherapy protocol*

VM (vinblastine, mitomycin) *chemotherapy protocol for breast cancer*

VM-26 [see: teniposide]

VM-26PP (teniposide, procarbazine, prednisone) *chemotherapy protocol* ⧉ VAMP; VMP

VMAD (vincristine, methotrexate, Adriamycin, actinomycin D) *chemotherapy protocol*

VMCP (vincristine, melphalan, cyclophosphamide, prednisone) *chemotherapy protocol for multiple myeloma* [also: VCMP]

VMP (VePesid, mitoxantrone, prednimustine) *chemotherapy protocol*

VOCAP (VP-16-213, Oncovin, cyclophosphamide, Adriamycin, Platinol) *chemotherapy protocol* ⧉ FCAP; FCP; VACP; VCAP; VCP

vofopitant dihydrochloride USAN *tachykinin NK₁ receptor antagonist; antiemetic*

voglibose USAN, INN *alpha-glucosidase inhibitor that delays the digestion of dietary carbohydrates* ⊡ Folpace; Phillips'

volatile nitrites *amyl nitrite, butyl nitrite, and isobutyl nitrite vapors that produce coronary stimulant effects, abused as street drugs* [see also: nitrous oxide; petroleum distillate inhalants]

volazocine USAN, INN *analgesic* ⊡ fluacizine

Volmax extended-release tablets (discontinued 2004) ℞ *sympathomimetic bronchodilator* [albuterol sulfate] 4, 8 mg ⊡ Flomax

Voltaren delayed-release tablets ℞ *analgesic; nonsteroidal anti-inflammatory drug (NSAID) for osteoarthritis, rheumatoid arthritis, and ankylosing spondylitis* [diclofenac sodium] 75 mg ⊡ Foltrin

Voltaren eye drops ℞ *analgesic; nonsteroidal anti-inflammatory drug (NSAID) for cataract extraction and corneal refractive surgery* [diclofenac sodium] 0.1% ⊡ Foltrin

Voltaren gel ℞ *analgesic; nonsteroidal anti-inflammatory drug (NSAID) for osteoarthritis* [diclofenac sodium] 1% ⊡ Foltrin

Voltaren-XR extended-release tablets ℞ *once-daily analgesic; nonsteroidal anti-inflammatory drug (NSAID) for osteoarthritis, rheumatoid arthritis, and ankylosing spondylitis* [diclofenac sodium] 100 mg

Voluven IV infusion ℞ *plasma volume expander for blood loss due to trauma or surgery* [hetastarch] 6 g/100 mL ⊡ valofane

von Willebrand factor (VWF) *antihemophilic for von Willebrand disease* (orphan)

Vopac caplets ℞ *narcotic antitussive; analgesic; antipyretic* [codeine phosphate; acetaminophen] 30•650 mg ⊡ VBC; VPCA

voriconazole *triazole antifungal for invasive aspergillosis, candidemia of the skin and internal organs, esophageal candidiasis, and other serious fungal infections*

vorinostat *histone deacetylase (HDAC) inhibitor; antineoplastic for cutaneous T-cell lymphoma (CTCL); investigational (orphan) for multiple myeloma, mesothelioma, and T-cell non-Hodgkin lymphoma*

vorozole USAN, INN, BAN *antineoplastic; aromatase inhibitor* ⊡ FeroSul

vortel [see: clorprenaline HCl]

VōSol HC Otic ear drops (discontinued 2006) ℞ *corticosteroidal anti-inflammatory; antiseptic* [hydrocortisone; acetic acid] 1%•2%

VōSol Otic ear drops (discontinued 2006) ℞ *antibacterial; antifungal; antiseptic* [acetic acid] 2%

VoSpire ER extended-release tablets ℞ *sympathomimetic bronchodilator* [albuterol sulfate] 4, 8 mg

votumumab USAN *monoclonal antibody for cancer imaging and therapy*

voxergolide INN

Voxsuprine tablets ℞ *peripheral vasodilator* [isoxsuprine HCl] 10, 20 mg

VP (vasopressin) [q.v.]

VP (VePesid, Platinol) *chemotherapy protocol for small cell lung cancer (SCLC)*

VP (vincristine, prednisone) *chemotherapy protocol*

VP + A (vincristine, prednisone, asparaginase) *chemotherapy protocol*

VP-16 [see: etoposide]

VPB (vinblastine, Platinol, bleomycin) *chemotherapy protocol*

VPBCPr (vincristine, prednisone, vinblastine, chlorambucil, procarbazine) *chemotherapy protocol*

VPCA (vincristine, prednisone, cyclophosphamide, ara-C) *chemotherapy protocol* ⊡ VBC; Vopac

VPCMF (vincristine, prednisone, cyclophosphamide, methotrexate, fluorouracil) *chemotherapy protocol*

VP-L-asparaginase (vincristine, prednisone, L-asparaginase) *chemotherapy protocol*

VPP (VePesid, Platinol) *chemotherapy protocol*

V-TAD (VePesid, thioguanine, ara-C, daunorubicin) *chemotherapy protocol for acute myelocytic leukemia (AML)*

V-Tann oral suspension ℞ *decongestant; antihistamine; sleep aid* [phenylephrine tannate; pyrilamine tannate] 12.5•30 mg/5 mL ⑨ Vytone

vulneraries *a class of agents that promote wound healing*

Vumon IV infusion ℞ *antineoplastic for acute lymphocytic leukemia (orphan) and bladder cancer* [teniposide] 50 mg (10 mg/mL)

Vusion ointment ℞ *diaper rash treatment; antifungal for candidiasis* [miconazole nitrate; zinc oxide] 0.25%•15% ⑨ Fuzeon; Visine

VWF (von Willebrand factor) [q.v.]

VX-175 *investigational (Phase III) protease inhibitor for HIV infections*

Vytone cream ℞ *corticosteroidal anti-inflammatory; antifungal; antibacterial* [hydrocortisone; iodoquinol] 1%•1% ⑨ V-Tann

Vytorin 10/10; Vytorin 10/20; Vytorin 10/40; Vytorin 10/80 caplets ℞ *combination intestinal cholesterol absorption inhibitor plus HMG-CoA reductase inhibitor to lower serum levels of LDL and total cholesterol* [ezetimibe; simvastatin] 10•10 mg; 10•20 mg; 10•40 mg; 10•80 mg

Vyvanse capsules ℞ *once-daily treatment for attention-deficit/hyperactivity disorder (ADHD)* [lisdexamfetamine dimesylate] 20, 30, 40, 50, 60, 70 mg

VZIG (varicella-zoster immune globulin) [q.v.]

wahoo (Euonymus atropurpureus) bark *medicinal herb used as a diuretic, expectorant, and laxative*

wakerobin *medicinal herb* [see: birthroot]

Wallette (trademarked packaging form) *patient compliance package for oral contraceptives* ⑨ violet

wallflower; western wallflower *medicinal herb* [see: dogbane]

walnut (Juglans spp.) *medicinal herb* [see: black walnut; butternut; English walnut]

walnut, lemon; white walnut *medicinal herb* [see: butternut]

Walpole tea *medicinal herb* [see: New Jersey tea]

wandering milkweed *medicinal herb* [see: dogbane]

warfarin INN, BAN *coumarin-derivative anticoagulant* [also: warfarin potassium]

warfarin potassium USP *coumarin-derivative anticoagulant* [also: warfarin]

warfarin sodium USP *coumarin-derivative anticoagulant for myocardial infarction, thromboembolic episodes, venous thrombosis, and pulmonary embolism* 1, 2, 2.5, 3, 4, 5, 6, 7.5, 10 mg oral

Wart Remover topical liquid OTC *keratolytic* [salicylic acid in flexible collodion] 17%

Wart-Off topical liquid OTC *keratolytic* [salicylic acid in flexible collodion] 17%

water, purified USP *solvent*

water, tritiated [see: tritiated water]

water cabbage *medicinal herb* [see: white pond lily]

water dock (Rumex aquaticus) *medicinal herb* [see: yellow dock]

water eryngo (Eryngium aquaticum) root *medicinal herb used as a diapho-*

retic, diuretic, emetic, expectorant, and stimulant

water fern medicinal herb [see: buckhorn brake]

water flag medicinal herb [see: blue flag]

water hemlock; water parsley medicinal herb [see: poison hemlock]

water lily medicinal herb [see: blue flag; white pond lily]

water lily, sweet; sweet-scented water lily; white water lily medicinal herb [see: white pond lily]

water moccasin snake antivenin [see: antivenin (Crotalidae) polyvalent]

water O 15 USAN radioactive diagnostic aid for vascular disorders

water pepper medicinal herb [see: knotweed]

water pimpernel; water purslain medicinal herb [see: brooklime]

water shamrock medicinal herb [see: buckbean]

water smartweed medicinal herb [see: knotweed]

[^{15}O] water [see: water O 15]

watercress (Nasturtium officinale) plant medicinal herb for anemia, cramps, kidney and liver disorders, nervousness, and rheumatism

water-d$_2$ [see: deuterium oxide]

wax, carnauba NF tablet-coating agent

wax, emulsifying NF emulsifying and stiffening agent

wax, microcrystalline NF stiffening and tablet-coating agent

wax, white NF stiffening agent [also: beeswax, white]

wax, yellow NF stiffening agent [also: beeswax, yellow]

wax cluster medicinal herb [see: wintergreen]

wax myrtle medicinal herb [see: bayberry]

weeping spruce medicinal herb [see: hemlock]

WelChol tablets ℞ nonabsorbable cholesterol-lowering polymer for hyperlipidemia and to improve glycemic control in type 2 diabetes [colesevelam HCl] 625 mg ⊘ Flagyl; Ful-Glo

Wellbutrin film-coated tablets ℞ aminoketone antidepressant; also used for attention-deficit/hyperactivity disorder (ADHD) [bupropion HCl] 75, 100 mg

Wellbutrin SR sustained-release (12-hour) film-coated tablets ℞ aminoketone antidepressant; also used for attention-deficit/hyperactivity disorder (ADHD), neuropathic pain, and weight loss [bupropion HCl] 100, 150, 200 mg

Wellbutrin XL sustained-release (24-hour) tablets ℞ aminoketone antidepressant for major depression and seasonal affective disorder (SAD); also used for attention deficit hyperactivity disorder (ADHD), neuropathic pain, and weight loss [bupropion HCl] 150, 300 mg

Wellcovorin powder for IV infusion (discontinued 2002) ℞ chemotherapy "rescue" agent (orphan) [leucovorin calcium] 100 mg/vial

Wellcovorin tablets (discontinued 2002) ℞ chemotherapy "rescue" agent (orphan); antidote to folic acid antagonist overdose [leucovorin calcium] 5, 25 mg

Wellements Organic Gripe Water oral liquid OTC natural product to relieve colic, stomach cramps, hiccups, and gas in infants [ginger; fennel; chamomile]

WellTuss EXP syrup (discontinued 2007) ℞ narcotic antitussive; decongestant; expectorant [dihydrocodeine bitartrate; pseudoephedrine HCl; guaifenesin] 7.5•15•100 mg/5 mL

Welltuss HC oral liquid ℞ narcotic antitussive; antihistamine; decongestant [hydrocodone bitartrate; chlorpheniramine maleate; pseudoephedrine HCl] 3•2•15 mg/5 mL ⊘ FluTuss HC

Westcort ointment, cream ℞ corticosteroidal anti-inflammatory [hydrocortisone valerate] 0.2%

western wallflower medicinal herb [see: dogbane]

Westhroid tablets ℞ natural thyroid replacement for hypothyroidism or thyroid cancer [thyroid, desiccated (porcine)] 32.4, 64.8, 129.6, 194.4 mg

Wet-N-Soak solution OTC *rewetting solution for rigid gas permeable contact lenses*

Wet-N-Soak Plus solution OTC *disinfecting/wetting/soaking solution for rigid gas permeable contact lenses* [note: RGP contact indication is different from hard contact indication for same product]

Wet-N-Soak Plus solution OTC *wetting/soaking solution for hard contact lenses* [note: hard contact indication is different from RGP contact indication for same product]

Wetting solution OTC *wetting solution for hard contact lenses*

Wetting & Soaking solution OTC *disinfecting/wetting/soaking solution for rigid gas permeable contact lenses* [note: one of two different products with the same name]

Wetting & Soaking solution OTC *wetting/soaking solution for hard contact lenses* [note: one of two different products with the same name]

wheat germ oil (octacosanol) *natural dietary supplement for increasing muscle endurance*

WHF Lubricating Gel OTC *vaginal antiseptic; moisturizer/lubricant* [chlorhexidine gluconate; glycerin]

white bay *medicinal herb* [see: magnolia]

white beeswax [see: beeswax, white]

White Cloverine Salve ointment OTC *skin protectant* [white petrolatum] 97%

White Cod Liver Oil Concentrate capsules, chewable tablets OTC *vitamin supplement* [vitamins A, D, and E] 10 000•400•$\frac{2}{2}$ IU; 4000•200•$\frac{2}{2}$ IU

White Cod Liver Oil Concentrate with Vitamin C chewable tablets OTC *vitamin supplement* [vitamins A, C, and D] 4000 IU•50 mg•200 IU

white cohosh (Actaea alba; A. pachypoda; A. rubra) plant and root *medicinal herb for arthritis, bowel evacuation, colds, cough, itching, promoting labor, reviving those near death,* rheumatism, stimulating menses, stomach disorders, and urogenital disorders

white endive *medicinal herb* [see: dandelion]

white fringe *medicinal herb* [see: fringe tree]

white hellebore (Veratrum album) [see: hellebore]

white horehound *medicinal herb* [see: horehound]

white lotion USP *astringent; topical protectant*

white mineral oil [see: petrolatum, white]

white mustard; white mustard seed *medicinal herb* [see: mustard]

white nettle *medicinal herb* [see: blind nettle]

white oak (Quercus alba) bark *medicinal herb for internal and external bleeding, menstrual disorders, mouth sores, skin irritation, toothache, strep throat, ulcers, and urinary bleeding*

white ointment [see: ointment, white]

white petrolatum [see: petrolatum, white]

white phenolphthalein [see: phenolphthalein]

white pine (Pinus strobus) bark *medicinal herb for bronchitis, dysentery, laryngitis, and mucous build-up*

white pond lily (Nymphaea odorata) root *medicinal herb used as an antiseptic, astringent, demulcent, discutient, and vulnerary*

white root *medicinal herb* [see: pleurisy root]

white sorrel *medicinal herb* [see: wood sorrel]

white walnut *medicinal herb* [see: butternut]

white water lily *medicinal herb* [see: white pond lily]

white wax [see: wax, white]

white willow (Salix alba) *medicinal herb* [see: willow]

whitethorn *medicinal herb* [see: hawthorn]

Whitfield's Ointment OTC *antifungal; keratolytic* [benzoic acid; salicylic acid] 6%•3%

Whitfield's ointment [see: benzoic & salicylic acids]

whole blood [see: blood, whole]

whole root rauwolfia [see: rauwolfia serpentina]

whole-cell pertussis vaccine [see: diphtheria & tetanus toxoids & whole-cell pertussis (DTwP) vaccine, adsorbed]

whorlywort *medicinal herb* [see: Culver root]

Wibi lotion OTC *moisturizer; emollient*

widow spider species antivenin [now: antivenin (Latrodectus mactans)]

Wigraine suppositories (discontinued 2005) ℞ *migraine-specific vasoconstrictor* [ergotamine tartrate; caffeine; tartaric acid] 2•100•21.5 mg ℞ IC-Green

Wigraine tablets (discontinued 2005) ℞ *migraine-specific vasoconstrictor* [ergotamine tartrate; caffeine] 1•100 mg ℞ IC-Green

wild bergamot (Monarda fistulosa) leaves *medicinal herb used as a carminative and stimulant*

wild black cherry (Prunus serotina) bark *medicinal herb used as an astringent, pectoral, sedative, and stimulant*

wild carrot *medicinal herb* [see: carrot]

wild cherry (Prunus virginiana) bark *medicinal herb for asthma, bronchitis, cough, fever, hypertension, and mucosal inflammation with discharge; also used as an expectorant*

wild cherry syrup USP

wild chicory *medicinal herb* [see: chicory]

wild clover *medicinal herb* [see: red clover]

wild cranesbill *medicinal herb* [see: alum root]

wild daisy (Bellis perennis) flowers and leaves *medicinal herb used as an analgesic, antispasmodic, demulcent, digestive, expectorant, laxative, and purgative*

wild endive *medicinal herb* [see: dandelion]

wild fennel *medicinal herb* [see: fennel]

wild geranium *medicinal herb* [see: alum root]

wild ginger (Asarum canadense) root *medicinal herb used as a carminative, diaphoretic, expectorant, and irritant; sometimes used as a substitute for ginger (Zingiber)*

wild hydrangea *medicinal herb* [see: hydrangea]

wild hyssop *medicinal herb* [see: blue vervain]

wild hyssop (Pycnanthemum virginianum) plant *medicinal herb used as an antispasmodic, carminative, diaphoretic, and stimulant*

wild indigo (Baptisia tinctoria) plant *medicinal herb used as an antiseptic, astringent, emetic, purgative, and stimulant*

wild jalap (Ipomoea pandurata) root *medicinal herb used as a strong cathartic*

wild lemon *medicinal herb* [see: mandrake]

wild lettuce (Lactuca virosa) leaves, flowers, and seeds *medicinal herb for asthma, bronchitis, chronic pain, circulatory disorders, cramps, laryngitis, nervous disorders, stimulating lactation, swollen genitals, and urinary tract infections*

wild marjoram *medicinal herb* [see: marjoram]

wild Oregon grape *medicinal herb* [see: Oregon grape]

wild pepper *medicinal herb* [see: mezereon; eleuthero]

wild potato; wild scammony; wild sweet potato vine *medicinal herb* [see: wild jalap]

wild red raspberry *medicinal herb* [see: red raspberry]

wild senna *medicinal herb* [see: senna]

wild snowball *medicinal herb* [see: New Jersey tea]

wild strawberry *medicinal herb* [see: strawberry]

wild tobacco medicinal herb [see: lobelia]

wild turkey pea medicinal herb [see: turkey corn]

wild valerian, great medicinal herb [see: valerian]

wild woodbine medicinal herb [see: American ivy]

wild yam (Dioscorea villosa) root medicinal herb for arthritis, bilious colic, bowel spasms, gas, menstrual cramps, morning sickness, and spasmodic asthma

Willard water natural remedy for acne, alopecia, anxiety, arthritis, hypertension, and stomach ulcers

willow (Salix alba; S. caprea; S. nigra; S. purpurea) bark and buds medicinal herb for analgesia, diuresis, eczema, fever, inducing diaphoresis, headache, nervousness, rheumatism, and ulcerations; also used as an anaphrodisiac, antiseptic, and astringent

wind root medicinal herb [see: pleurisy root]

wineberry medicinal herb [see: currant]

winged elm medicinal herb [see: slippery elm]

WinRho SDF liquid for IV or IM injection ℞ immunizing agent for antenatal or postpartum prophylaxis of Rh hemolytic disease of the newborn; treatment for immune thrombocytopenic purpura (orphan) [Rh$_O$(D) immune globulin, solvent/detergent treated] 600, 1500, 2500, 5000, 15 000 IU (120, 300, 500, 1000, 3000 mcg)

WinRho SDF powder for IV or IM injection (discontinued 2007) ℞ immunizing agent for antenatal or postpartum prophylaxis of Rh hemolytic disease of the newborn; treatment for immune thrombocytopenic purpura (orphan) [Rh$_O$(D) immune globulin, solvent/detergent treated] 600, 1500, 5000 IU (120, 300, 1000 mcg)

Winstrol tablets (discontinued 2005) ℞ anabolic steroid for hereditary angioedema [stanozolol] 2 mg ⑨ fenestrel

winter bloom medicinal herb [see: witch hazel]

winter clover medicinal herb [see: squaw vine]

winter marjoram; winter sweet medicinal herb [see: marjoram]

winter savory (Calamintha montana; Satureja montana; S. obovata) leaves and stems medicinal herb for diarrhea, nausea, promoting expectoration, relieving gas and flatulence, and stimulation of menstruation; also used as an aphrodisiac

winterberry (Ilex verticillata) bark and fruit medicinal herb used as an astringent, bitter tonic, and febrifuge ⑨ Entrobar

wintergreen (Gaultheria procumbens) leaves and oil medicinal herb for aches and pains, colds, gout, lumbago, and migraine headache; also used topically as an astringent and rubefacient

wintergreen, bitter; false wintergreen medicinal herb [see: pipsissewa]

wintergreen oil [see: methyl salicylate]

winterlein medicinal herb [see: flaxseed]

Wintersteiner's compound F [see: hydrocortisone]

winterweed medicinal herb [see: chickweed]

witch hazel (Hamamelis virginiana) bark medicinal herb for bruises, burns, colds, colitis, diarrhea, dysentery, eye irritations, hemorrhoids, internal and external bleeding, mucous membrane inflammation of mouth, gums, and throat, tuberculosis, and varicose veins

withania (Withania somnifera) fruit and roots medicinal herb for diuresis, inducing emesis, liver disorders, inflammation, sedation, tuberculosis, and tumors ⑨ V-Tann; Vytone

withe; withy medicinal herb [see: willow]

Wobe-Mugos investigational (orphan) enzyme combination adjunct to chemotherapy for multiple myeloma [papain; trypsin; chymotrypsin]

wolf claw medicinal herb [see: club moss]

Women's Daily Formula capsules OTC vitamin/calcium/iron supplement [multiple vitamins; calcium; iron; folic acid] ±•450•25•0.4 mg

Women's Gentle Laxative enteric-coated tablets OTC *stimulant laxative* [bisacodyl] 5 mg

Wonder Ice gel OTC *mild anesthetic; antipruritic; counterirritant* [menthol] 5.25%

Wondra lotion OTC *moisturizer; emollient* [lanolin]

wood betony *medicinal herb* [see: betony]

wood creosote [see: creosote carbonate]

wood sanicle *medicinal herb* [see: sanicle]

wood sorrel (*Oxalis acetosella*) plant *medicinal herb used as an anodyne, diuretic, emmenagogue, irritant, and stomachic*

wood strawberry *medicinal herb* [see: strawberry]

woodbine (*Clematis virginiana*) leaves *medicinal herb for bowel evacuation, cancer, edema, fever, hypertension, inflammation, insomnia, itching, kidney disorders, skin cuts and sores, tuberculous cervical lymphadenitis, tumors, and venereal eruptions; not generally regarded as safe and effective* 🖳 Iodopen

woodbine; American woodbine; wild woodbine *medicinal herb* [see: American ivy]

woodruff *medicinal herb* [see: sweet woodruff]

woody nightshade *medicinal herb* [see: bittersweet nightshade]

Woolley's antiserotonin [see: benanserin HCl]

wooly parsnip *medicinal herb* [see: masterwort]

wormwood (*Artemisia absinthium*) plant and leaves *medicinal herb for aiding digestion, constipation, debility, fever, intestinal worms, jaundice, labor pains, menstrual cramps, and stomach and liver disorders; not generally regarded as safe and effective*

wound weed *medicinal herb* [see: goldenrod]

woundwort (*Prunella vulgaris*) plant *medicinal herb used as an antispasmodic, astringent, bitter tonic, diuretic, hemostatic, vermifuge, and vulnerary* 🖳 Endrate

woundwort, soldier's *medicinal herb* [see: yarrow]

WOWtabs (trademarked dosage form) *quickly dissolving "without water" tablets*

Wyamine Sulfate IV or IM injection (discontinued 2005) ℞ *vasopressor for hypotensive shock* [mephentermine sulfate] 15, 30 mg/mL

Wyanoids Relief Factor rectal suppositories OTC *emollient* [cocoa butter; shark liver oil] 79%•3%

Wycillin IM injection ℞ *natural penicillin antibiotic* [penicillin G procaine] 600 000, 1 200 000 U/vial 🖳 Isolan

Wygesic tablets (discontinued 2004) ℞ *narcotic analgesic; antipyretic* [propoxyphene HCl; acetaminophen] 65•650 mg

wymote *medicinal herb* [see: marsh mallow]

Wyseal (trademarked dosage form) *film-coated tablet* 🖳 Feosol; Iosal II; PhosLo; VaZol

Wytensin tablets ℞ *antihypertensive* [guanabenz acetate] 4, 8 mg

Xalatan eye drops ℞ *prostaglandin agonist for glaucoma and ocular hypertension* [latanoprost] 0.005% 🖳 zileuton

xamoterol USAN, INN, BAN *cardiac stimulant* 🖳 cimaterol; Symmetrel

xamoterol fumarate USAN *cardiac stimulant*

Xanax tablets ℞ *benzodiazepine anxio-lytic; sedative; treatment for panic disor-ders and agoraphobia* [alprazolam] 0.25, 0.5, 1, 2 mg ⑤ Sancuso; Sina-12X

Xanax XR extended-release tablets ℞ *benzodiazepine anxiolytic for panic dis-order and agoraphobia* [alprazolam] 0.5, 1, 2, 3 mg

xanomeline USAN *cholinergic agonist for Alzheimer disease* ⑤ xinomiline

xanomeline tartrate USAN *cholinergic agonist for Alzheimer disease*

xanoxate sodium USAN *bronchodilator*

xanoxic acid INN

xanthan gum NF *suspending agent*

xanthines, xanthine derivatives *a class of bronchodilators*

xanthinol niacinate USAN *peripheral vasodilator* [also: xantinol nicotinate]

xanthiol INN ⑤ Santyl

xanthiol HCl [see: xanthiol]

xanthocillin BAN [also: xantocillin]

Xanthorhiza simplicissima medicinal herb [see: yellow root]

xanthotoxin [see: methoxsalen]

Xanthoxylum americanum; X. fraxi-neum medicinal herb [see: prickly ash]

xantifibrate INN

xantinol nicotinate INN *peripheral vasodilator* [also: xanthinol niacinate]

xantocillin INN [also: xanthocillin]

xantofyl palmitate INN

Xarelto *factor Xa coagulation inhibitor; investigational (NDA filed) once-daily oral antithrombotic for deep vein throm-bosis (DVT), venous thromboembolism (VTE), and stroke prevention* [riva-roxaban]

Xatral (foreign name for U.S. product **Uroxatral**)

Xcytrin injection *investigational (NDA filed, orphan) radiosensitizer for non–small cell lung cancer patients with brain metastases* [motexafin gadolinium]

^{127}**Xe** [see: xenon Xe 127]

^{133}**Xe** [see: xenon Xe 133]

Xedec; Xedec II extended-release tablets ℞ *decongestant; expectorant* [phenylephrine HCl; guaifenesin]

20•800 mg; 30•1100 mg ⑤ CyADIC; Cydec; Zodeac-100

Xeloda film-coated tablets ℞ *antineo-plastic for metastatic breast and colo-rectal cancer; investigational (Phase III) for pancreatic cancer* [capecitabine] 150, 500 mg

xemilofiban HCl USAN *antianginal*

Xenaderm ointment ℞ *proteolytic enzyme for debridement of necrotic tis-sue; vulnerary* [trypsin; Peruvian bal-sam] 90 U•87 mg

xenalamine [see: xenazoic acid]

xenaldial [see: xenygloxal]

xenalipin USAN, INN *hypolipidemic*

Xenazine tablets ℞ *selective dopamine depletor for chorea associated with Huntington disease (orphan)* [tetraben-azine] 12, 25 mg

xenazoic acid INN

xenbucin USAN, INN *antihypercholes-terolemic*

xenbuficin [see: xenbucin]

Xenical capsules ℞ *lipase inhibitor for weight loss in obese patients with a body mass index (BMI) of 27 or more; pre-ventative for type 2 diabetes* [orlistat] 120 mg ⑤ sanicle

xenipentone INN

xenogeneic hepatocytes *investiga-tional (orphan) for severe liver failure*

xenon *element (Xe)*

xenon (^{133}Xe) INN *radioactive agent* [also: xenon Xe 133]

xenon Xe 127 USP *diagnostic aid; medicinal gas; radioactive agent*

xenon Xe 133 USAN, USP *radioactive agent* [also: xenon (^{133}Xe)]

xenthiorate INN

xenygloxal INN

xenyhexenic acid INN

xenysalate INN, BAN *topical anesthetic; antibacterial; antifungal* [also: biphen-amine HCl]

xenysalate HCl [see: biphenamine HCl]

xenytropium bromide INN ⑤ sintro-pium bromide

Xerac AC topical liquid ℞ *cleanser for acne* [aluminum chloride; alcohol] 6.25%•96%

Xerecept *investigational (Phase I/II, orphan) agent for peritumoral brain edema* [corticotropin-releasing factor]

xibenolol INN

xibornol INN, BAN

Xibrom eye drops ℞ *long-acting nonsteroidal anti-inflammatory drug (NSAID) for pain and inflammation following cataract extraction surgery* [bromfenac sodium] 0.09%

Xifaxan film-coated tablets ℞ *broad-spectrum rifamycin antibiotic for traveler's diarrhea* [rifaximin] 200 mg

Xigris powder for IV infusion ℞ *thrombolytic/fibrinolytic for severe sepsis* [drotrecogin alfa] 5, 20 mg/vial ② sucrose

xilobam USAN, INN *muscle relaxant*

ximelagatran (discontinued 2006) *investigational (NDA filed) oral anticoagulant and direct thrombin inhibitor for the prevention of stroke due to atrial fibrillation and the prevention and treatment of a venous thromboembolic event (VTE); prodrug of melagatran*

ximoprofen INN

xinafoate USAN, INN, BAN *combining name for radicals or groups*

xinidamine INN ② Sandimmune

Xinlay *investigational (NDA filed) endothelin-A (EtA; ETA; ET_A) receptor antagonist to retard the progression of metastatic prostate cancer by reducing its proliferative effects in bone and prostate tissue* [atrasentan HCl]

xinomiline INN ② xanomeline

xipamide USAN, INN *antihypertensive; diuretic*

xipranolol INN

XiraHist DM Pediatric oral drops ℞ *antitussive; antihistamine; decongestant; for children 3–24 months* [dextromethorphan hydrobromide; carbinoxamine maleate; phenylephrine HCl] 3•2•2 mg/mL

XiraHist Pediatric oral drops ℞ *decongestant; antihistamine; for children 3–24 months* [phenylephrine HCl; carbinoxamine maleate] 2•2 mg/mL

Xiral sustained-release caplets (discontinued 2007) ℞ *decongestant; antihistamine; anticholinergic to dry mucosal secretions* [pseudoephedrine HCl; chlorpheniramine maleate; methscopolamine nitrate] 120•8•2.5 mg ② sorrel

Xodol caplets ℞ *narcotic analgesic; antipyretic* [hydrocodone bitartrate; acetaminophen] 5•300, 7.5•300, 10•300 mg ② Sudal 60/500

Xolair powder for subcu injection ℞ *immunoglobulin E (IgE) blocker for moderate to severe asthma* [omalizumab] 150 mg/1.2 mL dose ② celery; Sular

Xolegel gel ℞ *antifungal for seborrheic dermatitis in immunocompromised patients* [ketoconazole; dehydrated alcohol] 2%•34%

Xolegel Duo Convenience Pack gel + shampoo ℞ *antifungal for seborrheic dermatitis in immunocompromised patients* [(ketoconazole; dehydrated alcohol) + (pyrithione zinc)] 2%• 34% + 1%

XomaZyme-791 *investigational (orphan) for metastatic colorectal adenocarcinoma* [anti-TAP-72 immunotoxin]

XomaZyme-H65 *investigational (orphan) for graft vs. host disease following bone marrow transplants* [CD5-T lymphocyte immunotoxin]

Xopenex inhalation solution, inhalation solution concentrate ℞ *sympathomimetic bronchodilator* [levalbuterol HCl] 0.31, 0.63, 1.25 mg/3 mL dose; 1.25 mg/0.5 mL dose

Xopenex HFA inhalation aerosol ℞ *sympathomimetic bronchodilator* [levalbuterol tartrate] 45 mcg/actuation

xorphanol INN *analgesic* [also: xorphanol mesylate]

xorphanol mesylate USAN *analgesic* [also: xorphanol]

XPect-AT extended-release caplets ℞ *antitussive; expectorant* [carbetapentane citrate; guaifenesin] 60•600 mg

Xpect-HC extended-release tablets (discontinued 2007) ℞ *narcotic antitussive; expectorant* [hydrocodone bitartrate; guaifenesin] 5•600 mg

X-Prep oral liquid OTC *pre-procedure bowel evacuant* [senna extract] 74 mL ⊠ SuperEPA 1200

X-Prep Bowel Evacuant Kit-1 oral liquid + 2 tablets + 1 suppository OTC *pre-procedure bowel evacuant* [X-Prep liquid (q.v.); Senokot-S tablets (q.v.); Rectolax suppository (q.v.)]

XRT (x-ray therapy) *adjunct to chemotherapy* [not a pharmaceutical agent]

X-Seb shampoo OTC *antiseborrheic; keratolytic* [salicylic acid] 4%

X-Seb Plus shampoo OTC *antiseborrheic; keratolytic; antibacterial; antifungal* [salicylic acid; pyrithione zinc] 2%•1%

X-Seb T shampoo OTC *antiseborrheic; antipsoriatic; keratolytic* [coal tar; salicylic acid] 10%•4%

X-Seb T Plus shampoo OTC *antiseborrheic; antipsoriatic; keratolytic* [coal tar; salicylic acid] 10%•0.4%

xylamidine tosilate INN *serotonin inhibitor* [also: xylamidine tosylate]

xylamidine tosylate USAN *serotonin inhibitor* [also: xylamidine tosilate]

xylazine INN *analgesic; veterinary muscle relaxant* [also: xylazine HCl] ⊠ psilocin; salicin; Selsun

xylazine HCl USAN *analgesic; veterinary muscle relaxant* [also: xylazine]

xylitol NF *sweetened vehicle*

Xylocaine ointment (discontinued 2007) OTC *anesthetic* [lidocaine] 2.5% ⊠ Seloken; silicon; Solaquin

Xylocaine subcu and IV injection ℞ *local anesthetic (subcu); antiarrhythmic for acute ventricular arrhythmias (IV)* [lidocaine HCl] 0.5%, 1%, 2% ⊠ Seloken; silicon; Solaquin

Xylocaine topical liquid, oral ointment (discontinued 2007) ℞ *mucous membrane anesthetic* [lidocaine HCl] 5%; 2.5%, 5% ⊠ Seloken; silicon; Solaquin

Xylocaine topical solution, oral jelly ℞ *mucous membrane anesthetic* [lidocaine HCl] 4%; 2% ⊠ Seloken; silicon; Solaquin

Xylocaine 10% Oral throat spray (discontinued 2007) ℞ *mucous membrane anesthetic* [lidocaine HCl] 10%

Xylocaine HCl injection ℞ *local anesthetic* [lidocaine HCl; dextrose] 1.5%•7.5%

Xylocaine HCl injection ℞ *local anesthetic* [lidocaine HCl; epinephrine] 0.5%•1:200 000, 1%• 1:100 000, 1%•1:200 000, 2%• 1:50 000, 2%•1:100 000, 2%• 1:200 000

Xylocaine HCl IV for Cardiac Arrhythmias IV injection, IV admixture ℞ *antiarrhythmic* [lidocaine HCl] 1%, 2%, 4%, 20%

Xylocaine MPF injection ℞ *local anesthetic* [lidocaine HCl] 0.5%, 1%, 1.5%, 2%, 4%

Xylocaine MPF injection ℞ *local anesthetic* [lidocaine HCl; epinephrine] 1%•1:200 000, 1.5%• 1:200 000, 2%•1:200 000

Xylocaine MPF injection ℞ *local anesthetic* [lidocaine HCl; glucose] 5%•7.5%

Xylocaine Viscous topical solution ℞ *mucous membrane anesthetic* [lidocaine HCl] 2%

xylocoumarol INN

xylofilcon A USAN *hydrophilic contact lens material* ⊠ silafilcon A

xylometazoline INN, BAN *vasoconstrictor; nasal decongestant* [also: xylometazoline HCl]

xylometazoline HCl USP *vasoconstrictor; nasal decongestant* [also: xylometazoline]

Xylo-Pfan tablets (discontinued 2004) OTC *diagnostic aid for intestinal function* [xylose] 25 g

xylose (D-xylose) USP *diagnostic aid for intestinal function* ⊠ Cialis; Silace

xyloxemine INN

Xyntha powder for IV injection ℞ *systemic hemostatic; antihemophilic for the prevention and control of bleeding in classical hemophilia (hemophilia A)* [antihemophilic factor] 250, 500, 1000, 2000 IU/dose ☒ Sonata

Xyotax (name changed to **Opaxio** while in Phase III trials)

Xyralid cream ℞ *local anesthetic; corticosteroidal anti-inflammatory* [lidocaine HCl; hydrocortisone acetate] 3%•0.5%

Xyralid LP lotion ℞ *local anesthetic; corticosteroidal anti-inflammatory* [lidocaine HCl; hydrocortisone acetate] 3%•0.5%

Xyralid RC anorectal cream ℞ *local anesthetic and corticosteroidal anti-inflammatory for hemorrhoids* [lidocaine HCl; hydrocortisone acetate] 3%•1%

Xyrem oral solution ℞ *CNS depressant for narcolepsy (orphan), cataplexy, and excessive daytime sleepiness; also used for fibromyalgia and fatigue* [sodium oxybate] 500 mg/mL ☒ cerium

Xyvion *investigational (NDA filed) synthetic steroid for osteoporosis and other postmenopausal symptoms* [tibolone]

Xyzal film-coated tablets, oral solution ℞ *second-generation piperazine antihistamine for allergic rhinitis and chronic idiopathic urticaria* [levocetirizine dihydrochloride] 5 mg; 2.5 mg/5 mL ☒ Zazole

yam *medicinal herb* [see: wild yam]

yarrow (Achillea millefolium) flower *medicinal herb for bowel hemorrhage, colds, fever, flu, hypertension, inducing sweating, measles, mucosal inflammation with discharge, nosebleed, reducing heavy menstrual bleeding and pain, thrombosis, and topical hemostasis*

Yasmin film-coated tablets (in packs of 28) ℞ *monophasic oral contraceptive* [drospirenone; ethinyl estradiol] 3 mg•30 mcg × 21 days; counters × 7 days

yatren [see: chiniofon]

Yaz film-coated tablets (in packs of 28) ℞ *monophasic oral contraceptive in a novel 24-day regimen; also approved to treat premenstrual dysphoric disorder (PMDD) and acne vulgaris* [drospirenone; ethinyl estradiol] 3 mg•20 mcg × 24 days; counters × 4 days

169Yb [see: pentetate calcium trisodium Yb 169]

169Yb [see: ytterbium Yb 169 pentetate]

Y-Cof DM extended-release caplets ℞ *antitussive; antihistamine; decongestant* [dextromethorphan hydrobromide; dexbrompheniramine maleate; phenylephrine HCl] 30•6•20 mg

yeast, dried NF

yeast cell derivative *claimed to promote wound healing*

Yeast-Gard vaginal suppositories OTC *for irritation, itching, and burning* [pulsatilla 28x; Candida albicans 28x]

Yeast-Gard Medicated Disposable Douche Premix vaginal solution OTC *antifungal cleanser and deodorizer; acidity modifier* [sodium benzoate; lactic acid]

Yeast-Gard Medicated Douche; Yeast-Gard Medicated Disposable Douche vaginal solution OTC *antiseptic/germicidal cleanser and deodorizer* [povidone-iodine] 10%; 0.3%

Yeast-X vaginal suppositories OTC *for irritation, itching, and burning* [pulsatilla 28x]

Yelets tablets OTC *vitamin/mineral/iron supplement* [multiple vitamins & minerals; ferrous fumarate; folic acid] ≛•20•0.1 mg ☒ Altace

yellow bedstraw; yellow cleavers *medicinal herb* [see: bedstraw]

yellow beeswax [see: beeswax, yellow]

yellow dock (*Rumex crispus*) root *medicinal herb for anemia, blood cleansing, constipation, itching, liver congestion, rheumatism, skin problems, and eyelid ulcerations; also used as a dentifrice*

yellow ferric oxide [see: ferric oxide, yellow]

yellow fever vaccine USP *active immunizing agent for yellow fever*

yellow gentian *medicinal herb* [see: gentian]

yellow ginseng *medicinal herb* [see: blue cohosh]

yellow Indian paint *medicinal herb* [see: goldenseal]

yellow jessamine *medicinal herb* [see: gelsemium]

yellow mercuric oxide [see: mercuric oxide, yellow]

yellow ointment [see: ointment, yellow]

yellow paint root; yellow root *medicinal herb* [see: goldenseal]

yellow petrolatum JAN *ointment base; emollient/protectant* [also: petrolatum]

yellow phenolphthalein [see: phenolphthalein, yellow]

yellow precipitate [see: mercuric oxide, yellow]

yellow puccoon *medicinal herb* [see: goldenseal]

yellow root (*Xanthorhiza simplicissima*) *medicinal herb used for diabetes and hypertension* ② Alurate

yellow root; yellow paint root *medicinal herb* [see: goldenseal]

yellow wax [see: wax, yellow]

yellow wood; yellow wood berries *medicinal herb* [see: prickly ash]

Yentreve ⓔ (approved in Europe) *investigational (Phase II) selective serotonin and norepinephrine reuptake inhibitor (SSNRI) for stress urinary incontinence* [duloxetine HCl]

yerba maté (*Ilex paraguariensis*) leaves *medicinal herb used as a CNS stimulant, diuretic, and purifier*

yerba santa (*Eriodictyon californicum*) leaves *medicinal herb for asthma, bronchial congestion, colds, hay fever, inducing expectoration, inflammation, rheumatic pain, and tuberculosis*

yew (*Taxus bacatta* **and other species**) leaves *medicinal herb for liver disorders, rheumatism, and urinary tract disorders*

YF-Vax powder for subcu injection ℞ (available from designated Yellow Fever Vaccination Centers only) *active immunizing agent for yellow fever* [yellow fever vaccine] 0.5 mL

Yocon tablets ℞ *alpha₂-adrenergic blocker for impotence and orthostatic hypotension; sympatholytic; mydriatic; may have aphrodisiac activity; no FDA-approved indications* [yohimbine HCl] 5.4 mg ② A.C.N.

Yodoxin tablets, powder ℞ *amebicide for intestinal amebiasis* [iodoquinol] 210, 650 mg; 25 g

yohimbe (*Corynanthe johimbe; Pausinystalia johimbe*) bark *medicinal herb for angina, hypertension, and impotence and other sexual dysfunction; also used as an aphrodisiac*

yohimbic acid INN

yohimbine HCl *alpha₂-adrenergic blocker for impotence and orthostatic hypotension; sympatholytic; mydriatic; may have aphrodisiac activity; no FDA-approved indications* 5.4 mg oral

Yondelis ⓔ (available in Europe) *investigational (Phase III, orphan) tetrahydroisoquinoline alkaloid for soft tissue sarcoma and relapsed ovarian cancer* [ecteinascidin]

Your Choice Non-Preserved Saline solution OTC *rinsing/storage solution for soft contact lenses* [sodium chloride (saline solution)]

Your Choice Sterile Preserved Saline solution OTC *rinsing/storage solution for soft contact lenses* [sodium chloride (preserved saline solution)]

youthwort *medicinal herb* [see: masterwort]

ytterbium *element* (Yb)

ytterbium Yb 169 pentetate USP
   radioactive agent
yttrium *element* (Y)
yttrium Y 90 ibritumomab tiuxetan
   radioimmunotherapy for non-Hodgkin
   B-cell lymphoma (orphan)
yttrium Y 90 labetuzumab *monoclo-*
   nal antibody to carcinoembryonic anti-
gen (CEA); investigational (orphan)
   for ovarian cancer
yucca (*Yucca glauca*) *root medicinal*
   herb for arthritis, colitis, hypertension,
   migraine headache, and rheumatism
yuma *medicinal herb* [see: wild yam]
Yurelax ⓔⓤ (Spanish name for U.S.
   product **Flexeril**)

Z

zabicipril INN
zacopride INN *antiemetic; peristaltic*
   stimulant [also: zacopride HCl]
zacopride HCl USAN, INN *antiemetic;*
   peristaltic stimulant [also: zacopride]
Zactima *investigational (Phase III) anti-*
   neoplastic for advanced or metastatic
   non–small cell lung cancer [vandetanib]
Zadaxin ⓔⓤ (available in Italy) *vaccine*
   enhancer for hepatitis C, cancer, and
   infectious diseases; investigational (Phase
   III, orphan) for chronic active hepatitis
   B; investigational (orphan) for DiGeorge
   syndrome with immune defects and
   hepatocellular carcinoma; investigational
   (Phase II) for AIDS [thymalfasin]
Zaditen Ophthalmic ⓒⓐⓝ ⓔⓤ (foreign
   name for U.S. product **Zaditor**)
Zaditor eye drops OTC *antihistamine and*
   mast cell stabilizer for allergic conjunc-
   tivitis [ketotifen fumarate] 0.025%
zafirlukast USAN, INN, BAN *leukotriene*
   receptor antagonist (LTRA) for preven-
   tion and chronic treatment of asthma
zafuleptine INN
Zagam film-coated tablets (discontinued 2006) ℞ *once-daily broad-spec-*
   trum fluoroquinolone antibiotic for
   community-acquired respiratory infec-
   tions [sparfloxacin] 200 mg
zalcitabine USAN *nucleoside reverse*
   transcriptase inhibitor (NRTI); antivi-
   ral for advanced HIV infection (orphan)
zaleplon USAN *pyrazolopyrimidine hyp-*
   notic for the short-term treatment of
   insomnia 5, 10 mg oral

zalospirone INN *anxiolytic* [also: zalospirone HCl] ② Salazopyrin
zalospirone HCl USAN *anxiolytic* [also:
   zalospirone]
zaltidine INN, BAN *antagonist to hista-*
   mine H₂ receptors [also: zaltidine HCl]
zaltidine HCl USAN *antagonist to hista-*
   mine H₂ receptors [also: zaltidine]
zamifenacin INN, BAN *treatment for*
   irritable bowel syndrome
Zamyl *investigational (orphan) for acute*
   myelogenous leukemia [lintuzumab]
Zanaflex tablets, capsules ℞ *skeletal*
   muscle relaxant; antispasmodic for
   multiple sclerosis and spinal cord injury
   (orphan) [tizanidine HCl] 2, 4 mg; 2,
   4, 6 mg
zanamivir USAN *influenza neuramini-*
   dase inhibitor for the treatment of acute
   influenza types A and B
Zanfel cream, wash OTC *poison ivy*
   treatment [polyethylene granules]
zankiren HCl USAN *antihypertensive*
Zanosar powder for IV injection ℞
   nitrosourea-type alkylating antineoplastic
   for metastatic islet cell carcinoma of pan-
   creas [streptozocin] 1 g (100 mg/mL)
zanoterone USAN *antiandrogen*
Zantac film-coated tablets, syrup, IV
   or IM injection ℞ *histamine H₂*
   antagonist for gastric and duodenal
   ulcers [ranitidine HCl] 150, 300 mg;
   15 mg/mL; 1, 25 mg/mL
Zantac 75; Zantac 150 tablets OTC *his-*
   tamine H₂ antagonist for episodic heart-
   burn [ranitidine HCl] 75 mg; 150 mg

Zantac EFFERdose effervescent granules (discontinued 2005) ℞ *histamine H_2 antagonist for gastric and duodenal ulcers* [ranitidine HCl] 150 mg/pkt.

Zantac EFFERdose effervescent tablets ℞ *histamine H_2 antagonist for gastric and duodenal ulcers* [ranitidine HCl] 25, 150 mg

Zantac GELdose capsules (discontinued 2005) ℞ *histamine H_2 antagonist for gastric and duodenal ulcers* [ranitidine HCl] 150, 300 mg

Zanthorhiza apiifolia medicinal herb [see: yellow root]

Zanzibar aloe medicinal herb [see: aloe]

zapizolam INN

zaprinast INN, BAN

zardaverine INN

Zarnestra *investigational (NDA filed, orphan) antineoplastic for acute myeloid leukemia (AML)* [tipifarnib]

Zarontin capsules, syrup ℞ *anticonvulsant* [ethosuximide] 250 mg; 250 mg/5 mL

Zaroxolyn tablets ℞ *antihypertensive; diuretic* [metolazone] 2.5, 5, 10 mg

zatosetron INN, BAN *antimigraine* [also: zatosetron maleate]

zatosetron maleate USAN *antimigraine* [also: zatosetron]

Zavedos ⓔ (European name for U.S. product **Idamycin**)

Zavesca capsules ℞ *treatment for type I Gaucher disease (orphan)* [miglustat] 100 mg

Zazole vaginal cream ℞ *antifungal* [terconazole] 0.4%, 0.8% ⓢ Xyzal

Z-Bec tablets OTC *vitamin/zinc supplement* [multiple vitamins; zinc sulfate] ≜ •22.5 mg ⓢ Z-Pak

Z-Cof 12 DM oral suspension ℞ *antitussive; decongestant; expectorant* [dextromethorphan tannate; pseudoephedrine tannate; guaifenesin] 30•60•175 mg/5 mL

Z-Cof DM syrup (discontinued 2007) ℞ *antitussive; decongestant; expectorant* [dextromethorphan hydrobromide; pseudoephedrine HCl; guaifenesin] 30•80•400 mg/10 mL

Z-Cof DMX oral liquid (discontinued 2007) ℞ *antitussive; decongestant; expectorant* [dextromethorphan hydrobromide; pseudoephedrine HCl; guaifenesin] 15•36•200 mg/5 mL

Z-Cof HC oral liquid, syrup (discontinued 2007) ℞ *narcotic antitussive; antihistamine; decongestant* [hydrocodone bitartrate; chlorpheniramine maleate; phenylephrine HCl] 7•5•16 mg/10 mL; 7•5•20 mg/10 mL

Z-Cof HCX oral liquid ℞ *narcotic antitussive; expectorant* [hydrocodone bitartrate; guaifenesin] 7.5•200 mg/5 mL

Z-Cof LA; Z-Cof LAX sustained-release tablets (discontinued 2007) ℞ *antitussive; expectorant* [dextromethorphan hydrobromide; guaifenesin] 30•650 mg; 30•835 mg

Z-Dex Pediatric oral drops ℞ *antitussive; decongestant; expectorant; for children 6–18 months* [dextromethorphan hydrobromide; phenylephrine HCl; guaifenesin] 3•2.5•35 mg/mL

ZDV (zidovudine) [q.v.]

ZE Caps soft capsules OTC *dietary supplement* [vitamin E; zinc gluconate] 200•9.6 mg ⓢ Scopace

Zea mays medicinal herb [see: Indian corn]

Zeasorb powder OTC *absorbent* [microporous cellulose; talc]

Zeasorb-AF powder, gel OTC *antifungal for tinea pedis, tinea cruris, and tinea corporis* [miconazole nitrate] 2%

zeaxanthin *natural carotenoid used to prevent and treat age-related macular degeneration (AMD), retinitis pigmentosa (RP), and other retinal dysfunction*

Zebeta film-coated tablets ℞ *β-blocker for hypertension* [bisoprolol fumarate] 5, 10 mg

Zecnil *investigational (orphan) for secreting cutaneous gastrointestinal fistulas* [somatostatin]

Zee-Seltzer effervescent tablets OTC *antacid; analgesic; antipyretic* [sodium bicarbonate; citric acid; aspirin] 1916•1000•325 mg

Zefazone powder or frozen premix for IV injection (discontinued 2007) ℞ second-generation cephalosporin antibiotic [cefmetazole sodium] 1, 2 g ⑨ Cefzon

Zegerid capsules, powder for oral suspension ℞ combination antacid and proton pump inhibitor for gastric and duodenal ulcers, erosive esophagitis, gastroesophageal reflux disease (GERD), upper GI bleeding, and other gastroesophageal disorders [sodium bicarbonate; omeprazole] 1100•20, 1100•40 mg; 1680•20, 1680•40 mg/pkt. ⑨ Sucraid

Zegerid with Magnesium Hydroxide chewable tablets ℞ combination antacid and proton pump inhibitor for gastric and duodenal ulcers, erosive esophagitis, gastroesophageal reflux disease (GERD), upper GI bleeding, and other gastroesophageal disorders [sodium bicarbonate; magnesium hydroxide; omeprazole] 600•700•20, 600•700•40 mg

zein NF coating agent

Zelapar orally disintegrating tablets ℞ monoamine oxidase inhibitor (MAOI); dopaminergic for Parkinson disease [selegiline HCl] 1.25 mg

Zeldox ⓔᵁᴿ (European name for U.S. product Geodon) ⑨ Zoladex

Zelnorm tablets (discontinued 2007 due to safety concerns; limited availability through the manufacturer for specific cases) ℞ selective serotonin receptor antagonist for irritable bowel syndrome (IBS) with chronic constipation in women and chronic idiopathic constipation in all [tegaserod maleate] 2, 6 mg

Zemaira powder for IV infusion ℞ enzyme replacement therapy for hereditary alpha₁-proteinase inhibitor deficiency, which leads to progressive panacinar emphysema [alpha₁-proteinase inhibitor] 50 mg/mL (1000 mg/vial) ⑨ Swim-Ear; Zymar

Zemplar capsules, bolus injection during dialysis ℞ vitamin D therapy for hyperparathyroidism secondary to chronic kidney disease (CKD) [paricalcitol] 1, 2, 4 mcg; 2, 5 mcg/mL

Zemuron IV injection ℞ nondepolarizing neuromuscular blocking agent; muscle relaxant; adjunct to general anesthesia [rocuronium bromide] 10 mg/mL

Zenapax injection ℞ immunosuppressant; monoclonal antibody (MAb) to prevent acute rejection of organ and bone marrow transplants (orphan) [daclizumab] 25 mg/5 mL

zenarestat USAN aldose reductase inhibitor

Zenate, Advanced Formula film-coated tablets ℞ vitamin/iron supplement [multiple vitamins; iron; folic acid] ≛•65•1 mg

zenazocine mesylate USAN analgesic

Zenchent tablets (in packs of 28) ℞ monophasic oral contraceptive [norethindrone; ethinyl estradiol] 0.4 mg•35 mcg × 21 days; counters × 7 days

Zensana oral spray investigational (NDA filed) antiemetic for nausea and vomiting following chemotherapy, radiation, or surgery [ondansetron HCl]

Zenvia NMDA inhibitor plus sigma-1 agonist; investigational (NDA filed) treatment for involuntary emotional expression disorder; investigational (Phase III) treatment for diabetic neuropathic pain [dextromethorphan hydrobromide; quinidine sulfate]

zepastine INN

Zephiran Chloride tincture, tincture spray, aqueous solution, towelettes, disinfectant concentrate OTC antiseptic [benzalkonium chloride] 1:750; 1:750; 1:750; 1:750; 17%

zephirol [see: benzalkonium chloride]

Zephrex film-coated tablets (discontinued 2007) ℞ decongestant; expectorant [pseudoephedrine HCl; guaifenesin] 60•400 mg ⑨ sfericase; Zovirax

Zephrex LA extended-release tablets (discontinued 2007) ℞ decongestant; expectorant [pseudoephedrine HCl; guaifenesin] 120•600 mg

zeranol USAN, INN anabolic

Zerit capsules, powder for oral solution (discontinued 2006) ℞ *antiviral for HIV infection* [stavudine] 15, 20, 30, 40 mg; 1 mg/mL ⊠ XRT

Zerit XR extended-release capsules ℞ *antiviral for HIV infection* [stavudine] 37.5, 50, 75, 100 mg

Zestoretic tablets ℞ *antihypertensive; angiotensin-converting enzyme (ACE) inhibitor; diuretic* [lisinopril; hydrochlorothiazide] 10•12.5, 20•12.5, 20•25 mg

Zestra oil OTC *natural sexual lubricant; claimed to "increase female sexual sensation, arousal, and pleasure" when topically applied to the vaginal area* [borage oil; evening primrose oil; angelica seed oil; coleus extract; vitamins C and E] ⊠ Sustaire

Zestril tablets ℞ *antihypertensive; angiotensin-converting enzyme (ACE) inhibitor; adjunctive treatment for congestive heart failure (CHF)* [lisinopril] 2.5, 5, 10, 20, 30, 40 mg

Zetacet topical suspension, wash ℞ *antibiotic and keratolytic for acne* [sulfacetamide sodium; sulfur] 10%•5%

Zetar shampoo OTC *antiseborrheic; antipsoriatic; antipruritic; antibacterial* [coal tar] 1% ⊠ Cytra-2

Zetia caplets ℞ *antihyperlipidemic for primary hypercholesterolemia and mixed hyperlipidemia; intestinal cholesterol absorption inhibitor* [ezetimibe] 10 mg

zetidoline INN, BAN

Zevalin powder for IV infusion ℞ *radioimmunotherapy carrier; monoclonal antibody to treat non-Hodgkin B-cell lymphoma (orphan)* [indium In 111 ibritumomab tiuxetan; yttrium Y 90 ibritumomab tiuxetan] 3.2 mg

Zevalin therapeutic regimen "kit" (complete package for a one-week course of treatment) ℞ *multistep treatment protocol for non-Hodgkin B-cell lymphoma* [rituximab; indium In 111 ibritumomab tiuxetan; yttrium Y 90 ibritumomab tiuxetan]

Z-gen tablets OTC *vitamin/zinc supplement* [multiple vitamins; zinc] ≛• 22.5 mg ⊠ Cecon; Ziagen

Zhuzishen *(Panax pseudoginseng) medicinal herb* [see: ginseng]

Ziac tablets ℞ *antihypertensive; β-blocker; diuretic* [hydrochlorothiazide; bisoprolol fumarate] 6.25•2.5, 6.25•5, 6.25•10 mg

Ziagen film-coated caplets, oral solution ℞ *antiviral nucleoside reverse transcriptase inhibitor for HIV infection* [abacavir sulfate] 300 mg; 20 mg/mL ⊠ Cecon; Z-gen

Ziana gel ℞ *antibiotic/keratolytic combination for acne* [clindamycin phosphate; tretinoin] 1.2%•0.025%

ziconotide USAN *non-narcotic analgesic; calcium channel blocker*

ziconotide acetate *calcium-channel blocker; non-narcotic analgesic for intractable pain of cancer or AIDS*

zidapamide USAN, INN

zidometacin USAN, INN *anti-inflammatory*

zidovudine (ZDV) USAN, INN, BAN *nucleoside antiviral for AIDS and AIDS-related complex (orphan), HIV infection, and the prevention of maternal-fetal HIV transmission* 100, 300 mg oral; 50 mg/5 mL oral

zidovudine & abacavir sulfate & lamivudine *nucleoside reverse transcriptase inhibitor (NRTI) combination for HIV and AIDS* 300•300•150 mg oral

zifrosilone USAN *acetylcholinesterase inhibitor for Alzheimer disease*

Ziks cream OTC *analgesic; mild anesthetic; antipruritic; counterirritant* [methyl salicylate; menthol; capsaicin] 12%•1%•0.025% ⊠ Ziox 405

Zilactin oral gel OTC *antimicrobial throat preparation* [benzyl alcohol] 10%

Zilactin Medicated oral gel OTC *astringent and antiseptic for oral canker and herpes lesions* [tannic acid; alcohol 80%] 7%

Zilactin-B Medicated oral gel OTC *mucous membrane anesthetic; antiseptic* [benzocaine; alcohol 76%] 10%

Zilactin-L topical liquid OTC *anesthetic* [lidocaine] 2.5%

zilantel USAN, INN *anthelmintic* ⊉ salantel

zileuton USAN, INN, BAN *5-lipoxygenase inhibitor; leukotriene receptor inhibitor for the prophylaxis and chronic treatment of asthma* ⊉ Xalatan

zilpaterol INN

zimeldine INN, BAN *antidepressant* [also: zimeldine HCl]

zimeldine HCl USAN *antidepressant* [also: zimeldine]

zimelidine HCl [now: zimeldine HCl]

zimidoben INN

Zinacef powder or frozen premix for IV or IM injection R *second-generation cephalosporin antibiotic* [cefuroxime sodium] 0.75, 1.5, 7.5 g

zinc *element (Zn)* ⊉ Cena-K; senega

Zinc 15 tablets OTC *zinc supplement* [zinc sulfate] 66 mg ⊉ Cena-K; senega

zinc acetate USP *copper blocking/complexing agent for Wilson disease (orphan)*

zinc acetate, basic INN

zinc acetate dihydrate [see: zinc acetate]

zinc bacitracin [see: bacitracin zinc]

zinc caprylate *antifungal*

zinc carbonate USAN *dietary zinc supplement*

zinc chloride USP *astringent; dentin desensitizer; dietary zinc supplement*

zinc chloride Zn 65 USAN *radioactive agent*

zinc citrate *dietary zinc supplement; sore throat treatment (34% elemental zinc)*

zinc complex bacitracins [see: bacitracin zinc]

zinc DTPA [see: pentetate zinc trisodium]

zinc gelatin USP

zinc gluconate USP *dietary zinc supplement; sore throat treatment* 10, 15, 50, 78 mg oral

Zinc Lozenges OTC *antiseptic for sore throat* [zinc citrate and zinc gluconate] 23 mg

zinc oleate NF

zinc oxide USP, JAN *astringent; topical protectant; emollient; antiseptic* 20% topical

zinc peroxide, medicinal USP

zinc phenolsulfonate NF *not generally regarded as safe and effective as an antidiarrheal*

zinc propionate *antifungal*

zinc pyrithione [see: pyrithione zinc]

zinc stearate USP *dusting powder; tablet and capsule lubricant; antifungal*

zinc sulfate USP, JAN *ophthalmic astringent; dietary zinc supplement* 200, 220, 250 mg oral; 1, 5 mg/mL injection

zinc sulfate heptahydrate [see: zinc sulfate]

zinc sulfate monohydrate [see: zinc sulfate]

zinc sulfocarbolate [see: zinc phenolsulfonate]

zinc undecylenate USP *antifungal*

zinc valerate USP

Zinc-220 capsules OTC *zinc supplement* [zinc sulfate] 220 mg ⊉ Cena-K; senega

Zinca-Pak IV injection R *intravenous nutritional therapy* [zinc sulfate] 1, 5 mg/mL

Zincate capsules R *zinc supplement* [zinc sulfate] 220 mg ⊉ Cyanokit; Senokot

zinc-eugenol USP

Zincfrin Drop-Tainers (eye drops) OTC *decongestant; astringent* [phenylephrine HCl; zinc sulfate] 0.12%•0.25%

Zincon shampoo OTC *antiseborrheic; antibacterial; antifungal* [pyrithione zinc] 1% ⊉ Sinequan

Zincvit capsules R *vitamin/mineral supplement* [multiple vitamins & minerals; folic acid] ≙•1 mg

zindotrine USAN, INN *bronchodilator*

zindoxifene INN

Zinecard powder for IV drip or push R *cardioprotectant for doxorubicin-induced cardiomyopathy (orphan)* [dexrazoxane HCl] 294, 589 mg/vial (250, 500 mg base)

Zingiber officinale *medicinal herb* [see: ginger]

Zingo intradermal powder in a pre-filled, needle-free delivery system ℞ *fast-acting local anesthetic to reduce the pain of injections and blood draws in children 3–18 years* [lidocaine HCl] 0.5 mg ▣ Cena-K; senega

zinoconazole INN *antifungal* [also: zinoconazole HCl]

zinoconazole HCl USAN *antifungal* [also: zinoconazole]

zinostatin USAN, INN *antineoplastic*

zinterol INN *bronchodilator* [also: zinterol HCl] ▣ Center-Al

zinterol HCl USAN *bronchodilator* [also: zinterol]

zinviroxime USAN, INN *antiviral*

Zinx D-Tuss oral suspension ℞ *antitussive; decongestant* [carbetapentane tannate; phenylephrine tannate] 30•25 mg/5 mL

Zinx GCP oral solution ℞ *antitussive; decongestant; expectorant* [carbetapentane citrate; phenylephrine HCl; guaifenesin] 20•10•100 mg/5 mL

Zinx GP extended-release caplets ℞ *decongestant; expectorant* [phenylephrine HCl; guaifenesin] 30•1000 mg

Zinx PCM oral solution ℞ *decongestant; antihistamine; anticholinergic to dry mucosal secretions* [phenylephrine HCl; chlorpheniramine maleate; methscopolamine nitrate] 10•2•1.25 mg/5 mL

Ziox 405 ointment ℞ *proteolytic enzyme for debridement of necrotic tissue; vulnerary* [papain; urea] 405 900 IU/g•10% ▣ Ziks

zipeprol INN

ziprasidone HCl *oral novel (atypical) benzisoxazole antipsychotic for schizophrenia and manic episodes of a bipolar disorder; serotonin 5-HT$_2$ and dopamine D$_2$ antagonist*

ziprasidone mesylate USAN *novel (atypical) benzisoxazole antipsychotic injection for rapid control of acute agi-*

tation in schizophrenic patients; serotonin 5-HT$_2$ and dopamine D$_2$ antagonist

Ziradryl lotion OTC *antihistamine; astringent; protectant; antiseptic* [diphenhydramine HCl; zinc oxide; alcohol 2%] 1%•2%

zirconium *element (Zr)*

zirconium oxide *astringent*

Zithromax film-coated tablets, Tri-Pak (3 tablets), Z-Pak (6 tablets), powder for oral suspension, powder for IV or IM injection ℞ *macrolide antibiotic* [azithromycin] 250, 500, 600 mg; 500 mg; 250 mg; 100, 200 mg/5 mL, 1 g/pkt.; 500 mg

Zixoryn *investigational (orphan) agent for neonatal hyperbilirubinemia* [flumecinol]

Zmax powder for extended-release oral suspension ℞ *macrolide antibiotic* [azithromycin dihydrate] 167 mg/5 mL (2 g/dose)

^{65}Zn [see: zinc chloride Zn 65]

Zn-DTPA (zinc pentetate) [see: pentetate zinc trisodium]

ZNP cleansing bar OTC *antiseborrheic; antibacterial; antifungal* [pyrithione zinc] 2%

zocainone INN ▣ siccanin

Zocor film-coated tablets ℞ *HMG-CoA reductase inhibitor for hyperlipidemia, hypertriglyceridemia, and coronary heart disease (CHD)* [simvastatin] 5, 10, 20, 40, 80 mg

Zocor Heart-Pro film-coated tablets ℞ (available OTC in England) *HMG-CoA reductase inhibitor for hyperlipidemia, hypertriglyceridemia, and coronary heart disease* [simvastatin] 10 mg

Zodeac-100 tablets ℞ *hematinic; vitamin/mineral supplement* [ferrous fumarate; multiple vitamins & minerals; folic acid; biotin] 60 mg•≛•1 mg•300 mcg ▣ CyADIC; Cydec; Xedec

Zoderm gel, cream, liquid cleanser ℞ *keratolytic for acne* [benzoyl peroxide (in a urea base)] 4.5%, 5.75%, 6.5%, 8.5% ▣ Zyderm

zofenopril INN, BAN *antihypertensive; angiotensin-converting enzyme (ACE) inhibitor* [also: zofenopril calcium]

zofenopril calcium USAN *antihypertensive; angiotensin-converting enzyme (ACE) inhibitor* [also: zofenopril]

zofenoprilat INN *antihypertensive* [also: zofenoprilat arginine]

zofenoprilat arginine USAN *antihypertensive* [also: zofenoprilat]

zoficonazole INN

Zofran film-coated tablets, oral solution, IV infusion, IM injection ℞ *antiemetic to prevent nausea and vomiting following chemotherapy, radiation, or surgery* [ondansetron HCl (dihydrate)] 4, 8, 24 mg; 4 mg/5 mL; 32 mg/50 mL; 2 mg/mL ⚠ saffron; Zophren

Zofran ODT (orally disintegrating tablets) ℞ *antiemetic to prevent chemotherapy-induced nausea and vomiting (CINV)* [ondansetron HCl] 4, 8 mg ⚠ ceforanide

Zoladex subcu implant in preloaded syringe ℞ *hormonal antineoplastic for palliative treatment of prostatic carcinoma, breast cancer, and endometriosis* [goserelin acetate] 3.6 mg (1-month implant), 10.8 mg (3-month implant) ⚠ Slidecase; Zeldox

zolamine INN *antihistamine; topical anesthetic* [also: zolamine HCl]

zolamine HCl USAN *antihistamine; topical anesthetic* [also: zolamine]

zolazepam INN, BAN *sedative* [also: zolazepam HCl] ⚠ sulazepam

zolazepam HCl USAN *sedative* [also: zolazepam]

zoledronate disodium USAN *bone resorption inhibitor for osteoporosis*

zoledronate trisodium USAN *bone resorption inhibitor for osteoporosis*

zoledronic acid USAN *bisphosphonate bone resorption inhibitor for hypercalcemia of malignancy (HCM; orphan), multiple myeloma, bone metastases, and metabolic bone disorders such as Paget disease; once-yearly treatment for postmenopausal osteoporosis*

zolenzepine INN

zolertine INN *antiadrenergic; vasodilator* [also: zolertine HCl]

zolertine HCl USAN *antiadrenergic; vasodilator* [also: zolertine]

Zolicef powder for IV or IM injection (discontinued 2007) ℞ *first-generation cephalosporin antibiotic* [cefazolin sodium] 1 g

zolimidine INN

zolimomab aritox USAN *monoclonal antibody to pan T lymphocyte; investigational (orphan) for in vivo and ex vivo treatment of bone marrow transplants*

Zolinza capsules ℞ *antineoplastic for cutaneous T-cell lymphoma (CTCL)* [vorinostat] 100 mg ⚠ "cillins"

zoliprofen INN ⚠ Salprofen

zoliridine [see: zolimidine]

zolmitriptan USAN *vascular serotonin 5-HT$_{1B/1D}$ receptor agonist for the acute treatment of migraine*

Zoloft film-coated tablets, oral drops ℞ *selective serotonin reuptake inhibitor (SSRI) for depression, obsessive-compulsive disorder (OCD), panic disorder, post-traumatic stress disorder (PTSD), premenstrual dysmorphic disorder (PMDD), and social anxiety disorder* [sertraline HCl] 25, 50, 100 mg; 20 mg/mL ⚠ Solvet

zoloperone INN

zolpidem INN, BAN *imidazopyridine sedative/hypnotic* [also: zolpidem tartrate]

zolpidem tartrate USAN *imidazopyridine sedative/hypnotic for the short-term treatment of insomnia; investigational (NDA filed) oral spray delivery system* [also: zolpidem] 5, 10 mg oral

ZolpiMist oral spray *investigational (NDA filed) delivery system of a sedative/hypnotic for the short-term treatment of insomnia* [zolpidem tartrate]

Zomaril *investigational (Phase III) selective serotonin and dopamine antagonist for schizophrenia* [iloperidone]

zomebazam INN

zomepirac INN, BAN *analgesic; anti-inflammatory* [also: zomepirac sodium]

zomepirac sodium USAN, USP *analgesic; anti-inflammatory* [also: zomepirac]

Zometa IV infusion ℞ *bone resorption inhibitor for hypercalcemia of malig-*

nancy (orphan), multiple myeloma, and bone metastases; also used to treat postmenopausal osteoporosis [zoledronic acid] 4 mg

zometapine USAN antidepressant

Zomig film-coated tablets, nasal spray ℞ vascular serotonin 5-HT$_{1B/1D}$ receptor agonist for the acute treatment of migraine [zolmitriptan] 2.5, 5 mg; 5 mg/dose ② Sea-Omega; Simuc; sumach

Zomig-ZMT orally disintegrating tablets ℞ vascular serotonin 5-HT$_{1B/1D}$ receptor agonist for the acute treatment of migraine [zolmitriptan] 2.5 mg

Zonalon cream ℞ antihistamine; antipruritic [doxepin HCl] 5%

Zone-A Forte lotion ℞ corticosteroidal anti-inflammatory; anesthetic [hydrocortisone acetate; pramoxine] 2.5%•1%

Zonegran capsules ℞ sulfonamide anticonvulsant for partial seizures [zonisamide] 25, 50, 100 mg

zoniclezole INN anticonvulsant [also: zoniclezole HCl]

zoniclezole HCl USAN anticonvulsant [also: zoniclezole]

zonisamide USAN, INN, BAN sulfonamide anticonvulsant for partial seizures 25, 50, 100 mg oral

Zonite Douche vaginal solution concentrate OTC antiseptic cleanser and deodorizer; mild anesthetic; antipruritic; counterirritant [benzalkonium chloride; menthol; thymol]

Zophren ⓔᵁᴿ (European name for U.S. product Zofran) ② saffron

zopiclone INN, BAN, JAN sedative; hypnotic

zopolrestat USAN antidiabetic; aldose reductase inhibitor

zorbamycin USAN antibacterial

Zorbtive powder for subcu injection ℞ treatment for short bowel syndrome (SBS) in children (orphan) [somatropin (rDNA)] 8.8 mg (24.6 IU) per vial

ZORprin Zero Order Release tablets ℞ analgesic; antipyretic; anti-inflammatory; antirheumatic [aspirin] 800 mg

zorubicin INN antineoplastic [also: zorubicin HCl] ② Sorbsan

zorubicin HCl USAN antineoplastic [also: zorubicin]

Zostavax powder for subcu injection ℞ vaccine for adults ≥ 60 years to prevent herpes zoster infections; investigational for post-herpetic neuralgia and shingles-associated pain [varicella-zoster virus vaccine, live attenuated (Oka/Merck strain)] 19 400 PFU/ 0.65 mL dose

zoster vaccine, live [see: varicella-zoster virus vaccine, live]

Zostrix; Zostrix-HP cream OTC analgesic; counterirritant [capsaicin] 0.025%; 0.075%

zosuquidar trihydrochloride investigational (Phase III) p-glycoprotein inhibitor for acute myelogenous leukemia (AML)

Zosyn powder or frozen premix for IV injection ℞ extended-spectrum penicillin antibiotic plus synergist [piperacillin sodium; tazobactam sodium] 2•0.25, 3•0.375, 4•0.5, 36•4.5 g ② Saizen; Susano

zotepine INN, JAN antipsychotic ② cetaben

Zotex GPX extended-release tablets ℞ decongestant; expectorant [phenylephrine HCl; guaifenesin] 8.5•550 mg

Zotex Pediatric oral drops ℞ antitussive; decongestant; expectorant; for children 6–18 months [dextromethorphan hydrobromide; phenylephrine HCl; guaifenesin] 3•2.5•35 mg/mL

Zotex-G syrup (discontinued 2007) ℞ antitussive; decongestant; expectorant [dextromethorphan hydrobromide; phenylephrine HCl; guaifenesin] 15•10•133 mg/5 mL

Zotex-PE extended-release tablets ℞ decongestant; antihistamine [phenylephrine HCl; brompheniramine maleate] 30•6 mg

Zoto-HC ear drops ℞ corticosteroidal anti-inflammatory; antiseptic; anesthetic [hydrocortisone; chloroxylenol;

pramoxine HCl] 10%•1%•10% ☒
Stay Awake

Zovia 1/35E; Zovia 1/50E tablets (in packs of 21 or 28) ℞ *monophasic oral contraceptive* [ethynodiol diacetate; ethinyl estradiol] 1 mg•35 mcg; 1 mg•50 mcg

Zovirax capsules, tablets, oral suspension ℞ *antiviral for herpes simplex, herpes zoster, and adult-onset chickenpox* [acyclovir] 200 mg; 400, 800 mg; 200 mg/5 mL ☒ sfericase; Zephrex

Zovirax cream ℞ *antiviral for recurrent herpes labialis* [acyclovir] 5% ☒ sfericase; Zephrex

Zovirax ointment ℞ *antiviral for herpes genitalis and mucocutaneous herpes simplex infections* [acyclovir] 5% ☒ sfericase; Zephrex

Zovirax powder for IV infusion ℞ *antiviral for herpes infections* [acyclovir sodium] 500 mg/vial ☒ sfericase; Zephrex

zoxazolamine NF, INN

Z-Pak (trademarked packaging form) *6-tablet pack of* **Zithromax** ☒ Z-Bec

ZTuss Expectorant oral liquid ℞ *narcotic antitussive; decongestant; antihistamine; expectorant* [hydrocodone bitartrate; pseudoephedrine HCl; chlorpheniramine maleate; guaifenesin] 2.5•15•2•100 mg/5 mL

ZTuss ZT caplets (discontinued 2007) ℞ *narcotic antitussive; expectorant* [hydrocodone bitartrate; guaifenesin] 5•300 mg

Zucapsaicin *investigational (orphan) agent for postherpetic neuralgia of the trigeminal nerve* [civamide]

zucapsaicin USAN *topical analgesic*

zuclomifene INN

zuclomiphene USAN

zuclopenthixol INN, BAN *thioxanthene antipsychotic*

Zurase *investigational (orphan) agent for cancer-related tumor lysis syndrome and hyperuricemia due to cancer or severe gout* [PEG-uricase]

Z-Xtra lotion OTC *anesthetic; antihistamine; emollient* [pyrilamine maleate;

benzocaine; zinc oxide] 2.07•2.08• 41.35 mg/mL

Zyban sustained-release film-coated tablets ℞ *non-nicotine aid to smoking cessation* [bupropion HCl] 150 mg

Zycose tablets ℞ *vitamin B supplement* [folic acid; benfotiamine; Benzamine (q.v.)] 1•150•850 mg

Zyderm gel for subcu injection ℞ *dermal filler for fine-to-moderate scars and wrinkles* [collagen, purified bovine] 35, 65 mg/mL ☒ Zoderm

Zydis (trademarked dosage form) *orally disintegrating tablets*

Zydone tablets, capsules ℞ *narcotic analgesic; antipyretic* [hydrocodone bitartrate; acetaminophen] 5•400, 7.5•400, 10•400 mg; 5•500 mg

Zyflo film-coated tablets ℞ *leukotriene receptor inhibitor for the prophylaxis and chronic treatment of asthma* [zileuton] 600 mg ☒ Cefol

Zyflo CR extended-release film-coated tablets ℞ *twice-daily leukotriene receptor inhibitor for the prophylaxis and chronic treatment of asthma* [zileuton] 600 mg

Zylet eye drop suspension ℞ *corticosteroidal anti-inflammatory; aminoglycoside antibiotic* [loteprednol etabonate; tobramycin] 0.5%•0.3% ☒ Saleto; SLT

zylofuramine INN

Zyloprim tablets ℞ *xanthine oxidase inhibitor for gout and hyperuricemia; antineoplastic adjunct for reducing uric acid levels following chemotherapy for leukemia, lymphoma, and solid-tumor malignancies (orphan)* [allopurinol] 100, 300 mg

Zymacap capsules OTC *vitamin supplement* [multiple vitamins; folic acid] ±•0.4 mg

Zymar eye drops ℞ *broad-spectrum fluoroquinolone antibiotic* [gatifloxacin] 0.3% ☒ Swim-Ear; Zemaira

Zymine oral liquid ℞ *antihistamine* [triprolidine HCl] 1.25 mg/5 mL ☒ Cyomin

Zymine DXR oral suspension ℞ *decongestant; antihistamine* [pseudoephedrine HCl; triprolidine HCl] 45•2.5 mg/5 mL

Zymine HC oral liquid (discontinued 2008) ℞ *narcotic antitussive; antihistamine; decongestant* [hydrocodone bitartrate; triprolidine HCl; pseudoephedrine HCl] 2.5•1.25•30 mg/5 mL

Zymine XR oral suspension ℞ *antihistamine* [triprolidine HCl] 2.5 mg/5 mL

Zyplast gel for subcu injection ℞ *dermal filler for deep scars and wrinkles* [collagen, purified bovine, cross-linked] 35 mg/mL

Zyprexa film-coated tablets, Zydis (orally disintegrating tablets) ℞ *novel (atypical) thienobenzodiazepine antipsychotic for schizophrenia and manic episodes of a bipolar disorder* [olanzapine] 2.5, 5, 7.5, 10, 15, 20 mg; 5, 10, 15, 20 mg ⊠ Suprax

Zyprexa Adhera long-acting IM injection *investigational 2- to 4-week dosing; novel (atypical) antipsychotic for control of psychomotor agitation due to schizophrenia or bipolar disorder* [olanzapine]

Zyprexa IntraMuscular powder for IM injection ℞ *novel (atypical) antipsychotic for rapid control of psychomotor agitation due to schizophrenia or bipolar disorder* [olanzapine] 5 mg/mL (10 mg/vial)

Zyrtec chewable tablets, syrup (name changed to **Zyrtec Children's Allergy** upon status change to OTC in 2007) ⊠ Psoriatec; Saratoga

Zyrtec film-coated tablets (name changed to **Zyrtec Allergy** upon status change to OTC in 2007) ⊠ Psoriatec; Saratoga

Zyrtec Allergy; Zyrtec Hives Relief tablets OTC *nonsedating antihistamine for allergic rhinitis and chronic idiopathic urticaria* [cetirizine HCl] 5, 10 mg

Zyrtec Children's Allergy chewable tablets, oral solution OTC *nonsedating antihistamine for allergic rhinitis* [cetirizine HCl] 5, 10 mg; 1 mg/mL

Zyrtec Children's Hives Relief oral solution OTC *nonsedating antihistamine for hives* [cetirizine HCl] 1 mg/mL

Zyrtec-D 12 Hour extended-release tablets OTC *nonsedating antihistamine and decongestant for allergic rhinitis* [cetirizine HCl; pseudoephedrine HCl] 5•120 mg

Zyvox film-coated tablets, powder for oral suspension, IV infusion ℞ *oxazolidinone antibiotic for gram-positive bacterial infections* [linezolid] 400, 600 mg; 100 mg/5 mL; 200, 400, 600 mg/bag

APPENDIX A
Sound-Alikes

Below are 1785 drug names that may be confused in transcription, followed by one or more possible "sound-alike" names. The list below includes only ℞, OTC, and generic drugs available in the U.S. The main section of the book includes all of these, plus sound-alikes for chemotherapy protocols, medicinal herbs and natural remedies, foreign drugs, and more. Look for the "ear" icon (🔊) on over 2100 entries in the main list.

A1cNOW 🔊 A.C.N.; Yocon
Abenol 🔊 Epinal
Accolate 🔊 Equilet
Aceon 🔊 Aczone; Ocean
aceperone 🔊 aspirin; azaperone; Easprin; esuprone
Acephen 🔊 Asaphen; Ucephan
aciclovir 🔊 acyclovir
acifran 🔊 Isovorin
Aclaro 🔊 Acular
A.C.N. 🔊 A1cNOW; Yocon
Acno 🔊 A1cNOW; Yocon
aconitine 🔊 Akineton
ActHIB 🔊 AK-Tob
Acthrel 🔊 AK-Trol
actisomide 🔊 octazamide
Acular 🔊 Aclaro
acyclovir 🔊 aciclovir
Aczone 🔊 Aceon; Ocean
Adavite 🔊 Advate
ADEKs 🔊 Adoxa; Edex; Iodex
Adoxa 🔊 ADEKs; Edex; Iodex
Advate 🔊 Adavite
Aerius 🔊 Ear-Eze; Oracea; Urso 250
Aeroaid 🔊 Aredia; Euro-D
AeroBid 🔊 EryPed
AeroCaine 🔊 argon; Ircon
Aerodine 🔊 Arduan
AeroSpan 🔊 erizepine
AeroTuss 12 🔊 Artiss; Ertaczo
AeroZoin 🔊 Orasone; Ureacin-10
A/G Pro 🔊 AKPro
agar 🔊 Icar
Agoral 🔊 Aquoral
*Medicinal herbs/natural remedies.

AK-Chlor 🔊 OcuClear
AK-Cide 🔊 Axid
Akineton 🔊 aconitine
aklomide 🔊 iogulamide
AKPro 🔊 A/G Pro
AK-Spore 🔊 Exubera
AK-Sulf 🔊 Ocusulf-10
AK-Tracin 🔊 Ocutricin
Ala-Quin 🔊 Alcaine; Elocon; elucaine
AlaSTAT 🔊 Elestat
Alasulf 🔊 alusulf
Albay 🔊 Eye-Lube-A
Alcaine 🔊 Ala-Quin; Elocon; elucaine
Alcare 🔊 Allegra
Aleve 🔊 olive*
alexidine 🔊 aloxidone
alfadolone 🔊 alphadolone
alfaxalone 🔊 alphaxalone
Alfenta 🔊 Alphanate
Alimta 🔊 Elimite
Alinia 🔊 aloin
Allegra 🔊 agar; Alcare; Icar
Allegra ODT 🔊 Eligard
AlleRx 🔊 Alrex
Allfen 🔊 Alophen
aloin 🔊 Align*
Alophen 🔊 Allfen
alosetron 🔊 Elestrin
Aloxi 🔊 I-L-X; Olux
aloxidone 🔊 alexidine
alphadolone 🔊 alfadolone
Alphanate 🔊 Alfenta
alphaxalone 🔊 alfaxalone
Alrex 🔊 AlleRx
Altace 🔊 Yelets

Altazine ▢ Ilotycin
Altinac ▢ eltenac
Alurate ▢ yellow root*
alusulf ▢ Alasulf
amalgucin ▢ imiloxan
amanozine ▢ Aminess N
ambazone ▢ amipizone; ampyzine
Ambi 10; Ambi 60/580; Ambi 60/580/30; Ambi 80/700/40; Ambi 600; Ambi 1000/5; Ambi 1000/55 ▢ AMPA
Amcort ▢ Emo-Cort
amedalin ▢ imidoline; omidoline
amezepine ▢ amicibone
amfecloral ▢ amphecloral
amfetamine ▢ amphetamine
amfomycin ▢ amphomycin
amicibone ▢ amezepine
amikhelline ▢ Amoclan
Aminess N ▢ amanozine
Aminosyn 3.5%; Aminosyn 7% ▢ amanozine
amiperone ▢ Empirin
amipizone ▢ ambazone; ampyzine
amiterol ▢ Emetrol
amitivir ▢ emitefur
Amitone ▢ emetine; iometin
amixetrine ▢ amogastrin
Amoclan ▢ amikhelline
amogastrin ▢ amixetrine
Amosan ▢ E-Mycin
AMPA ▢ Ambi 10
amphecloral ▢ amfecloral
amphetamine ▢ amfetamine
amphomycin ▢ amfomycin
ampyrimine ▢ embramine; imipramine
ampyzine ▢ ambazone; amipizone
Anacin ▢ Enzone; inosine; Unasyn
Anadrol-50 ▢ Inderal
Anatrast ▢ IntraSite
Anatrofin ▢ Entrophen
ancitabine ▢ enocitabine
Android ▢ Inderide 40/25
Androxy ▢ Ondrox
anethole ▢ Intal
anisatil ▢ inositol
anise oil ▢ Enisyl; Unisol
Antiox ▢ Entex
Anturane ▢ Intron A
* Medicinal herbs/natural remedies.

Aosept + Aodisc ▢ Azopt
Apetil ▢ Epitol
Aphrodyne ▢ avridine
Aphthasol ▢ efetozole
A.P.L. ▢ apple*; E-Pilo-1; IPOL
Apo-K ▢ Epi-C; iboga
Apokyn ▢ Opcon-A
Aquabase ▢ Equipoise; ICaps
Aquanil ▢ Equanil
AquaSite ▢ wax, white
Aquasol A; Aquasol E ▢ wax, yellow
Aquavit-E ▢ Ocuvite
Aquoral ▢ Agoral
ara-G ▢ ERYC
Aramine ▢ Orimune
Arduan ▢ Aerodine
Aredia ▢ Aeroaid; Euro-D
Argesic ▢ Urogesic
argon ▢ AeroCaine; Ircon
Aricept ▢ Orasept
arsenic ▢ Orazinc
Artha-G ▢ Oretic; Wartec
Artiss ▢ AeroTuss 12; Ertaczo
Asacol ▢ Isocal; Os-Cal 500
Asaphen ▢ Acephen; Ucephan
Ascor L 500 ▢ ozagrel
Aseptone 1 ▢ azapetine; isobutane
asparagine ▢ esproquine
A-Spas S/L ▢ isobuzole
aspirin ▢ aceperone; azaperone; Easprin; esuprone
Astroglide ▢ Oystercal-D 250
atevirdine ▢ etofuradine
atosiban ▢ etazepine
Atralin ▢ iotrolan
A/T/S ▢ oats*
Auro Ear Drops ▢ E-R-O Ear Drops
Auro-Dri ▢ Ear-Dry
Aveeno ▢ Aviane; Iophen
Avelox ▢ Euflex; I-Valex-1
Aviane ▢ Aveeno; Iophen
avridine ▢ Aphrodyne
Axid ▢ AK-Cide
Aygestin ▢ Extina
azabon ▢ Isopan
azaconazole ▢ isoconazole
azamulin ▢ azumolene
azaperone ▢ aceperone; aspirin; Easprin; esuprone
azapetine ▢ Aseptone 1; isobutane

azaprocin ⧉ isoprazone
azaquinzole ⧉ isoconazole
azarole ⧉ acerola*
azatepa ⧉ azetepa
azetepa ⧉ azatepa
azithromycin ⧉ astromicin
Azopt ⧉ Aosept + Aodisc
azumolene ⧉ azamulin
BAL in Oil ⧉ bolenol
bamethan ⧉ pimetine
bamifylline ⧉ pimefylline
bamnidazole ⧉ pimonidazole
Bancap HC ⧉ Pancof-HC
Baraclude ⧉ pergolide
Baricon ⧉ Paracaine; procaine; Pure-gon; pyrrocaine
Baridium ⧉ Perdiem; Prodium; Pyridium
barium ⧉ broom*
barnidipine ⧉ pranidipine
Barobag ⧉ Boropak; Propac
Baro-cat ⧉ Pro-Cute
batoprazine ⧉ butaperazine
Bayer Plus ⧉ propolis*
BCAD 2 ⧉ pokeweed*
B-Complex ⧉ B Complex + C
B-Complex with B-12 ⧉ B Complex with C and B-12
Bear-E-Yum GI ⧉ Promega
befunolol ⧉ pafenolol
befuraline ⧉ bufrolin
belarizine ⧉ plauracin
Belganyl ⧉ Plaquenil
Bellacane ⧉ bulaquine; Pilagan; Polo-caine
Bellatal ⧉ Pletal
benaxibine ⧉ pinoxepin
bendazol ⧉ panidazole
Benicar ⧉ Penecare
Ben-Tann ⧉ Panitone-500
Bentyl ⧉ peanut oil
Benuryl ⧉ pennyroyal*
Benza ⧉ Pannaz
berefrine ⧉ Proviron
berkelium ⧉ brooklime*
Berocca ⧉ Pro-Q
Betagen ⧉ butacaine
Betaxon ⧉ butikacin
Biaxin ⧉ Bicozene; pecazine
*Medicinal herbs/natural remedies.

Bicitra ⧉ Posture
Bicozene ⧉ Biaxin; pecazine
Bidex-A ⧉ Pediox
Bidhist; Bidhist-D ⧉ PD-Hist D
binedaline ⧉ pinadoline
binifibrate ⧉ ponfibrate
biotin ⧉ betony*; Bitin; butane; P-Tanna 12
bisobrin ⧉ buspirone
Bite Rx ⧉ Pitrex
bithionol ⧉ Botanol; Patanol
Bitin ⧉ betony*; biotin; butane; P-Tanna 12
bizelesin ⧉ pecilocin
bleomycin ⧉ paulomycin; peliomycin
Bluboro ⧉ bilberry*
Blue Ice ⧉ Boil-Ease; PALS
Boil-Ease ⧉ Blue Ice; PALS
bolandiol ⧉ Plendil
bolenol ⧉ BAL in Oil
bometolol ⧉ pamatolol
Boost ⧉ Bucet
boric acid ⧉ BrachySeed I-125
bornaprine ⧉ pirenperone
bornelone ⧉ pyrinoline
Boropak ⧉ Barobag; Propac
Botanol ⧉ Patanol
BrachySeed I-125 ⧉ boric acid
Brethine ⧉ Pre-Attain; protein A
Brevicon ⧉ parvaquone; porofocon A
brimonidine ⧉ bromindione
Brite Eyes II ⧉ Pretz; protease
bromazepam ⧉ premazepam
bromazine ⧉ Pramosone; primycin; promazine; puromycin
bromhexine ⧉ pramoxine
bromindione ⧉ brimonidine
bromofos ⧉ Premphase
Bronchial ⧉ periwinkle*
Brovana ⧉ paraffin; Preven; Privine; Profen II
Bucet ⧉ Boost
bufrolin ⧉ befuraline
bufylline ⧉ Pavulon
bulaquine ⧉ Bellacane; Pilagan; Polo-caine
buniodyl ⧉ Panadol
buquiterine ⧉ picotrin
buramate ⧉ PowerMate
burodiline ⧉ Predalone 50

Buro-Sol ⊡ parsley*; ProSol 20%
buspirone ⊡ bisobrin
butane ⊡ betony*; biotin; Bitin; P-Tanna 12
butaperazine ⊡ batoprazine
buterizine ⊡ Pitressin
butikacin ⊡ Betaxon
butirosin ⊡ Pitressin
butoprozine ⊡ batoprazine
Byclomine ⊡ picolamine
cacao butter ⊡ cocoa butter
Caelyx ⊡ glucose
caffeine ⊡ C-Phen; Kuvan
Calafol ⊡ clove oil
Cala-gen ⊡ collagen; Glaucon; Glyquin; Qualaquin
calamine ⊡ Chlo-Amine; gallamine
Calan ⊡ Clenia; kaolin*; khellin
Cal-Cee ⊡ Colace; K-Lease
Calcet ⊡ Gelhist; Glyset
Calcionate ⊡ Cleocin T
Calcium 600 + D ⊡ galosemide
Caldesene ⊡ clodazon
Cal-Nate ⊡ kola nut*
Calphosan ⊡ clofezone
Calphron ⊡ Claforan; Kolephrin
Caltro ⊡ coal tar; Kaletra
Campath ⊡ Compete
camphor ⊡ comfrey*
Candin ⊡ quinidine
Capex ⊡ Copegus
Capitrol ⊡ Gabitril
Capsin ⊡ Cubicin; kebuzone; quipazine
capuride ⊡ Key-Pred 25
Carac ⊡ Coreg; Kuric
Carafate ⊡ Geravite
caramel ⊡ Gerimal
caraway oil ⊡ coral*; Kerol
carazolol ⊡ Kerasal AL
Cardec-S ⊡ Kerodex #51
Cardene SR ⊡ Gordon's Urea 40%
carfimate ⊡ crufomate
Carmol 10; Carmol 20; Carmol 40 ⊡ Gerimal
CarraFoam ⊡ Geravim; Kerafoam
Carrasyn ⊡ chrysin*; garcinia*
carticaine ⊡ Corticaine
carumonam ⊡ germanium
* Medicinal herbs/natural remedies.

cathine ⊡ Kao-Tin; K-Tan
cathinone ⊡ cotinine
Cedax ⊡ ciadox; Cidex; Sudex
cefalexin ⊡ cephalexin
cefaloglycin ⊡ cephaloglycin
cefalonium ⊡ cephalonium
cefaloram ⊡ cephaloram
cefaloridine ⊡ cephaloridine
cefamandole ⊡ cephamandole
cefamandole nafate ⊡ cephamandole nafate
cefazolin ⊡ cephazolin
cefazolin sodium ⊡ cephazolin sodium
cefixime ⊡ Zyvoxam
Cefobid ⊡ Cevi-Bid
Cefol ⊡ Zyflo
ceforanide ⊡ Zofran ODT
cefoxazole ⊡ cephoxazole
cefpiramide ⊡ sevopramide
cefradine ⊡ cephradine
Celexa ⊡ Cylex; Salex
Cena-K ⊡ senega*; zinc
Center-Al ⊡ zinterol
cephalexin ⊡ cefalexin
cephaloglycin ⊡ cefaloglycin
cephalonium ⊡ cefalonium
cephaloram ⊡ cefaloram
cephaloridine ⊡ cefaloridine
cephalothin ⊡ cefalotin
cephamandole ⊡ cefamandole
cephamandole nafate ⊡ cefamandole nafate
cephazolin ⊡ cefazolin
cephazolin sodium ⊡ cefazolin sodium
cephoxazole ⊡ cefoxazole
cephradine ⊡ cefradine
Ceprotin ⊡ sparteine
Cerebyx ⊡ Surbex
cerium ⊡ Xyrem
Ceron ⊡ Sereine
Cerovite ⊡ Syrvite
cetaben ⊡ zotepine
Cetacort ⊡ S-T Cort
Cetafen ⊡ Cytovene
cetiedil ⊡ Stadol
cetirizine ⊡ Storzine 2
Cevi-Bid ⊡ Cefobid
Chlo-Amine ⊡ calamine; gallamine
chlophedianol ⊡ clofedanol
chloral betaine ⊡ cloral betaine

chlorindanol ⬚ clorindanol
chlorine ⬚ Klaron 10%
chloroquine ⬚ Klor-Con
Cholac ⬚ shellac
Choron-10 ⬚ Creon 5; guarana*
ciadox ⬚ Cedax; Cidex; Sudex
Cialis ⬚ Silace; xylose
ciclacillin ⬚ cyclacillin
ciclindole ⬚ cyclindole
cicliomenol ⬚ cyclomenol
ciclobendazole ⬚ cyclobendazole
cicloheximide ⬚ cycloheximide
cicloprolol ⬚ cycloprolol
ciclosporin ⬚ cyclosporin
cideferron ⬚ Pseudofrin
Cidex ⬚ Cedax; ciadox; Sudex
cilostamide ⬚ salacetamide
cimaterol ⬚ Symmetrel; xamoterol
cioteronel ⬚ citronella*; soterenol;
   SteriNail
cipionate ⬚ cypionate
Cipro I.V. ⬚ Spiriva
ciprofloxacin; ciprofloxacin HCl ⬚
   sparfloxacin
ciproquinate ⬚ cyproquinate
ciproximide ⬚ cyproximide
Citralax ⬚ Starlix
citric acid ⬚ stearic acid
Claforan ⬚ Calphron; Kolephrin
Claravis ⬚ Klorvess
clazuril ⬚ Clozaril; glycerol
clemastine ⬚ galamustine
Clenia ⬚ Calan; kaolin*; khellin
Cleocin ⬚ Galzin; glycine; Quelicin
Cleocin T ⬚ Calcionate
clodazon ⬚ Caldesene
clofedanol ⬚ chlophedianol
clofezone ⬚ Calphosan
clomocycline ⬚ colimecycline
cloprothiazole ⬚ glyprothiazol
cloral betaine ⬚ chloral betaine
cloramfenicol pantotenate complex ⬚
   chloramphenicol
clorindanol ⬚ chlorindanol
clostebol ⬚ colestipol
clove oil ⬚ Calafol
Clozaril ⬚ clazuril; glycerol
coal tar ⬚ Caltro; Kaletra
cocoa butter ⬚ cacao butter
*Medicinal herbs/natural remedies.

codeine ⬚ Kadian; Quad Tann
Cognex ⬚ Kionex
Colace ⬚ Cal-Cee; K-Lease
Colazal ⬚ Gelusil
colestipol ⬚ clostebol
colimecycline ⬚ clomocycline
colistin ⬚ glycitein*
collagen ⬚ Cala-gen; Glaucon;
   Glyquin; Qualaquin
colterol ⬚ glutaral
CoLyte ⬚ Klout; K-Lyte
Copegus ⬚ Capex
copper ⬚ Keppra
Coreg ⬚ Carac; Kuric
Corque ⬚ Carac; Kuric
Corticaine ⬚ carticaine
CPB WC ⬚ K-Pek
C-Phen ⬚ caffeine; Kuvan
C-Phen DM ⬚ G Phen DM; GFN
   1000/DM 50; Guaifen DM
Creon 5; Creon 25 ⬚ Choron-10;
   guarana*
cresol ⬚ Cryselle; Kerasal
crufomate ⬚ carfimate
Cryselle ⬚ cresol; Kerasal
CTAB ⬚ K-Tab; Q-Tapp
Cubicin ⬚ Capsin; kebuzone;
   quipazine
cumetharol ⬚ coumetarol
Cyanokit ⬚ Senokot; Zincate
cyclacillin ⬚ ciclacillin
cyclindole ⬚ ciclindole
cyclizine ⬚ seclazone
cyclobendazole ⬚ ciclobendazole
cycloheximide ⬚ cicloheximide
cyclomenol ⬚ cicliomenol
cycloprolol ⬚ cicloprolol
cyclosporin ⬚ ciclosporin
Cycrin ⬚ Secran
Cydec ⬚ Xedec; Zodeac-100
Cylex ⬚ Celexa; Salex
Cymbalta ⬚ Simplet
Cyomin ⬚ Zymine
cypionate ⬚ cipionate
cyproquinate ⬚ ciproquinate
cyproximide ⬚ ciproximide
cyromazine ⬚ Seromycin
cystine ⬚ Sustain; Systane
Cytovene ⬚ Cetafen
Cytra-2; Cytra-3 ⬚ Zetar

dacemazine ⬚ duazomycin
Dacex-A ⬚ Desoxi
Dairy Ease ⬚ Diurese; Dry Eyes
Dallergy ⬚ Dolorac
Dalmane ⬚ Dilomine; diolamine
Darvon; Darvon-N ⬚ Duraphen II
Dayhist-1 ⬚ Duohist DH
Daypro ⬚ Dopar
Debrisan ⬚ Diprosone
Decholin ⬚ Dyclone
decil ⬚ Dicel
Deconsal II ⬚ doconazole
Degas ⬚ Doxy 100
Denaze ⬚ Doan's
Depacon ⬚ dibucaine
Depakene ⬚ dibucaine
Deponit ⬚ Dibent
Depopred-40 ⬚ dobupride
deprodone ⬚ diperodon
deprostil ⬚ dipyrocetyl
Dequasine ⬚ Dexone
Derifil ⬚ Duraflu
Dermolin ⬚ Dramilin
desipramine ⬚ diisopromine
Desogen ⬚ Diascan
Desoxi ⬚ Dacex-A
de-Stat 3 ⬚ Diastat
Detane ⬚ Dytan
Dexameth ⬚ dioxamate
Dexodryl ⬚ dioxadrol
Dexone ⬚ Dequasine
Dexone LA ⬚ docosanol
Dex-Tuss DM ⬚ docusate sodium
DHC Plus ⬚ DOK-Plus
D-Hist D ⬚ Duocet
Diamox ⬚ DMax
Diastat ⬚ de-Stat 3
Dibent ⬚ Deponit
dibucaine ⬚ Depacon
dibunate ⬚ Deponit
Dicel ⬚ decil
diethazine ⬚ Detussin
difenidol ⬚ diphenidol
Difil-G ⬚ Duphalac
Di-Gel ⬚ Dical
diisopromine ⬚ desipramine
Dilomine ⬚ Dalmane; diolamine
dimethazan ⬚ duometacin
Dinate ⬚ D-Tann AT; Duonate-12
* Medicinal herbs/natural remedies.

dinsed ⬚ Donna-Sed
diolamine ⬚ Dalmane; Dilomine
diotyrosine I 125; diotyrosine I 131 ⬚ dotarizine
Diovan ⬚ D-Phen 1000
dioxadrol ⬚ Dexodryl
diperodon ⬚ deprodone
diphenidol ⬚ difenidol
Diprosone ⬚ Debrisan
dipyrocetyl ⬚ deprostil
dipyrone ⬚ duoperone
dithranol ⬚ deterenol
Diurese ⬚ Dairy Ease; Dry Eyes
Diurigen ⬚ DuraGen
Diuril ⬚ Doral
DMax ⬚ Diamox
Doan's ⬚ Denaze
dobupride ⬚ Depopred-40
doconazole ⬚ Deconsal II
docosanol ⬚ Dexone LA
docusate sodium ⬚ Dex-Tuss DM
DOK-Plus ⬚ DHC Plus
Donnagel ⬚ Denquel
Donna-Sed ⬚ dinsed
Dopar ⬚ Daypro
Doral ⬚ Diuril
Doryx ⬚ Droxia
dotarizine ⬚ diotyrosine I 125
Doxy 100 ⬚ Degas
D-Phen 1000 ⬚ Diovan
Dramilin ⬚ Dermolin
DroTuss ⬚ Duratuss
Droxia ⬚ Doryx
Dry Eyes ⬚ Dairy Ease; Diurese
Drysol ⬚ Durasal II
D-Tann AT ⬚ Dinate; Duonate-12
duazomycin ⬚ dacemazine
Duocet ⬚ D-Hist D
Duohist DH ⬚ Dayhist-1
Duonate-12 ⬚ Dinate; D-Tann AT
duoperone ⬚ dipyrone
Duphalac ⬚ Difil-G
Duraflu ⬚ Derifil
DuraGen ⬚ Diurigen
Duraphen II ⬚ Darvon
Durasal II ⬚ Drysol
Duratuss; Duratuss A ⬚ DroTuss
Durezol ⬚ Drysol
dymanthine HCl ⬚ dimantine HCl
Dytan ⬚ Detane

Ear-Dry ▣ Auro-Dri
Ear-Eze ▣ Aerius; Oracea; Urso 250
Easprin ▣ aceperone; aspirin; azaperone; esuprone
Easy A1C ▣ Oysco 500
ebastine ▣ epostane
ebselen ▣ epicillin
Edex ▣ ADEKs; Adoxa; Iodex
elanzepine ▣ olanzapine
Elavil ▣ olive oil
Elestat ▣ AlaSTAT
Elestrin ▣ alosetron
Eligard ▣ Allegra ODT
Elimite ▣ Alimta
Elocon ▣ Ala-Quin; Alcaine; elucaine
eltenac ▣ Altinac
elucaine ▣ Ala-Quin; Alcaine; Elocon
embramine ▣ ampyrimine; imipramine
Emend ▣ Immun-Aid
emetine ▣ Amitone; iometin
Emetrol ▣ amiterol
emitefur ▣ amitivir
EMLA ▣ Emollia; emu oil*
Emo-Cort ▣ Amcort
Emollia ▣ EMLA; emu oil*
Empirin ▣ amiperone
E-Mycin ▣ Amosan
Endagen-HD ▣ indecainide
Endrate ▣ woundwort*
Enfalyte ▣ Infalyte
Enisyl ▣ anise oil; Unisol
Enlive! ▣ One-Alpha
Enlon ▣ inulin
enocitabine ▣ ancitabine
Entex ▣ Antiox
Entex ER ▣ Uni-Tex 120/10 ER
Entrobar ▣ winterberry*
Entrophen ▣ Anatrofin
Enzone ▣ Anacin; inosine; Unasyn
Eovist ▣ Evista
eperisone ▣ euprocin
Epi-C ▣ Apo-K; iboga
epicillin ▣ ebselen
Epifrin ▣ ibuverine
E-Pilo-1 ▣ A.P.L.; apple*; IPOL
Epinal ▣ Abenol
Epitol ▣ Apetil
Epogen ▣ Apokyn; Opcon-A
epostane ▣ ebastine
*Medicinal herbs/natural remedies.

Equanil ▣ Aquanil
Equilet ▣ Accolate
Equipoise ▣ Aquabase; ICaps
erbium ▣ europium
erizepine ▣ AeroSpan
E-R-O Ear Drops ▣ Auro Ear Drops
Errin ▣ iron
Ertaczo ▣ AeroTuss 12; Artiss
ERYC ▣ ara-G
Erygel ▣ Orajel
EryPed; EryPed 200 ▣ AeroBid
erythrityl tetranitrate ▣ eritrityl tetranitrate
Eryzole ▣ Orasol; uracil
Esclim ▣ Oesclim
esilate ▣ esylate; Isolyte E
Esimil ▣ Isomil
estradiol ▣ oestradiol
estradiol benzoate ▣ oestradiol benzoate
estradiol valerate ▣ oestradiol valerate
estriol succinate ▣ oestriol succinate
estrone ▣ isoetarine; oestrone
esuprone ▣ aceperone; aspirin; azaperone; Easprin
esylate ▣ esilate; Isolyte E
etafenone ▣ etifenin
etamivan ▣ ethamivan
etamsylate ▣ ethamsylate
etasuline ▣ etozolin
etazepine ▣ atosiban
ethacrynic acid ▣ etacrynic acid
ethamivan ▣ etamivan
ethamsylate ▣ etamsylate
ethebenecid ▣ etebenecid
ethenzamide ▣ etenzamide
ether ▣ water O 15
ethiazide ▣ Atuss HD
ethisterone ▣ itasetron
ethoglucid ▣ etoglucid
ethosalamide ▣ etosalamide
ethybenztropine ▣ etybenzatropine
ethylene ▣ Atolone
ethynodiol ▣ etynodiol
etifenin ▣ etafenone
etofuradine ▣ atevirdine
etorphine ▣ Etrafon; Otrivin
etozolin ▣ etasuline
Etrafon ▣ etorphine; Otrivin
Euflex ▣ Avelox; I-Valex-1

Euflexxa ⑨ Avelox; I-Valex-1
eugenol ⑨ Aquanil; Equanil
euprocin ⑨ eperisone
Eurax ⑨ Urex
Euro-D ⑨ Aeroaid; Aredia
europium ⑨ erbium
Evista ⑨ Eovist
E-Vitamin ⑨ iofetamine
Evoclin ⑨ ivoqualine
Excedrin Extra Strength ⑨ oxidronic acid
Exelon ⑨ ioxilan
Exsel ⑨ Oxizole; Oxycel
Exubera ⑨ AK-Spore
Eye-Lube-A ⑨ Albay
EZFE 200 ⑨ Isovue-200
Factive ⑨ Viactiv
farnesil ⑨ Fer-In-Sol
FazaClo ⑨ Visicol
felypressin ⑨ fluprazine
fenadiazole ⑨ Vandazole
fenamole ⑨ Venomil
fenbenicillin ⑨ phenbenicillin
fenbutrazate ⑨ phenbutrazate
fencarbamide ⑨ phencarbamide
fendosal ⑨ Vandazole
Fenesin ⑨ phenazone; Vanocin
fenethazine ⑨ phenothiazine
fenethylline ⑨ phenythilone; Ventolin
fenetylline ⑨ Ventolin
fenharmane ⑨ pheniramine
fenimide ⑨ Vanamide
fenoterol ⑨ Phentrol 2
fenoxypropazine ⑨ phenoxypropazine
fenquizone ⑨ Vancocin
fenthion ⑨ phenytoin; Vantin
Feocyte ⑨ P-Hist
FeoGen ⑨ Phicon
FeoGen FA ⑨ Phicon F
Feosol ⑨ PhosLo; VaZol
Fer-Gen-Sol ⑨ voriconazole
Fergon ⑨ Vergon
Fer-In-Sol ⑨ farnesil
FeroSul ⑨ vorozole
Ferretts ⑨ Fortaz
filipin ⑨ fleabane*; Velban
Finac ⑨ Fung-O; Vaniqa
Finacea ⑨ Phenazo; Vanos
Flagyl ⑨ Ful-Glo
* Medicinal herbs/natural remedies.

Flarex ⑨ Fluarix
flazalone ⑨ flusalan
Fleet ⑨ violet*
Flexon ⑨ Floxin; fluquazone
Flomax ⑨ Volmax
Florone; Florone E ⑨ fluorine; valerian*
floverine ⑨ Fluvirin
Floxin ⑨ Flexon; fluquazone
fluacizine ⑨ volazocine
Fluarix ⑨ Flarex
fluconazole ⑨ valconazole
fluorine ⑨ Florone; valerian*
fluperamide ⑨ valpromide
fluprazine ⑨ felypressin
fluquazone ⑨ Flexon; Floxin
Flurox ⑨ Flarex
flusalan ⑨ flazalone
Flutex ⑨ Foltx
fluticasone ⑨ Valtaxin
Fluvirin ⑨ floverine
Fluzone ⑨ Valisone
Foamicon ⑨ fomocaine
Focalin ⑨ viqualine
Folpace ⑨ Phillips'
Foltrin ⑨ Voltaren
Foltx ⑨ Flutex
Folvite ⑨ Velivet
fomocaine ⑨ Foamicon
Forane ⑨ Fourneau 309
Fortaz ⑨ Ferretts
Fostril ⑨ Vistaril
Fourneau 309 ⑨ Forane
FreAmine III 3%; FreAmine III 8.5% ⑨ furomine; Viramune
Freezone ⑨ Furacin
frusemide ⑨ furosemide
Fucidin; Fucidin H ⑨ Visudyne
Ful-Glo ⑨ Flagyl
Funduscein-10 ⑨ vindesine
fungimycin ⑨ vancomycin
Fungi-Nail ⑨ vincanol
Fungizone ⑨ fenquizone; Vancocin
Fung-O ⑨ Finac; Vaniqa
fuprazole ⑨ Vaprisol
Furacin ⑨ Freezone
furafylline ⑨ verofylline
Furalan ⑨ Verelan; Virilon
furomine ⑨ FreAmine III 3%; Viramune

furosemide ▣ frusemide

Furoxone ▣ Viroxyn

Fuzeon ▣ Visine; Vusion

G Phen DM ▣ C-Phen DM; GFN 1000/DM 50; Guaifen DM

Gabarone ▣ gepirone; Quibron

Gabitril ▣ Capitrol

galamustine ▣ clemastine

gallamine ▣ calamine; Chlo-Amine

gallic acid ▣ Gly-Oxide

gallium ▣ Kolyum

galosemide ▣ Calcium 600 + D

Galzin ▣ Cleocin; glycine; Quelicin

Gas-Ban ▣ Kao-Spen

Gelhist ▣ Calcet; Glyset

Gelusil ▣ Colazal

Genac ▣ Gonak; Kank-a

Genaphed ▣ Confide

Genasal ▣ Goniosol; Gynazole-1; Konsyl

Gendex 75 ▣ Quinidex

Generet-500 ▣ Kineret

GenESA ▣ Canasa

Gen-K ▣ Gonak; Kank-a

Genpril ▣ quinapril

GenTeal ▣ Cantil

Gentran 40; Gentran 70 ▣ Contrin

Geodon ▣ codeine; Kadian; Quad Tann

gepirone ▣ Gabarone; Quibron

Geravim ▣ CarraFoam; Kerafoam

Geravite ▣ Carafate

Geref ▣ Kariva

Geridium ▣ Karidium

Gerimal ▣ caramel

Geriot ▣ carrot*

Gerivite ▣ Carafate

germanium ▣ carumonam

Gets-It ▣ QTest

GFN 1000/DM 50; GFN 1000/DM 60 ▣ C-Phen DM; G Phen DM; Guaifen DM

B>Giltuss ▣ Glutose

giparmen ▣ Cuprimine

gitalin ▣ guaietolin

Glaucon ▣ Glyquin; Qualaquin

glucalox ▣ glycalox

Glucerna ▣ glycerin

glucose ▣ Caelyx

glutaral ▣ colterol

Glutarex-1; Glutarex-2 ▣ Klotrix

Glutose ▣ Giltuss

glybuthiazol ▣ clobetasol

glycalox ▣ glucalox

glycerin ▣ Glucerna

glycerol ▣ clazuril; Clozaril

glycine ▣ Cleocin; Galzin; Quelicin

GlycoLax ▣ glucalox

Gly-Oxide ▣ gallic acid

glyprothiazol ▣ cloprothiazole

Glyquin ▣ Glaucon; Qualaquin

Glyset ▣ Calcet; Gelhist

Gonak ▣ Kank-a

Gonic ▣ Kank-a

Goniosol ▣ Gynazole-1; Konsyl

Gordon's Urea 40% ▣ Cardene SR

guaiacol ▣ guggul*

Guaifen DM ▣ C-Phen DM; G Phen DM; GFN 1000/DM 50

guaimesal ▣ Kemsol

guanisoquine ▣ quinisocaine

guar gum ▣ karaya gum*

Guiatuss AC ▣ cat's claw*

Gynazole-1 ▣ Genasal; Goniosol; Konsyl

halothane ▣ Hylutin

Hemopad ▣ Humibid

Hemotene ▣ Humatin

hibenzate ▣ hybenzate

Hivid ▣ Hyphed

Humalog ▣ hemlock*

Humatin ▣ Hemotene

Humibid; Humibid E ▣ Hemopad

hybenzate ▣ hibenzate

Hyphed ▣ Hivid

Iberet ▣ eyebright*

iboga ▣ Apo-K; Epi-C

Ibudone ▣ Iopidine

ibuverine ▣ Epifrin

ICaps ▣ Aquabase; Equipoise

Icar ▣ agar

IC-Green ▣ Wigraine

icospiramide ▣ oxiperomide

Ilotycin ▣ Altazine

I-L-X ▣ Aloxi; Olux

imafen ▣ Imovane

Imdur ▣ imidurea

imidoline ▣ amedalin; omidoline

imidurea ▣ Imdur

*Medicinal herbs/natural remedies.

imiloxan ▨ amalgucin
imipramine ▨ ampyrimine; embramine
Immun-Aid ▨ Emend
Imovane ▨ imafen
Inapsine ▨ InhibiZone
Inderal; Inderal LA ▨ Anadrol-50
Inderide 40/25; Inderide 80/25 ▨ Android
Infalyte ▨ Enfalyte
INFeD ▨ Unifed
InhibiZone ▨ Inapsine
InnoLet ▨ Ionil T
inosine ▨ Anacin; Enzone; Unasyn
inositol ▨ anisatil
Intergel ▨ Antrocol
IntraSite ▨ Anatrast
Intron A ▨ Anturane
inulin ▨ Enlon
Iodex ▨ ADEKs; Adoxa; Edex
Iodopen ▨ woodbine*
iofendylate ▨ iophendylate
iofetamine ▨ E-Vitamin
iogulamide ▨ aklomide
iomethin I 125; iomethin I 131 ▨ Amitone; emetine
iometin ▨ Amitone; emetine
Ionil T ▨ InnoLet
Iophen ▨ Aveeno; Aviane
iophendylate ▨ iofendylate
Iophylline ▨ Avolean*
Iopidine ▨ Ibudone
iopydone ▨ Ibudone
iosulamide ▨ osalmid
iotrolan ▨ Atralin
ioxilan ▨ Exelon
IPOL ▨ A.P.L.; apple*; E-Pilo-1
Ircon ▨ AeroCaine; argon
iron ▨ Errin
Irrigate ▨ ergot*
isobutane ▨ Aseptone 1; azapetine
isobuzole ▨ A-Spas S/L
Isocal ▨ Asacol; Os-Cal 500
isoconazole ▨ azaconazole
isoetarine ▨ estrone; oestrone
isoetharine ▨ estrone; oestrone
Isolan ▨ Wycillin
Isolyte E ▨ esilate; esylate
Isomil ▨ Esimil
Isopan ▨ azabon
* Medicinal herbs/natural remedies.

isoprazone ▨ azaprocin
Isovorin ▨ acifran
Isovue-200 ▨ EZFE 200
I-Valex-1; I-Valex-2 ▨ Avelox; Euflex
ivoqualine ▨ Evoclin
Ivy Soothe ▨ Eovist; Evista
Ivy-Dry ▨ ephedra*
Jay-Phyl ▨ Avail
Jets ▨ A/T/S; oats*
Jevity ▨ Avita
Jolessa ▨ Alesse
J-Tan ▨ Attain
Junel Fe 1/20; Junel Fe 1.5/30 ▨ Enlive!; One-Alpha
Just Tears ▨ Estrace
Kadian ▨ codeine; Quad Tann
Kaletra ▨ Caltro; coal tar
Kank-a ▨ Gonak
Kao-Spen ▨ Gas-Ban
Kao-Tin ▨ K-Tan
Karidium ▨ Geridium
Kariva ▨ Geref
kasal ▨ Kay Ciel
Kay Ciel ▨ kasal
kebuzone ▨ Capsin; Cubicin; quipazine
Kemsol ▨ guaimesal
Keppra ▨ copper
Kerafoam ▨ CarraFoam; Geravim
Keralac ▨ garlic*
Kerasal ▨ cresol; Cryselle
Kerasal AL ▨ carazolol
Kerodex #51; Kerodex #71 ▨ Cardec-S
Kerol ▨ caraway oil; coral*
ketocaine ▨ quatacaine
Key-Pred 25 ▨ capuride
khellin ▨ Calan; Clenia; kaolin*
Kionex ▨ Cognex
Klaron 10% ▨ chlorine
KLB6 ▨ kelp*
K-Lease ▨ Cal-Cee; Colace
Klor-Con ▨ chloroquine
Klorvess ▨ Claravis
Klotrix ▨ Glutarex-1
Klout ▨ CoLyte; K-Lyte
K-Lyte ▨ CoLyte; Klout
Kof-Eze ▨ Coughtuss
Kolephrin ▨ Calphron; Claforan
Kolyum ▨ gallium

Konsyl ▣ Goniosol; Gynazole-1
K-Pek; K-Pek II ▣ CPB WC
K-Tab ▣ CTAB; Q-Tapp
K-Tan; K-Tan 4 ▣ Kao-Tin
Kuric ▣ Carac; Coreg
Kuvan ▣ caffeine; C-Phen
Lagesic ▣ Luxiq
Lanacane ▣ lignocaine
Lanacort 5; Lanacort 10 ▣ lungwort*
Lanoxin ▣ Lincocin
Lessina ▣ leucine; lysine*
leucine ▣ Lessina; lysine*
levamisole ▣ lofemizole
levamisole HCl ▣ lofemizole HCl
Levlen ▣ Lufyllin
Levlite ▣ Lypholyte
Levolet ▣ Lypholyte
liarozole ▣ Lioresal
Librax ▣ Loprox
Librium ▣ Lipram 4500
lidimycin ▣ lydimycin
lignocaine ▣ Lanacane
Lincocin ▣ Lanoxin
Lioresal ▣ liarozole
Lipram 4500 ▣ Librium
Liquadd ▣ Locoid
Listerine ▣ Loestrin 21 1/20
lisuride ▣ lysuride
Lithane ▣ lutein
litracen ▣ Lotrisone
Locoid ▣ Liquadd
Loestrin 21 1/20 ▣ Listerine
lofemizole ▣ levamisole
lofemizole HCl ▣ levamisole HCl
Logen ▣ Leukine
Loprox ▣ Librax
Lotrisone ▣ litracen
Lubrin ▣ Lupron
Lufyllin; Lufyllin 400 ▣ Levlen
Lupron ▣ Lubrin
lydimycin ▣ lidimycin
Lypholyte ▣ Levlite
lysuride ▣ lisuride
Macugen ▣ Mycogen II
mafilcon A ▣ mefloquine
Magnacal ▣ Monocal
Magnacet ▣ Menest
Magnaprin ▣ minaprine
Magnox ▣ Minox
*Medicinal herbs/natural remedies.

Magsal ▣ Mucosil-10
maitansine ▣ maytansine
Malarone ▣ Myleran
malathion ▣ Miltown
malotilate ▣ Multilyte-20
Maolate ▣ Multi 75
Maox 420 ▣ Megace; M-oxy
Marezine ▣ morazone
Marinol ▣ Moranyl
Maxidone ▣ mixidine
maytansine ▣ maitansine
meclocycline ▣ meglucycline
meclozine ▣ Miacalcin
Medacote ▣ Modecate
Medicone ▣ Modicon
mefloquine ▣ mafilcon A
Megace ▣ Maox 420; M-oxy
Megaton ▣ Micatin
meglucycline ▣ meclocycline
meglutol ▣ miglitol
menadione ▣ Minidyne
Menest ▣ Magnacet
Mentax ▣ Mintox
menthol ▣ Mynatal
mequinol ▣ Micanol; Myconel
Mersol ▣ Murocel
Meruvax II ▣ M-R-Vax II
mesalamine ▣ mezilamine; muzolimine
metetoin ▣ mitotane
methazolamide ▣ mitozolomide
methetoin ▣ mitotane
MET-Rx ▣ Mytrex
mezilamine ▣ mesalamine; muzolimine
Mezlin ▣ Mysoline
Miacalcin ▣ meclozine
Micanol ▣ mequinol; Myconel
Micatin ▣ Megaton
Miconal ▣ mequinol; Myconel
Midrin ▣ Mudrane
miglitol ▣ meglutol
minaprine ▣ Magnaprin
Minidyne ▣ menadione
Minizide 1 ▣ Monocid
Minox ▣ Magnox
Mintox ▣ Mentax
Mirena ▣ Murine
mitotane ▣ metetoin
mixidine ▣ Maxidone
Modecate ▣ Medacote
Modicon ▣ Medicone

Monocal ⧆ Magnacal
Monocid ⧆ Minizide 1
monteplase ⧆ Mynate 90 Plus
Moranyl ⧆ Marinol
morazone ⧆ Marezine
morphine ⧆ myrophine
M-oxy ⧆ Maox 420; Megace
M-R-Vax II ⧆ Meruvax II
MSIR ⧆ mouse ear*
Mucosil-10 ⧆ Magsal
Mudrane ⧆ Midrin
Multi-12; Multi 75 ⧆ Maolate
Multilyte-20 ⧆ malotilate
Murine ⧆ Mirena
Murocel ⧆ Mersol
muzolimine ⧆ mesalamine; mezil-
   amine
Mycogen II ⧆ Macugen
Myconel ⧆ mequinol; Micanol
Myleran ⧆ Malarone
Mynate 90 Plus ⧆ monteplase
Myolin ⧆ mullein*
Myozyme ⧆ MSM; MZM
myrophine ⧆ morphine
Mysoline ⧆ Mezlin
Mytrex ⧆ MET-Rx
nafcillin ⧆ naphazoline
nafomine ⧆ Novamine
naphazoline ⧆ nafcillin
Naphcon; Naphcon-A ⧆ nefocon A;
   Novocain
Naprosyn ⧆ niaprazine
naproxen ⧆ nibroxane
naranol ⧆ Norinyl 1 + 35
narasin ⧆ Norzine
NāSal ⧆ Neosol
Nasarel ⧆ Nizoral
Naturalyte ⧆ Nutrilyte
nefocon A ⧆ Naphcon; Novocain
Neocate One + ⧆ nicotine
Neo-fradin ⧆ nifuradene
Neofrin ⧆ Nephron
neomycin ⧆ nimazone; Numoisyn
Neoral ⧆ Norel LA
Neosol ⧆ NāSal
Neotrace-4 ⧆ Nu-Tears
Nephron ⧆ Neofrin
Nephrox ⧆ Niferex
Nesacaine ⧆ New-Skin
* Medicinal herbs/natural remedies.

Neutra-Caine ⧆ Nutricon
Neutrogena Moisture ⧆ nitrogen mustard
New-Skin ⧆ Nesacaine
niaprazine ⧆ Naprosyn
nibroxane ⧆ naproxen
nicotine ⧆ Neocate One +
Niferex; Niferex-150 ⧆ Nephrox
nifuradene ⧆ Neo-fradin
nilestriol ⧆ nylestriol
nimazone ⧆ neomycin; Numoisyn
niometacin ⧆ Pneumotussin
nitrogen ⧆ Neutra-Caine; Nutricon
nitrogen mustard ⧆ Neutrogena Mois-
   ture
Nitrolan ⧆ Nutrilan
nivazol ⧆ Novasal
Nizoral ⧆ Nasarel
NoHist; NoHist A ⧆ Nuhist
Norel LA ⧆ Neoral
Norinyl 1 + 35; Norinyl 1 + 50 ⧆
   naranol
Norzine ⧆ narasin
Novamine ⧆ nafomine
Novasal ⧆ nivazol
Novocain ⧆ Naphcon; nefocon A
Nuhist ⧆ NoHist
Numoisyn ⧆ neomycin; nimazone
Nu-Tears; Nu-Tears II ⧆ Neotrace-4
Nutricon ⧆ Neutra-Caine
Nutrilan ⧆ Nitrolan
Nutrilyte ⧆ Naturalyte
nylestriol ⧆ nilestriol
Nytol ⧆ nettle*
Occucoat ⧆ OcuCoat
Ocean ⧆ Aceon; Aczone
octazamide ⧆ actisomide
OcuCoat ⧆ Occucoat
Ocusulf-10 ⧆ AK-Sulf
Ocutricin ⧆ AK-Tracin
Ocuvite ⧆ Aquavit-E
Oesclim ⧆ Esclim
Oesto-Mins ⧆ Osteo-Mins
oestradiol ⧆ estradiol
oestradiol benzoate ⧆ estradiol benzo-
   ate
oestradiol valerate ⧆ estradiol valerate
oestriol succinate ⧆ estriol succinate
oestrone ⧆ estrone; isoetarine
Ogen ⧆ A1cNOW; A.C.N.; Yocon

Ogestrel 0.5/50 ⧄ Oxytrol
olanzapine ⧄ elanzepine
olive oil ⧄ Elavil
Olux ⧄ Aloxi; I-L-X
omidoline ⧄ amedalin; imidoline
Ondrox ⧄ Androxy
One Touch ⧄ Ontak
One-Alpha ⧄ Enlive!
Ontak ⧄ One Touch
Opcon-A ⧄ Apokyn
Optigene; Optigene 3 ⧄ aptocaine
Oracea ⧄ Aerius; Ear-Eze; Urso 250
Orajel ⧄ Erygel
Orasept ⧄ Aricept
Orasol ⧄ Eryzole; uracil
Orasone ⧄ AeroZoin; Ureacin-10
Orazinc ⧄ arsenic
Orencia ⧄ Orinase
Oretic ⧄ Wartec
Orimune ⧄ Aramine
Orinase ⧄ Orencia
ornithine ⧄ aranotin
Ortho 0.5/35; Ortho 7/7/7 ⧄ Airet
Oruvail ⧄ Ureaphil
osalmid ⧄ iosulamide
Os-Cal 500 ⧄ Asacol; Isocal
Osteo-Mins ⧄ Oesto-Mins
Oticair ⧄ Outgro
Otic-Care ⧄ Outgro
Otrivin ⧄ etorphine; Etrafon
Outgro ⧄ Oticair
oxazorone ⧄ oxisuran
oxethazaine ⧄ oxytocin
oxidronic acid ⧄ Excedrin Extra
  Strength
oxiperomide ⧄ icospiramide
oxipurinol ⧄ oxypurinol
oxisuran ⧄ oxazorone
Oxizole ⧄ Exsel; Oxycel
Oxycel ⧄ Exsel; Oxizole
oxypurinol ⧄ oxipurinol
Oysco 500 ⧄ Easy A1C
Oystercal-D 250 ⧄ Astroglide
ozagrel ⧄ Ascor L 500
pafenolol ⧄ befunolol
Pain-X ⧄ Panokase; Pin-X
Paladin ⧄ belladonna*; Polydine
Palladone ⧄ belladonna*; Polydine
PALS ⧄ Blue Ice; Boil-Ease
*Medicinal herbs/natural remedies.

pamatolol ⧄ bometolol
Panacet 5/500 ⧄ boneset*; poinsettia*
Panadol ⧄ buniodyl
Pancof-HC ⧄ Bancap HC
Pandel ⧄ buniodyl
panidazole ⧄ bendazol
Panitone-500 ⧄ Ben-Tann
Pannaz ⧄ Benza
Panokase ⧄ Pain-X; Pin-X
Pap-Urea ⧄ bayberry*
Paracaine ⧄ Baricon; procaine; Pure-
  gon; pyrrocaine
paraffin ⧄ Brovana; Preven; Privine;
  Profen II
Parafon Forte DSC ⧄ Profen Forte
  DM
ParaGard T 380A ⧄ PerioGard; Pro-
  cardia
Paral ⧄ barley*; perilla*; Prelu-2
paramethasone ⧄ perimetazine; pro-
  methazine
parbendazole ⧄ propenidazole
parconazole ⧄ pirquinozol
Paredrine ⧄ pyridarone
Paremyd ⧄ PerioMed; ProMod
pargolol ⧄ pyrogallol
pargyline ⧄ Percolone; piriqualone
paridocaine ⧄ piridocaine
Par-Natal Plus 1 Improved ⧄ Prena-
  tal Plus
Parnate ⧄ burnet*; Pronto
parvaquone ⧄ Brevicon; porofocon A
Patanol ⧄ Botanol
paulomycin ⧄ bleomycin; peliomycin
Pavulon ⧄ bufylline
Paxil ⧄ piquizil
PC Tar ⧄ beech tree*
PD-Hist D ⧄ Bidhist
peanut oil ⧄ Bentyl
pecazine ⧄ Biaxin; Bicozene
pecilocin ⧄ bizelesin
Pedameth ⧄ padimate
Pediox ⧄ Bidex-A
peliomycin ⧄ bleomycin; paulomycin
Penecare ⧄ Benicar
Pen-Kera ⧄ Benicar
pentaquine ⧄ Pontocaine
perastine ⧄ prazitone; Prostin E2
Percocet ⧄ Pyrroxate
Percolone ⧄ piriqualone

Perdiem ⧉ Baridium; Prodium; Pyridium

pergolide ⧉ Baraclude

Pergonal ⧉ proguanil

perhexiline ⧉ pyroxylin

periciazine ⧉ prazosin

pericyazine ⧉ prazosin

PerioChip ⧉ Parcopa

PerioGard ⧉ ParaGard T 380A; Procardia

PerioMed ⧉ Paremyd; ProMod

Periostat ⧉ Pro-Stat 64

Perlane ⧉ Prelone; proline

Perloxx ⧉ Pyrlex

Permapen ⧉ prampine

pethidine ⧉ Betadine

phanquone ⧉ phenacaine

phenacaine ⧉ phanquone

Phenazo ⧉ Finacea; Vanos

phenazone ⧉ Fenesin; Vanocin

phenbenicillin ⧉ fenbenicillin

phenbutrazate ⧉ fenbutrazate

phencarbamide ⧉ fencarbamide

pheniramine ⧉ fenharmane

phenobarbital ⧉ vinbarbital

phenobarbital sodium ⧉ vinbarbital sodium

phenobarbitone ⧉ vinbarbitone

phenol ⧉ fennel*; vanilla

phenothiazine ⧉ fenethazine

phenoxypropazine ⧉ fenoxypropazine

Phentrol 2 ⧉ fenoterol

phenythilone ⧉ fenethylline; Ventolin

phenytoin ⧉ Vantin

Phillips' ⧉ Folpace

P-Hist ⧉ Feocyte

P-Hist DM ⧉ Fosteum*

PhosLo ⧉ Feosol; VaZol

phthalofyne ⧉ ftalofyne

piberaline ⧉ piperylone

picolamine ⧉ Byclomine

picotrin ⧉ buquiterine

pifexole ⧉ pivoxil

Pilagan ⧉ Bellacane; bulaquine; Polocaine

pimefylline ⧉ bamifylline

pimonidazole ⧉ bamnidazole

pinadoline ⧉ binedaline

pinoxepin ⧉ benaxibine

* Medicinal herbs/natural remedies.

Pin-X ⧉ Pain-X; Panokase

pioglitazone ⧉ Baltussin

piperylone ⧉ piberaline

piquizil ⧉ Paxil

pirazofurin ⧉ pyrazofurin

pirenperone ⧉ bornaprine

pirenzepine ⧉ Principen

pirfenidone ⧉ pyrophendane

piribedil ⧉ Prepidil

piridocaine ⧉ paridocaine

piriqualone ⧉ Percolone

pirmenol ⧉ Prominol

pirolate ⧉ Prialt

piroximone ⧉ pyroxamine

pirquinozol ⧉ parconazole

Pitressin ⧉ buterizine

Pitrex ⧉ Bite Rx

pivoxil ⧉ pifexole

Plaquenil ⧉ Belganyl

platinum ⧉ plutonium

plauracin ⧉ belarizine

Plax ⧉ Polycose

Plendil ⧉ bolandiol

Pletal ⧉ Bellatal

plutonium ⧉ platinum

Pneumotussin ⧉ niometacin

Polocaine ⧉ Bellacane; bulaquine; Pilagan

Polycose ⧉ Plax

Polydine ⧉ belladonna*; Paladin

ponfibrate ⧉ binifibrate

Pontocaine ⧉ pentaquine

porofocon A ⧉ Brevicon; parvaquone

Portia ⧉ birch*

Posture ⧉ Bicitra

PowerMate ⧉ buramate

pramocaine ⧉ primaquine

Pramosone ⧉ bromazine; primycin; promazine; puromycin

pramoxine ⧉ bromhexine

prampine ⧉ Permapen

pranidipine ⧉ barnidipine

Prax ⧉ Precose

prazepine ⧉ prozapine

prazitone ⧉ perastine; Prostin E2

prazosin ⧉ periciazine

Pre-Attain ⧉ protein A

Precose ⧉ Prax

Predalone 50 ⧉ burodiline

Pred-G ⧉ burdock*

Pregnyl ⏺ Pergonal; proguanil
Prelone ⏺ Perlane; proline
Prelu-2 ⏺ barley*; Paral; perilla*
premazepam ⏺ bromazepam
Premphase ⏺ bromofos
Prenatal 19 ⏺ pyrantel
Prenatal Plus; Prenatal Plus Improved; Prenatal Plus Iron; Prenatal Plus with Betacarotene ⏺ Par-Natal Plus 1 Improved
Prenatal-H ⏺ pyrantel
Prepcat ⏺ Probec-T
Pre-Pen ⏺ propane
Prepidil ⏺ piribedil
Pretz ⏺ Brite Eyes II; protease
Pretz-D ⏺ Protuss-D
Preven ⏺ Brovana; paraffin; Privine; Profen II
Prialt ⏺ pirolate
pridefine ⏺ proadifen
prifelone ⏺ Prophyllin
primaquine ⏺ pramocaine
primycin ⏺ bromazine; Pramosone; promazine; puromycin
Principen ⏺ pirenzepine
Privigen ⏺ Brevicon; parvaquone; porofocon A
Privine ⏺ Brovana; paraffin; Preven; Profen II
proadifen ⏺ pridefine
Probec-T ⏺ Prepcat
procaine ⏺ Baricon; Paracaine; Puregon; pyrrocaine
Procardia ⏺ ParaGard T 380A; PerioGard
Pro-Cute ⏺ Baro-cat
Prodium ⏺ Baridium; Perdiem; Pyridium
Profen II ⏺ Brovana; paraffin; Preven; Privine
Profen Forte DM ⏺ Parafon Forte DSC
proguanil ⏺ Pergonal
proline ⏺ Perlane; Prelone
promazine ⏺ bromazine; Pramosone; primycin; puromycin
promethazine ⏺ paramethasone; perimetazine
Prominol ⏺ pirmenol
*Medicinal herbs/natural remedies.

ProMod ⏺ Paremyd; PerioMed
Pronto ⏺ burnet*; Parnate
Propac ⏺ Barobag; Boropak
propane ⏺ Pre-Pen
propenidazole ⏺ parbendazole
Prophyllin ⏺ prifelone
Propine ⏺ Pre-Pen
propiram ⏺ pyrabrom
Pro-Q ⏺ Berocca
ProSol 20% ⏺ Buro-Sol; parsley*
Pro-Stat 64 ⏺ Periostat
Prostin E2 ⏺ perastine; prazitone
protease ⏺ Brite Eyes II; Pretz
protein A ⏺ Pre-Attain
Protuss ⏺ Brite Eyes II; Pretz
Protuss-D ⏺ Pretz-D
Provigil ⏺ Pravachol
Proviron ⏺ berefrine
prozapine ⏺ prazepine
Prudoxin ⏺ pyridoxine
Pseudofrin ⏺ cideferron
psilocin ⏺ salicin; Selsun; xylazine
Psoriatec ⏺ Saratoga
PsoriGel ⏺ Seroquel; Surgel
psyllium husk ⏺ Sulmasque
P-Tanna 12 ⏺ betony*; biotin; Bitin; butane
Puregon ⏺ Baricon; Paracaine; procaine; pyrrocaine
Purge ⏺ Berocca; borage*; Pro-Q
Purinethol ⏺ Prenatal 19; pyrantel
puromycin ⏺ bromazine; Pramosone; primycin; promazine
pyrabrom ⏺ propiram
pyrantel ⏺ Prenatal 19
pyrazofurin ⏺ pirazofurin
pyridarone ⏺ Paredrine
Pyridium ⏺ Baridium; Perdiem; Prodium
pyridoxine ⏺ Prudoxin
pyrinoline ⏺ bornelone
Pyrlex ⏺ Perloxx
pyrogallol ⏺ pargolol
pyrophendane ⏺ pirfenidone
pyroxamine ⏺ piroximone
pyroxylin ⏺ perhexiline
pyrrocaine ⏺ Baricon; Paracaine; procaine; Puregon
Pyrroxate ⏺ Percocet
Q-Pap ⏺ cubeb*

Q-Tapp ▣ CTAB; K-Tab
QTest ▣ Gets-It
Quad Tann ▣ codeine; Kadian
Qualaquin ▣ Glaucon; Glyquin
quatacaine ▣ ketocaine
Quelicin ▣ Cleocin; Galzin; glycine
Quibron ▣ Gabarone; gepirone
quinidine ▣ Candin
quinisocaine ▣ guanisoquine
quipazine ▣ Capsin; Cubicin; kebu-zone
radium ▣ rhodium
Ralix ▣ RuLox
Ranexa ▣ Renax; Ryna-12X
Rgain ▣ Rogaine
Regitine ▣ Reactine
Renax ▣ Ranexa; Ryna-12X
Repan ▣ Rheaban; Riopan
Resol ▣ rose oil
Re-Tann ▣ R-Tanna; rutin
Retin-A ▣ R-Tanna; rutin
Rv-Eyes ▣ Rivasa
R-Gen ▣ Rgain; Rogaine
R-gene 10 ▣ Rgain; Rogaine
Rheaban ▣ Repan; Riopan
Rhinall ▣ ronnel
rhodium ▣ radium
Rid-A-Pain ▣ riodipine
Rimso-50 ▣ RMS
riodipine ▣ Rid-A-Pain
Riopan ▣ Repan; Rheaban
Rivasa ▣ Rv-Eyes
Rogaine ▣ Rgain
ronnel ▣ Rhinall
rose oil ▣ Resol
Rosula ▣ Resol
R-Tanna; R-Tanna 12 ▣ Re-Tann; rutin
RuLox; RuLox #1 ▣ Ralix
rutin ▣ Re-Tann; R-Tanna
Ryna-12X ▣ Ranexa; Renax
Saizen ▣ Susano; Zosyn
SalAc ▣ Slow-K; Soyalac
salacetamide ▣ cilostamide
Salagen ▣ silicon; Solaquin; Xylocaine
salantel ▣ zilantel
Saleto ▣ SLT; Zylet
Salex ▣ Celexa; Cylex
Salflex ▣ Sulfolax
* Medicinal herbs/natural remedies.

salicin ▣ psilocin; Selsun; xylazine
Salofalk ▣ Sulpho-Lac
Sal-Plant ▣ Sleepwell 2-nite
Sal-Tropine ▣ sulotroban
Sancuso ▣ Sina-12X; Xanax
Sandimmune ▣ xinidamine
SangCya ▣ Sina-12X; Xanax
Saratoga ▣ Psoriatec
Scopace ▣ ZE Caps
Sea-Omega 30 ▣ Simuc; sumach*; Zomig
seclazone ▣ cyclizine
Secran ▣ Cycrin
Selsun ▣ psilocin; salicin; xylazine
Senna-Gen ▣ Sinequan; Zincon
Senokot ▣ Cyanokit; Zincate
Ser-Ap-Es ▣ Surpass
Sereine ▣ Ceron
Serevent ▣ Survanta
serine ▣ Ceron
Seromycin ▣ cyromazine
Serutan ▣ Soriatane
sevopramide ▣ cefpiramide
sfericase ▣ Zephrex; Zovirax
shellac ▣ Cholac
siccanin ▣ zocainone
Silace ▣ Cialis; xylose
silafilcon A ▣ xylofilcon A
silicon ▣ Solaquin; Xylocaine
silicone ▣ Solaquin; Xylocaine
silver ▣ sulphaurea
Simplet ▣ Cymbalta
Simuc ▣ Sea-Omega 30; sumach*; Zomig
Sina-12X ▣ Sancuso; Xanax
Sinequan ▣ Zincon
sintropium bromide ▣ xenytropium bromide
Sitrex ▣ storax
Sleepwell 2-nite ▣ Sal-Plant
Slo-phyllin ▣ sulfalene
Slow Fe ▣ Sulf-10
Slow-K ▣ Cholac; SalAc; shellac; Soyalac
Solagé ▣ SalAc; Slow-K; Soyalac
Solaquin ▣ silicon; Xylocaine
Soothe XP ▣ Zotex-PE
Soriatane ▣ Serutan
soterenol ▣ cioteronel; citronella*; SteriNail

Soyalac ⬚ SalAc; Slow-K
sparfloxacin ⬚ ciprofloxacin
sparteine ⬚ Ceprotin
spirazine ⬚ Sprayzoin
spirilene ⬚ Supprelin
Spiriva ⬚ Cipro I.V.
Sprayzoin ⬚ spirazine
S-T Cort ⬚ Cetacort
Stadol ⬚ cetiedil
Stagesic ⬚ Zotex-G
starch ⬚ Cytra-K
Starlix ⬚ Citralax
Stay Awake ⬚ Zoto-HC
stearic acid ⬚ citric acid
SteriNail ⬚ cioteronel; citronella*; soterenol
storax ⬚ Sitrex
Storzine 2 ⬚ cetirizine
subathizone ⬚ sopitazine
sucrose ⬚ Xigris
Sudal-12; Sudal 60/500 ⬚ Xodol
Sudex ⬚ Cedax; ciadox; Cidex
Sular ⬚ celery*; Xolair
sulazepam ⬚ zolazepam
Sulf-10 ⬚ Slow Fe
sulfalene ⬚ Slo-phyllin
Sulfolax ⬚ Salflex
Sulmasque ⬚ psyllium husk
sulotroban ⬚ Sal-Tropine
sulphaurea ⬚ silver
Sulpho-Lac ⬚ Salofalk
SuperEPA 1200 ⬚ X-Prep
Supprelin ⬚ spirilene
Suprane ⬚ Syprine
Suprax ⬚ Zyprexa
Surbex ⬚ Cerebyx
Surgel ⬚ PsoriGel; Seroquel
Surpass ⬚ Ser-Ap-Es
Survanta ⬚ Serevent
Susano ⬚ Saizen; Zosyn
Sustagen ⬚ Cystagon
Sustain ⬚ cystine; Systane
Sustaire ⬚ Zestra
Swim-Ear ⬚ Zemaira; Zymar
Symmetrel ⬚ cimaterol; xamoterol
Synagis ⬚ Sancuso; Sina-12X; Xanax
Syprine ⬚ Suprane
Syrvite ⬚ Cerovite
Systane ⬚ cystine; Sustain
*Medicinal herbs/natural remedies.

Talacen ⬚ tylosin
Tanac ⬚ Ten-K; Ting; Twin-K
tannic acid ⬚ tung seed*
Tannic-12 ⬚ Ten-K; Ting; Twin-K
Tannic-12 S ⬚ TNKase
Tarka ⬚ Touro CC; Tri-K
Tarlene ⬚ Trilone
Tasigna ⬚ tisoquone; Tussigon; Tyzine
tauromustine ⬚ trimustine
Tazidime ⬚ Tuss-DM
TearGard ⬚ terguride
Teargen ⬚ tarragon*; Torecan; Trocaine; Trugene
Tearisol ⬚ Terazol 3
Tears Again ⬚ triaziquone
tefazoline ⬚ tofisoline
telbivudine ⬚ tolpovidone I 131
Ten-K ⬚ Tanac; Ting; Twin-K
tenoate ⬚ 20/20
Tensilon ⬚ tinazoline; Tonsaline
Tenuate ⬚ 20/20
teprenone ⬚ tiopronin; toborinone
Tequin ⬚ Ticon; Tigan
Tera-Gel ⬚ Trocal
Terazol 3; Terazol 7 ⬚ Tearisol
terguride ⬚ TearGard
terizidone ⬚ trazodone
teroxalene ⬚ trixolane
Terramycin ⬚ Trimo-San
Terrell ⬚ Touro LA
Tessalon ⬚ tiosalan
T-Gen ⬚ Tequin; Ticon; Tigan
thallium ⬚ thulium
thebacon ⬚ tebuquine
thenalidine ⬚ tenylidone
Theochron ⬚ tacrine
theoclate ⬚ teoclate
Theolate ⬚ Twilite
Theovent ⬚ thiophanate
Theo-X ⬚ Tucks
Therabid ⬚ Tripedia
Therac ⬚ Tarka; Touro CC; Tri-K
Thera-M ⬚ thiram; thorium; Triam-A
Theravee ⬚ Thrive
Thermazene ⬚ Terramycin; Trimo-San
thiamiprine ⬚ timiperone
thiamylal ⬚ timolol
thiocarlide ⬚ tiocarlide
thioguanine ⬚ tioguanine
thiomesterone ⬚ tiomesterone

thiophanate ⑨ Theovent
thiosalan ⑨ Tessalon; tiosalan
thiothixene ⑨ tiotixene
thiouracil ⑨ Tearisol; Terazol 3
thioxolone ⑨ tioxolone
thiram ⑨ Thera-M; thorium; Triam-A
thonzonium bromide ⑨ tonzonium bromide
Thorazine ⑨ Trisan; tyrosine
thorium ⑨ Thera-M; thiram; Triam-A
thozalinone ⑨ tozalinone
Thrive ⑨ Theravee
thulium ⑨ thallium
Thyrogen ⑨ tarragon*; Torecan; Trocaine
thyroid ⑨ Triad
Ticon ⑨ Tequin; Tigan
tiformin ⑨ tyformin
Tigan ⑨ Tequin; Ticon
Tikosyn ⑨ toquizine
tinazoline ⑨ Tensilon; Tonsaline
Ting ⑨ Tanac; Ten-K; Twin-K
tioperidone ⑨ tipredane
tiopronin ⑨ teprenone; toborinone
tiosalan ⑨ Tessalon
tiospirone ⑨ tisopurine; tizabrin
tipredane ⑨ tioperidone
TiSol ⑨ Tussall
tisopurine ⑨ tiospirone; tizabrin
tisoquone ⑨ Tussigon
tizabrin ⑨ tiospirone; tisopurine
TNKase ⑨ Tannic-12 S
tobacco ⑨ Topic
toborinone ⑨ teprenone; tiopronin
tofisoline ⑨ tefazoline
tolpovidone I 131 ⑨ telbivudine
Tonsaline ⑨ Tensilon; tinazoline
Topic ⑨ tobacco
toquizine ⑨ Tikosyn
Toradol ⑨ Tridal
Torecan ⑨ tarragon*; Trocaine
tosulur ⑨ Tussall-ER
Touro CC ⑨ Tarka; Tri-K
Touro CC-LD ⑨ Triglide
Touro Ex ⑨ Tyrex-2
Touro HC ⑨ Tarka; Tri-K
Touro LA ⑨ Terrell
Travasol 3.5%; Travasol 5.5% ⑨ Triphasil

* Medicinal herbs/natural remedies.

trazitiline ⑨ trestolone
trazodone ⑨ terizidone
trestolone ⑨ trazitiline
Trexall ⑨ Tricosal
Triacet ⑨ Trycet
triaziquone ⑨ Tears Again
Tri-Biozene ⑨ Trobicin
tribuzone ⑨ Trobicin
Tri-Chlor ⑨ Tracleer
Tricosal ⑨ Trexall
Tridal ⑨ Toradol
Tridil ⑨ Toradol
Triglide ⑨ Touro CC-LD
Tri-K ⑨ Tarka; Touro CC
Trilone ⑨ Tarlene
Trimo-San ⑨ Terramycin
Trimox ⑨ Tyromex-1
trimustine ⑨ tauromustine
Trinalin ⑨ Tronolane
triolein I 125; triolein I 131 ⑨ Tarlene
Triphasil ⑨ Travasol 3.5%
Trisan ⑨ tyrosine
Tri-Vi-Sol ⑨ Travasol 3.5%
trixolane ⑨ teroxalene
Trobicin ⑨ Tri-Biozene
Trocaine ⑨ tarragon*; Torecan
Tronolane ⑨ Trinalin
Tronothane HCl ⑨ trientine HCl
Trugene ⑨ tarragon*; Teargen; Torecan; Trocaine
Trycet ⑨ Triacet
T-Stat ⑨ Tusstat
Tussall ⑨ TiSol
Tussall-ER ⑨ tosulur
Tuss-DM ⑨ Tazidime
Tussigon ⑨ tisoquone
Tusso DM ⑨ Tazidime
Tusso HC ⑨ Tyzeka
Tusstat ⑨ T-Stat
20/20 ⑨ tenoate
Twin-K ⑨ Tanac; Ten-K; Ting
tyformin ⑨ tiformin
tylosin ⑨ Talacen
Tyrex-2 ⑨ Touro Ex
Tyromex-1 ⑨ Trimox
tyrosine ⑨ Trisan
Tyzeka ⑨ Tusso HC
Tyzine ⑨ Tasigna
Ucephan ⑨ Acephen; Asaphen

Unasyn ☒ Anacin; Enzone; inosine
Uni-Ace ☒ anise*
Unifed ☒ INFeD
Unisol ☒ anise oil; Enisyl
Uni-Tex 120/10 ER ☒ Entex ER
Uracid ☒ Urised
uracil ☒ Eryzole; Orasol
Ureacin-10; Ureacin-20 ☒ AeroZoin; Orasone
Ureaphil ☒ Oruvail
urethan ☒ Uritin
urethane ☒ Uritin
Urex ☒ Eurax
Urised ☒ Uracid
Urogesic ☒ Argesic
Urso 250 ☒ Aerius; Ear-Eze; Oracea
Vagisil ☒ Vexol
valconazole ☒ fluconazole
Valisone ☒ Fluzone
valofane ☒ Voluven
Valorin ☒ Florone; fluorine
valpromide ☒ fluperamide
Valtaxin ☒ fluticasone
Vanamide ☒ fenimide
Vancocin ☒ fenquizone
Vandazole ☒ fenadiazole
vanilla ☒ fennel*; phenol
Vaniqa ☒ Finac; Fung-O
Vanocin ☒ Fenesin; phenazone
Vanos ☒ Finacea; Phenazo
Vantin ☒ phenytoin
Vaprisol ☒ fuprazole
Vasocon-A ☒ Visken
VaZol ☒ Feosol; PhosLo
Velban ☒ filipin; fleabane*
Velivet ☒ Folvite
Venomil ☒ fenamole
Ventolin ☒ fenetylline
Veregen ☒ Fergon
Verelan ☒ Furalan; Virilon
Vergon ☒ Fergon
verofylline ☒ furafylline
Viactiv ☒ Factive
vinbarbital ☒ phenobarbital
vinbarbital sodium ☒ phenobarbital sodium
vinbarbitone ☒ phenobarbitone
vindesine ☒ Funduscein-10
Viogen-C ☒ Vicon-C
*Medicinal herbs/natural remedies.

viqualine ☒ Focalin
Viramune ☒ FreAmine III 3%; furomine
Virilon ☒ Furalan; Verelan
Viroxyn ☒ Furoxone
Visicol ☒ FazaClo
Visine; Visine-A ☒ Fuzeon; Vusion
Visken ☒ Vasocon-A
Vistaril ☒ Fostril
Visudyne ☒ Fucidin
voglibose ☒ Folpace; Phillips'
volazocine ☒ fluacizine
Volmax ☒ Flomax
Voltaren ☒ Foltrin
Voluven ☒ valofane
vorozole ☒ FeroSul
V-Tann ☒ Vytone
Vusion ☒ Fuzeon; Visine
Vytone ☒ V-Tann
Wartec ☒ Fruit C 100; Oretic
wax, white ☒ AquaSite
wax, yellow ☒ Aquasol A
WelChol ☒ Flagyl; Ful-Glo
Welltuss HC ☒ FluTuss HC
Wetting ☒ Fe-Tinic 150
Wigraine ☒ IC-Green
Winstrol ☒ fenestrel
Wycillin ☒ Isolan
Xalatan ☒ zileuton
xamoterol ☒ cimaterol; Symmetrel
Xanax ☒ Sancuso; Sina-12X
xanomeline ☒ xinomiline
xanthiol ☒ Santyl
Xedec ☒ Cydec; Zodeac-100
Xenical ☒ sanicle*
xenytropium bromide ☒ sintropium bromide
Xigris ☒ sucrose
xinidamine ☒ Sandimmune
xinomiline ☒ xanomeline
Xiral ☒ sorrel*
Xodol ☒ Sudal 60/500
Xolair ☒ celery*; Sular
X-Prep ☒ SuperEPA 1200
xylazine ☒ psilocin; salicin; Selsun
Xylocaine ☒ silicon; Solaquin
xylofilcon A ☒ silafilcon A
xylose ☒ Cialis; Silace
Xyntha ☒ Sonata
Xyrem ☒ cerium

Xyzal ⑨ Zazole
Yelets ⑨ Altace
Yocon ⑨ A1cNOW; A.C.N.
Zazole ⑨ Xyzal
ZE Caps ⑨ Scopace
Zegerid ⑨ Sucraid
Zemaira ⑨ Swim-Ear; Zymar
Zephrex ⑨ sfericase; Zovirax
Zerit ⑨ XRT
Zestra ⑨ Sustaire
Zetar ⑨ Cytra-2
Z-gen ⑨ Cecon; Ziagen
Ziagen ⑨ Cecon; Z-gen
Ziks ⑨ Ziox 405
zilantel ⑨ salantel
zileuton ⑨ Xalatan
zinc; Zinc 15; Zinc-220 ⑨ Cena-K; senega*
Zincate ⑨ Cyanokit; Senokot
Zincon ⑨ Sinequan
Zingo ⑨ Cena-K; senega*

zinterol ⑨ Center-Al
Ziox 405 ⑨ Ziks
zocainone ⑨ siccanin
Zodeac-100 ⑨ Cydec; Xedec
Zoderm ⑨ Zyderm
Zofran ⑨ saffron*
Zofran ODT ⑨ ceforanide
zolazepam ⑨ sulazepam
Zomig ⑨ Sea-Omega·30; Simuc; sumach*
Zosyn ⑨ Saizen; Susano
zotepine ⑨ cetaben
Zoto-HC ⑨ Stay Awake
Zovirax ⑨ sfericase; Zephrex
Zyderm ⑨ Zoderm
Zyflo ⑨ Cefol
Zylet ⑨ Saleto; SLT
Zymar ⑨ Swim-Ear; Zemaira
Zymine ⑨ Cyomin
Zyprexa ⑨ Suprax
Zyvoxam ⑨ cefixime

* Medicinal herbs/natural remedies.

Abbreviations Used with Medications and Dosages

Abbreviation/Term	Literally	Meaning
a.c.	ante cibum	before meals or food
ad	ad	to, up to
A.D., AD	auris dextra	right ear
ad lib.	ad libitum	at pleasure
A.L.	auris laeva	left ear
a.m., A.M.	ante meridiem	morning
Aq.	aqua	water
A.S., AS	auris sinistra	left ear
A.U., AU*	auris uterque	each ear
b.i.d.	bis in die	twice daily
b.m.	bowel movement	
cc, cm^3	cubic centimeter	
CFU	colony-forming unit(s)	
d.	die	day
EL.U.	ELISA unit(s)	
et	et	and
g	gram(s)	
gt. (plural gtt.)	gutta (plural guttae)	a drop (drops)
h.	hora	hour
HAU	hemagglutinating unit(s)	
h.s.	hora somni	at bedtime
IM†	intramuscular	
IU	international unit(s)	
IV†	intravenous	
LfU	limes flocculating unit(s)	
	limit of flocculation unit(s)	
mcg, μg	microgram(s)	
mg	milligram(s)	
mEq	milliequivalent(s)	
mkat	millikatal unit(s)	
mL, ml	milliliter(s)	
mU, mIU	milliunit(s)	
MU, MIU	megaunit(s)	one million (10^6) IU
μg, mcg	microgram(s)	
nkat	nanokatal unit(s)	
O.D.	oculus dexter	right eye
O.L.	oculus laevus	left eye
O.S.	oculus sinister	left eye
O.U.§	oculus uterque	each eye

Abbreviation/Term	Literally	Meaning
p.c.	post cibum	after meals
p.m., P.M.	post meridiem	afternoon or evening
p.o.	per os	by mouth
p.r.n.	pro re nata	as needed
q.d.	quaque die	every day
q.h.	quaque hora	every hour
q.i.d.	quater in die	four times a day
q.o.d.		every other day
q.s.	quantum satis	sufficient quantity
q.s. ad	quantum satis ad	a sufficient quantity to make
℞, Rx	recipe	take; a recipe
Sig.	signetur	label
s.o.s.	si opus sit	if there is need
stat	statim	at once, immediately
subcu, subq, SQ	subcutaneous	beneath the skin
t.i.d.	ter in die	three times a day
tsp.	teaspoonful	
μg, mcg	microgram(s)	

---

* Although some references have aures unitas (Latin, both ears), this cannot be justified by classical Latin.

† Some references suggest that IM and IV be typed with periods to distinguish from Roman numerals, but we believe context is sufficient to make this distinction.

§ Although some references have oculi unitas (Latin, both eyes), this cannot be justified by classical Latin.

APPENDIX C
Therapeutic Drug Levels

Drug	Class	Serum Levels metric units (SI units)
amantadine	antiviral	300 ng/mL
amikacin	aminoglycoside	16–32 μg/mL
amiodarone	antiarrhythmic	0.5–2.5 μg/mL
amitriptyline	antidepressant	110–250 ng/mL
amoxapine	antidepressant	200–500 ng/mL
amrinone	cardiotonic	3.7 μg/mL
bretylium	antiarrhythmic	0.5–1.5 μg/mL
bupropion	antidepressant	25–100 ng/mL
carbamazepine	anticonvulsant	4–12 μg/mL (17–51 μmol/L)
chloramphenicol	antibiotic	10–20 μg/mL (31–62 μmol/L)
chlorpromazine	antipsychotic	30–500 ng/mL
clomipramine	antidepressant	80–100 ng/mL
cyclosporine	immunosuppressive	250–800 ng/mL (whole blood, RIA*)
trough values:		50–300 ng/mL (plasma, RIA*)
desipramine	antidepressant	125–300 ng/mL
digitoxin	antiarrhythmic	9–25 μg/L (11.8–32.8 nmol/L)
digoxin	antiarrhythmic	0.5–2.2 ng/mL (0.6–2.8 nmol/L)
disopyramide	antiarrhythmic	2–8 μg/mL (6–18 μmol/L)
doxepin	antidepressant	100–200 ng/mL
flecainide	antiarrhythmic	0.2–1 μg/mL
fluphenazine	antipsychotic	0.13–2.8 ng/mL
gentamicin	aminoglycoside	4–8 μg/mL
haloperidol	antipsychotic	5–20 ng/mL
hydralazine	antihypertensive	100 ng/mL
imipramine	antidepressant	200–350 ng/mL
kanamycin	aminoglycoside	15–40 μg/mL
lidocaine	antiarrhythmic	1.5–6 μg/mL (4.5–21.5 μmol/L)
lithium	antipsychotic	0.5–1.5 mEq/L (0.5–1.5 mmol/L)
maprotiline	antidepressant	200–300 ng/mL
mexiletine	antiarrhythmic	0.5–2 μg/mL
netilmicin	aminoglycoside	6–10 μg/mL

Drug	Class	Serum Levels metric units (SI units)
nortriptyline	antidepressant	50–150 ng/mL
perphenazine	antipsychotic	0.8–1.2 ng/mL
phenobarbital	anticonvulsant	15–40 μg/mL (65–172 μmol/L)
phenytoin	anticonvulsant	10–20 μg/mL (40–80 μmol/L)
primidone	anticonvulsant	5–12 μg/mL (25–46 μmol/L)
procainamide	antiarrhythmic	4–8 μg/mL (17–34 μmol/L)
propranolol	antiarrhythmic	50–200 ng/mL (190–770 nmol/L)
protriptyline	antidepressant	100–200 ng/mL
quinidine	antiarrhythmic	2–6 μg/mL (4.6–9.2 μmol/L)
salicylate	analgesic	100–200 mg/L (725–1448 μmol/L)
streptomycin	aminoglycoside	20–30 μg/mL
sulfonamide	antibiotic	5–15 mg/dL
terbutaline	bronchodilator	0.5–4.1 ng/mL
theophylline	bronchodilator	10–20 μg/mL (55–110 μmol/L)
thiothixene	antipsychotic	2–57 ng/mL
tobramycin	aminoglycoside	4–8 μg/mL
tocainide	antiarrhythmic	4–10 μg/mL
trazodone	antidepressant	800–1600 ng/mL
valproic acid	anticonvulsant	50–100 μg/mL (350–700 μmol/L)
vancomycin	antibiotic	30–40 ng/mL (peak)
verapamil	antiarrhythmic	0.08–0.3 μg/mL

* radioimmunoassay

The Most Prescribed Drugs

Drug	Class/Indication(s)
Abilify (aripiprazole)	quinolinone antipsychotic, antimanic
acetaminophen with codeine	analgesic, anti-inflammatory
Aciphex (rabeprazole sodium)	proton pump inhibitor for GERD
Actonel (risedronate sodium)	osteoporosis prevention and treatment
Actos (pioglitazone HCl)	oral antidiabetic
acyclovir	antiviral
Adderall XR (mixed amphetamines)	CNS stimulant for ADHD
Advair Diskus (salmeterol xinafoate, fluticasone propionate)	bronchodilator and corticosteroidal anti-inflammatory for asthma
albuterol; albuterol sulfate	bronchodilator for asthma
Allegra-D 12-Hour (fexofenadine HCl, pseudoephedrine HCl)	nonsedating antihistamine and decongestant for allergy
allopurinol	treatment for gout and hyperuricemia
alprazolam	anxiolytic, sedative
Altace (ramipril)	antihypertensive, ACE inhibitor
Ambien; Ambien CR (zolpidem tartrate)	sedative, hypnotic
amitriptyline HCl	tricyclic antidepressant
amlodipine besylate	antianginal, antihypertensive
amlodipine besylate & benazepril HCl	antihypertensive, ACE inhibitor, calcium channel blocker
amoxicillin	aminopenicillin antibiotic
amoxicillin & clavulanate potassium	aminopenicillin antibiotic
amphetamines, mixed	CNS stimulant for ADHD
Aricept (donepezil HCl)	cognition enhancer for dementia
Armour Thyroid (thyroid, desiccated)	thyroid hormone
aspirin, enteric coated	analgesic, antipyretic, NSAID
Astelin (azelastine HCl)	nasal antihistamine/mast cell stabilizer
atenolol	β-blocker for hypertension
atenolol & chlorthalidone	β-blocker and diuretic for hypertension
Avalide (irbesartan, hydrochlorothiazide)	antihypertensive, angiotensin II blocker, diuretic
Avandia (rosiglitazone maleate)	antidiabetic; decreases insulin resistance
Avapro (irbesartan)	antihypertensive
Avelox (moxifloxacin HCl)	fluoroquinolone antibiotic
Aviane (levonorgestrel, ethinyl estradiol)	monophasic oral contraceptive
azithromycin	macrolide antibiotic
baclofen	skeletal muscle relaxant
benazepril HCl	antihypertensive, ACE inhibitor
Benicar (olmesartan medoxomil)	antihypertensive, angiotensin II blocker
Benicar HCT (olmesartan medoxomil, hydrochlorothiazide)	antihypertensive, angiotensin II blocker, diuretic

Drug	Class/Indication(s)
benzonatate	antitussive
bisoprolol & hydrochlorothiazide	β-blocker and diuretic for hypertension
Boniva (ibandronate sodium)	osteoporosis prevention and treatment
Budeprion XL or SR (bupropion HCl)	aminoketone antidepressant
bupropion HCl [sustained-release form]	aminoketone antidepressant
buspirone HCl	anxiolytic
butalbital & acetaminophen & caffeine	barbiturate sedative, analgesic
carisoprodol	skeletal muscle relaxant
Cartia XT (diltiazem HCl)	antihypertensive, antianginal
carvedilol	α- and β-blocker for hypertension and congestive heart failure
cefdinir	cephalosporin antibiotic
Celebrex (celecoxib)	antiarthritic, NSAID, COX-2 inhibitor
cephalexin	cephalosporin antibiotic
Chantix (varenicline tartrate)	non-nicotine smoking cessation aid
chlorhexidine gluconate	broad-spectrum antimicrobial, antiseptic
Cialis (tadalafil)	vasodilator for erectile dysfunction
ciprofloxacin; ciprofloxacin HCl	fluoroquinolone antibiotic
citalopram hydrobromide	SSRI antidepressant
Clarinex (desloratadine)	nonsedating antihistamine for allergy
clarithromycin	macrolide antibiotic
clindamycin	lincosamide antibiotic
clobetasol propionate	topical steroidal anti-inflammatory
clonazepam	anticonvulsant
clonidine	antihypertensive
clotrimazole & betamethasone dipropionate	broad-spectrum antifungal, corticosteroidal anti-inflammatory
colchicine	gout suppressant
Combivent (ipratropium bromide, albuterol sulfate)	bronchodilator for COPD
Concerta (methylphenidate HCl)	CNS stimulant for ADHD
Coreg (carvedilol)	α- and β-blocker for hypertension and congestive heart failure
Coumadin (warfarin sodium)	anticoagulant
Cozaar (losartan potassium)	antihypertensive, angiotensin II blocker
Crestor (rosuvastatin potassium)	antihyperlipidemic
cyclobenzaprine HCl	skeletal muscle relaxant
Cymbalta (duloxetine HCl)	SSRI antidepressant
Depakote; Depakote ER (divalproex sodium)	anticonvulsant
Detrol LA (tolterodine tartrate)	treatment for urinary frequency
diazepam	anxiolytic, skeletal muscle relaxant
diclofenac sodium	antiarthritic, analgesic, NSAID
dicyclomine HCl	anticholinergic, GI antispasmodic
Digitek (digoxin)	antiarrhythmic
digoxin	antiarrhythmic
diltiazem HCl	antihypertensive, antianginal
Diovan (valsartan)	antihypertensive, angiotensin II blocker

Drug	Class/Indication(s)
Diovan HCT (valsartan, hydrochloro-thiazide)	antihypertensive, angiotensin II blocker, diuretic
doxazosin mesylate	α-blocker for hypertension and BPH
doxycycline hyclate	tetracycline antibiotic
Effexor XR (venlafaxine)	SSNRI antidepressant, anxiolytic
enalapril maleate	antihypertensive, ACE inhibitor
Endocet (oxycodone HCl; acetamino-phen)	narcotic analgesic
estradiol	oral estrogen for postmenopausal HRT
etodolac	analgesic, antiarthritic, NSAID
Evista (raloxifene HCl)	postmenopausal osteoporosis treatment
famotidine	histamine antagonist for gastric ulcers
felodipine [sustained-release form]	antihypertensive, calcium channel blocker
fentanyl [transdermal form]	narcotic analgesic
ferrous sulfate	hematinic, iron supplement
fexofenadine HCl	nonsedating antihistamine for allergy
finasteride	androgen hormone inhibitor for BPH
Flomax (tamsulosin HCl)	benign prostatic hypertrophy treatment
Flovent HFA (fluticasone propionate)	steroidal anti-inflammatory
fluconazole	systemic antifungal
fluoxetine HCl	SSRI antidepressant
fluticasone propionate	steroidal anti-inflammatory
folic acid	hematopoietic, prevents birth defects
Fosamax (alendronate sodium)	postmenopausal osteoporosis treatment
furosemide	diuretic, antihypertensive
gabapentin	anticonvulsant
gemfibrozil	antihyperlipidemic
glimepiride	oral antidiabetic
glipizide	oral antidiabetic
glyburide	oral antidiabetic
Glycolax (polyethylene glycol 3350)	laxative, pre-procedure bowel evacuant
Humalog (insulin lispro)	parenteral antidiabetic
hydrochlorothiazide	diuretic, antihypertensive
hydrocodone & acetaminophen	antitussive, analgesic
hydroxychloroquine sulfate	antimalarial
hydroxyzine HCl	anxiolytic, minor tranquilizer
hyoscyamine sulfate	anticholinergic
Hyzaar (losartan potassium, hydro-chlorothiazide)	antihypertensive, angiotensin II blocker, diuretic
ibuprofen	analgesic, antiarthritic, NSAID
Imitrex [oral] (sumatriptan succinate)	migraine headache treatment
isosorbide mononitrate	coronary vasodilator, antianginal
Klor-Con (potassium chloride)	potassium supplement
Lamictal (lamotrigine)	anticonvulsant, antimanic
Lantus (insulin glargine)	parenteral antidiabetic
Levaquin (levofloxacin)	fluoroquinolone antibiotic
levothyroxine sodium	thyroid hormone

Drug	Class/Indication(s)
Levoxyl (levothyroxine sodium)	thyroid hormone
Lexapro (escitalopram oxalate)	SSRI antidepressant
Lidoderm (lidocaine) [transdermal]	anesthetic for post-herpetic neuralgia
Lipitor (atorvastatin calcium)	antihyperlipidemic
lisinopril	antihypertensive, ACE inhibitor
lisinopril & hydrochlorothiazide	antihypertensive, ACE inhibitor, diuretic
lithium carbonate	antipsychotic, antimanic
lorazepam	anxiolytic, tranquilizer
Lotrel (amlodipine besylate, benazepril HCl)	antihypertensive, ACE inhibitor, calcium channel blocker
lovastatin	antihyperlipidemic
Lunesta (eszopiclone)	nonbarbiturate sedative and hypnotic
Lyrica (pregabalin)	anticonvulsant; neuropathy agent
meclizine HCl	antiemetic for motion sickness, vertigo
meloxicam	analgesic, antiarthritic, NSAID
metformin HCl	oral antidiabetic
metformin HCl & glyburide	oral antidiabetic
methadone HCl	narcotic analgesic; addiction detoxicant
methocarbamol	skeletal muscle relaxant
methotrexate	antineoplastic, antipsoriatic, anti-rheumatic
methylprednisolone	corticosteroidal anti-inflammatory
metoclopramide HCl	antiemetic for chemotherapy
metoprolol tartrate/succinate	antianginal, antihypertensive
metronidazole	oral antibiotic, antiprotozoal
minocycline HCl	broad-spectrum antibiotic
mirtazapine	tetracyclic antidepressant
mupirocin	topical antibiotic
nabumetone	analgesic, antiarthritic, NSAID
Namenda (memantine HCl)	cognition enhancer for dementia
naproxen; naproxen sodium	analgesic, antiarthritic, NSAID
Nasacort AQ (triamcinolone acetonide)	nasal steroid for allergic rhinitis
Nasonex (mometasone furoate)	nasal steroid for allergic rhinitis
Nexium (esomeprazole magnesium)	proton pump inhibitor for GERD
Niaspan (niacin)	vasodilator, antihyperlipidemic
nifedipine [extended-release form]	antianginal, antihypertensive
nitrofurantoin	urinary antibiotic
nitroglycerin	antianginal, coronary vasodilator
Nitroquick (nitroglycerin)	antianginal, coronary vasodilator
nortriptyline HCl	tricyclic antidepressant
Norvasc (amlodipine besylate)	antianginal, antihypertensive
NovoLog (insulin aspart)	parenteral antidiabetic
NuvaRing (ethinyl estradiol, etonogestrel)	contraceptive vaginal insert
omeprazole	proton pump inhibitor for GERD
Omnicef (cefdinir)	cephalosporin antibiotic

Drug	Class/Indication(s)
Ortho Tri-Cyclen Lo (norgestimate, ethinyl estradiol)	triphasic oral contraceptive
oxycodone HCl	narcotic analgesic
oxycodone HCl & acetaminophen	narcotic analgesic, NSAID
paroxetine HCl	SSRI antidepressant
Patanol (olopatadine HCl)	ophthalmic antihistamine for allergy
penicillin VK (penicillin V potassium)	natural antibiotic
phenazopyridine HCl	urinary analgesic
phentermine HCl	CNS stimulant for weight loss
phenytoin sodium	anticonvulsant
Plavix (clopidogrel bisulfate)	platelet aggregation inhibitor
potassium chloride	potassium supplement
pravastatin sodium	antihyperlipidemic
prednisolone sodium phosphate	corticosteroidal anti-inflammatory
prednisone	corticosteroidal anti-inflammatory
Premarin (conjugated estrogens)	estrogen replacement
Prevacid (lansoprazole)	antisecretory, antiulcer
ProAir HFA (albuterol sulfate)	bronchodilator for asthma
promethazine HCl	antihistamine, antiemetic
promethazine with codeine	narcotic antitussive, antihistamine
propoxyphene napsylate/acetaminophen	narcotic analgesic, NSAID
propranolol HCl	antihypertensive, antiarrhythmic
Protonix (pantoprazole sodium)	proton pump inhibitor for GERD
Proventil HFA (albuterol sulfate)	bronchodilator for asthma
quinapril HCl	antihypertensive, ACE inhibitor
ranitidine HCl	histamine antagonist for gastric ulcers
Requip (ropinirole HCl)	dopamine agonist for Parkinson disease
Risperdal (risperidone)	antipsychotic
Seroquel (quetiapine fumarate)	antipsychotic
sertraline HCl	SSRI antidepressant
simvastatin	antihyperlipidemic
Singulair (montelukast sodium)	antiasthmatic
Skelaxin (metaxalone)	skeletal muscle relaxant
Spiriva (tiotropium bromide)	bronchodilator for emphysema, COPD
spironolactone	antihypertensive, diuretic
Strattera (atomoxetine HCl)	nonstimulant ADHD treatment
sulfamethoxazole & trimethoprim	anti-infective, antibacterial
Synthroid (levothyroxine sodium)	thyroid replacement
temazepam	tranquilizer, hypnotic
terazosin HCl	α-blocker for hypertension and BPH
tizanidine HCl	skeletal muscle relaxant
Topamax (topiramate)	anticonvulsant
Toprol XL (metoprolol succinate)	antihypertensive, antianginal
tramadol HCl	central analgesic
tramadol HCl & acetaminophen	central analgesic, NSAID
trazodone HCl	tetracyclic antidepressant
triamcinolone acetonide	topical steroidal anti-inflammatory
triamterene & hydrochlorothiazide	diuretic, antihypertensive

Drug	Class/Indication(s)
Tricor (fenofibrate)	antihyperlipidemic
trimethoprim & sulfamethoxazole	anti-infective, antibacterial
Trinessa (norgestimate, ethinyl estradiol)	triphasic oral contraceptive
Tri-Sprintec (norgestimate, ethinyl estradiol)	triphasic oral contraceptive
Tussionex (hydrocodone polistirex, chlorpheniramine polistirex)	narcotic antitussive, antihistamine
Valtrex (valacyclovir HCl)	antiviral for herpes infections
verapamil HCl [sustained-release form]	antianginal, antiarrhythmic, calcium channel blocker
Viagra (sildenafil citrate)	vasodilator for erectile dysfunction
Vigamox (moxifloxacin HCl)	fluoroquinolone antibiotic
Vytorin (simvastatin, ezetimibe)	antihyperlipidemic
warfarin sodium	anticoagulant
Wellbutrin XL (bupropion HCl)	aminoketone antidepressant
Xalatan (latanoprost)	topical antiglaucoma agent
Yasmin (drospirenone, ethinyl estradiol)	monophasic oral contraceptive
Yaz (drospirenone, ethinyl estradiol)	monophasic oral contraceptive
Zetia (ezetimibe)	antihyperlipidemic
zolpidem tartrate	sedative, hypnotic
Zyprexa (olanzapine)	antipsychotic, antimanic
Zyrtec (cetirizine HCl)	antihistamine
Zyrtec-D (cetirizine HCl, pseudoephedrine HCl)	antihistamine, nasal decongestant

Dropped from the previous year's list:

Drug	Class/Indication(s)
clopidogrel bisulfate**	platelet aggregation inhibitor
fosinopril sodium	antihypertensive, ACE inhibitor
Flonase (fluticasone propionate)*/**	steroidal anti-inflammatory
Kariva (desogestrel, ethinyl estradiol)	biphasic oral contraceptive
Levothroid (levothyroxine sodium)*/**	thyroid hormone
Mobic (meloxicam)*	analgesic, antiarthritic, NSAID
morphine sulfate (MS)	narcotic analgesic
Ortho Evra (norelgestromin, ethinyl estradiol)	once-weekly contraceptive patch
Paxil CR (paroxetine HCl)*	SSRI antidepressant
phenobarbital	anticonvulsant, sedative, hypnotic
polyethylene glycol**	laxative, pre-procedure bowel evacuant
Pravachol (pravastatin sodium)*	antihyperlipidemic
Prempro (conjugated estrogens, medroxyprogesterone acetate)	hormone replacement therapy
quinine sulfate	antimalarial
Rhinocort Aqua (budesonide)	nasal steroid for allergic rhinitis
Zithromax (azithromycin)*	macrolide antibiotic
Zocor (simvastatin)*	antihyperlipidemic
Zoloft (sertraline HCl)*	SSRI antidepressant

*On this list as a generic drug.   **On this list as a (different) brand.